NCLEX-RN® Questions & Answers made Incredibly Easy!®

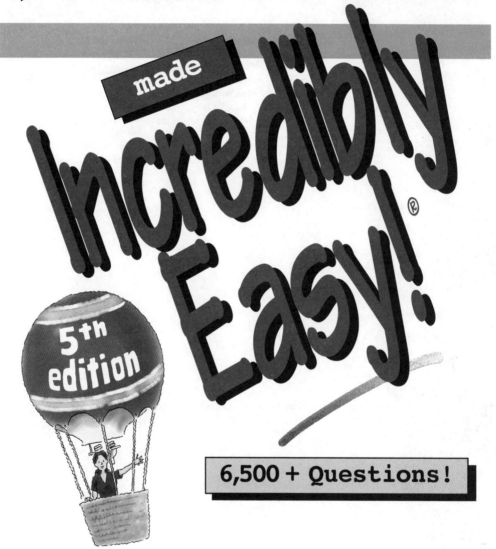

5th edition

6,500 + Questions!

Wolters Kluwer Health | Lippincott Williams & Wilkins

Philadelphia • Baltimore • New York • London
Buenos Aires • Hong Kong • Sydney • Tokyo

Staff

Publisher
Chris Burghardt

Clinical Director
Joan M. Robinson, RN, MSN

Clinical Project Manager
Beverly Ann Tscheschlog, RN, MS

Clinical Editor
Pamela Kovach, RN, BSN

Acquisitions Editor
Bill Lamsback

Product Director
David Moreau

Product Manager
Jennifer K. Forestieri

Art Director
Elaine Kasmer

Illustrator
Bot Roda

Design Assistant
Kate Zulak

Vendor Manager
Beth Martz

Associate Manufacturing Manager
Beth J. Welsh

Editorial Assistants
Karen J. Kirk, Jeri O'Shea, Linda K. Ruhf

Q&AIE5E010710

Library of Congress Cataloging-in-Publication Data

NCLEX-RN questions & answers made incredibly easy! : 6,500 + questions!—5th ed.
p. ; cm.
Other title: NCLEX-RN questions and answers made incredibly easy!
Includes index.
ISBN 978-1-60831-291-7 (alk. paper)
1. Nursing—Examinations, questions, etc. 2. National Council Licensure Examination for Registered Nurses—Study guides. I. Title: NCLEX-RN questions and answers made incredibly easy!
[DNLM: 1. Nursing Care—Examination Questions. 2. Nursing—Examination Questions. WY 18.2 N33652 2011]
RT55.N44 2011
610.73076—dc22

2010012803

RRS1004

Contents

Part IV Maternal-neonatal care

Part V Care of the child

Part VI Issues in nursing

Appendices and index

Contributors and consultants

Vicky H. Becherer, RN, MSN
Assistant Teaching Professor
College of Nursing at the University of Missouri
St. Louis, MO

Julie Calvery Carman, APN, FNP-BC, MS
Nurse Practitioner
River Valley Musculoskeletal
Ft. Smith, AR

Marsha L. Conroy, RN, MSN
Nurse Educator
Chamberlain College of Nursing
Columbus, OH

Maggie Thurmond Dorsey, RN, EdD
Associate Professor of Nursing
University of South Carolina–Aiken
Aiken, SC

Sally E. Erdel, RN, MS, CNE
Assistant Professor of Nursing
Bethel College
Mishawaka, IN

Margaret Fried, RN, MA
Instructional Faculty
Pima Community College
Tucson, AZ

Kathy Henley Haugh, RN, PhD
Assistant Professor
University of Virginia School of Nursing
Charlottesville, VA

Corlis Hayden, RN, MSN
Assistant Professor
Nebraska Methodist College
Omaha, NE

Connie S. Heflin, RN, MSN, CNE
Professor of Nursing
West Kentucky Community and Technical College
Paducah, KY

Soosannamma Joseph, RN, MS
Professor
Cochran School of Nursing
Yonkers, NY

Carolyn Kingston, RN, MSN
Instructor/Coordinator Nursing Resource Center
St. Francis Medical Center College of Nursing
Peoria, IL

Kathleen Lehmann, RN, BSN, BA, Med
Charge Nurse
Edith Nourse Rogers VAMC
Bedford, MA

Marilyn Little, APRN, BS, MSN
Professor
Salt Lake Community College
Salt Lake City, UT

Jennifer McWha, RN, MSN
Associate Professor of Nursing
Del Mar College
Corpus Christi, TX

Susan A. Moore, RN, BSN, MS, MSN
Assistant Clinical Professor
University of Memphis
Memphis, TN

Noel C., Piano, RN, MS
Instructor/Director
Lafayette School of Practical Nursing
Williamsburg, VA
Adjunct Faculty
Thomas Nelson Community College
Hampton, VA

Elizabeth R. Pratt, RNC-INP, BSN, MSN
Assistant Professor of Nursing
Southern Arkansas University
Magnolia, AR

Nan C. Riedé, RN, MSN, CPN, PLNC
Assistant Professor
Baptist College of Health Sciences
Memphis, TN

Ora V. Robinson, RN, PhD
Assistant Professor of Nursing
California State University
San Bernardino, CA

Mary Frances Schneider, RN, BSN, MS
Assistant Professor
The Christ College of Nursing and Health Sciences
Cincinnati, OH

Lisa A. Seldomridge, RN, PhD
Chair and Professor
Salisbury University
Salisbury, MD

Barbara Selvek, RN, MSN, CCRN
Associate Professor
Finger Lakes Community College
Canandaigua, NY

Allison J. Terry, RN, MSN, PhD
Director, Center for Nursing
Alabama Board of Nursing
Montgomery, AL

Mary L. Terwilliger, RN, MSN
Associate Professor
Clarion University of Pennsylvania
Oil City, PA

Peggy Thweatt, RN, BSN, MSN
Nursing Faculty
Medical Careers Institute, LPN Program
Newport News, VA

Sandra K. Voll, RNC, MS, WHNP, CNM, FNP
Clinical Assistant Professor
Virginia Commonwealth University School of Nursing
Richmond, VA

Karen A. Wolf, APRN-BC, FNAP, PhD
Associate Professor & Coordinator for Faculty Development
Samuel Merritt University
Oakland, CA
Nurse Practitioner
Lifelong Medical
Berkeley, CA

Michele Woodbeck, RN, MS
Professor, Nursing
Hudson Valley Community College
Troy, NY

Patricia Zrelak, CNRN, CNAA-BC, PhD
Administrative Nurse, Department of Neurology
University of California at Davis Medical Center

Advisory board

Susan Barnason, RN, PhD, CEN, CCRN, CS
Associate Professor
University of Nebraska Medical Center
College of Nursing
Lincoln

Michael A. Carter, APRN-BC, DNSc, FAAN
University Distinguished Professor
University of Tennessee Health Science Center
College of Nursing
Memphis

Caroline Dorsen, APRN-BC, FNP, MSN,
Clinical Instructor and Coordinator, Adult Nurse Practitioner Program
New York University College of Nursing

Stephen Gilliam, APRN-BC, FNP, PhD
Assistant Professor,
Medical College of Georgia
School of Nursing
Athens

Margaret Mary Hansen, RN, MSN, EdD, NI Certificate
Associate Professor
University of San Francisco

Kathy Henley Haugh, RN, PhD
Assistant Professor
University of Virginia
School of Nursing
Charlottesville

Janice J. Hoffman, RN, PhD, CCRN
Assistant Professor and Vice Chair
Organizational Systems and Adult Health
University of Maryland School of Nursing
Baltimore

Linda Honan Pellico, APRN, MSN, PhD
Assistant Professor
Yale University
School of Nursing
New Haven, Conn.

Susan L. Woods, RN, PhD, FAAN, FAHA
Professor and Associate Dean for Academic Programs
University of Washington
Seattle

Foreword

As a nurse for more than 20 years, I will be the first to tell you that nursing is far from easy. Nursing is one of the most complex and challenging careers that you will find; it is also one of the most rewarding. If you are looking at this book, you may very well be a new nurse, almost ready to begin your career. Or, you may be a nurse returning to practice with perhaps some trepidation and uncertainty. Regardless, you will find the fifth edition of *NCLEX-RN Questions & Answers Made Incredibly Easy* to be a breath of fresh air. This book acknowledges that you already have learned what you need to know to be successful; it does not present outlines or summarize content. Instead, this book provides you with thousands of exemplary questions and answers, which are designed to help you discover those areas in which you are particularly strong and those areas in which some degree of review might be in order.

These questions are exemplary because they are consistent with the format of the National Council Licensure Examination for Registered Nurses (NCLEX-RN®), a format that challenges you to be the best nurse you can be through thoughtful analysis and reflection. Part I provides an excellent overview of the NCLEX. This presentation is straightforward, entertaining and, most importantly, reassuring. Chapter 1 presents sensible strategies for approaching different types of NCLEX questions. Chapter 2 provides guidance on how to study for the NCLEX and how to be at your best.

Parts II through VI are built on the familiar. You will see systems (cardiovascular, respiratory), populations (adults, maternal-neonatal), and issues (leadership, ethics), just as you learned in school. This familiarity helps you to organize your thoughts and to work your way easily and confidently through what may seem like an insurmountable amount of material. Fortunately, the fifth edition of *NCLEX-RN Questions & Answers Made Incredibly Easy* also includes lighthearted cartoons that provide useful information, as well as humor and encouragement. They serve to remind us not to take ourselves too seriously, but to enjoy learning and nursing. At the end of the book, several comprehensive tests, which simulate the actual NCLEX format, help to build confidence in your test-taking skills.

Having so many questions in one offering is truly a gift. But equally helpful are the answers you will find in the fifth edition of *NCLEX-RN Questions & Answers Made Incredibly Easy.* Each answer includes not only the rationale for the correct response, but also information as to which aspects of nursing are being evaluated by that particular question. Thus, you will discover which parts of the nursing process are more problematic for you and which client needs categories are most challenging for you. Knowing this can help you focus on the further review needed for you to be successful.

The fifth edition of *NCLEX-RN Questions & Answers Made Incredibly Easy* is an excellent, user-friendly resource that provides exactly what is needed in NCLEX text preparation: questions, answers, rationales, and self-analysis. Whether you are preparing to take the NCLEX for the first time or preparing for reentry into the profession of nursing, I am convinced that challenging yourself with these thoughtful questions will do your heart and brain (and patients) good. Good luck!

Kathy Henley Haugh, RN, PhD
Assistant Professor
University of Virginia School of Nursing
Charlottesville

Part I Surviving the NCLEX®

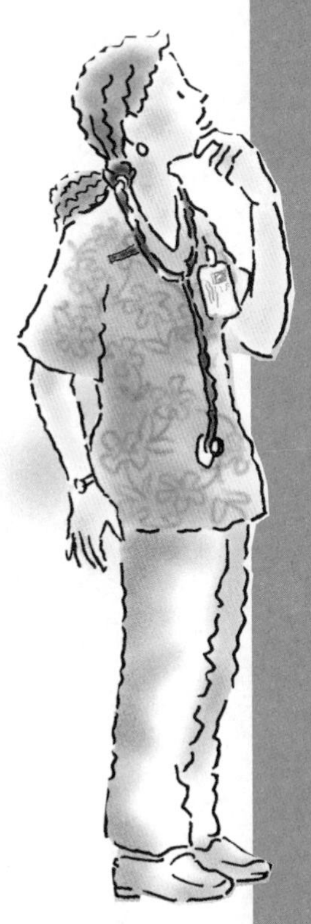

Understanding the NCLEX goals and structure is an important first step in proper preparation for the test. This chapter explains how best to prepare for this important examination.

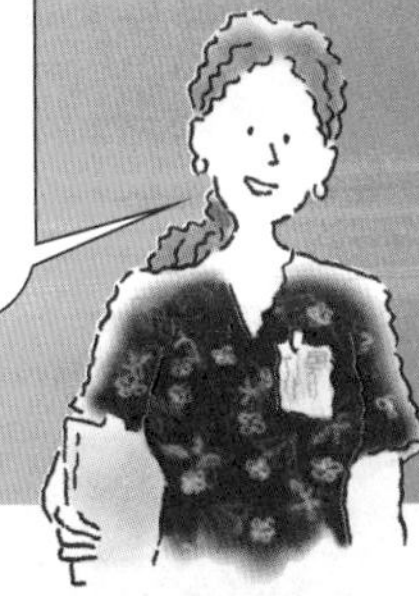

Chapter 1 Preparing for the NCLEX®

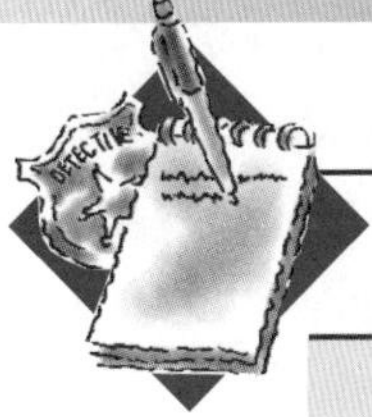

Just the facts

In this chapter, you'll learn:

- about the NCLEX® and why you must take it
- what you need to know about taking the NCLEX by computer
- strategies to use when answering NCLEX questions
- how to recognize and answer alternate-format questions
- how to avoid common mistakes when taking the NCLEX.

NCLEX basics

Passing the National Council Licensure Examination (NCLEX®) is an important landmark in your career as a nurse. The first step on your way to passing the NCLEX is to understand what it is and how it's administered.

All your experience with testing means you're ready to do battle with this exam!

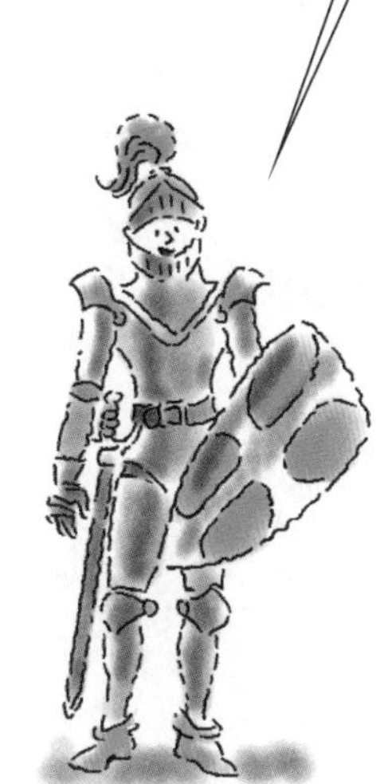

NCLEX structure

The NCLEX is a test written by nurses who, like most of your nursing instructors, have an advanced degree and clinical expertise in a particular area. Only one small difference distinguishes nurses who write NCLEX questions: They're trained to write questions in a style particular to the NCLEX.

If you've completed an accredited nursing program, you've already taken numerous tests written by nurses with backgrounds and experiences similar to those of the nurses who write for the NCLEX. The test-taking experience you've already gained will help you pass the NCLEX. So your NCLEX review should be just that—a review.

What's the point of it all?

The NCLEX is designed for one purpose: to determine whether it's appropriate for you to receive a license to practice as a nurse. By passing the NCLEX, you demonstrate that you possess the minimum level of knowledge necessary to practice nursing safely.

Studying abroad

If you completed your nursing education in a foreign country, you must follow certain guidelines to be eligible to work as a registered nurse in the United States. (See *Guidelines for international nurses.*)

Mix 'em up

In nursing school, you probably took courses that were separated into such subjects as pharmacology; nursing leadership; health assessment; adult health; and pediatric, maternal-neonatal, and psychiatric nursing. In contrast, the NCLEX is integrated, meaning that different subjects are mixed together.

As you answer NCLEX questions, you may encounter patients in any stage of life, from neonatal to geriatric. These patients—clients, in NCLEX terminology—may be of any background, and may be completely well or extremely ill, and may have any of a variety of disorders.

Client needs, front and center

The NCLEX draws questions from four categories of client needs that were developed by the *National Council of State Boards of Nursing* (NCSBN), the organization that sponsors and manages the NCLEX. *Client needs categories* ensure that a wide variety of topics appears on every NCLEX examination.

The NCSBN developed client needs categories after conducting a practice analysis of new nurses. All aspects of nursing care observed in the study were broken down into four main categories, some of which were broken down further into subcategories. (See *Client needs categories,* page 6.)

What's the plan?

The categories and subcategories are used to develop the *NCLEX test plan*, the content guidelines for the distribution of test questions. Question writers and the people who put the NCLEX together use the test plan and client needs categories to make sure that a full spectrum of nursing activities is covered in the NCLEX. Client needs categories appear in most NCLEX review and question-and-answer books, including this one. As a test-taker you don't have to concern yourself with client needs categories. You'll see those categories for each question and answer in this book, but they'll be invisible on the actual NCLEX.

Guidelines for international nurses

In order to become eligible to work as a registered nurse (RN) in the United States, you will need to complete several steps. In addition to passing the NCLEX-RN, you may need to obtain a certificate and credentials evaluation from the Commission on Graduates of Foreign Nursing Schools (CGFNS®) and acquire a visa. Since requirements differ from state to state, it's important that you first contact the Board of Nursing in the state where you want to practice nursing.

CGFNS Certification Program

Most states require that you obtain CGFNS certification. This certification requires:

- a review and authentication of your credentials, including your nursing education, registration, and licensure
- a passing score on the CGFNS Qualifying Examination of nursing knowledge
- a passing score on an English language proficiency test.

In order to be eligible to take the CGFNS Qualifying Examination, you must complete a minimum number of classroom and clinical practice hours in medical-surgical nursing, maternal-neonatal nursing, pediatric nursing, and psychiatric and mental health nursing from a government-approved nursing school. You must also be registered as a first-level nurse in your country of education, and currently hold a license as an RN in some jurisdiction.

The CGFNS Qualifying Examination is a paper and pencil test that includes 260 multiple-choice questions. It's administered under controlled testing conditions. Because the test is designed to predict your likelihood of successfully passing the NCLEX-RN exam, it's based on the NCLEX-RN test plan.

You may select from three English proficiency examinations, Test of English as a Foreign Language (TOEFL®), Test of English for International Communication (TOEIC®), or International English Language Testing System (IELTS). Each test has different passing scores and the scores are valid for up to 2 years.

CGFNS credentials evaluation service

This evaluation is a comprehensive report that analyzes and compares your education and licensure with U.S. standards. It's prepared by the CGFNS for a state board of nursing, an immigration office, an employer, or a university. It requires that you complete an application, submit appropriate documentation, and pay a fee.

More information about the CGFNS certification program and credentials evaluation service is available at *www.cgfns.org*.

Visa

You can't legally immigrate to work in the United States without an occupational visa (temporary or permanent) from the United States Citizenship and Immigration Services (USCIS). The visa process is separate from the CGFNS certification process, although some of the same steps are involved. Some visas require prior CGFNS certification and a *VisaScreen*™ Certificate from the International Commission on Healthcare Professions. The *VisaScreen* program involves:

- a credentials review of your nursing education and current registration or licensure
- successful completion of either the CGFNS certification program or the NCLEX-RN to provide proof of nursing knowledge
- a passing score on an approved English language proficiency examination.

Once you successfully complete all parts of the *VisaScreen* program, you will receive a certificate to present to the USCIS. The visa-granting process can take up to a year.

You can obtain more detailed information about visa application at *www.uscis.gov*.

Client needs categories

Each question on the NCLEX is assigned a category based on client needs. This chart lists client needs categories and subcategories and the percentages of each type of question that appears on an NCLEX examination.

Category	Subcategories	Percentage of NCLEX questions
Safe, effective care environment	• Management of care • Safety and infection control	16% to 22% 8% to 14%
Health promotion and maintenance		6% to 12%
Psychosocial integrity		6% to 12%
Physiological integrity	• Basic care and comfort • Pharmacological and parenteral therapies • Reduction of risk potential • Physiological adaptation	6% to 12% 13% to 19% 10% to 16% 11% to 17%

Testing by computer

Like many standardized tests today, the NCLEX is administered by computer. That means you won't be filling in empty circles, sharpening pencils, or erasing frantically. It also means that you must become familiar with computer tests, if you aren't already. Fortunately, the skills required to take the NCLEX on a computer are simple enough to allow you to focus on the questions, not the keyboard.

Q&A

When you take the test, depending on the question format, you'll be presented with a question and four or more possible answers, a blank space in which to enter your answer, a figure on which you'll click the mouse to select the correct area of the figure, a series of charts or exhibits to view in order to select the correct response, items you must prioritize by dragging and dropping them in place, an audio recording to listen to in order to select the correct response, or a question and four graphic options.

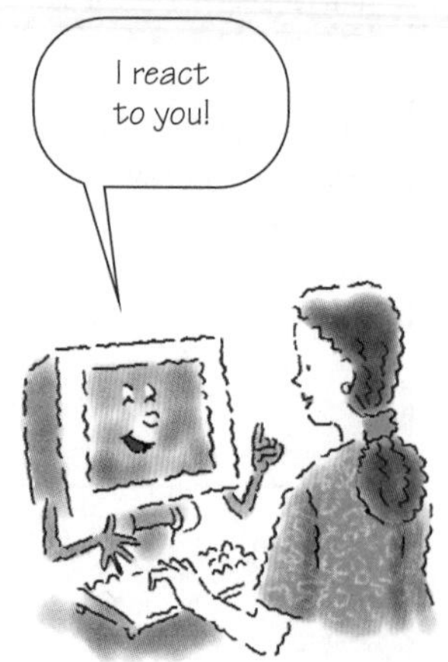

Feeling smart? Think hard!

The NCLEX is a *computer-adaptive test*, meaning that the computer reacts to the answers you give, supplying more difficult questions if you answer correctly, and slightly easier questions if you answer incorrectly. Each test is thus uniquely adapted to the individual test-taker.

A matter of time

You have a great deal of flexibility with the amount of time you spend on individual questions. The examination lasts a maximum of 6 hours, however, so don't waste time. If you fail to answer a set number of questions within 6 hours, the computer will determine that you lack minimum competency.

Most students have plenty of time to complete the test, so take as much time as you need to get the question right without wasting time. Keep moving at a decent pace to help maintain concentration.

Difficult items = Good news

If you find as you progress through the test that the questions seem to be increasingly difficult, it's a good sign. The more questions you answer correctly, the more difficult the questions become.

Some students, though, knowing that questions get progressively harder, focus on the degree of difficulty of subsequent questions to try to figure out if they're answering questions correctly. Avoid the temptation to do this, as this may get you off track.

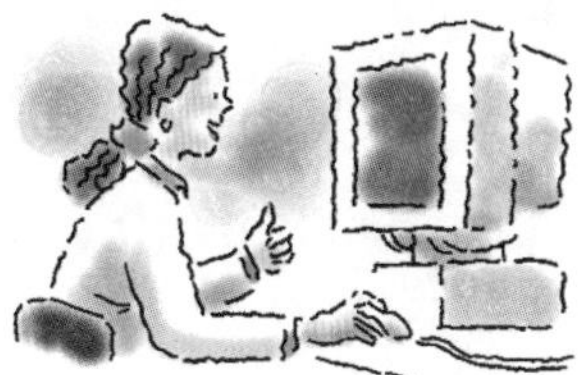
The harder it gets, the better I do.

The finish line

The computer test finishes when one of these events occurs:

- You demonstrate minimum competency, according to the computer program, which does so with 95% certainty that your ability exceeds the passing standard.
- You demonstrate a lack of minimum competency, according to the computer program.
- You've answered the maximum number of questions (265 total questions).
- You've used the maximum time allowed (6 hours).

Unlocking the NCLEX mystery

In April of 2004, the NCSBN added alternate-format items to the exam. However, most of the questions on the NCLEX are four-option, multiple-choice items with only one correct answer. Certain strategies can help you understand and answer any type of NCLEX question.

Alternate formats

The first type of alternate-format item is the ***multiple-response, multiple-choice question***. Unlike a traditional multiple-choice question, each multiple-response, multiple-choice question has more than one correct answer for every question, and it may contain more than four possible answer options. You'll recognize this type of question because it will ask you to select *all* answers that apply—not just the best answer (as may be requested in the more traditional multiple-choice questions).

No points for partials

Keep in mind that for each multiple-response, multiple-choice question, you must select at least one answer and you must select all correct answers for the item to be counted as correct. On the NCLEX, there's no partial credit in the scoring of these items.

Don't go blank!

The second type of alternate-format item is the *fill-in-the-blank*. These questions require you to provide the answer yourself, rather than select it from a list of options. You will perform a calculation, then type your answer (a number without any words, units of measurement, commas, or spaces) in the blank space provided after the question. Rules for rounding are included in the question stem if appropriate. A calculator button is provided so you can easily do your calculations electronically.

Master that mouse!

The third type of alternate-format item is a question that asks you to identify an area on an illustration or graphic. For these so-called *"hotspot"* questions, the computerized exam will ask you to place your cursor and click over the correct area on an illustration. Try to be as precise as possible when marking the location. As with the fill-in-the-blanks, the identification questions on the computerized exam may require extremely precise answers to be considered correct.

Chart smarts

The fourth type of alternate-format item is the *chart/exhibit* format. Here you'll be given a problem, then a series of small screens containing additional information you'll need in order to answer the question. By clicking on the Tab button, you can access each screen in turn. Your answer can then be chosen from four multiple-choice answer options.

All in order

The fifth type of alternate-format item involves prioritizing or placing in correct order a series of statements, using a *drag-and-drop* technique. You'll decide which of the given options is first, click and hold it with the mouse, then drag it into the first box given underneath and drop it into place. You'll repeat this process until you've placed all the available options in the lower boxes.

Now hear this!

The sixth alternate-format item type is the *audio item* format. You'll be given a set of headphones and you'll be asked to listen to an audio clip and select the correct answer from four options. You'll need to select the correct answer on the computer screen as you would with the traditional multiple-choice questions.

Picture perfect

The final alternate-format item type is the *graphic option* question. This varies from the exhibit format type because in the graphic option, your answer choices will be graphics, such as ECG strips. You'll have to select the appropriate graphic to answer the question presented.

The standard's still the standard

The NCSBN hasn't yet established a percentage of alternate-format items to be administered to each candidate. In fact, your exam may contain only one alternate-format item. So relax; the standard, four-option, multiple-choice format questions compose the bulk of the test. (See *Sample NCLEX questions,* pages 10–12.)

Understanding the question

NCLEX questions are usually long. As a result, it's easy to feel overwhelmed with information. To focus on the question, apply proven strategies for answering NCLEX questions, including:

- determining what the question is asking
- determining relevant facts about the client
- rephrasing the question in your mind
- choosing the best option(s) before entering your answer.

Determine what the question is asking

Read the question twice. If the answer isn't apparent, rephrase the question in simpler, more personal terms. Breaking down the question into easier, less intimidating terms may help you to focus more accurately on the correct answer.

Give it a try

For example, a question might be, "A 74-year-old client with a history of heart failure is admitted to the coronary care unit with pulmonary edema. He's intubated and placed on a mechanical ventilator. Which parameter should the nurse monitor closely to assess the client's response to a bolus dose of furosemide (Lasix) I.V.?"

The options for this question—numbered from 1 to 4—may be:

1. Daily weight
2. 24-hour intake and output
3. Serum sodium levels
4. Hourly urine output

Sample NCLEX questions

Sometimes, getting used to the test format is as important as knowing the material covered. Try your hand at these sample questions and you'll have a leg up when you take the real test!

Sample four-option, multiple-choice question

A client's arterial blood gas (ABG) results are as follows: pH, 7.16; $Paco_2$, 80 mm Hg; Pao_2, 46 mm Hg; HCO_3^-, 24 mEq/L; Sao_2, 81%. This ABG result represents which condition?

1. Metabolic acidosis
2. Metabolic alkalosis
3. Respiratory acidosis
4. Respiratory alkalosis

Correct answer: 3

Sample multiple-response, multiple-choice question

The nurse is caring for a 45-year-old married client who has undergone hemicolectomy for colon cancer. The client has two children. Which concepts about families should the nurse keep in mind when providing care for this client? Select all that apply:

1. Illness in one family member can affect all members.
2. Family roles don't change because of illness.
3. A family member may have more than one role in the family.
4. Children typically aren't affected by adult illness.
5. The effects of an illness on a family depend on the stage of the family's life cycle.
6. Changes in sleeping and eating patterns may be signs of stress in a family.

Correct answer: 1, 3, 5, 6

Sample fill-in-the-blank calculation question

An infant who weighs 8 kg is to receive ampicillin 25 mg/kg I.V. every 6 hours. How many milligrams should the nurse administer per dose? Record your answer using a whole number.

______________________ milligrams

Correct answer: 200

Sample hotspot question

A client has a history of aortic stenosis. Identify the area where the nurse should place the stethoscope to best hear the murmur.

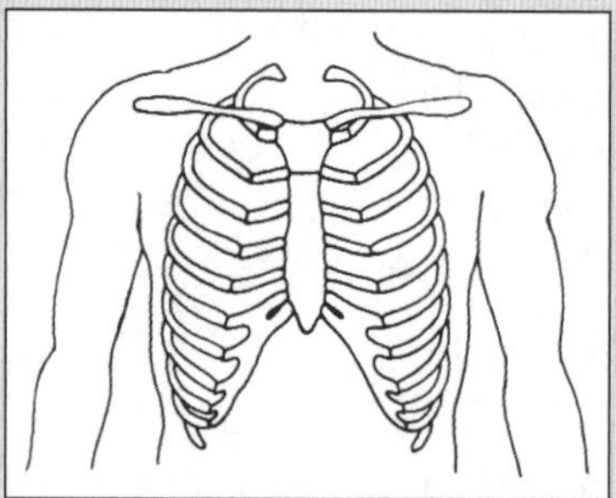

Correct answer:

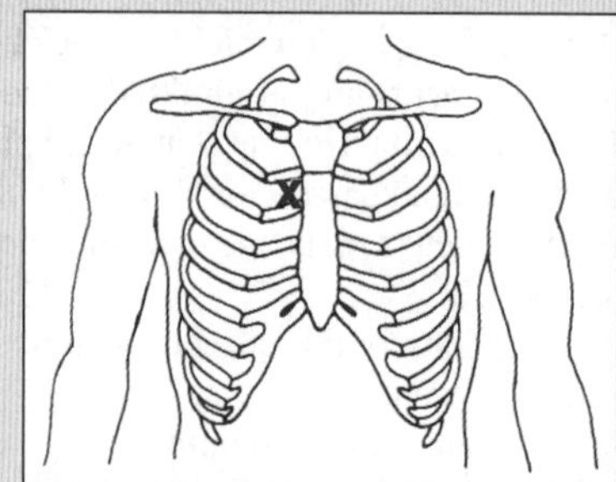

Sample NCLEX questions *(continued)*

Sample chart/exhibit question

A 3-year-old client is being treated for severe status asthmaticus. After reviewing the progress notes (shown below), the nurse should determine that this client is being treated for which condition?

Progress notes

4/5/10	Pt. was acutely restless, diaphoretic, and with
0600	dyspnea at 0530. Dr. T. Smith notified and
	ordered ABG analysis. ABG drawn from (R)
	radial artery. Stat results as follows: pH 7.28,
	$Paco_2$ 55 mm Hg, HCO_3^- 26 mEq/L. Dr. Smith
	with pt. now. ——— J. Collins, RN

1. Metabolic acidosis
2. Respiratory alkalosis
3. Respiratory acidosis
4. Metabolic alkalosis

Correct answer: 3

Sample drag-and-drop question

When teaching an antepartal client about the passage of the fetus through the birth canal during labor, the nurse describes the cardinal mechanisms of labor. Place these events in the sequence in which they occur. Use all the options.

1. Flexion
2. External rotation
3. Descent
4. Expulsion
5. Internal rotation
6. Extension

Correct answer:

3. Descent
1. Flexion
5. Internal rotation
6. Extension
2. External rotation
4. Expulsion

Sample NCLEX questions *(continued)*

Sample audio item question

Listen to the audio clip. What sound do you hear in the bases of this client with heart failure?

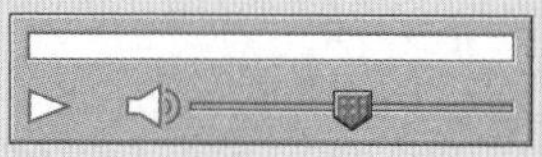

1. Crackles
2. Rhonchi
3. Wheezes
4. Pleural friction rub

Correct answer: 1

Sample graphic option question

Which electrocardiogram strip should the nurse document as sinus tachycardia?

1.

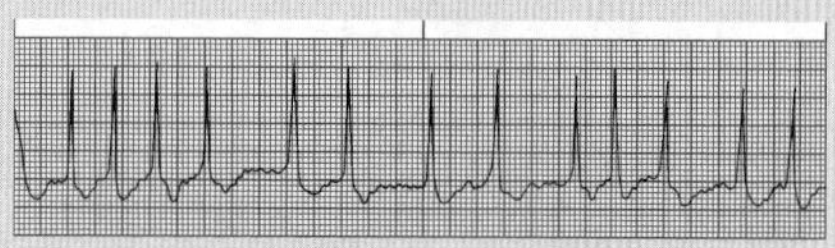

2.

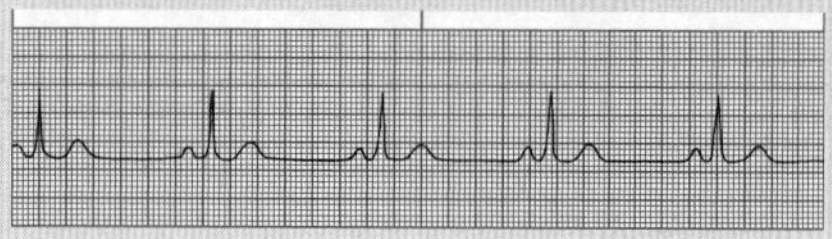

3.

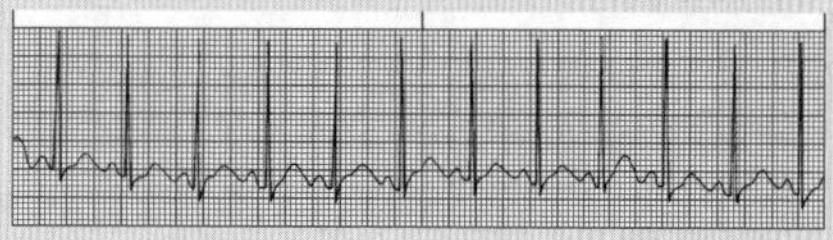

4.

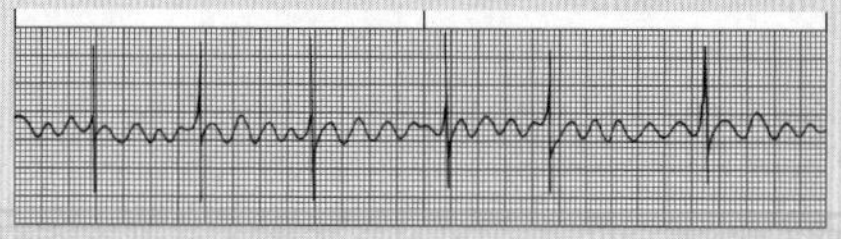

Correct answer: 3

Hocus, focus on the question

Read the question again, ignoring all details except what's being asked. Focus on the last line of the question. It asks you to select the appropriate assessment for monitoring a client who received a bolus of furosemide I.V.

Determine what facts about the client are relevant

Next, sort out the relevant client information. Start by asking whether any of the information provided about the client isn't relevant. For instance, do you need to know that the client has been admitted to the coronary care unit? Probably not; his reaction to I.V. furosemide won't be affected by his location in the hospital.

Determine what you do know about the client. In the example, you know that:

- he just received an I.V. bolus of furosemide, a crucial fact
- he has pulmonary edema, the most fundamental aspect of the client's underlying condition
- he's intubated and placed on a mechanical ventilator, suggesting that his pulmonary edema is serious
- he's 74 years old and has a history of heart failure, a fact that may or may not be relevant.

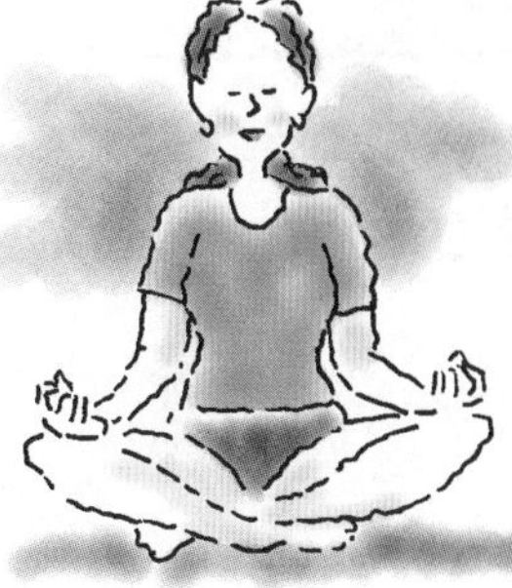

Focusing on what the question is really asking can help you choose the correct answer.

Rephrase the question

After you've determined relevant information about the client and the question being asked, consider rephrasing the question to make it more clear. Eliminate jargon and put the question in simpler, more personal terms. Here's how you might rephrase the question in the example: "My client has pulmonary edema. He requires intubation and mechanical ventilation. He's 74 years old and has a history of heart failure. He received an I.V. bolus of furosemide. What assessment parameter should I monitor?"

Choose the best option

Armed with all the information you now have, it's time to select an option. You know that the client received an I.V. bolus of furosemide, a diuretic. You know that monitoring fluid intake and output is a key nursing intervention for a client taking a diuretic, a fact that eliminates options 1 and 3 (daily weight and serum sodium levels), narrowing the answer down to option 2 or 4 (24-hour intake and output or hourly urine output).

Can I use a lifeline?

You also know that the drug was administered by I.V. bolus, suggesting a rapid effect. (In fact, furosemide administered by I.V. bolus takes effect almost immediately.) Monitoring the client's 24-hour intake and output would be appropriate for assessing the effects of repeated doses of furosemide. Hourly urine output, however, is most appropriate in this situation because it monitors the immediate effect of this rapid-acting drug.

Key strategies

Regardless of the type of question, four key strategies will help you determine the correct answer for each question. These strategies are:

 considering the nursing process

 referring to Maslow's hierarchy of needs

 reviewing patient safety

 reflecting on principles of therapeutic communication.

Nursing process

One of the ways to answer a question is to apply the nursing process. Steps in the nursing process include:

- assessment
- diagnosis
- planning
- implementation
- evaluation.

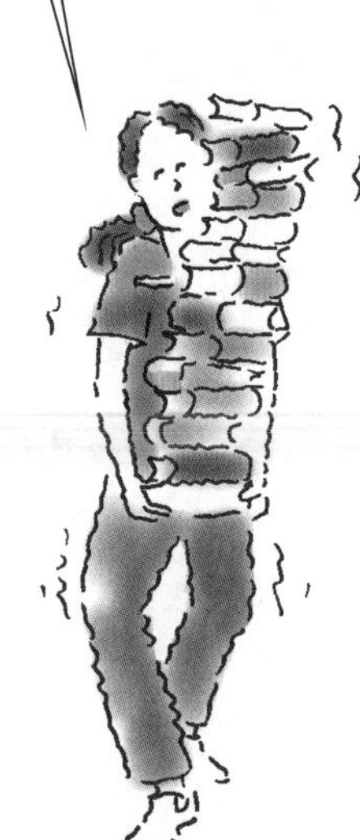

Say it 1,000 times: Studying for the NCLEX is fun . . . studying for the NCLEX is fun . . .

Process pointers

The nursing process may provide insights that help you analyze a question. According to the nursing process, assessment comes before analysis, which comes before planning, which comes before implementation, which comes before evaluation.

You're halfway to the correct answer when you encounter a four-option, multiple-choice question that asks you to assess the situation and then provides two assessment options and two implementation options. You can immediately eliminate the implementation options, which then gives you, at worst, a 50-50 chance of selecting the correct answer. Use the following sample question to apply the nursing process:

A client returns from an endoscopic procedure during which he was sedated. Before offering the client food, which action should the nurse take?

1. Assess the client's respiratory status.
2. Check the client's gag reflex.
3. Place the client in a side-lying position.
4. Have the client drink a few sips of water.

Assess before intervening

According to the nursing process, the nurse must assess a client before performing an intervention. Does the question indicate that the client has been properly assessed? No, it doesn't. Therefore, you can eliminate options 3 and 4 because they're both interventions.

That leaves options 1 and 2, both of which are assessments. Your nursing knowledge should tell you the correct answer—in this case, option 2. The sedation required for an endoscopic procedure may impair the client's gag reflex, so you would assess the gag reflex before giving food to the client to reduce the risk of aspiration and airway obstruction.

Watch phrasing

Why not select option 1, assessing the client's respiratory status? You might select this option but the question is specifically asking about offering the client food, an action that wouldn't be taken if the client's respiratory status was at all compromised. In this case, you're making a judgment based on the phrase, "Before offering the client food." If the question was trying to test your knowledge of respiratory depression following an endoscopic procedure, it probably wouldn't mention a function—such as giving food to a client—that clearly occurs only after the client's respiratory status has been stabilized.

Maslow's hierarchy

Knowledge of Maslow's hierarchy of needs can be a vital tool for establishing priorities on the NCLEX. Maslow's theory states that physiologic needs are the most basic human needs of all. Only after physiologic needs have been met can safety concerns be addressed. Only after safety concerns are met can concerns involving love and belonging be addressed, and so forth. Apply the principles of Maslow's hierarchy of needs to the following sample question:

A client complains of severe pain 2 days after surgery. Which action should the nurse perform first?

1. Offer reassurance to the client that he will feel less pain tomorrow.
2. Allow the client time to verbalize his feelings.
3. Check the client's vital signs.
4. Administer an analgesic.

Phys before psych

In this example, two of the options—3 and 4—address physiologic needs. Options 1 and 2 address psychosocial concerns. According to Maslow, physiologic needs must be met before psychosocial needs, so you can eliminate options 1 and 2.

Final elimination

Now, use your nursing knowledge to choose the best answer from the two remaining options. In this case, option 3 is correct because the client's vital signs should be checked before administering an analgesic (assessment before intervention). When prioritizing according to Maslow's hierarchy, remember your ABCs—airway, breathing, circulation—to help you further prioritize. Check for a patent airway before addressing breathing. Check breathing before checking the health of the cardiovascular system.

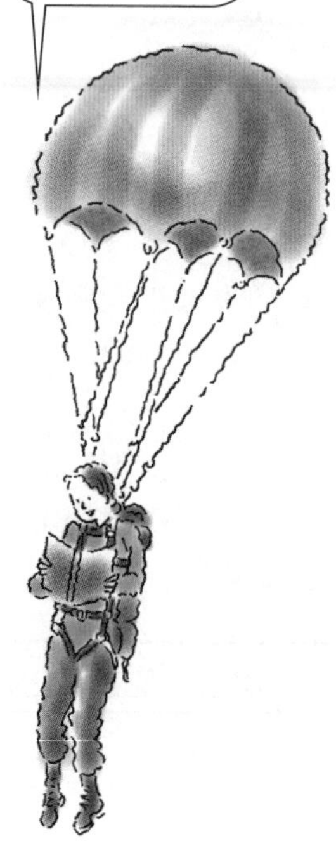
Patient safety takes high priority on the NCLEX.

Tricky, tricky

Just because an option appears on the NCLEX doesn't mean it's a viable choice for the client referred to in the question. Always examine your choice in light of your knowledge and experience. Ask yourself, "Does this choice make sense for this client?" Allow yourself to eliminate choices—even ones that might normally take priority—if they don't make sense for a particular client's situation.

Patient safety

As you might expect, patient safety takes high priority on the NCLEX. You'll encounter many questions that can be answered by asking yourself, "Which answer will best ensure the safety of this client?" Use patient safety criteria for situations involving laboratory values, drug administration, activities of daily living, or nursing care procedures.

Client first, equipment second

You may encounter a question in which some options address the client and others address the equipment. When in doubt, select an option relating to the client; never place equipment before a client.

For instance, suppose a question asks what the nurse should do first when entering a client's room where an infusion pump alarm is sounding. If two options deal with the infusion pump, one with the infusion tubing, and another with the client's catheter insertion site, select the one relating to the client's catheter insertion site. Always check the client first; the equipment can wait.

Therapeutic communication

Some NCLEX questions focus on the nurse's ability to communicate effectively with the client. Therapeutic communication incorporates verbal or nonverbal responses and involves:

- listening to the client
- understanding the client's needs
- promoting clarification and insight about the client's condition.

Room for improvement

Like other NCLEX questions, those dealing with therapeutic communication require choosing the best response. First, eliminate options that indicate the use of poor therapeutic communication techniques, such as those in which the nurse:

- tells the client what to do without regard to the client's feelings or desires (the "do this" response)
- asks a question that can be answered "yes" or "no," or with another one-syllable response
- seeks reasons for the client's behavior
- implies disapproval of the client's behavior
- offers false reassurances
- attempts to interpret the client's behavior rather than allowing the client to verbalize his own feelings
- offers a response that focuses on the nurse, not the client.

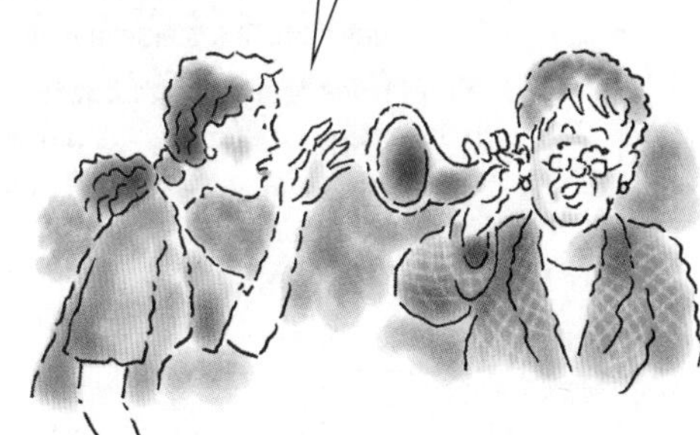

I said that some exam questions will focus on good therapeutic COMMUNICATION!

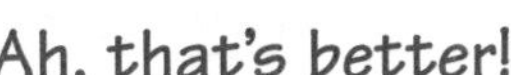

Ah, that's better!

When answering NCLEX questions, look for responses that:

- allow the client time to think and reflect
- encourage the client to talk
- encourage the client to describe a particular experience
- reflect that the nurse has listened to the client, such as through paraphrasing the client's response.

Avoiding pitfalls

Even the most knowledgeable students can get tripped up on certain NCLEX questions. (See *A tricky question*.) Students commonly cite three areas that can be difficult for unwary test-takers:

 knowing the difference between the NCLEX and the "real world"

 delegating care

 knowing laboratory values.

NCLEX versus the real world

Some students who take the NCLEX have extensive practical experience in health care. For example, many test-takers have

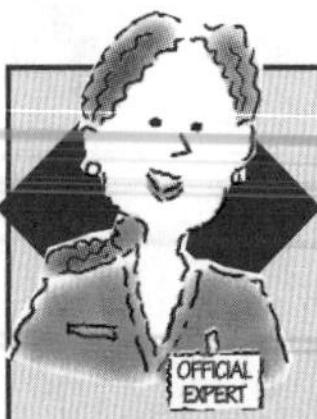

Advice from the experts

A tricky question

The NCLEX occasionally asks a particular kind of question called the "further teaching" question, which involves patient-teaching situations. These questions can be tricky. You'll have to choose the response that suggests that the patient has *not* learned the correct information. Here's an example:

37. A client undergoes a total hip replacement. Which statement by the client indicates that he requires further teaching?

1. "I'll need to keep several pillows between my legs at night."
2. "I'll need to remember not to cross my legs. It's such a bad habit."
3. "The occupational therapist is showing me how to use a 'sock puller' to help me get dressed."
4. "I don't know if I'll be able to get off that low toilet seat at home by myself."

The answer you should choose here is option 4 because it indicates that the client has a poor understanding of the precautions required after a total hip replacement and that he needs further teaching. *Remember:* If you see the phrase *further teaching* or *further instruction,* you're looking for a wrong answer by the patient.

worked as licensed practical nurses or nursing assistants. In one of those capacities, test-takers might have been exposed to less than optimum clinical practice and may carry those experiences over to the NCLEX.

However, the NCLEX is a textbook examination—not a test of clinical skills. Take the NCLEX with the understanding that what happens in the real world may differ from what the NCLEX and your nursing school say should happen.

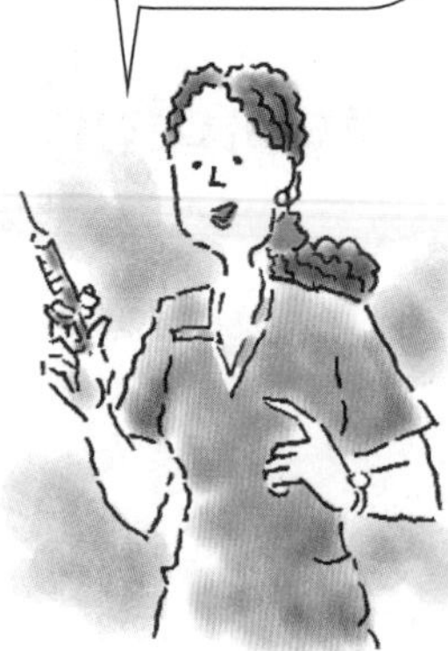

Remember, this is the real world. The NCLEX may not always reflect what happens in it.

Don't take shortcuts

If you've had practical experience in health care, you may know a quicker way to perform a procedure or tricks to get by when you don't have the right equipment. Situations such as staff shortages may force you to improvise. On the NCLEX, such scenarios can lead to trouble. Always check your practical experiences against textbook nursing care, taking care to select the response that follows the textbook.

Delegating care

On the NCLEX, you may encounter questions that assess your ability to delegate care. Delegating care involves coordinating the efforts of other health care workers to provide effective care for your client. On the NCLEX, you may be asked to assign duties to:

- licensed practical nurses or licensed vocational nurses
- direct care workers, such as nursing assistants and personal care aides
- other support staff, such as nutrition assistants and housekeepers.

In addition, you'll be asked to decide when to notify a physician, a social worker, or another hospital staff member. In each case, you'll have to decide when, where, and how to delegate.

Shoulds and shouldn'ts

As a general rule, it's okay to delegate actions that involve stable clients or standard, unchanging procedures. Bathing, feeding, dressing, and transferring clients are examples of procedures that can be delegated.

Be careful not to delegate complicated or complex activities. In addition, don't delegate activities that involve assessment, evaluation, or your own nursing judgment. On the NCLEX and in the real world, these duties fall squarely on your shoulders. Make sure that you take primary responsibility for assessing and evaluating the client and for making decisions about the client's care. Never hand off those responsibilities to someone with less training.

Calling in reinforcements

Deciding when to notify a physician, a social worker, or another hospital staff member is an important element of nursing care. On the NCLEX, however, choices that involve notifying the physician are usually incorrect. Remember that the NCLEX wants to see you, the nurse, at work.

If you're sure the correct answer is to notify the physician, though, make sure the client's safety has been addressed before notifying a physician or another staff member. On the NCLEX, the client's safety has a higher priority than notifying other health care providers.

Normal laboratory values

- Blood urea nitrogen: 8 to 25 mg/dl
- Creatinine: 0.6 to 1.5 mg/dl
- Sodium: 135 to 145 mmol/L
- Potassium: 3.5 to 5.5 mEq/L
- Chloride: 97 to 110 mmol/L
- Glucose (fasting plasma): 70 to 110 mg/dl
- Hemoglobin
  Male: 13.8 to 17.2 g/dl
  Female: 12.1 to 15.1 g/dl
- Hematocrit
  Male: 40.7% to 50.3%
  Female: 36.1% to 44.3%

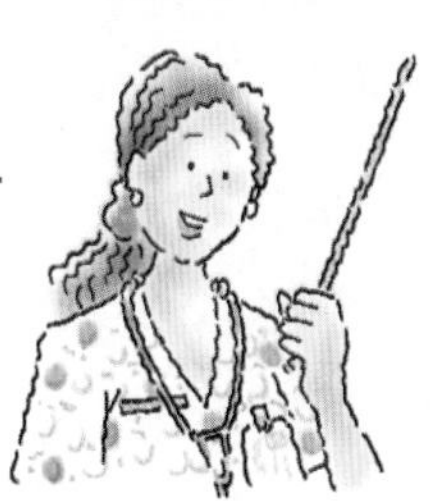

Knowing laboratory values

Some NCLEX questions supply laboratory results without indicating normal levels. As a result, answering questions involving laboratory values requires you to have the normal range of the most common laboratory values memorized to make an informed decision. (See *Normal laboratory values.*)

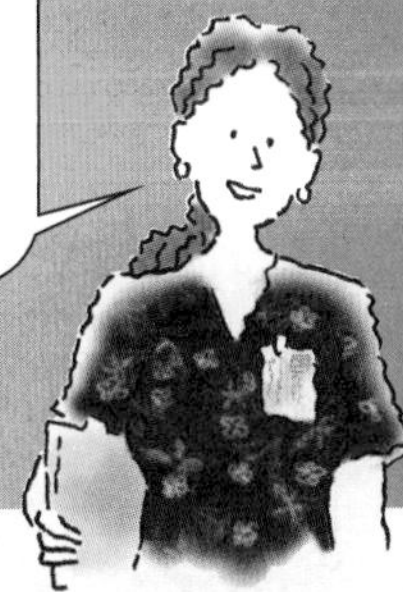

As you count down the weeks, days, and finally hours to the NCLEX, refer back to the information in this chapter. It's a recipe for NCLEX success!

Chapter 2
Passing the NCLEX

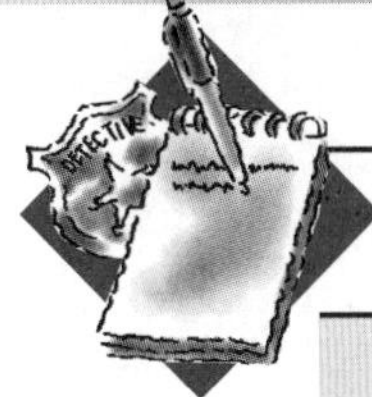

Just the facts

In this chapter, you'll learn:

- ♦ how to properly prepare for the NCLEX
- ♦ how to concentrate during difficult study times
- ♦ ways to make more effective use of your time
- ♦ why creative studying strategies can enhance learning
- ♦ how to get the most out of NCLEX practice tests.

Study preparations

If you're like most people preparing to take the test, you're probably feeling nervous, anxious, or concerned. Keep in mind that most test-takers pass the NCLEX the first time around.

Passing the test won't happen by accident, though; you'll need to prepare carefully and efficiently. To help jump-start your preparations:

- determine your strengths and weaknesses
- create a study schedule
- set realistic goals
- find an effective study space
- think positively
- start studying sooner rather than later.

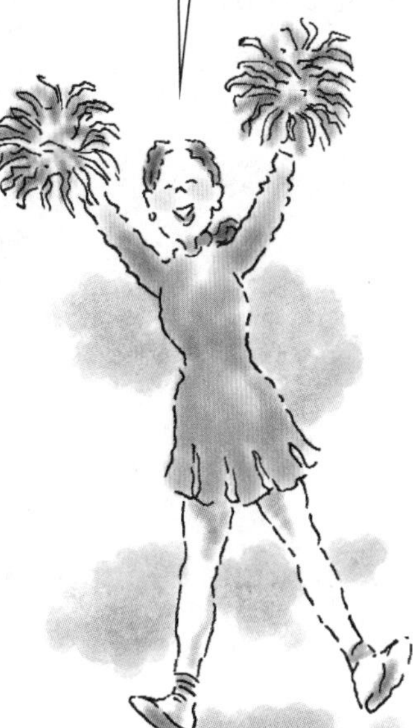

Most students pass the NCLEX on the first try. I know you can, too!

Strengths and weaknesses

Most students recognize that, even at the end of their nursing studies, they know more about some topics than others. Because the NCLEX covers a broad range of material, you should make some decisions about how intensively you'll review each topic.

Make a list

Base those decisions on a list. Divide a sheet of paper in half vertically. On one side, list topics you think you know well. On the other side, list topics you need to review. Pay no attention if one side is longer than the other. When you're done studying, you'll feel strong in every area.

Where the list comes from

To make sure your list reflects a comprehensive view of all the areas you studied in school, look at the contents page in the front of this book. For each topic listed, place it in the "know well" column or "needs review" column. Separating content areas this way shows immediately which topics need less study time and which need more time.

I'll cover difficult topics in the morning when I'm more alert.

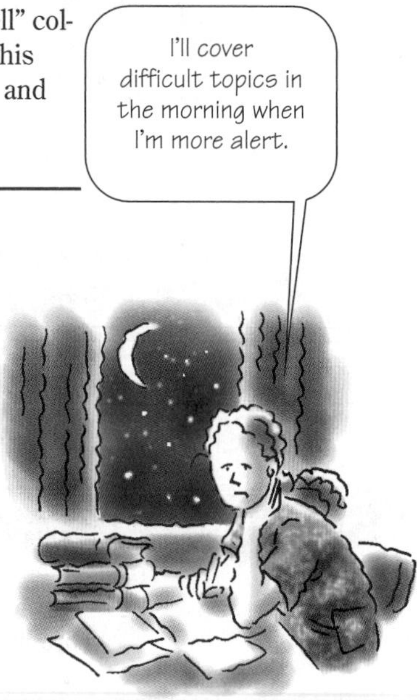

Scheduling study time

Study when you're most alert. Most people can identify a period of the day when they feel most alert. If you feel most alert and energized in the morning, for example, set aside sections of time in the morning for topics that need a lot of review. Then you can use the evening, a time of lesser alertness, for topics that need some refreshing. The opposite is true as well; if you're more alert in the evening, study difficult topics at that time.

What and when

Set up a basic schedule for studying. Using a calendar or organizer, determine how much time remains before you'll take the NCLEX. (See *2 to 3 months before the NCLEX.*) Fill in the remaining days with specific times and topics to be studied. For example, you might schedule the respiratory system on a Tuesday morning and the GI system that afternoon. Remember to schedule difficult topics during your most alert times.

Keep in mind that you shouldn't fill each day with studying. Be realistic and set aside time for normal activities. Try to create ample study time before the NCLEX and then stick to the schedule. Allow some extra time in the schedule in case you get behind or come across a topic that requires extra review.

Keep goals manageable

Part of creating a schedule means setting goals you can accomplish. You no doubt studied a great deal in nursing school, and by now you have a sense of your own capabilities. Ask yourself, "How much can I cover in a day?" Set that amount of time aside and then stay on task. You'll feel better about yourself—and your

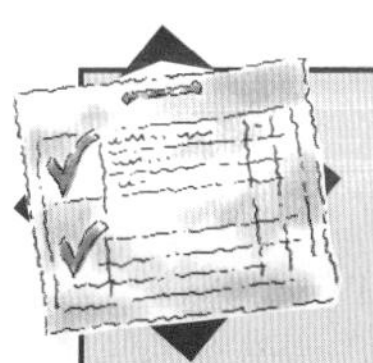

To-do list

2 to 3 months before the NCLEX

With 2 to 3 months remaining before you plan to take the examination, take these steps:
- Establish a study schedule. Set aside ample time to study but also leave time for social activities, exercise, family or personal responsibilities, and other matters.
- Become knowledgeable about the NCLEX-RN examination, its content, the types of questions it asks, and the testing format.
- Begin studying your notes, texts, and other study materials.
- Take some NCLEX practice questions to help you diagnose strengths and weaknesses as well as to become familiar with NCLEX-style questions.

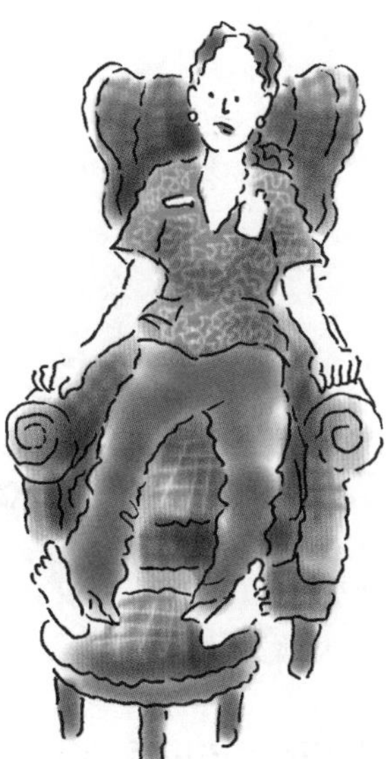
This chair invites slacking, not studying! You should find a chair that encourages good posture instead.

chances of passing the NCLEX—when you meet your goals regularly.

Study space

Find a space conducive to effective learning and then study there. Whatever you do, don't study with a television on in the room. Instead, find a quiet, inviting study space that:
- is located in a quiet, convenient place, away from normal traffic patterns
- contains a solid chair that encourages good posture (Avoid studying in bed; you'll be more likely to fall asleep and not accomplish your goals.)
- uses comfortable, soft lighting with which you can see clearly without eye strain
- has a temperature between 65° and 70° F
- contains flowers or green plants, familiar photos or paintings, and easy access to soft, instrumental background music.

Accentuate the positive

Consider taping positive messages around your study space. Make signs with words of encouragement, such as, "You can do it!" "Keep studying!" and "Remember the goal!" These upbeat messages can help keep you going when your attention begins to waver.

Maintaining concentration

When you're faced with reviewing the amount of information covered by the NCLEX, it's easy to become distracted and lose your concentration. When you lose concentration, you make less effective use of valuable study time. To help stay focused, keep these tips in mind:

- Alternate the order of the subjects you study during the day to add variety to your study. Try alternating between topics you find most interesting and those you find least interesting.
- Approach your studying with enthusiasm, sincerity, and determination.
- Once you've decided to study, begin immediately. Don't let anything interfere with your thought processes once you've begun.
- Concentrate on accomplishing one task at a time, to the exclusion of everything else.
- Don't try to do two things at once, such as studying and watching television or conversing with friends.
- Work continuously without interruption for a while, but don't study for such a long period that the whole experience becomes grueling or boring.
- Allow time for periodic breaks to give yourself a change of pace. Use these breaks to ease your transition into studying a new topic.
- When studying in the evening, wind down from your studies slowly. Don't progress directly from studying to sleeping.

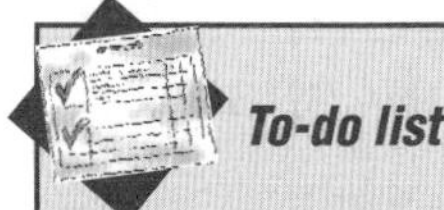

4 to 6 weeks before the NCLEX

With 4 to 6 weeks remaining before you plan to take the examination, take these steps:

- Focus on your areas of weakness. That way, you'll have time to review these areas again before the test date.
- Find a study partner or form a study group.
- Take a practice test to gauge your skill level early.
- Take time to eat, sleep, exercise, and socialize to avoid burnout.

Taking care of yourself

Never neglect your physical and mental well-being in favor of longer study hours. Maintaining physical and mental health is critical for success in taking the NCLEX. (See *4 to 6 weeks before the NCLEX*.)

A few simple rules

You can increase your likelihood of passing the test by following these simple health rules:

- Get plenty of rest. You can't think deeply or concentrate for long periods when you're tired.
- Drink enough noncaffeinated beverages. Mild dehydration increases the effort required to concentrate and reason while distracting attention through feelings of fatigue and thirst.
- Eat nutritious meals. Maintaining your energy level is impossible when you're undernourished.

• Exercise regularly. Regular exercise, preferably 30 minutes daily, helps you work harder and think more clearly. As a result, you'll study more efficiently and increase the likelihood of success.

Memory powers, activate!

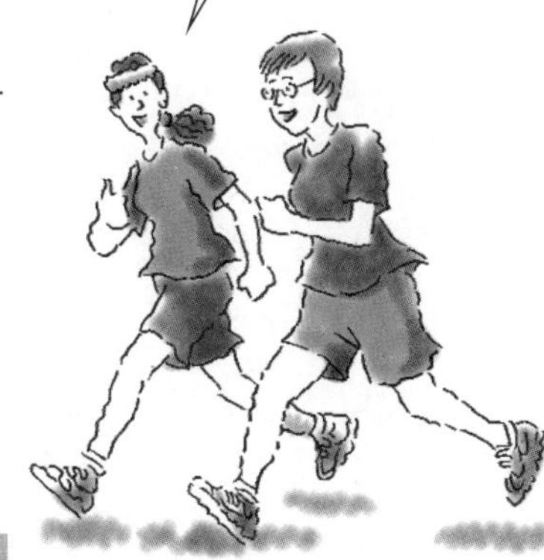

A short jog now will help us concentrate later.

If you're having trouble concentrating but would rather push through than take a break, try making your studying more active by reading out loud. Active studying can renew your powers of concentration. By reading review material out loud to yourself, you're engaging your ears as well as your eyes—and making your studying a more active process. Hearing the material out loud also fosters memory and subsequent recall.

You can also rewrite in your own words a few of the more difficult concepts you're reviewing. Explaining these concepts in writing forces you to think through the material and can jump-start your memory.

Study schedule

When you were creating your schedule, you might have asked yourself, "How long should I study? One hour at a stretch? Two hours? Three?" To make the best use of your study time, you'll need to answer those questions.

Optimum study time

Consider studying in 20- to 30-minute intervals with a short break in-between. You remember the material you study at the beginning and end of a session best and tend to remember less material studied in the middle of the session. The total length of time in each study session depends on you and the amount of material you need to cover.

To thine own self be true

So what's the answer? It doesn't matter as long as you determine what's best for *you*. At the beginning of your NCLEX study schedule, try study periods of varying lengths. Pay close attention to those that seem more successful.

Remember that you're a trained nurse who is competent at assessment. Think of yourself as a patient, and assess your own progress. Then implement the strategy that works best for you.

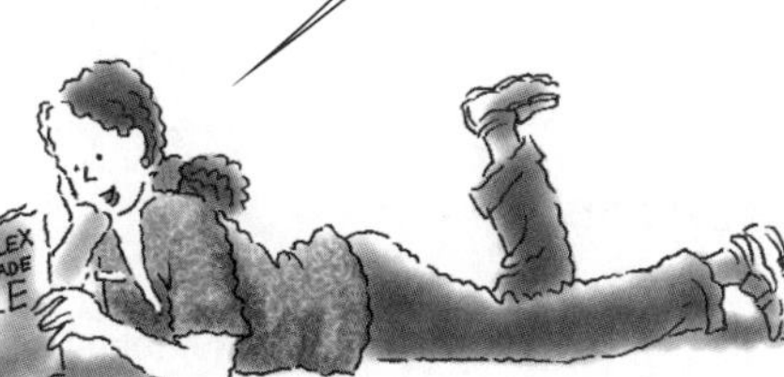

I've found that hour-and-a-half sessions work best for me.

Finding time to study

So does that mean that short sections of time are useless? Not at all. We all have spaces in our day that might otherwise be dead time. (See *1 week before the NCLEX.*) These are perfect times to review for the NCLEX but not to cover new material because by the time you get deep into new material, your time will be over. Always keep some flashcards or a small notebook handy for situations when you have a few extra minutes.

You'll be amazed how many short sessions you can find in a day and how much reviewing you can do in 5 minutes. The following places offer short stretches of time you can use:

- eating breakfast
- waiting for, or riding on, a train or bus
- waiting in line at the bank, post office, bookstore, or other places
- using exercise equipment, such as a treadmill.

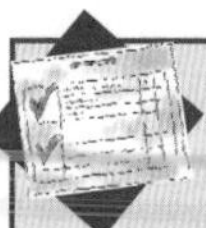

To-do list

1 week before the NCLEX

With 1 week remaining before the NCLEX examination, take these steps:

- Take a review test to measure your progress.
- Record key ideas and principles on note cards or audiotapes.
- Rest, eat well, and avoid thinking about the examination during nonstudy times.
- Treat yourself to one special event. You've been working hard, and you deserve it!

Creative studying

Even when you study in a perfect study space and concentrate better than ever, studying for the NCLEX can get a little, well, dull. Even people with terrific study habits occasionally feel bored or sluggish. That is why it's important to have some creative tricks in your study bag to liven up your studying during those down times.

Creative studying doesn't have to be hard work. It involves making efforts to alter your study habits a bit. Some techniques that might help include studying with a partner or group and creating flash cards or other audiovisual study tools.

Study partners

Studying with a partner or group of students (3 or 4 students at most) can be an excellent way to energize your studying. Working with a partner allows you to test each other on the material you've reviewed. Your partner can give you encouragement and motivation. Perhaps most important, working with a partner can provide a welcome break from solitary studying.

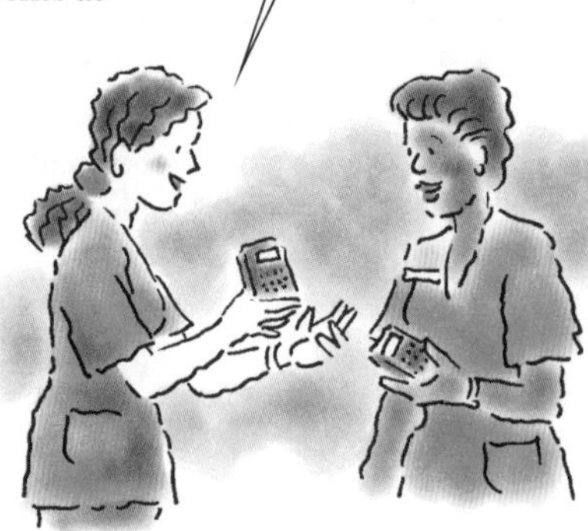

Find a partner with similar goals and strengths. But remember to stay focused!

Be choosy

Exercise some care when choosing a study partner or assembling a study group. A partner who doesn't fit your needs won't help you make the most of your study time. Look for a partner who:

• possesses similar goals to yours. For example, someone taking the NCLEX at approximately the same date who feels the same sense of urgency as you do might make an excellent partner.

• possesses about the same level of knowledge as you. Tutoring someone can sometimes help you learn, but partnering should be give-and-take so both partners can gain knowledge.

• can study without excess chatting or interruptions. Socializing is an important part of creative study, but remember, you've still got to pass the NCLEX—so stay serious!

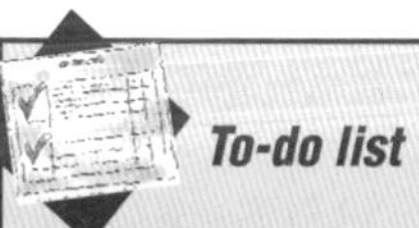

To-do list

The day before the NCLEX

With 1 day before the NCLEX examination, take these steps:

• Drive to the test site, review traffic patterns, and find out where to park. If your route to the test site occurs during heavy traffic or if you're expecting bad weather, set aside extra time to ensure prompt arrival.

• Do something relaxing during the day.

• Avoid concentrating on the test.

• Eat and drink well and avoid dwelling on the NCLEX during nonstudy periods.

• Call a supportive friend or relative for some last-minute words of encouragement.

• Get plenty of rest the night before and allow for plenty of time in the morning.

Audiovisual tools

Flash cards and other audiovisual tools foster retention and make learning and reviewing fun.

Flash Gordon? No, it's Flash Card!

Flash cards can provide you with an excellent study tool. The process of writing material on a flash card will help you remember it. In addition, flash cards are small and easily portable, perfect for those 5-minute slivers of time that show up during the day.

Creating a flash card should be fun. Use magic markers, highlighters, and other colorful tools to make them visually stimulating. The more effort you put into creating your flash cards, the better you'll remember the material contained on the cards.

Other visual tools

Flowcharts, drawings, diagrams, and other image-oriented study aids can also help you learn material more effectively. Substituting images for text can be a great way to give your eyes a break and recharge your brain. Remember to use vivid colors to make your creations visually engaging.

Hear's the thing

If you learn more effectively when you hear information rather than see it, consider recording key ideas using a handheld tape recorder. Recording information helps promote memory because you say the information aloud when taping and then listen to it when playing it back. Like flash cards, tapes are portable and perfect for those short study periods during the day. (See *The day before the NCLEX.*)

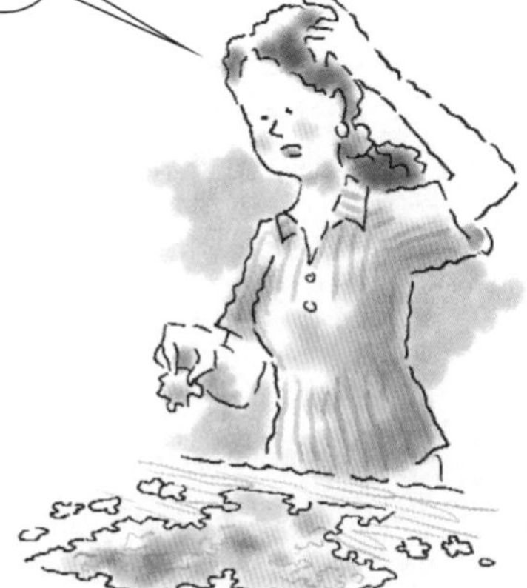

Charts, drawings, and diagrams make concepts less puzzling.

Practice tests

Practice questions should constitute an important part of your NCLEX study strategy. Practice questions can improve your studying by helping you review material and familiarizing yourself with the exact style of questions you'll encounter on the NCLEX.

Practice at the beginning

Consider working through some practice questions as soon as you begin studying for the NCLEX. For example, you might try a half-dozen questions from each chapter in this book.

If you score well, you probably know the material contained in that chapter fairly well and can spend less time reviewing that particular topic. If you have trouble with the questions, spend extra study time on that topic.

You're getting there

Practice questions can also provide an excellent means of marking your progress. Don't worry if you have trouble answering the first few practice questions you take; you'll need time to adjust to the way the questions are asked. Eventually you'll become accustomed to the question format and begin to focus more on the questions themselves.

If you make practice questions a regular part of your study regimen, you'll be able to notice areas in which you're improving. You can then adjust your study time accordingly.

Practice makes perfect

As you near the examination date, continue to answer practice questions, but also set aside time to take an entire NCLEX practice test. (We've included six at the back of this book.) That way, you'll know exactly what to expect. (See *The day of the NCLEX*.) The more you know ahead of time, the better you're likely to do on the NCLEX.

Taking an entire practice test is also a way to gauge your progress. When you find yourself answering questions correctly, it will give you the confidence you need to conquer the real NCLEX.

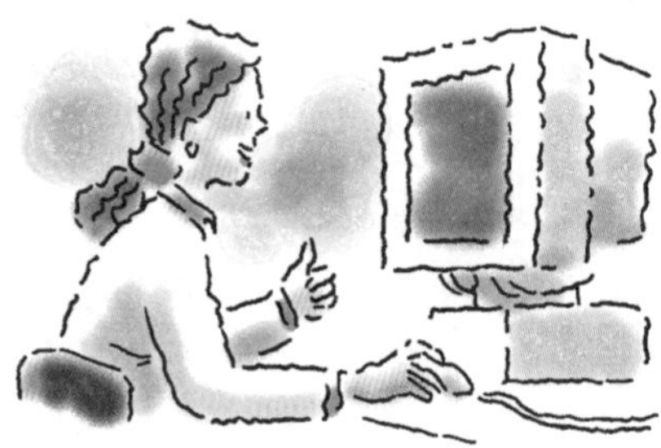

Because I've taken lots of practice tests, I understand how the questions work.

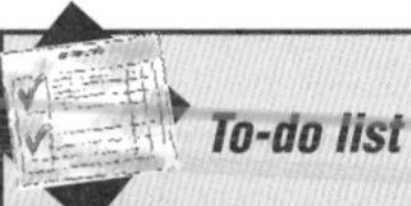

To-do list

The day of the NCLEX

On the day of the NCLEX examination, take these steps:

- Get up early.
- Wear comfortable clothes, preferably with layers you can adjust to fit the room temperature.
- Drink a glass of water and eat a small nutritious breakfast.
- Leave your house early.
- Arrive at the test site early with the required paperwork in hand.
- Avoid looking at your notes as you wait for your computer test.
- Listen carefully to the instructions given before entering the test room.
- Succeed, succeed, *succeed!*

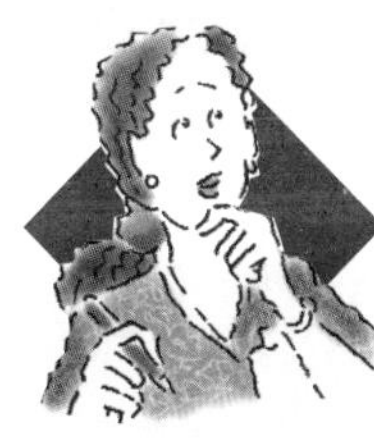

Quick quiz

1. The best time to study is:

A. in the morning.
B. early in the evening.
C. after eating a full meal.
D. when you feel most alert.

Answer: D. Study when you're most alert. If you feel most alert and energized in the morning, for example, set aside sections of time in the morning for topics that need a lot of review.

2. The temperature of the ideal study area should be between:

A. 60° and 65° F.
B. 65° and 70° F.
C. 70° and 75° F.
D. 75° and 80° F.

Answer: B. The ideal study area has a temperature between 65° and 70° F.

3. To help you maintain concentration during long study periods, recommended study strategies include:

A. Study the topics you find most interesting first, followed by the topics you find least interesting.
B. Study the topics you find least interesting first, followed by the topics you find most interesting.
C. Alternate the order of the subjects you study during the day.
D. Study only the topics you find least interesting; you'll remember the others.

Answer: C. Alternating the order of the subjects you study during the day adds variety to your study and helps you remain focused and make the most of your study time.

4. When selecting a study partner, choose one who:

A. possesses similar goals as you.
B. is highly social and will keep you entertained.
C. isn't as knowledgeable as you so you can tutor him.
D. likes to take a lot of breaks.

Answer: A. A partner who doesn't fit your needs won't help you make the most of your study time. Look for a partner who has similar goals to yours, possesses about the same level of knowledge as you, and won't spend too much time socializing.

Scoring

☆☆☆ If you answered all four questions correctly, wow! We hope the exam is ready for *you!*

☆☆ If you answered three questions correctly, terrific! You're cruising toward an exam day victory!

☆ If you answered fewer than three questions correctly, fear not. By the time you're done practicing, you'll be an NCLEX success!

Part II Care of the adult

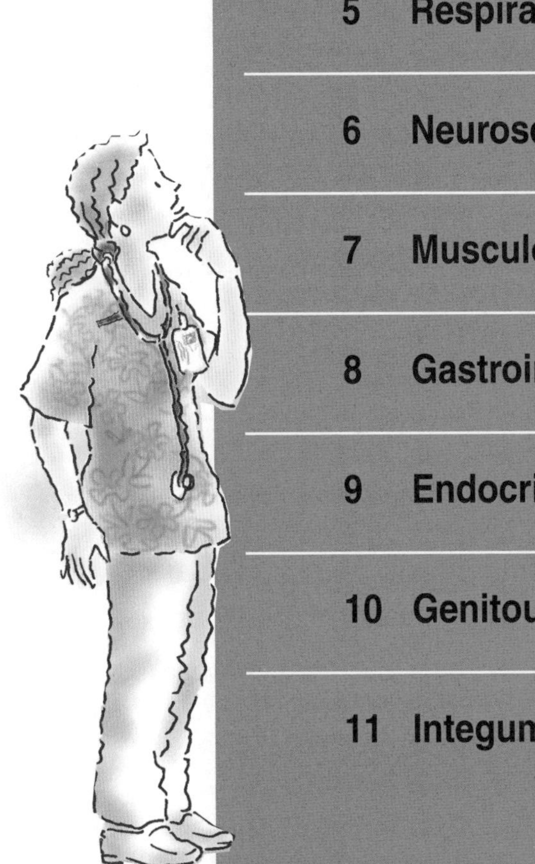

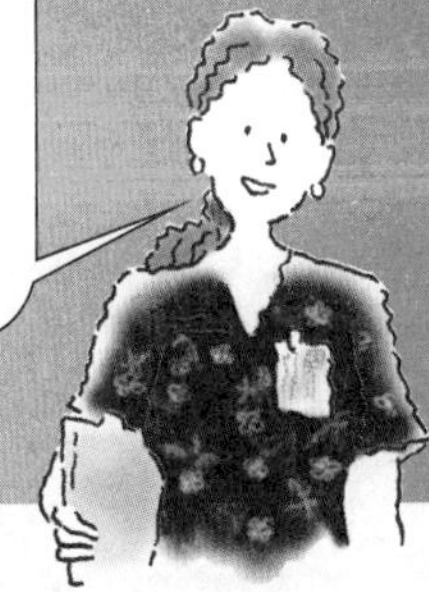

Chapter 3 Cardiovascular disorders

1. A client's electrocardiogram (ECG) is showing ST elevation in Leads V_2, V_3, and V_4. Which artery is most likely to be occluded?
1. Circumflex artery
2. Internal mammary artery
3. Left anterior descending artery
4. Right coronary artery

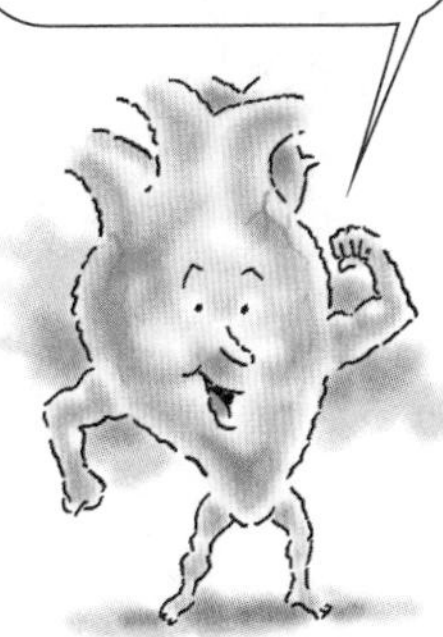

Different arteries supply my different sections with the blood I need to stay healthy.

1. 3. The client's ECG changes suggest an anterior-wall myocardial infarction. The left anterior descending artery is the primary source of blood for the anterior wall of the heart. The circumflex artery supplies the lateral wall, the internal mammary artery supplies the mammary, and the right coronary artery supplies the inferior wall of the heart.
CN: Physiological integrity; CNS: Physiological adaptation; CL: Analysis

2. A nurse on a telemetry unit teaches a student nurse how coronary arteries primarily receive blood flow. It would be most important for the nurse to emphasize that most of the blood flow to coronary arteries is supplied during which of the following?
1. During inspiration
2. During diastole
3. During expiration
4. During systole

2. 2. Although the coronary arteries may receive a minute portion of blood during systole, most of the blood flow to coronary arteries is supplied during diastole. Breathing patterns are irrelevant to blood flow.
CN: Physiological integrity; CNS: Physiological adaptation; CL: Application

3. Which of the following illnesses, if stated by a client, would indicate that he understands the leading cause of death in the United States?
1. Cancer
2. Coronary artery disease (CAD)
3. Liver failure
4. Renal failure

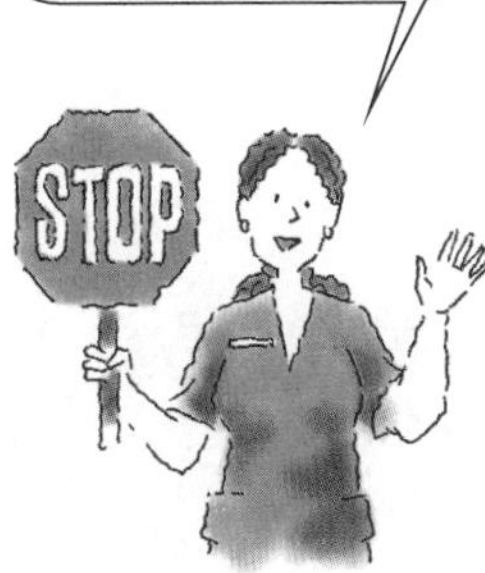

Stop and think! Although all of the answers relate to CAD, only one answer is correct.
STOP

3. 2. CAD accounts for 30% of all deaths in the United States. Cancer accounts for approximately 20%. Liver failure and renal failure account for less than 10% of all deaths in the United States.
CN: Health promotion and maintenance; CNS: None; CL: Analysis

4. Which condition most commonly <u>results</u> in <u>coronary</u> artery disease (CAD)?
1. Atherosclerosis
2. Diabetes mellitus
3. Myocardial infarction (MI)
4. Renal failure

4. 1. Atherosclerosis, or plaque formation, is the leading cause of CAD. Diabetes mellitus is a risk factor for CAD but it isn't the most common cause. Renal failure doesn't cause CAD, but the two conditions are related. MI is commonly a result of CAD.
CN: Physiological integrity; CNS: Physiological adaptation; CL: Analysis

CN: Client needs category CNS: Client needs subcategory CL: Cognitive level

5. A nurse describes atherosclerosis for client education. Which of the following statements, if made by the client, requires additional teaching?

1. Plaques obstruct the coronary artery.
2. Plaques obstruct the vein.
3. Hardened vessels can't dilate to allow blood to flow through.
4. Atherosclerosis can cause angina.

5. 2. Arteries, not veins, supply the coronary arteries with oxygen and other nutrients. Atherosclerosis is a direct result of plaque formation in the artery. Hardened vessels can't dilate properly and, therefore, constrict blood flow and oxygen, causing angina.

CN: Physiological integrity; CNS: Physiological adaptation; CL: Analysis

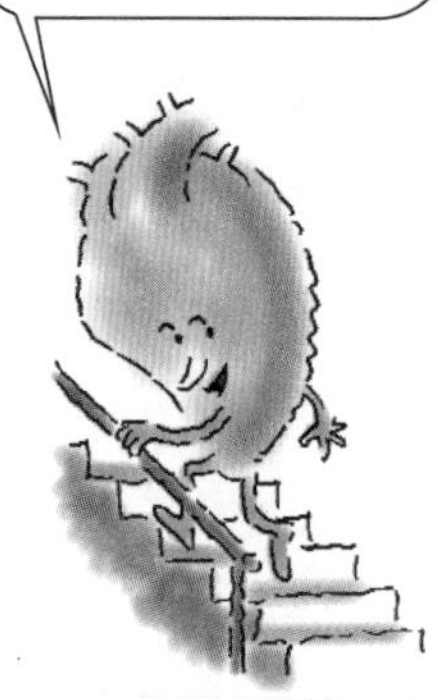

Exercise does wonders for me!

6. Which risk factor for coronary artery disease is non-modifiable?

1. Cigarette smoking
2. Diabetes mellitus
3. Heredity
4. Hypertension

6. 3. Because *heredity* refers to our genetic makeup, it can't be modified. Cigarette smoking cessation is a lifestyle change that involves behavior modification. Diabetes mellitus is a risk factor that can be controlled with diet, exercise, and medication. Altering one's diet, exercise, and medication can correct hypertension.

CN: Physiological integrity; CNS: Reduction of risk potential; CL: Analysis

7. Exceeding which serum cholesterol level significantly increases the risk of coronary artery disease (CAD)?

1. 100 mg/dl
2. 150 mg/dl
3. 175 mg/dl
4. 240 mg/dl

7. 4. Cholesterol levels above 240 mg/dl are considered excessive. They require dietary restriction and perhaps medication. Exercise also helps reduce cholesterol levels. The other levels listed are all below the nationally accepted levels for cholesterol and carry a lesser risk of CAD.

CN: Physiological integrity; CNS: Reduction of risk potential; CL: Comprehension

8. Which action is the <u>first</u> priority of care for a client exhibiting signs and symptoms of coronary artery disease?

1. Decrease anxiety.
2. Enhance myocardial oxygenation.
3. Administer sublingual nitroglycerin.
4. Educate the client about his symptoms.

8. 2. Enhancing myocardial oxygenation is always the first priority when a client exhibits signs or symptoms of cardiac compromise. Without adequate oxygen, the myocardium suffers damage. Sublingual nitroglycerin is administered to treat acute angina, but its administration isn't the first priority. Although educating the client and decreasing anxiety are important in care delivery, neither are priorities when a client is compromised.

CN: Physiological integrity; CNS: Physiological adaptation; CL: Application

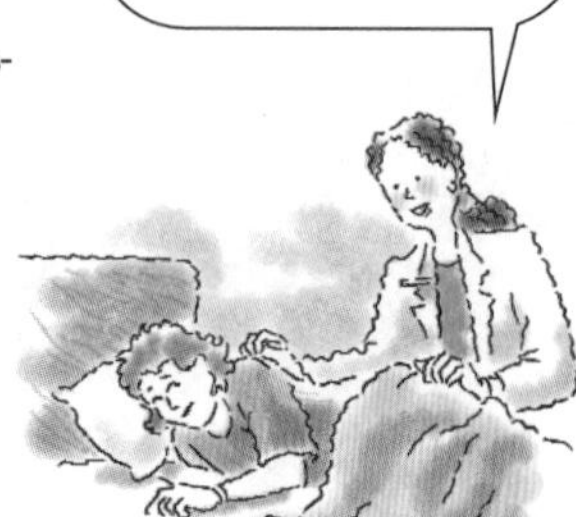

Conservative methods of treatment should always be your first course of action.

9. Medical treatment of coronary artery disease (CAD) includes which procedure?

1. Cardiac catheterization
2. Coronary artery bypass surgery
3. Oral medication administration
4. Percutaneous transluminal coronary angioplasty

9. 3. Oral medication administration is a noninvasive, medical treatment for CAD. Cardiac catheterization isn't a treatment but a diagnostic tool. Coronary artery bypass surgery and percutaneous transluminal coronary angioplasty are invasive, surgical treatments.

CN: Physiological integrity; CNS: Physiological adaptation; CL: Analysis

CN: Client needs category CNS: Client needs subcategory CL: Cognitive level

10. A client's electrocardiogram shows ST elevation in leads II, III, and aV_F, suggesting occlusion of the right coronary artery. Which area of the heart is experiencing an infarction?

1. Anterior
2. Apical
3. Inferior
4. Lateral

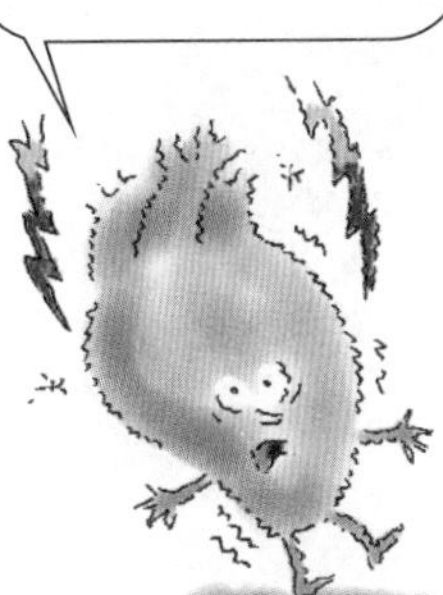

I may experience many symptoms during a heart attack, but which one are you most likely to see?

11. Which is the most common symptom of myocardial infarction (MI)?

1. Chest pain
2. Dyspnea
3. Edema
4. Palpitations

12. Which landmark is the correct one for obtaining an apical pulse?

1. Left fifth intercostal space, midaxillary line
2. Left fifth intercostal space, midclavicular line
3. Left second intercostal space, midclavicular line
4. Left seventh intercostal space, midclavicular line

13. Which system is the most likely origin of pain the client describes as knifelike chest pain that increases in intensity with inspiration?

1. Cardiac
2. Gastrointestinal
3. Musculoskeletal
4. Pulmonary

14. While assessing a client's heart sounds, a murmur is heard at the second left intercostal space along the left sternal border. Which valve is most likely involved?

1. Aortic
2. Mitral
3. Pulmonic
4. Tricuspid

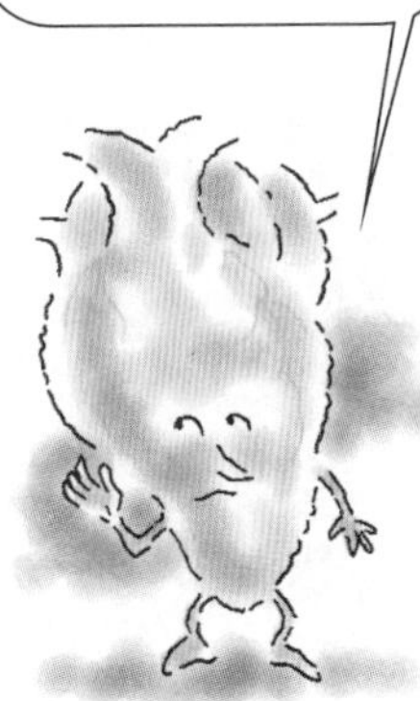

Did someone murmur something?

10. 3. The right coronary artery supplies the right ventricle, or the inferior portion of the heart. Therefore, occlusion could produce an infarction in that area. The right coronary artery doesn't supply the anterior portion (left ventricle), lateral portion (some of the left ventricle and the left atrium), or the apical portion (left ventricle) of the heart.

CN: Physiological integrity; CNS: Physiological adaptation; CL: Application

11. 1. The most common symptom of an MI is chest pain, resulting from deprivation of oxygen to the heart. Dyspnea is the second most common symptom, related to an increase in the metabolic needs of the body during an MI. Edema is a later sign of heart failure, commonly seen after an MI. Palpitations may result from reduced cardiac output, producing arrhythmias.

CN: Safe, effective care environment; CNS: Management of care; CL: Analysis

12. 2. The correct landmark for obtaining an apical pulse is the left fifth intercostal space in the midclavicular line. This is the point of maximum impulse and the location of the left ventricular apex. The left second intercostal space in the midclavicular line is where pulmonic sounds are auscultated. Normally, heart sounds aren't heard in the midaxillary line or the seventh intercostal space in the midclavicular line.

CN: Physiological integrity; CNS: Basic care and comfort; CL: Application

13. 4. Pulmonary pain is generally described by these symptoms. Musculoskeletal pain only increases with movement. Cardiac and GI pains don't change with respiration.

CN: Physiological integrity; CNS: Physiological adaptation; CL: Analysis

14. 3. Abnormalities of the pulmonic valve are auscultated at the second left intercostal space along the left sternal border. Aortic valve abnormalities are heard at the second intercostal space, to the right of the sternum. Mitral valve abnormalities are heard at the fifth intercostal space in the midclavicular line. Tricuspid valve abnormalities are heard at the third and fourth intercostal spaces along the sternal border.

CN: Physiological integrity; CNS: Physiological adaptation; CL: Application

15. Which blood test is the best indicator for myocardial injury?
1. Lactate dehydrogenase (LD)
2. Complete blood count (CBC)
3. Troponin I
4. Creatine kinase (CK)

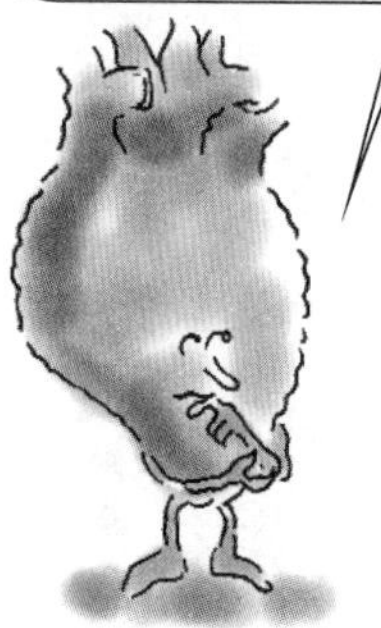

Think of what happens when cardiac tissue is damaged.

15. 3. Troponin I levels rise rapidly and are detectable within 1 hour of myocardial injury. Troponin I levels aren't detectable in people without cardiac injury. LD is present in almost all body tissues and not specific to heart muscle. LD isoenzymes may be useful in diagnosing cardiac injury. CBC is obtained to review blood counts, and a complete chemistry is obtained to review electrolytes. Because CK levels may rise with skeletal muscle injury, CK isoenzymes are required to detect cardiac injury.
CN: Health promotion and maintenance; CNS: None; CL: Analysis

16. What is the primary reason for administering morphine to a client with a myocardial infarction?
1. To sedate the client
2. To decrease the client's pain
3. To decrease the client's anxiety
4. To decrease oxygen demand on the client's heart

16. 4. Morphine is administered because it decreases myocardial oxygen demand. Morphine will also decrease pain and anxiety while causing sedation, but it isn't primarily given for those reasons.
CN: Physiological integrity; CNS: Pharmacological and parenteral therapies; CL: Application

17. In caring for a client with cardiac problems, the nurse must know that the condition most likely responsible for myocardial infarction (MI) is which of the following?
1. Aneurysm
2. Heart failure
3. Coronary artery thrombosis
4. Renal failure

17. 3. Coronary artery thrombosis causes an occlusion of the artery, leading to myocardial death. An aneurysm is an outpouching of a vessel and doesn't cause an MI. Heart failure is usually the result of an MI. Renal failure can be associated with MI but isn't a direct cause.
CN: Physiological integrity; CNS: Physiological adaptation; CL: Analysis

18. What supplemental medication is most frequently ordered in conjunction with furosemide (Lasix)?
1. Chloride
2. Digoxin
3. Potassium
4. Sodium

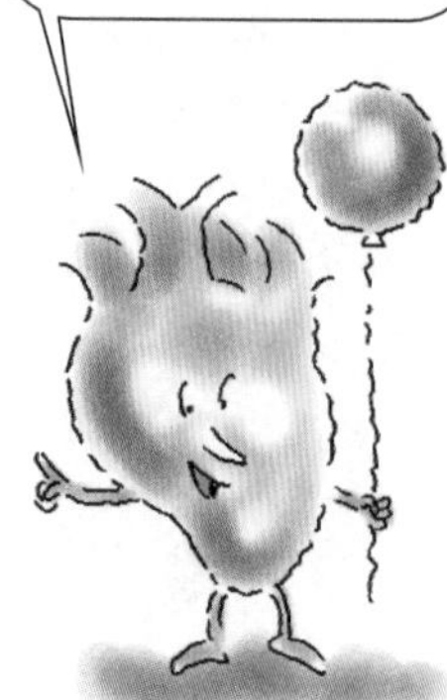

It's important to know what physiologic changes occur in your client after a heart attack.

18. 3. Supplemental potassium is given with furosemide because of the potassium loss that occurs as a result of this diuretic. Chloride and sodium aren't lost during diuresis. Digoxin acts to increase contractility but isn't given routinely with furosemide.
CN: Physiological integrity; CNS: Pharmacological and parenteral therapies; CL: Analysis

19. In order to anticipate problems in a client following a myocardial infarction (MI), the nurse should understand that which type of physiological changes will increase serum glucose levels and free fatty acid production?
1. Electrophysiologic
2. Hematologic
3. Mechanical
4. Metabolic

19. 4. Both glucose and fatty acids are metabolites whose levels increase after an MI. Mechanical changes are those that affect the pumping action of the heart, and electrophysiologic changes affect conduction. Hematologic changes would affect the blood.
CN: Physiological integrity; CNS: Physiological adaptation; CL: Application

20. Which complication is indicated by a third heart sound (S_3)?

1. Ventricular dilation
2. Systemic hypertension
3. Aortic valve malfunction
4. Increased atrial contractions

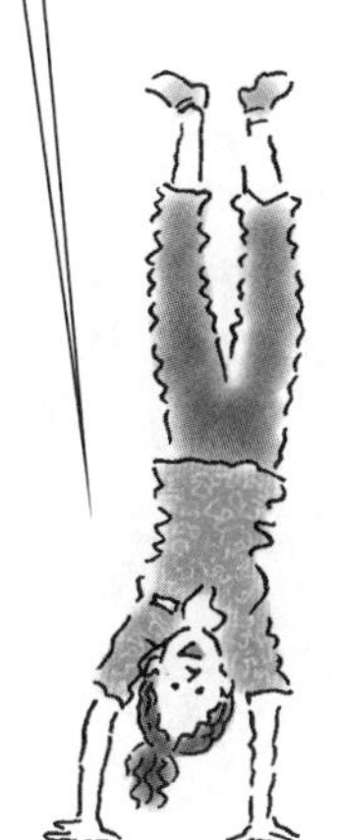
Twenty questions done! Good job!

20. 1. Rapid filling of the ventricle causes vasodilation that is auscultated as S_3. Systemic hypertension or increased atrial contraction can result in a fourth heart sound. Aortic valve malfunction is heard as a murmur.

CN: Health promotion and maintenance; CNS: None; CL: Analysis

21. After an anterior-wall myocardial infarction (MI), which problem is indicated by auscultation of crackles in the lungs?

1. Left-sided heart failure
2. Pulmonic valve malfunction
3. Right-sided heart failure
4. Tricuspid valve malfunction

21. 1. The left ventricle is responsible for most of the cardiac output. An anterior-wall MI may result in a decrease in left ventricular function. When the left ventricle doesn't function properly, resulting in left-sided heart failure, fluid accumulates in the interstitial and alveolar spaces in the lungs and causes crackles. Pulmonic and tricuspid valve malfunction causes right-sided heart failure.

CN: Physiological integrity; CNS: Physiological adaptation; CL: Analysis

22. A client who is being evaluated for myocardial infarction (MI) asks the nurse which diagnostic tool is most commonly used to determine the location of myocardial damage. Which of the following would be the best response by the nurse?

1. Cardiac catheterization
2. Cardiac enzymes
3. Echocardiogram
4. Electrocardiogram (ECG)

22. 4. The ECG is the quickest, most accurate, and most widely used tool to determine the location of myocardial infarction (MI). Cardiac catheterization is an invasive study for determining coronary artery disease and may also indicate the location of myocardial damage, but the study may not be performed immediately. Cardiac enzymes are used to diagnose MI but can't determine the location. An echocardiogram is used most widely to view myocardial wall function after an MI has been diagnosed.

CN: Physiological integrity; CNS: Reduction of risk potential; CL: Application

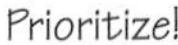
Prioritize!

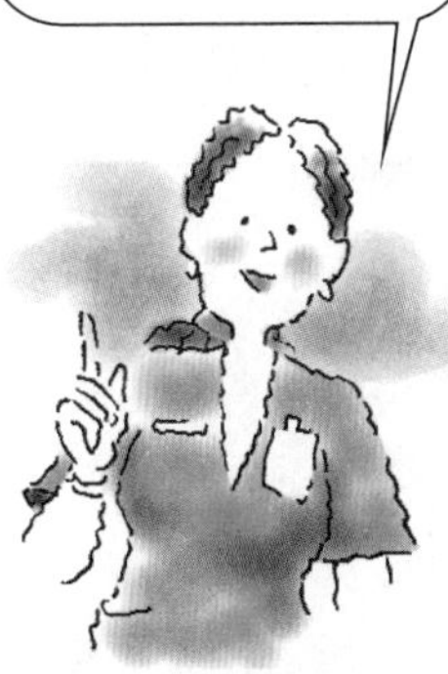

23. What is the first intervention for a client experiencing myocardial infarction (MI)?

1. Administer morphine.
2. Administer oxygen.
3. Administer sublingual nitroglycerin.
4. Obtain an electrocardiogram (ECG).

23. 2. Administering supplemental oxygen to the client is the first priority of care. The myocardium is deprived of oxygen during an infarction, so additional oxygen is administered to assist in oxygenation and prevent further damage. Morphine and sublingual nitroglycerin are also used to treat MI, but they're more commonly administered after the oxygen. An ECG is the most common diagnostic tool used to evaluate MI.

CN: Safe, effective care environment; CNS: Management of care; CL: Analysis

24. What is the most appropriate nursing response to a myocardial infarction (MI) client who is fearful of dying?

1. "Tell me about your feelings right now."
2. "When the doctor arrives, everything will be fine."
3. "This is a bad situation, but you'll feel better soon."
4. "Please be assured we're doing everything we can to make you feel better."

24. 1. Validation of a client's feelings is the most appropriate response. It gives the client a feeling of comfort and safety. The other three responses give the client false hope. No one can determine if a client experiencing an MI will feel or get better and, therefore, these responses are inappropriate.
CN: Psychosocial integrity; CNS: None; CL: Comprehension

25. Which class of medications protects the ischemic myocardium by blocking catecholamines and sympathetic nerve stimulation?

1. Beta-adrenergic blockers
2. Calcium channel blockers
3. Opioids
4. Nitrates

25. 1. Beta-adrenergic blockers work by blocking beta receptors in the myocardium, reducing the response to catecholamines and sympathetic nerve stimulation. They protect the myocardium, helping to reduce the risk of another infarction by decreasing the workload of the heart and decreasing myocardial oxygen demand. Calcium channel blockers reduce the workload of the heart by decreasing the heart rate. Opioids reduce myocardial oxygen demand, promote vasodilation, and decrease anxiety. Nitrates reduce myocardial oxygen consumption by decreasing left ventricular end-diastolic pressure (preload) and systemic vascular resistance (afterload).
CN: Physiological integrity; CNS: Pharmacological and parenteral therapies; CL: Application

26. What is the most common complication of a myocardial infarction (MI)?

1. Cardiogenic shock
2. Heart failure
3. Arrhythmias
4. Pericarditis

26. 3. Arrhythmias, caused by oxygen deprivation to the myocardium, are the most common complication of an MI. Cardiogenic shock, another complication of MI, is defined as the end stage of left ventricular dysfunction. The condition occurs in approximately 15% of clients with MI. Because the pumping function of the heart is compromised by an MI, heart failure is the second most common complication. Pericarditis most commonly results from a bacterial or viral infection but may occur after MI.
CN: Physiological integrity; CNS: Physiological adaptation; CL: Application

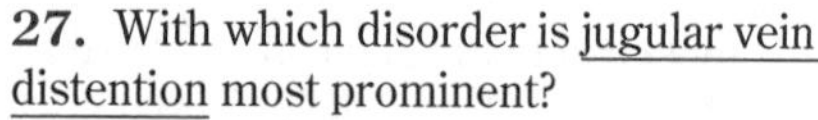

27. With which disorder is jugular vein distention most prominent?

1. Abdominal aortic aneurysm
2. Heart failure
3. Myocardial infarction (MI)
4. Pneumothorax

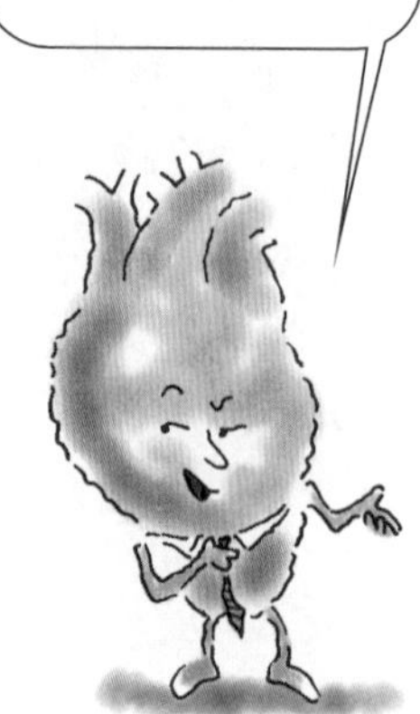

This question wasn't asked in vein. (Hah! Get it?)

27. 2. Elevated venous pressure, exhibited as jugular vein distention, indicates a failure of the heart to pump. Jugular vein distention isn't a symptom of abdominal aortic aneurysm or pneumothorax. An MI, if severe enough, can progress to heart failure; however, in and of itself, an MI doesn't cause jugular vein distention.
CN: Physiological integrity; CNS: Physiological adaptation; CL: Analysis

28. In what position should the nurse place the head of the bed to obtain the most accurate reading of jugular vein distention?

1. High Fowler's
2. Raised 10 degrees
3. Raised 30 degrees
4. Supine

28. 3. Jugular venous pressure is measured with a centimeter ruler to obtain the vertical distance between the sternal angle and the point of highest pulsation with the head of the bed inclined between 15 and 30 degrees. Increased pressure can't be seen when the client is supine or when the head of the bed is raised 10 degrees because the point that marks the pressure level is above the jaw (therefore, not visible). In high Fowler's position, the veins would be barely discernible above the clavicle.
CN: Physiological integrity; CNS: Reduction of risk potential; CL: Analysis

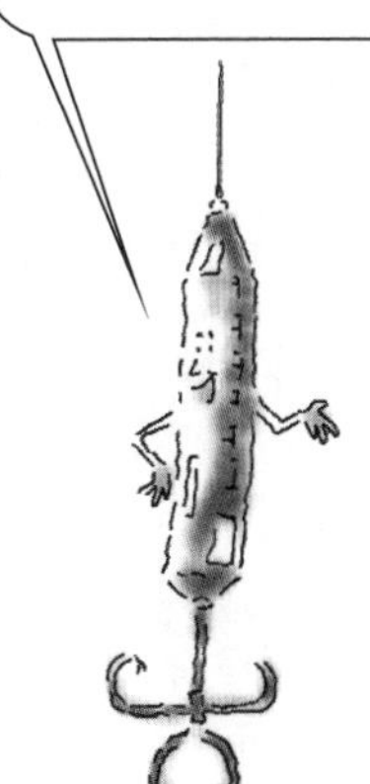

Keep in mind that digoxin strengthens myocardial contraction.

29. A client is ordered to start receving digoxin 0.25 mg P.O. Which parameter should be checked first before administering digoxin?

1. Apical pulse
2. Blood pressure
3. Radial pulse
4. Respiratory rate

29. 1. An apical pulse is essential for accurately assessing the client's heart rate before administering digoxin. The apical pulse is the most accurate pulse point in the body. Blood pressure is usually only affected if the heart rate is too low, in which case the nurse would withhold digoxin. The radial pulse can be affected by cardiac and vascular disease and, therefore, won't always accurately depict the heart rate. Digoxin has no effect on respiratory function.
CN: Physiological integrity; CNS: Pharmacological and parenteral therapies; CL: Application

30. A client complains that he sees a green halo around lights. Upon reviewing the client's medication list, the nurse determines that this is most likely caused by a high level of which medication?

1. Digoxin
2. Furosemide (Lasix)
3. Metoprolol (Lopressor)
4. Enalapril (Vasotec)

30. 1. One of the most common signs of digoxin toxicity is the visual disturbance known as the *green halo sign.* The other medications aren't associated with such an effect.
CN: Physiological integrity; CNS: Pharmacological and parenteral therapies; CL: Analysis

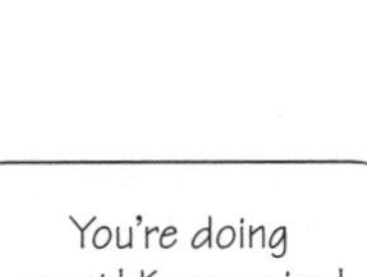

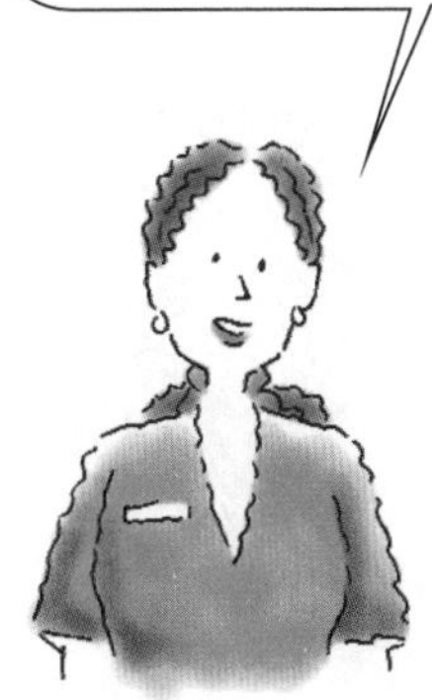

31. Which symptom is most commonly associated with left-sided heart failure?

1. Crackles
2. Arrhythmias
3. Hepatic engorgement
4. Hypotension

31. 1. Crackles in the lungs are a classic sign of left-sided heart failure. These sounds are caused by fluid backing up into the pulmonary system. Arrhythmias can be associated with both right- and left-sided heart failure. Hepatic engorgement is associated with right-sided heart failure. Left-sided heart failure causes hypertension secondary to an increased workload on the system.
CN: Physiological integrity; CNS: Physiological adaptation; CL: Application

32. In which disorder would the nurse expect to assess sacral edema in a bedridden client?

1. Diabetes mellitus
2. Pulmonary emboli
3. Chronic kidney disease
4. Right-sided heart failure

32. 4. The most accurate area on the body to assess dependent edema in a bedridden client is the sacral area. Sacral, or dependent, edema is secondary to right-sided heart failure. Diabetes mellitus, pulmonary emboli, and chronic kidney disease aren't directly linked to sacral edema.
CN: Physiological integrity; CNS: Physiological adaptation; CL: Analysis

33. Which symptom might a client with right-sided heart failure exhibit?

1. Adequate urine output
2. Polyuria
3. Oliguria
4. Polydipsia

33. 3. Inadequate deactivation of aldosterone by the liver after right-sided heart failure leads to fluid retention, which causes oliguria. Adequate urine output, polyuria, and polydipsia aren't associated with right-sided heart failure.
CN: Physiological integrity; CNS: Physiological adaptation; CL: Application

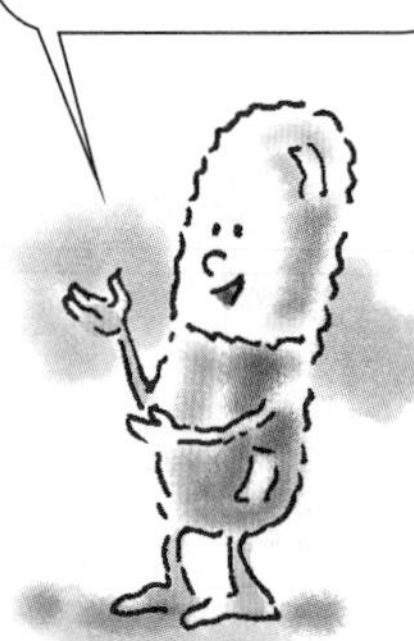

Make sure you understand how these different drugs work to benefit the heart.

34. Which of the following drug classes should be administered to a client with heart failure to maximize cardiac performance by increasing ventricular contractility?

1. Beta-adrenergic blockers
2. Calcium channel blockers
3. Diuretics
4. Inotropic agents

34. 4. Inotropic agents are administered to increase the force of the heart's contractions, thereby increasing ventricular contractility and ultimately increasing cardiac output. Beta-adrenergic blockers and calcium channel blockers decrease the heart rate and ultimately decrease the workload of the heart. Diuretics are administered to decrease the overall vascular volume, also decreasing the workload of the heart.
CN: Physiological integrity; CNS: Pharmacological and parenteral therapies; CL: Application

35. The heart rhythm of a client who has experienced cardiac arrest and is receiving cardiopulmonary resuscitation (CPR) deteriorates to ventricular fibrillation. Which action should the nurse perform first?

1. Administer 1 mg of epinephrine I.V.
2. Defibrillate with 360 joules.
3. Continue CPR.
4. Administer vasopressin 40 units I.V.

35. 2. To attempt to convert the rhythm, the nurse should first defibrillate the client with 360 joules. If this is unsuccessful, she would then continue CPR for five cycles and attempt to defibrillate again. Epinephrine and vasopressin may be given but not until after the first two defibrillation attempts.
CN: Physiological integrity; CNS: Physiological adaptation; CL: Analysis

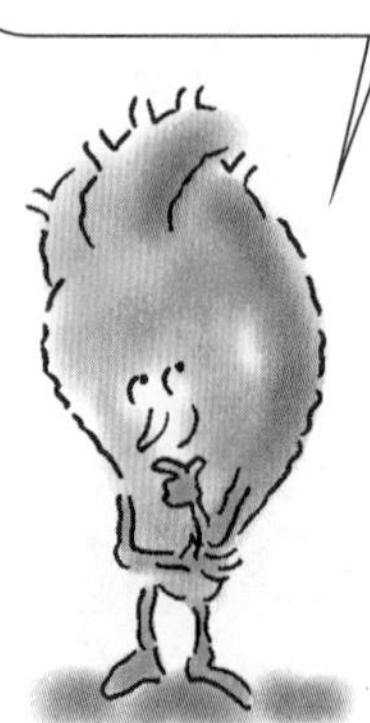

This question asks you to distinguish between symptoms of left- and right-sided heart failure.

36. Which condition is most closely associated with weight gain, nausea, and a decrease in urine output?

1. Angina pectoris
2. Cardiomyopathy
3. Left-sided heart failure
4. Right-sided heart failure

36. 4. Weight gain, nausea, and a decrease in urine output are secondary effects of right-sided heart failure. Cardiomyopathy is usually identified as a symptom of left-sided heart failure. Left-sided heart failure causes primarily pulmonary symptoms rather than systemic ones. Angina pectoris doesn't cause weight gain, nausea, or a decrease in urine output.
CN: Physiological integrity; CNS: Physiological adaptation; CL: Application

37. A client's rhythm strip shows a regular rhythm with atrial and ventricular rates of 70 beats/minute, a PR interval of 0.24, and a QRS duration of 0.08 second. The nurse interprets this rhythm as:

1. normal sinus rhythm (NSR).
2. NSR with 1-degree atrioventricular (AV) block.
3. sinus arrhythmia.
4. accelerated junctional rhythm.

37. 2. An increased PR interval is indicative of a 1-degree AV block. NSR and sinus arrhythmia have normal PR intervals. The PR interval (if present) is less than 0.12 second in accelerated junctional rhythm.

CN: Physiological integrity; CNS: Reducation of risk potential; CL: Analysis

38. A client with abdominal aortic aneurysm asks the nurse in which area are abdominal aortic aneurysms most commonly located. Which of the following would be the nurse's best response?

1. Distal to the iliac arteries
2. Distal to the renal arteries
3. Adjacent to the aortic arch
4. Proximal to the renal arteries

38. 2. The portion of the aorta distal to the renal arteries is more prone to an aneurysm because the vessel isn't surrounded by stable structures, unlike the proximal portion of the aorta. Distal to the iliac arteries, the vessel is again surrounded by stable vasculature, making this an uncommon site for an aneurysm. There is no area adjacent to the aortic arch, which bends into the thoracic (descending) aorta.

CN: Physiological integrity; CNS: Physiological adaptation; CL: Application

39. While palpating a client's abdomen, the nurse notes a pulsating abdominal mass. This may indicate which condition?

1. Abdominal aortic aneurysm
2. Enlarged spleen
3. Gastric distention
4. Gastritis

39. 1. The presence of a pulsating mass in the abdomen is an abnormal finding, usually indicating an outpouching in a weakened vessel, as in abdominal aortic aneurysm. The finding, however, can be normal on a thin person. Neither an enlarged spleen, gastric distention, nor gastritis causes pulsation.

CN: Health promotion and maintenance; CNS: None; CL: Application

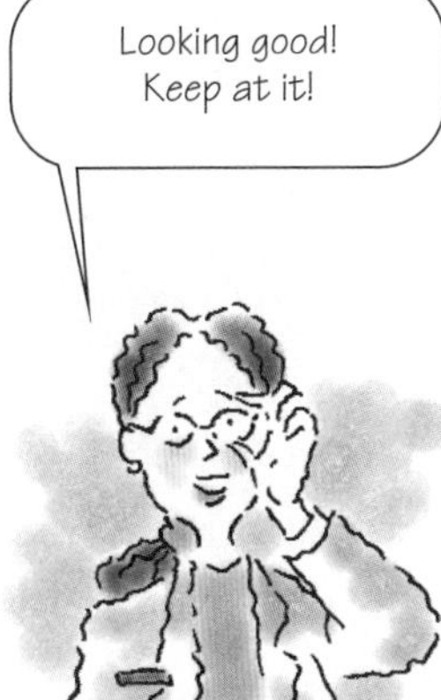

40. What is the most common symptom in a client with abdominal aortic aneurysm?

1. Abdominal pain
2. Diaphoresis
3. Headache
4. Upper back pain

40. 1. Abdominal pain in a client with an abdominal aortic aneurysm results from the disruption of normal circulation in the abdominal region. Diaphoresis and headache aren't associated with abdominal aortic aneurysm. Lower back pain, not upper, is a common symptom, usually signifying expansion and impending rupture of the aneurysm.

CN: Physiological integrity; CNS: Basic care and comfort; CL: Application

41. Which symptom usually signifies rapid expansion and impending rupture of an abdominal aortic aneurysm?

1. Abdominal pain
2. Absent pedal pulses
3. Angina
4. Lower back pain

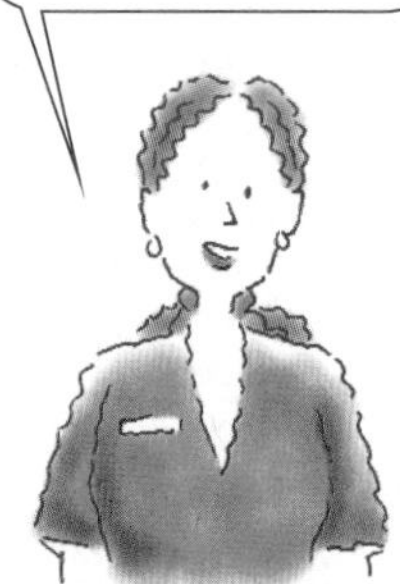

Knowing which symptom relates to which complication will help you to make a more accurate diagnosis.

41. 4. Lower back pain results from expansion of the aneurysm. The expansion applies pressure in the abdominal cavity, and the pain is referred to the lower back. Abdominal pain is the most common symptom resulting from impaired circulation. Absent pedal pulses are a sign of no circulation and would occur after a ruptured aneurysm or in peripheral vascular disease. Angina is associated with atherosclerosis of the coronary arteries.

CN: Physiological integrity; CNS: Basic care and comfort; CL: Application

42. What is the definitive test used to diagnose an abdominal aortic aneurysm?

1. Abdominal X-ray
2. Aortogram
3. Computed tomography (CT) scan
4. Ultrasound

42. 2. An aortogram accurately and directly depicts the vasculature; therefore, it clearly delineates the vessels and any abnormalities. An abdominal aneurysm would only be visible on an X-ray if it were calcified. CT scan and ultrasound don't give a direct view of the vessels and don't yield as accurate a diagnosis as the aortogram.

CN: Health promotion and maintenance; CNS: None; CL: Application

43. Which complication is of greatest concern when caring for a preoperative abdominal aortic aneurysm client?

1. Hypertension
2. Aneurysm rupture
3. Cardiac arrhythmias
4. Diminished pedal pulses

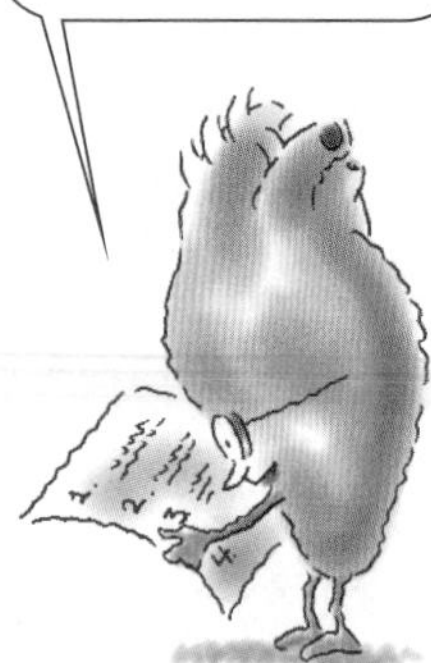

This question is asking you to prioritize, once again.

43. 2. Rupture of the aneurysm is a life-threatening emergency and is of the greatest concern for the nurse caring for this type of client. Hypertension should be avoided and controlled because it can cause the weakened vessel to rupture. Cardiac arrhythmias aren't directly linked to an aneurysm. Diminished pedal pulses, a sign of poor circulation to the lower extremities, are associated with an aneurysm but aren't life-threatening.

CN: Physiological integrity; CNS: Basic care and comfort; CL: Analysis

44. Which precaution should a nurse take when caring for a client with a myocardial infarction who has received a thrombolytic agent?

1. Avoid puncture wounds
2. Monitor potassium levels.
3. Maintain a supine position.
4. Encourage fluids.

44. 1. Thrombolytic agents are declotting agents that place the client at risk for hemorrhage from puncture wounds. All unnecessary needle sticks and invasive procedures should be avoided. The potassium level should be monitored in all cardiac clients, not just those receiving a thrombolytic agent. Although no specific position is required, most cardiac clients seem more comfortable in semi-Fowler's position. The client's fluid balance must be carefully monitored, so it may be inappropriate to encourage fluids at this time.

CN: Physiological integrity; CNS: Reduction of risk potential; CL: Application

45. When assessing a client for an abdominal aortic aneurysm, which area of the abdomen is most commonly palpated?

1. Right upper quadrant
2. Directly over the umbilicus
3. Middle lower abdomen to the left of the midline
4. Middle lower abdomen to the right of the midline

45. 3. The aorta lies directly left of the umbilicus; therefore, any other region is inappropriate for palpation.

CN: Physiological integrity; CNS: Basic care and comfort; CL: Application

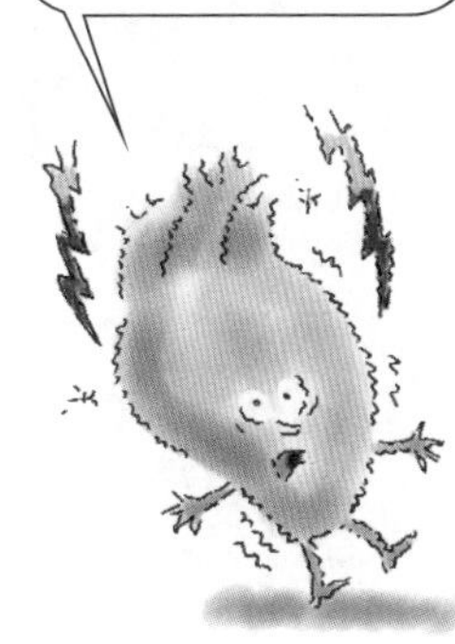

I'm suddenly feeling a little tense, a little hyper. (Get it?)

46. Which condition is linked to more than 50% of clients with abdominal aortic aneurysms?

1. Diabetes mellitus
2. Hypertension
3. Peripheral vascular disease
4. Syphilis

46. 2. Continuous pressure on the vessel walls from hypertension causes the walls to weaken and an aneurysm to occur. Diabetes mellitus doesn't have a direct link to aneurysm. Atherosclerotic changes can occur with peripheral vascular diseases and are linked to aneurysms, but the link isn't as strong as it is with hypertension. Only 1% of clients with syphilis experience an aneurysm.

CN: Health promotion and maintenance; CNS: None; CL: Application

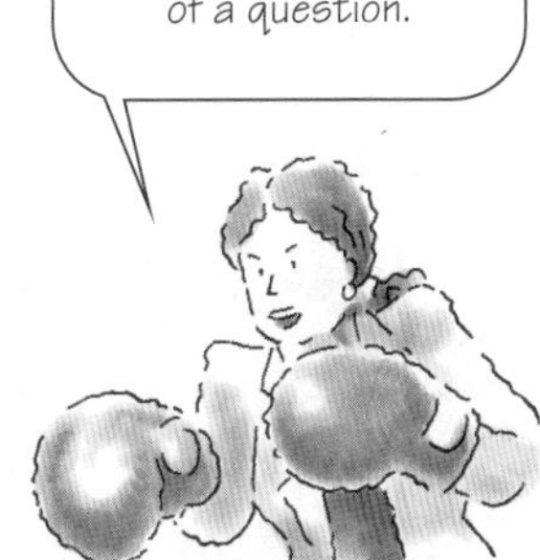

This is a real bruit of a question.

47. When auscultating the abdominal region of a client with abdominal aortic aneurysm, the nurse hears a bruit. Which of the following indicates the significance of this finding?

1. It is a normal finding.
2. It reflects a partial arterial occlusion.
3. It indicates a collection of fluid in the lungs.
4. It shows an inflammation of the peritoneal surface.

47. 2. A bruit is a vascular sound that reflects partial arterial occlusion. It is not a normal finding. Fluid in the lungs is called crackles and inflammation of the peritoneal surface produces a friction rub.

CN: Physiological integrity; CNS: Basic care and comfort; CL: Analysis

48. Which group of symptoms indicates a ruptured abdominal aortic aneurysm?

1. Lower back pain, increased blood pressure, decreased red blood cell (RBC) count, increased white blood cell (WBC) count
2. Severe lower back pain, decreased blood pressure, decreased RBC count, increased WBC count
3. Severe lower back pain, decreased blood pressure, decreased RBC count, decreased WBC count
4. Intermittent lower back pain, decreased blood pressure, decreased RBC count, increased WBC count

48. 2. Severe lower back pain indicates an aneurysm rupture, secondary to pressure being applied within the abdominal cavity. When rupture occurs, the pain is constant because it can't be alleviated until the aneurysm is repaired. Blood pressure decreases due to the loss of blood. After the aneurysm ruptures, the vasculature is interrupted and blood volume is lost, so blood pressure wouldn't increase. For the same reason, the RBC count is decreased. The WBC count increases as cells migrate to the site of injury.

CN: Physiological integrity; CNS: Physiological adaptation; CL: Application

49. Which complication of an abdominal aortic repair is indicated by detection of a hematoma in the perineal area?

1. Hernia
2. Stage 1 pressure ulcer
3. Retroperitoneal rupture at the repair site
4. Rapid expansion of the aneurysm

49. 3. Blood collects in the retroperitoneal space and is exhibited as a hematoma in the perineal area. This rupture is most commonly caused by leakage at the repair site. A hernia doesn't cause vascular disturbances, nor does a pressure ulcer. Because no bleeding occurs with rapid expansion of the aneurysm, a hematoma won't form.

CN: Physiological integrity; CNS: Physiological adaptation; CL: Comprehension

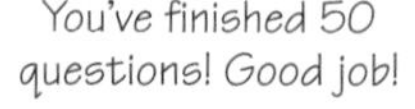

You've finished 50 questions! Good job!

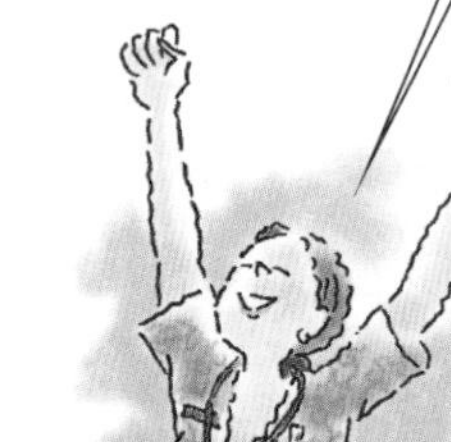

50. Which genetic disease is most closely linked to aneurysm?

1. Cystic fibrosis
2. Hemophilia
3. Marfan's syndrome
4. Sickle cell anemia

50. 3. Marfan's syndrome results in the degeneration of the elastic fibers of the aortic media. Therefore, clients with the syndrome are more likely to develop an aneurysm. Although cystic fibrosis, hemophilia, and sickle cell anemia are all genetic diseases, they haven't been linked to aneurysms.

CN: Health promotion and maintenance; CNS: None; CL: Application

51. What is the <u>best</u> treatment for a ruptured aneurysm?

1. Antihypertensive medication administration
2. Aortogram
3. Beta-adrenergic blocker administration
4. Surgical intervention

51. 4. When the vessel ruptures, surgery is the only intervention that can repair it. Administration of antihypertensive medications and beta-adrenergic blockers can help control hypertension, reducing the risk of rupture. An aortogram is a diagnostic tool used to detect an aneurysm.

CN: Physiological integrity; CNS: Basic care and comfort; CL: Application

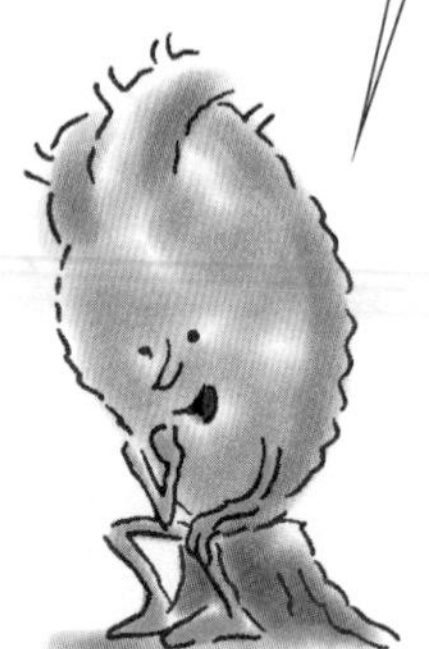

Think! This question is asking for a treatment, not a preventive measure.

52. When teaching a client about cardiomyopathy, which statement by the client indicates that further teaching is needed related to the causes of cardiomyopathy?

1. "It is caused by a plaque in the arteries."
2. "It is caused by a virus."
3. "It is caused by bacteria."
4. "It is caused by certain drugs."

52. 1. Cardiomyopathy isn't usually caused by plaque in the arteries or atherosclerosis. The etiology in most cases is viral or bacterial infection or cardiotoxic effects of drugs or alcohol.

CN: Physiological integrity; CNS: Physiological adaptation; CL: Application

53. The nurse is counseling a client on types of cardiomyopathy associated with childbirth. The nurse should teach the client about which of the following?

1. Dilated
2. Hypertrophic obstructive
3. Myocarditis
4. Restrictive

53. 1. Although the cause isn't entirely known, cardiac dilation and heart failure may develop during the last month of pregnancy or the first few months after birth. The condition may result from a preexisting cardiomyopathy not apparent prior to pregnancy. Hypertrophic obstructive cardiomyopathy is an abnormal symmetry of the ventricles that has an unknown etiology but a strong familial tendency. Myocarditis isn't a form of cardiomyopathy; it's an inflammation of the cardiac muscle. Restrictive cardiomyopathy indicates constrictive pericarditis; the underlying cause is usually myocardial.

CN: Physiological integrity; CNS: Physiological adaptation; CL: Application

54. The nurse is reviewing a client's echocardiogram, which states, "hypertrophy of the ventricular septum." The client should be further evaluated for which type of cardiomyopathy?
1. Congestive
2. Dilated
3. Hypertrophic obstructive
4. Restrictive

55. Which recurring condition most commonly occurs in clients with cardiomyopathy?
1. Heart failure
2. Diabetes mellitus
3. Myocardial infarction (MI)
4. Pericardial effusion

56. While assessing a client with dilated cardiomyopathy, the nurse notices that the electrocardiogram (ECG) rhythm no longer has any P waves, only a fine wavy line. The ventricular rhythm is irregular with a QRS duration of 0.08 second. The heart rate is 110 beats/minute. The nurse interprets this rhythm as:
1. atrial fibrillation.
2. ventricular fibrillation.
3. atrial flutter.
4. sinus tachycardia.

57. Dyspnea, cough, weight gain, weakness, and edema are classic signs and symptoms of which condition?
1. Pericarditis
2. Hypertension
3. Myocardial infarction (MI)
4. Heart failure

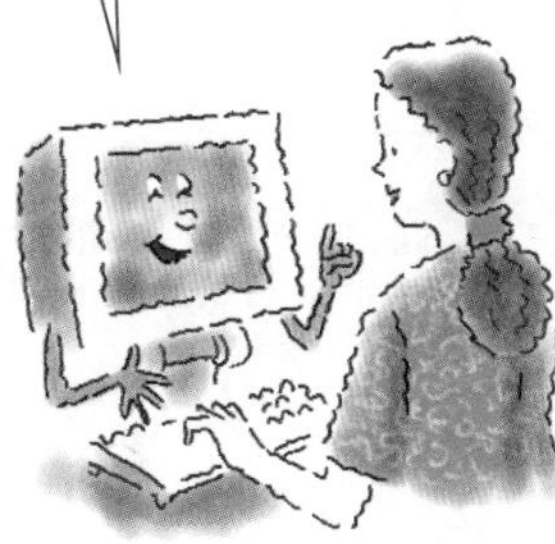

This is a tough one! Keep plugging along!

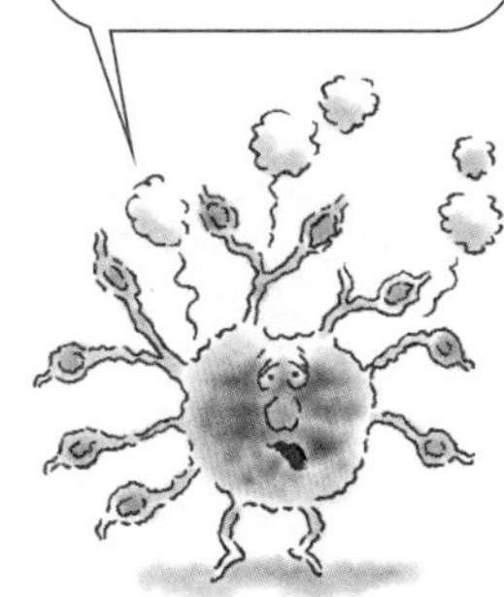

I don't know about you, but along about now, I'm getting kinda fried.

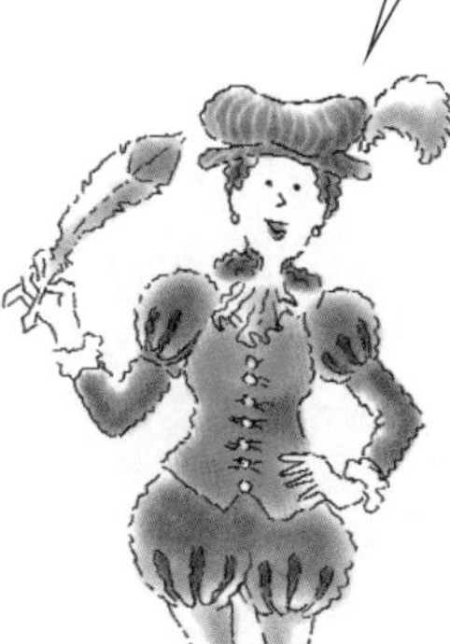

This question is a classic one, if you catch my drift.

54. 3. In hypertrophic obstructive cardiomyopathy, hypertrophy of the ventricular septum—not the ventricle chambers—is apparent. This abnormality isn't seen in other types of cardiomyopathy. Congestive isn't a form of cardiomyopathy.
CN: Physiological integrity; CNS: Physiological adaptation; CL: Analysis

55. 1. Because the structure and function of the heart muscle is affected, heart failure most commonly occurs in clients with cardiomyopathy. Diabetes mellitus is unrelated to cardiomyopathy. MI results from prolonged myocardial ischemia due to reduced blood flow through one of the coronary arteries. Pericardial effusion is most predominant in clients with pericarditis.
CN: Physiological integrity; CNS: Physiological adaptation; CL: Comprehension

56. 1. Atrial fibrillation is defined as chaotic, asynchronous, electrical activity in the atrial tissue. On an ECG, uneven baseline fibrillating waves appear rather than distinguishable P waves. Ventricular fibrillation is a chaotic rhythm with no QRS complexes. In atrial flutter there are flutter waves that are "saw-tooth" in appearance. P waves are present in sinus tachycardia.
CN: Physiological integrity; CNS: Physiological adaptation; CL: Analysis

57. 4. These are the classic symptoms of heart failure. Pericarditis is exhibited by a feeling of fullness in the chest and auscultation of a pericardial friction rub. Hypertension is usually exhibited by headaches, visual disturbances, and a flushed face. MI is usually exhibited by chest pain and diaphoresis.
CN: Physiological integrity; CNS: Reduction of risk potential; CL: Application

58. In which type of cardiomyopathy does cardiac output remain normal?

1. Dilated
2. Hypertrophic obstructive
3. Obliterative
4. Restrictive

58. 2. Cardiac output isn't affected by hypertrophic obstructive cardiomyopathy because the size of the ventricle remains relatively unchanged. Dilated cardiomyopathy and restrictive cardiomyopathy decrease cardiac output. Obliterative isn't a form of cardiomyopathy.
CN: Physiological integrity; CNS: Physiological adaptation; CL: Comprehension

59. Which cardiac condition does a fourth heart sound (S_4) indicate?

1. Dilated aorta
2. Normally functioning heart
3. Decreased myocardial contractility
4. Failure of the ventricle to eject all the blood during systole

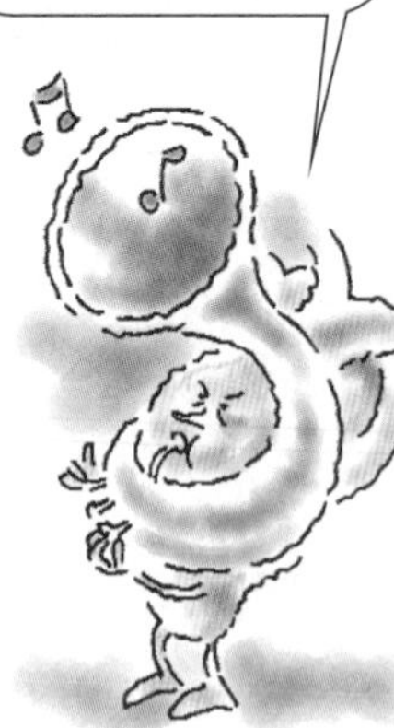

It's important to know what the different sounds I make indicate.

59. 4. An S_4 occurs as a result of increased resistance to ventricular filling after atrial contraction. This increased resistance is related to decreased compliance of the ventricle. A dilated aorta doesn't cause an extra heart sound, though it does cause a murmur. Decreased myocardial contractility is heard as a third heart sound. An S_4 isn't heard in a normally functioning heart.
CN: Physiological integrity; CNS: Physiological adaptation; CL: Application

60. Which class of drugs is most widely used in the treatment of cardiomyopathy?

1. Anticoagulants
2. Beta-adrenergic blockers
3. Calcium channel blockers
4. Nitrates

60. 2. By decreasing the heart rate and contractility, beta-adrenergic blockers improve myocardial filling and cardiac output, which are primary goals in the treatment of cardiomyopathy. Anticoagulants may sometimes be used to reduce the risk of emboli, but this practice is considered controversial. Calcium channel blockers are sometimes used for the same reasons as beta-adrenergic blockers; however, they aren't as effective as beta-adrenergic blockers and cause increased hypotension. Nitrates aren't used because of their dilating effects, which would further compromise the myocardium.
CN: Physiological integrity; CNS: Pharmacological and parenteral therapies; CL: Comprehension

61. If medical treatment for cardiomyopathy fails, the nurse should prepare the client for which of the following procedures?

1. Cardiac catheterization
2. Coronary artery bypass graft (CABG)
3. Heart transplantation
4. Intra-aortic balloon pump (IABP)

61. 3. The only definitive treatment for cardiomyopathy that can't be controlled medically is a heart transplant because the damage to the heart muscle is irreversible. Cardiac catheterization is an invasive diagnostic procedure for coronary artery disease. CABG is a surgical intervention used for atherosclerotic vessels. An IABP is an invasive treatment that assists the failing heart; however, it's only a temporary solution.
CN: Physiological integrity; CNS: Physiological adaptation; CL: Application

62. Which condition is associated with a predictable level of pain that occurs as a result of physical or emotional stress?
1. Anxiety
2. Stable angina
3. Unstable angina
4. Variant angina

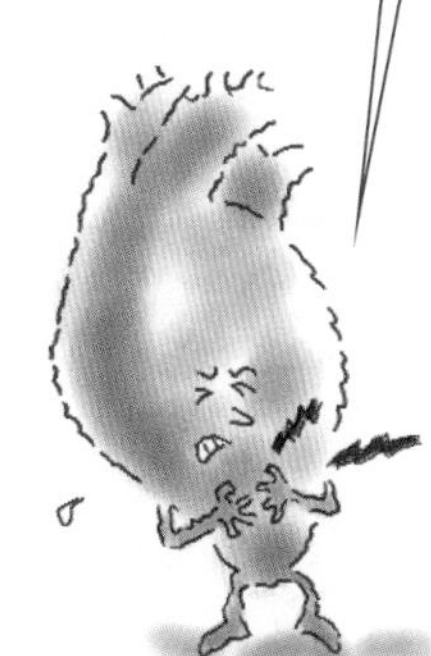

Stress can be a real pain in the heart.

62. 2. The pain of stable angina is predictable in nature, builds gradually, and quickly reaches maximum intensity. Anxiety generally isn't described as painful. Unstable angina doesn't always need a trigger, is more intense, and lasts longer than stable angina. Variant angina usually occurs at rest—not as a result of exertion or stress.

CN: Physiological integrity; CNS: Physiological adaptation; CL: Analysis

63. After undergoing a cardiac catheterization, a client has a large puddle of blood under his buttocks. Which step should the nurse take first?
1. Call for help.
2. Obtain vital signs.
3. Ask the client to "lift up."
4. Apply gloves and assess the groin site.

63. 4. Observing standard precautions is the first priority when dealing with any body fluid. Assessment of the groin site is the second priority. This establishes where the blood is coming from and determines how much blood has been lost. The goal in this situation is to stop the bleeding. The nurse would call for help if it were warranted after the assessment of the situation. After determining the extent of the bleeding, vital signs assessment is important. The nurse should never move the client, in case a clot has formed. Moving can disturb the clot and cause rebleeding.

CN: Safe, effective care environment; CNS: Management of care; CL: Analysis

64. A client with angina pectoris has an electrocardiogram (ECG) performed during an episode of chest pain. Which change on the ECG indicates myocardial ischemia?
1. Increased QRS duration
2. Shortened PR interval
3. Pathological Q-wave formation
4. T-wave inversion

64. 4. Ischemic changes are represented on an ECG by T-wave inversion. An increased QRS duration suggests a bundle-branch block. A shortened PR interval indicates a junctional rhythm. Pathological Q waves are present with myocardial infarction.

CN: Physiological integrity; CNS: Physiological adaptation; CL: Analysis

65. Which type of angina is most closely associated with an impending myocardial infarction (MI)?
1. Variant angina
2. Chronic stable angina
3. Microvascular angina
4. Unstable angina

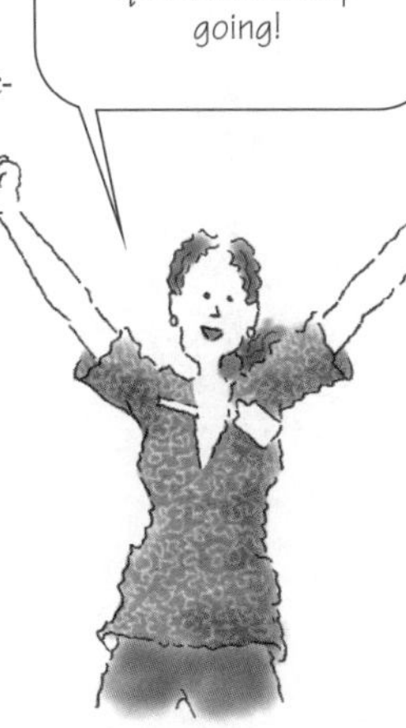

You've finished 65 questions! Keep going!

65. 4. Unstable angina progressively increases in frequency, intensity, and duration and is related to an increased risk of MI within 3 to 18 months. Variant angina is related to coronany artery spasm, chronic stable angina is predictable and relieved by rest and nitrates, and microvascular angina is related to impairment of vasodilator reserve in normal coronary arteries.

CN: Physiological integrity; CNS: Physiological adaptation; CL: Application

66. A client with angina pectoris comes to the emergency room. Which of the following drugs can the nurse expect to administer as the drug of choice?

1. Aspirin
2. Furosemide (Lasix)
3. Nitroglycerin
4. Nifedipine (Procardia)

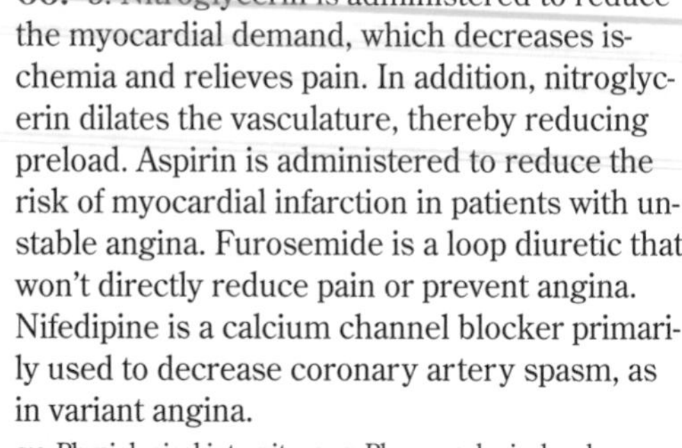

66. 3. Nitroglycerin is administered to reduce the myocardial demand, which decreases ischemia and relieves pain. In addition, nitroglycerin dilates the vasculature, thereby reducing preload. Aspirin is administered to reduce the risk of myocardial infarction in patients with unstable angina. Furosemide is a loop diuretic that won't directly reduce pain or prevent angina. Nifedipine is a calcium channel blocker primarily used to decrease coronary artery spasm, as in variant angina.

CN: Physiological integrity; CNS: Pharmacological and parenteral therapies; CL: Analysis

67. While assessing a client diagnosed with angina, the client asks what causes it. Which of the following responses by the nurse would be the most appropriate?

1. Increased preload
2. Decreased afterload
3. Coronary artery spasm
4. Inadequate oxygen supply to the myocardium

67. 4. Inadequate oxygen supply to the myocardium is responsible for the pain accompanying angina. Increased preload would be responsible for right-sided heart failure. Decreased afterload causes increased cardiac output. Coronary artery spasm is responsible for variant angina.

CN: Physiological integrity; CNS: Physiological adaptation; CL: Analysis

68. A nurse is preparing a client for cardiac catheterization. Which assessment is most important prior to the procedure?

1. Weight and height
2. Allergy to iodine or shellfish
3. Apical heart rate
4. Cardiac rhythm

68. 2. Since cardiac catheterization involves the injection of a radiopaque dye, it's most important for the nurse to determine if the client has allergies to iodine or shellfish. The other three parameters are also part of the assessment, but none is the most critical assessment.

CN: Physiological integrity; CNS: Reduction of risk potential; CL: Analysis

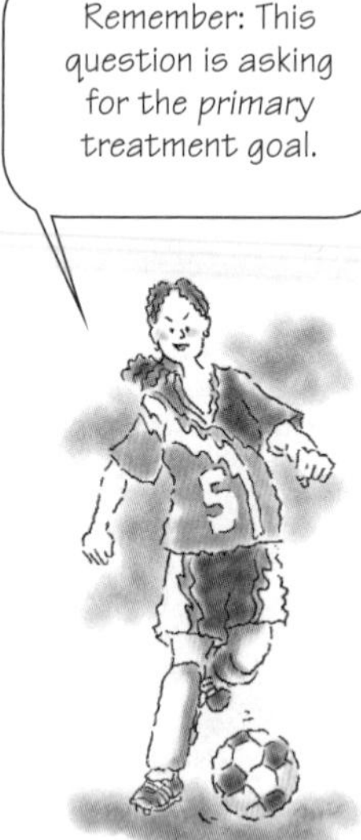
Remember: This question is asking for the primary treatment goal.

69. The nurse is teaching a client about angina. Which statement by the nurse would be most accurate regarding the primary treatment goal?

1. Reversal of ischemia
2. Reversal of infarction
3. Reduction of stress and anxiety
4. Reduction of associated risk factors

69. 1. Reversal of the ischemia is the primary goal, achieved by reducing oxygen consumption and increasing oxygen supply. An infarction is permanent and can't be reversed. Reduction of associated risk factors, such as stress and anxiety, is a progressive, long-term treatment goal that has cumulative effects. Reduction of these factors will decrease the risk for angina but this usually isn't an immediate goal.

CN: Physiological integrity; CNS: Physiological adaptation; CL: Application

70. A 59-year-old female client is experiencing chest pain at rest that is unresponsive to nitroglycerine. The physician diagnoses unstable angina and alerts the nurse that the client will require treatment with immediate surgical intervention. Which treatment is most suitable?

1. Cardiac catheterization
2. Echocardiogram
3. Heart transplantation
4. Percutaneous transluminal coronary angioplasty (PTCA)

70. 4. PTCA can alleviate the blockage and restore blood flow and oxygenation. Cardiac catheterization is a diagnostic tool—not a treatment. An echocardiogram is a noninvasive diagnostic test. Heart transplantation involves replacing the client's heart with a donor heart and is the treatment for end-stage cardiac disease.

CN: Physiological integrity; CNS: Physiological adaptation; CL: Application

71. Which intervention should be the first priority when treating a client experiencing chest pain while walking?

1. Sit the client down.
2. Get the client back to bed.
3. Obtain an electrocardiogram (ECG).
4. Administer sublingual nitroglycerin.

71. 1. The initial priority is to decrease the oxygen consumption; this would be achieved by sitting the client down. When the client's condition is stabilized, he can be returned to bed. An ECG can be obtained after the client is sitting down. After the ECG, sublingual nitroglycerin would be administered.

CN: Physiological integrity; CNS: Basic care and comfort; CL: Analysis

72. The nurse is assessing a client with heart failure. The client is experiencing tachycardia, decreased blood pressure, and decreased peripheral pulses. The nurse interprets these symptoms as indicating which condition?

1. Anaphylactic shock
2. Cardiogenic shock
3. Distributive shock
4. Myocardial infarction (MI)

72. 2. Cardiogenic shock is shock related to reduced cardiac output and ineffective pumping of the heart. Anaphylactic shock results from an allergic reaction. Distributive shock results from changes in the intravascular volume distribution and is usually associated with increased cardiac output. MI isn't a shock state, though a severe MI can lead to shock.

CN: Physiological integrity; CNS: Physiological adaptation; CL: Analysis

73. Which of the following conditions may result in cardiogenic shock?

1. Acute myocardial infarction (MI)
2. Coronary artery disease (CAD)
3. Decreased hemoglobin level
4. Hypotension

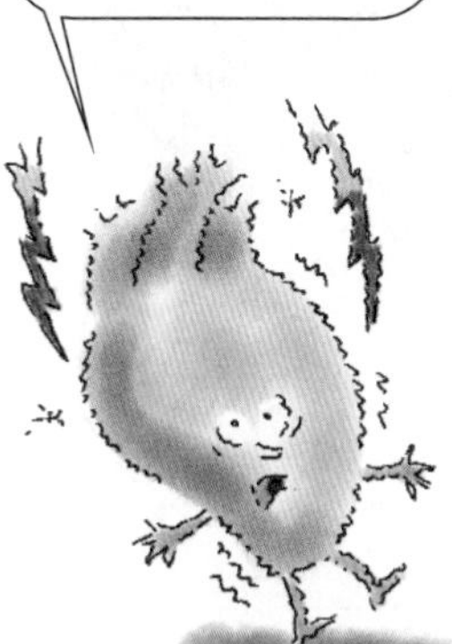

Pay attention. This info could really shock you!

73. 1. Of all clients with an acute MI, 15% suffer cardiogenic shock secondary to the myocardial damage and decreased function. CAD causes MI. A decreased hemoglobin level is a result of bleeding. Hypotension is the result of a reduced cardiac output produced by the shock state.

CN: Physiological integrity; CNS: Reduction of risk potential; CL: Analysis

74. Which percentage represents the amount of damage the myocardium must sustain before signs and symptoms of cardiogenic shock develop?
1. 10%
2. 25%
3. 40%
4. 90%

74. 3. At least 40% of the heart muscle must be involved for cardiogenic shock to develop. In most circumstances, the heart can compensate for up to 25% damage. An infarction involving 90% of the heart would result in death.

CN: Physiological integrity; CNS: Physiological adaptation; CL: Comprehension

75. Which of the following parameters increases as myocardial oxygen consumption increases?
1. Preload, afterload, and cerebral blood flow
2. Preload, afterload, and renal blood flow
3. Preload, afterload, contractility, and heart rate
4. Preload, afterload, cerebral blood flow, and heart rate

75. 3. Myocardial oxygen consumption increases as preload, afterload, contractility, and heart rate increase. Cerebral blood flow and renal blood flow don't directly affect myocardial oxygen consumption.

CN: Physiological integrity; CNS: Physiological adaptation; CL: Application

76. Which factor would be most useful in detecting a client's risk of developing cardiogenic shock?
1. Decreased heart rate
2. Decreased cardiac index
3. Decreased blood pressure
4. Decreased cerebral blood flow

76. 2. The cardiac index, a figure derived by dividing the cardiac output by the client's body surface area, is used for identifying whether the cardiac output is meeting a client's needs. Heart rate, blood pressure, and decreased cerebral blood flow are less useful in detecting the risk of cardiogenic shock.

CN: Physiological integrity; CNS: Physiological adaptation; CL: Analysis

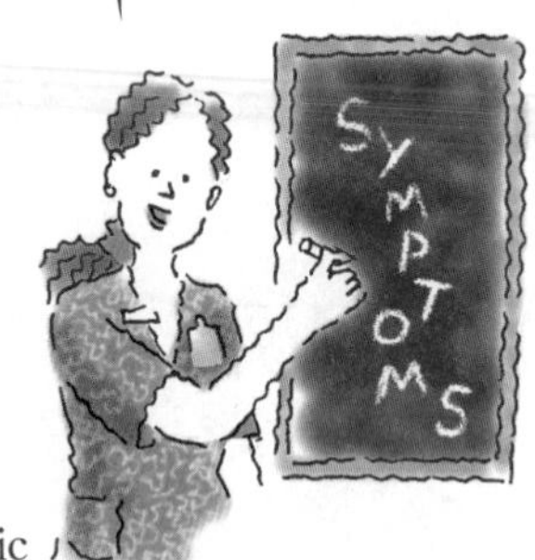

Pay attention. This question involves assessing the order of symptoms.
SYMPTOMS

77. Which symptom is one of the earliest signs of cardiogenic shock?
1. Cyanosis
2. Decreased urine output
3. Presence of fourth heart sound (S_4)
4. Altered level of consciousness

77. 4. Initially, the decrease in cardiac output results in a decrease in cerebral blood flow that causes restlessness, agitation, or confusion. Cyanosis, decreased urine output, and presence of an S_4 are all later signs of shock.

CN: Physiological integrity; CNS: Basic care and comfort; CL: Application

78. Which diagnostic study can determine when cellular metabolism becomes anaerobic and when pH decreases?
1. Arterial blood gas (ABG) levels
2. Complete blood count (CBC)
3. Electrocardiogram (ECG)
4. Lung scan

78. 1. ABG levels reflect cellular metabolism and indicate hypoxia. A CBC is performed to determine various constituents of venous blood. An ECG shows the electrical activity of the heart. A lung scan is performed to view functionality of the lungs.

CN: Health promotion and maintenance; CNS: None; CL: Analysis

79. What is the <u>first</u> treatment goal for cardiogenic shock?
1. Correct hypoxia
2. Prevent infarction
3. Correct metabolic acidosis
4. Increase myocardial oxygen supply

79. 4. A balance must be maintained between oxygen supply and demand. In a shock state, the myocardium requires more oxygen. If it can't get more oxygen, the shock worsens. Increasing the oxygen will also play a large role in correcting metabolic acidosis and hypoxia. Infarction typically causes the shock state, so prevention isn't an appropriate goal for this condition.

CN: Physiological integrity; CN: Physiological adaptation; CL: Analysis

80. Which drug is <u>most commonly</u> used to treat cardiogenic shock?
1. Dopamine
2. Enalapril (Vasotec)
3. Furosemide (Lasix)
4. Metoprolol (Lopressor)

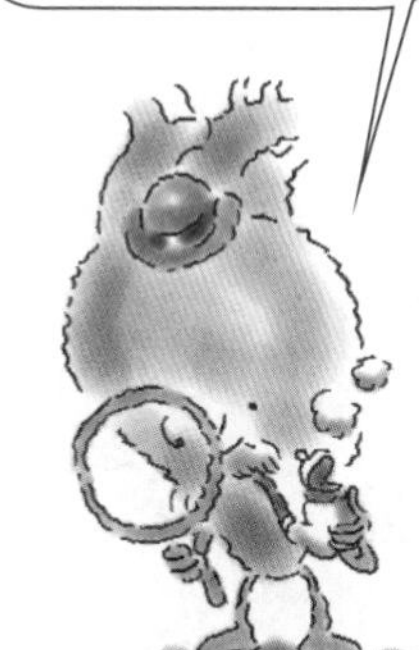

When answering questions, look for phrases such as most commonly. These are often clues.

80. 1. Dopamine, a sympathomimetic drug, improves myocardial contractility and blood flow through vital organs by increasing perfusion pressure. Enalapril is an angiotensin-converting enzyme inhibitor that directly lowers blood pressure. Furosemide is a diuretic and doesn't have a direct effect on contractility or tissue perfusion. Metoprolol is a beta-adrenergic blocker that slows heart rate and lowers blood pressure; neither is a desired effect in the treatment of cardiogenic shock.

CN: Physiological integrity; CNS: Pharmacological and parenteral therapies; CL: Application

81. Which is the most important instrument used as a diagnostic and monitoring tool for determining the severity of a shock state?
1. Arterial line
2. Indwelling urinary catheter
3. Electrocardiogram (ECG) monitor
4. Pulmonary artery catheter

81. 4. A pulmonary artery catheter is used to give accurate pressure measurements within the heart, which aids in determining the course of treatment. An arterial line, an indwelling urinary catheter, and an ECG monitor all provide valuable information related to the severity of a shock state but aren't the most important instrument.

CN: Physiological integrity; CNS: Pharmacological and parenteral therapies; CL: Analysis

82. A client has a continuous blood pressure reading of 142/90 mm Hg. Into which classification does this reading fall according to the Seventh Joint National Committee (JNC 7) on the Prevention, Detection, Evaluation, and Treatment of High Blood Pressure?
1. Stage 2 hypertension
2. Prehypertension
3. Stage 1 hypertension
4. Normal

82. 3. According to the JNC 7, a systolic blood pressure of 140 to 159 mm Hg or a diastolic pressure of 90 to 99 mm Hg represents stage 1 hypertension. A systolic pressure greater than or equal to 160 mm Hg or diastolic pressure greater than or equal to 100 mm Hg represents stage 2 hypertension. A systolic pressure of 120 to 139 mm Hg or diastolic pressure of 80 to 89 mm Hg represents prehypertension. A systolic pressure less than 120 mm Hg and diastolic pressure less than 80 mm Hg are considered normal.

CN: Health promotion and maintenance; CNS: None; CL: Application

83. Which sound will be heard during the first phase of Korotkoff's sounds?

1. Disappearance of sounds
2. Faint, clear tapping sounds
3. A murmur or swishing sounds
4. Soft, muffling sounds

83. 2. In phase I, auscultation produces a faint, clear tapping sound that gradually increases in intensity. Phase II produces a murmur sound, and precedes Phase III, the phase marked by an increased intensity of sound. Phase IV produces a muffling sound that gives a soft blowing noise. Phase V, the final phase, is marked by the disappearance of sounds.

CN: Physiological integrity; CNS: Basic care and comfort; CL: Application

84. Which of the following is a key point to include when teaching the nursing assistant about the major determinant of diastolic blood pressure?

1. Baroreceptors
2. Cardiac output
3. Renal function
4. Vascular resistance

84. 4. Vascular resistance is the impedance of blood flow by the arterioles that most predominantly affects the diastolic pressure. Baroreceptors are nerve endings that are embedded in the blood vessels and respond to the stretching of vessel walls. They don't directly affect diastolic blood pressure. Cardiac output determines systolic blood pressure. Renal function helps control blood volume and indirectly affects diastolic blood pressure.

CN: Physiological integrity; CNS: Physiological adaptation; CL: Application

How would I respond to a rise in blood pressure?

85. A nurse knows that kidneys play an important role in regulating blood pressure. When hypertension occurs, which responses by the kidneys help normalize blood pressure?

1. The kidneys retain sodium and excrete water.
2. The kidneys excrete sodium and excrete water.
3. The kidneys retain sodium and retain water.
4. The kidneys excrete sodium and retain water.

85. 2. The kidneys respond to a rise in blood pressure by excreting sodium and excess water. This response ultimately affects systolic blood pressure by regulating blood volume. Sodium or water retention would only further increase blood pressure. Sodium and water travel together across the membrane in the kidneys; one can't travel without the other.

CN: Physiological integrity; CNS: Physiological adaptation; CL: Application

86. Which change would indicate the baroreceptors in the carotid artery walls and aorta are functioning?

1. Changes in blood pressure
2. Changes in arterial oxygen tension
3. Changes in arterial carbon dioxide tension
4. Changes in heart rate

86. 1. Baroreceptors located in the carotid arteries and aorta sense pulsatile pressure. Peripheral chemoreceptors in the aorta and carotid arteries are primarily stimulated by oxygen. Chemoreceptors in the medulla are primarily stimulated by carbon dioxide. Decreases in pulsatile pressure cause a reflex increase in heart rate.

CN: Physiological integrity; CNS: Physiological adaptation; CL: Analysis

87. The nurse is teaching a client about blood pressure and hormones. Which of the following responses indicates the client understands which hormone raises arterial pressure and promotes venous return?
1. Angiotensin I
2. Angiotensin II
3. Thyroid hormone
4. Insulin

87. 2. Angiotensin II is a potent vasoconstrictor, thereby promoting venous return. Angiotensin I is a precursor that is converted in the pulmonary vasculature to angiotensin II. Neither thyroid hormone nor insulin has vasoconstrictive properties.
CN: Physiological integrity; CNS: Physiological adaptation; CL: Analysis

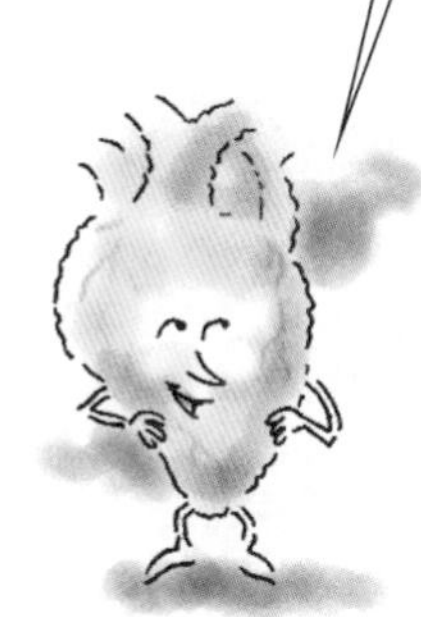

Don't get two tense to answer this question. (Oh, I am just two, er, too clever for words.)

88. Which term is used to describe persistently elevated blood pressure with an unknown cause that accounts for approximately 90% of hypertension cases?
1. Accelerated hypertension
2. Malignant hypertension
3. Primary hypertension
4. Secondary hypertension

88. 3. Characterized by a progressive, usually asymptomatic blood pressure increase over several years, primary hypertension is the most common type. Malignant hypertension, also known as *accelerated hypertension,* is rapidly progressive, uncontrollable, and causes a rapid onset of complications. Secondary hypertension occurs secondary to a known, correctable cause.
CN: Physiological integrity; CNS: Reduction of risk potential; CL: Analysis

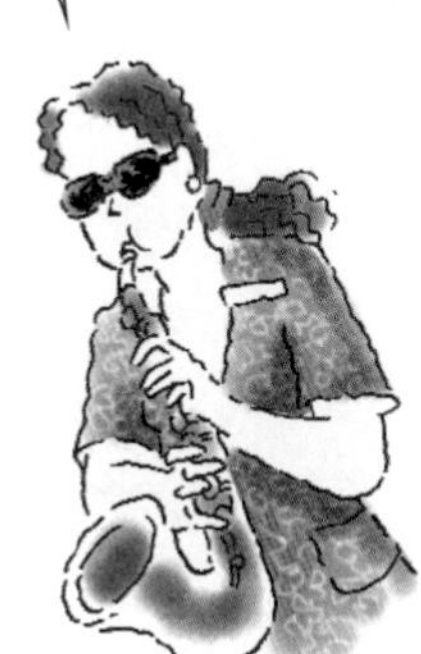

"Note" the words most common in this question. That's a hint.

89. The nurse is assessing a client with hypertension. The nurse should be alert for which of the most common symptoms of hypertension?
1. Blurred vision
2. Epistaxis
3. Headache
4. Peripheral edema

89. 3. An occipital headache is typical of hypertension secondary to continued increased pressure on the cerebral vasculature. Blurred vision can result from hypertension due to the arteriolar changes in the eye. Epistaxis (nosebleed) occurs far less frequently than a headache but can also be a diagnostic sign of hypertension. Peripheral edema can also occur from an increase in sodium and water retention but is usually a latent sign.
CN: Health promotion and maintenance; CNS: None; CL: Application

90. The bell of the stethoscope is most commonly placed over which artery to obtain a blood pressure measurement?
1. Brachial
2. Brachiocephalic
3. Radial
4. Ulnar

90. 1. The brachial artery is most commonly used due to its easy accessibility and location. The brachiocephalic artery isn't accessible for blood pressure measurement. The radial and ulnar arteries can be used in extraordinary circumstances, but the measurement may not be as accurate.
CN: Physiological integrity; CNS: Basic care and comfort; CL: Application

91. Which of the following statements, if made by the client, indicates an understanding of why furosemide (Lasix) is administered to treat hypertension?

1. It dilates peripheral blood vessels.
2. It decreases sympathetic cardioacceleration.
3. It inhibits the angiotensin-converting enzyme.
4. It inhibits reabsorption of sodium and water in the loop of Henle.

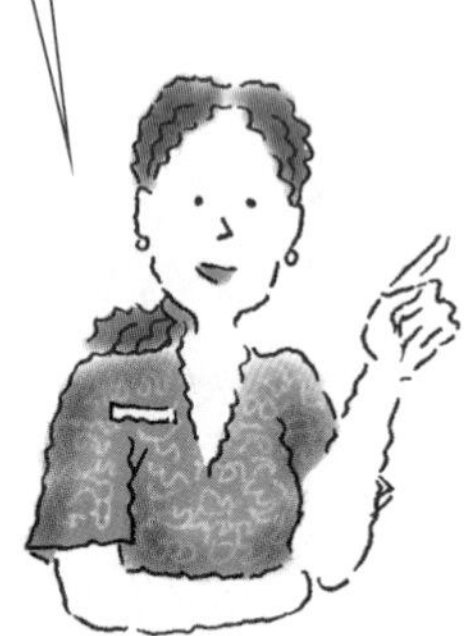

This question is asking for the mechanism of action of furosemide.

91. 4. Furosemide is a loop diuretic that inhibits sodium and water reabsorption in the loop of Henle, thereby causing a decrease in blood pressure. Vasodilators cause dilation of peripheral blood vessels, directly relaxing vascular smooth muscle and decreasing blood pressure. Adrenergic blockers decrease sympathetic cardioacceleration and decrease blood pressure. Angiotensin-converting enzyme inhibitors decrease blood pressure due to their action on angiotensin.

CN: Physiological integrity; CNS: Pharmacological and parenteral therapies; CL: Analysis

92. A 52-year-old client with a history of hypertension has just had a total hip replacement. The physician orders hydrochlorothiazide 35 mg oral solution by mouth, once per day. The label on the solution reads hydrochlorothiazide 50 mg/5 milliliters. To administer the correct dose, how many milliliters should the nurse pour? Record your answer using one decimal place. ________ ml

92. 3.5. The correct formula to calculate a drug dosage is:

Dose on hand/quantity on hand = dose desired/X.

In this example, the equation is:

50 mg/5 ml = 35 mg/X

X = 3.5 ml.

CN: Physiological integrity; CNS: Pharmacological and parenteral therapies; CL: Application

93. Which statement by the nurse accurately explains the need for a client with hypertension to obtain an annual eye exam?

1. "By examining your corneas, an ophthalmologist can visualize microvascular hemorrhages in your eyes."
2. "By examining the fovea in your eyes, an ophthalmologist can visualize microvascular venous occlusions in your eyes."
3. "By examining the retina in your eyes, an ophthalmologist can detect changes in the arteries in your eyes."
4. "By examining the sclera of your eyes, an ophthalmologist can detect changes in the arteries in your eyes."

93. 3. The retina is the only site in the body where arteries can be seen without invasive techniques. Changes in the retinal arteries signal similar damage to vessels elsewhere. The cornea is the nonvascular, transparent fibrous coat where the iris can be seen. The fovea is the point of central vision. The sclera is the fibrous tissue that forms the outer protective covering over the eyeball.

CN: Health promotion and maintenance; CNS: None; CL: Application

94. Based on which of the following conditions would the nurse suspect the client has varicose veins?

1. Tunica media tear
2. Intraluminal occlusion
3. Intraluminal valvular compression
4. Intraluminal valvular incompetence

94. 4. Varicose veins, dilated tortuous surface veins engorged with blood, result from intraluminal valvular incompetence. An intraluminal occlusion would result from plaque or thrombosis. The valves aren't outside the lumen (intraluminal) and a tear would result in a hematoma.

CN: Physiological integrity; CNS: Physiological adaptation; CL: Analysis

95. A nurse determines that a client with varicose veins understands the factor causing primary varicose veins when the client states which of the following?

1. Hypertension
2. Pregnancy
3. Thrombosis
4. Trauma

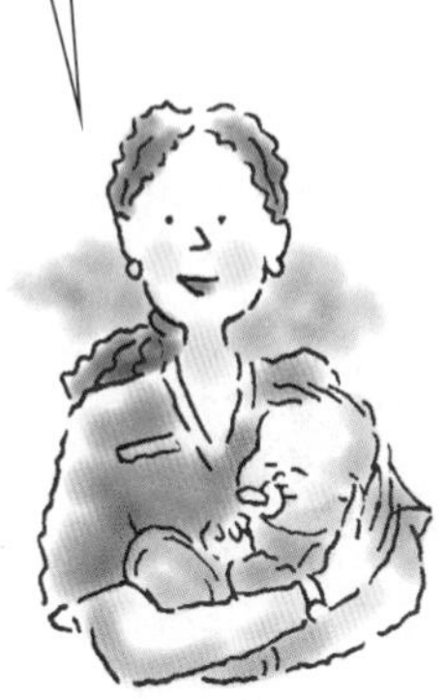

I love babies, but not the varicose veins that go with them!

95. 2. Primary varicose veins have a gradual onset and progressively worsen. In pregnancy, the expanding uterus and increased vascular volume impede blood return to the heart. The pressure places increased stress on the veins. Hypertension has no role in varicose vein formation. Thrombosis and trauma cause valvular incompetence and so are secondary causes of varicosities—not primary.

CN: Health promotion and maintenance; CNS: None; CL: Analysis

96. The nurse assessing a client for varicose veins would look for which commonly occurring symptom?

1. Fatigue and pressure
2. Fatigue and cool feet
3. Sharp pain and fatigue
4. Sharp pain and cool feet

96. 1. Fatigue and pressure are classic signs of varicose veins, secondary to increased blood volume and edema. Sharp pain and cool feet are symptoms of alteration in arterial blood flow.

CN: Physiological integrity; CNS: Physiological adaptation; CL: Application

97. While planning to teach a client with varicose veins, the nurse should include in the teaching plan that varicose veins most commonly occur in which type of vein?

1. Brachial
2. Femoral
3. Renal
4. Saphenous

97. 4. Varicose veins occur most commonly in the saphenous veins of the lower extremities. They don't develop in the brachial, femoral, or renal veins.

CN: Physiological integrity; CNS: Physiological adaptation; CL: Analysis

98. Which condition is caused by increased hydrostatic pressure and chronic venous stasis?

1. Venous occlusion
2. Cool extremities
3. Nocturnal calf muscle cramps
4. Diminished blood supply to the feet

98. 3. Calf muscle cramps result from increased pressure and venous stasis secondary to varicose veins. An occlusion is a blockage of blood flow. Cool extremities and diminished blood supply to the feet are symptoms of arterial blood flow changes.

CN: Health promotion and maintenance; CNS: None; CL: Analysis

99. The nurse is providing discharge instructions for a client with varicose veins. The nurse determines the need for further teaching when the client states which of the following?

1. "Exercise will make me feel better."
2. "I have to elevate my legs."
3. "Lying down can relieve my symptoms."
4. "Wearing tight clothes will not affect me."

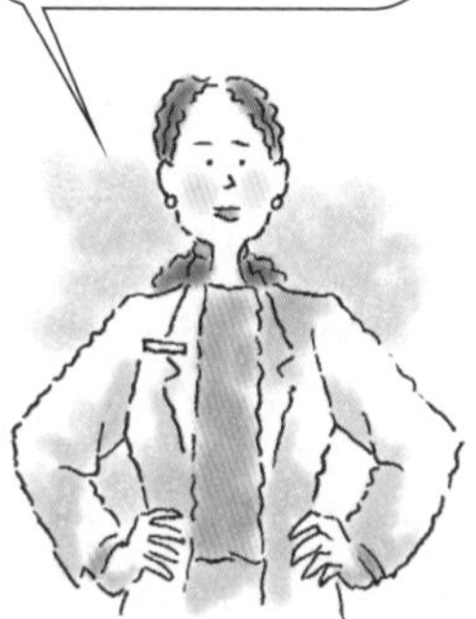

Be careful. This question could put you in a tight squeeze.

99. 4. Tight clothing, especially below the waist, increases vascular volume and impedes blood return to the heart. Exercise, leg elevations, and lying down usually relieve symptoms of varicose veins.

CN: Health promotion and maintenance; CNS: None; CL: Analysis

100. Which test demonstrates the backward flow of blood through incompetent valves of superficial veins?

1. Trendelenburg's test
2. Manual compression test
3. Perthes' test
4. Plethysmography

100. 1. Trendelenburg's test is the most accurate tool used to determine retrograde venous filling. The manual compression test is a quick, easy test done by palpation and usually isn't diagnostic of the backward flow of blood. Perthes' test easily indicates whether the deeper venous system and communicating veins are competent. Plethysmography allows measurement of changes in venous blood volume.

CN: Health promotion and maintenance; CNS: None; CL: Application

101. The nurse should assess for what signs and symptoms in a client with <u>secondary</u> varicose veins?

1. Pallor and severe pain
2. Severe pain and edema
3. Edema and pigmentation
4. Absent hair growth and pigmentation

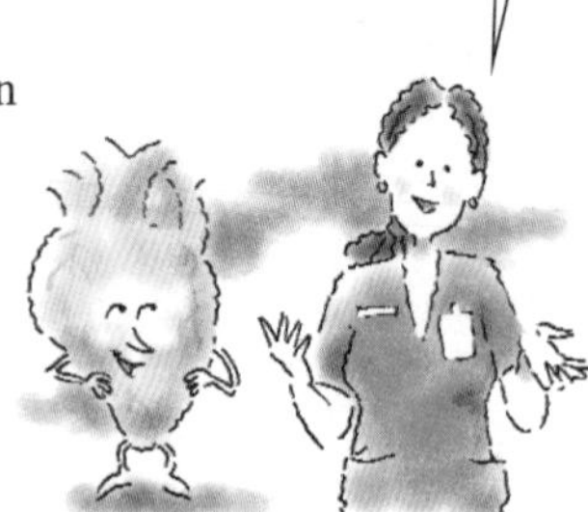

Congratulations! You've finished 100 questions! You're almost there!

101. 3. Secondary varicose veins result from an obstruction of the deep veins. Incompetent valves lead to impaired blood flow, and edema and pigmentation result from venous stasis. Severe pain, pallor, and absent hair growth are symptoms of an altered arterial blood flow.

CN: Physiological integrity; CNS: Physiological adaptation; CL: Application

102. The nurse should prepare a client for which treatment to eliminate varicose veins?

1. Ablation therapy
2. Cold therapy
3. Ligation and stripping
4. Radiation

102. 3. Ligation and stripping of the vein can rid the vein of varicosity. This invasive procedure will take care of current varicose veins only; it won't prevent others from forming. The other procedures aren't used for varicose veins.

CN: Physiological integrity; CNS: Pharmacological and parenteral therapies; CL: Application

103. Which treatment is recommended for postoperative management of a client who has undergone ligation and stripping?

1. Sitting
2. Bed rest
3. Ice packs
4. Elastic leg compression

103. 4. Elastic leg compression helps venous return to the heart, thereby decreasing venous stasis. Sitting and bed rest are contraindicated because both promote decreased blood return to the heart and venous stasis. Although ice packs would help reduce edema, they would also cause vasoconstriction and impede blood flow.

CN: Physiological integrity; CNS: Basic care and comfort; CL: Application

104. Which client is <u>most</u> at risk for developing deep vein thrombosis (DVT)?

1. A 62-year-old female recovering from a total hip replacement.
2. A 35-year-old female 2 days postpartum.
3. A 33-year-old male runner with Achilles tendonitis.
4. An ambulatory 70-year-old male who's recovering from pneumonia.

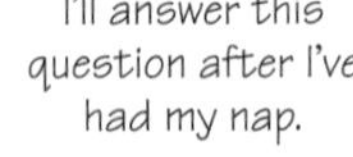

I'll answer this question after I've had my nap.

104. 1. DVT is more common in immobilized clients who have had surgical procedures such as total hip replacement. Pregnancy can cause varicose veins, which can lead to venous stasis, but it isn't a primary cause of DVT. Clients who are recovering from an injury or pneumonia may have decreased mobility, but these clients don't have the highest risk of developing DVT.

CN: Physiological integrity; CNS: Reduction of risk potential; CL: Analysis

105. Which complication of lower extremity deep vein thrombosis is manifested by dyspnea, chest pain, and diminished breath sounds?
1. Hemothorax
2. Pneumothorax
3. Pulmonary embolism
4. Pulmonary hypertension

105. 3. A pulmonary embolism is a blood clot that forms in a vein, travels to the lungs, and lodges in the pulmonary vasculature. A hemothorax refers to blood in the pleural space. A pneumothorax is caused by an opening in the pleura. Pulmonary hypertension is an increase in pulmonary artery pressure, which increases the workload of the right ventricle.
CN: Physiological integrity; CNS: Physiological adaptation; CL: Analysis

106. Which term refers to the condition of blood coagulating faster than normal, causing thrombin and other clotting factors to multiply?
1. Embolus
2. Hypercoagulability
3. Venous stasis
4. Venous wall injury

106. 2. Hypercoagulability is the condition of blood coagulating faster than normal, causing thrombin and other clotting factors to multiply. This condition, along with venous stasis and venous wall injury, accounts for the formation of deep vein thrombosis. An embolus is a blood clot or fatty globule that formed in one area and is carried through the bloodstream to another area.
CN: Physiological integrity; CNS: Physiological adaptation; CL: Application

107. Which characteristic is <u>typical</u> of the pain associated with deep vein thrombosis (DVT)?
1. Dull ache
2. No pain
3. Sudden onset
4. Tingling

I see ... This question is asking you to characterize the type of pain experienced during deep vein thrombosis.

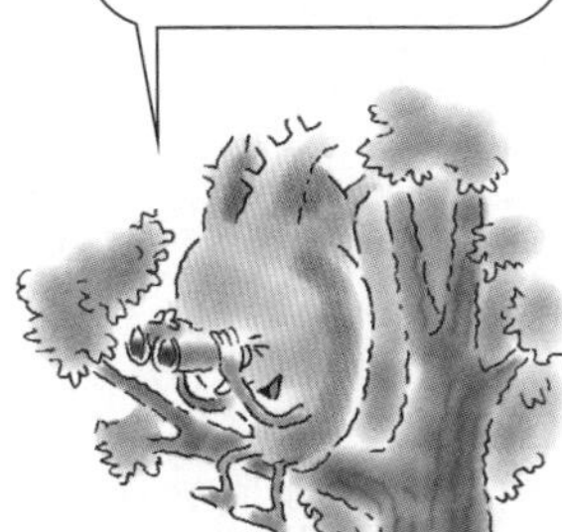

107. 3. DVT is associated with deep leg pain of sudden onset, which occurs secondary to the occlusion. A dull ache is more commonly associated with varicose veins. If the thrombus is large enough, it will cause pain. A tingling sensation is associated with an alteration in arterial blood flow.
CN: Physiological integrity; CNS: Basic care and comfort; CL: Analysis

108. A client is admitted with deep vein thrombosis (DVT). Which of the following treatments would be <u>most</u> appropriate to relieve the pain?
1. Application of heat
2. Bed rest
3. Exercise
4. Leg elevation

108. 4. Leg elevation alleviates the pressure caused by thrombosis and occlusion by assisting venous return. The application of heat would dilate the vessels and pool blood in the area of the thrombus, increasing the risk of further thrombus formation. Bed rest adds to venous stasis by increasing the risk of thrombosis formation. When DVT is diagnosed, exercise isn't recommended until the clot has dissolved.
CN: Physiological integrity; CNS: Basic care and comfort; CL: Application

109. Which term best describes the findings on cautious palpation of the vein in typical superficial thrombophlebitis?
1. Dilated
2. Knotty
3. Smooth
4. Tortuous

109. 2. The knotty feeling is secondary to the emboli adhering to the vein wall. Varicose veins may be described as dilated and tortuous. Normal veins feel smooth.
CN: Physiological integrity; CNS: Physiological adaptation; CL: Application

110. While assessing a client with deep vein thrombosis (DVT), which of the following terms indicates calf pain experienced by the client due to sharp dorsiflexion of the foot?

1. Dyskinesia
2. Eversion
3. Positive Babinski's reflex
4. Positive Homans' sign

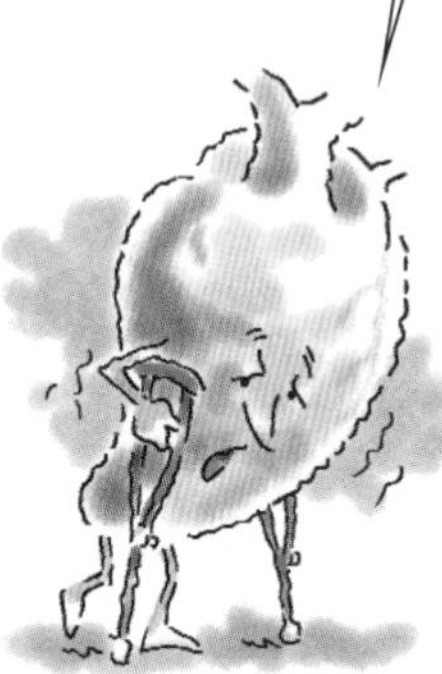

I have a pain in my foot. I'm going to go Homan rest it.

110. 4. A positive Homans' sign (elicited by quickly dorsiflexing the foot), when accompanied by other findings, is diagnostic of DVT. Alone, however, Homans' sign can't be used to diagnose DVT because other conditions of the calf can produce a positive Homans' sign. Dyskinesia is the inability to perform voluntary movement. Eversion is the outward movement of the transverse tarsal joint. A positive Babinski's reflex is an extensor plantar response.

CN: Health promotion and maintenance; CNS: None; CL: Application

111. A client is admitted to the unit with intermittent claudication (cramplike pain in the calves). Which of the following responses by the nurse would most accurately explain the cause of the condition to the client?

1. Inadequate blood supply
2. Elevated leg position
3. Dependent leg position
4. Inadequate muscle oxygenation

111. 4. When a muscle is starved of oxygen, it produces pain much like that of angina. Inadequate blood supply would cause necrosis. Leg position either alleviates or aggravates the condition.

CN: Physiological integrity; CNS: Physiological adaptation; CL: Application

112. The nurse should prepare a client with intermittent claudication to receive which medical treatment?

1. Analgesics
2. Warfarin (Coumadin)
3. Heparin
4. Pentoxifylline (Trental)

112. 4. Pentoxifylline decreases blood viscosity, increases red blood cell flexibility, and improves flow through small vessels. Analgesics are administered for pain relief. Warfarin and heparin are anticoagulants.

CN: Physiological integrity; CNS: Pharmacological and parenteral therapies; CL: Analysis

113. Which oral medication is administered to prevent further thrombus formation?

1. Warfarin (Coumadin)
2. Heparin
3. Furosemide (Lasix)
4. Metoprolol (Lopressor)

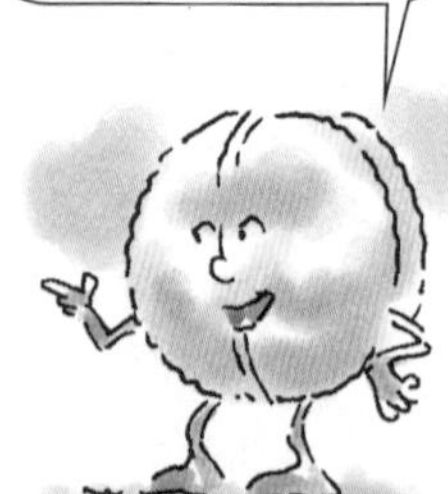

This question requires you to know how certain drugs are administered.

113. 1. Warfarin prevents vitamin K from synthesizing certain clotting factors. This oral anticoagulant can be given long-term. Heparin is a parenteral anticoagulant that interferes with coagulation by readily combining with antithrombin; it can't be given by mouth. Neither furosemide nor metoprolol affects anticoagulation.

CN: Physiological integrity; CNS: Pharmacological and parenteral therapies; CL: Application

CN: Client needs category CNS: Client needs subcategory CL: Cognitive level

114. A nurse should place the client with pulmonary edema in which position to facilitate breathing?

1. Lying flat in bed
2. Left side-lying
3. In high Fowler's position
4. In semi-Fowler's position

114. 3. A high Fowler's position promotes ventilation and facilitates breathing by reducing venous return. Lying flat and side-lying positions worsen the breathing and increase workload of the heart. Semi-Fowler's position won't reduce the workload of the heart as well as high Fowler's position will.

CN: Physiological integrity; CNS: Basic care and comfort; CL: Application

115. Which blood gas abnormality is initially most suggestive of pulmonary edema?

1. Anoxia
2. Hypercapnia
3. Hyperoxygenation
4. Hypocapnia

115. 4. In an attempt to compensate for increased work of breathing due to hyperventilation, carbon dioxide (CO_2) decreases, causing hypocapnia. If the condition persists, CO_2 retention occurs and hypercapnia results. Although oxygenation is relatively low, the client isn't anoxic. Hyperoxygenation would result if the client was given oxygen in excess. However, secondary to fluid build-up, the client would have a low oxygenation level.

CN: Physiological integrity; CNS: Physiological adaptation; CL: Analysis

116. A nurse is caring for a 78-year-old female client with sick sinus syndrome who's awaiting permanent pacemaker placement. Given this client's risk of decreased cardiac output, what assessment findings would indicate that she's experiencing an initial drop in cardiac output?

1. Decreased blood pressure
2. Alteration in level of consciousness (LOC)
3. Decreased blood pressure and diuresis
4. Increased blood pressure and fluid volume

116. 4. The body compensates for a decrease in cardiac output with a rise in blood pressure, due to the stimulation of the sympathetic nervous system and an increase in blood volume as the kidneys retain sodium and water. Blood pressure doesn't initially drop in response to the compensatory mechanism of the body. Alteration in LOC will occur only if the decreased cardiac output persists.

CN: Physiological integrity; CNS: Physiological adaptation; CL: Analysis

117. Which action is the appropriate initial response to a client coughing up pink, frothy sputum?

1. Call for help.
2. Call the physician.
3. Start an I.V. line.
4. Suction the client.

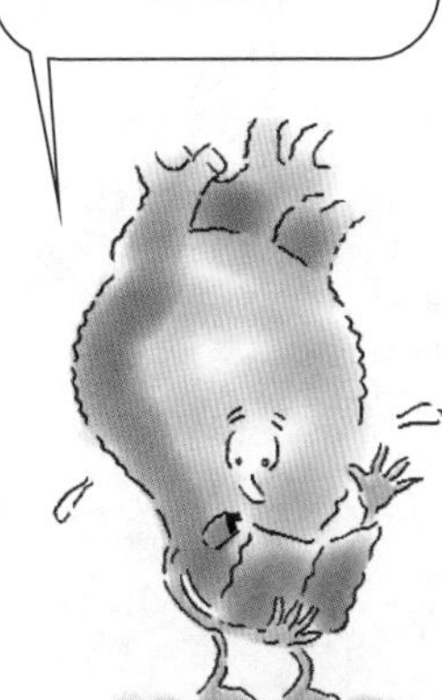

Don't panic! Just think about what to do first.

117. 1. Production of pink, frothy sputum is a classic sign of acute pulmonary edema. Because the client is at high risk for decompensation, the nurse should call for help but not leave the room. The other three interventions should immediately follow.

CN: Physiological integrity; CNS: Physiological adaptation; CL: Analysis

118. Which precaution should a client be instructed to take after an episode of acute pulmonary edema?

1. Limit caloric intake.
2. Restrict carbohydrates.
3. Measure weight twice per day.
4. Call the physician if there is weight gain of more than 3 lb (1.5 kg) in 1 day.

118. 4. Gaining 3 lb in 1 day is indicative of fluid retention that would increase the workload of the heart, thereby putting the client at risk for acute pulmonary edema. Limiting caloric intake doesn't influence fluid status. Restricting carbohydrates wouldn't affect fluid status. The body needs carbohydrates for energy and healing. The client must be weighed in the morning after the first urination. If the client is weighed later in the day, the finding wouldn't be accurate because of fluid intake during the day.

CN: Physiological integrity; CNS: Reduction of risk potential; CL: Application

119. The nurse knows that a 45-year-old client with severe hypertension will experience increased workload of the heart due to which of the following?

1. Increased afterload
2. Increased cardiac output
3. Overload of the heart
4. Increased preload

119. 1. *Afterload* refers to the resistance normally maintained by the aortic and pulmonic valves, the condition and tone of the aorta, and the resistance offered by the systemic and pulmonary arterioles. Hypertension increases afterload, as the left ventricle has to work harder to eject blood against vasoconstriction. *Cardiac output* is the amount of blood expelled from the heart per minute. *Overload* refers to an abundance of circulating volume. *Preload* is the volume of blood in the ventricle at the end of diastole.

CN: Physiological integrity; CNS: Physiological adaptation; CL: Analysis

120. A client with acute pulmonary edema has been taking an angiotensin-converting enzyme (ACE) inhibitor. The nurse teaches him that this medication has been ordered for which reason?

1. To promote diuresis
2. To increase contractility
3. To decrease contractility
4. To reduce blood pressure

This is another question that tests your knowledge of what certain drugs do.

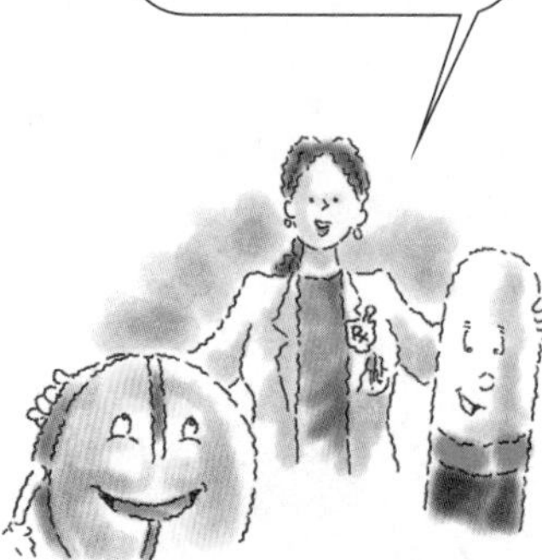

120. 4. ACE inhibitors are given to reduce blood pressure by inhibiting aldosterone production, which in turn decreases sodium and water reabsorption. ACE inhibitors also reduce production of angiotensin II, a potent vasoconstrictor. Diuretics are given to promote diuresis. Inotropic agents increase contractility. Negative inotropic agents decrease contractility.

CN: Physiological integrity; CNS: Pharmacological and parenteral therapies; CL: Application

121. A client with acute pulmonary edema caused by heart failure asks the nurse which area of the heart is usually damaged. The best response by the nurse would be which of the following?

1. Left atrium
2. Right atrium
3. Left ventricle
4. Right ventricle

121. 3. The left ventricle is responsible for the majority of force for cardiac output. If the left ventricle is damaged, the output decreases and fluid accumulates in the interstitial and alveolar spaces, causing pulmonary edema. Damage to the left atrium would contribute to heart failure but wouldn't affect cardiac output or, therefore, the onset of pulmonary edema. If the right atrium and right ventricle were damaged, right-sided heart failure would result.

CN: Physiological integrity; CNS: Physiological adaptation; CL: Application

122. Which statement by a nurse to the health care aide best explains the need to promptly report changes in respiratory rate for a client diagnosed with heart failure?

1. "Pulmonary edema, a life-threatening condition, can develop in minutes."
2. "Severe acute respiratory syndrome (SARS) is a complication of heart failure."
3. "Pneumonia is a consequence of inadequate ventilation with heart failure."
4. "Pneumothorax, a life-threatening condition, can develop in minutes."

122. 1. Pulmonary edema, a life threatening complication of heart failure, can develop in minutes, secondary to a sudden fluid shift from the pulmonary vasculature to the lung interstitial alveoli. SARS and pneumonia are caused by infections. Pneumothorax is a collection of air or gas in the plueral space, causing the lung to collapse.

CN: Physiological Integrity; CNS: Reduction of risk potential; CL: Application

123. The nurse evaluates her teaching by asking the student nurse which term is used to describe the amount of stretch on the myocardium at the end of diastole. Which of the following is most accurate?

1. Afterload
2. Cardiac index
3. Cardiac output
4. Preload

123. 4. Preload is the amount of stretch of the cardiac muscle fibers at the end of diastole. The volume of blood in the ventricle at the end of diastole determines preload. Afterload is the force against which the ventricle must expel blood. Cardiac index is the individualized measurement of cardiac output, based on the client's body surface area. Cardiac output is the amount of blood the heart is expelling per minute.

CN: Physiological integrity; CNS: Physiological adaptation; CL: Application

124. Which action should a nurse take when administering a new blood pressure medication to a client?

1. Administer the medication to the client without explanation.
2. Inform the client of the new drug only if he asks about it.
3. Inform the client of the new medication, its name, use, and the reason for the change in medication.
4. Administer the medication, and inform the client that the physician will later explain the medication.

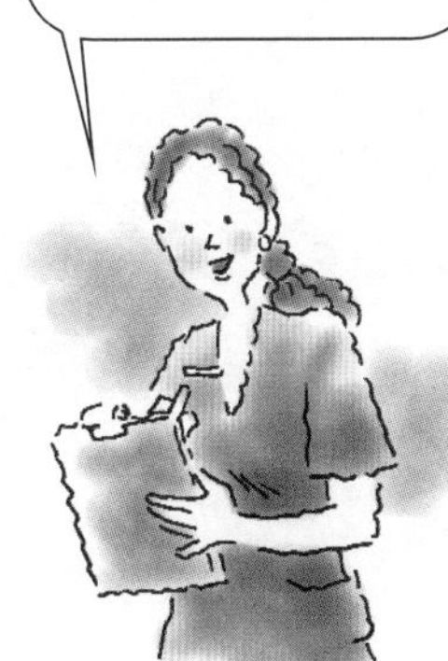
Which answer best promotes compliance?

124. 3. Informing the client of the medication, its use, and the reason for the medication change is important to the care of the client. Teaching the client about his treatment regimen promotes compliance. The other responses are inappropriate.

CN: Safe, effective care environment; CNS: Management of care; CL: Application

125. Antihypertensives should be used cautiously in clients already taking which other drug?

1. Ibuprofen (Advil)
2. Diphenhydramine (Benadryl)
3. Thioridazine
4. Vitamins

125. 3. Thioridazine affects the neurotransmitter norepinephrine, which causes hypotension and other cardiovascular effects. Administering an antihypertensive to a client who already has hypotension could have serious adverse effects. Ibuprofen is an anti-inflammatory that doesn't interfere with the cardiovascular system. Although diphenhydramine does have histaminic effects such as sedation, it isn't known to decrease blood pressure. Vitamins aren't drugs and don't interfere with cardiovascular function.

CN: Physiological integrity; CNS: Pharmacological and parenteral therapies; CL: Application

126. A 57-year-old client with a history of bronchial asthma is prescribed propranolol (Inderal) to control hypertension. Before administering propranolol, which action should the nurse take first?

1. Monitor apical pulse rate.
2. Instruct the client to take the medication with food.
3. Question the physician about the order.
4. Caution the client to rise slowly when standing.

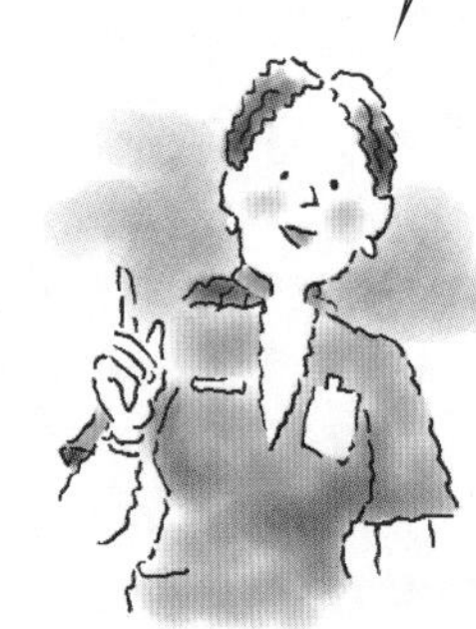
Note the first in question 126. It's the key to the right answer.

126. 3. Propranolol and other beta-adrenergic blockers are contraindicated in a client with bronchial asthma, so the nurse should question the physician before giving the dose. The other responses are appropriate actions for a client receiving propranolol, but questioning the physician takes priority. The client's apical pulse should always be checked before giving propranolol; if the pulse rate is extremely low, the nurse should withhold the drug and notify the physician. Taking propranolol with food enhances its absorption. Because propranolol can cause light-headedness, the client should be told to rise slowly when standing.

CN: Physiological integrity; CNS: Pharmacological and parenteral therapies; CL: Application

127. One hour after I.V. furosemide (Lasix) is administered to a client with heart failure, a short burst of ventricular tachycardia appears on the cardiac monitor. Which electrolyte imbalance should the nurse suspect?

1. Hypocalcemia
2. Hypermagnesemia
3. Hypokalemia
4. Hypernatremia

127. 3. Furosemide is a potassium-depleting diuretic that can cause hypokalemia. In turn, hypokalemia increases myocardial excitability, leading to ventricular tachycardia. Hypocalcemia, which slows conduction through the atrioventricular junction, can cause such bradyarrhythmias as atrioventricular block. Hypermagnesemia may lead to bradycardia, not tachycardia. Hypernatremia may cause sinus tachycardia as a result of water loss.

CN: Physiological integrity; CNS: Physiological adaptation; CL: Analysis

128. A client has a reduced serum high-density lipoprotein (HDL) level and an elevated low-density lipoprotein (LDL) level. Which dietary modification is appropriate for this client?

1. Fiber intake of less than 10% of total calories daily
2. Less than 40% of calories from fat
3. Cholesterol intake of less than 300 mg daily
4. Less than 7% of calories from saturated fat

128. 4. A client with low serum HDL and high serum LDL levels should get less than 7% of daily calories from saturated fat. Fiber intake should be at least 15% of total daily calories, total fat intake should be only 25% to 35% of daily calories, and cholesterol intake should be less than 200 mg daily.

CN: Physiological integrity; CNS: Reduction of risk potential; CL: Application

129. A paradoxical pulse occurs in a client who had coronary artery bypass graft (CABG) surgery 2 days ago. Which surgical complication should the nurse suspect?

1. Left-sided heart failure
2. Aortic regurgitation
3. Complete heart block
4. Pericardial tamponade

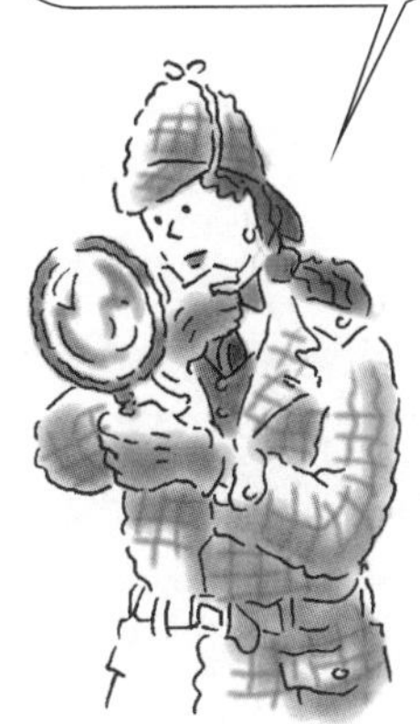

Just as I suspected—a pericardial paradox!

129. 4. A *paradoxical pulse* (a palpable decrease in pulse amplitude on quiet inspiration) signals pericardial tamponade, a complication of CABG surgery. Left-sided heart failure can cause *pulsus alternans* (pulse amplitude alternation from beat to beat, with a regular rhythm). Aortic regurgitation may cause *bisferious pulse* (an increased arterial pulse with a double systolic peak). Complete heart block may cause a *bounding pulse* (a strong pulse with increased pulse pressure).

CN: Physiological integrity; CNS: Physiological adaptation; CL: Application

130. A 35-year-old client was admitted to the coronary care unit (CCU) 2 days ago with an acute myocardial infarction. Which action would breach client confidentiality?

1. The CCU nurse gives a verbal report to the nurse on the telemetry unit before transferring the client to that unit.
2. The CCU nurse notifies the on-call physician about a change in the client's condition.
3. The emergency department (ED) nurse calls up the latest electrocardiogram results to check the client's progress.
4. At the client's request, the CCU nurse updates the client's wife on his condition.

130. 3. The ED nurse is no longer directly involved with the client's care and thus has no legal right to information about his present condition. Anyone directly involved in his care (such as the telemetry nurse and the on-call physician) has the right to information about his condition. Because the client requested that the nurse update his wife on his condition, doing so doesn't breach confidentiality.

CN: Safe, effective care environment; CNS: Management of care; CL: Application

131. A client arriving in the emergency department (ED) is receiving cardiopulmonary resuscitation from paramedics, who are giving ventilations through an endotracheal (ET) tube that they placed in the client's home. During a pause in compressions, the cardiac monitor shows narrow QRS complexes and a heart rate of 55 beats/minute with a palpable pulse. Which action should the nurse take <u>first</u>?

1. Start an I.V. line and administer amiodarone, 300 mg I.V. over 10 minutes.
2. Check ET tube placement.
3. Obtain an arterial blood gas (ABG) sample.
4. Administer atropine, 1 mg I.V.

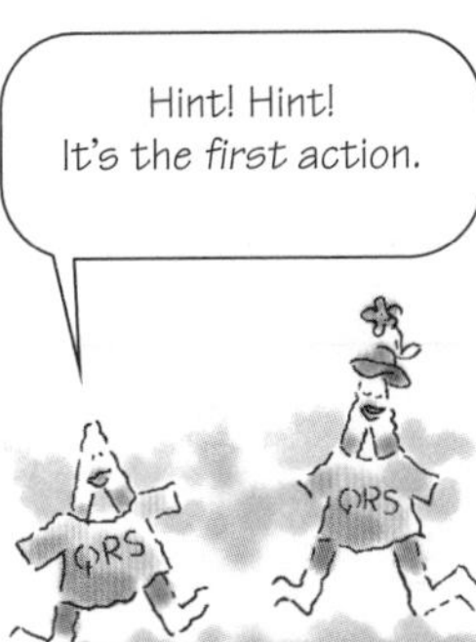

Hint! Hint!
It's the first action.
QRS
QRS

131. 2. ET tube placement should be confirmed as soon as the client arrives in the ED. Once the airway is secured, oxygenation and ventilation should be confirmed using an end-tidal carbon dioxide monitor and pulse oximetry. Next, the nurse should make sure I.V. access is established. If the client experiences symptomatic bradycardia, atropine is administered as ordered, 0.5 to 1 mg every 3 to 5 minutes to a total of 3 mg. Then the nurse should try to find the cause of the client's arrest by obtaining an ABG sample. Amiodarone is indicated for ventricular tachycardia, ventricular fibrillation, and atrial flutter—not symptomatic bradycardia.

CN: Physiological integrity; CNS: Physiological adaptation; CL: Application

132. After unsuccessful cardiopulmonary resuscitation efforts, the nurse must prepare an Islamic client for the morgue. Which nursing action should the nurse take?

1. Allowing the client's family to perform the ritualistic washing
2. Doing nothing; the Burial Society will perform a ritual cleansing
3. Doing nothing; only the family and close friends may touch the body
4. Providing routine postmortem care

132. 1. Physical care at death for a person of the Islamic faith consists of ritualistic washing by the family, with the client's body positioned toward Mecca. The Burial Society may perform ritual cleansing for clients of the Jewish faith. Hindu clients believe that only family and close friends should touch the body. Routine postmortem care is appropriate for Christian clients.

CN: Psychosocial integrity; CNS: None; CL: Application

133. A 63-year-old client has Prinzmetal's angina. To reduce the risk of coronary artery spasms, which type of medication is the physician most likely to prescribe?

1. Beta-adrenergic blocker
2. Angiotensin-converting enzyme (ACE) inhibitor
3. Inotropic vasodilator
4. Calcium channel blocker

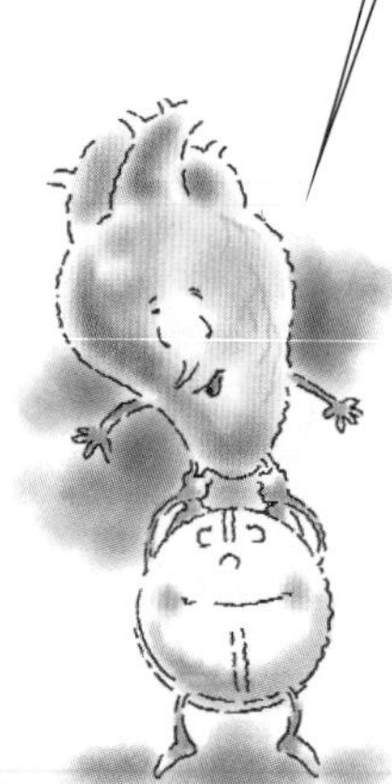

133. 4. A calcium channel blocker, such as diltiazem (Cardizem), is indicated in managing Prinzmetal's angina because it reduces the incidence of coronary artery spasm. A beta-adrenergic blocker, such as metoprolol (Lopressor), treats angina by decreasing myocardial oxygen needs and has no effect on coronary artery spasms. An ACE inhibitor, such as enalapril (Vasotec), is used to manage hypertension. An inotropic vasodilator, such as milrinone, is indicated for short-term I.V. therapy in heart failure.

CN: Physiological integrity; CNS: Pharmacological and parenteral therapies; CL: Application

134. An 86-year-old client with heart failure is receiving furosemide (Lasix), 40 mg I.V. The physician orders 40 mEq of potassium chloride in 100 ml of dextrose 5% in water, to infuse over 4 hours. The client's most recent serum potassium level is 3.0 mEq/L. At which infusion rate should the nurse set the I.V. pump?

1. 25 ml/hour
2. 10 ml/hour
3. 100 ml/hour
4. 50 ml/hour

134. 1. Use this formula to determine the infusion rate:

$$\text{ml/hour} = \frac{\text{total volume (in ml) to be infused}}{\text{total time of infusion in hours}}$$

$$\text{ml/hour} = \frac{100 \text{ ml}}{4 \text{ hours}}$$

$$\text{ml/hour} = 25$$

CN: Physiological integrity; CNS: Pharmacological and parenteral therapies; CL: Application

135. A nurse is planning discharge instructions for a client who is being treated for ventricular tachycardia. Which of the following rationales for including bananas in the client's diet would be most accurate?

1. Because bananas are high in carbohydrate
2. Because bananas are high in potassium
3. Because bananas are low in sodium
4. Because bananas are high in fiber

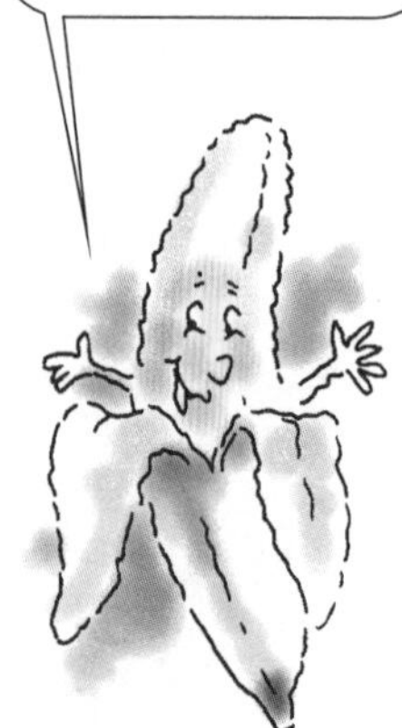

I'm good for the heart. Can you guess why?

135. 2. A low serum potassium level increases the risk of ventricular tachycardia. Therefore, the client should be instructed to eat potassium-rich foods such as bananas.

CN: Health promotion and maintenance; CNS: None; CL: Analysis

CN: Client needs category CNS: Client needs subcategory CL: Cognitive level

136. After cardiac surgery, a client's blood pressure measures 126/80 mm Hg. The nurse determines that mean arterial pressure (MAP) is:

1. 46 mm Hg.
2. 80 mm Hg.
3. 95 mm Hg.
4. 90 mm Hg.

136. 3. Use this formula to calculate MAP:

$$MAP = \frac{\text{systolic} + 2\ (\text{diastolic})}{3}$$

$$MAP = \frac{126\ \text{mm Hg} + 2\ (80\ \text{mm Hg})}{3}$$

$$MAP = \frac{286\ \text{mm Hg}}{3}$$

$$MAP = 95\ \text{mm Hg}$$

CN: Physiological integrity; CNS: Reduction of risk potential; CL: Analysis

137. A charge nurse is preparing client care assignments for the next shift. A client who underwent femoral-popliteal bypass surgery is scheduled to return from the postanesthesia care unit. Which staff member should receive this client?

1. Registered nurse with 1 year of experience
2. Licensed practical nurse (LPN) with 5 years of experience
3. Nursing assistant with 15 years of experience
4. Charge nurse with 10 years of experience

137. 1. Because this client requires frequent neurovascular assessments, a registered nurse should receive him. An LPN, although she's experienced and can collect data, doesn't have the education to perform the physical assessment required by this client. The nursing assistant lacks the necessary assessment skills. The charge nurse needs to be available to direct the care of other clients.

CN: Safe, effective care environment; CNS: Management of care; CL: Analysis

138. An 18-year-old client who recently had an upper respiratory infection is admitted with suspected rheumatic fever. Which assessment findings confirm this diagnosis?

1. Erythema marginatum, subcutaneous nodules, and fever
2. Tachycardia, finger clubbing, and a loud second heart sound (S_2)
3. Dyspnea, cough, and palpitations
4. Dyspnea, fatigue, and syncope

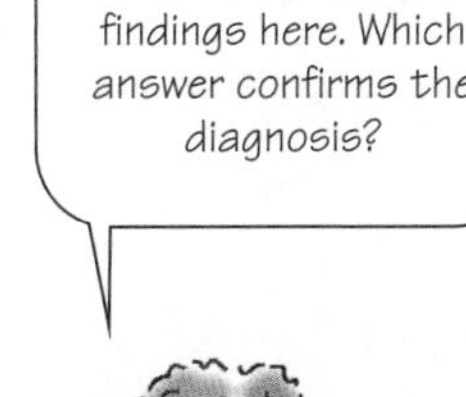

There are several findings here. Which answer confirms the diagnosis?

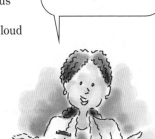

138. 1. Diagnosis of rheumatic fever requires that the client have either two major Jones criteria or one minor criterion plus evidence of a previous streptococcal infection. Major criteria include carditis, polyarthritis, Sydenham's chorea, subcutaneous nodules, and erythema marginatum (transient, nonpruritic macules on the trunk or inner aspects of the upper arms or thighs). Minor criteria include fever, arthralgia, elevated levels of acute phase reactants, and a prolonged PR interval on electrocardiography. Tachycardia, finger clubbing, and a loud S_2 suggest transposition of the great arteries (a cyanotic congenital heart defect). Dyspnea, cough, and palpitations occur with mitral insufficiency. Dyspnea, fatigue, and syncope indicate aortic insufficiency.

CN: Physiological integrity; CNS: Physiological adaptation; CL: Application

139. A client with new onset of atrial fibrillation is receiving warfarin (Coumadin) to help prevent thromboemboli. The warfarin dosage will reach therapeutic levels when the International Normalized Ratio (INR) falls within which range?

1. 1 to 2
2. 1.5 to 2.5
3. 2 to 3
4. 2.5 to 3.5

139. 3. In a client with atrial fibrillation, warfarin reaches therapeutic levels when the INR is 2 to 3. Lower ratios are below the therapeutic range. A range of 2.5 to 3.5 is too high for a client on warfarin and increases the hemorrhage risk.

CN: Physiological integrity; CNS: Reduction of risk potential; CL: Application

140. A 38-year-old client comes to the emergency department complaining that his heart "suddenly began to race." After attaching him to the cardiac monitor, the nurse observes atrial tachycardia. Which rhythm strip characteristics indicate this arrhythmia?

1. Atrial rate greater than the ventricular rate, sawtooth P waves
2. Irregular rhythm, indiscernible atrial rate, absent P waves
3. Regular atrial and ventricular rhythms, rate of 123 beats/minute
4. Regular atrial and ventricular rhythms, P wave hidden in the T wave, rate of 210 beats/minute

140. 4. With atrial tachycardia, the rhythm is regular, the P wave is hidden in the preceding T wave, and the rate ranges from 140 to 250 beats/minute. A ventricular rate that varies with the degree of atrioventricular block, along with sawtooth P waves, characterizes atrial flutter. Irregular ventricular response and absent P waves characterize atrial fibrillation. Regular and equal atrial and ventricular rhythms and a rate of 100 to 160 beats/minute characterize sinus tachycardia.

CN: Physiological integrity; CNS: Physiological adaptation; CL: Application

141. A client is receiving spironolactone to treat hypertension. Which instruction should the nurse provide?

1. "Eat foods high in potassium."
2. "Take daily potassium supplements."
3. "Discontinue sodium restrictions."
4. "Avoid salt substitutes."

141. 4. Because spironolactone is a potassium-sparing diuretic, the client should avoid salt substitutes because of their high potassium content. The client should also avoid potassium-rich foods and potassium supplements. To reduce fluid volume overload, sodium restrictions should continue.

CN: Physiological integrity; CNS: Pharmacological and parenteral therapies; CL: Application

142. A 23-year-old client develops cardiac tamponade when the car he was driving hits a telephone pole; he wasn't wearing a seat belt. The nurse helps the physician perform pericardiocentesis. Which outcome would indicate that pericardiocentesis has been effective?

1. Neck vein distention
2. Pulsus paradoxus
3. Increased blood pressure
4. Muffled heart sounds

142. 3. Cardiac tamponade is associated with decreased cardiac output, which in turn reduces blood pressure. By removing a small amount of blood, pericardiocentesis increases blood pressure. Neck vein distention, pulsus paradoxus, and muffled heart sounds indicate persistent cardiac tamponade, meaning that pericardiocentesis hasn't been effective.

CN: Physiological integrity; CNS: Physiological adaptation; CL: Application

143. A client admitted with angina complains of severe chest pain and suddenly becomes unresponsive. After establishing unresponsiveness, which action should the nurse take first?

1. Activate the resuscitation team.
2. Open the client's airway.
3. Check for breathing.
4. Check for signs of circulation.

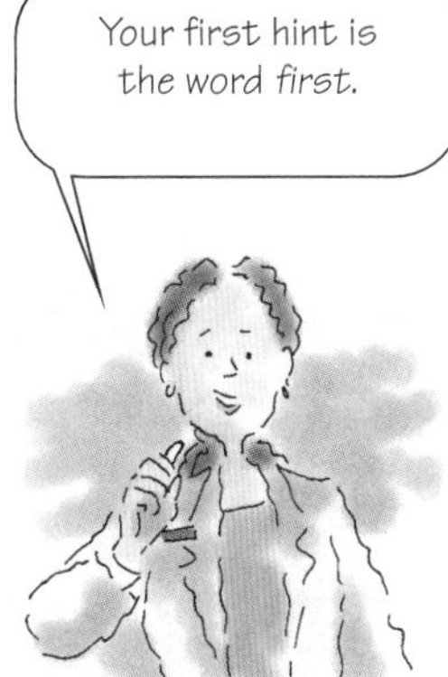
Your first hint is
the word first.

143. 1. Immediately after establishing unresponsiveness, the nurse should activate the resuscitation team. The next step is to open the airway using the head-tilt, chin-lift maneuver and check for breathing (looking, listening, and feeling for no more than 10 seconds). If the client isn't breathing, give two slow breaths using a bag mask or pocket mask. Next, check for signs of circulation by palpating the carotid pulse.

CN: Physiological integrity; CNS: Physiological adaptation; CL: Application

144. A 54-year-old client is admitted with an acute inferior-wall myocardial infarction (MI). During the admission interview, he says he stopped taking his metoprolol (Lopressor) 5 days ago because he was feeling better. Which nursing diagnosis takes priority for this client?

1. *Anxiety*
2. *Risk for decreased cardiac tissue perfusion*
3. *Acute pain*
4. *Ineffective family therapeutic regimen management*

144. 2. MI results from prolonged myocardial ischemia caused by reduced blood flow through the coronary arteries. Therefore, the priority nursing diagnosis for this client is *Risk for decreased cardiac tissue perfusion. Anxiety, Acute pain,* and *Ineffective family therapeutic regimen management* are appropriate but don't take priority.

CN: Safe, effective care environment; CNS: Management of care; CL: Analysis

145. A client comes to the emergency department with acute shortness of breath and a cough that produces pink, frothy sputum. Admission assessment reveals crackles and wheezes, a blood pressure of 82/45 mm Hg, a heart rate of 120 beats/minute, and a respiratory rate of 38 breaths/minute. The client's medical history includes diabetes mellitus, hypertension, and heart failure. Which disorder should the nurse suspect?

1. Pulmonary edema
2. Pneumothorax
3. Cardiac tamponade
4. Pulmonary embolus

145. 1. Shortness of breath, tachypnea, low blood pressure, tachycardia, diffuse crackles, and a cough producing pink, frothy sputum are late signs of pulmonary edema. Pneumothorax causes sudden, sharp pleuritic pain exacerbated by chest movement, breathing, and coughing; shortness of breath; and absent breath sounds on the affected side. Cardiac tamponade produces muffled heart sounds, pulsus paradoxus, and jugular vein distention. Pulmonary embolus may cause fever, cough, hemoptysis, and a pleural friction rub.

CN: Physiological integrity; CNS: Physiological adaptation; CL: Application

146. A 57-year-old client with acute arterial occlusion of the left leg undergoes an emergency embolectomy. Six hours later, the nurse isn't able to obtain pulses in his left foot using Doppler ultrasound. She immediately notifies the physician, who asks her to prepare the client for surgery. As the nurse enters the client's room to prepare him, he states that he won't have any more surgery. Which action is the best initial response by the nurse?

1. Explaining the risks of not having the surgery
2. Notifying the physician immediately
3. Notifying the nursing supervisor
4. Recording the client's refusal in the nurses' notes

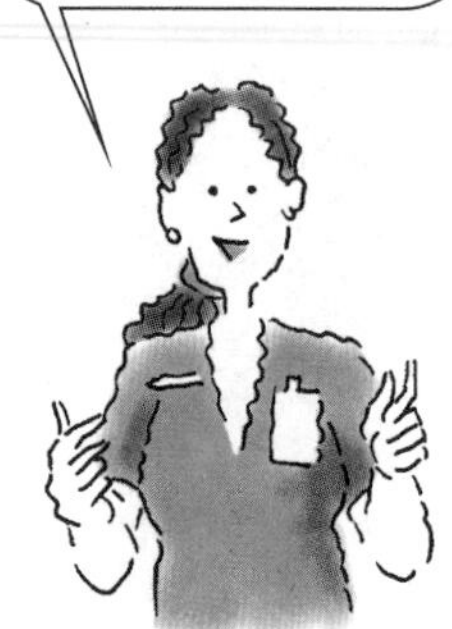
Here you're looking for the best initial response.

146. 1. The best initial response is to explain the risks of not having the surgery. If the client understands the risks but still refuses, the nurse should notify the physician and the nursing supervisor and then record the client's refusal in the nurses' notes.

CN: Safe, effective care environment; CNS: Management of care; CL: Analysis

147. The nurse coming on duty receives the report from the nurse going off duty. Which client should the on-duty nurse assess first?

1. The 58-year-old client who was admitted 2 days ago with heart failure, blood pressure of 126/76 mm Hg, and a respiratory rate of 22 breaths/minute
2. The 89-year-old client with end-stage right-sided heart failure, blood pressure of 78/50 mm Hg, and a "Do not resuscitate" order
3. The 62-year-old client who was admitted 1 day ago with thrombophlebitis and is receiving I.V. heparin
4. The 75-year-old client who was admitted 1 hour ago with new-onset atrial fibrillation and is receiving I.V. diltiazem (Cardizem)

147. 4. The client with atrial fibrillation has the greatest potential to become unstable and is on I.V. medication that requires close monitoring. After assessing this client, the nurse should assess the 62-year-old client with thrombophlebitis who is receiving a heparin infusion, and then the 58-year-old client admitted 2 days ago with heart failure (his signs and symptoms are resolving and don't require immediate attention). The lowest priority is the 89-year-old with end-stage right-sided heart failure, who requires time-consuming supportive measures.

CN: Safe, effective care environment; CNS: Management of care; CL: Analysis

148. When developing a teaching plan for a client with endocarditis, which point is most essential for the nurse to include?

1. "Report fever, anorexia, and night sweats to the physician."
2. "Take prophylactic antibiotics after dental work and invasive procedures."
3. "Include potassium-rich foods in your diet."
4. "Monitor your pulse rate daily."

148. 1. The most essential teaching point is to report signs of relapse, such as fever, anorexia, and night sweats, to the physician. To prevent further endocarditis episodes, prophylactic antibiotics are taken before and sometimes after dental work, childbirth, or genitourinary, GI, or gynecologic procedures. A potassium-rich diet and daily pulse monitoring aren't necessary for a client with endocarditis.

CN: Health promotion and maintenance; CNS: None; CL: Application

149. Which finding suggests that fluid resuscitation has been effective for a 23-year-old client admitted in hypovolemic shock?

1. Urine output of 15 ml/hour
2. Urine output of 20 ml/hour
3. Urine output of 25 ml/hour
4. Urine output of 30 ml/hour

149. 4. In an adult, urine output below 30 ml/hour indicates inadequate blood flow to the kidneys. Therefore, urine output of 30 ml/hour or greater reflects adequate fluid resuscitation.
CN: Physiological integrity; CNS: Physiological adaptation; CL: Analysis

150. A client is being monitored via telemetry using a 3 lead system. Which graphic shows the correct electrode positions to monitor modified chest lead 1 (MCL1)?

1. 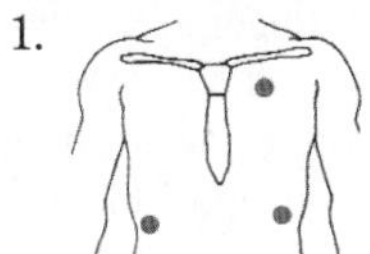
2. 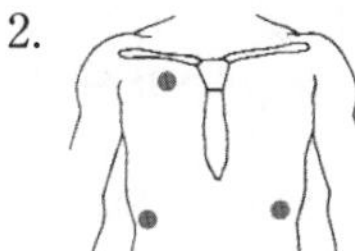
3. 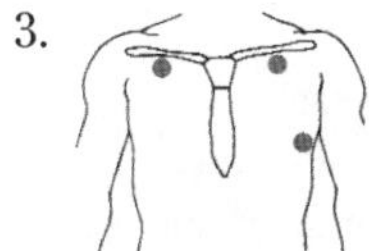
4. 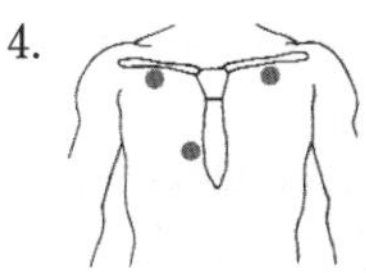

150. 4. Option four shows the correct electrode placement for MCL1. Option one shows the correct placement to monitor Lead III. Option two shows the correct placement to monitor MCL6. Option three shows the correct placement to monitor Lead II.
CN: Physiological integrity; CNS: Reduction of risk potential; CL: Application

151. An elderly client has a history of aortic stenosis. Identify the area where the nurse should place the stethoscope to best hear the murmur.

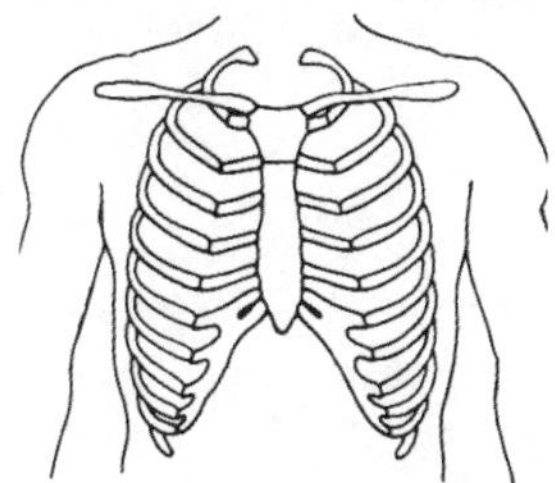

151. The murmur of aortic stenosis is low-pitched, rough, and rasping. It's heard loudest in second intercostal space to right of sternum.
CN: Physiological integrity; CNS: Physiological adaptation; CL: Application

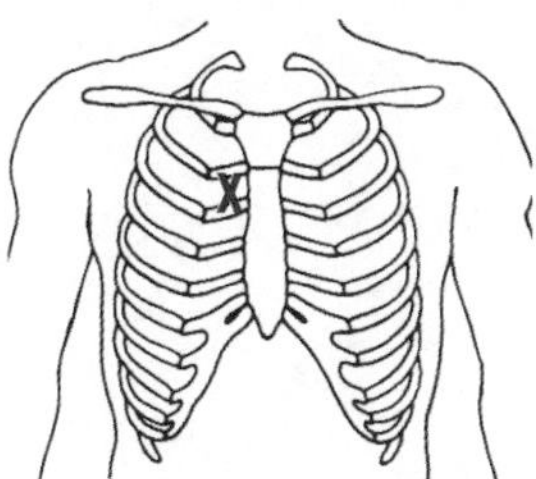

152. A client with deep vein thrombosis has an I.V. infusion of heparin sodium infusing at 1,500 units/hour. The concentration in the bag is 25,000 units/500 ml. How many milliliters should the nurse document as intake from this infusion for an 8-hour shift? Record your answer using a whole number.

_______________ milliliters

152. 240. First, calculate how many units are in each milliliter of the medication: 25,000 units/500 ml = 50 units/ml. Next, calculate how many milliliters the client receives each hour: 1 ml/50 units × 1,500 units/hour = 30 ml/hour. Lastly, multiply by 8 hours: 30 ml × 8 hours = 240 ml.

CN: Physiological integrity; CNS: Pharmacological and parenteral therapies; CL: Application

153. The nurse suspects that her client is in cardiac arrest. According to the American Heart Association (AHA), she should perform the actions listed below. Order these actions in the sequence that the nurse should perform them.

1. Activate the emergency response team.
2. Assess responsiveness.
3. Call for a defibrillator.
4. Provide two slow breaths.
5. Assess pulse.
6. Assess breathing.

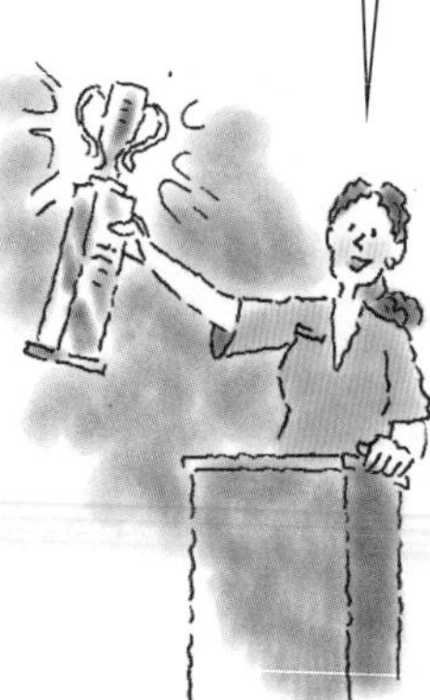
Congratulations!
You did it!

153. According to the AHA, the nurse should first assess responsiveness. If the client is unresponsive, she should activate the emergency response system, then call for a defibrillator. Next, she should assess breathing by opening the airway and then look, listen, and feel for respirations. If respirations aren't present, she should administer two slow breaths, then assess carotid pulse. If no pulse is present, she should start chest compressions.

CN: Physiological integrity; CNS: Physiological adaptation; CL: Application

2. Assess responsiveness.
1. Activate the emergency response team.
3. Call for a defibrillator.
6. Assess breathing.
4. Provide two slow breaths.
5. Assess pulse.

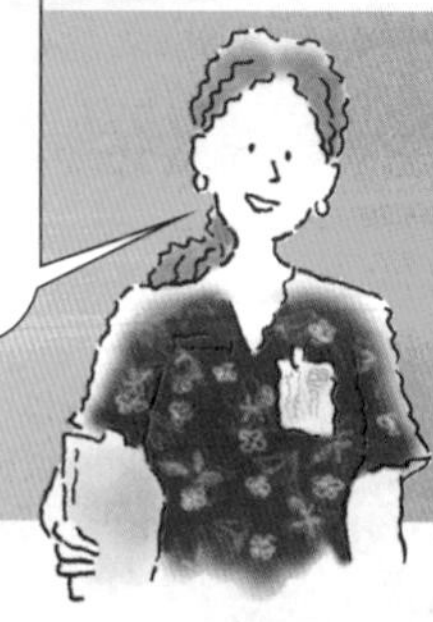

This challenging chapter covers HIV infection, AIDS, rheumatoid arthritis, ITP, and lots of other complex disorders. You can handle it, though, I know you can. Go for it!

Chapter 4 Hematologic & immune disorders

1. For an adult client to be diagnosed with acquired immunodeficiency syndrome (AIDS), which condition must be present?

1. Infection with human immunodeficiency virus (HIV), tuberculosis, and cytomegalovirus infection
2. Infection with HIV, an alternative lifestyle, and a T-cell count above 200 cells/µl
3. Infection with HIV, $CD4^+$ count below 200 cells/µl, and a T-cell count above 400 cells/µl
4. Infection with HIV, a history of acute HIV infection, and a $CD4^+$ T-cell count below 200 cells/µl

1. 4. Three criteria must be met for an adult client to be diagnosed with AIDS. He must be HIV-positive, have a $CD4^+$ T-cell count below 200 cells/µl, and have one or more specific conditions that include acute infection with HIV. Because HIV attaches to the $CD4^+$ receptor sites of the T cell, a T-cell value alone is incorrect.

CN: Physiological integrity; CNS: Physiological adaptation; CL: Application

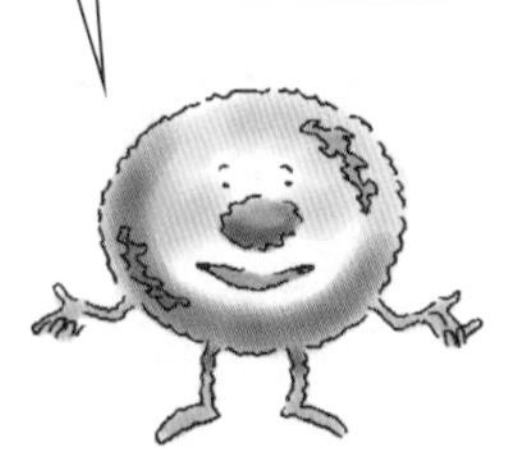

More than one answer may seem correct. Be careful to choose the best answer.

2. Which body substances most easily transmit human immunodeficiency virus (HIV)?

1. Feces and saliva
2. Blood and semen
3. Breast milk and tears
4. Vaginal secretions and urine

2. 2. HIV is most easily transmitted in blood, semen, and vaginal secretions. However, it has also been found in urine, feces, saliva, tears, and breast milk.

CN: Health promotion and maintenance; CNS: None; CL: Analysis

3. Immediately after giving an injection, a nurse is accidentally stuck with the needle when a client becomes agitated. When is the best time for the employer to test the nurse for human immunodeficiency virus (HIV) antibodies to determine if she became infected as a result of the needle stick?

1. Immediately and then again in 6 weeks
2. Immediately and then again in 3 months
3. In 2 weeks and then again in 6 months
4. In 2 weeks and then again in 1 year

3. 2. The employer will want to test the nurse immediately to determine whether a preexisting infection is present, and then again in 3 months to detect seroconversion as a result of the needle stick. Waiting 2 weeks to perform the first test is too late to detect preexisting infection. Testing sooner than 3 months may yield false-negative results.

CN: Health promotion and maintenance; CNS: None; CL: Application

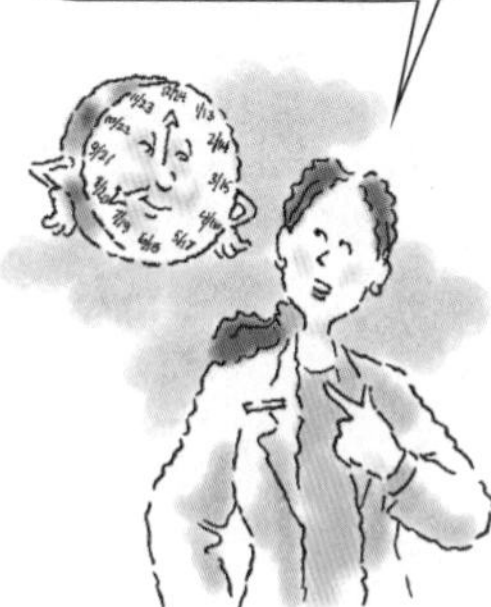

Time is often a crucial element in testing for HIV.

CN: Client needs category CNS: Client needs subcategory CL: Cognitive level

4. Which blood test is used <u>first</u> to identify a response to human immunodeficiency virus (HIV) infection?
1. Western blot
2. CD4+ T-cell count
3. Erythrocyte sedimentation rate
4. Enzyme-linked immunosorbent assay (ELISA)

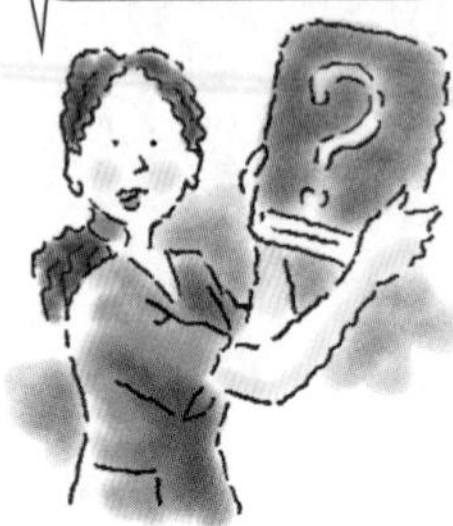
Question 4 is asking you to prioritize.

4. 4. The ELISA is the first screening test for HIV. A Western blot test confirms a positive ELISA test. Other blood tests that support the diagnosis of HIV include $CD4^+$ and $CD8^+$ counts, complete blood counts, immunoglobulin levels, p24 antigen assay, and quantitative ribonucleic acid assays.
CN: Health promotion and maintenance; CNS: None; CL: Analysis

5. The nurse would instruct a client with human immunodeficiency virus who has frequent bouts of diarrhea to avoid consuming which of the following?
1. Milk
2. Red licorice
3. Chicken soup
4. Broiled meat

5. 1. Clients with chronic diarrhea may develop intolerance to lactose, which may worsen the diarrhea. Although red licorice may be eaten, black licorice should be avoided. Other foods that the client should avoid include fatty foods, other lactose-containing foods, caffeine, and sugar. Chicken soup and broiled meat may be consumed.
CN: Physiological integrity; CNS: Reduction of risk potential; CL: Application

6. A nurse is preparing a teaching plan for a client with rheumatoid arthritis. Which dietary recommendation may help this client reduce inflammation?
1. Fish oil
2. Vitamin D
3. Iron-rich foods
4. Calcium carbonate

6. 1. The therapeutic effect of fish oil suppresses inflammatory mediator production (such as prostaglandins); how it works is unknown. Iron-rich foods are recommended to decrease the anemia associated with rheumatoid arthritis. Vitamin D and calcium supplements may help reduce bone resorption.
CN: Physiological integrity; CNS: Physiological adaptation; CL: Application

7. Which is a nonsteroidal anti-inflammatory drug (NSAID) used <u>most often</u> to treat rheumatoid arthritis?
1. Furosemide
2. Haloperidol
3. Ibuprofen
4. Methotrexate

7. 3. Ibuprofen, fenoprofen, naproxen, piroxicam, and indomethacin are NSAIDs used for clients with rheumatoid arthritis. Furosemide is a loop diuretic and haloperidol is an antipsychotic agent, neither of which is used to treat rheumatoid arthritis. Methotrexate is an immunosuppressant used in the *early* treatment of rheumatoid arthritis.
CN: Physiological integrity; CNS: Pharmacological and parenteral therapies; CL: Application

8. The nurse is teaching a client about the method of transmission that has the most risk for exposure to human immunodeficiency virus (HIV). Which of the following statements by the client best demonstrates that he understands the teaching about exposure risks?

1. "I can have routine teeth cleaning at the dentist's office."
2. "I may have intercourse with my spouse."
3. "I may engage in unprotected, noninsertive sexual contact."
4. "I should not engage in intercourse with a new partner without a condom."

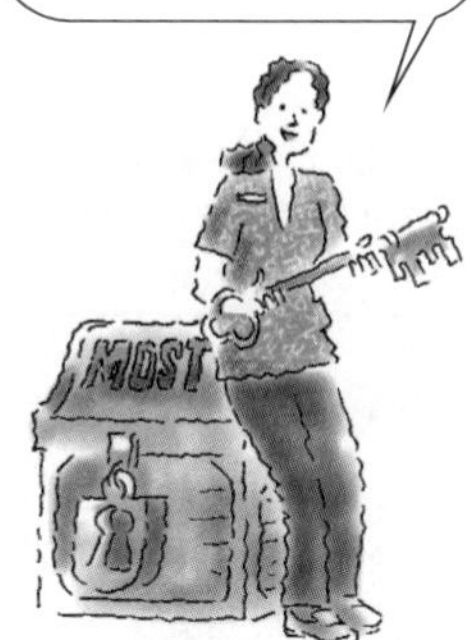

The key word in question 8 is most.
MOST

8. 4. Having intercourse with a new partner is risky because of the unknown I.V. drug use and sexual history. Use of a condom may increase the protection against HIV exposure. Absolutely safe sex practices include autosexual activities, abstinence, and intercourse within a monogamous uninfected couple. Very safe practices include noninsertive sexual contact. Having your teeth cleaned isn't a risk factor if the dental office properly sterilizes the equipment.
CN: Health promotion and maintenance; CNS: None; CL: Analysis

9. Which client is most at risk for developing rheumatoid arthritis?

1. A 25-year-old woman
2. A 40-year-old man
3. A 65-year-old woman
4. A 70-year-old man

9. 3. Rheumatoid arthritis affects women three times more often than men. The average age of onset is 55.
CN: Health promotion and maintenance; CNS: None; CL: Analysis

10. While caring for a client with acquired immunodeficiency syndrome (AIDS) who is receiving zidovudine, the nurse is asked, "How does this drug work?" After teaching the client, the nurse interprets which response by the client to indicate an understanding of the medication?

1. "It kills the human immunodeficiency (HIV) virus."
2. "It suppresses the HIV virus."
3. "I won't infect anyone else when I take this drug."
4. "It's the only drug for HIV I need to take."

10. 2. Zidovudine is an antiviral drug that suppresses the replication of the HIV virus. It is most commonly used for HIV clients in conjunction with other antiretroviral drugs. It also helps prevent maternal-fetal transmission of HIV. However, it is not a cure, it doesn't kill the HIV virus, and clients taking this medication remain infectious.
CN: Physiological integrity; CNS: Pharmacological therapies; CL: Analysis

11. Which precaution must a nurse take when taking the blood pressure of an HIV-positive client?

1. Wearing gloves
2. Wearing a gown
3. Using contact precautions
4. Washing hands

11. 4. Since taking a client's blood pressure doesn't involve contact with his blood or secretions, washing hands is all that is necessary.
CN: Safe, effective care environment; CNS: Safety and infection control; CL: Application

12. Which group or factor is linked to higher morbidity and mortality in human immunodeficiency virus (HIV)–infected clients?

1. Homosexual men
2. Lower socioeconomic status
3. Treatment in a large teaching hospital
4. Treatment by a physician who specializes in HIV infection

12. 2. Morbidity and mortality have been associated with lower socioeconomic status, receiving care in a community hospital or by a physician without much experience with HIV infections, or lack of access to adequate health care.
CN: Physiological integrity; CNS: Physiological adaptation; CL: Analysis

13. After teaching a client about rheumatoid arthritis, which statement indicates the client understands the disease process?

1. "It will get better and worse again."
2. "Once it clears up, it will never come back."
3. "I will definitely have to have surgery for this."
4. "It will never get any better than it is right now."

13. 1. The client with rheumatoid arthritis needs to understand it is a somewhat unpredictable disease characterized by periods of exacerbation and remission. There's no cure, but symptoms can be managed at times. Surgery may be indicated in some cases but not always.

CN: Psychosocial integrity; CNS: None; CL: Application

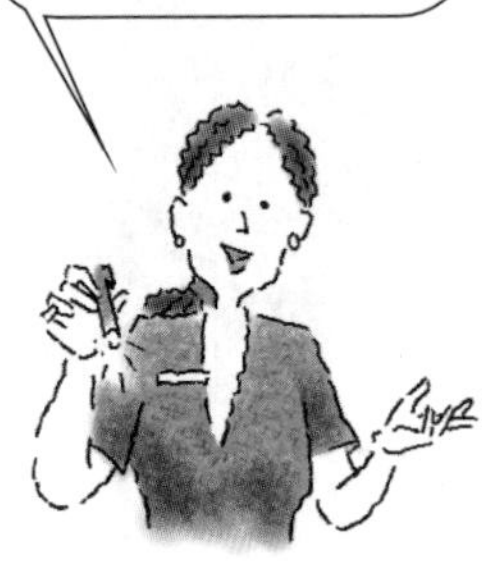

The word first should shed some light on the answer.

14. Which medication would <u>first</u> be prescribed for a client with rheumatoid arthritis?

1. Aspirin
2. Cytoxan
3. Ferrous sulfate
4. Prednisone

14. 1. Nonsteroidal anti-inflammatory drugs (NSAIDs) such as aspirin are considered first-line therapy by some physicians. Cytoxan may be used in cases of severe synovitis, rather than as first-line therapy. Ferrous sulfate isn't used to treat rheumatoid arthritis. Prednisone may be used to control inflammation when NSAIDs aren't tolerated.

CN: Physiological integrity; CNS: Pharmacological and parenteral therapies; CL: Application

15. A client with acquired immunodeficiency syndrome is admitted with *pneumocystis carinii* pneumonia. During the admission assessment, the nurse notes a 3-cm foot ulcer on his left great toe. Which is the most critical nusing diagnosis?

1. *Impaired tissue integrity*
2. *Risk for compromised human dignity*
3. *Imbalanced nutrition: Less than body requirement*
4. *Impaired gas exchange*

15. 4. The respiratory status of the client is the priority. Although the other nursing diagnoses are appropriate, none of them is the priority.

CN: Physiological integrity; CNS: Reduction of risk potential; CL: Analysis

16. A nurse is reviewing the laboratory results of a client with anemia. In which blood component would she expect to see a reduced value?

1. Erythrocytes
2. Granulocytes
3. Leukocytes
4. Platelets

16. 1. Anemia is defined as a decreased number of erythrocytes (red blood cells). Leukopenia is a decreased number of leukocytes (white blood cells [WBCs]). Thrombocytopenia is a decreased number of platelets. Lastly, granulocytopenia is a decreased number of granulocytes (a type of WBC).

CN: Health promotion and maintenance; CNS: None; CL: Application

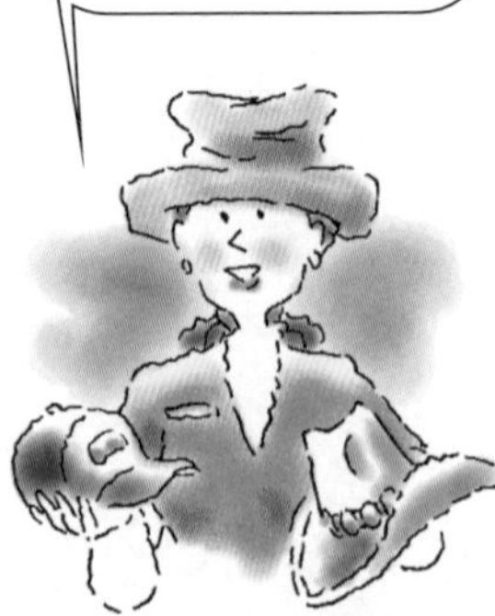

Put your thinking cap on! Remember: assessment before intervention.

17. A middle-aged client arrives at the emergency department complaining of chest and stomach pain. He also reports passing black stools for a month. Which intervention should be done <u>first</u>?

1. Give nasal oxygen.
2. Take his vital signs.
3. Begin cardiac monitoring.
4. Draw blood for laboratory analysis.

17. 2. The client's vital signs will show hemodynamic stability, and monitoring his heart rhythm may be indicated based on assessment findings. Giving nasal oxygen and drawing blood require a physician's order and shouldn't be part of a screening evaluation.

CN: Safe, effective care environment; CNS: Management of care; CL: Analysis

18. A client arrives at the emergency department with chest and stomach pain and a report of black, tarry stools for several months. Which order should the nurse anticipate?
1. Cardiac monitor, oxygen, creatine kinase, and lactate dehydrogenase (LD) levels
2. Prothrombin time (PT), partial thromboplastin time (PTT), fibrinogen, and fibrin split product values
3. ECG, complete blood count, testing for occult blood, and comprehensive serum metabolic panel
4. EEG, alkaline phosphatase and aspartate aminotransferase levels, and basic serum metabolic panel

18. 3. An ECG evaluates the complaint of chest pain, laboratory tests determine anemia, and the test for occult blood determines blood in the stool. Cardiac monitoring, oxygen, and creatine kinase and LD levels are appropriate for a cardiac primary problem. A basic metabolic panel and alkaline phosphatase and aspartate aminotransferase levels assess liver function. PT, PTT, fibrinogen and fibrin split products are measured to verify bleeding dyscrasias. An EEG evaluates brain electrical activity.
CN: Physiological integrity; CNS: Reduction of risk potential; CL: Analysis

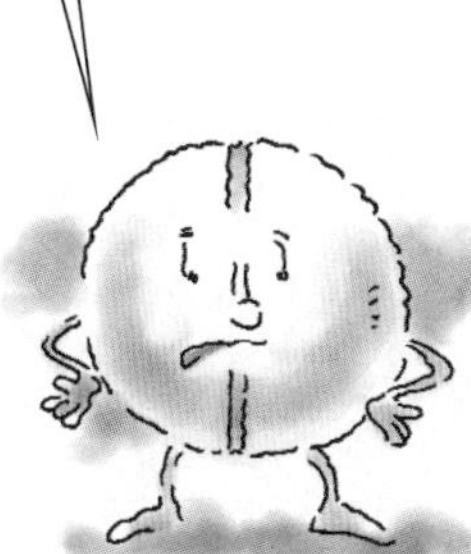

Make sure you know the action of the drug before you administer it.

19. What is the primary goal for medications prescribed to treat rheumatoid arthritis?
1. To cure the disease
2. To prevent osteoporosis
3. To control inflammation
4. To encourage bone regeneration

19. 3. The primary goal of medications in the treatment of rheumatoid arthritis is to control inflammation. There is no cure for rheumatoid arthritis. Rheumatoid arthritis causes bone erosion at the joints, not osteoporosis. Medications aren't available to replace bone lost through erosion.
CN: Physiological integrity; CNS: Pharmacological and parenteral therapies; CL: Application

20. A client with anemia may be tired due to a tissue deficiency of which substance?
1. Carbon dioxide
2. Factor VIII
3. Oxygen
4. T-cell antibodies

20. 3. Anemia stems from a decreased number of red blood cells and the resulting deficiency in oxygen in body tissues. Clotting factors, such as factor VIII, relate to the body's ability to form blood clots and aren't related to anemia, nor is carbon dioxide or T-cell antibodies.
CN: Physiological integrity; CNS: Physiological adaptation; CL: Application

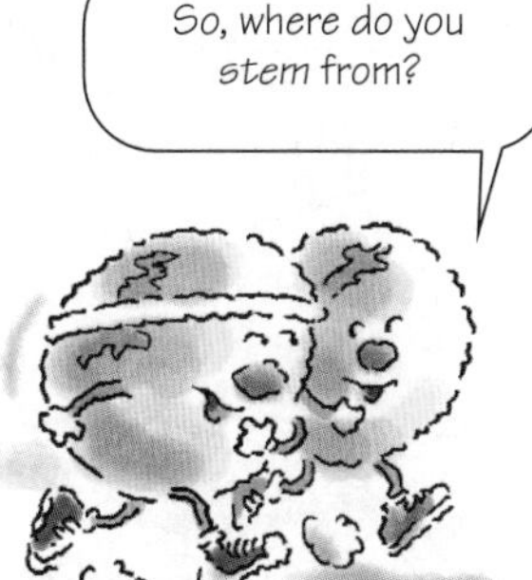

So, where do you stem from?

21. Which client has the highest risk of developing anemia?
1. A client with a colostomy following colon resection
2. A client with gastroesophageal reflux disease (GERD)
3. A client who has had a gastrectomy
4. A client with frequent bouts of dumping syndrome

21. 3. Lack of intrinsic factor following gastrectomy would cause pernicious anemia due to the client's inability to absorb Vitamin B_{12}. The presence of a colostomy, GERD, or dumping syndrome would not place a client at risk for developing anemia.
CN: Physiological integrity; CNS: Physiological adaptation; CL: Application

22. A nurse is teaching a client with microcytic anemia about choosing combinations of foods to increase non-heme iron absorbtion. She should include:
1. enriched breakfast cereal and hot tea.
2. eggs and yogurt.
3. chicken and brown rice.
4. split pea soup with ham.

22. 4. Combining a non-heme iron source (split pea soup) with a heme iron source (ham) increases absorption of non-heme iron. Tea, calcium (in yogurt), and phytates (brown rice) block iron absorption.
CN: Physiological integrity; CNS: Basic care and comfort; CL: Analysis

23. Which diagnostic test should the nurse expect to see ordered as a screening tool for rheumatoid arthritis (RA)?
1. Antinuclear antibody (ANA) titer
2. Complete blood count (CBC)
3. Erythrocyte sedimentation rate (ESR)
4. Rheumatoid factor (RF)

23. 1. ANA is commonly used as a screening tool rather than a diagnostic tool for RA because many people without RA can have elevated titers. CBC, ESR, and RF are all used as diagnostic tools and to monitor progress of the disease or response to therapy.
CN: Health promotion and maintenance; CNS: None; CL: Analysis

24. Which symptom is expected with a hemoglobin level of 10 g/dl?
1. None
2. Pallor
3. Palpitations
4. Shortness of breath

24. 1. Mild anemia usually has no clinical signs. Pallor, palpitations, and shortness of breath are associated with *severe* anemia.
CN: Physiological adaptation; CNS: Reduction of risk potential; CL: Application

25. Which factor is a common cause of anemia?
1. Lack of dietary iron
2. Vitamin C deficiency
3. Virus
4. Hereditary disorders of the red blood cells

25. 1. Anemia can commonly be caused by a lack of vitamin B_{12}, iron, and folic acid, as well as inflammation caused by some chronic diseases. Vitamin C deficiency doesn't cause anemia. Viruses and hereditary disorders are less common causes of anemia.
CN: Physiological integrity; CNS: Physiological adaptation; CL: Analysis

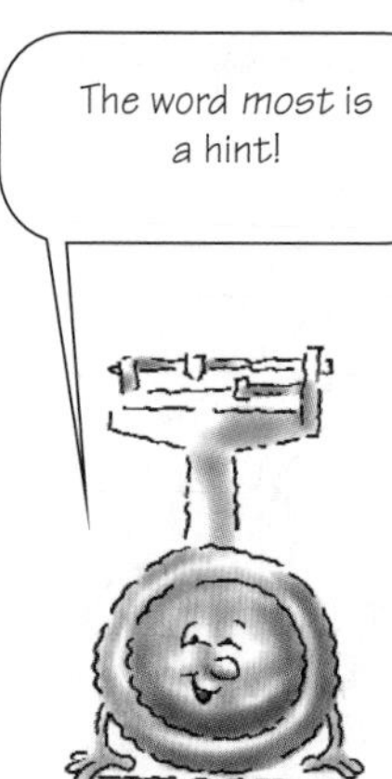

26. Which age-group is most at risk for developing anemia?
1. Younger than 24 months
2. 18 to 30 years
3. 30 to 65 years
4. 65 years and older

26. 4. Elderly people are most at risk for developing anemia, often due to financial concerns affecting protein intake or poor dentition that interferes with chewing meat.
CN: Health promotion and maintenance; CNS: None; CL: Analysis

27. A client is experiencing an anaphylactic reaction to an antibiotic infusion. Which action should the nurse take first?
1. Administer a bolus of normal saline solution.
2. Maintain a patent airway.
3. Administer epinephrine.
4. Monitor vital signs.

27. 2. The first priority is to maintain a patent airway. The client will require an epinephrine injection next. If hypotension develops, a saline bolus may be given. His vital signs should be monitored, but not as the first action.
CN: Safe, effective care environment; CNS: Management of care; CL: Analysis

28. For which condition is a client who has just had an appendectomy most at risk?
1. Anemia
2. Polycythemia
3. Purpura
4. Thrombocytopenia

28. 1. Surgery is a risk factor for anemia. Polycythemia can occur from severe hypoxia due to congenital heart and pulmonary disease. Purpura and thrombocytopenia may result from decreased bone marrow production of platelets and doesn't result from surgery.
CN: Physiological integrity; CNS: Reduction of risk potential; CL: Analysis

29. The nurse is reviewing a 52-year-old client's laboratory values. The platelet count is 75,000/µl. This value indicates which of the following conditions?

1. Normal platelet count
2. Thrombocytopenia
3. Thrombocytopathy
4. Thrombocytosis

29. 2. Thrombocytopenia is a decreased number of platelets. In adults, this would be less than 100,000/µl. Normal platelet count ranges from 140,000/µl to 400,000/µl. Thrombocytopathy is platelet dysfunction, and thrombocytosis is an excess number of platelets.

CN: Physiological integrity; CNS: Reduction of risk potential; CL: Application

30. Which symptoms are classic for thrombocytopenia?

1. Weakness and fatigue
2. Dizziness and vomiting
3. Bruising and petechiae
4. Light-headedness and nausea

30. 3. Platelets are necessary for clot formation, so petechiae and bruising are classic signs of a decreased number of platelets. Weakness and fatigue are signs of anemia. Light-headedness, nausea, dizziness, and vomiting are *not* classic signs of thrombocytopenia.

CN: Physiological integrity; CNS: Physiological adaptation; CL: Analysis

31. The nurse is planning care for a 67-year-old client who recently had abdominal aortic aneurysm repair surgery. The client has developed disseminated intravascular coagulation (DIC). Which is the most critical nursing diagnosis for this client?

1. *Ineffective breathing pattern*
2. *Risk for aspiration*
3. *Risk for infection*
4. *Risk for ineffective cerebral tissue perfusion*

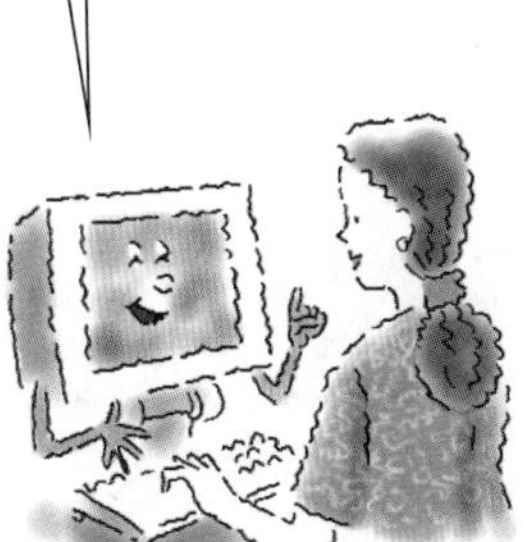

Pay close attention to the word *most critical* before choosing an answer.

31. 4. DIC affects cerebral, cardiopulmonary, and peripheral tissues with clotting that obstructs tissue perfusion. This can result in damage to these tissues. Although risk for infection is a problem for this client following surgery, it is not the most critical diagnosis. Ineffective breathing pattern and risk for aspiration would not be problems initially.

CL: Physiological integrity; CNS: Reduction of risk potential; CL: Analysis

32. A client had coronary artery bypass graft (CABG) surgery 3 days ago. Which condition is suspected when a decrease in platelet count from 230,000 µl to 5,000 µl is noted?

1. Pancytopenia
2. Idiopathic thrombocytopenic purpura (ITP)
3. Disseminated intravascular coagulation (DIC)
4. Heparin-associated thrombosis and thrombocytopenia (HATT)

32. 4. HATT may occur after CABG surgery due to heparin use during surgery. Pancytopenia is a reduction in all blood cells. Although ITP and DIC cause platelet aggregation and bleeding, neither is common in a client after revascularization surgery.

CN: Physiological integrity; CNS: Physiological adaptation; CL: Application

33. Which explanation about the action of heparin should the nurse provide to a client who has just started being administered this drug?

1. It slows the time it takes for the blood to clot.
2. It stops the blood from clotting.
3. It thins the blood.
4. It dissolves clots in the arteries of the heart.

33. 1. Heparin prolongs the time needed for blood to clot; however, it doesn't thin the blood. If given in large doses, heparin may stop the blood from clotting; however, this isn't why heparin is usually given. Heparin doesn't dissolve clots.

CN: Physiological integrity; CNS: Pharmacological and parenteral therapies; CL: Application

34. A pregnant client arrives at the emergency department with abruptio placentae at 34 weeks' gestation. She is at risk for which blood dyscrasia?

1. Thrombocytopenia
2. Idiopathic thrombocytopenic purpura (ITP)
3. Disseminated intravascular coagulation (DIC)
4. Heparin-associated thrombosis and thrombocytopenia (HATT)

34. 3. Abruptio placentae is a cause of DIC because of activation of the clotting cascade after hemorrhage. Thrombocytopenia results from decreased bone marrow production. ITP can result in DIC but isn't associated with abruptio placentae. A client with abruptio placentae wouldn't receive heparin and, as a result, wouldn't be at risk for HATT.
CN: Physiological integrity; CNS: Reduction of risk potential; CL: Application

35. While assessing a client with disseminated intravascular coagulation (DIC), the nurse suspects the client has developed internal bleeding. Which of the following symptoms would indicate this condition?

1. Hypertension
2. Petechiae
3. Increasing abdominal girth
4. Bradycardia

35. 3. As blood collects in the peritoneal cavity, dilation and distention of the abdomen occur. This is reflected by an increase in abdominal girth. The client with DIC would have hypotension and tachycardia. Petechiae are a result of the leaking of blood from tiny blood vessels into the skin.
CN: Physiological integrity; CNS: Physiological adaptation; CL: Analysis

36. A 36-year-old client complains of fatigue, weight loss, and a low-grade fever. He also has pain in his fingers, elbows, and ankles. Which condition is suspected?

1. Anemia
2. Leukemia
3. Rheumatic arthritis
4. Systemic lupus erythematosus (SLE)

36. 3. Fatigue, weight loss, and a low-grade fever are all early signs of many immune system diseases, including anemia, leukemia, and SLE. However, only rheumatic arthritis is associated with pain in the fingers, elbows, wrists, ankles, and knees.
CN: Physiological integrity; CNS: Physiological adaptation; CL: Application

37. Which laboratory test, besides a platelet count, <u>best</u> confirms the diagnosis of essential thrombocytopenia?

1. Bleeding time
2. White blood cell (WBC) count
3. Immunoglobulin (Ig) G level
4. Prothrombin time (PT) and International Normalized Ratio (INR)

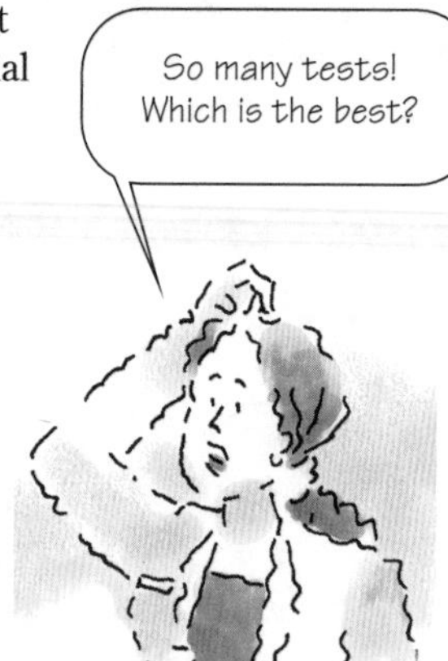
So many tests!
Which is the best?

37. 1. After a platelet count, the best test to determine thrombocytopenia is a bleeding time. The platelet count is decreased and bleeding time is prolonged. IgG assays are nonspecific but may help determine the diagnosis. A WBC count shows WBC values, and the PT and INR evaluate the effect of warfarin therapy.
CN: Physiological integrity; CNS: Reduction of risk potential; CL: Application

38. Which drug would be ordered to improve the platelet count in a client with idiopathic thrombocytopenic purpura?

1. Acetylsalicylic acid (ASA)
2. Corticosteroids
3. Methotrexate
4. Vitamin K

38. 2. Corticosteroid therapy can decrease antibody production and phagocytosis of the antibody-coated platelets, retaining more functioning platelets. ASA decreases platelet aggregation. Methotrexate can cause thrombocytopenia. Vitamin K is used to treat an excessive anticoagulable state from warfarin overload.
CN: Physiological integrity; CNS: Pharmacological and parenteral therapies; CL: Application

39. Which statement by a client with sickle cell disease indicates further teaching is needed to reinforce the therapeutic regimen?

1. "I should avoid vacationing or traveling in areas of high altitude."
2. "Cigarette smoking can cause a sickle cell crisis."
3. "I should drink 4 to 6 liters of fluid each day."
4. "I should take one baby aspirin daily to help prevent sickle cell crisis."

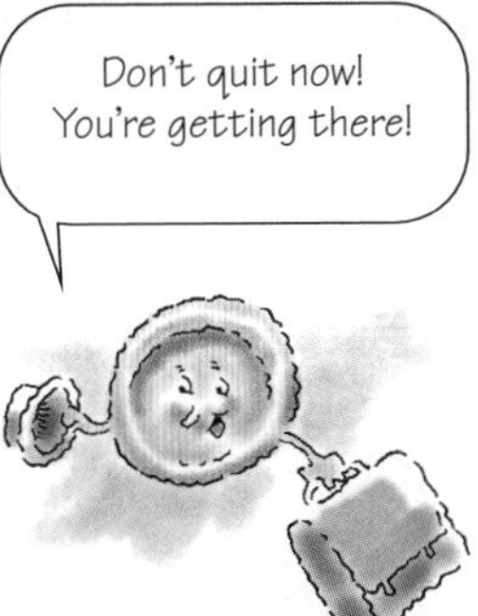
Don't quit now!
You're getting there!

39. 4. Aspirin inhibits platelet aggregation and won't help prevent sickle cell crisis. Hydroxyurea is prescribed for some people to help prevent sickle cell crisis. High altitude increases oxygen demand and therefore can also precipitate a crisis. Tobacco, alcohol, and dehydration can precipitate a sickle cell crisis and should be avoided.
CN: Health promotion and maintenance; CNS: None; CL: Analysis

40. A nurse is preparing to teach a client about the immune system. Which statement best explains the function of the thymus gland?

1. The thymus gland is a reservoir for blood cells.
2. The thymus gland stores blood cells until they mature.
3. The thymus gland protects the body against ingested pathogens.
4. The thymus gland removes bacteria and toxins from the circulatory system.

40. 2. Bone marrow produces immature blood cells (stem cells). Those that become lymphocytes migrate to the bone marrow for maturation (to B lymphocytes) or to the thymus for maturation (to T lymphocytes). These lymphocytes are responsible for cell-mediated immunity. The spleen is a reservoir for blood cells. The tonsils shield against airborne and ingested pathogens, and the lymph nodes remove bacteria and toxins from the bloodstream.
CN: Physiological integrity; CNS: Physiological adaptation; CL: Application

41. A client with thrombocytopenia, secondary to leukemia, develops epistaxis. The nurse should instruct the client to do which of the following?

1. Lie supine with his neck extended.
2. Sit upright, leaning slightly forward.
3. Blow his nose and then put lateral pressure on it.
4. Hold his nose while bending forward at the waist.

41. 2. The upright position, leaning slightly forward, avoids increasing the vascular pressure in the nose and helps the client avoid aspirating blood. Lying supine won't prevent aspiration of blood. Nose blowing can dislodge any clotting that has occurred. Bending at the waist increases vascular pressure and promotes bleeding rather than stopping it.
CN: Physiological integrity; CNS: Physiological adaptation; CL: Application

42. The nurse is teaching a client scheduled to receive a heart valve replacement with a porcine valve. Which statement by the client indicates an understanding of what type transplant they will receive?

1. Allogeneic
2. Autologous
3. Syngeneic
4. Xenogeneic

42. 4. A xenogeneic transplant is between humans and another species. An allogeneic transplant is between two humans, a syngeneic transplant is between identical twins, and autologous is a transplant from the same individual.
CN: Physiological integrity; CNS: Physiological adaptation; CL: Analysis

43. Which client is <u>most</u> at risk for developing malignant lymphoma?

1. A 22-year-old man with a history of mononucleosis
2. A 25-year-old man who smokes a pack of cigarettes a day
3. A 33-year-old man with a cousin with Hodgkin's lymphoma
4. A 40-year-old woman with a history of human immunodeficiency virus (HIV) infection

43. 1. Malignant lymphoma has a peak incidence between ages 20 and 30 and after age 50. It's more common in men than women and is associated with a history of Epstein-Barr virus (which causes mononucleosis). There is also an increased incidence of the disease among siblings. There is no reported association between malignant lymphoma and smoking or HIV infection.

CN: Health promotion and maintenance; CNS: None; CL: Application

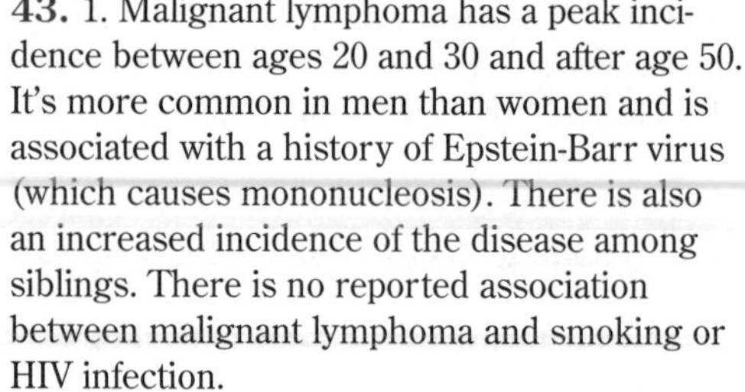

44. A nurse is teaching a client about idiopathic thrombocytopenia. What should she tell the client is the normal life span for platelets?

1. The normal life span is 1 to 3 days.
2. The normal life span is 3 to 5 days.
3. The normal life span is 7 to 10 days.
4. The normal life span is 3 to 4 months.

44. 3. The normal life span of a platelet is 7 to 10 days. However, in idiopathic thrombocytopenia, the platelet life span is reduced to 1 to 3 days.

CN: Physiological integrity; CNS: Physiological adaptation; CL: Application

45. A nurse is documenting care for a client with iron deficiency anemia. Which nursing diagnosis is <u>most appropriate</u>?

1. *Impaired gas exchange*
2. *Deficient fluid volume*
3. *Ineffective airway clearance*
4. *Ineffective breathing pattern*

45. 1. Iron is necessary for hemoglobin synthesis. Hemoglobin is responsible for oxygen transport in the body. Iron deficiency anemia causes subnormal hemoglobin levels, which impair tissue oxygenation and warrants a nursing diagnosis of impaired gas exchange. Iron deficiency anemia doesn't cause a deficient fluid volume and is less directly related to ineffective airway clearance and ineffective breathing pattern than it is to ineffective gas exchange.

CN: Physiological integrity; CNS: Physiological adaptation; CL: Analysis

46. Which statement indicates that a client with thrombocytopenia understands the function of platelets in her body?

1. "Platelets regulate acid-base balance."
2. "Platelets regulate the immune response."
3. "Platelets protect the body from infection."
4. "Platelets stop the bleeding when arteries and veins are injured."

46. 4. Platelets clump together to plug small breaks in blood vessels. They also initiate the clotting cascade by releasing thromboplastin, which (in the presence of calcium) converts prothrombin into thrombin. Platelets don't perform the other functions listed.

CN: Physiological integrity; CNS: Reduction of risk potential; CL: Application

Make sure you observe this.

47. The nurse is caring for a 43-year-old client undergoing colon cancer treatment. The client has developed thrombocytopenia. Which of the following observations can the nurse expect?

1. Diarrhea
2. Thin, brittle hair
3. Bruises on the skin
4. Urinary urgency

47. 3. With thrombocytopenia, there's an abnormal decrease in the number of blood platelets, which can result in bruises and bleeding. The client may have constipation, but usually not diarrhea. Thin, brittle hair isn't a sign of thrombocytopenia, but could be a sign of hypothyroidism. Urinary urgency could be a sign of urinary tract infection, but not thrombocytopenia.

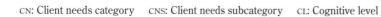

CN: Physiological integrity; CNS: Reduction of risk potential; CL: Application

48. A 16-year-old client involved in a motor vehicle collision arrives in the emergency department unconscious and severely hypotensive. He is suspected to have several fractures (pelvis and legs). Which parenteral fluid is the best choice for his current condition?

1. Fresh frozen plasma
2. Normal saline solution
3. Lactated Ringer's solution
4. Packed red blood cells (RBCs)

48. 4. In a trauma situation, the first blood product given is unmatched (O negative) packed RBCs. Fresh frozen plasma is often used to replace clotting factors. Normal saline or lactated Ringer's solution is used to increase volume and blood pressure, but too much colloid will hemodilute the blood and won't improve oxygen-carrying capacity, as RBCs would.

CN: Physiological integrity; CNS: Physiological adaptation; CL: Application

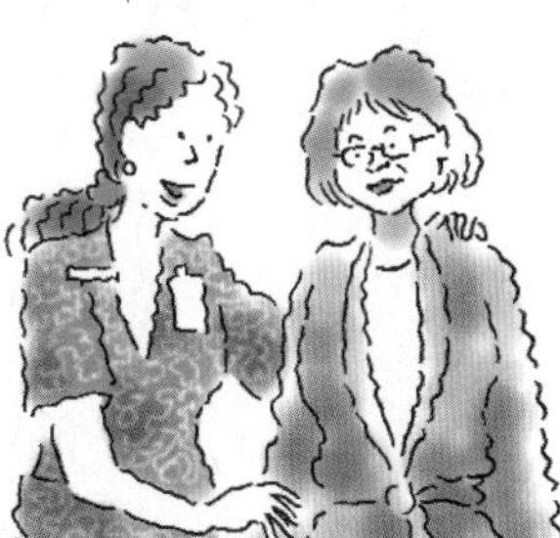
Client teaching is important.

49. Instructions for a client with systemic lupus erythematosus (SLE) would include information about which blood dyscrasia?

1. Dressler's syndrome
2. Polycythemia
3. Essential thrombocytopenia
4. von Willebrand's disease

49. 3. Essential thrombocytopenia is linked to immunologic disorders, such as SLE and human immunodeficiency virus. Dressler's syndrome is pericarditis that occurs after a myocardial infarction and isn't linked to SLE. Moderate to severe anemia is associated with SLE, not polycythemia. The disorder known as *von Willebrand's disease* is a type of hemophilia and isn't linked to SLE.

CN: Health promotion and maintenance; CNS: None; CL: Application

50. Which client is <u>most</u> at risk for systemic lupus erythematosus (SLE)?

1. A 20-year-old White man
2. A 25-year-old Black woman
3. A 45-year-old Hispanic man
4. A 65-year-old Black woman

50. 2. SLE affects women eight times more often than men and usually strikes during childbearing age. It's three times more common in Black women than in White women.

CN: Health promotion and maintenance; CNS: None; CL: Analysis

51. The nurse is teaching a client with systemic lupus erythematosus (SLE). Which response by the client indicates understanding about which tissues in the body are <u>primarily</u> attacked by SLE?

1. Connective
2. Heart
3. Lung
4. Nerve

51. 1. SLE is a chronic, inflammatory, autoimmune disorder that primarily affects connective tissue. It also affects the skin and kidneys and may affect the pulmonary, cardiac, neural, and renal systems.

CN: Physiological integrity; CNS: Physiological adaptation; CL: Application

52. Which <u>symptom</u> is most commonly an early indication of stage I Hodgkin's disease?

1. Pericarditis
2. Night sweats
3. Splenomegaly
4. Persistent hypothermia

52. 2. In stage I, symptoms include a single enlarged lymph node (usually), unexplained fever, night sweats, malaise, and generalized pruritis. Although splenomegaly may be present in some clients, night sweats are generally more prevalent. Pericarditis isn't associated with Hodgkin's disease. Moreover, splenomegaly and pericarditis aren't symptoms. Persistent hypothermia is associated with Hodgkin's but isn't an early sign of the disease.

CN: Health promotion and maintenance; CNS: None; CL: Application

53. Which statement shows that a client needs further teaching about the cause of an exacerbation of systemic lupus erythematosus (SLE)?
1. "I need to stay away from sunlight."
2. "I don't have to worry if I get a strep throat."
3. "I need to work on managing stress in my life."
4. "I don't have to worry about changing my diet."

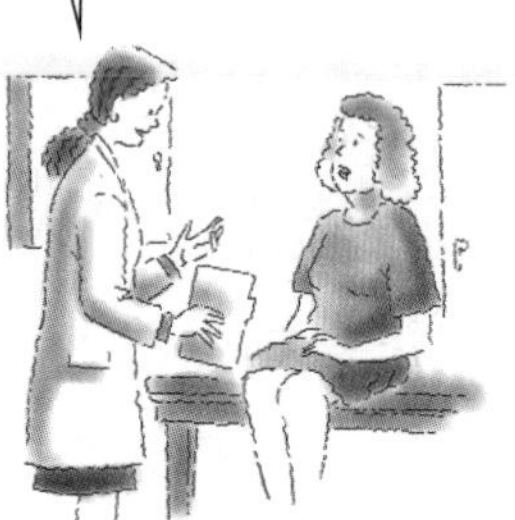
Hmm... I think some more teaching is in order.

53. 2. Infection may cause an exacerbation of SLE. Other factors that can precipitate an exacerbation are immunizations, sunlight exposure, and stress.
CN: Health promotion and maintenance; CNS: None; CL: Application

54. Which complication of systemic lupus erythematosus (SLE) is <u>most common</u> and <u>life-threatening</u>?
1. Arthritis
2. Nephritis
3. Pericarditis
4. Pleural effusion

54. 2. About 50% of the clients with SLE have some type of nephritis, and kidney failure is the most common cause of death for clients with SLE. Pericarditis is the most common cardiovascular manifestation of SLE, but it isn't usually life-threatening. Arthritis is very common (95%), as are pleural effusions (50%), but neither is life-threatening.
CN: Physiological integrity; CNS: Physiological adaptation; CL: Analysis

55. Which condition is a sign of neurologic involvement in systemic lupus erythematosus (SLE)?
1. Facial tic
2. Psychosis
3. Extremity weakness
4. Cerebrovascular accidents

55. 2. Neurologic involvement may be shown by psychosis, seizures, and headaches. Tics and cerebrovascular accidents aren't related to SLE. Weakness may be present, but it's usually related to muscle atrophy, not neurologic involvement.
CN: Physiological integrity; CNS: Physiological adaptation; CL: Application

56. A nurse is reviewing the physician's orders for a client with systemic lupus erythamatosus (SLE). Which medication does she expect to see prescribed?
1. Morphine
2. Ketoconazole
3. Hydroxychloroquine
4. Dimenhydrinate

56. 3. Treatment of SLE involves nonsteroidal anti-inflammatory drugs, antimalarial drugs such as hydroxychloroquine, corticosteroids, and immunosuppresive agents. Morphine is an opioid analgesic, ketoconazole is an antifungal agent, and dimenhydrinate is an antiemetic.
CN: Physiological integrity; CNS: Pharmacological and parenteral therapies; CL: Analysis

57. Which symptom is a <u>classic</u> sign of systemic lupus erythematosus (SLE)?
1. Vomiting
2. Weight loss
3. Difficulty urinating
4. Superficial lesions over the cheeks and nose

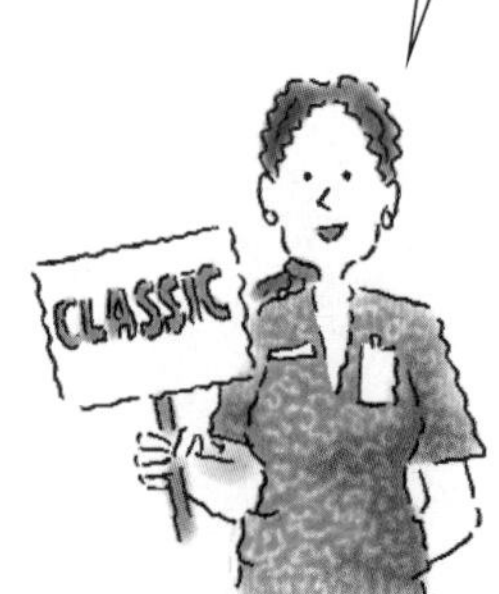
This question is a classic.
CLASSIC

57. 4. Although all of these symptoms can be signs of SLE, the classic sign is the butterfly rash over the cheeks and nose.
CN: Physiological integrity; CNS: Physiological adaptation; CL: Application

58. Which laboratory test result supports the diagnosis of systemic lupus erythematosus (SLE)?

1. Elevated serum complement level
2. Thrombocytosis, elevated sedimentation rate
3. Pancytopenia, elevated antinuclear antibody (ANA) titer
4. Leukocytosis, elevated blood urea nitrogen (BUN) and creatinine levels

58. 3. Laboratory findings for clients with SLE usually show pancytopenia, elevated ANA titer, and decreased serum complement levels. Clients may have elevated BUN and creatinine levels from nephritis, but the increase does *not* indicate SLE.

CN: Physiological integrity; CNS: Reduction of risk potential; CL: Application

59. The nurse is reviewing a client's laboratory values. Which of the following results would most likely be present in a client recently diagnosed with chronic lymphocytic leukemia?

1. Elevated sedimentation rate
2. Uncontrolled proliferation of granulocytes
3. Thrombocytopenia and increased lymphocytes
4. Elevated aspartate aminotransferase and alanine aminotransferase levels

59. 3. Chronic lymphocytic leukemia shows a proliferation of small abnormal mature B lymphocytes and decreased antibody response. Thrombocytopenia also is often present. Uncontrolled proliferation of granulocytes occurs in myelogenous leukemia. Aspartate aminotransferase, alanine aminotransferase, and erythrocyte sedimentation rate values are *not* affected.

CN: Physiological integrity; CNS: Reduction of risk potential; CL: Application

60. A nurse is assessing a client newly diagnosed with Stage I Hodgkin's lymphoma. Which area of the body would the nurse most likely find involved?

1. Back
2. Chest
3. Groin
4. Neck

60. 4. At the time of diagnosis of stage I Hodgkin's lymphoma, a painless cervical lesion is often present. The back, chest, and groin areas may be involved in later stages.

CN: Physiological integrity; CNS: Physiological adaptation; CL: Application

61. According to a standard staging classification of Hodgkin's disease, which criterion reflects stage II?

1. Involvement of extralymphatic organs or tissues
2. Involvement of a single lymph node region or structure
3. Involvement of two or more lymph node regions or structures
4. Involvement of lymph node regions or structures on both sides of the diaphragm

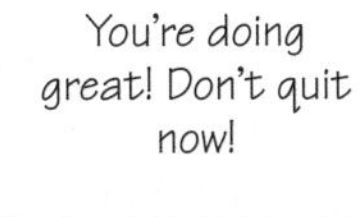
You're doing great! Don't quit now!

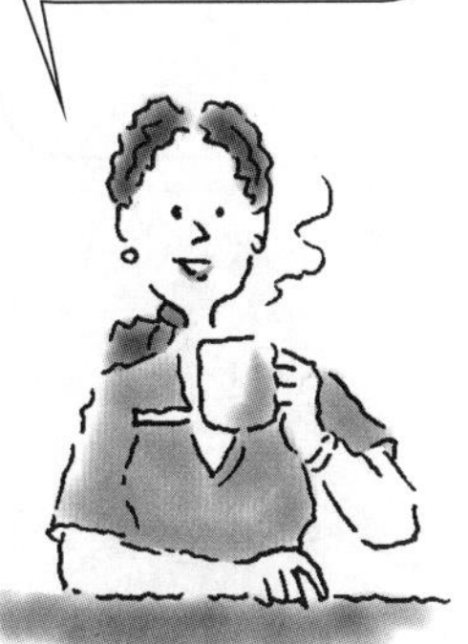

61. 3. Stage II involves two or more lymph node regions. Stage I involves only one lymph node region; stage III involves nodes on both sides of the diaphragm; and stage IV involves extralymphatic organs or tissues.

CN: Physiological integrity; CNS: Physiological adaptation; CL: Analysis

62. A client is about to start chemotherapy for acute lymphocytic leukemia. Which statement shows that he requires further teaching about this phase of chemotherapy?
1. "I'll have treatments only once a month."
2. "I'll be getting high doses of chemotherapy."
3. "I won't get sick at this stage of the treatment."
4. "The purpose of these treatments is to induce a remission."

62. 1. The initial phase of chemotherapy is called the induction phase and is designed to put the client into remission by giving high doses of the drugs; however, treatments will be closer together than once each month. Monthly treatments usually occur during the maintenance phase of chemotherapy. The other options indicate that the client understands chemotherapy.
CN: Physiological integrity; CNS: Basic care and comfort; CL: Application

63. Which statement is correct about the rate of cell growth in relation to chemotherapy?
1. Faster growing cells are less susceptible to chemotherapy.
2. Nondividing cells are more susceptible to chemotherapy.
3. Faster growing cells are more susceptible to chemotherapy.
4. Slower growing cells are more susceptible to chemotherapy.

63. 3. The faster the cell grows, the more susceptible it is to chemotherapy and radiation therapy. Slow-growing and nondividing cells are less susceptible to chemotherapy. Repeated cycles of chemotherapy are used to destroy nondividing cells as they begin active cell division.
CN: Physiological integrity; CNS: Physiological adaptation; CL: Application

64. A client receiving chemotherapy is considered at high risk for developing lysis syndrome. Which tests would the nurse expect to monitor for 48 to 72 hours after the infusion?
1. Complete blood count, prothrombin time, and partial thromboplastin time
2. Myoglobin, troponin, and creatine kinase
3. Glucose, bilirubin, and alanine aminotransferase
4. Electrolytes, blood urea nitrogen (BUN), and creatinine

64. 4. Because the client is at high risk for electrolyte imbalances and acute renal failure, electrolyte, BUN, and creatinine levels should be measured prior to treatment and for 48 to 72 hours afterward. The other tests wouldn't be indicated.
CN: Physiological integrity; CNS: Reduction of risk potential; CL: Application

65. Which treatment is most appropriate for the client with tumor lysis syndrome?
1. Give antibiotics.
2. Give I.V. hydration.
3. Give packed red blood cells (RBCs).
4. Give potassium chloride I.V.

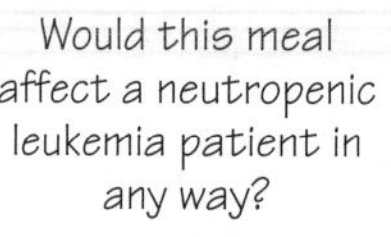

Would this meal affect a neutropenic leukemia patient in any way?

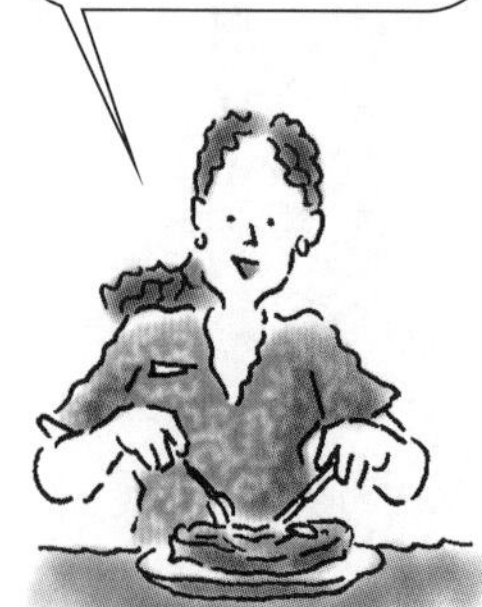

65. 2. The treatment for tumor lysis syndrome is I.V. hydration, allopurinol, and alkalizing the urine. Antibiotics are given when infection is first detected. Transfusions of RBCs aren't given until the body can produce mature cells. The potassium level is often elevated in tumor lysis syndrome, so potassium chloride wouldn't be indicated.
CN: Physiological integrity; CNS: Pharmacological and parenteral therapies; CL: Analysis

66. Which food should a neutropenic client with leukemia avoid?
1. White bread
2. Carrot sticks
3. Stewed apples
4. Medium rare steak

66. 2. A low-bacteria diet would be indicated, which excludes raw fruits and vegetables.
CN: Safe, effective care environment; CNS: Safety and infection control; CL: Application

67. A client with leukemia has neutropenia. Which function must be frequently assessed?
1. Blood pressure
2. Bowel sounds
3. Heart sounds
4. Breath sounds

67. 4. Pneumonia, both viral and fungal, is a common cause of death in clients with neutropenia, so frequent assessment of respiratory rate and breath sounds is required. Although assessing blood pressure, bowel sounds, and heart sounds is important, it won't help detect pneumonia.
CN: Physiological integrity; CNS: Physiological adaptation; CL: Application

68. When protective isolation isn't indicated, which activity is recommended for a client receiving chemotherapy?
1. Bed rest
2. Activity as tolerated
3. Walk to bathroom only
4. Out of bed for brief periods

68. 2. It's important that the client be able to engage in activities that are of interest and to maintain as much independence and autonomy as possible. Bed rest isn't necessary, nor is it necessary to limit the client's activity to only walks to the bathroom or out of bed for brief periods.
CN: Health promotion and maintenance; CNS: None; CL: Application

69. Which client is most at risk for developing multiple myeloma?
1. A 20-year-old Asian woman
2. A 30-year-old White man
3. A 50-year-old Hispanic woman
4. A 60-year-old Black man

69. 4. Multiple myeloma is more common in middle-aged and older clients (the median age at diagnosis is 60 years) and is twice as common in Blacks as Whites. It occurs most often in Black men.
CN: Health promotion and maintenance; CNS: None; CL: Analysis

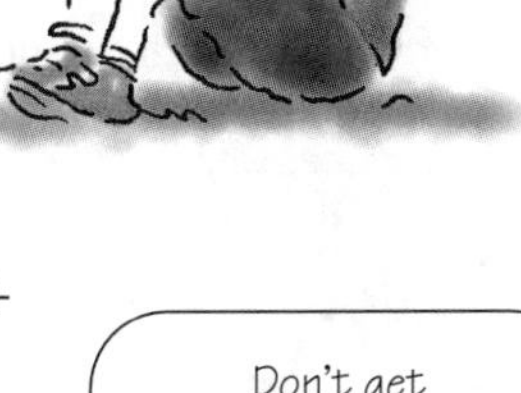

Forget the weights. Keep an eye on those "abs."

70. Which substance has abnormal values early in the course of multiple myeloma?
1. Immunoglobulins
2. Platelets
3. Red blood cells (RBCs)
4. White blood cells (WBCs)

70. 1. Multiple myeloma is characterized by malignant plasma cells that produce an increased amount of immunoglobulin that isn't functional. As more malignant plasma cells are produced, there's less space in the bone marrow for RBC production. In late stages, platelets and WBCs are reduced as the bone marrow is infiltrated by malignant plasma cells.
CN: Health promotion and maintenance; CNS: None; CL: Analysis

71. For which condition is a client with multiple myeloma monitored?
1. Hypercalcemia
2. Hyperkalemia
3. Hypernatremia
4. Hypermagnesemia

71. 1. Calcium is released when bone is destroyed. This causes an increase in serum calcium levels. Multiple myeloma doesn't affect potassium, sodium, or magnesium levels.
CN: Physiological integrity; CNS: Physiological adaptation; CL: Application

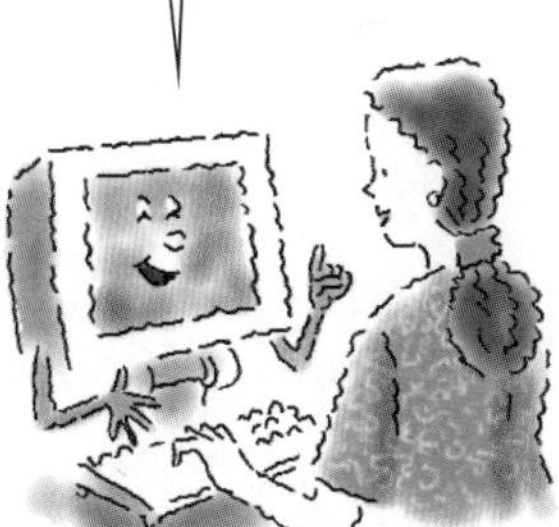

Don't get confused by this prefix! (Tee-hee!)

72. Which symptom commonly occurs with hypercalcemia?
1. Tremors
2. Headache
3. Confusion
4. Muscle weakness

72. 3. Signs of hypercalcemia include confusion, anorexia, nausea, vomiting, abdominal pain, ileus, constipation, and eventually impaired renal function. Tremors, headache, and muscle weakness aren't common symptoms of hypercalcemia.
CN: Physiological integrity; CNS: Physiological adaptation; CL: Application

73. A client with multiple myeloma has developed hypercalcemia. The nurse should monitor the client for which complication secondary to hypercalcemia?

1. Pneumonia
2. Muscle spasms
3. Renal dysfunction
4. Myocardial irritability

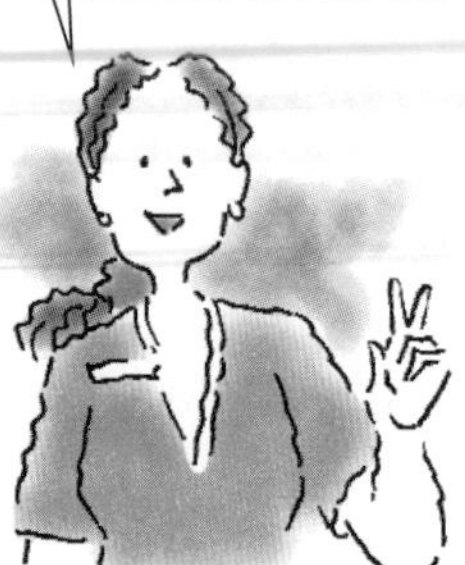
Wait a second!
Here's a hint for you!

73. 3. Twenty percent of multiple myeloma clients with hypercalcemia and hyperuricemia develop renal insufficiency. Pneumonia doesn't result from hypercalcemia. Hypocalcemia causes muscle spasms and hypokalemia causes myocardial irritability.
CN: Physiological integrity; CNS: Physiological adaptation; CL: Application

74. The neurologic complications of multiple myeloma usually involve which body system?

1. Brain
2. Spinal column
3. Autonomic nervous system
4. Parasympathetic nervous system

74. 2. Back pain or paresthesia in the lower extremities may indicate impending spinal cord compression from a spinal tumor. This should be recognized and treated promptly as progression of the tumor may result in paraplegia. The other options, which reflect parts of the nervous system, aren't usually affected by multiple myeloma.
CN: Physiological integrity; CNS: Physiological adaptation; CL: Application

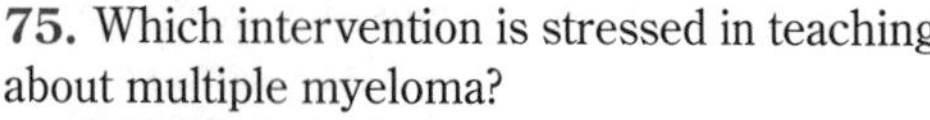

75. Which intervention is stressed in teaching about multiple myeloma?

1. Maintain bed rest.
2. Enforce fluid restriction.
3. Drink 3 qt (3 L) of fluid daily.
4. Keep the lower extremities elevated.

75. 3. The client needs to drink 3 to 5 qt (3 to 5 L) of fluid each day to dilute calcium and uric acid to try to reduce the risk of renal dysfunction. Walking is encouraged to prevent further bone demineralization. The lower extremities don't need to be elevated.
CN: Physiological integrity; CNS: Basic care and comfort; CL: Application

76. Although a client's physiologic response to a health crisis is important to the health outcome, which nursing intervention also must be addressed?

1. Teach the family how to care for the client.
2. Help the client effectively cope with the crisis.
3. Maintain I.V. access, medications, and diet.
4. Teach the client basic information about the illness.

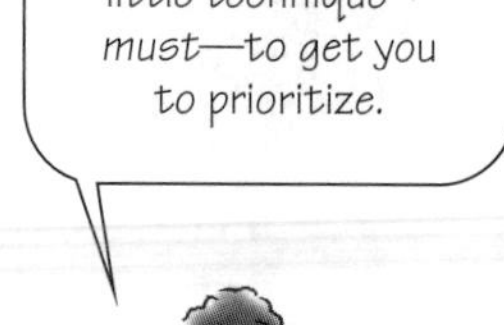
Here's a question that uses a clever little technique—must—to get you to prioritize.

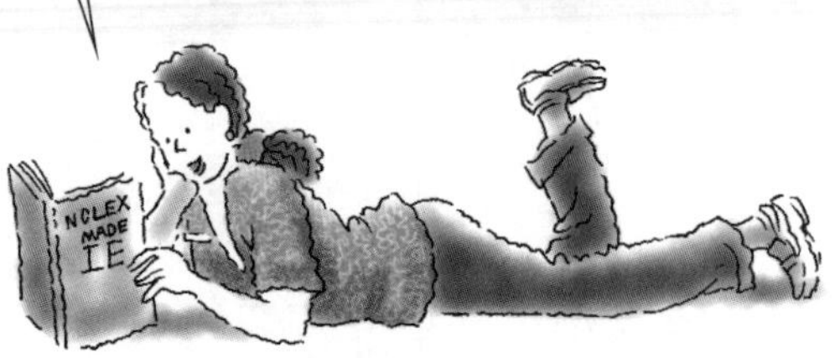

76. 2. Although all of the answers are important in the care of the client, if the individual isn't able to cope with the emotional, spiritual, and psychological aspects of his crisis, the other components of care may be ineffective as well.
CN: Psychosocial integrity; CNS: None; CL: Application

CN: Client needs category CNS: Client needs subcategory CL: Cognitive level

77. To promote healing of a laceration, which intervention is correct?

1. Elevate the body part.
2. Monitor blood pressure.
3. Apply a pressure dressing and heat.
4. Apply a pressure dressing and ice pack.

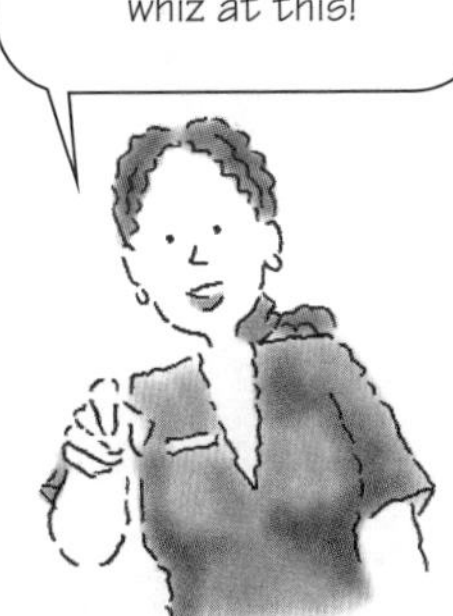

Only 29 more questions! You're a whiz at this!

77. 4. Pressure dressings help clotting by promoting the localization of microorganisms and the development of meshwork for repair and healing. Ice decreases blood flow to the site, slowing the bleeding. Elevating the body part helps reduce edema but doesn't directly promote healing. Monitoring blood pressure is important when the individual is bleeding but does nothing to promote clotting. Heat increases blood flow to the site, increasing the bleeding.

CN: Physiological integrity; CNS: Physiological adaptation; CL: Application

78. An elderly client has a wound that isn't healing normally. Interventions should be based on which principle or test results?

1. Laboratory test results
2. Kidney function test results
3. Poor wound healing expected as part of the aging process
4. Diminished immune function interfering with ability to fight infection

78. 4. Immune function is important in the healing process and diminished response may slow or prevent the healing process from taking place. Laboratory results and kidney function are important but are *not* solely responsible for health outcomes. Although immune function declines with age, there are healthy behaviors that will enhance the elderly individual's response to tissue trauma (nutrition, exercise).

CN: Physiological integrity; CNS: Physiological adaptation; CL: Analysis

79. Which response to an antigen is an appropriate therapeutic immune system response?

1. Widespread histamine release
2. Autoimmune response
3. Inflammation and increased body temperature
4. Antibody production by T cells

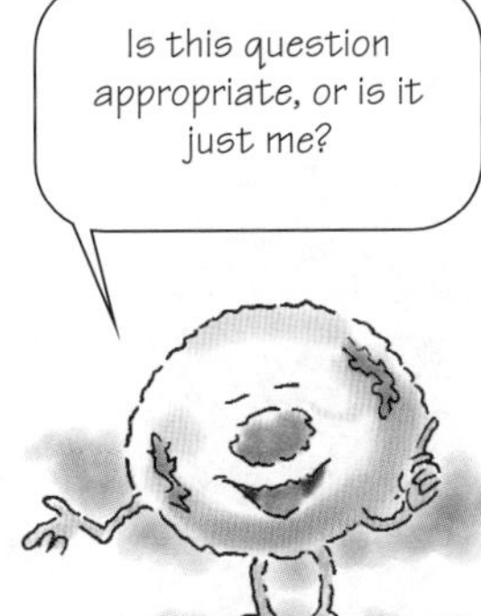

Is this question appropriate, or is it just me?

79. 3. Inflammation and increased body temperature are normal immune responses to detected antigens. Allergies are heightened responses to antigens. Widespread histamine release is an exaggerated response that can lead to anaphylaxis. Autoimmune response is one in which the immune system forms antibodies against the body's own tissues, resulting in disease. Antibodies are produced by B cells, not T cells.

CN: Physiological integrity; CNS: Reduction of risk potential; CL: Analysis

80. Which intervention has the most impact in delaying the development of acquired immunodeficiency syndrome (AIDS) once a client has been infected with human immunodeficiency virus (HIV)?

1. Monthly plasmapheresis
2. Eating a balanced, nutritious diet
3. Compliance with complete therapeutic regimen
4. Getting adequate rest and sleep

80. 3. Compliance with the complete therapeutic regimen includes adhering to a healthy lifestyle, taking prescribed medications, and reducing risks from other infections and is the most important intervention in delaying the onset of AIDS. Eating a balanced diet and getting adequate rest and sleep are part of the overall therapeutic regimen. Plasmapheresis isn't a treatment for HIV/AIDS.

CN: Health promotion and maintenance; CNS: None; CL: Analysis

81. Which condition or factor may cause an acquired immune deficiency?

1. Age
2. Genetics
3. Environment
4. Medical treatments

81. 4. Immune deficiencies may result from medical treatments, such as medications, radiation, or transplants. Immune function may decline with age, but it isn't considered the cause of acquired immune deficiency. Genetics and environment haven't been shown to be factors in acquired immune deficiency.
CN: Physiological integrity; CNS: Physiological adaptation; CL: Analysis

82. The nurse is teaching a client about stress management. Which of the following statements best explains the reason for using stress management?

1. Everyone is stressed.
2. It has become an accepted practice.
3. Eastern health practices have shown its effectiveness.
4. Prolonged psychological stress may contribute to the development of physical illness.

82. 4. Psychological and emotional stress stimulate the central nervous system, increasing the levels of corticotropin and cortisol, which results in harmful effects on immune, cardiac, neural, and endocrine function. Many people report high levels of stress, but not everyone would claim to be stressed. Although stress management may be a common therapy for stressed individuals, and Eastern countries may promote its use, nursing interventions must have research-based rationales.
CN: Psychosocial integrity; CNS: None; CL: Application

83. During discharge teaching for corticosteroids, the client asks the nurse what the drugs suppress. Which of the following responses by the nurse would be the most accurate?

1. Sympathetic response
2. Pain receptors
3. Immune response
4. Neural transmission

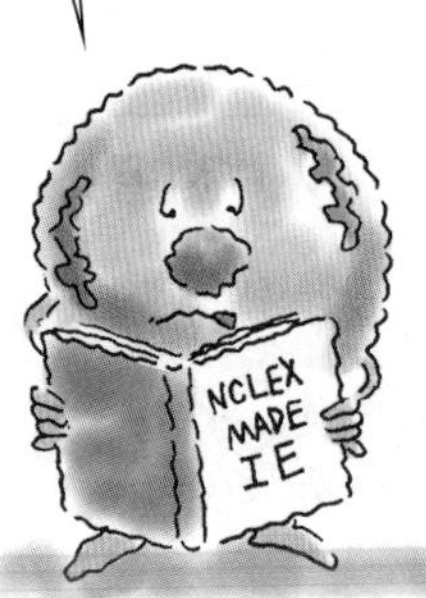
Don't suppress your response here.
NCLEX MADE IE

83. 3. Corticosteroids suppress eosinophils, lymphocytes, natural-killer cells, and other microorganisms, inhibiting the natural inflammatory process in an infected or injured part of the body. This promotes resolution of inflammation, stabilizes lysosomal membranes, decreases capillary permeability, and depresses phagocytosis of tissues by white blood cells, thus blocking the release of more inflammatory materials. Corticosteroids don't affect the sympathetic response, pain receptors, or neural transmission.
CN: Physiological integrity; CNS: Pharmacological and parenteral therapies; CL: Application

84. Which statement made by a client indicates that he understands the results of a negative human immunodeficiency virus (HIV) antibody test?

1. "I'm not infected with HIV."
2. "I haven't produced antibodies to HIV."
3. "I'm immune to HIV."
4. "I have antibodies to HIV."

84. 2. A negative HIV antibody test means that HIV antibodies weren't in the client's blood at the time the test was performed. Antibodies may take 3 weeks to 6 months or longer to develop. A negative test result doesn't indicate immunity. If antibodies to HIV are present, the test result is positive.
CN: Physiological integrity; CNS: Reduction of risk potential; CL: Application

85. In community health and epidemiologic studies, which definition of disease prevalence is correct?

1. The number of individuals affected by a particular disease at a specific time
2. The rate at which individuals without a specific disease develop that disease
3. The proportion of individuals affected by the disease who live for a particular period of time
4. The proportion of individuals without the disease who eventually develop the disease within a specific period of time

85. 1. Prevalence is the number of individuals affected by the disease at a specific time. Incidence rate is the rapidity with which individuals without the disease contract it. Survival is the proportion of individuals affected by the disease who live for a particular length of time. Risk is the proportion of individuals without the disease who develop the disease within a particular time period.
CN: Health promotion and maintenance; CNS: None; CL: Analysis

86. A 73-year-old client is about to receive a blood transfusion to treat severe anemia. She asks the nurse how long the procedure will take. Which of the following statements by the nurse is the most correct?

1. 8 hours
2. At least 12 hours
3. At least 24 hours
4. No longer than 4 hours

86. 4. The American Association of Blood Banks recommends that blood or blood components should be transfused within 4 hours. If they aren't, they should be divided and stored appropriately in the blood bank. Any length of time over 4 hours would compromise the integrity of the transfusion components.
CN: Safe, effective care environment; CNS: Safety and infection control; CL: Application

87. Which additional physician order should a nurse anticipate for a client who has been prescribed corticosteroids?

1. Perform blood glucose checks every 6 hours.
2. Restrict fluids to 1000 ml in 24 hours.
3. Administer lactulose 40 g in 4 oz. of water daily
4. Obtain serum platelet counts with hemoglobin and hematocrit levels every 12 hours.

87. 1. Corticosteroids cause elevated blood glucose levels; insulin may be necessary to maintain normal blood glucose levels. Corticosteroids can cause edema but fluid restrictions are generally unnecessary unless the client also has renal or cardiac disease. Lactulose is given for constipation and to treat hepatic encephalopathy. Hematologic studies, such as platelet counts, hemoglobin, and hematocrit levels, aren't usually necessary when monitoring clients undergoing corticosteroid therapy.
CN: Physiological integrity; CNS: Pharmacological therapies; CL: Application

88. A 32-year-old client is admitted with a tentative diagnosis of acquired immunodeficiency syndrome (AIDS). The preliminary report of biopsies done on his facial lesions indicates Kaposi's sarcoma. Which approach would be most appropriate?

1. Tell the client that Kaposi's sarcoma is common in people with AIDS.
2. Pretend not to notice the lesions on the client's face.
3. Inform the client of the biopsy results and support him emotionally.
4. Explore the client's feelings about his facial disfigurement.

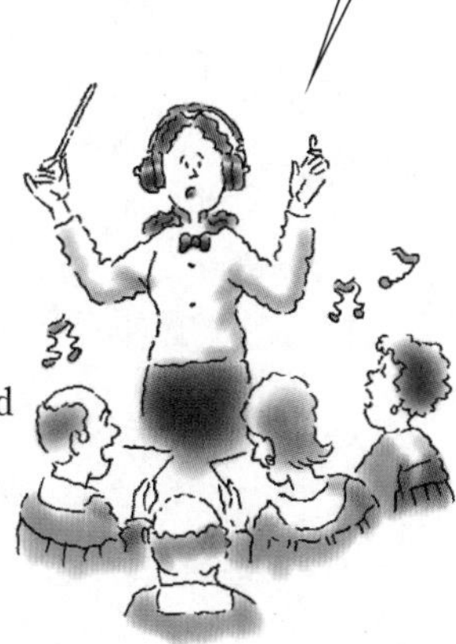
"Note" the words most appropriate in question 88. They're a key to the right answer.

88. 4. Facial lesions can contribute to decreased self-esteem and an altered body image. Discussing AIDS with a client whose diagnosis isn't final may be inappropriate and doesn't provide emotional support. Pretending not to notice visible lesions ignores the client's concerns. The physician—not the nurse—should inform the client of the biopsy results.
CN: Psychosocial integrity; CNS: None; CL: Application

89. During the recovery phase of a surgical client's hospitalization, a nurse notes that the client's immune status appears to be altered. Although there's no obvious rationale for the immunocompromise, which area should be further investigated?

1. Nutrition
2. Acquired immune disorder
3. Family history of immune problems
4. Personal history of substance abuse or use

89. 4. Substance abuse, including alcohol consumption and tobacco or marijuana use, influences immunocompetence and overall health status. Although nutrition is important for immunocompetence, it would be part of the client's daily assessment. A family history would have been assessed initially. Assessing the client for an acquired immune disorder would be a joint effort with the physician and wouldn't be conducted independently.

CN: Health promotion and maintenance; CNS: None; CL: Application

90. For a client with acquired immunodeficiency syndrome (AIDS), the nurse should follow standard precautions and take which action to protect herself when performing mouth care on the client?

1. Use reverse isolation.
2. Place the client in a private room.
3. Put on a mask, gloves, and a gown.
4. Wear gloves.

90. 4. Standard precautions stipulate that a health care worker who anticipates coming into contact with a client's blood or body fluids must wear gloves. Reverse isolation is used to protect the client from the health care worker, not the other way around. A private room doesn't provide barrier protection, an essential step in standard precautions. A mask and gloves are needed only for anticipated contact with airborne droplets of blood or body fluids; a gown is needed only for anticipated contact with splashes of blood or body fluids. Neither is the case when performing oral hygiene.

CN: Safe, effective care environment; CNS: Safety and infection control; CL: Application

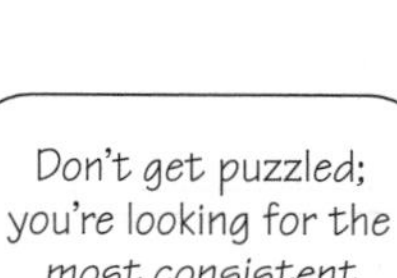

Don't get puzzled; you're looking for the most consistent answer.

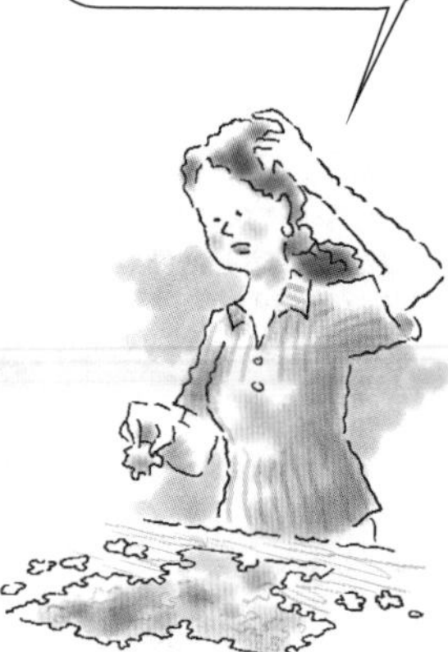

91. The nurse is reviewing a client's laboratory values. Which of the following is most consistent with a diagnosis of aplastic anemia?

1. Decreased production of T-helper cells
2. Decreased levels of white blood cells (WBCs), red blood cells (RBCs), and platelets
3. Increased levels of WBCs, RBCs, and platelets
4. Reed-Sternberg cells and lymph node enlargement

91. 2. In aplastic anemia, the diagnostic findings are decreased levels of all the cellular elements of the blood (pancytopenia). T-helper cell production doesn't decrease in aplastic anemia. Reed-Sternberg cells and lymph node enlargement occur with Hodgkin's disease.

CN: Physiological integrity; CNS: Physiological adaptation; CL: Analysis

92. A client with iron deficiency anemia is scheduled for discharge. Which instruction about prescribed ferrous gluconate therapy should the nurse include in the teaching plan?

1. "Take the medication with an antacid."
2. "Take the medication with a glass of milk."
3. "Take the medication with whole-grain cereal."
4. "Take the medication on an empty stomach."

92. 4. Preferably, ferrous gluconate should be taken on an empty stomach. Ferrous gluconate shouldn't be taken with antacids, milk, or whole-grain cereals because these foods reduce iron absorption.

CN: Physiological integrity; CNS: Pharmacological and parenteral therapies; CL: Application

93. The nurse is assessing a client with ankylosing spondylitis. Which of the following initial symptoms would the nurse most likely assess in this client?

1. Red, painful, swollen joints
2. Fatigue and night sweats
3. Low back pain
4. Neck pain and stiffness

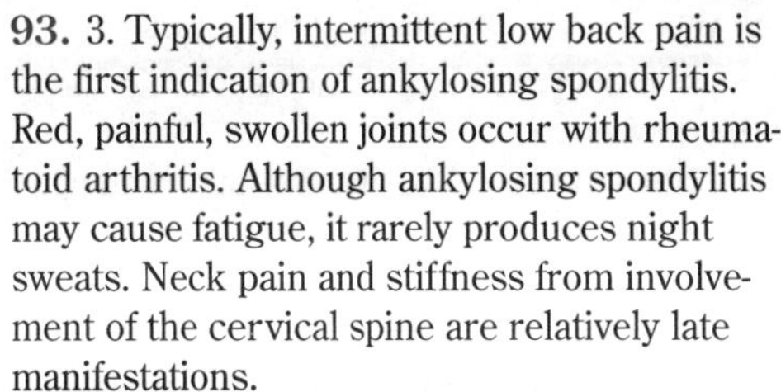

93. 3. Typically, intermittent low back pain is the first indication of ankylosing spondylitis. Red, painful, swollen joints occur with rheumatoid arthritis. Although ankylosing spondylitis may cause fatigue, it rarely produces night sweats. Neck pain and stiffness from involvement of the cervical spine are relatively late manifestations.

CN: Physiological integrity; CNS: Physiological adaptation; CL: Analysis

94. A female client with the beta-thalassemia trait plans to marry a man of Italian ancestry who also has the trait. Which client statement would indicate that she understands the teaching provided by the nurse?

1. "Thalassemia is treated with iron supplements."
2. "I need to learn how to give myself vitamin B_{12} injections."
3. "I'll see a genetic counselor before starting a family."
4. "If my fiancé were of Middle Eastern descent, I wouldn't be worried about having children."

94. 3. Two people with the beta-thalassemia trait have a 25% chance of having a child with thalassemia major, a potentially life-threatening disease. Iron supplements aren't used to treat thalassemia; in fact, they could contribute to iron overload. Vitamin B_{12} injections are used to treat pernicious anemia, not thalassemia. Thalassemia occurs primarily in people of Italian, Greek, African, Asian, Middle Eastern, East Indian, and Caribbean descent.

CN: Health promotion and maintenance; CNS: None; CL: Application

95. A young, African-American, female client with a history of sickle cell disease is complaining of severe abdominal pain. Which nursing intervention is the most important for this client?

1. Obtaining a history of the sequence of symptoms
2. Keeping the client nothing by mouth (NPO)
3. Administering I.V. fluids
4. Preparing the client for a computed tomography (CT) scan of the abdomen

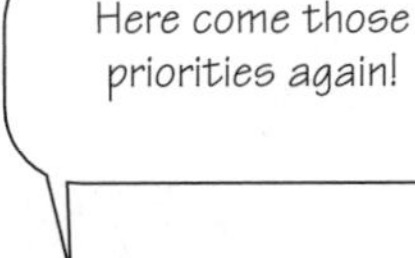
Here come those priorities again!

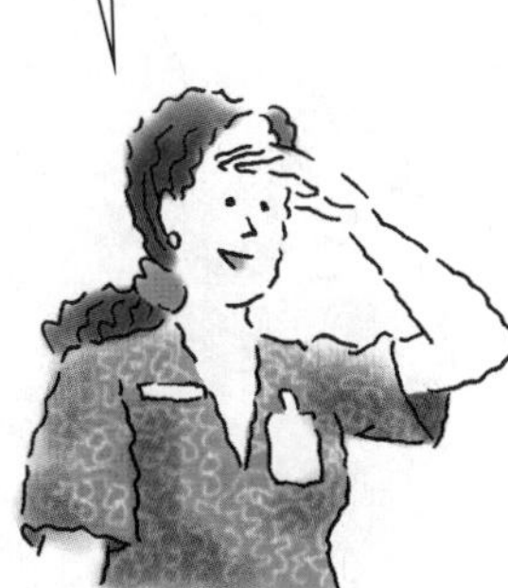

95. 1. Although the client may be in a sickle cell crisis and experiencing acute abdominal pain caused by sickling in the mesenteric circulation, it's important to remember that clients with sickle cell disease aren't spared from appendicitis or other intra-abdominal events. The history obtained from the client outlining the sequence of symptoms provides the most important assessment information. Other nursing interventions would include preparing the client for possible surgery by keeping her NPO and for diagnostic studies such as CT scanning. Administering I.V. fluids will help replenish fluid volume.

CN: Physiological integrity; CNS: Reduction of risk potential; CL: Application

96. Which precautions should the nurse include in the care plan for a neutropenic client with lymphoma?

1. Have the client use a soft toothbrush and electric razor, avoid using enemas, and watch for signs of bleeding.
2. Put on a mask, gown, and gloves when entering the client's room.
3. Provide a clear liquid, low-sodium diet.
4. Eliminate fresh fruits and vegetables, avoid using enemas, and practice frequent hand washing.

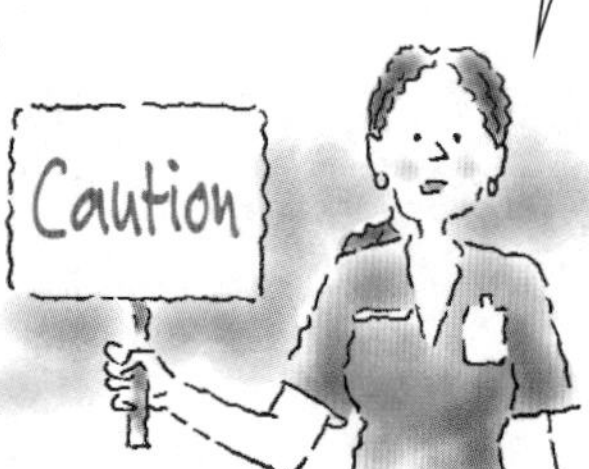

96. 4. Neutropenia occurs when the absolute neutrophil count falls below 1,000/mm^3, reflecting a severe risk for infection. The nurse should provide a low-bacterial diet, which means eliminating fresh fruits and vegetables; avoid invasive procedures, such as enemas, because they increase the infection risk; and practice frequent hand washing to lower the infection risk. Using a soft toothbrush, avoiding straight-edged razors and enemas, and monitoring for bleeding are thrombocytopenia precautions. Putting on a mask, gown, and gloves when entering the client's room are reverse isolation measures. A neutropenic patient doesn't need a clear liquid diet or sodium restrictions.

CN: Safe, effective care environment; CNS: Safety and infection control; CL: Application

97. The nurse is reviewing a client's laboratory values and notes a deficiency of factor VIII. Which of the following conditions is most consistent with this result?

1. Sickle cell disease
2. Christmas disease
3. Hemophilia A
4. Hemophilia B

97. 3. Hemophilia A results from a deficiency of factor VIII. Sickle cell disease is caused by a defective hemoglobin molecule. Christmas disease, also called *hemophilia B,* results from a factor IX deficiency.

CN: Physiological integrity; CNS: Physiological adaptation; CL: Analysis

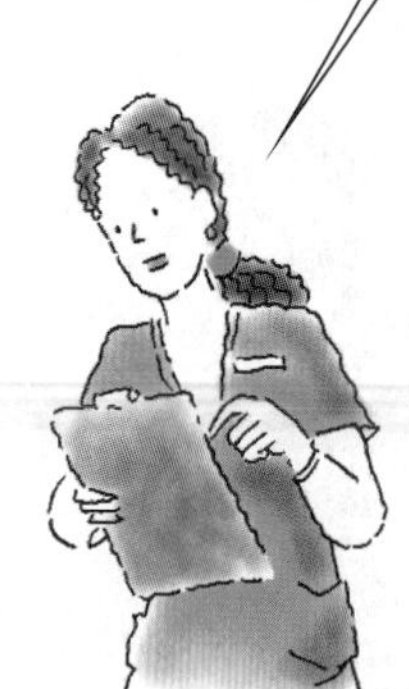

We're most consistent with these hints, aren't we?

98. A 19-year-old client admitted with heat stroke begins to show signs of disseminated intravascular coagulation (DIC). Which laboratory finding is most consistent with DIC?

1. Low platelet count
2. Elevated fibrinogen levels
3. Low levels of fibrin degradation products
4. Reduced prothrombin time (PT)

98. 1. In DIC, platelets and clotting factors are consumed, resulting in microthrombi and excessive bleeding. As clots form, fibrinogen levels decrease and the PT increases. Fibrin degradation products increase as fibrinolysis takes place.

CN: Physiological integrity; CNS: Physiological adaptation; CL: Analysis

99. A client comes to the clinic complaining of fever, drenching night sweats, and unexplained weight loss over the past 3 months. Physical examination reveals a single enlarged supraclavicular lymph node. Which illness is the most probable diagnosis?

1. Influenza
2. Sickle cell anemia
3. Leukemia
4. Hodgkin's disease

99. 4. Hodgkin's disease typically causes fever, night sweats, weight loss, and lymph node enlargement. Influenza doesn't last for months. Clients with sickle cell anemia manifest signs and symptoms of chronic anemia with pallor of the mucous membranes, fatigue, and decreased tolerance for exercise; they don't show fever, night sweats, weight loss, or lymph node enlargement. Leukemia doesn't cause lymph node enlargement.

CN: Health promotion and maintenance; CNS: None; CL: Application

100. A client learns from the physician that he has Hodgkin's disease. After the physician leaves the room, the client tells the nurse he's afraid of dying. Which response by the nurse is appropriate?

1. "Don't worry, many people survive this disease."
2. "Hodgkin's disease is very treatable."
3. "You're afraid of dying?"
4. "You should speak with your minister."

100. 3. Repeating what the client has said (or describing his feelings) encourages the client to elaborate on his thoughts and feelings. Telling him not to worry and saying that Hodgkin's disease is very treatable ignores his feelings and offers false reassurance. Telling a client what to do, such as calling his minister, also ignores his feelings.

CN: Psychosocial integrity; CNS: None; CL: Application

101. Before starting treatment for leukemia, a client receives I.V. fluids and allopurinol (Zyloprim). The goal of these interventions is to reduce the risk of which complication of chemotherapy?

1. Disseminated intravascular coagulation (DIC)
2. Pancytopenia
3. Tumor lysis syndrome
4. Mucositis

101. 3. During chemotherapy for leukemia, tumor lysis syndrome may occur as cell destruction releases intracellular components, resulting in hyperuricemia. Large fluid quantities and allopurinol therapy help reduce the amount of uric acid as a result of tumor lysis syndrome, but don't stop the cell lysis. Although DIC, pancytopenia, and mucositis are possible chemotherapy complications, they're not treated with I.V. fluids and allopurinol.

CN: Physiological integrity; CNS: Pharmacological and parenteral therapies; CL: Application

102. A client with a gunshot wound requires an emergency blood transfusion. His blood type is AB negative. Which blood type would be the <u>safest</u> for him to receive?

1. AB Rh-positive
2. A Rh-positive
3. A Rh-negative
4. O Rh-positive

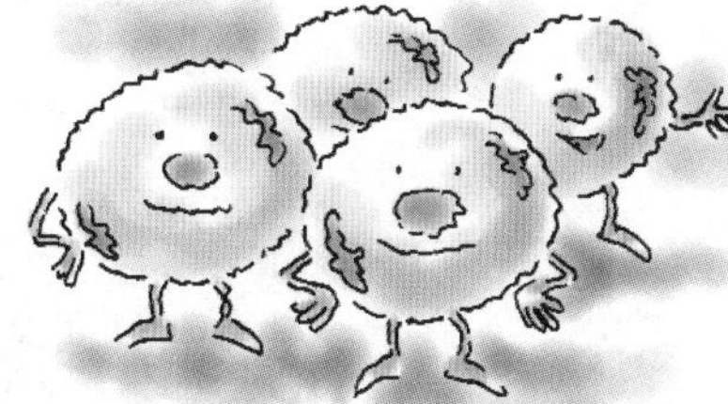

Be on the safe side and choose the safest type.

102. 3. Human blood can sometimes contain an inherited D antigen. Persons with the D antigen have Rh-positive blood type; those lacking the antigen have Rh-negative blood. It's important that a person with Rh-negative blood receives Rh-negative blood. If Rh-positive blood is administered to an Rh-negative person, the recipient develops anti-Rh agglutinins, and subsequent transfusions with Rh-positive blood may cause serious reactions with clumping and hemolysis of red blood cells.

CN: Physiological integrity; CNS: Pharmacological and parenteral therapies; CL: Application

103. Which client is <u>most</u> at risk for developing acute lymphocytic leukemia?

1. 25-year-old black male
2. 4-year-old white female
3. 44-year-old white male
4. 51-year-old Asian female

103. 2. Acute lymphocytic leukemia is most common in young children and in adults age 65 and older. It's also more common in Whites than in Blacks or Asians.

CN: Health promotion and maintenance; CNS: None; CL: Analysis

104. A client with Hodgkin's disease who weighs 143 lb is to receive vincristine 25 mcg/kg I.V. What is the correct dose in micrograms that the client should receive? Record your answer using a whole number.

____________________ micrograms

104. 1625. First, convert the client's weight from pounds to kilograms:

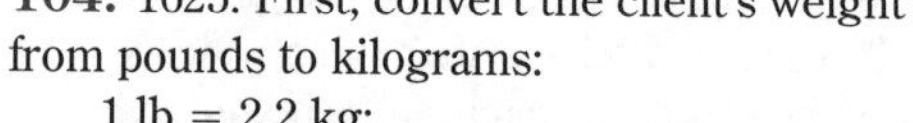

1 lb = 2.2 kg;

143 lb = X kg; 143 lb/2.2 kg = 65 kg.

Next, multiply the weight in kilograms by the number of micrograms desired per kilogram:

65 kg × 25 = 1625 mcg.

CN: Physiological integrity; CNS: Pharmacological and parenteral therapies; CL: Application

105. A client has a viral infection and swollen lymph nodes. Identify the area where the nurse should place her hand to palpate the submandibular lymph nodes.

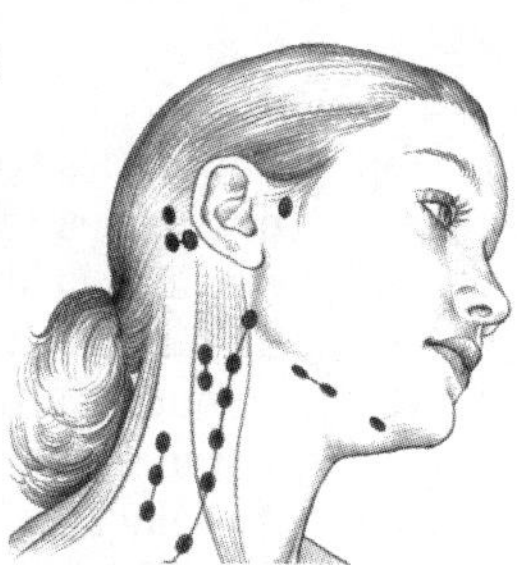

105. The submandibular lymph nodes are found halfway between the angle and tip of the mandible.

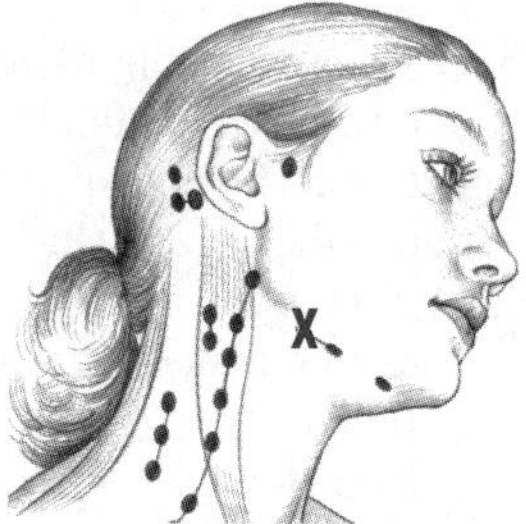

CN: Physiological integrity; CNS: Physiological adaptation; CL: Application

106. Which nonpharmacologic interventions should the nurse include in the care plan for a client who has moderate rheumatoid arthritis? Select all that apply:

1. Massaging inflamed joints
2. Avoiding range-of-motion (ROM) exercises
3. Applying splints to inflamed joints
4. Using assistive devices at all times
5. Selecting clothing that has Velcro fasteners
6. Applying moist heat to joints

106. 3, 5, 6. Supportive, nonpharmacologic measures for the client with rheumatoid arthritis include applying splints to rest inflamed joints, using Velcro fasteners on clothes to aid dressing, and applying moist heat to joints to relax muscles and relieve pain. Inflamed joints should never be massaged because doing so can aggravate inflammation. A physical therapy program including ROM exercises and carefully individualized therapeutic exercises prevents loss of joint function. Assistive devices should be used only when marked loss of ROM occurs.

CN: Physiological integrity; CNS: Basic care and comfort; CL: Application

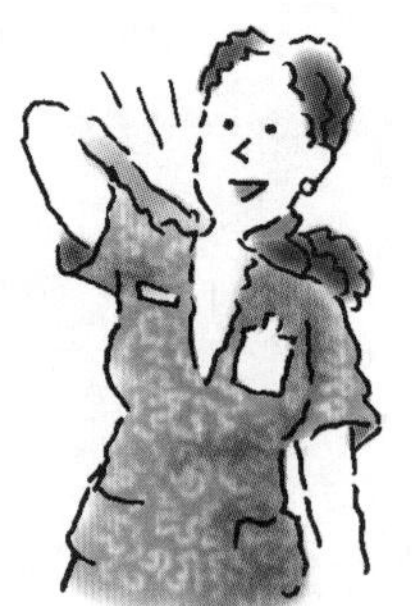

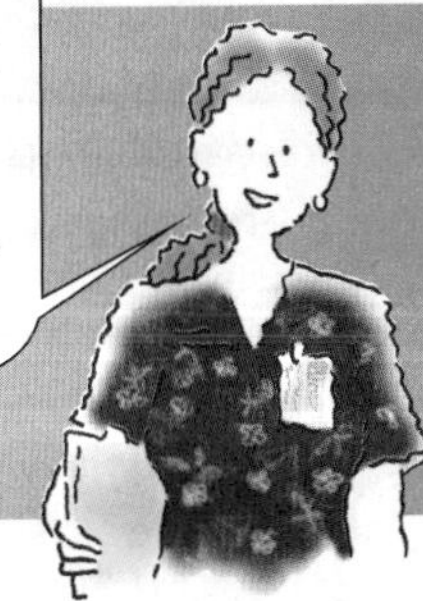

Looking for the latest information about respiratory disorders? Check out the American Association for Respiratory Care's Web site at **www.aarc.org**. It will respire—er, inspire—you.

Chapter 5
Respiratory disorders

1. Which factor will most contribute to a client's development of pneumonia in conjunction with a chronic illness?

1. Dehydration
2. Group living
3. Malnutrition
4. Severe periodontal disease

1. 2. Clients with chronic illnesses generally have poor immune systems. Often, residing in group living situations increases the chance of disease transmission. Adequate fluid intake, adequate nutrition, and proper oral hygiene help maintain normal defenses and can reduce the incidence of getting such diseases as pneumonia.

CN: Physiological integrity; CNS: Physiological adaptation; CL: Analysis

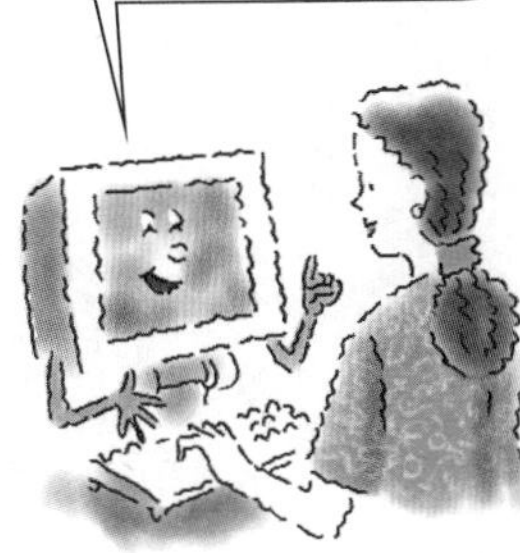

In question 1, the terms most contribute are a hint for finding the correct answer.

2. Which pathophysiological mechanism will be expected to develop as a secondary response to pneumonia after development of the primary causative organism?

1. Atelectasis
2. Bronchiectasis
3. Effusion
4. Inflammation

2. 4. The common feature of all types of pneumonia is an inflammatory pulmonary response to the offending organism or agent. Atelectasis and bronchiectasis indicate a collapse of a portion of the airway that doesn't occur in pneumonia. An effusion is an accumulation of excess pleural fluid in the pleural space, which may be a secondary response to pneumonia.

CN: Physiological integrity; CNS: Physiological adaptation; CL: Application

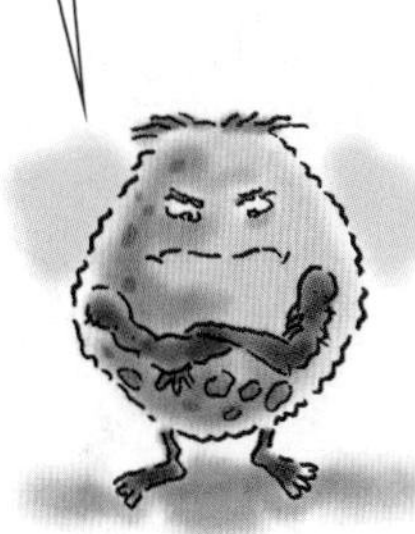

Pssst. Yeah, I'm talking to you. You'd better strep lively—er, I mean, step lively. Got it?

3. The nurse is reviewing the chart of a 58-year-old male client with community-acquired pneumonia. Which of the following will most likely be reported as a causative organism?

1. *Haemophilus influenzae*
2. *Klebsiella pneumoniae*
3. *Streptococcus pneumoniae*
4. *Staphylococcus aureus*

3. 3. Pneumococcal or streptococcal pneumonia, caused by *Streptococcus pneumoniae,* is the most common cause of community-acquired pneumonia. *Haemophilus influenzae* is the most common cause of infection in children. *Klebsiella* species is the most common gram-negative organism found in the hospital setting. *Staphylococcus aureus* is the most common cause of hospital-acquired pneumonia.

CN: Physiological integrity; CNS: Reduction of risk potential; CL: Application

4. An elderly client with pneumonia may appear with which symptoms first?

1. Altered mental status and dehydration
2. Fever and chills
3. Hemoptysis and dyspnea
4. Pleuritic chest pain and cough

4. 1. Fever, chills, hemoptysis, dyspnea, cough, and pleuritic chest pain are the common symptoms of pneumonia, but elderly clients may first appear with only an altered mental status and dehydration due to a blunted immune response.

CN: Physiological integrity; CNS: Physiological adaptation; CL: Application

CN: Client needs category CNS: Client needs subcategory CL: Cognitive level

5. When auscultating the chest of a client with pneumonia, the nurse should expect to hear which type of sounds over areas of consolidation?

1. Bronchial
2. Bronchovesicular
3. Tubular
4. Vesicular

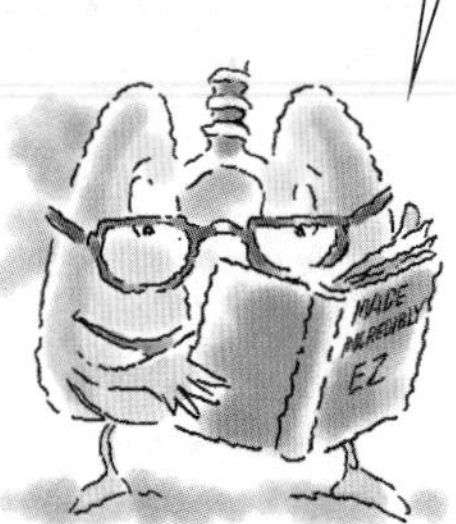

For question 5, think of where you normally hear each type of breath sound.
MADE INCREDIBLY EZ

5. 1. Chest auscultation reveals bronchial breath sounds over areas of consolidation. Bronchovesicular breath sounds are normal over midlobe lung regions, tubular sounds are commonly heard over large airways, and vesicular breath sounds are commonly heard in the bases of the lung fields.

CN: Physiological integrity; CNS: Reduction of risk potential; CL: Application

6. A diagnosis of pneumonia is typically achieved by which diagnostic test?

1. Arterial blood gas (ABG) analysis
2. Chest X-ray
3. Blood cultures
4. Sputum culture and sensitivity

6. 4. Sputum culture and sensitivity is the best way to identify the organism causing the pneumonia. ABG analysis will determine the extent of hypoxia present due to the pneumonia. Chest X-ray will show the area of lung consolidation. Blood cultures will help determine if the infection is systemic.

CN: Physiological integrity; CNS: Reduction of risk potential; CL: Application

7. A 78-year-old client is admitted with a diagnosis of dehydration and change in mental status. He's being hydrated with I.V. fluids. When the nurse takes his vital signs, she notes he has a fever of 103° F (39.4° C), a cough producing yellow sputum, and pleuritic chest pain. The nurse suspects this client may have which condition?

1. Acute respiratory distress syndrome (ARDS)
2. Myocardial infarction (MI)
3. Pneumonia
4. Tuberculosis (TB)

7. 3. Fever, productive cough, and pleuritic chest pain are common signs and symptoms of pneumonia. The client with ARDS has dyspnea and hypoxia, with worsening hypoxia over time if not treated aggressively. Pleuritic chest pain varies with respiration, unlike the constant chest pain during an MI, so this client most likely isn't having an MI. The client with TB typically has a cough producing blood-tinged sputum. A sputum culture should be obtained to confirm the nurse's suspicions.

CN: Physiological integrity; CNS: Physiological adaptation; CL: Analysis

8. A client with pneumonia develops dyspnea with a respiratory rate of 32 breaths/minute and difficulty expelling his secretions. The nurse auscultates his lung fields and hears bronchial sounds in the left lower lobe. The nurse determines that the client requires which treatment first?

1. Antibiotics
2. Bed rest
3. Oxygen
4. Nutritional intake

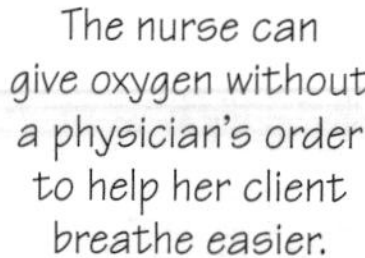

The nurse can give oxygen without a physician's order to help her client breathe easier.

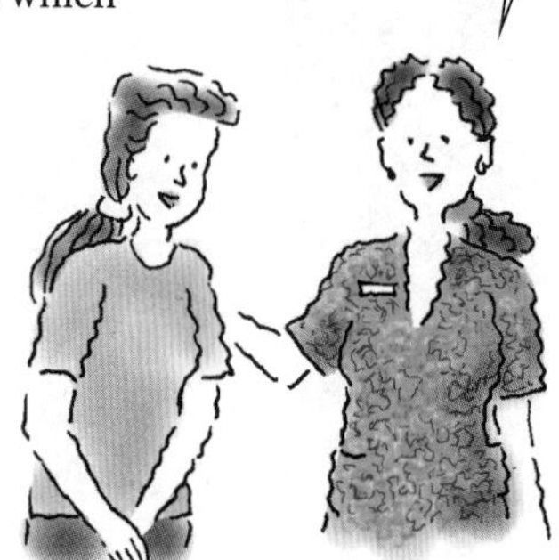

8. 3. The client is having difficulty breathing and is probably becoming hypoxic. As an emergency measure, the nurse can provide oxygen without waiting for a physician's order. Antibiotics may be warranted, but this isn't a nursing decision. The client should be maintained on bed rest if he's dyspneic to minimize his oxygen demands, but providing additional oxygen will deal more immediately with his problem. The client will need nutritional support, but while dyspneic, he may be unable to spare the energy needed to eat and at the same time maintain adequate oxygenation.

CN: Safe, effective care environment; CNS: Management of care; CL: Analysis

9. A client has been treated with antibiotic therapy for right lower-lobe pneumonia for 10 days and will be discharged today. Which physical finding would lead the nurse to believe it's appropriate to discharge this client?

1. Continued dyspnea
2. Fever of 102° F (38.9° C)
3. Respiratory rate of 32 breaths/minute
4. Vesicular breath sounds in right base

9. 4. If the client still has pneumonia, the breath sounds in the right base will be bronchial, not the normal vesicular breath sounds. If the client still has dyspnea, fever, and increased respiratory rate, he should be examined by the physician before discharge because he may have another source of infection or still have pneumonia.

CN: Physiological integrity; CNS: Physiological adaptation; CL: Analysis

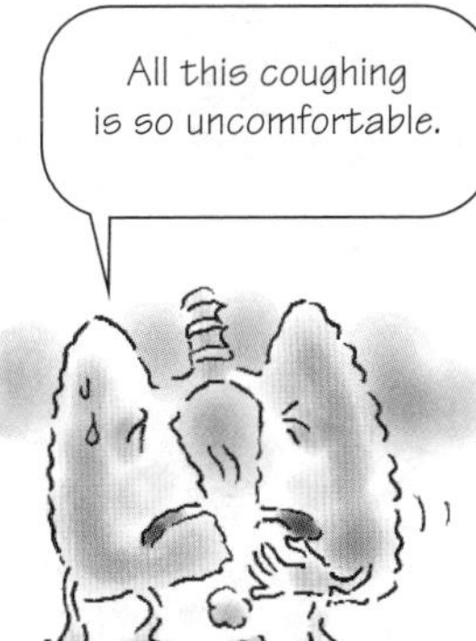
All this coughing
is so uncomfortable.

10. A 20-year-old client is being treated for pneumonia. He has a persistent cough and complains of severe pain on coughing. What type of instruction should be given to help the client reduce the discomfort he's having?

1. "Hold in your cough as much as possible."
2. "Place the head of your bed flat to help with coughing."
3. "Restrict fluids to help decrease the amount of sputum."
4. "Splint your chest wall with a pillow for comfort."

10. 4. Showing this client how to splint his chest wall will help decrease discomfort when coughing. Holding in his coughs will only increase the amount of pain he has. Placing the head of the bed flat may increase the frequency of his cough and require more work; a 45-degree angle may help him cough more efficiently and with less pain. Increasing fluid intake will help thin his secretions, making it easier for him to clear them. Promoting fluid intake is appropriate in this situation.

CN: Physiological integrity; CNS: Basic care and comfort; CL: Application

11. A client in a long-term care facility has been receiving tube feedings around the clock. The nurse notices he has a cough producing tan sputum, much like the content of his tube feedings, and is now febrile to 102° F (38.9° C). The nurse auscultates his lung fields and hears bronchial breath sounds in his right middle lobe. The nurse suspects he may have developed which condition?

1. Atelectasis
2. Bronchitis
3. Pneumonia
4. Pulmonary embolism

11. 3. The client probably has aspirated the contents of his tube feedings and developed aspiration pneumonia. This is the most common cause of pneumonia in clients with tube feedings. Atelectasis wouldn't be associated with a productive cough, and breath sounds would be decreased in the areas of atelectasis. The client most likely hasn't developed bronchitis because in that condition, he may have a nonproductive or productive cough but secretions are usually clear. A client with a pulmonary embolism wouldn't have a cough producing tan sputum, and pulmonary embolisms aren't typically associated with high fever.

CN: Physiological integrity; CNS: Physiological adaptation; CL: Analysis

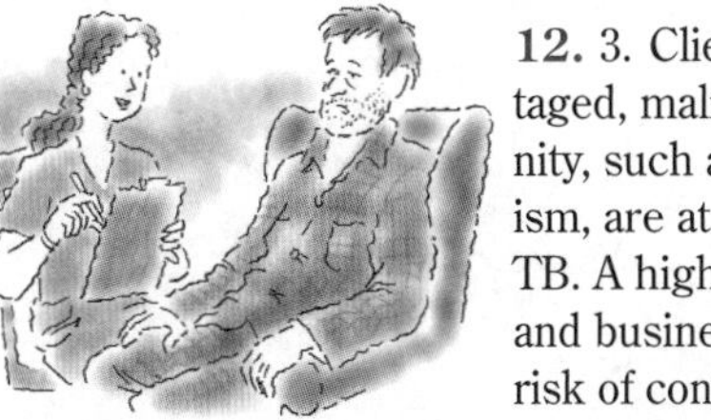
Asking a client
questions will help
determine his
degree of risk.

12. A nurse is working in a walk-in clinic. She has been alerted that there is an outbreak of tuberculosis (TB). Which client is *most* at risk for developing TB?

1. A 16-year-old female high school student
2. A 33-year-old day-care worker
3. A 43-year-old homeless man with a history of alcoholism
4. A 54-year-old businessman

12. 3. Clients who are economically disadvantaged, malnourished, and have reduced immunity, such as a client with a history of alcoholism, are at extremely high risk for developing TB. A high school student, day-care worker, and businessman probably have a much lower risk of contracting TB.

CN: Physiological integrity; CNS: Physiological adaptation; CL: Application

13. The nurse is conducting a class for family members of clients diagnosed with tuberculosis (TB). Which of the following should the nurse teach family members regarding transmission of the disease?

1. It is transmitted by sexual contact.
2. It is transmitted by contaminated needles.
3. It is transmitted through contaminated eating utensils.
4. It is transmitted by droplets exhaled from an infected person.

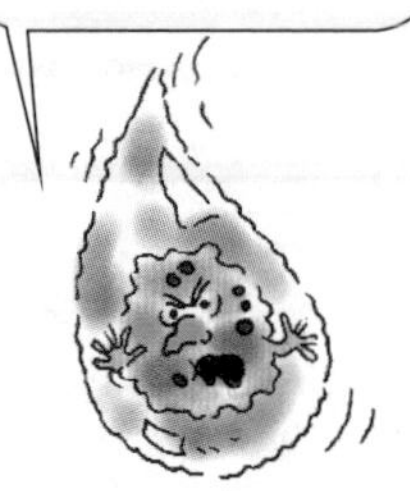

This droplet transmission stuff sure beats the subway! Wheeee!

13. 4. The TB bacillus is airborne and carried in droplets exhaled by an infected person who is coughing, sneezing, laughing, or singing. Sexual contact and contaminated needles don't spread the TB bacillus, but may spread other communicable diseases. It's never advisable to use contaminated utensils, but if they're cleaned normally, it isn't necessary to dispose of eating utensils used by someone infected with TB.

CN: Safe, effective care environment; CNS: Safety and infection control; CL: Application

14. An adult client is being screened in the clinic today for tuberculosis. He reports having negative purified protein derivative (PPD) test results in the past. The nurse performs a PPD test on his right forearm today. When should he return to have the test read?

1. Immediately after performing the test
2. 24 hours after performing the test
3. 48 hours after performing the test
4. 1 week after performing the test

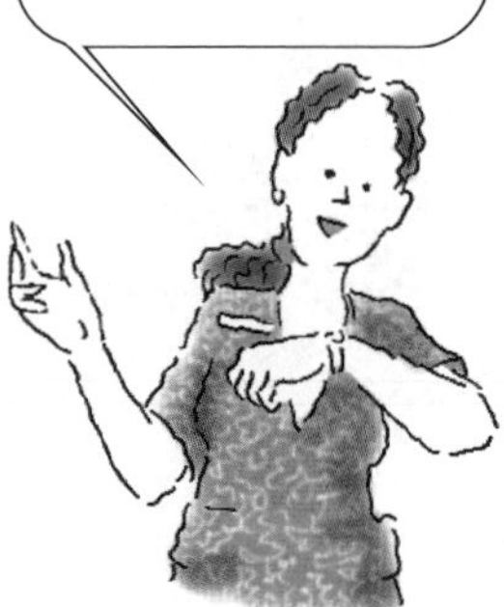

The timing is the clue!

14. 3. PPD tests should be read in 48 to 72 hours. If read too early or too late, the results won't be accurate.

CN: Physiological integrity; CNS: Reduction of risk potential; CL: Application

15. The right forearm of a client who had a purified protein derivative (PPD) test for tuberculosis (TB) is reddened and raised about 3 mm where the test was given. This PPD should be read as having which result?

1. Indeterminate
2. Needs to be redone
3. Negative
4. Positive

15. 3. This test would be classed as negative. A 3-mm raised area would be a positive result if the client had recent close contact with someone diagnosed with or suspected of having infectious TB. Follow-up should be done with this client, and a chest X-ray should be ordered. *Indeterminate* isn't a term used to describe results of a PPD test. The test can be redone in 6 months to see if the client's test results change. If the PPD test is reddened and raised 10 mm or more, it's considered positive according to the Centers for Disease Control and Prevention.

CN: Physiological integrity; CNS: Reduction of risk potential; CL: Analysis

16. A client with a primary tuberculosis (TB) infection can expect to develop:

1. active TB within 2 weeks.
2. active TB within 1 month.
3. a fever that requires hospitalization.
4. a positive skin test.

16. 4. A primary TB infection occurs when the bacillus has successfully invaded the entire body after entering through the lungs. At this point, the bacilli are walled off and skin tests read positive. The general population has a 10% risk of developing active TB over their lifetime, in many cases because of a break in the body's immune defenses. The active stage shows the classic symptoms of TB: fever, hemoptysis, and night sweats.

CN: Physiological integrity; CNS: Physiological adaptation; CL: Analysis

17. A client was infected with tuberculosis (TB) bacillus 10 years ago but never developed the disease. He's now being treated for cancer. The client begins to develop signs of TB. This is known as which type of infection?

1. Active infection
2. Latent infection
3. Superinfection
4. Tertiary infection

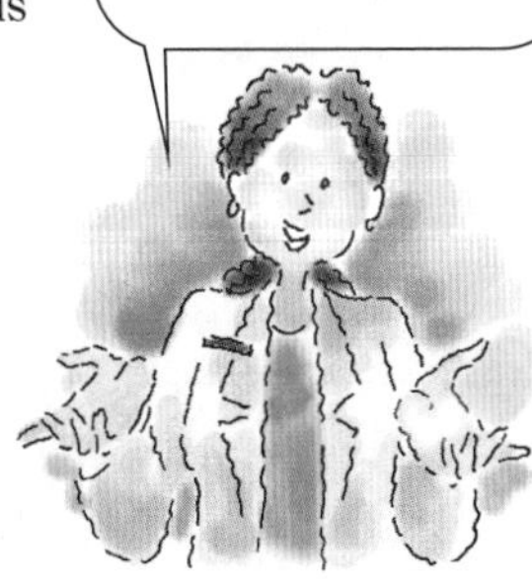

Think: How does cancer affect the immune system?

17. 1. Some people carry dormant TB infections that may develop into active disease. If there's no active infection, it's called a *latent infection.* The TB bacilli may remain latent for years and then activate when the client's resistance is lowered, as when a client is being treated for cancer. Superinfection doesn't apply in this case, and there's no such thing as tertiary infection.

CN: Physiological integrity; CNS: Physiological adaptation; CL: Application

18. A client has active tuberculosis (TB). Which symptoms will he exhibit?

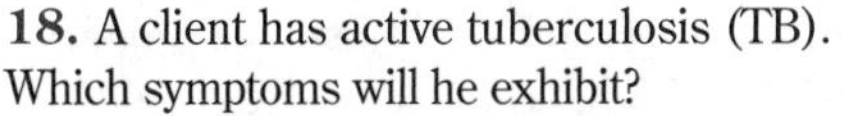

1. Chest and lower back pain
2. Chills, fever, night sweats, and hemoptysis
3. Fever of more than 104° F (40° C) and nausea
4. Headache and photophobia

18. 2. Typical signs and symptoms are chills, fever, night sweats, and hemoptysis. Chest pain may be present from coughing, but isn't usual. Clients with TB typically have low-grade fevers, not higher than 102° F (38.9° C). Nausea, headache, and photophobia aren't usual TB symptoms.

CN: Physiological integrity; CNS: Physiological adaptation; CL: Application

19. A client has received a preliminary diagnosis of tuberculosis. In order to obtain a definitive diagnosis, which test will the nurse expect to see ordered?

1. Chest X-ray
2. Mantoux test
3. Sputum culture
4. Tuberculin test

19. 3. The sputum culture for *Mycobacterium tuberculosis* is the only method of confirming the diagnosis. Lesions in the lung may not be big enough to be seen on X-ray. Skin tests may be falsely positive or falsely negative.

CN: Physiological integrity; CNS: Reduction of risk potential; CL: Application

20. A client with a positive Mantoux test result will be sent for a chest X-ray. For which reason is this done?

1. To confirm the diagnosis
2. To determine if a repeat skin test is needed
3. To determine the extent of lesions
4. To determine if this is a primary or secondary infection

20. 3. If the lesions are large enough, the chest X-ray will show their presence in the lungs. Sputum culture confirms the diagnosis. There can be false-positive and false-negative skin test results. A chest X-ray can't determine if this is a primary or secondary infection.

CN: Physiological integrity; CNS: Reduction of risk potential; CL: Application

21. A chest X-ray shows a client's lungs to be clear. His Mantoux test is positive, with 10 mm of induration. His previous test was negative. These test results are possible because:

1. he had tuberculosis (TB) in the past and no longer has it.
2. he was successfully treated for TB, but skin tests always stay positive.
3. he's a "seroconverter," meaning the TB has gotten to his bloodstream.
4. he's a "tuberculin converter," which means he has been infected with TB since his last skin test.

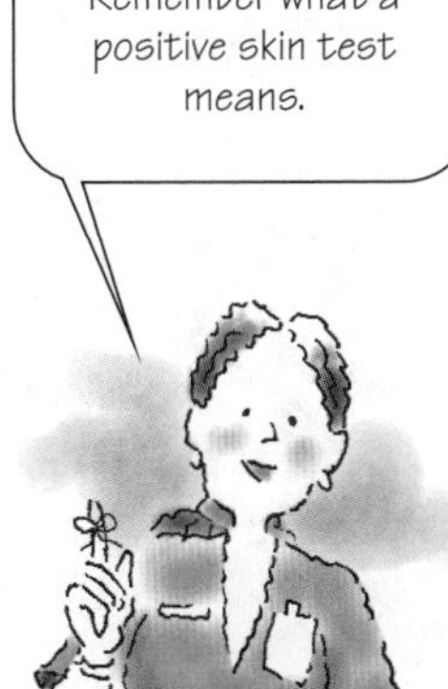

21. 4. A tuberculin converter's skin test will be positive, meaning he has been exposed to and infected with TB and now has a cell-mediated immune response to the skin test. The client's blood and X-ray results may stay negative. It doesn't mean the infection has advanced to the active stage. Because his X-ray is negative, he should be monitored every 6 months to see if he develops changes in his chest X-ray or pulmonary examination. Being a seroconverter doesn't mean the TB has gotten into his bloodstream; it means it can be detected by a blood test.

CN: Physiological integrity; CNS: Physiological adaptation; CL: Analysis

22. A client with a positive skin test for tuberculosis (TB) isn't showing signs of active disease. To help prevent the development of active TB, the client should be treated with isoniazid, 300 mg daily, for how long?

1. 10 to 14 days
2. 2 to 4 weeks
3. 3 to 6 months
4. 9 to 12 months

22. 4. Because of the increasing incidence of resistant strains of TB, the disease must be treated for up to 24 months in some cases, but treatment typically lasts from 9 to 12 months. Isoniazid is the most common medication used for the treatment of TB, but other antibiotics are added to the regimen to obtain the best results.

CN: Physiological integrity; CNS: Pharmacological and parenteral therapies; CL: Application

23. A client with a productive cough, chills, and night sweats is suspected of having active tuberculosis (TB). The physician should take which action?

1. Admit him to the hospital in respiratory isolation.
2. Prescribe isoniazid and tell him to go home and rest.
3. Give a tuberculin test and tell him to come back in 48 hours to have it read.
4. Give a prescription for isoniazid, 300 mg daily for 2 weeks, and send him home.

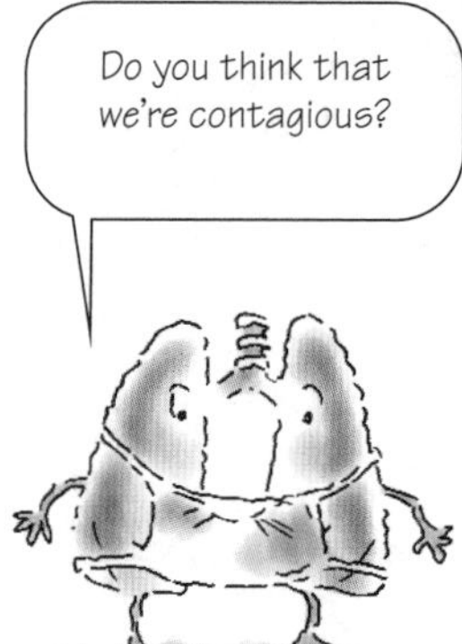
Do you think that we're contagious?

23. 1. This client is showing signs and symptoms of active TB and, because of the productive cough, is highly contagious. He should be admitted to the hospital, placed in respiratory isolation, and three sputum cultures should be obtained to confirm the diagnosis. He would most likely be given isoniazid and two or three other antitubercular antibiotics until the diagnosis is confirmed, and then isolation and treatment would continue if the cultures were positive for TB. After 7 to 10 days, three more consecutive sputum cultures will be obtained. If they're negative, he would be considered noncontagious and may be sent home, although he'll continue to take the antitubercular drugs for 9 to 12 months.

CN: Physiological integrity; CNS: Physiological adaptation; CL: Application

24. A client is diagnosed with active tuberculosis and started on triple antibiotic therapy. What sign or symptom should the client show if therapy is <u>inadequate</u>?

1. Decreased shortness of breath
2. Improved chest X-ray
3. Nonproductive cough
4. Positive acid-fast bacilli in a sputum sample after 2 months of treatment

24. 4. Continuing to have acid-fast bacilli in the sputum after 2 months indicates continued infection. The other choices would all indicate improvement with therapy.

CN: Physiological integrity; CNS: Physiological adaptation; CL: Application

25. Which instruction should the nurse give a client about his active tuberculosis (TB)?

1. "It's OK to miss a dose every day or two."
2. "If side effects occur, stop taking the medication."
3. "Only take the medication until you feel better."
4. "You must comply with the medication regimen to treat TB."

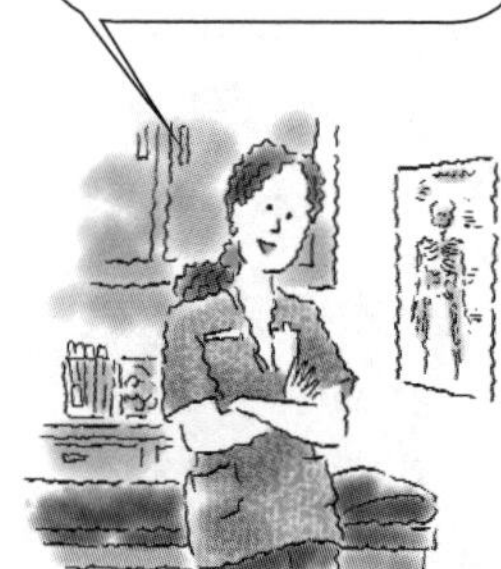
Hmmm. Is it OK to miss a dose of an antitubercular drug?

25. 4. The regimen may last up to 24 months. It's essential that the client comply with therapy during that time or resistance will develop. At no time should he stop taking the medications before his physician tells him to.

CN: Safe, effective care environment; CNS: Management of care; CL: Analysis

CN: Client needs category CNS: Client needs subcategory CL: Cognitive level

26. A client diagnosed with active tuberculosis (TB) would be hospitalized primarily for which reason?

1. To evaluate his condition
2. To determine his compliance
3. To prevent spread of the disease
4. To determine the need for antibiotic therapy

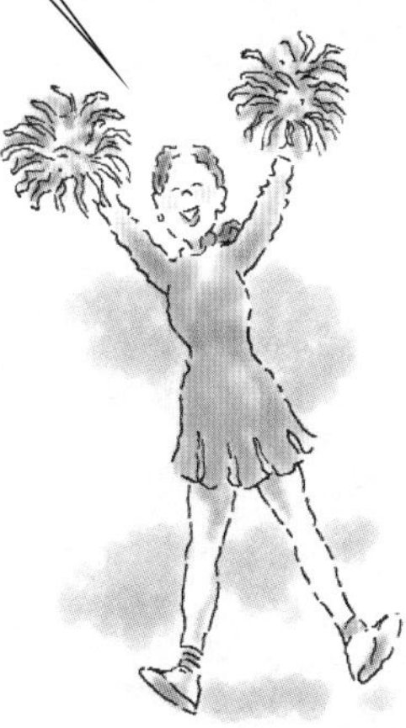

You're doing great! Keep it up!

26. 3. The client with active TB is highly contagious until three consecutive sputum cultures are negative, so he's put in respiratory isolation in the hospital. Neither assessment of physical condition, determinations of compliance, nor antibiotic therapy is a primary reason for hospitalization in this case.

CN: Safe, effective care environment; CNS: Safety and infection control; CL: Application

27. A 7-year-old is brought to the emergency department. He's tachypneic and afebrile and has a respiratory rate of 36 breaths/minute and a nonproductive cough. He recently had a cold. From this history, the child may have which condition?

1. Acute asthma
2. Bronchial pneumonia
3. Chronic obstructive pulmonary disease (COPD)
4. Emphysema

27. 1. Based on the child's history and symptoms, acute asthma is the most likely diagnosis. He's unlikely to have bronchial pneumonia without a productive cough and fever and he's too young to have developed COPD and emphysema.

CN: Physiological integrity; CNS: Physiological adaptation; CL: Analysis

28. Which assessment finding helps confirm a diagnosis of asthma in a client suspected of having the disorder?

1. Circumoral cyanosis
2. Increased forced expiratory volume
3. Inspiratory and expiratory wheezing
4. Normal breath sounds

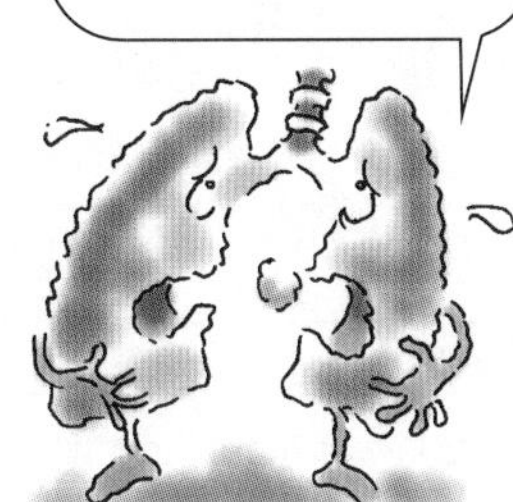

Listen to how we sound—any changes from normal are clues.

28. 3. Inspiratory and expiratory wheezes are typical findings in asthma. Circumoral cyanosis may be present in extreme cases of respiratory distress. The nurse would expect the client to have a decreased forced expiratory volume because asthma is an obstructive pulmonary disease. Breath sounds will be "tight"-sounding or markedly decreased; they won't be normal.

CN: Physiological integrity; CNS: Physiological adaptation; CL: Analysis

29. The client has recently had a common cold and subsequently experiences an asthma attack. Which type of asthma is the client <u>most likely</u> experiencing?

1. Emotional
2. Allergic
3. Non-allergic
4. Mediated

29. 3. Non-allergic asthma doesn't have an easily identifiable allergen and can be triggered by the common cold. Asthma caused by emotional reasons is considered to be in the extrinsic category. Allergic asthma is caused by dust, molds, and pets—easily identifiable allergens. Mediated asthma doesn't exist.

CN: Physiological integrity; CNS: Physiological adaptation; CL: Analysis

30. A client with acute asthma showing inspiratory and expiratory wheezes and a decreased forced expiratory volume should be treated with which class of medication <u>right away</u>?

1. Beta-adrenergic blockers
2. Bronchodilators
3. Inhaled steroids
4. Oral steroids

30. 2. Bronchodilators are the first line of treatment for asthma because bronchoconstriction is the cause of reduced airflow. Beta-adrenergic blockers aren't used to treat asthma and can cause bronchoconstriction. Inhaled or oral steroids may be given to reduce the inflammation but aren't used for emergency relief.

CN: Physiological integrity; CNS: Pharmacological and parenteral therapies; CL: Application

31. A 19-year-old client comes to the emergency department with acute asthma. His respiratory rate is 44 breaths/minute, and he appears in acute respiratory distress. Which action should be taken <u>first</u>?

1. Take a full medical history.
2. Give a bronchodilator by nebulizer.
3. Apply a cardiac monitor to the client.
4. Provide emotional support to the client.

31. 2. The client having an acute asthma attack needs to increase oxygen delivery to the lung and body. Nebulized bronchodilators open airways and increase the amount of oxygen delivered. First resolve the acute phase of the attack, then obtain a full medical history to determine the cause of the attack and how to prevent attacks in the future. It may not be necessary to place the client on a cardiac monitor because he's only 19 years old, unless he has a past medical history of cardiac problems.

CN: Physiological integrity; CNS: Physiological adaptation; CL: Application

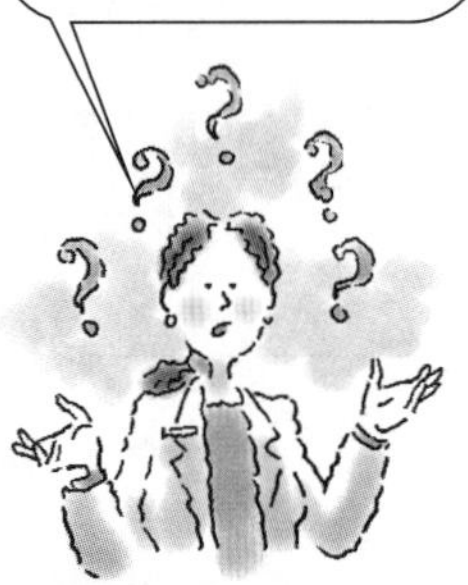

32. A client is found to be allergic to Chinese food, which causes acute asthma. Which instruction should the nurse give the client?

1. "Only eat Chinese food once per month."
2. "Use your inhalers before eating Chinese food."
3. "Avoid Chinese food because this is a trigger for you."
4. "Determine other causes because Chinese food wouldn't cause such a violent reaction."

32. 3. If the trigger of an acute asthma attack is known, this trigger should be avoided at all times. Using an inhaler before eating wouldn't prevent the attack, and food is commonly a trigger for an acute asthma attack.

CN: Physiological integrity; CNS: Physiological adaptation; CL: Application

33. A 58-year-old client with a 40-year history of smoking one to two packs of cigarettes per day has a chronic cough producing thick sputum and peripheral edema. He also has cyanotic nail beds. Based on this information, he most likely has which condition?

1. Acute respiratory distress syndrome (ARDS)
2. Asthma
3. Chronic obstructive bronchitis
4. Emphysema

33. 3. Because of his extensive smoking history and symptoms, the client most likely has chronic obstructive bronchitis. Clients with ARDS have acute symptoms of hypoxia and typically need large amounts of oxygen. Clients with asthma and emphysema tend not to have a chronic cough or peripheral edema.

CN: Physiological integrity; CNS: Physiological adaptation; CL: Application

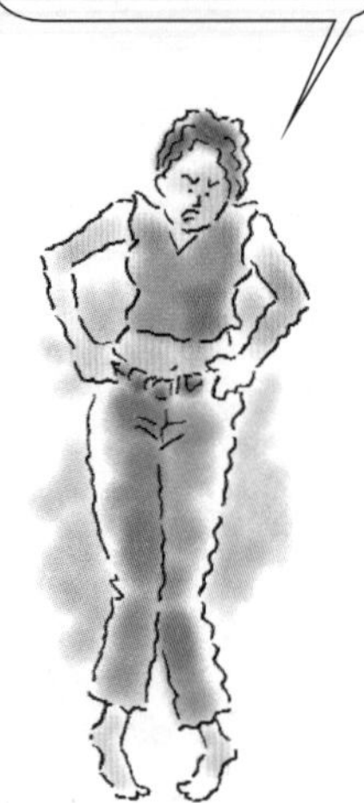

Terms such as blue bloater can help you remember the symptoms of some diseases.

34. The term "blue bloater" refers to which condition?

1. Acute respiratory distress syndrome (ARDS)
2. Asthma
3. Chronic obstructive bronchitis
4. Emphysema

34. 3. Clients with chronic obstructive bronchitis appear bloated; they have large barrel chests and peripheral edema, cyanotic nail beds and, at times, circumoral cyanosis. Clients with ARDS are acutely short of breath and frequently need intubation for mechanical ventilation and large amounts of oxygen. Clients with asthma don't exhibit characteristics of chronic disease, and clients with emphysema appear pink and cachectic.

CN: Physiological integrity; CNS: Physiological adaptation; CL: Application

35. The term "pink puffer" refers to a client with which condition?

1. Acute respiratory distress syndrome (ARDS)
2. Asthma
3. Chronic obstructive bronchitis
4. Emphysema

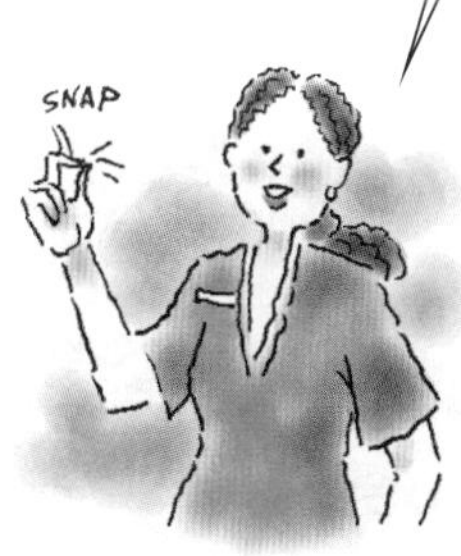

Terms like these make remembering symptoms a snap!
SNAP

35. 4. Because of the large amount of energy it takes to breathe, clients with emphysema are usually cachectic. They're pink and usually breathe through pursed lips, hence the term "puffer." Clients with ARDS are usually acutely short of breath. Clients with asthma don't have any particular characteristics, and clients with chronic obstructive bronchitis are bloated and cyanotic in appearance.
CN: Physiological integrity; CNS: Physiological adaptation; CL: Application

36. A 66-year-old client has marked dyspnea at rest, is thin, and uses accessory muscles to breathe. He's tachypneic, with a prolonged expiratory phase. He has no cough. He leans forward with his arms braced on his knees to support his chest and shoulders for breathing. This client has symptoms of which respiratory disorder?

1. Acute respiratory distress syndrome (ARDS)
2. Asthma
3. Chronic obstructive bronchitis
4. Emphysema

36. 4. These are classic signs and symptoms of a client with emphysema. Clients with ARDS are acutely short of breath and require emergency care; those with asthma are also acutely short of breath during an attack and appear very frightened. Clients with chronic obstructive bronchitis are bloated and cyanotic in appearance.
CN: Physiological integrity; CNS: Physiological adaptation; CL: Application

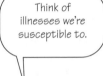

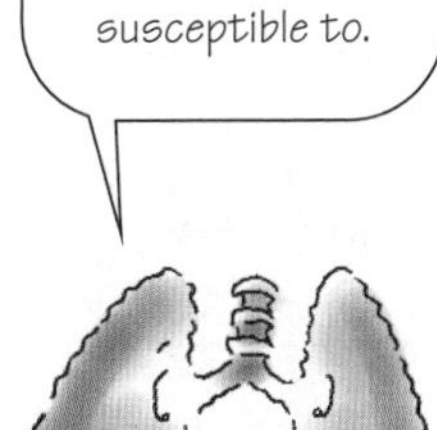

Think of illnesses we're susceptible to.

37. It's highly recommended that clients with asthma, chronic bronchitis, and emphysema have Pneumovax and flu vaccinations for which reason?

1. These vaccines are recommended for all clients.
2. These vaccines produce bronchodilation and improve oxygenation.
3. These vaccines help reduce the tachypnea these clients experience.
4. Respiratory infections can cause severe hypoxia and possibly death in these clients.

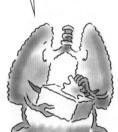

37. 4. It's highly recommended that clients with respiratory disorders be given vaccines to protect against respiratory infection. Infections can cause these clients to need intubation and mechanical ventilation, and it may be difficult to wean these clients from the ventilator. The vaccines have no effect on bronchodilation or respiratory rate.
CN: Health promotion and maintenance; CNS: None; CL: Application

38. Exercise has which effect on clients with asthma, chronic bronchitis, and emphysema?

1. It enhances cardiovascular fitness.
2. It improves respiratory muscle strength.
3. It reduces the number of acute attacks.
4. It worsens respiratory function and is discouraged.

38. 1. Exercise can improve cardiovascular fitness and help the client tolerate periods of hypoxia better, perhaps reducing the risk of heart attack. Most exercise has little effect on respiratory muscle strength, and these clients can't tolerate the type of exercise necessary to do this. Exercise won't reduce the number of acute attacks. In some instances, exercise may be contraindicated, and the client should check with his physician before starting any exercise program.
CN: Health promotion and maintenance; CNS: None; CL: Application

39. Clients with chronic obstructive bronchitis are given diuretic therapy. Which reason best explains why?

1. Reducing fluid volume reduces oxygen demand.
2. Reducing fluid volume improves clients' mobility.
3. Reducing fluid volume reduces sputum production.
4. Reducing fluid volume improves respiratory function.

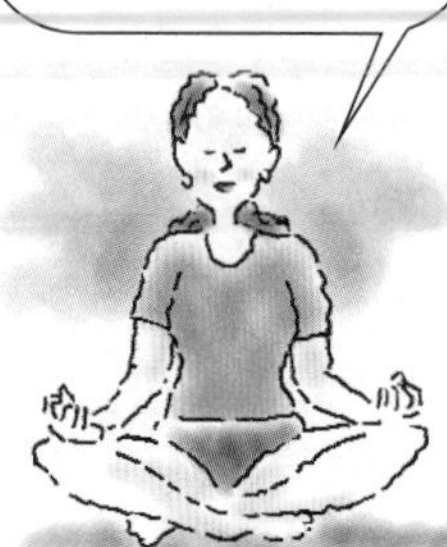

39. 1. Reducing fluid volume reduces the workload of the heart, which reduces oxygen demand and, in turn, reduces the respiratory rate. It also may reduce edema and improve mobility a little, but exercise tolerance will still be poor. Sputum may get thicker and make it harder to clear airways. Reducing fluid volume won't improve respiratory function, but may improve oxygenation.

CN: Physiological integrity; CNS: Physiological adaptation; CL: Application

40. A 69-year-old client appears thin and cachectic. He's short of breath at rest and his dyspnea increases with the slightest exertion. His breath sounds are diminished even with deep inspiration. These signs and symptoms fit which condition?

1. Acute respiratory distress syndrome (ARDS)
2. Asthma
3. Chronic obstructive bronchitis
4. Emphysema

40. 4. In emphysema, the wall integrity of the individual air sacs is damaged, reducing the surface area available for gas exchange. Very little air movement occurs in the lungs because of bronchiole collapse, as well. In ARDS, the client's condition is more acute and typically requires mechanical ventilation. In asthma and bronchitis, wheezing is prevalent.

CN: Physiological integrity; CNS: Physiological adaptation; CL: Application

41. A client with emphysema should receive only 1 to 3 L/minute of oxygen, if needed, or he may lose his hypoxic drive. Which statement is correct about hypoxic drive?

1. The client doesn't notice he needs to breathe.
2. The client breathes only when his oxygen levels climb above a certain point.
3. The client breathes only when his oxygen levels dip below a certain point.
4. The client breathes only when his carbon dioxide level dips below a certain point.

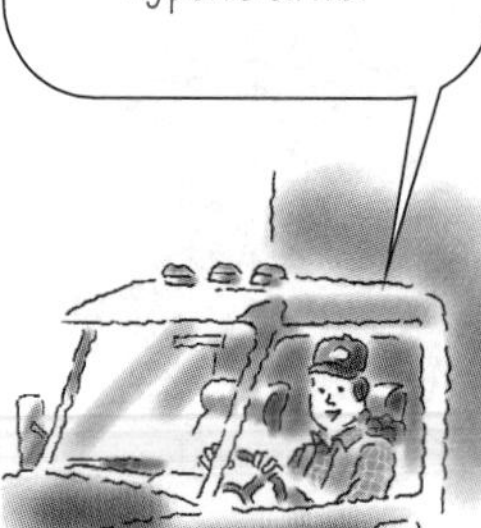

We keep moving
thanks to our
hypoxic drive!

41. 3. Clients with emphysema breathe when their oxygen levels drop to a certain level; this is known as the *hypoxic drive.* They don't take a breath when their levels of carbon dioxide are higher than normal, as do those with healthy respiratory physiology. If too much oxygen is given, the client has little stimulus to take another breath. In the meantime, his carbon dioxide levels continue to climb, and the client will pass out, leading to respiratory arrest.

CN: Physiological integrity; CNS: Physiological adaptation; CL: Analysis

42. Teaching for a client with chronic obstructive pulmonary disease should include which topic?

1. How to listen to his own lungs
2. How to change his oxygen therapy
3. How to treat respiratory infections without going to the physician
4. How to recognize the signs of an impending respiratory infection

42. 4. Respiratory infection in clients with a respiratory disorder can be fatal. It's important that the client understands how to recognize the signs and symptoms of an impending respiratory infection. It isn't appropriate to teach a client how to listen to his own lungs or change his oxygen therapy regimen. If the client has signs and symptoms of an infection, he should contact his physician at once.

CN: Health promotion and maintenance; CNS: None; CL: Application

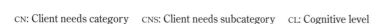

43. Which respiratory disorder is most common in the first 24 to 48 hours after surgery?
1. Atelectasis
2. Bronchitis
3. Pneumonia
4. Pneumothorax

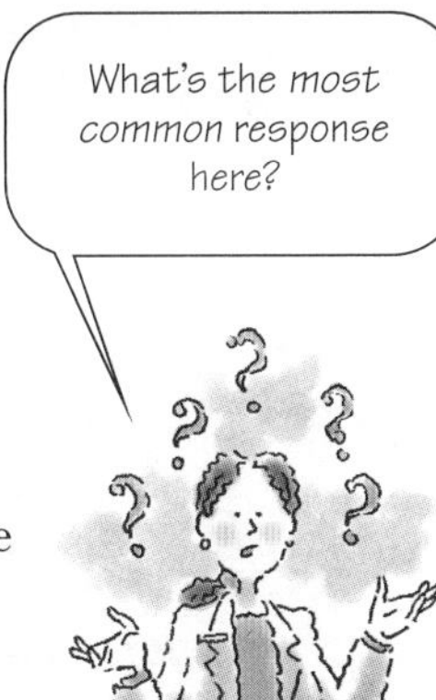
What's the *most common* response here?

43. 1. Atelectasis develops when there's interference with the normal negative pressure that promotes lung expansion. Clients in the postoperative phase often splint their breathing because of pain and positioning, which causes hypoxia. It's uncommon for any of the other respiratory disorders to develop.
CN: Physiological integrity; CNS: Reduction of risk potential; CL: Application

44. Which measure can reduce or prevent the incidence of atelectasis in a postoperative client?
1. Chest physiotherapy
2. Mechanical ventilation
3. Reducing oxygen requirements
4. Use of an incentive spirometer

44. 4. Using an incentive spirometer requires the client to take deep breaths and promotes lung expansion. Chest physiotherapy helps mobilize secretions but won't prevent atelectasis. Reducing oxygen requirements or placing someone on mechanical ventilation doesn't affect the development of atelectasis.
CN: Physiological integrity; CNS: Reduction of risk potential; CL: Application

45. Initial emergency treatment of a client in status asthmaticus includes which medications?
1. Inhaled beta-adrenergic agents
2. Inhaled corticosteroids
3. I.V. beta-adrenergic agents
4. Oral corticosteroids

45. 1. Inhaled beta-adrenergic agents help promote bronchodilation, which improves oxygenation. I.V. beta-adrenergic agents can be used but have to be monitored because of their greater systemic effects. They're typically used when the inhaled beta-adrenergic agents don't work. Corticosteroids are slow-acting, so their use won't reduce hypoxia in the acute phase.
CN: Physiological integrity; CNS: Physiological adaptation; CL: Application

For question 46, you need to choose the *best* out of several possible goals.

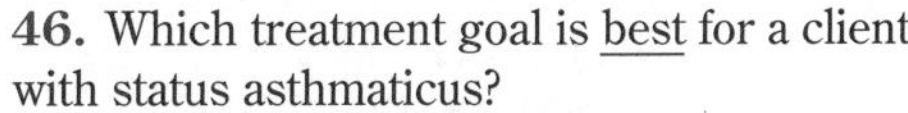

46. Which treatment goal is best for a client with status asthmaticus?
1. Avoiding intubation
2. Determining the cause of the attack
3. Improving exercise tolerance
4. Reducing secretions

46. 1. Inhaled beta-adrenergic agents, I.V. corticosteroids, and supplemental oxygen are used to reduce bronchospasm, improve oxygenation, and avoid intubation. Determining the trigger for the client's attack and improving exercise tolerance are later goals. Typically, secretions aren't a problem in status asthmaticus.
CN: Physiological integrity; CNS: Physiological adaptation; CL: Application

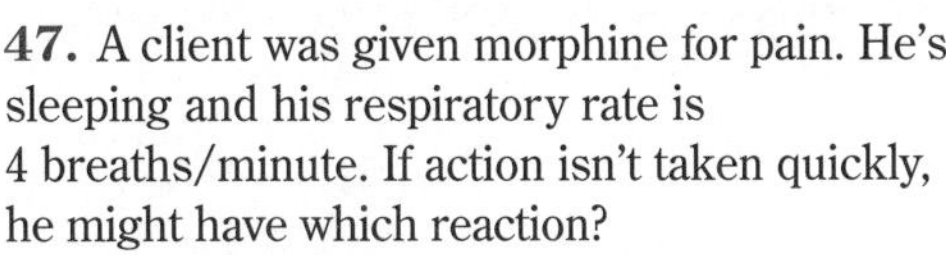

47. A client was given morphine for pain. He's sleeping and his respiratory rate is 4 breaths/minute. If action isn't taken quickly, he might have which reaction?
1. Asthma attack
2. Respiratory arrest
3. Seizure
4. Wake up on his own

47. 2. Opioids such as morphine can cause respiratory arrest if given in large quantities. It's unlikely the client will have an asthma attack or a seizure or wake up on his own.
CN: Physiological integrity; CNS: Pharmacological and parenteral therapies; CL: Analysis

48. Which additional assessment data should <u>immediately</u> be gathered to determine the status of a client with a respiratory rate of 4 breaths/minute?

1. Arterial blood gas (ABG) and breath sounds
2. Level of consciousness and a pulse oximetry value
3. Breath sounds and reflexes
4. Pulse oximetry value and heart sounds

48. 2. First, the nurse should attempt to rouse the client because this should increase the client's respiratory rate. If available, a spot pulse oximetry check should be done and breath sounds should be checked. The physician should be notified immediately of the findings. He'll probably order ABG analysis to determine specific carbon dioxide and oxygen levels, which will indicate the effectiveness of ventilation. Reflexes and heart sounds will be part of the more extensive examination done after these initial actions are completed.

CN: Physiological integrity; CNS: Physiological adaptation; CL: Application

49. A client is in danger of respiratory arrest following the administration of an opioid analgesic. An arterial blood gas value is obtained. The nurse should expect the $Paco_2$ to be which value?

1. 15 mm Hg
2. 30 mm Hg
3. 40 mm Hg
4. 80 mm Hg

49. 4. A client about to go into respiratory arrest will have inefficient ventilation and will be retaining carbon dioxide. The value expected would be around 80 mm Hg. All other values are lower than expected.

CN: Physiological integrity; CNS: Physiological adaptation; CL: Analysis

50. A client's arterial blood gas (ABG) results are as follows: pH, 7.16; $Paco_2$, 80 mm Hg; Pao_2, 46 mm Hg; HCO_3^-, 24 mEq/L; Sao_2, 81%. These ABG results represent which condition?

1. Metabolic acidosis
2. Metabolic alkalosis
3. Respiratory acidosis
4. Respiratory alkalosis

50. 3. Because the $Paco_2$ is high at 80 mm Hg and the metabolic measure, HCO_3^-, is normal, the client has respiratory acidosis. The pH is less than 7.35, acidemic, which eliminates metabolic and respiratory alkalosis as possibilities. If the HCO_3^- was below 22 mEq/L the client would have metabolic acidosis.

CN: Physiological integrity; CNS: Physiological adaptation; CL: Application

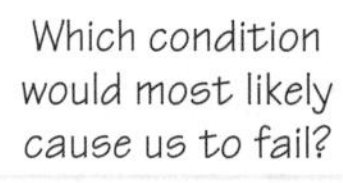
Which condition
would most likely
cause us to fail?

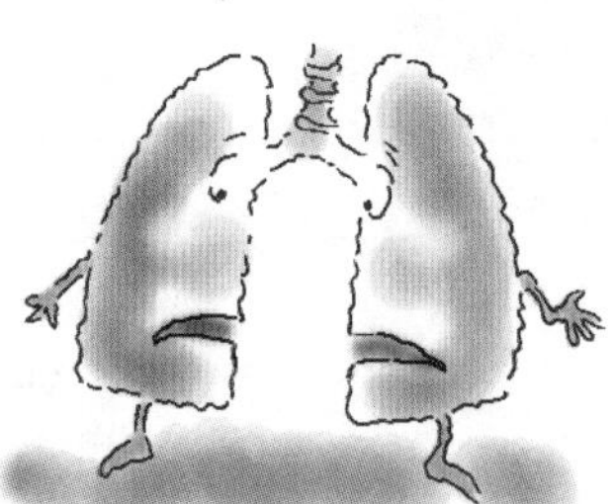

51. Clients at <u>high risk</u> for respiratory failure include those with which diagnosis?

1. Breast cancer
2. Cervical sprains
3. Fractured hip
4. Guillain-Barré syndrome

51. 4. Guillain-Barré syndrome is a progressive neuromuscular disorder that can affect the respiratory muscles and cause respiratory failure. The other conditions typically don't affect the respiratory system.

CN: Physiological integrity; CNS: Physiological adaptation; CL: Analysis

52. A client has started a new drug for hypertension. Thirty minutes after he takes the drug, he develops chest tightness and becomes short of breath and tachypneic. He has a decreased level of consciousness. These signs indicate which condition?

1. Asthma attack
2. Pulmonary embolism
3. Respiratory failure
4. Rheumatoid arthritis

52. 3. The client was reacting to the drug with respiratory signs of impending anaphylaxis, which could lead to eventual respiratory failure. Although the signs are also related to an asthma attack or a pulmonary embolism, consider the new drug first. Rheumatoid arthritis doesn't manifest these signs.

CN: Physiological integrity; CNS: Pharmacological and parenteral therapies; CL: Analysis

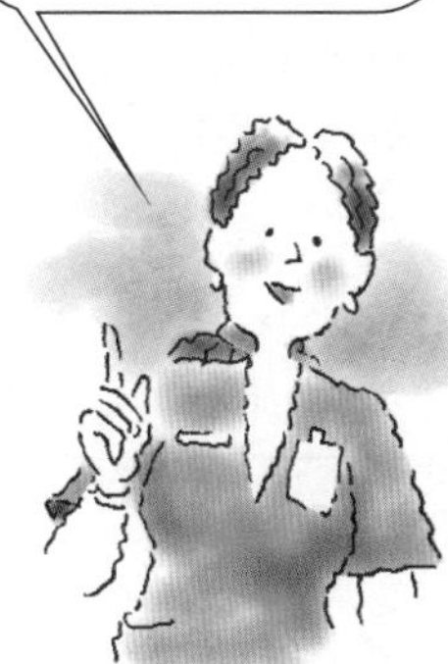

Set your priorities properly. What should be done first?

53. Emergency treatment for a client with impending anaphylaxis secondary to hypersensitivity to a drug should include which action first?

1. Administering oxygen
2. Inserting an I.V. catheter
3. Obtaining a complete blood count (CBC)
4. Taking vital signs

53. 1. Giving oxygen would be the best first action in this case. Vital signs should then be checked and the physician immediately notified. If the client doesn't already have an I.V. catheter, one may be inserted now if anaphylactic shock is developing. Obtaining a CBC wouldn't help the emergency situation.

CN: Physiological integrity; CNS: Physiological adaptation; CL: Analysis

54. Following the initial care of a client with asthma and impending anaphylaxis from hypersensitivity to a drug, the nurse should take which emergency treatment step next?

1. Administer beta-adrenergic blockers.
2. Administer bronchodilators.
3. Obtain serum electrolyte levels.
4. Have the client lie flat in the bed.

54. 2. Bronchodilators would help open the client's airway and improve his oxygenation status. Beta-adrenergic blockers aren't indicated in the management of asthma because they may cause bronchospasm. Obtaining laboratory values wouldn't be done on an emergency basis, and having the client lie flat in bed could worsen his ability to breathe.

CN: Physiological integrity; CNS: Physiological adaptation; CL: Analysis

55. A 19-year-old client went to a party, took "some pills," and drank beer. He's brought to the emergency department because he won't wake up. When assessing him, the nurse should expect to find which reaction?

1. Hyperreflexive reflexes
2. Muscle spasms
3. Shallow respirations
4. Tachypnea

55. 3. The client probably can't be roused from the combination of pills and alcohol he has taken. This has probably caused him to breathe shallowly, which, if not monitored closely, could lead to respiratory arrest. The nurse wouldn't expect to find tachypnea and doesn't have enough information about which drugs he took to expect muscle spasms or hyperreflexia.

CN: Physiological integrity; CNS: Physiological adaptation; CL: Application

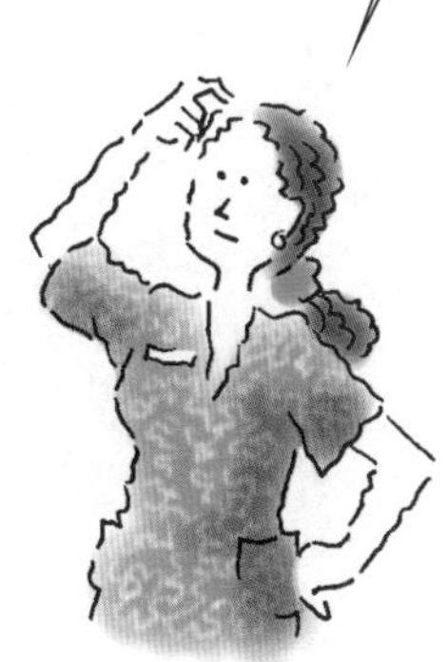

In a drug overdose, you'll want to do only one of these first. Which one?

56. Which action should be taken first in response to an initial assessment of probable opioid overdose complicated by alcohol ingestion?

1. Administer I.V. fluids.
2. Administer I.V. naloxone (Narcan).
3. Continue close monitoring of vital signs.
4. Draw blood for a drug screen.

56. 2. If the client took opioids, giving naloxone could reverse the effects and awaken the client. I.V. fluids will most likely be administered, and he'll be closely monitored over a period of several hours to several days. A drug screen should be drawn but results may not come back for several hours.

CN: Physiological integrity; CNS: Physiological adaptation; CL: Analysis

57. An unconscious client who overdosed on an opioid while consuming alcohol receives naloxone (Narcan) to reverse the overdose. After he awakens, which action by the nurse would be the best?

1. Feed the client.
2. Teach the client about the effects of taking pills and alcohol together.
3. Discharge the client from the hospital.
4. Admit the client to a psychiatric facility.

57. 2. This client needs information about the dangers of taking pills and alcohol together. It may not be advisable to feed the client at first in case his level of consciousness decreases again, increasing the possibility of aspiration. Discharge at this point is inappropriate. Unless the client was trying to commit suicide, admission to a psychiatric facility isn't necessary.
CN: Physiological integrity; CNS: Physiological adaptation; CL: Analysis

58. A firefighter was involved in extinguishing a house fire and is being treated for smoke inhalation. He develops severe hypoxia 48 hours after the incident, requiring intubation and mechanical ventilation. He most likely has developed which condition?

1. Acute respiratory distress syndrome (ARDS)
2. Atelectasis
3. Bronchitis
4. Pneumonia

58. 1. Severe hypoxia after smoke inhalation is typically related to ARDS. The other conditions listed aren't typically associated with smoke inhalation and severe hypoxia.
CN: Physiological integrity; CNS: Physiological adaptation; CL: Application

Crackle, wheeze, or rattle? Each sound is another clue.

59. In a client with smoke inhalation who develops pulmonary edema, the nurse should expect to hear which breath sound?

1. Crackles
2. Decreased breath sounds
3. Inspiratory and expiratory wheezing
4. Upper airway rhonchi

59. 1. In pulmonary edema, the most frequently heard sounds are crackles. Decreased breath sounds or inspiratory and expiratory wheezing are associated with asthma, and rhonchi are heard when there's sputum in the airways.
CN: Physiological integrity; CNS: Physiological adaptation; CL: Application

60. Which nursing diagnosis would be the priority for a client with acute respiratory distress syndrome (ARDS)?

1. *Impaired gas exchange*
2. *Risk for infection*
3. *Imbalanced nutrition: Less than body requirements*
4. *Impaired skin integrity*

60. 1. *Impaired gas exchange* is the priority nursing diagnosis. A client with ARDS usually requires intubation and mechanical ventilation. The other diagnoses are appropriate but not priority.
CN: Safe, effective care environment; CNS: Management of care; CL: Analysis

61. Which statement best describes what happens to the alveoli in acute respiratory distress syndrome (ARDS)?

1. Alveoli are overexpanded.
2. Alveoli increase perfusion.
3. Alveolar spaces are filled with fluid.
4. Alveoli improve gaseous exchange.

61. 3. In ARDS, the alveolar membranes are more permeable and the spaces are fluid-filled. Alveoli collapse, impairing gas exchange. The fluid interferes with gas exchange and reduces perfusion.
CN: Physiological integrity; CNS: Physiological adaptation; CL: Application

62. A 69-year-old client develops acute shortness of breath and progressive hypoxia requiring mechanical ventilation after repair of a fractured right femur. The hypoxia was probably caused by which condition?

1. Asthma attack
2. Atelectasis
3. Bronchitis
4. Fat embolism

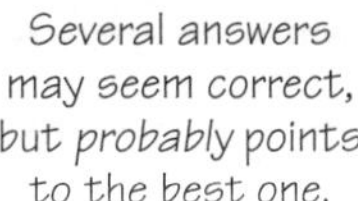

Several answers may seem correct, but *probably* points to the best one.

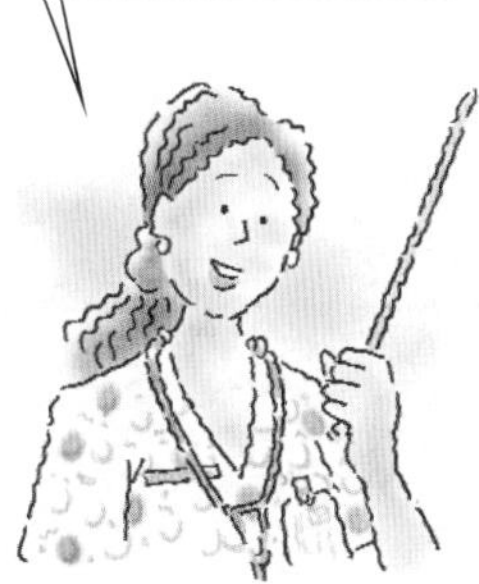

62. 4. Long bone fractures are correlated with fat emboli, which cause shortness of breath and hypoxia. It's unlikely that the client has developed asthma or bronchitis without a previous history. He could develop atelectasis, but it typically doesn't produce progressive hypoxia.
CN: Physiological integrity; CNS: Physiological adaptation; CL: Analysis

63. A client with a fat embolism is receiving 100% FIO_2 on a mechanical ventilator and continues to be hypoxic. Which measure can improve his oxygenation?

1. Add positive end-expiratory pressure (PEEP).
2. Give beta-adrenergic blockers.
3. Give diuretics.
4. Increase the FIO_2 on the ventilator.

63. 1. PEEP can be added to open up alveoli and keep them open. There's no reason to give the client beta-adrenergic blockers. He may benefit from diuresis, but in the meantime, PEEP should be added to improve oxygenation. The highest amount of oxygen that can be delivered is 100% FIO_2.
CN: Physiological integrity; CNS: Physiological adaptation; CL: Application

64. If a client with a fat embolism continues to be hypoxic following therapy with positive end-expiratory pressure, what can be done to reduce oxygen demand?

1. Give diuretics.
2. Give neuromuscular blockers.
3. Put the head of the bed flat.
4. Use bronchodilators.

64. 2. Neuromuscular blockers cause skeletal muscle paralysis, reducing the amount of oxygen used by the restless skeletal muscles. This should improve oxygenation. Diuretics can be administered to reduce pulmonary congestion and the head of the bed should be partially elevated to facilitate diaphragm movement. Bronchodilators may be used, but they typically don't have enough of an effect to reduce the amount of hypoxia present. However, diuretics, head elevation, and bronchodilators would improve oxygen delivery, not reduce oxygen demand.
CN: Physiological integrity; CNS: Physiological adaptation; CL: Application

65. Positive end-expiratory pressure (PEEP) therapy has which initial effect on the heart?

1. Bradycardia
2. Tachycardia
3. Increased blood pressure
4. Reduced cardiac output

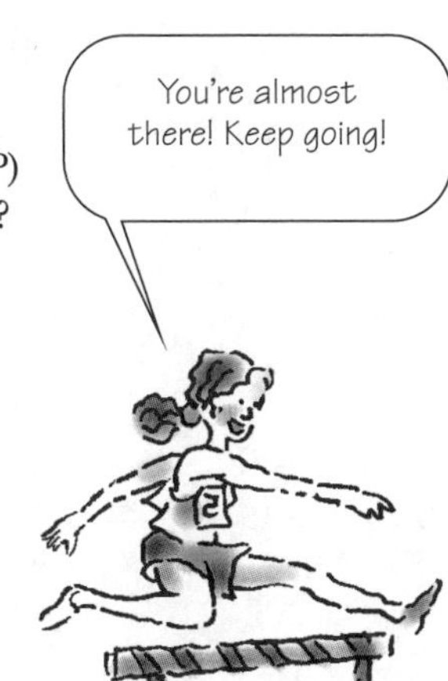

You're almost there! Keep going!

65. 4. PEEP reduces cardiac output by increasing intrathoracic pressure and reducing the amount of blood delivered to the left side of the heart, thereby reducing cardiac output. It doesn't affect heart rate, but a decrease in cardiac output may reduce blood pressure, commonly causing a compensatory tachycardia.
CN: Physiological integrity; CNS: Physiological adaptation; CL: Application

66. Occasionally, clients with acute respiratory distress syndrome (ARDS) are placed in the prone position. How does this position help the client?

1. It improves cardiac output.
2. It makes the client more comfortable.
3. It prevents skin breakdown.
4. It recruits more alveoli.

66. 4. A supine position may reduce the ability of posterior alveoli to open and remain open. Turning the client to the prone position may recruit new alveoli in the posterior region of the lung and improve oxygenation status. Cardiac output shouldn't be affected by the prone position. The prone position doesn't make the client more comfortable and he often requires sedation to tolerate it. Skin breakdown can still occur over the new pressure points.
CN: Physiological integrity; CNS: Physiological adaptation; CL: Application

67. Which condition could lead to acute respiratory distress syndrome (ARDS)?

1. Appendicitis
2. Massive trauma
3. Receiving conscious sedation
4. Right meniscus injury

67. 2. The client with massive trauma will require multiple transfusions. Blood products are preserved with citrate, which causes increased permeability in the lungs, the defect that allows ARDS to develop. Appendicitis, unless it causes overwhelming sepsis, won't lead to ARDS. Conscious sedation and injuries to the meniscus don't lead to ARDS.
CN: Physiological integrity; CNS: Physiological adaptation; CL: Analysis

68. Which indicators would show if the condition of a client with acute respiratory distress syndrome (ARDS) is improving?

1. Arterial blood gas (ABG) values
2. Bronchoscopy results
3. Increased blood pressure
4. Sputum culture and sensitivity results

68. 1. Improved ABG results would indicate that the client's oxygenation status is improved. Hypoxia is the problem in ARDS, so bronchoscopy and sputum culture results may have no bearing on the improvement of ARDS. Increased blood pressure isn't relative to the client's respiratory condition.
CN: Physiological integrity; CNS: Physiological adaptation; CL: Analysis

69. A high level of oxygen exerts which effect on the lung?

1. Improves oxygen uptake
2. Increases carbon dioxide levels
3. Stabilizes carbon dioxide levels
4. Reduces the amount of functional alveolar surface area

69. 4. Oxygen toxicity causes direct pulmonary trauma, reducing the amount of alveolar surface area available for gaseous exchange, which results in increased carbon dioxide levels and decreased oxygen uptake.
CN: Physiological integrity; CNS: Physiological adaptation; CL: Application

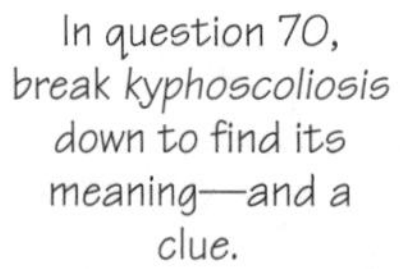

In question 70, break kyphoscoliosis down to find its meaning—and a clue.

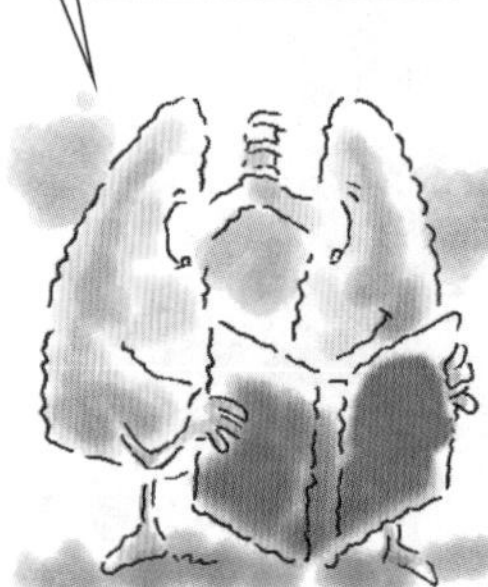

70. Which effect can thoracic kyphoscoliosis have on lung function?

1. Improves lung expansion
2. Obstructs lung deflation
3. Reduces alveolar compression during expiration
4. Restricts lung expansion

70. 4. Thoracic kyphoscoliosis causes lung compression, restricts lung expansion, and results in more rapid and shallow respiration. It doesn't improve lung expansion because of the compression. It also doesn't cause obstruction or reduce alveolar compression during expiration.
CN: Physiological integrity; CNS: Physiological adaptation; CL: Application

71. A 24-year-old client comes into the clinic complaining of right-sided chest pain and shortness of breath. He reports that it started suddenly. The assessment should include which intervention?

1. Auscultation of breath sounds
2. Chest X-ray
3. Echocardiogram
4. Electrocardiogram (ECG)

71. 1. Because the client is short of breath, listening to breath sounds is a good idea. He may need a chest X-ray and an ECG, but a physician must order these tests. Unless a cardiac source for the client's pain is identified, he won't need an echocardiogram.
CN: Physiological integrity; CNS: Physiological adaptation; CL: Application

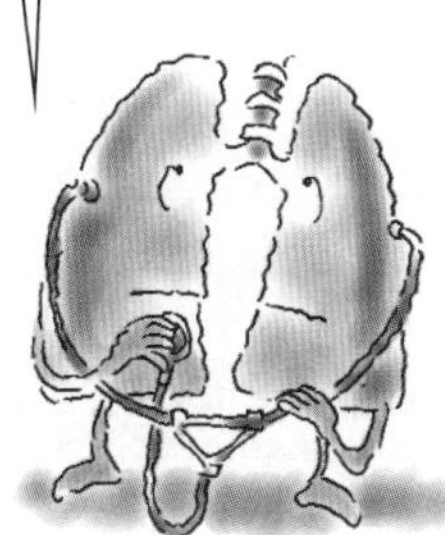
Listening to breath sounds sure helps diagnose a lot of conditions, doesn't it?

72. A client with shortness of breath has decreased-to-absent breath sounds on the right side, from the apex to the base. Which condition best explains this?

1. Acute asthma
2. Chronic bronchitis
3. Pneumonia
4. Spontaneous pneumothorax

72. 4. A spontaneous pneumothorax occurs when the client's lung collapses, causing an acute decrease in the amount of functional lung used in oxygenation. The sudden collapse was the cause of his chest pain and shortness of breath. An asthma attack would show wheezing breath sounds, and bronchitis would have rhonchi. Pneumonia would have bronchial breath sounds over the area of consolidation.
CN: Physiological integrity; CNS: Physiological adaptation; CL: Analysis

73. Which treatment should a nurse expect for a client with spontaneous pneumothorax?

1. Antibiotics
2. Bronchodilators
3. Chest tube placement
4. Hyperbaric chamber

73. 3. The only way to reexpand the lung is to place a chest tube on the right side so the air in the pleural space can be removed and the lung reexpanded. Antibiotics and bronchodilators would have no effect on lung reexpansion, nor would the hyperbaric chamber.
CN: Physiological integrity; CNS: Physiological adaptation; CL: Application

74. A 60-year-old client was in a motor vehicle collision as an unrestrained driver. He's now in the emergency department complaining of difficulty breathing and chest pain. On auscultation of his lung fields, no breath sounds are present in the left upper lobe. This client may have which condition?

1. Bronchitis
2. Pneumonia
3. Pneumothorax
4. Tuberculosis (TB)

74. 3. The client may have a left pneumothorax from the trauma he experienced. Auscultation would reveal rhonchi with bronchitis, bronchial breath sounds with pneumonia, and rhonchorous breath sounds with TB.
CN: Physiological integrity; CNS: Physiological adaptation; CL: Application

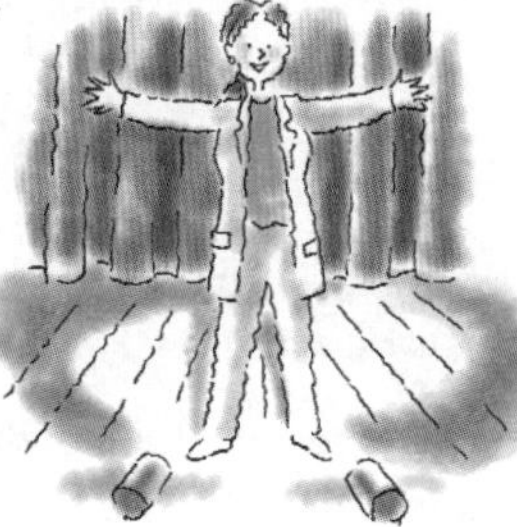
You're a natural! Keep going!

75. Which method is the best way to confirm the diagnosis of a pneumothorax?

1. Auscultate for breath sounds.
2. Have the client use an incentive spirometer.
3. Take a chest X-ray.
4. Stick a needle in the area of the decreased breath sounds.

75. 3. A chest X-ray will show the area of collapsed lung if a pneumothorax is present as well as the volume of air in the pleural space. Listening to breath sounds won't confirm a diagnosis. An incentive spirometer is used to encourage deep breathing. A needle thoracostomy is done only in an emergency and only by someone trained to do it.
CN: Physiological integrity; CNS: Physiological adaptation; CL: Application

76. After a motor vehicle collision, a client has a chest tube inserted in the left upper chest. When the tube is inserted, it begins to drain a large amount of dark red fluid. Which explanation best describes what caused this?

1. The chest tube was inserted improperly.
2. This always happens when a chest tube is inserted.
3. An artery was nicked when the chest tube was placed.
4. The client had a hemothorax instead of a pneumothorax.

76. 4. Because of the traumatic cause of injury, the client had a hemothorax, in which blood collection causes the collapse of the lung. The placement of the chest tube will drain the blood from the space and reexpand the lung. There's a very slight chance of nicking an intercostal artery during insertion, but it's fairly unlikely if the person placing the chest tube has been trained. The initial chest X-ray would help confirm whether there was blood in the pleural space or just air.

CN: Physiological integrity; CNS: Physiological adaptation; CL: Application

77. A hospitalized client needs a central I.V. catheter inserted. The physician places the catheter in the subclavian vein. Shortly afterward, the client develops shortness of breath and appears restless. Which action should the nurse perform first?

1. Administer a sedative.
2. Advise the client to calm down.
3. Auscultate for breath sounds.
4. Check to see if the client can have medication.

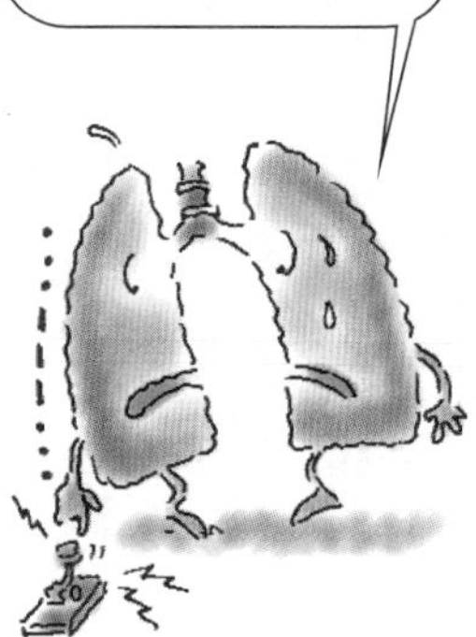

When I'm in distress, what should you do first?

77. 3. Because this is an acute episode, listen to the client's lungs to see if anything has changed. Don't give this client medication, especially sedatives, if he's having difficulty breathing. Give the client emotional support and contact the physician who placed the central venous access.

CN: Physiological integrity; CNS: Physiological adaptation; CL: Analysis

78. Which measure would be ordered for a client who recently had a central venous catheter inserted and who now appears short of breath and anxious?

1. Chest X-ray
2. Electrocardiogram
3. Laboratory tests
4. Sedation

78. 1. Inserting an I.V. catheter in the subclavian vein can result in a pneumothorax, so a chest X-ray should be done. If it's negative, then other tests should be done but they aren't appropriate as the first intervention. Sedation may depress respirations.

CN: Physiological integrity; CNS: Reduction of risk potential; CL: Application

79. A client needs to have a chest tube inserted in the right upper chest. Which action is part of the nurse's role?

1. The nurse isn't needed.
2. Prepare the chest tube drainage system.
3. Bring the chest X-ray to the client's room.
4. Insert the chest tube.

79. 2. The nurse must anticipate that a drainage system is required and set this up before insertion so the tube can be directly connected to the drainage system. The chest X-ray need not be brought to the client's room. A physician will insert the chest tube.

CN: Physiological integrity; CNS: Physiological adaptation; CL: Application

80. The nurse is auscultating the lungs of a client following chest tube insertion. Which of the following results indicates to the nurse correct chest tube placement?

1. Bronchial sounds heard at both bases
2. Vesicular sounds heard over upper lung fields
3. Bronchovesicular sounds heard over both lung fields
4. Crackles heard on the affected side

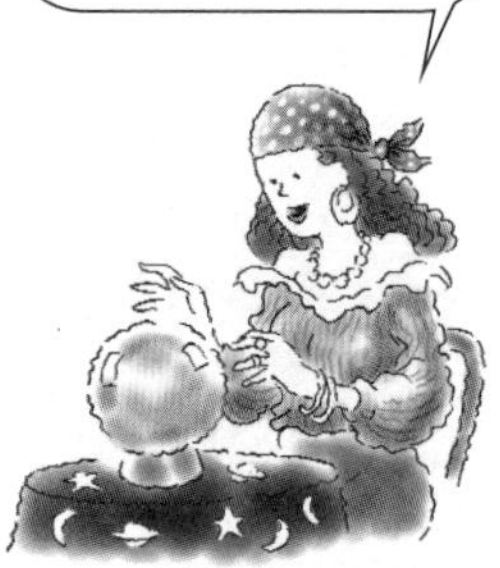

Which breath sounds do I predict hearing after chest tube insertion?

80. 3. If the chest tube is inserted correctly, normal bronchovesicular breath sounds in that area will be heard and the client's oxygenation status will improve. A chest X-ray should be done to ensure reexpansion. All other sounds noted are abnormal.

CN: Physiological integrity; CNS: Reduction of risk potential; CL: Analysis

81. Which measure <u>best</u> determines that a chest tube is no longer needed for a client who had a pneumothorax?

1. The drainage from the chest tube is minimal.
2. Arterial blood gas (ABG) levels are obtained to ensure proper oxygenation.
3. It's removed and the client is assessed to see if he's breathing adequately.
4. No fluctuation in the water seal chamber occurs when no suction is applied.

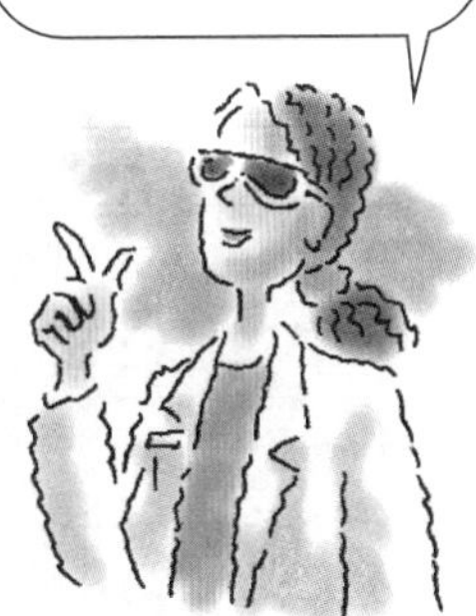

Go for the best!

81. 4. One indication of reexpansion is the cessation of fluctuation in the water seal chamber when suction isn't applied. Drainage should be minimal before the chest tube is removed. An ABG analysis may be done to ensure proper oxygenation but isn't necessary if clinical assessment criteria are met. The chest tube isn't removed until it's determined the client's lung has adequately reexpanded and will stay that way. After the lung stays expanded, the chest tube is removed.

CN: Physiological integrity; CNS: Physiological adaptation; CL: Analysis

82. Which intervention should be done <u>before</u> a chest tube is removed?

1. Disconnect the drainage system from the tube.
2. Obtain a chest X-ray to document reexpansion.
3. Obtain an arterial blood gas level to document oxygen status.
4. Sedate the client, and the physician will slip the tube out without warning the client.

82. 2. A chest X-ray should be done to ensure and document that the lung is reexpanded and has remained expanded since suction was discontinued. The drainage system shouldn't be disconnected from the tube while still in the client because that could cause a pneumothorax to recur. A pulse oximetry measurement is sufficient to track oxygenation before the tube is removed. Client cooperation is desirable; if the client can hold his breath while the chest tube is removed, there's less chance that air will be drawn back into the pleural space during removal.

CN: Physiological integrity; CNS: Reduction of risk potential; CL: Application

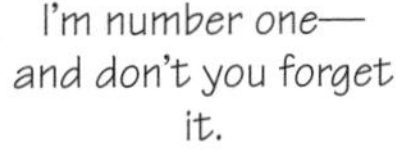

I'm number one—
and don't you forget it.

83. The nurse is teaching a client about lung cancer. The client indicates an understanding of the number one cause of lung cancer when he makes which of the following responses?

1. Genetics
2. Occupational exposures
3. Smoking a pipe
4. Smoking cigarettes

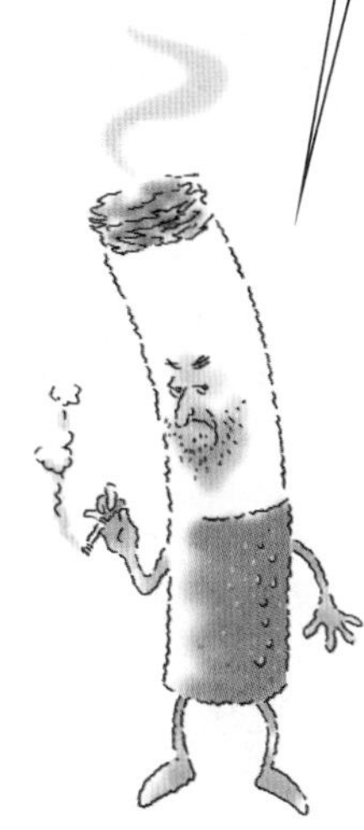

83. 4. As many as 90% of clients with lung cancer smoke cigarettes. Cigarette smoke contains several organ-specific carcinogens. There may be a genetic predisposition for the development of cancer. Occupational hazards such as pollutants can cause cancer. Pipe smokers inhale less often than cigarette smokers and tend to develop cancers of the lip and mouth.

CN: Health promotion and maintenance; CNS: None; CL: Application

84. A nurse is preparing to reinforce the teaching plan for a client who has recently been diagnosed with squamous cell carcinoma of the left lung. Which statement by the nurse is correct?

1. "You have a slow-growing cancer that rarely spreads."
2. "In terms of prognosis, you may have only a few months to live."
3. "Squamous cell cancer is a very rapid-growing cancer."
4. "The cancer has generally metastasized by the time diagnosis is made."

84. 1. Squamous cell carcinoma is a slow-growing, rarely metastasizing type of cancer. It has the best prognosis of all lung cancer types.

CN: Physiological integrity; CNS: Physiological adaptation; CL: Analysis

85. A client is exhibiting the symptoms listed below. Which one should be investigated first as a potential symptom of lung cancer?
1. Dizziness
2. Generalized weakness
3. Hypotension
4. Recurrent pleural effusions

85. 4. Recurring episodes of pleural effusions can be caused by the tumor and should be investigated. Dizziness, generalized weakness, and hypotension aren't typically considered warning signals, but may occur in advanced stages of cancer.
CN: Physiological integrity; CNS: Physiological adaptation; CL: Application

Centrally located. That's your clue for question 86.

86. The nurse is assessing a client with a centrally located lung tumor. Which of the following symptoms would the client most likely have?
1. Coughing
2. Hemoptysis
3. Pleuritic pain
4. Shoulder pain

86. 1. Centrally located lung tumors are found in the upper airway and usually produce such symptoms as coughing, wheezing, and stridor. Small cell tumors tend to be located in the lower airways and often cause hemoptysis. Tumors invading the pleural space may cause pleuritic pain. Pancoast tumors that occur in the apices may cause shoulder pain.
CN: Physiological integrity; CNS: Physiological adaptation; CL: Analysis

87. A definitive diagnosis of lung cancer is obtained by which evaluation?
1. Bronchoscopy
2. Chest X-ray
3. Computed tomography (CT) scan of the chest
4. Surgical biopsy

87. 4. Only surgical biopsy with cytologic examination of the cells can give a definitive diagnosis of cancer and type. Bronchoscopy gives positive results in only 30% of the cases. Chest X-ray and CT scan can identify location of abnormal tissue but not confirm cancer.
CN: Physiological integrity; CNS: Physiological adaptation; CL: Application

88. Which statements are true about staging lung cancer tumors? Select all that apply:
1. Staging describes the severity of the cancer.
2. Staging helps the physician plan appropriate treatment.
3. Staging systems don't change over time.
4. Surgical biopsy with cytologic cell examination is the only data collection method used to perform staging.
5. Staging helps to determine whether the cancer has spread to distant areas of the body.

88. 1, 2, 5. Staging describes the extent and severity of the cancer and helps the physician determine the most appropriate therapy. Staging systems continue to evolve as cancer is better understood. Multiple data collection methods, such as laboratory results, physical examinations, and imaging results, are used to determine the stage of a cancer.
CN: Physiological integrity; CNS: Physiological adaptation; CL: Analysis

89. Which intervention is the key to increasing the survival rates of clients with lung cancer?
1. Early bronchoscopy
2. Early detection
3. High-dose chemotherapy
4. Smoking cessation

89. 2. Early detection of cancer when the cells may be premalignant and potentially curable would be most beneficial. However, a tumor must be 1 cm in diameter before it's detectable on a chest X-ray. A bronchoscopy may help early identification but is often not ordered until an abnormal X-ray is seen. High-dose chemotherapy has minimal effect on long-term survival. Smoking cessation won't reverse the process but may prevent further decompensation.
CN: Health promotion and maintenance; CNS: None; CL: Application

CN: Client needs category CNS: Client needs subcategory CL: Cognitive level

90. A client with a chest tube has accidentally removed it. What action should the nurse perform first?

1. Position the client on his left side.
2. Position the client on his right side.
3. Apply an occlusive dressing over the site.
4. Reinsert the chest tube that fell out.

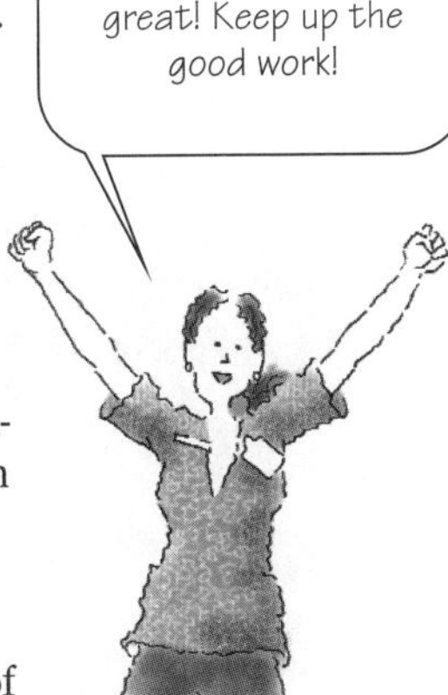

You're doing great! Keep up the good work!

90. 3. To prevent the client from sucking air into the pleural space and causing a pneumothorax, an occlusive dressing should be put over the hole where the tube came out. The physician should be called and the client checked for signs of respiratory distress. Positioning the client on either the left or right side won't make a difference. It isn't advisable for the physician to reinsert the old tube because it's no longer sterile.

CN: Physiological integrity; CNS: Reduction of risk potential; CL: Application

91. A client has been diagnosed with lung cancer and requires a wedge resection. How much of the lung is removed?

1. One entire lung
2. A lobe of the lung
3. A small, localized area near the surface of the lung
4. A segment of the lung, including a bronchiole and its alveoli

91. 3. A small area of tissue close to the surface of the lung is removed in a wedge resection. An entire lung is removed in a pneumonectomy. A lobe is removed in a lobectomy, and a segment of the lung is removed in a segmental resection.

CN: Physiological integrity; CNS: Physiological adaptation; CL: Application

92. When a client has a lobectomy, what fills the space where the lobe was?

1. The space stays empty.
2. The surgeon fills the space with a gel.
3. The lung space fills up with serous fluid.
4. The remaining lobe or lobes overexpand to fill the space.

92. 4. The remaining lobe or lobes overexpand slightly to fill the space previously occupied by the removed tissue. The diaphragm is carried higher on the operative side to further reduce the empty space. The space can't remain "empty" because truly empty would imply a vacuum, which would interfere with the intrathoracic pressure changes that allow breathing. The surgeon doesn't use gel to fill the space. Serous fluid overproduction would compress the remaining lobes, diminish their function, and, possibly, cause a mediastinal shift.

CN: Physiological integrity; CNS: Physiological adaptation; CL: Application

93. If a client requires a pneumonectomy, what fills the area of the thoracic cavity?

1. The space remains filled with air only.
2. The surgeon fills the space with a gel.
3. Serous fluid fills the space and consolidates the region.
4. The tissue from the other lung grows over to the other side.

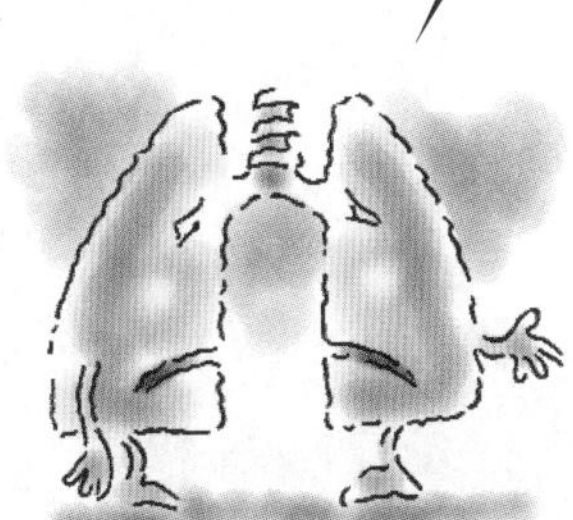

What happens when there is only one of me?

93. 3. Serous fluid fills the space and eventually consolidates, preventing extensive mediastinal shift of the heart and remaining lung. Air can't be left in the space. There's no gel that can be placed in the pleural space. The tissue from the other lung can't cross the mediastinum, although a temporary mediastinal shift exists until the space is filled.

CN: Physiological integrity; CNS: Physiological adaptation; CL: Application

94. During a pneumonectomy, the phrenic nerve on the surgical side is usually cut to cause hemidiaphragm paralysis. Why is this done?

1. Paralyzing the diaphragm reduces oxygen demand.
2. Cutting the phrenic nerve reduces postoperative pain.
3. It will increase the capacity of the remaining lung.
4. It will reduce the space left by the pneumonectomy.

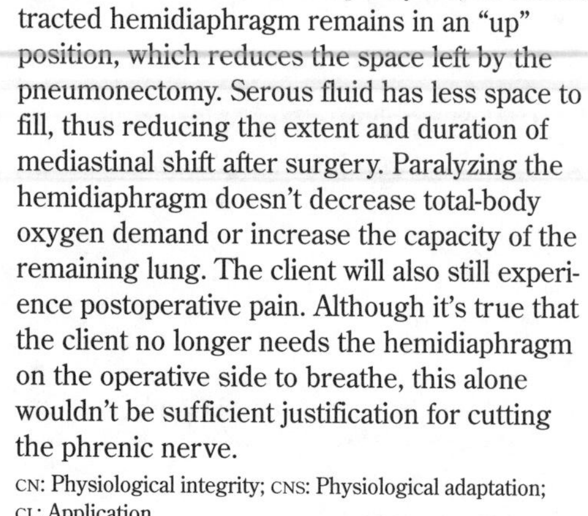

94. 4. Because the hemidiaphragm is a muscle that doesn't contract when paralyzed, an uncontracted hemidiaphragm remains in an "up" position, which reduces the space left by the pneumonectomy. Serous fluid has less space to fill, thus reducing the extent and duration of mediastinal shift after surgery. Paralyzing the hemidiaphragm doesn't decrease total-body oxygen demand or increase the capacity of the remaining lung. The client will also still experience postoperative pain. Although it's true that the client no longer needs the hemidiaphragm on the operative side to breathe, this alone wouldn't be sufficient justification for cutting the phrenic nerve.

CN: Physiological integrity; CNS: Physiological adaptation; CL: Application

95. Which result is the <u>primary</u> goal of surgical resection for lung cancer?

1. To remove the tumor and all surrounding tissue
2. To remove the tumor and as little surrounding tissue as possible
3. To remove all the tumor and any collapsed alveoli in the same region
4. To remove as much of the tumor as possible, without removing any alveoli

95. 2. The goal of surgical resection is to remove the lung tissue that has a tumor in it while saving as much surrounding tissue as possible. It may be necessary to remove alveoli and bronchioles, but care is taken to make sure only what's absolutely necessary is removed.

CN: Physiological integrity; CNS: Physiological adaptation; CL: Application

96. If a client with lung cancer also has preexisting pulmonary disease, which statement best describes how this affects the extent of surgery that can be performed?

1. It doesn't affect it.
2. It may require a whole lung to be removed.
3. The entire tumor may not be able to be removed.
4. It may prevent surgery if the client can't tolerate lung tissue removal.

96. 4. If the client's preexisting pulmonary disease is restrictive and advanced, it may be impossible to perform surgery, and the client may have to be treated with only chemotherapy and radiation.

CN: Physiological integrity; CNS: Physiological adaptation; CL: Application

97. Preoperative teaching for the client having surgery should focus on which area?

1. Deciding if the client should have the surgery
2. Giving emotional support to the client and his family
3. Giving minute details of the surgery to the client and his family
4. Providing general information to reduce client and family anxiety

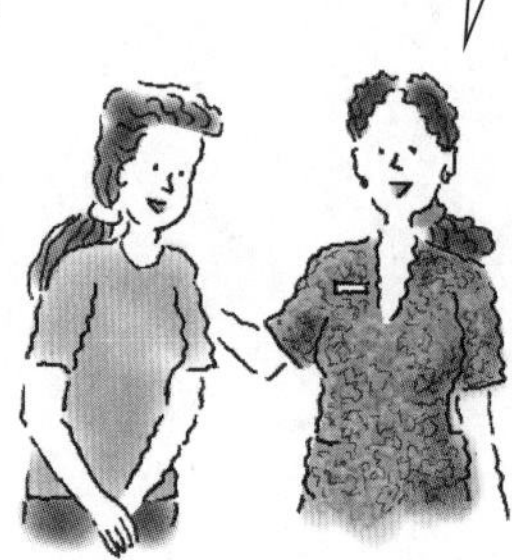

The nurse does a lot of teaching but in this case, what would be the main focus?

97. 4. The nurse's role is to provide general information about the surgery and what to expect before and after surgery, and to give emotional support during this time. The nurse's role isn't to decide if the client should have surgery or to give minute details of the surgery unless the client or family requests them, in which case the surgeon should answer the questions. Emotional support alone during this time isn't sufficient.

CN: Physiological integrity; CNS: Reduction of risk potential; CL: Application

98. A client with a benign lung tumor is treated in which way?

1. The tumor is treated with radiation only.
2. The tumor is treated with chemotherapy only.
3. The tumor is left alone unless symptoms are present.
4. The tumor is removed, involving the least possible amount of tissue.

98. 4. The tumor is removed to prevent further compression of lung tissue as the tumor grows, which could lead to respiratory decompensation. If for some reason it can't be removed, then radiation or chemotherapy may be used to try to shrink the tumor.

CN: Physiological integrity; CNS: Physiological adaptation; CL: Application

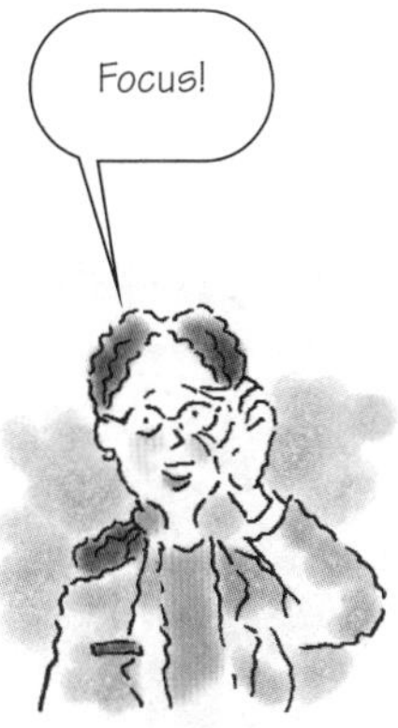

99. In a client with terminal lung cancer, the primary focus of nursing care is on which nursing intervention?

1. Provide emotional support.
2. Provide nutritional support.
3. Provide pain control.
4. Prepare the client's will.

99. 3. The client with terminal lung cancer may have extreme pleuritic pain and should be treated to reduce his discomfort. Preparing the client and his family for the impending death and providing emotional support is also important but shouldn't be the primary focus until pain is under control. Nutritional support may be provided, but as the terminal phase advances, the client's nutritional needs greatly decrease. Nursing care doesn't focus on helping the client prepare a will.

CN: Physiological integrity; CNS: Basic care and comfort; CL: Analysis

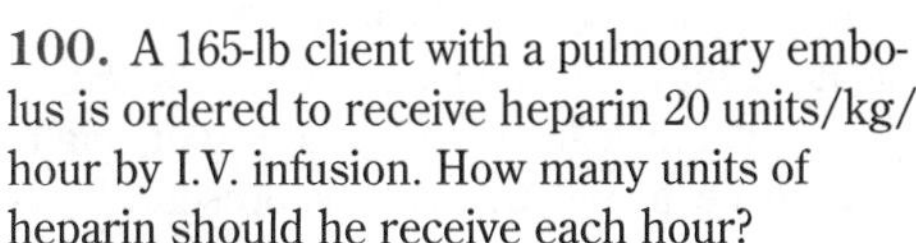

100. A 165-lb client with a pulmonary embolus is ordered to receive heparin 20 units/kg/hour by I.V. infusion. How many units of heparin should he receive each hour?

1. 1,000
2. 1,200
3. 1,500
4. 1,700

100. 3. A 165-lb client weighs 75 kg (2.2 lbs = 1 kg). 20 units × 75 kg × 1 hour = 1,500 units/hour.

CN: Physiological integrity; CNS: Pharmacological and parenteral therapies; CL: Application

101. Which of the following is the most common origin for a pulmonary embolism?

1. Amniotic fluid
2. Bone marrow
3. Septic thrombi
4. Venous thrombi

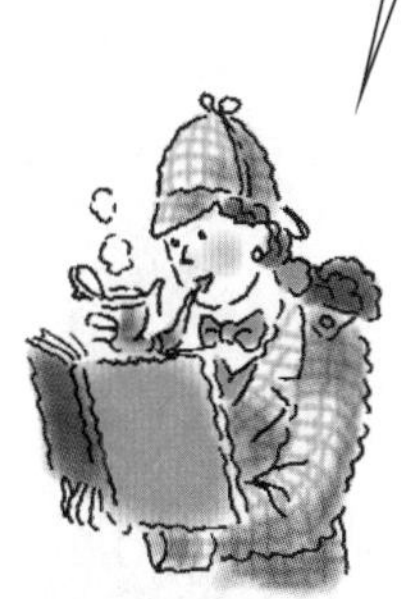

This clue asks you to select the most common, even when all answers are correct.

101. 4. Venous thrombi in the thigh and pelvis are the most common sources for pulmonary emboli. Clients who are immobile form clots from this source. When dislodged, the clots are carried through the bloodstream and lodge in the pulmonary vasculature. The other options are also sources, but not the most common.

CN: Physiological integrity; CNS: Physiological adaptation; CL: Application

102. Which client is at highest risk for developing a pulmonary embolism?

1. An ambulatory client with an inflammatory joint disease
2. An ambulatory client who has type I diabetes
3. A healthy client who's 6 months pregnant
4. A client who has fractures of his pelvis and right femur

102. 4. Thrombosis formation is caused by abnormalities in blood flow, vein wall integrity, and blood coagulation. The client with pelvic and femur fractures will be immobilized and probably have edema which leads to venous stasis and predisposes him to the development of deep vein thrombosis. A pulmonary embolus commonly arises from clots in the deep veins of the leg that break off and travel to the pulmonary arteries. The risk of developing venous thrombosis isn't as high with the other conditions.

CN: Physiological integrity; CNS: Physiological adaptation; CL: Application

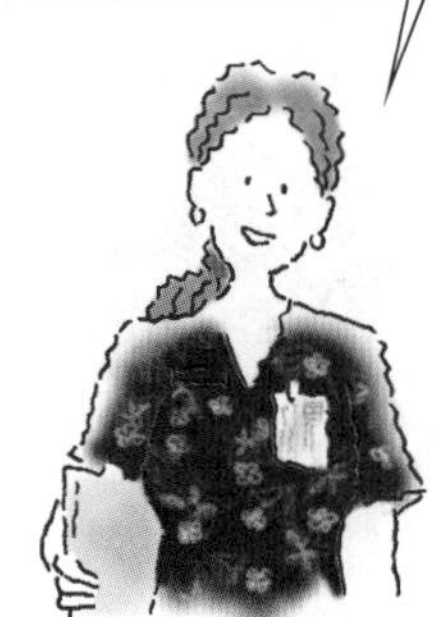

Hint! Check out the word best!

103. Which intervention to prevent pulmonary embolism after lower extremity surgery is the best?

1. Early ambulation
2. Frequent chest X-rays to find a pulmonary embolism
3. Frequent lower extremity scans
4. Intubation of the client

103. 1. Early ambulation helps reduce pooling of blood, which reduces the tendency of the blood to form a clot that could then dislodge. Frequent chest X-rays or lower extremity scans don't prevent pulmonary embolism. Intubation of the client won't prevent the occurrence of a pulmonary embolism.

CN: Physiological integrity; CNS: Reduction of risk potential; CL: Application

104. Which physiologic effects of a pulmonary embolism would initially affect oxygenation?

1. A blood clot blocks ventilation; perfusion is unaffected.
2. A blood clot blocks ventilation, producing hypoxia despite normal perfusion.
3. A blood clot blocks perfusion and ventilation, producing profound hypoxia.
4. A blood clot blocks perfusion, producing hypoxia despite normal or supernormal ventilation.

104. 4. The blood clot blocks blood flow to a region of the lung tissue. That area remains ventilated, but because blood flow is blocked, no gas exchange can occur in that region and a ventilation-perfusion mismatch is present. Ventilation isn't initially affected by a blood clot because air can still move normally through the bronchial tree.

CN: Physiological integrity; CNS: Physiological adaptation; CL: Application

105. Which statement best describes the ventilation-perfusion mismatch that occurs with a pulmonary embolism?

1. The area of the lung being ventilated isn't being perfused.
2. The area of the lung being perfused isn't being ventilated.
3. The area of the lung being ventilated is also being perfused.
4. The amount of ventilation occurring doesn't equal perfusion.

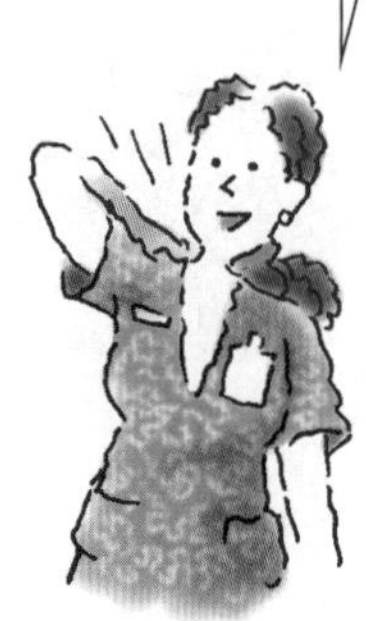

Pat yourself on the back and keep going. Good job!

105. 1. A pulmonary embolism blocks the flow of blood past a region of the lung tissue, which is still being ventilated because no disorder of the bronchial tree exists. A pulmonary embolism blocks the pulmonary vasculature, not allowing blood to flow to the distal region of the lung and interfering with gas exchange. Blood must flow around each alveolus, or perfuse, for the exchange of carbon dioxide and oxygen to occur across the alveolar-capillary membrane. When an area of lung is ventilated but not perfused, there is a ventilation-perfusion mismatch specific to pulmonary embolism. A mismatch that shows impaired ventilation but normal perfusion indicates a pathological state in the bronchial tree, such as pneumonia or atelectasis.

CN: Physiological integrity; CNS: Physiological adaptation; CL: Application

CN: Client needs category CNS: Client needs subcategory CL: Cognitive level

106. When a client has a pulmonary embolism, he may develop chest pain caused by which condition?

1. Costochondritis
2. Myocardial infarction (MI)
3. Inflammatory reaction
4. Referred pain from the pelvis to the chest

106. 3. Pleuritic pain is caused by the inflammatory reaction of the lung parenchyma. The pain isn't associated with costochondritis, MI, or referred pain from the pelvis to the chest.

CN: Physiological integrity; CNS: Physiological adaptation; CL: Application

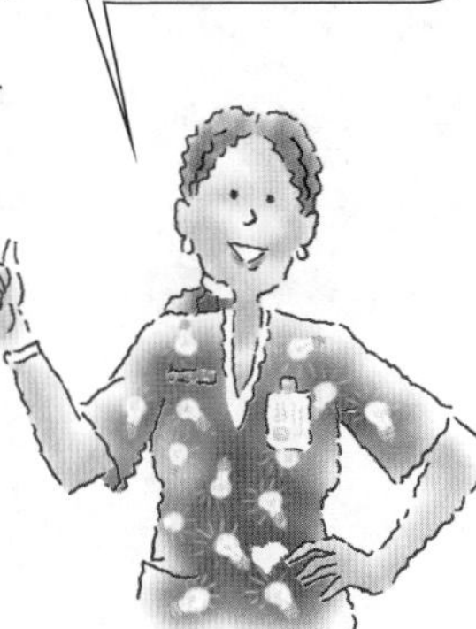

Here's a hint for question 107: Think about what causes the condition.

107. A client with a pulmonary embolism frequently feels apprehension or a sense of "impending doom" because of which reason?

1. Inflammatory reaction in the lung parenchyma
2. Loss of chest expansion
3. Loss of lung tissue
4. Sudden reduction in adequate oxygenation

107. 4. The client with a pulmonary embolism has a portion of the lung not involved in oxygenation, causing the client to feel apprehensive. If the area involved is large, the apprehension can be great, giving the client the feeling of "impending doom." The inflammatory reaction in the lung causes chest pain. There's no actual loss of lung tissue, and chest expansion isn't affected.

CN: Physiological integrity; CNS: Physiological adaptation; CL: Application

108. A client with pulmonary embolism has developed hemoptysis. Which of the following responses would best explain this symptom?

1. Alveolar damage in the infarcted area
2. Involvement of major blood vessels where the clot formed
3. Loss of lung parenchyma
4. Loss of lung tissue

108. 1. The infarcted area produces alveolar damage that can lead to the production of bloody sputum, sometimes in massive amounts. Clot formation usually occurs in the legs. There's a loss of lung parenchyma and subsequent scar tissue formation, but these don't cause hemoptysis.

CN: Physiological integrity; CNS: Physiological adaptation; CL: Application

109. A client with a massive pulmonary embolism will have an arterial blood gas analysis performed to determine the extent of hypoxia. Which acid-base disorder may be present?

1. Metabolic acidosis
2. Metabolic alkalosis
3. Respiratory acidosis
4. Respiratory alkalosis

109. 4. A client with a massive pulmonary embolism will have a large region of lung tissue unavailable for perfusion. This causes the client to hyperventilate and blow off large amounts of carbon dioxide, which crosses the unaffected alveolar-capillary membrane more readily than does oxygen and results in respiratory alkalosis.

CN: Physiological integrity; CNS: Physiological adaptation; CL: Analysis

110. A ventilation-perfusion ($\dot{V}/\dot{Q}$) scan is commonly performed to diagnose a pulmonary embolism. This test provides what type of information?

1. Amount of perfusion present in the lung
2. Extent of the occlusion and amount of perfusion lost
3. Location of the pulmonary embolism
4. Location and size of the pulmonary embolism

110. 2. The $\dot{V}/\dot{Q}$ scan provides information on the extent of occlusion caused by the pulmonary embolism and the amount of lung tissue involved in the area not perfused.

CN: Physiological integrity; CNS: Physiological adaptation; CL: Application

111. Which test definitively diagnoses a pulmonary embolism?

1. Arterial blood gas (ABG) analysis
2. Chest X-ray
3. Pulmonary angiogram
4. Ventilation-perfusion ($\dot{V}/\dot{Q}$) scan

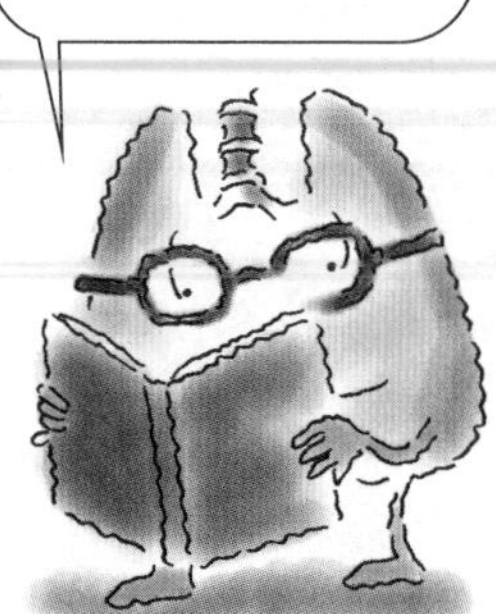

Watch that word, definitively.

111. 3. A pulmonary angiogram is used to definitively diagnose a pulmonary embolism. A catheter is passed through the circulation to the region of the occlusion; the region can be outlined with an injection of contrast medium and viewed by fluoroscopy. This shows the location of the clot, as well as the extent of the perfusion defect. ABG levels can define the amount of hypoxia present. A chest X-ray can't provide a definitive diagnosis of pulmonary embolism. The $\dot{V}/\dot{Q}$ scan can report whether there's a $\dot{V}/\dot{Q}$ mismatch present and define the amount of tissue involved.

CN: Physiological integrity; CNS: Reduction of risk potential; CL: Application

112. Which medication is prescribed after a pulmonary embolism is diagnosed?

1. Warfarin (Coumadin)
2. Heparin
3. Streptokinase (Streptase)
4. Acyclovir (Zovirax)

112. 2. Heparin is started I.V. once a pulmonary embolism is diagnosed to reduce further clot formation. When a therapeutic level of heparin is established, warfarin is started. It can take up to 3 days before a therapeutic level of warfarin is achieved. Streptokinase is a fibrinolytic, and its usefulness in the management of pulmonary embolism is unclear. Acyclovir is an antiviral and is not prescribed after a pulmonary embolism.

CN: Physiological integrity; CNS: Pharmacological and parenteral therapies; CL: Application

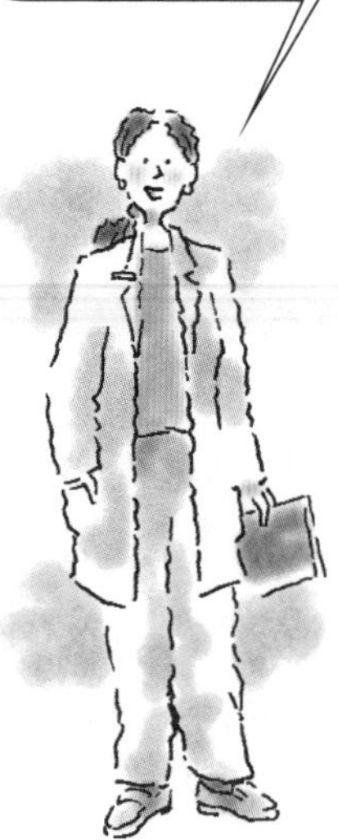

Knowing what a treatment should achieve will help you monitor the response.

113. I.V. heparin is given to clients with pulmonary embolism for which reason?

1. To dissolve the clot
2. To break up the pulmonary embolism
3. To slow the development of other clots
4. To prevent clots from breaking off and embolizing to the lung

113. 3. Heparin slows the development of other clots. It doesn't break up pulmonary embolisms or dissolve clots already formed. Heparin doesn't stop clots from going to the lung.

CN: Physiological integrity; CNS: Pharmacological and parenteral therapies; CL: Application

114. A client who was hospitalized for pulmonary embolism is being discharged on warfarin (Coumadin) therapy. Which teaching by the nurse about warfarin therapy is correct?

1. It inhibits the formation of blood clots.
2. It's given to continue to reduce the size of the pulmonary embolism.
3. It will reduce blood pressure and prevent venous stasis.
4. Coagulation studies to monitor bleeding times will be necessary every 6 months.

114. 1. Warfarin inhibits clot formation by interfering with clotting factors that are dependent on Vitamin K. Warfarin doesn't dissolve clots and won't reduce the size of the pulmonary embolus. It doesn't reduce blood pressure and won't prevent venous stasis. Coagulation studies will be performed every 2 to 4 weeks while the client is receiving warfarin.

CN: Physiological integrity; CNS: Pharmacological and parenteral therapies; CL: Application

CN: Client needs category CNS: Client needs subcategory CL: Cognitive level

115. The goal of oxygen therapy for a client with a pulmonary embolism is to obtain which value?

1. $Paco_2$ greater than 40 mm Hg
2. $Paco_2$ less than 40 mm Hg
3. Pao_2 greater than 60 mm Hg
4. Pao_2 less than 60 mm Hg

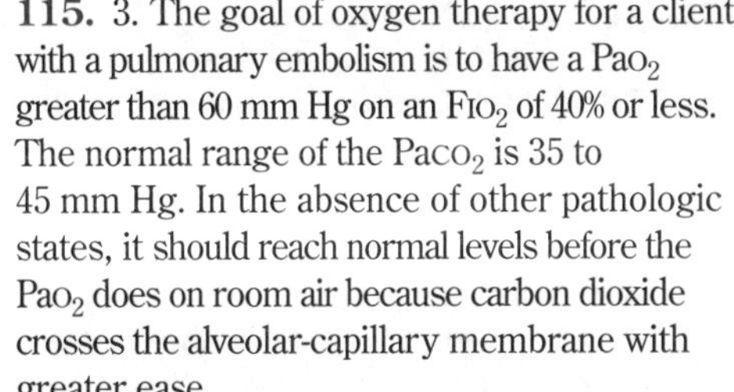

Remember, hypo and hyper are opposites.
HYPER
HYPO

115. 3. The goal of oxygen therapy for a client with a pulmonary embolism is to have a Pao_2 greater than 60 mm Hg on an Fio_2 of 40% or less. The normal range of the $Paco_2$ is 35 to 45 mm Hg. In the absence of other pathologic states, it should reach normal levels before the Pao_2 does on room air because carbon dioxide crosses the alveolar-capillary membrane with greater ease.

CN: Physiological integrity; CNS: Reduction of risk potential; CL: Analysis

116. A client may develop hypotension caused by a pulmonary embolism that produces which result?

1. Pressure on the heart and reduced cardiac output
2. Reduced blood flow to the lung, which causes hypotension
3. Reduced blood return to the right side of the heart leading to lower blood pressure
4. Increased pulmonary vascular resistance and reduced blood delivery to the left side of the heart

116. 4. Blood meets resistance and can't perfuse the pulmonary vasculature because of the embolism. Pulmonary vascular resistance is increased, which reduces the amount of blood returned to the left side of the heart, lowers the cardiac output of the heart, and reduces blood pressure, sometimes significantly.

CN: Physiological integrity; CNS: Physiological adaptation; CL: Application

117. A client with a pulmonary embolism typically has chest pain and apprehension. Which of the following would be the <u>best</u> treatment method?

1. Administering analgesics
2. Using guided imagery
3. Positioning the client on his left side
4. Providing emotional support

117. 1. Once the pulmonary embolism has been diagnosed and the amount of hypoxia determined, chest pain and the accompanying apprehension can be treated with analgesics as long as respiratory status isn't compromised. Using guided imagery and providing emotional support can be used as alternatives. Positioning the client on his left side when a pulmonary embolism is suspected may prevent a clot that has extended through the capillaries and into the pulmonary veins from breaking off and traveling through the heart into the arterial circulation, leading to a massive stroke.

CN: Physiological integrity; CNS: Physiological adaptation; CL: Application

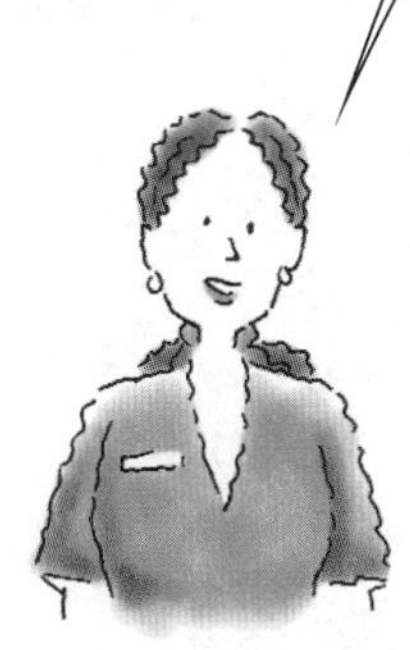

Always know the whys of a condition, especially the most common ones, like this one.

118. A client with a pulmonary embolism may have an umbrella filter placed in the vena cava for which reason?

1. The filter prevents further clot formation.
2. The filter collects clots so they don't go to the lung.
3. The filter breaks up clots into insignificantly small pieces.
4. The filter contains anticoagulants that are slowly released, dissolving any clots.

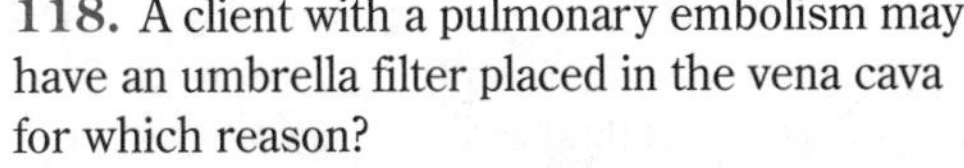

118. 3. The umbrella filter is placed in a client at high risk for the formation of more clots that could potentially become pulmonary emboli. The filter breaks the clots into small pieces that won't significantly occlude the pulmonary vasculature. The filter doesn't prevent further clot formation and doesn't release anticoagulants. The filter doesn't collect the clots, because if it did, it would have to be emptied periodically, causing the client to require surgery in the future.

CN: Physiological integrity; CNS: Physiological adaptation; CL: Application

119. The nurse is teaching a client with a pulmonary embolism who may need an embolectomy. Which of the following statements by the nurse would most accurately describe this procedure?

1. "It is done to remove an embolism in the lower extremity."
2. "It sucks an embolism out of the lung by bronchoscopy."
3. "It surgically removes the embolism source in the pelvis."
4. "It surgically removes the embolism in the pulmonary vasculature."

119. 4. If the pulmonary embolism is large and doesn't respond to treatment, surgical removal may be necessary to restore perfusion to the area of the lung. This is rarely done because of the associated high mortality risk. It's impossible to remove a pulmonary embolism through bronchoscopy because the defect isn't in the bronchial tree. A thrombectomy can be performed at other sources of clot, but when a pulmonary embolism has already occurred, it would have little effect on oxygenation.

CN: Physiological integrity; CNS: Physiological adaptation; CL: Analysis

120. Nursing management of a client with a pulmonary embolism focuses on which action?

1. Assessing oxygenation status
2. Monitoring the oxygen delivery device
3. Monitoring for other sources of clots
4. Determining whether the client requires another ventilation-perfusion ($\dot{V}/\dot{Q}$) scan

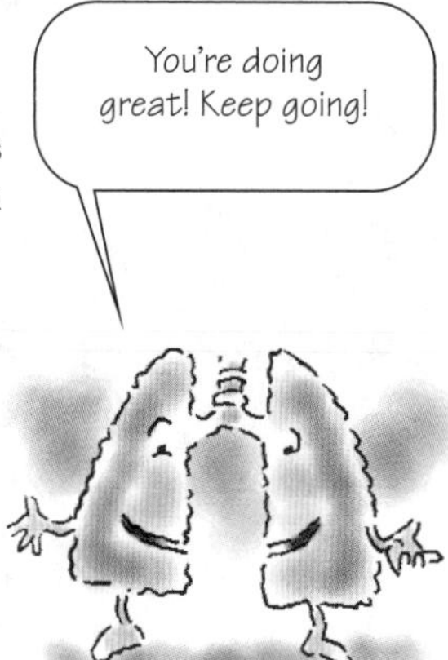
You're doing great! Keep going!

120. 1. Nursing management of a client with a pulmonary embolism focuses on assessing oxygenation status and ensuring that treatment is adequate. If the client's status begins to deteriorate, it's the nurse's responsibility to contact the physician and attempt to improve oxygenation. Ensuring that the oxygen delivery device is working properly and monitoring for other clot sources are other nursing responsibilities, but they aren't the focus of care. The physician would determine if the client required another $\dot{V}/\dot{Q}$ scan.

CN: Physiological integrity; CNS: Reduction of risk potential; CL: Application

121. Pulse oximetry gives what type of information about a client?

1. Amount of carbon dioxide in the blood
2. Amount of oxygen in the blood
3. Percentage of hemoglobin carrying oxygen
4. Respiratory rate

121. 3. Pulse oximetry determines the percentage of hemoglobin carrying oxygen. This doesn't ensure that the oxygen being carried through the bloodstream is actually being taken up by the tissue. Pulse oximetry doesn't provide information about the amount of carbon dioxide or oxygen in the blood or the client's respiratory rate.

CN: Physiological integrity; CNS: Physiological adaptation; CL: Application

122. What effect does hemoglobin level have on oxygenation status?

1. It has no effect.
2. More hemoglobin reduces the client's respiratory rate.
3. Low hemoglobin levels cause reduced oxygen-carrying capacity.
4. Low hemoglobin levels cause increased oxygen-carrying capacity.

122. 3. Hemoglobin carries oxygen to all tissues in the body. If the hemoglobin level is low, the amount of oxygen-carrying capacity is also low. More hemoglobin will increase oxygen-carrying capacity and thus increase the total amount of oxygen available in the blood. If the client has been tachypneic during exertion, or even at rest, because oxygen demand is higher than the available oxygen content, then an increase in hemoglobin may decrease the respiratory rate to normal levels.

CN: Physiological integrity; CNS: Reduction of risk potential; CL: Application

CN: Client needs category CNS: Client needs subcategory CL: Cognitive level

123. How does positive end-expiratory pressure (PEEP) improve oxygenation?

1. It provides more oxygen to the client.
2. It opens up bronchioles and allows oxygen to get in the lungs.
3. It opens up collapsed alveoli and helps keep them open.
4. It adds pressure to the lung tissue, which improves gaseous exchange.

123. 3. PEEP delivers positive pressure to the lung at the end of expiration. This helps open collapsed alveoli and helps them stay open so gas exchange can occur in these newly opened alveoli, improving oxygenation. The bronchioles don't participate in gas exchange except to act as a conduit for inspired and expired air. The walls are rigid enough they generally don't collapse. PEEP doesn't directly add pressure to the lung tissue or provide more oxygen to the client.
CN: Physiological integrity; CNS: Physiological adaptation; CL: Application

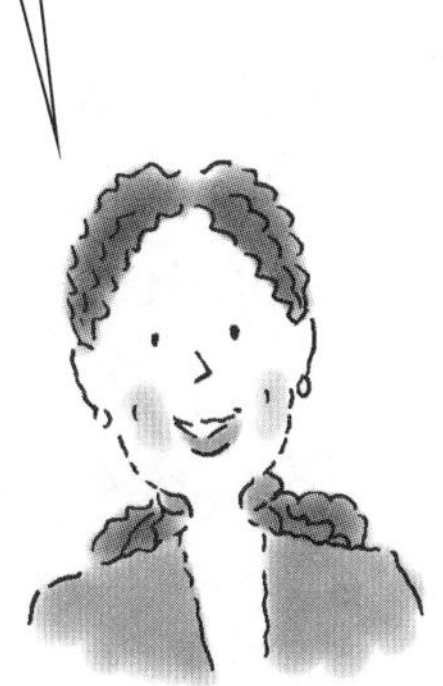

You're the best for catching these hints!

124. Which statement best explains how opening up collapsed alveoli improves oxygenation?

1. Alveoli need oxygen to live.
2. Alveoli have no effect on oxygenation.
3. Collapsed alveoli increase oxygen demand.
4. Gaseous exchange occurs in the alveolar membrane.

124. 4. Gaseous exchange occurs in the alveolar membrane, so if the alveoli collapse, no exchange occurs. Collapsed alveoli receive oxygen, as well as other nutrients, from the bloodstream. Collapsed alveoli have no effect on oxygen demand, though by decreasing the surface area available for gas exchange, they decrease oxygenation of the blood.
CN: Physiological integrity; CNS: Physiological adaptation; CL: Application

125. Continuous positive airway pressure (CPAP) can be provided through an oxygen mask to improve oxygenation in hypoxic clients by which method?

1. The mask provides 100% oxygen to the client.
2. The mask provides continuous air that the client can breathe.
3. The mask provides pressurized oxygen so the client can breathe more easily.
4. The mask provides pressurized oxygen at the end of expiration to open collapsed alveoli.

125. 3. The mask provides pressurized oxygen continuously through both inspiration and expiration. The mask can be set to deliver any amount of oxygen needed. By providing a client with pressurized oxygen, the client has less resistance to overcome in taking in his next breath, making it easier to breathe. Pressurized oxygen delivered at the end of expiration is positive end-expiratory pressure, not CPAP.
CN: Physiological integrity; CNS: Physiological adaptation; CL: Application

126. Bilevel positive airway pressure (BiPAP) is delivered though a special oxygen mask that performs which function?

1. The mask provides 100% oxygen at both inspiration and expiration.
2. The mask provides pressurized oxygen so the client can breathe more easily.
3. The mask provides pressurized oxygen at the end of expiration to open collapsed alveoli.
4. The mask provides both continuous positive airway pressure (CPAP) and positive end-expiratory pressure (PEEP) to provide optimal oxygenation and ventilation.

126. 4. BiPAP delivers both CPAP and PEEP. It provides the differing pressures throughout the respiratory cycle, attempting to optimize a client's oxygenation and ventilation. It's used in an effort to avoid intubation for mechanical ventilation. Inspiratory and expiratory pressures are set separately to optimize the client's ventilatory status, and the fraction of inspired oxygen is adjusted to optimize oxygenation. The second choice describes only the CPAP component of BiPAP, and the third choice describes the PEEP component.
CN: Physiological integrity; CNS: Physiological adaptation; CL: Application

127. The nurse is caring for a client with a pleural effusion. The client asks, "What is a pleural effusion?" Which of the following responses would be appropriate for the nurse to make?

1. "It is the collapse of alveoli."
2. "It is the collapse of a bronchiole."
3. "It is the fluid in the alveolar space."
4. "It is the accumulation of fluid between the linings of the pleural space."

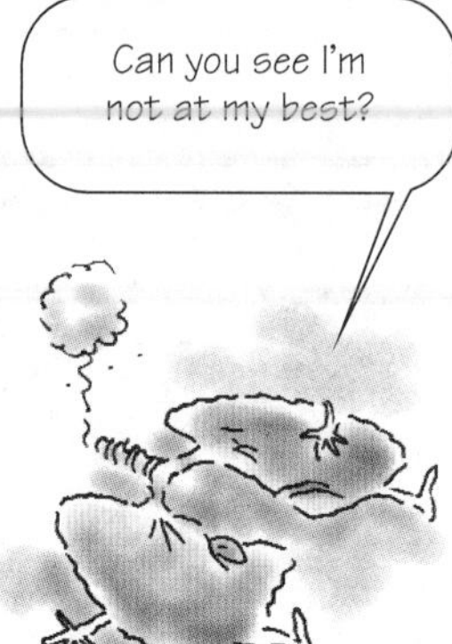
Can you see I'm not at my best?

127. 4. Pleural fluid normally seeps continually into the pleural space from the capillaries lining the parietal pleura and is reabsorbed by the visceral pleural capillaries and lymphatics. Any condition that interferes with either the secretion or drainage of this fluid will lead to a pleural effusion. The collapse of alveoli or a bronchiole has no particular name. Fluid within the alveolar space can be caused by heart failure or adult respiratory distress syndrome.

CN: Physiological integrity; CNS: Physiological adaptation; CL: Application

128. If a client develops a pleural effusion, which treatment would the nurse anticipate the physician to perform?

1. Inserting a chest tube
2. Performing thoracentesis
3. Performing paracentesis
4. Allowing the pleural effusion to drain by itself

128. 2. Thoracentesis is used to remove excess pleural fluid and restore proper lung status. The fluid is then analyzed to determine if it's transudative or exudative. Transudates are substances that have passed through a membrane and usually occur in low protein states. Exudates are substances that have escaped from blood vessels. They contain an accumulation of cells and have a high specific gravity and a high lactate dehydrogenase level. Exudates usually occur in response to a malignancy, infection, or inflammatory process. A chest tube is rarely necessary because the amount of fluid typically isn't large enough to warrant such a measure. Paracentesis is the removal of fluid from the abdomen. Pleural effusions can't drain by themselves.

CN: Physiological integrity; CNS: Physiological adaptation; CL: Application

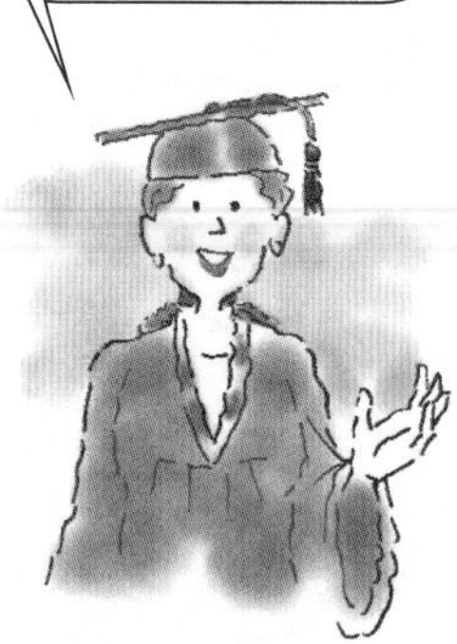
I bet you were voted most likely to pick the most likely choice.

129. After a motor vehicle collision, an 18-year-old client is admitted with a pneumothorax. The surgeon inserts a chest tube and attaches it to a chest drainage system. Bubbling soon appears in the water seal chamber. Which factor is the most likely cause of the bubbling?

1. Air leak
2. Adequate suction
3. Inadequate suction
4. Kinked chest tube

129. 1. Bubbling in the water seal chamber of a chest drainage system stems from an air leak. In pneumothorax, an air leak can occur as air is pulled from the pleural space. Bubbling doesn't normally occur with either adequate or inadequate suction. A kinked chest tube can stop the suction and any preexisting bubbling in the water seal chamber.

CN: Physiological integrity; CNS: Reduction of risk potential; CL: Application

CN: Client needs category CNS: Client needs subcategory CL: Cognitive level

130. A comatose client needs a nasopharyngeal airway for suctioning. After the airway is inserted, he gags and coughs. Which action should the nurse take?

1. Remove the airway and insert a shorter one.
2. Reposition the airway.
3. Leave the airway in place until the client gets used to it.
4. Remove the airway and attempt suctioning without it.

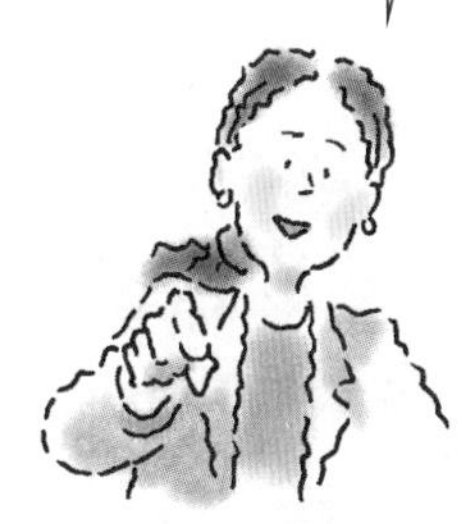

It's time to take action with this client. What's first?

130. 1. If the client gags or coughs after nasopharyngeal airway placement, the tube may be too long. The nurse should remove it and insert a shorter one. Simply repositioning the airway won't solve the problem. The client won't get used to the tube because it's the wrong size. Suctioning without a nasopharyngeal airway causes trauma to the natural airway.

CN: Physiological integrity; CNS: Reduction of risk potential; CL: Application

131. An 87-year-old client requires long-term ventilator therapy. He has a tracheostomy in place and requires frequent suctioning. Which technique is correct?

1. Using intermittent suction while advancing the catheter
2. Using continuous suction for no longer than 10 seconds while withdrawing the catheter
3. Using continuous suction for no longer than 20 seconds while withdrawing the catheter
4. Using continuous suction while advancing the catheter

131. 2. To prevent hypoxia, continuous suctioning shouldn't last more than 10 seconds at a time during catheter withdrawal. Suction shouldn't be applied while the catheter is being advanced.

CN: Physiological integrity; CNS: Reduction of risk potential; CL: Application

132. A client's arterial blood gas (ABG) analysis reveals a pH of 7.18, $Paco_2$ of 73 mm Hg, Pao_2 of 77 mm Hg, and HCO_3^- of 24 mEq/L. What do these values indicate?

1. Metabolic acidosis
2. Respiratory alkalosis
3. Metabolic alkalosis
4. Respiratory acidosis

132. 4. Normal ABG values include a pH of 7.35 to 7.45; $Paco_2$ of 35 to 45 mm Hg; Pao_2 of 75 to 100 mm Hg; and HCO_3^- of 22 to 26 mEq/L. This client has a below-normal pH, an elevated $Paco_2$, and normal HCO_3^-, indicating respiratory acidosis. With metabolic acidosis, pH and HCO_3^- are low and $Paco_2$ is normal. In respiratory alkalosis, pH is elevated and $Paco_2$ is low. In metabolic alkalosis, both pH and HCO_3^- are elevated.

CN: Physiological integrity; CNS: Reduction of risk potential; CL: Analysis

What position will promote my expansion?

133. A 67-year-old client is in distress after being admitted with an exacerbation of chronic obstructive pulmonary disease. In which position should the nurse put the client to promote optimal lung expansion?

1. Prone
2. Semi-Fowler's
3. Reverse Trendelenburg's
4. Supine

133. 2. Semi-Fowler's position (with the head of the bed elevated 30 degrees) promotes optimal lung expansion. A prone position (lying on the abdomen) improves oxygenation in a client with acute respiratory distress syndrome who's receiving mechanical ventilation by recruiting new alveoli in the posterior region of the lung. Reverse Trendelenburg's position (in which the entire bed is raised to a 45-degree angle) may improve lung expansion but is less effective than semi-Fowler's position. Supine positioning (lying flat on the back) doesn't aid lung expansion.

CN: Physiological integrity; CNS: Reduction of risk potential; CL: Application

134. A nursing home client is transferred to the hospital with dehydration and pneumonia. After receiving the client from the emergency department, the nurse notices that his I.V. infusion has been infiltrated. Which action is the best initial response by the nurse?

1. Stop the infusion, remove the I.V. catheter, and restart the infusion in another site.
2. Remove the I.V. catheter and apply a cool compress to the site.
3. Apply moist heat to the site.
4. Gently massage the site.

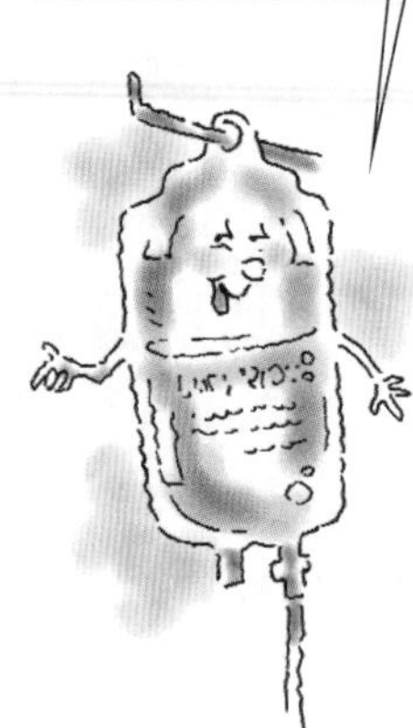

I've been infiltrated. What's the nurse's best initial response?

134. 1. Immediately after discovering an I.V. infiltration, the nurse should stop the infusion, remove the I.V. catheter, restart the infusion in another site, and apply a warm compress to the infiltrated site. A cool compress doesn't promote fluid absorption. Moist heat shouldn't be applied until the infusion is stopped, the catheter is removed, and another catheter is inserted at a different site. Massaging the site is likely to cause pain and isn't effective in treating an infiltration.

CN: Physiological integrity; CNS: Pharmacological and parenteral therapies; CL: Application

135. A police officer brings a 45-year-old homeless client to the emergency department. A chest X-ray suggests he has tuberculosis. The physician orders an intradermal injection of 5 tuberculin units/0.1 ml of tuberculin purified protein derivative. Which needle is appropriate for this injection?

1. ⅝″ to ½″ 25G to 27G needle
2. 1″ to 3″ 20G to 25G needle
3. ½″ to ⅜″ 26G or 27G needle
4. 1″ 20G needle

135. 3. Intradermal injections like those used in tuberculin skin tests are administered in small volumes (usually 0.5 ml or less) into the outer skin layers to produce a local effect. A tuberculin syringe with a ½″ to ⅜″ 26G or 27G needle should be inserted about ⅛″ below the epidermis. A ⅝″ to ½″ 25G to 27G needle is appropriate for a subcutaneous injection; a 1″ to 3″ 20G to 25G needle, for an I.M. injection; and a 1″ 20G needle, for an I.V. bolus injection.

CN: Physiological integrity; CNS: Pharmacological and parenteral therapies; CL: Application

136. After a right lower lobectomy for lung cancer, a client returns to her room with a chest tube in place. The nurse formulates a care plan with a primary nursing diagnosis of *Impaired gas exchange related to lung surgery.* Which expected outcome is appropriate for this diagnosis?

1. The client will sit upright, leaning slightly forward.
2. The client will request pain medication as needed.
3. The client will maintain a pulse oximetry level above 93%.
4. The client will be pain-free.

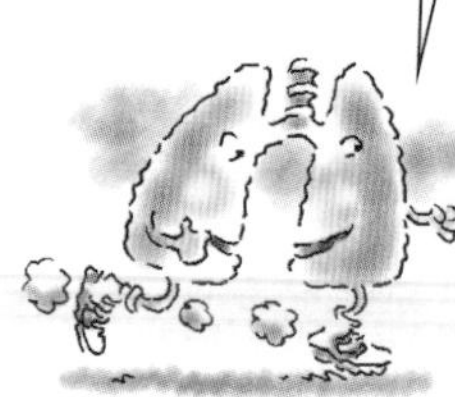

What outcome are we headed toward?

136. 3. A pulse oximetry level above 93% and a normal respiratory rate demonstrate probable lung expansion and normal chest tube functioning. Sitting upright and leaning slightly forward suggests that the client has impaired gas exchange because this position increases lung expansion. Requesting pain medication as needed and remaining pain-free are expected outcomes associated with a nursing diagnosis of *Acute pain.*

CN: Physiological integrity; CNS: Physiological adaptation; CL: Analysis

CN: Client needs category CNS: Client needs subcategory CL: Cognitive level

137. An unrestrained passenger is thrown 20′ (6.1 m) from a car. On admission to the emergency department, he has a heart rate of 130 beats/minute, shallow respirations at a rate of 32 breaths/minute, and a blood pressure of 90/60 mm Hg. His skin is pale and cool, and capillary refill is delayed. Breath sounds are diminished on the right side and paradoxical chest-wall movement appears on the right side. A chest X-ray reveals a right pneumothorax with multiple rib fractures (4th to 7th right ribs). Which diagnosis is the most probable?

1. Tension pneumothorax
2. Flail chest
3. Ruptured diaphragm
4. Massive hemothorax

137. 2. Multiple rib fractures and paradoxical chest-wall movement confirm a diagnosis of flail chest. Tension pneumothorax causes severe respiratory distress, hypotension, diminished breath sounds over the affected area, hyperresonance, distended neck veins, eventual tracheal shift, and, possibly, paradoxical chest-wall movement on the injured side. A ruptured diaphragm leads to hyperresonance on percussion, hypotension, dyspnea, dysphagia, and shifting of heart and bowel sounds in the lower to middle chest. A massive hemothorax produces signs of shock (such as tachycardia and hypotension), dullness on percussion on the injured side, decreased breath sounds on the injured side, respiratory distress, and, possibly, mediastinal shift.

CN: Physiological integrity; CNS: Physiological adaptation; CL: Analysis

138. A healthy client comes to the clinic for a routine examination. When auscultating his lower lung lobes, the nurse should expect to hear which type of breath sound?

1. Bronchial
2. Tracheal
3. Vesicular
4. Bronchovesicular

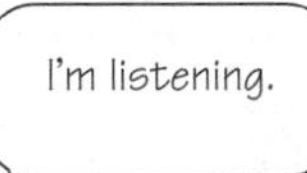

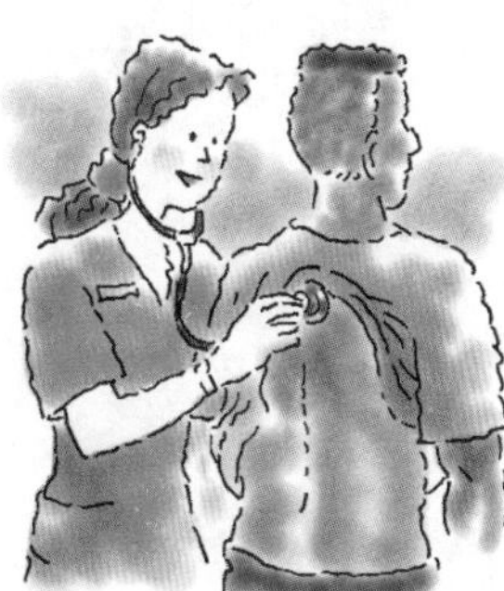

138. 3. Vesicular breath sounds are soft, low-pitched sounds normally heard over the lower lobes of the lung. They're prolonged on inhalation and shortened on exhalation. Bronchial breath sounds are loud, high-pitched sounds normally heard next to the trachea; discontinuous, they're loudest during exhalation. Tracheal breath sounds are harsh, discontinuous sounds heard over the trachea during inhalation or exhalation. Bronchovesicular breath sounds are medium-pitched, continuous sounds that occur during inhalation or exhalation and are best heard over the upper third of the sternum and between the scapulae.

CN: Health promotion and maintenance; CNS: None; CL: Application

139. A 76-year-old client is admitted for elective knee surgery. Physical examination reveals shallow respirations but no signs of respiratory distress. Which finding is a normal physiologic change related to aging?

1. Increased elastic recoil of the lungs
2. Increased number of functional capillaries in the alveoli
3. Decreased residual volume
4. Decreased vital capacity

139. 4. Reduction in vital capacity is a normal physiologic change in the older adult. Other normal physiologic changes include decreased elastic recoil of the lungs, fewer functional capillaries in the alveoli, and an increase in residual volume.

CN: Health promotion and maintenance; CNS: None; CL: Application

140. A 79-year-old client is admitted with pneumonia. Which nursing diagnosis should take priority?

1. *Acute pain related to lung expansion secondary to lung infection*
2. *Risk for imbalanced fluid volume related to increased insensible fluid losses secondary to fever*
3. *Anxiety related to dyspnea and chest pain*
4. *Ineffective airway clearance related to retained secretions*

140. 4. Pneumonia is an acute infection of the lung parenchyma. The inflammatory reaction may cause an outpouring of exudate into the alveolar spaces, leading to *Ineffective airway clearance related to retained secretions.* Pneumonia also can cause *Acute pain related to lung expansion* and *Anxiety related to dyspnea and chest pain.* However, these diagnoses take lower priority than *Ineffective airway clearance.* Fever associated with pneumonia places the client at risk for imbalanced fluid volume—but this diagnosis also doesn't take priority.

CN: Physiological integrity; CNS: Physiological adaptation; CL: Analysis

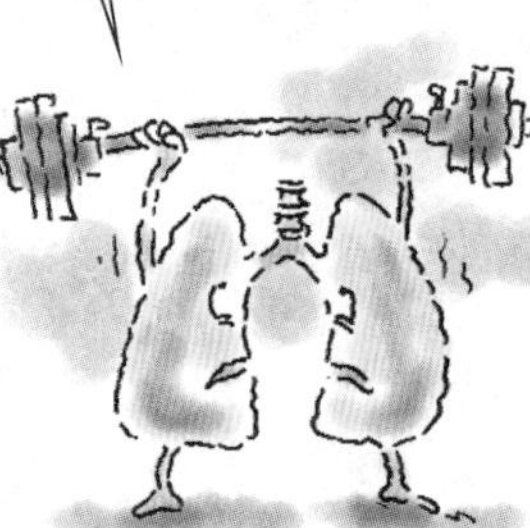

What's effective when it comes to exercise and asthma medication?

141. An asthmatic client is being discharged on a new asthma medication. Teaching about cromolyn (Intal inhaler) is effective when the client makes which statement?

1. "I should use my inhaler no more than 1 hour before I exercise."
2. "I should use my inhaler whenever I feel an asthma attack coming on."
3. "I should stop taking steroids if I need a dose of my inhaler."
4. "I should avoid gargling and rinsing my mouth after using my inhaler."

141. 1. The client should verbalize the need to use the inhaler no more than 1 hour before exercise when indicated for exercise-induced asthma. Cromolyn is contraindicated during an acute asthma attack. A client who is taking steroids should continue to take them during cromolyn therapy, if appropriate. Gargling and rinsing the mouth after cromolyn administration can reduce mouth dryness.

CN: Physiological integrity; CNS: Pharmacological and parenteral therapies; CL: Analysis

142. Sputum analysis is ordered when a client with pneumonia expectorates green sputum. Which guideline should the nurse include in the teaching plan?

1. Fluids will be restricted the night before the test.
2. The client will be asked to take several deep abdominal breaths and then to take one more breath, bend forward, and cough into the provided sterile container.
3. If bronchoscopy is required for specimen collection, the client will have no oral intake for 12 hours before the procedure.
4. After bronchoscopy, the client will receive a drink of water.

142. 2. If the specimen will be collected by expectoration, the client should be instructed to take several deep abdominal breaths; when he's ready to cough, he should take one more deep abdominal breath, bend forward, and cough into the provided sterile container. He should be instructed to drink plenty of fluids the night before the test. If the specimen will be collected during bronchoscopy, the client should fast for 6 hours before the procedure. After bronchoscopy, he's observed for possible complications. He can have liquids when his gag reflex returns.

CN: Physiological integrity; CNS: Reduction of risk potential; CL: Application

143. A 57-year-old client is admitted with acute bronchitis. During the admission interview, he tells the nurse he's allergic to bananas. Based on this statement, he may also have an allergy to which drug or substance?

1. Iodine-containing drugs
2. Cephalosporins
3. Penicillins
4. Latex

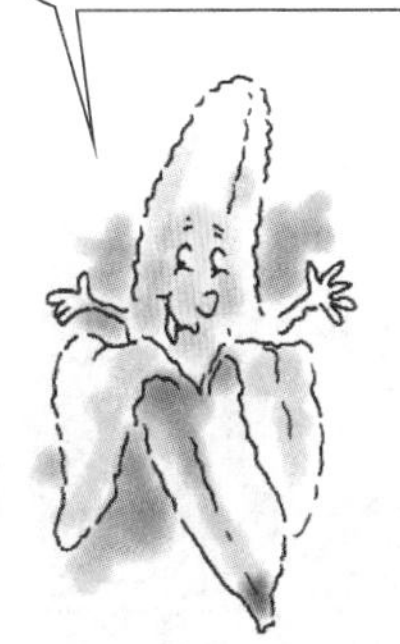

An allergy to bananas can cause which other allergy?

143. 4. Clients who are allergic to certain cross-reactive foods—including apricots, avocados, bananas, cherries, chestnuts, grapes, kiwis, passion fruit, peaches, and tomatoes—may also be allergic to latex. When exposed to latex, they may have an allergic response similar to the one these foods produce. Clients with allergies to shellfish may be allergic to iodine-containing drugs. Hypersensitivity reactions to cephalosporins are more common in clients with penicillin allergy. There's no link between food allergies and penicillin.

CN: Physiological integrity; CNS: Reduction of risk potential; CL: Application

144. The care plan for a 42-year-old client with deep vein thrombosis (DVT) includes monitoring the client for complications. Which pulmonary complication is the client <u>most</u> at risk for developing?

1. Pulmonary embolism
2. Pneumothorax
3. Pulmonary edema
4. Pneumonia

144. 1. The most common etiology of pulmonary embolism is thromboembolism from a distant site, particularly from deep veins of the legs and pelvis (90% to 95%). Moreover, the immobilization used to treat DVT is an additional clinical risk factor for pulmonary embolism. Pneumothorax and pulmonary edema aren't complications of DVT. Although immobility also places the client at risk for pneumonia, the risk isn't as great for this client.

CN: Physiological integrity; CNS: Reduction of risk potential; CL: Application

145. A 20-year-old client with cystic fibrosis is being discharged with a high-frequency chest wall oscillating vest. Which statement by the client indicates that she understands how to use the vest?

1. "I'll wear the vest for 5 minutes each time a treatment is due."
2. "I'll lie down to use the vest."
3. "I'll require help in applying the vest."
4. "I can be in any position to use the vest."

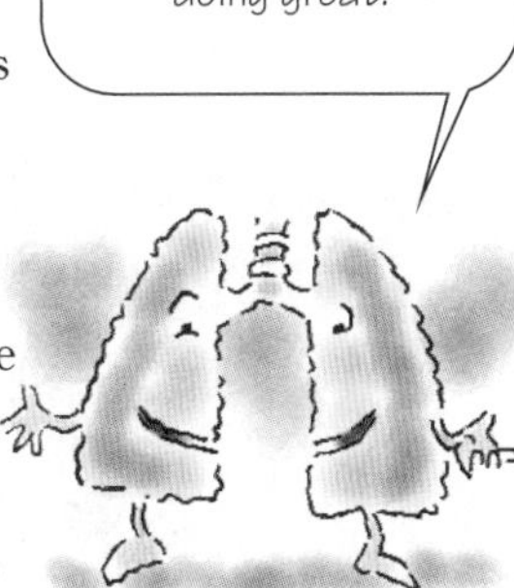

No sweat! You're doing great!

145. 4. The vest system doesn't require special positioning or breathing to be effective. In most cases, treatments last 15 to 20 minutes and clients can manage therapy without any assistance.

CN: Safe, effective care environment; CNS: Safety and infection control; CL: Analysis

146. To obtain an arterial blood sample from a client's radial artery, which action should the nurse perform first?
1. Perform Allen's test.
2. Place a rolled towel under the client's wrist.
3. Clean the puncture site with an alcohol or povidone-iodine pad.
4. Palpate the artery with the index and middle fingers of one hand.

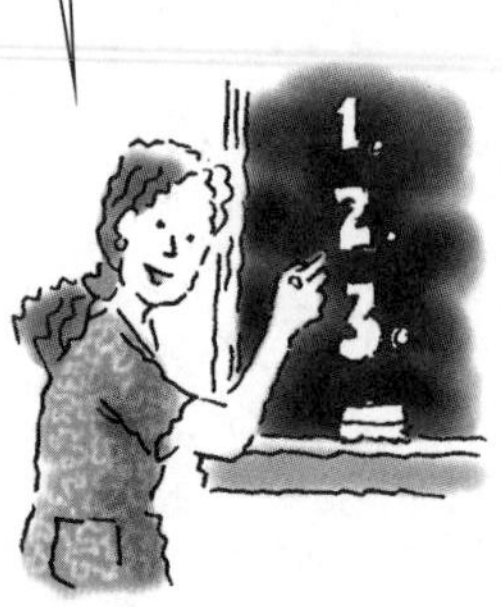
Question 146
asks for the first
action.
1.
2.
3.

146. 1. First, perform Allen's test to assess circulation. Next, wash your hands, put on gloves, and place a rolled towel under the client's wrist for support. Then locate the artery and palpate it for a strong pulse. Next, clean the puncture site with an alcohol or povidone-iodine pad. Then palpate the artery with the index and middle fingers of one hand while holding the syringe over the puncture site with the other hand. Holding the needle bevel at a 30- to 45-degree angle, puncture the skin and arterial wall in one smooth motion, watch for blood backflow in the syringe, and fill it to the 5-ml mark. After collecting the sample, press a gauze pad over the puncture site for at least 5 minutes.
CN: Physiological integrity; CNS: Reduction of risk potential; CL: Application

147. After receiving radiation treatment for lung cancer, a client complains that he has lost his appetite. The nurse should provide which instruction?
1. "Drink plenty of fluids."
2. "Eat hot meats with spices to improve the taste."
3. "Limit activities immediately before and after meals."
4. "Consume food high in calories."

147. 4. The client should consume high-calorie foods whenever he can eat, to help compensate for the times when he can't eat. Consuming large amounts of fluids creates a feeling of fullness, which can limit food intake. Hot meats tend to cause taste aversions during radiation therapy. Activity increases the appetite.
CN: Physiological integrity; CNS: Physiological adaptation; CL: Application

148. Three days after an abdominal aortic aneurysm repair, a client develops a pulmonary embolus. Which nursing diagnosis takes priority?
1. *Ineffective peripheral tissue perfusion*
2. *Impaired physical mobility*
3. *Ineffective airway clearance*
4. *Risk for aspiration*

148. 1. Pulmonary embolus occurs when a thrombus lodges in a branch of the pulmonary artery, partially or totally occluding it. The lung is adequately ventilated but can't be perfused, resulting in ineffective peripheral tissue perfusion. Although *Impaired physical mobility* is an appropriate nursing diagnosis for this client, it doesn't take priority over *Ineffective peripheral tissue perfusion*. A pulmonary embolus doesn't increase secretions, so *Ineffective airway clearance* isn't an appropriate diagnosis. It also doesn't place the client at *Risk for aspiration*.
CN: Physiological integrity; CNS: Physiological adaptation; CL: Analysis

149. After experiencing an anxiety attack, a client comes to the emergency department complaining of dizziness and light-headedness. Arterial blood gas (ABG) analysis reveals a pH of 7.62, $Paco_2$ of 22 mm Hg, Pao_2 of 96 mm Hg, and HCO_3^- of 24 mEq/L. Which action should the nurse take?

1. Do nothing; these ABG values are normal.
2. Encourage the client to breathe into a paper bag.
3. Notify the physician and prepare to give sodium bicarbonate.
4. Notify the physician and prepare to give supplemental oxygen.

149. 2. These ABG values reveal respiratory alkalosis (elevated pH, decreased $Paco_2$, and normal Pao_2 and HCO_3^- levels), so the client is most likely hyperventilating from anxiety. Breathing into a paper bag can stop the hyperventilation by increasing carbon dioxide. Doing nothing or giving sodium bicarbonate could worsen respiratory alkalosis. The client has a normal Pao_2 level and doesn't need supplemental oxygen.

CN: Physiological integrity; CNS: Reduction of risk potential; CL: Analysis

150. After a nurse teaches a group of police officers about the spread of tuberculosis (TB), which statement by an officer indicates that teaching has been effective?

1. "I could get TB by being in close proximity for a brief time with someone who has the disease."
2. "I could get TB if I inhale infected droplets when an infected individual coughs."
3. "I could get TB if I search the home of someone infected with TB."
4. "I could get TB if I come in contact with blood from an infected person."

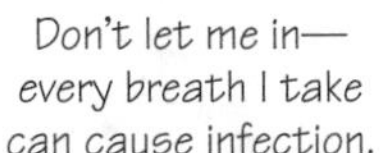

Don't let me in—
every breath I take
can cause infection.

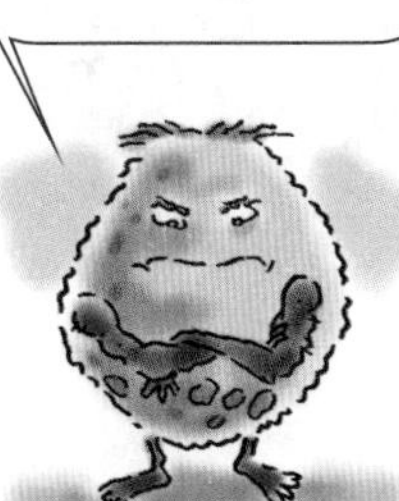

150. 2. TB infection typically occurs from inhaling infected droplets after a person with TB coughs. Transmission usually requires close, frequent, prolonged contact. Human immunodeficiency virus—not TB—is spread through contact with an infected person's blood.

CN: Safe, effective care environment; CNS: Safety and infection control; CL: Analysis

151. A client receives midazolam, 2 mg I.V., as sedation before bronchoscopy. Five minutes after he receives the drug, his respiratory rate drops to 4 breaths/minute. Which agent should the nurse administer to reverse the effects of midazolam?

1. Naloxone
2. Protamine sulfate
3. Phentolamine (Regitine)
4. Flumazenil (Romazicon)

151. 4. Flumazenil reverses the effects of benzodiazepines such as midazolam. Naloxone is used to reverse opioids, such as morphine. Protamine sulfate reverses the effects of heparin. Phentolamine is injected into the tissues to reverse the damaging effects of a dopamine infiltration.

CN: Physiological integrity; CNS: Pharmacological and parenteral therapies; CL: Application

152. A physician places an order in the computer for a nurse to change a client's chest drainage system from suction to gravity drainage. How should the nurse proceed?

1. Detach the tubing from the suction port to provide a vent.
2. Clamp the client's drainage tube.
3. Question the physician's order.
4. Turn off the suction source and leave the tubing connected.

152. 1. When the suction source is turned off, the drainage system should be opened to the atmosphere so intrapleural air can escape from the system. Detaching the tubing from the suction port provides an exit vent for the air and, thus, reduces the risk of tension pneumothorax. Clamping the tube may cause air to accumulate in the pleural space, rapidly leading to tension pneumothorax. There's no need to question the order.

CN: Physiological integrity; CNS: Physiological adaptation; CL: Application

153. A client with cancer develops pleural effusion. During chest auscultation, which breath sounds should the nurse expect to hear?

1. Crackles
2. Rhonchi
3. Diminished breath sounds
4. Wheezes

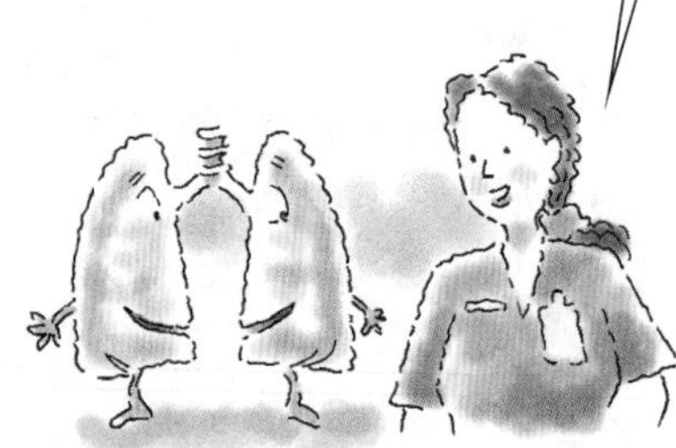
What? I can barely hear you.

153. 3. In pleural effusion, fluid accumulates in the pleural space, impairing transmission of normal breath sounds. Because of the acoustic mismatch, breath sounds are diminished. Crackles (short explosive or popping sounds) commonly accompany atelectasis, interstitial fibrosis, and left-sided heart failure. Rhonchi (low-pitched sounds with a snoring quality) suggest secretions in the large airways. Wheezes (high-pitched, hissing sounds) result from narrowed airways, as in asthma, chronic obstructive pulmonary disease, or bronchitis.

CN: Physiological integrity; CNS: Physiological adaptation; CL: Application

154. An employee-health nurse who performs annual purified protein derivative (PPD) testing instructs the staff that their results must be read within how many hours after administration?

1. 6 to 12 hours
2. 12 to 24 hours
3. 24 to 48 hours
4. 48 to 72 hours

154. 4. To ensure accurate results, a PPD test must be read 48 to 72 hours after administration.

CN: Health promotion and maintenance; CNS: None; CL: Application

155. A 79-year-old client suddenly develops pulmonary edema. The physician prescribes furosemide (Lasix), 40 mg I.V., and use of a nonrebreather mask. Which oxygen concentrations does this mask deliver?

1. 60% to 80%
2. 80% to 100%
3. 36%
4. 44%

155. 2. The nonrebreather mask delivers oxygen concentrations of 80% to 100%. It's reserved for emergency situations. A partial rebreather mask delivers concentrations of 60% to 80%. A nasal cannula delivers oxygen at flow rates of 1 to 6 L/minute. A flow rate of 4 L/minute delivers an oxygen concentration of 36%; a rate of 6 L/minute delivers an oxygen concentration of 44%.

CN: Physiological integrity; CNS: Physiological adaptation; CL: Application

156. A nurse passes by a neighbor's swimming pool and notices an adult at the bottom of the pool. She immediately calls for help and tries to rescue the person. When she pulls him out, he's unresponsive and breathless. How should the nurse proceed?

1. By opening the airway and beginning rescue breathing immediately
2. By immobilizing the cervical spine
3. By starting chest compressions
4. By performing abdominal thrust

157. A client with newly diagnosed chronic obstructive pulmonary disease (COPD) presents to the clinic for a routine examination. The nurse teaches him strategies for preventing airway irritation and infection. Which statement by the client indicates that teaching was successful?

1. "I should avoid enclosed, crowded areas during the summer."
2. "I'm glad I only need to get the flu vaccine."
3. "I should use products with aerosol sprays."
4. "I should avoid using powders."

158. A client with a suspected pulmonary embolus is brought to the emergency department. He complains of shortness of breath and pleuritic chest pain. Which other signs and symptoms would support this diagnosis? Select all that apply:

1. Low-grade fever
2. Thick green sputum
3. Bradycardia
4. Frothy sputum
5. Tachycardia
6. Blood-tinged sputum

159. A physician prescribes normal saline solution to infuse at a rate of 125 ml/hour for a client admitted with dehydration and pneumonia. How many liters of solution will the client receive during an 8-hour shift? Record your answer using a whole number.

_______________________ liters

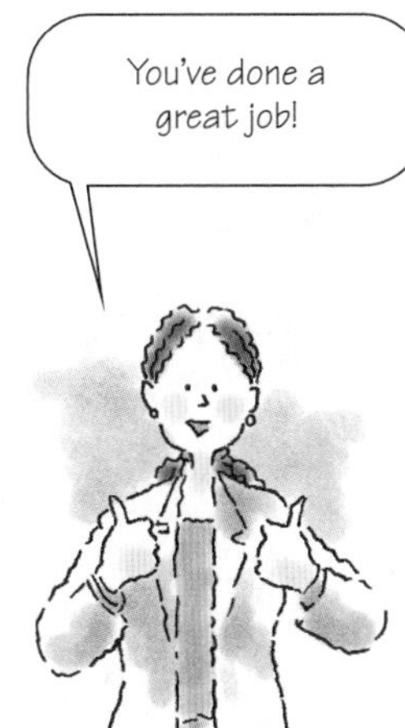

156. 1. The nurse should open the airway and begin rescue breathing immediately—while still in the water, if possible. Immobilizing the cervical spine won't provide the needed oxygenation. Chest compressions should be delivered only if circulation is absent. Performing abdominal thrust in an attempt to remove water from the lungs would delay the start of rescue breathing.

CN: Physiological integrity; CNS: Physiological adaptation; CL: Application

157. 4. A client with COPD should verbalize the need to avoid exposure to powders, dusts, and smoke from cigarettes, pipes, and cigars. He should stay indoors when the humidity, temperature, and pollen counts are high; avoid enclosed, crowded areas during cold and flu season; and avoid aerosol sprays. He should obtain immunizations against pneumococcal pneumonia as well as influenza.

CN: Health promotion and maintenance; CNS: None; CL: Analysis

158. 1, 5, 6. In addition to pleuritic chest pain and dyspnea, a client with a pulmonary embolus may also present with a low-grade fever, tachycardia, and blood-tinged sputum. Thick green sputum would indicate infection, and frothy sputum would indicate pulmonary edema. A client with a pulmonary embolus is tachycardic (to compensate for decreased oxygen supply), not bradycardic.

CN: Physiological integrity; CNS: Physiological adaptation; CL: Application

159. 1. The client is to receive the solution at an infusion rate of 125 ml/hour. 125 ml × 8 hours = 1,000 ml, the total volume in milliliters the client will receive during an 8-hour shift. Convert milliliters to liters by dividing by 1,000. The total volume in liters of normal saline solution that the client will receive in 8 hours is 1 L.

CN: Physiological integrity; CNS: Pharmacological and parenteral therapies; CL: Application

160. A nurse begins her shift by reading the following shift report note on a client.

Miscellaneous reports
H.B. age 78
Hyperventilating, RR 36
bpm. C/O dizziness,
shortness of breath,
tingling in hands and feet,
weakness. Anxious.
ABG: pH 7.48
$Paco_2$: 33 mm Hg

Without further information, the nurse plans to reevaluate the client's status for which problem?

1. Metabolic acidosis
2. Acute respiratory failure
3. Respiratory alkalosis
4. Anxiety reaction

161. The nurse is assessing a client's respiratory pattern. Which graphic illustrates Cheyne-Stokes respirations?

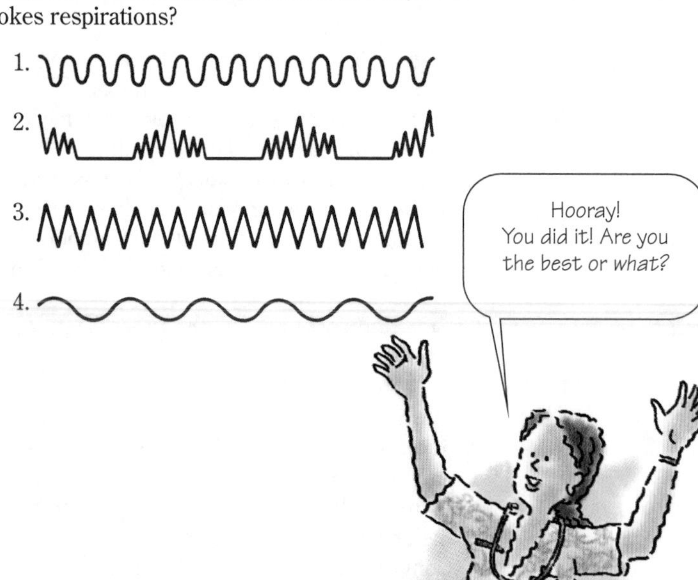

1.
2.
3.
4.
Hooray!
You did it! Are you the best or what?

160. 3. Respiratory alkalosis is defined by a pH greater than 7.45 and $Paco_2$ less than 35 mm Hg, and generally is associated with deep, rapid breathing; light-headedness or dizziness; circumoral and peripheral paresthesia; and carpopedal spasms, twitching, and muscle weakness as it progresses. Metabolic acidosis is defined as a pH less than 7.3, $Paco_2$ less than or equal to 34 mm Hg depending on respiratory compensation, and HCO_3^- less than 22 mEq/L, and is caused by an underlying nonrespiratory disorder. Acute respiratory failure is characterized by a pH less than 3, $Paco_2$ greater than 50 mm Hg, and markedly diminished oxygen saturation levels. Although the client may be anxious, the abnormal blood gas levels and corresponding symptoms indicate that treatment of respiratory alkalosis is the primary concern, and may greatly reduce the client's anxiety level.

CN: Physiological integrity; CNS: Physiological adaptation; CL: Analysis

161. 2. In Cheyne-Stokes respirations, breaths gradually become faster and deeper than normal and then slower during a 30- to 170-second period with intermittent periods of apnea (option 2). Option 1 shows tachypnea—shallow breathing with an increased respiratory rate. Option 3 shows Kussmaul's breathing—rapid, deep breathing without pauses. Option 4 shows bradypnea—regular breathing at a decreased rate.

CN: Physiological integrity; CNS: Reduction of risk potential; CL: Analysis

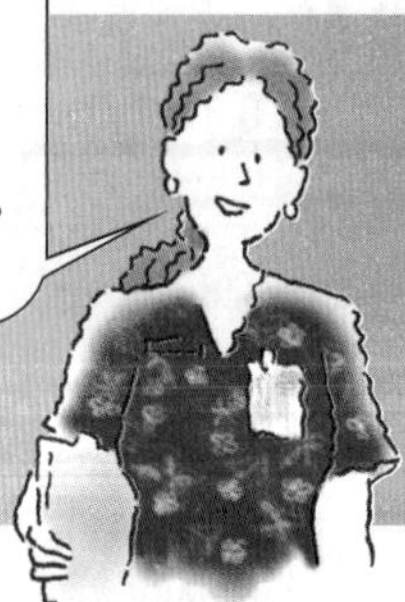

Stroke, subdural hematoma, laminectomy—they're all here in this comprehensive chapter on neurosensory disorders in adults. I've got a sixth sense, you're going to do great!

Chapter 6 Neurosensory disorders

1. An elderly client had a stroke and can only see the nasal visual field on one side and the temporal portion on the opposite side. Which term correctly describes this condition?

1. Astereognosis
2. Homonymous hemianopia
3. Oculogyric crisis
4. Receptive aphasia

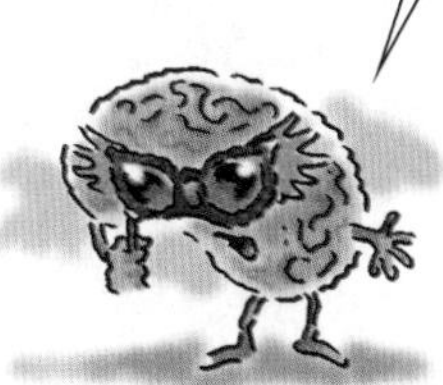

A stroke can change my normal views.

1. 2. Homonymous hemianopia describes the loss of visual field on the nasal side and the opposite temporal side due to damage of the optic nerves. Astereognosis is the inability to identify common objects through touch. Oculogyric crisis, a fixed position of the eyeballs that can last for minutes or hours, occurs in response to antipsychotic medications. Receptive aphasia is the inability to understand words or word meaning.

CN: Physiological integrity; CNS: Physiological adaptation; CL: Application

2. A client had an embolic stroke. Which condition places him at risk for thromboembolic stroke?

1. Atrial fibrillation
2. Bradycardia
3. Deep vein thrombosis (DVT)
4. History of myocardial infarction (MI)

2. 1. Atrial fibrillation occurs with the irregular and rapid discharge from multiple ectopic atrial foci that causes quivering of the atria without atrial systole. This asynchronous atrial contraction predisposes to mural thrombi, which may embolize, leading to a stroke. Bradycardia, DVT, or past MI won't lead to arterial embolization.

CN: Physiological integrity; CNS: Physiological adaptation; CL: Application

3. A 65-year-old client with a stroke in evolution has ordered t-PA, a thrombolytic agent. The order is for 0.9 mg/kg over 1 hour. The client weighs 110 lbs. What is the total dose in milligrams (mg) the client will receive?

1. 35 mg
2. 40 mg
3. 45 mg
4. 50 mg

3. 3. First, convert lbs to kg (2.2 lbs = 1 kg) by dividing: $110 \div 2.2 = 50$ kg. Next, multiply 0.9 mg $\times$ 50 kg = 45 mg. The total dose the client will receive is 45 mg.

CN: Physiological integrity; CNS: Pharmacological and parenteral therapies; CL: Application

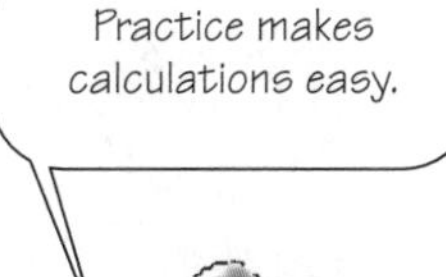

Practice makes calculations easy.

4. A client is admitted with thromboembolic stroke. Which medication should be started by day 2?

1. Acetaminophen
2. Aspirin
3. Tenecteplase
4. Methylprednisolone

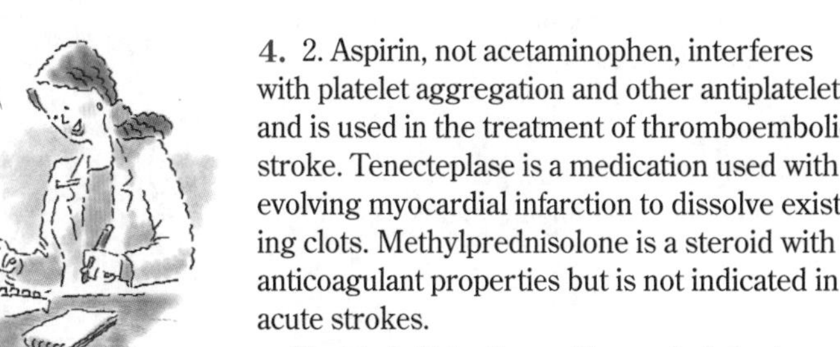

4. 2. Aspirin, not acetaminophen, interferes with platelet aggregation and other antiplatelets, and is used in the treatment of thromboembolic stroke. Tenecteplase is a medication used with evolving myocardial infarction to dissolve existing clots. Methylprednisolone is a steroid with anticoagulant properties but is not indicated in acute strokes.

CN: Physiological integrity; CNS: Pharmacological and parenteral therapies; CL: Application

CN: Client needs category CNS: Client needs subcategory CL: Cognitive level

5. To maintain airway patency during a stroke in evolution, which nursing intervention is appropriate?

1. Thicken all dietary liquids.
2. Restrict dietary and parenteral fluids.
3. Place the client on oxygen.
4. Have tracheal suction available at all times.

5. 4. Because of a potential loss of the gag reflex and potential altered level of consciousness, tracheal suction should be available at all times. Thickening dietary liquids isn't done until the gag reflex returns or the stroke has evolved and the deficit can be assessed. Unless heart failure is present, restricting fluids isn't indicated. Oxygen is based on saturation results and oxygen alone will not maintain an airway.

CN: Physiological integrity; CNS: Reduction of risk potential; CL: Application

6. For a client with a stroke, which criterion must be fulfilled before the client is fed?

1. The gag reflex returns.
2. Speech returns to normal.
3. Cranial nerves III, IV, and VI are intact.
4. The client swallows small sips of water without coughing.

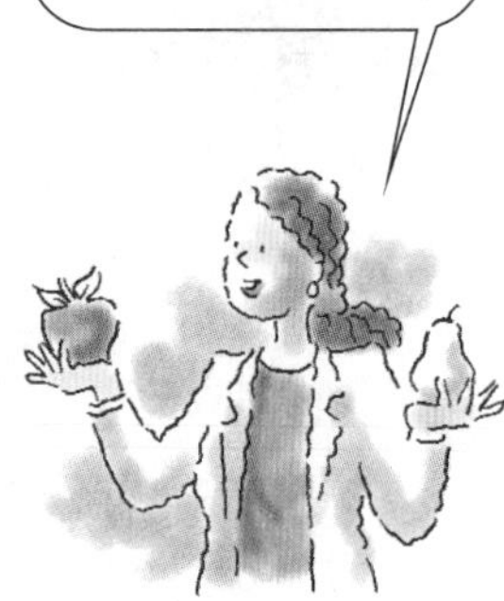

Think: How well can a dysphagic client chew and swallow?

6. 1. An intact gag reflex shows a properly functioning cranial nerve IX (glossopharyngeal). Speech may be normal while the gag reflex is absent. Cranial nerves III, IV, and VI evaluate eye movement and accommodation. A nurse shouldn't offer food or fluids without assessing for an intact gag reflex.

CN: Physiological integrity; CNS: Reduction of risk potential; CL: Application

7. Which diet would be least likely to lead to aspiration in a client who had a stroke with residual dysphagia?

1. Clear liquid
2. Full liquid
3. Mechanical soft
4. Thickened liquid

7. 4. Thickened liquids are easiest to form into a bolus and swallow. Clear and full liquids are amorphous and can't easily form a bolus. A mechanical soft diet may be too hard to chew and too dry to swallow when dysphagia is present.

CN: Physiological integrity; CNS: Reduction of risk potential; CL: Application

8. A 77-year-old client had a thromboembolic right stroke; his left arm is swollen. Which condition may cause swelling after a stroke?

1. Elbow contracture secondary to spasticity
2. Loss of muscle contraction decreasing venous return
3. Deep vein thrombosis (DVT) due to immobility of the ipsilateral side
4. Hypoalbuminemia due to protein escaping from an inflamed glomerulus

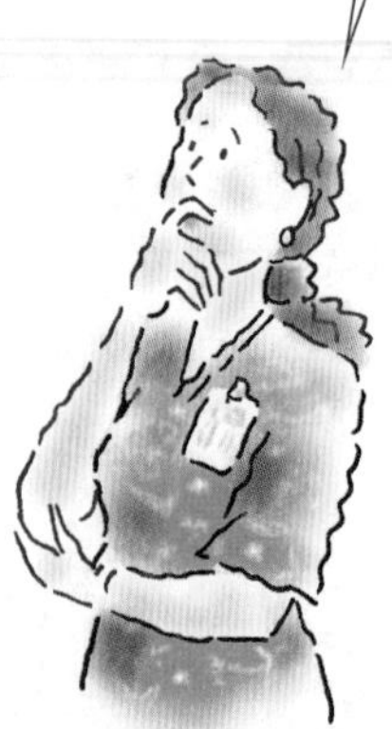

Where is the hemiplegia in a right stroke?

8. 2. In clients with hemiplegia or hemiparesis, loss of muscle contraction decreases venous return and may cause swelling of the affected extremity. Contractures, or bony calcifications, may occur with a stroke, but don't appear with swelling. DVT may develop in clients with a stroke but is more likely to occur in the lower extremities. A stroke isn't linked to protein loss.

CN: Physiological integrity; CNS: Physiological adaptation; CL: Analysis

9. After a brain stem infarction, a nurse should observe for which condition?

1. Aphasia
2. Bradypnea
3. Contralateral hemiplegia
4. Numbness and tingling to the face or arm

9. 2. The brain stem contains the medulla and the vital cardiac, vasomotor, and respiratory centers. A brain stem infarction leads to vital sign changes such as bradypnea. Contralateral hemiplegia, and numbness or tingling in the face or arm may occur, depending on the level of injury. Aphasia is associated with lobar strokes in the cerebral hemispheres.

CN: Physiological integrity; CNS: Physiological adaptation; CL: Application

10. Which condition is a risk factor for the development of cataracts in a 40-year-old client?

1. History of frequent streptococcal throat infections
2. Maternal exposure to rubella during pregnancy
3. Increased intraocular pressure
4. Prolonged use of steroidal anti-inflammatory agents

10. 4. Prolonged use of steroidal anti-inflammatory agents is a risk factor for cataracts. The other risk factors don't contribute to the development of cataracts.

CN: Health promotion and maintenance; CNS: None; CL: Application

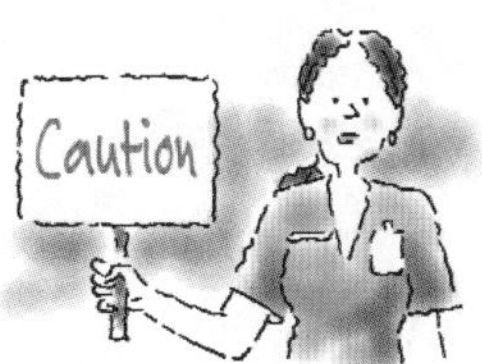

Which symptom would spell danger?
Caution

11. In caring for a client after cataract surgery, the nurse should notify a physician if the client has which of the following conditions?

1. Blurred vision
2. Eye pain
3. Glare
4. Itching

11. 2. Pain shouldn't be present after cataract surgery. Pain may be an indication of hyphema, or clouding in the anterior chamber, and infection. The other symptoms might be present.

CN: Physiological integrity; CNS: Physiological adaptation; CL: Application

12. Clear fluid is draining from the nose of a client who had a head trauma 3 hours ago. This may indicate which condition?

1. Basilar skull fracture
2. Cerebral concussion
3. Cerebral palsy
4. Sinus infection

12. 1. Clear fluid draining from the ear or nose of a client may mean a cerebrospinal fluid leak, which is common in basilar skull fractures. Concussion is associated with a brief loss of consciousness, cerebral palsy is associated with nonprogressive paralysis present since birth, and sinus infection is associated with facial pain and pressure with or without nasal drainage.

CN: Physiological integrity; CNS: Physiological adaptation; CL: Analysis

13. A 19-year-old client with a mild concussion is discharged from the emergency department. Before discharge, he complains of a headache. When offered acetaminophen, his mother tells the nurse the headache is severe and she would like her son to have something stronger. Which response by the nurse is appropriate?

1. "Your son had a mild concussion; acetaminophen is strong enough."
2. "Aspirin is avoided because of the danger of Reye's syndrome in children or young adults."
3. "Opioids are avoided after a head injury because they may hide a worsening condition."
4. "Stronger medications may lead to vomiting, which increases the intracranial pressure (ICP)."

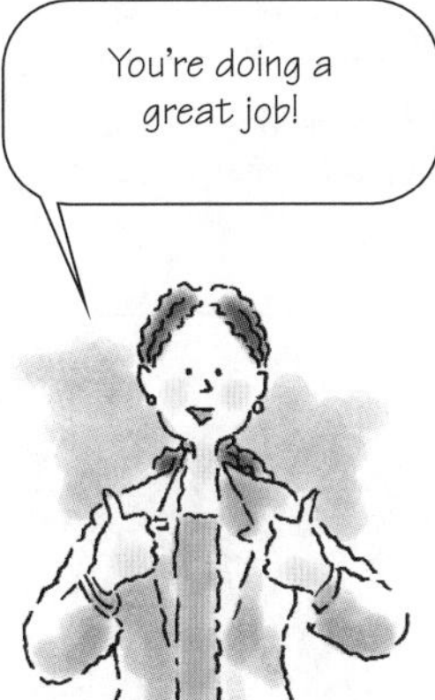

You're doing a great job!

13. 3. Opioids may mask changes in the level of consciousness (LOC) that indicate increased ICP and shouldn't be given as a first-line drug. Saying acetaminophen is strong enough ignores the mother's question and therefore isn't appropriate. Aspirin is contraindicated in conditions that may have bleeding, such as trauma, and for children or young adults with viral illnesses due to the danger of Reye's syndrome. Stronger medications may not necessarily lead to vomiting but will sedate the client, thereby masking changes in his LOC.

CN: Physiological integrity; CNS: Reduction of risk potential; CL: Application

14. A client admitted to the hospital with a subarachnoid hemorrhage has complaints of severe headache, nuchal rigidity, and projectile vomiting. The nurse knows lumbar puncture (LP) would be contraindicated in this client in which circumstance?

1. Vomiting continues.
2. Intracranial pressure (ICP) is increased.
3. The client needs mechanical ventilation.
4. Blood is anticipated in the cerebrospinal fluid (CSF).

14. 2. Sudden removal of CSF results in pressures lower in the lumbar area than the brain and favors herniation of the brain; therefore, LP is contraindicated with increased ICP. An LP is performed if brain imaging is negative or inconclusive in the presence of subarachnoid hemorrhage-type symptoms. Vomiting may be caused by reasons other than increased ICP; therefore, LP isn't strictly contraindicated. An LP may be performed on clients needing mechanical ventilation. Blood in the CSF is diagnostic for subarachnoid hemorrhage.

CN: Physiological integrity; CNS: Physiological adaptation; CL: Application

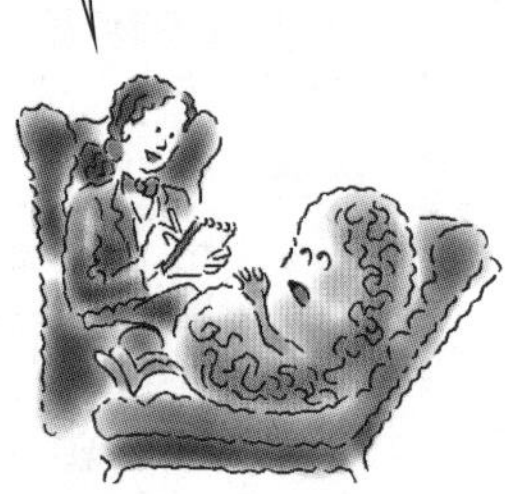

15. A client with head trauma develops a urine output of 300 ml/hour, dry skin, and dry mucous membranes. Which nursing intervention is the most appropriate to perform immediately?

1. Evaluate urine specific gravity.
2. Anticipate treatment for renal failure.
3. Provide emollients to the skin to prevent breakdown.
4. Slow the I.V. fluids and notify the physician.

15. 1. Urine output of 300 ml/hour may indicate diabetes insipidus, which is a failure of the pituitary to produce antidiuretic hormone. This condition may occur with increased intracranial pressure and head trauma; the nurse evaluates for low urine specific gravity, increased serum osmolarity, and dehydration. There's no evidence that the client is experiencing renal failure. Providing emollients to prevent skin breakdown is important, but doesn't need to be performed immediately. Slowing the rate of I.V. fluid would contribute to dehydration when polyuria is present.

CN: Physiological integrity; CNS: Physiological adaptation; CL: Analysis

16. Stool softeners would be given to a client after a repair of a cerebral aneurysm for which reason?

1. To stimulate the bowel due to loss of nerve innervation
2. To prevent straining, which increases intracranial pressure (ICP)
3. To prevent the Valsalva maneuver, which may lead to bradycardia
4. To prevent constipation when osmotic diuretics are used

16. 2. Straining when having a bowel movement, sneezing, coughing, and suctioning may lead to increased ICP and should be avoided when potential increased ICP exists. Stool softeners don't stimulate the bowel and aren't used in combination with osmotic diuretics. Although the Valsalva maneuver may lead to bradycardia and reflex tachycardia, this rationale doesn't apply to this client.

CN: Physiological integrity; CNS: Reduction of risk potential; CL: Application

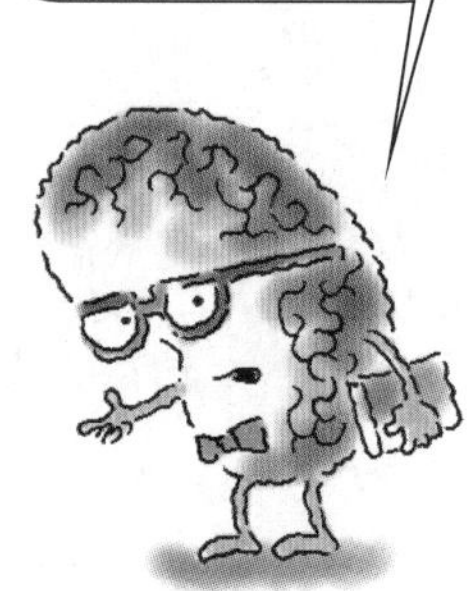

Knowing why you do something can help prevent errors.

17. A client with a subdural hematoma becomes restless and confused, with dilation of the ipsilateral pupil. The physician orders mannitol for which reason?

1. To reduce intraocular pressure
2. To prevent acute tubular necrosis
3. To promote osmotic diuresis to decrease intracranial pressure (ICP)
4. To draw water into the vascular system to increase blood pressure

17. 3. Mannitol promotes osmotic diuresis by increasing the pressure gradient, drawing fluid from intracellular to intravascular spaces. Although mannitol is used for all the reasons described, the reduction of ICP in this client is of greatest concern.

CN: Physiological integrity; CNS: Pharmacological and parenteral therapies; CL: Application

18. A client with a subdural hematoma was given mannitol to decrease intracranial pressure (ICP). Which result would best show the mannitol was effective?

1. Urine output increases.
2. Pupils are 8 mm and nonreactive.
3. Systolic blood pressure remains at 150 mm Hg.
4. Blood urea nitrogen (BUN) and creatinine levels return to normal.

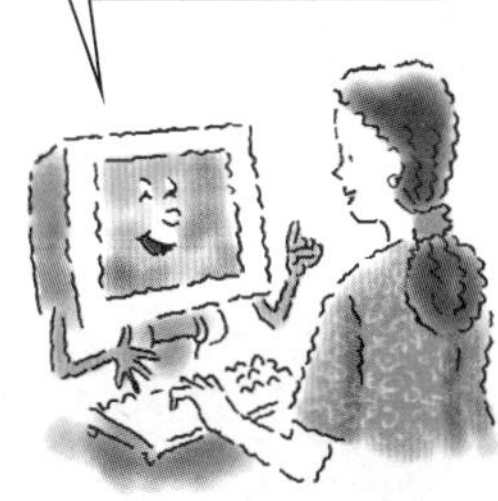
Choose the best response.

18. 1. Mannitol promotes osmotic diuresis by increasing the pressure gradient in the renal tubules, thus increasing urine output. Fixed and dilated pupils are symptoms of increased ICP or cranial nerve damage. No information is given about abnormal BUN and creatinine levels or that mannitol is being given for renal dysfunction or blood pressure maintenance.

CN: Physiological integrity; CNS: Physiological adaptation; CL: Application

19. When evaluating an arterial blood gas from a client with a subdural hematoma, the nurse notes the $Paco_2$ is 30 mm Hg. Which response best describes this result?

1. Appropriate; lowering carbon dioxide (CO_2) may reduce intracranial pressure (ICP)
2. Emergent; the client is poorly oxygenated
3. Normal
4. Significant; the client has alveolar hypoventilation

19. 1. A normal $Paco_2$ value is 35 to 45 mm Hg. CO_2 has vasodilating properties; therefore, lowering $Paco_2$ through hyperventilation in some clients may lower ICP caused by dilated cerebral vessels. Oxygenation is evaluated through Pao_2 and oxygen saturation. Alveolar hypoventilation would be reflected in an increased $Paco_2$.

CN: Physiological integrity; CNS: Physiological adaptation; CL: Analysis

20. Which nursing intervention should be used to prevent footdrop and contractures in a client recovering from a subdural hematoma?

1. High-topped sneakers
2. Low-dose heparin therapy
3. Physical therapy consultation
4. Sequential compression device

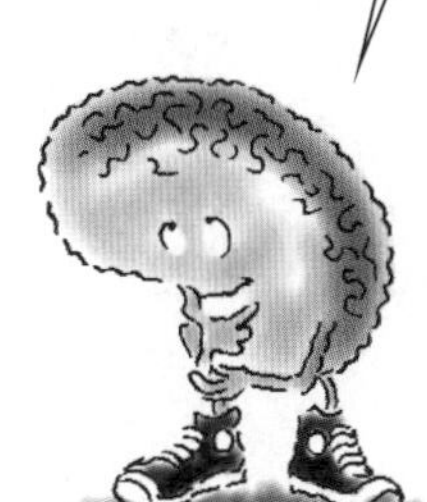
Hmmm, does health insurance cover high-topped sneakers?

20. 1. High-topped sneakers are used to prevent footdrop and contractures in neurologic clients. Low-dose heparin therapy and sequential compression boots will prevent deep vein thrombosis. Although a physical therapy consultation is important to initiate other interventions to prevent footdrop, a nurse may use high-topped sneakers independently.

CN: Physiological integrity; CNS: Basic care and comfort; CL: Application

21. A client who had a transsphenoidal hypophysectomy should be watched carefully for hemorrhage, which may be shown by which sign?

1. Bloody drainage from the ears
2. Frequent swallowing
3. Guaiac-positive stools
4. Hematuria

21. 2. Frequent swallowing after brain surgery may indicate fluid or blood leaking from the sinuses into the oropharynx. Blood or fluid draining from the ear may indicate a basilar skull fracture, guaiac-positive stools indicate GI bleeding, and hematuria may result from cystitis or other urologic complications.

CN: Physiological integrity; CNS: Physiological adaptation; CL: Analysis

22. After a hypophysectomy, vasopressin is given for which reason?

1. To treat growth failure
2. To prevent syndrome of inappropriate antidiuretic hormone (SIADH)
3. To reduce cerebral edema and lower intracranial pressure
4. To replace antidiuretic hormone (ADH) normally secreted from the pituitary

22. 4. After hypophysectomy, or removal of the pituitary gland, the body can't synthesize ADH. Somatropin or growth hormone, not vasopressin, is used to treat growth failure. SIADH results from excessive ADH secretion. Mannitol or corticosteroids are used to reduce cerebral edema.

CN: Physiological integrity; CNS: Pharmacological and parenteral therapies; CL: Application

23. A client's intracranial pressure (ICP) is fluctuating between 20 and 25 mm Hg. Which of the following nursing interventions is the most appropriate?

1. Ensure that the mean arterial pressure (MAP) is less than 90 mm Hg.
2. Lower the head of the bed to less than 15 degrees.
3. Encourage visitation.
4. Reassess the client's ABC's (airway, breathing, and circulation).

23. 4. The nurse should always reassess the client's ABC's when the ICP is elevated (normal is between 0 and15 mm Hg.). MAP should be maintained at or above 90 mm Hg. The head of the bed should be elevated between 15 and 30 degrees to facilitate venous drainage. External stimulation, such as visitors, should be limited as it may increase ICP.

CN: Physiological integrity; CNS: Physiological adaptation; CL: Application

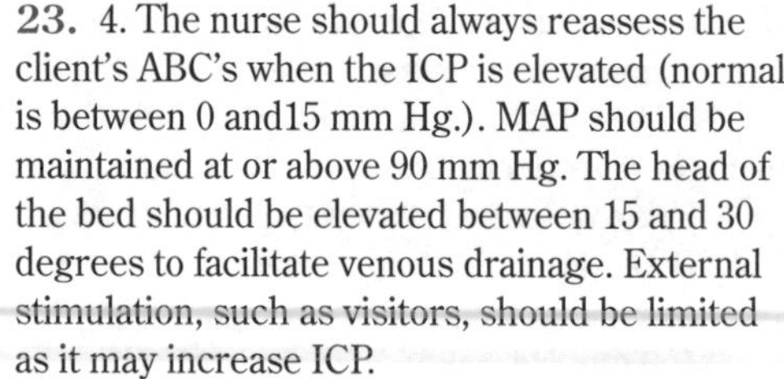

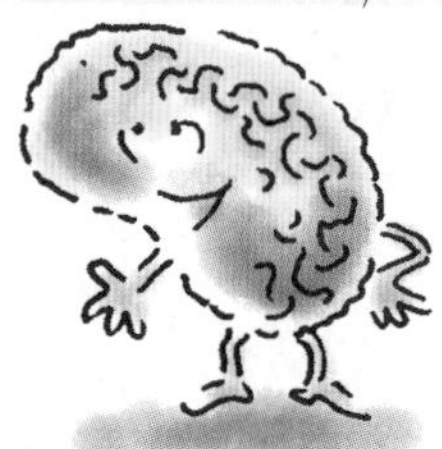

Be familiar with normal values to recognize an abnormal result.

24. A 33-year-old client undergoes an L4–L5 laminectomy. Which method would be best to prevent postoperative complications?

1. Encourage the client to be out of bed the first postoperative day.
2. Maximize bracing while in bed.
3. Limit movement in bed and reposition only when necessary.
4. Use a soft mattress.

24. 1. In most cases, clients should be out of bed the first postoperative day. Frequent repositioning, use of a chair-like brace for the lower back when out of bed, and a firm mattress will help minimize complications.

CN: Physiological integrity; CNS: Reduction of risk potential; CL: Application

25. Frequent voiding of small amounts of urine after a lumbar laminectomy may indicate which condition?

1. Diabetes insipidus
2. Diabetic ketoacidosis
3. Urine retention
4. Urinary tract infection (UTI)

25. 3. Swelling or pressure on the peripheral nerves controlling micturition, anesthesia, or use of an indwelling urinary catheter may lead to urine retention with frequent overflow of small amounts of urine. Diabetes insipidus and diabetic ketoacidosis are shown by polyuria. UTI may be shown by dysuria and frequent voiding of small amounts of urine, but would be less likely in this situation.

CN: Physiological integrity; CNS: Basic care and comfort; CL: Analysis

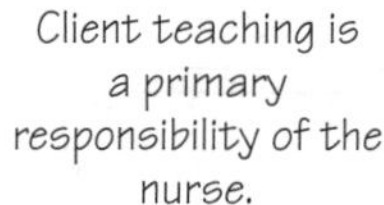

Client teaching is a primary responsibility of the nurse.

26. A client with lower back pain and a herniated nucleus pulposus should be taught that strengthening which muscle after laminectomy will prevent lower back pain?

1. Abdominal
2. Diaphragm
3. Gluteus
4. Rectus femoris

26. 1. Strengthening abdominal muscles will support the back, preventing lower back pain. Strengthening the diaphragm, the gluteus, or the rectus femoris won't prevent lower back pain.

CN: Physiological integrity; CNS: Reduction of risk potential; CL: Application

27. When preparing a client with suspected lumbar herniated nucleus pulposus for magnetic resonance imaging (MRI), which nursing intervention should be done before the test?

1. Question the client about allergy to iodine.
2. Mark distal pulses on the foot in indelible ink.
3. Teach the client relaxation techniques.
4. Tell the client he may be asked to cough or pant to clear the dye.

27. 3. The MRI scanner is a narrow tube that contains a magnet. The client lies on a platform and is placed in the tube. Some clients may become claustrophobic during the test; teaching relaxation techniques may help to alleviate this. Radiopaque dyes, used in myelography and cardiac catheterization, are usually iodine-based and may cause a reaction in those clients who are allergic. No dyes are used in MRI. During cardiac catheterization, a client is asked to cough or pant to clear the dye, and before cardiac catheterization or arteriogram, the nurse marks pedal pulses in ink.

CN: Physiological integrity; CNS: Reduction of risk potential; CL: Application

28. A client is scheduled for chemonucleolysis with chymopapain to relieve the pain of a herniated disk. Which factor should be assessed before the procedure?

1. Allergy to meat tenderizers
2. Allergy to shellfish
3. Ability to lie flat during the procedure
4. Range of motion (ROM) on the affected side

28. 1. Chymopapain, derived from papaya, is an ingredient in meat tenderizers. Sensitivity to this substance may preclude the use of chymopapain. Allergy to shellfish may be a contraindication to tests using iodine-based dyes. The client may be positioned on the side in a "C" position to allow access to the intervertebral area. Full ROM isn't needed for this procedure.

CN: Physiological integrity; CNS: Pharmacological and parenteral therapies; CL: Application

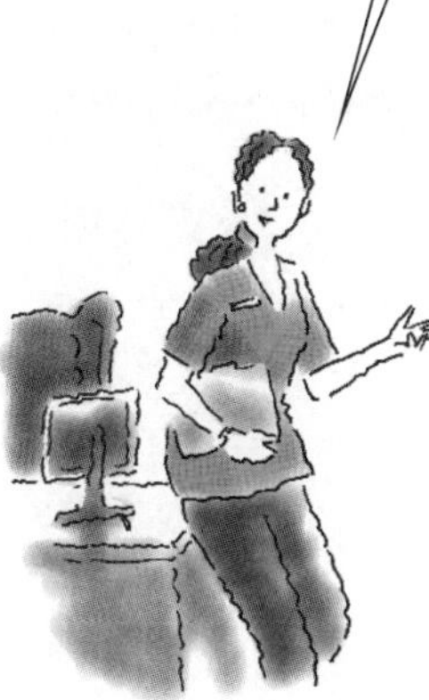

Here's a test-taking hint: prioritize.

29. When prioritizing care, which client should the nurse assess <u>first</u>?

1. A 17-year-old client 24 hours postappendectomy
2. A 33-year-old client with a recent diagnosis of Guillain-Barré syndrome
3. A 50-year-old client 3 days postmyocardial infarction
4. A 50-year-old client with diverticulitis

29. 2. Guillain-Barré syndrome is characterized by ascending paralysis and potential respiratory failure. The order of client assessment should follow client priorities, with disorders of airway, breathing, and then circulation. There's no information to suggest the postmyocardial infarction client has an arrhythmia or other complication. There's no evidence to suggest hemorrhage or perforation for the remaining clients as a priority of care.

CN: Safe, effective care environment; CNS: Management of care; CL: Analysis

30. A client is newly diagnosed with myasthenia gravis. The nurse is teaching the client about the cause of this disease. Which of the following responses by the client indicates that the teaching has been effective?

1. A postviral illness characterized by ascending paralysis
2. Loss of the myelin sheath surrounding peripheral nerves
3. Inability of basal ganglia to produce sufficient dopamine
4. Destruction of acetylcholine receptors causing muscle weakness

30. 4. Myasthenia gravis, an autoimmune disorder, is caused by the destruction of acetylcholine receptors. Guillain-Barré syndrome is a postviral illness characterized by ascending paralysis, multiple sclerosis is caused by loss of the myelin sheath, and Parkinson's disease is caused by the inability of basal ganglia to produce sufficient dopamine.

CN: Health promotion and maintenance; CNS: None; CL: Analysis

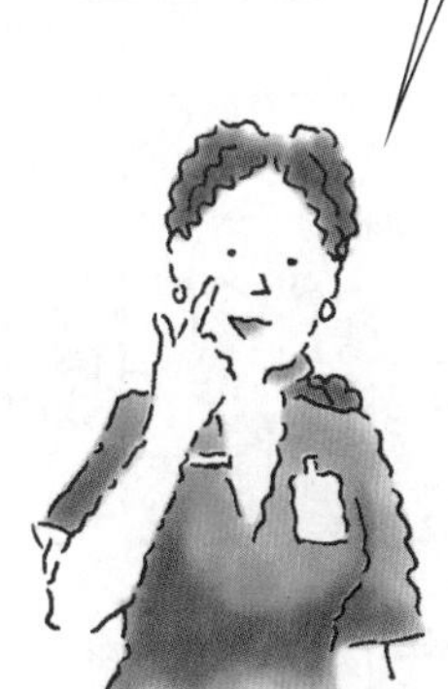

Keep your eyes open for clues.

31. Which condition is an <u>early</u> symptom commonly seen in myasthenia gravis?

1. Dysphagia
2. Fatigue improving at the end of the day
3. Ptosis
4. Respiratory distress

31. 3. Ptosis and diplopia are early signs of myasthenia gravis; dysphagia and respiratory distress occur later. Symptoms are typically milder in the morning and may be exacerbated by stress or lack of rest.

CN: Health promotion and maintenance; CNS: None; CL: Application

32. One hour after receiving pyridostigmine bromide (Mestinon), a client reports difficulty swallowing and excessive respiratory secretions. The nurse notifies the physician and prepares to administer which medication?

1. Additional pyridostigmine bromide (Mestinon)
2. Atropine
3. Edrophonium (Tensilon)
4. Acyclovir (Zovirax)

32. 2. These symptoms suggest cholinergic crisis or excessive acetylcholinesterase medication, typically appearing 45 to 60 minutes after the last dose of acetylcholinesterase inhibitor. Atropine, an anticholinergic drug, is used to antagonize acetylcholinesterase inhibitors. The other drugs are acetylcholinesterase inhibitors. Edrophonium is used for the diagnosis and pyrostigmine bromide is used for the treatment of myasthenia gravis and would worsen these symptoms. Acyclovir is an antiviral and would not be used to treat these symptoms.

CN: Physiological integrity; CNS: Pharmacological and parenteral therapies; CL: Analysis

33. A client with suspected myasthenia gravis is to undergo a Tensilon test. Tensilon is used to diagnose—but not treat—myasthenia gravis. Why isn't it used for treatment?

1. It isn't available in an oral form.
2. With repeated use, immunosuppression may occur.
3. Dry mouth and abdominal cramps may be intolerable adverse effects.
4. The short half-life of Tensilon makes it impractical for long-term use.

33. 4. The duration of action of Tensilon is 1 to 2 minutes, making it impractical for the long-term management of myasthenia gravis. Even though Tensilon isn't available in an oral form, its short half-life makes its use impractical. Immunosuppression with repeated use is an adverse effect of steroid administration, a medication used to treat myasthenia gravis. Dry mouth and abdominal cramps are adverse effects of increased acetylcholine in the parasympathetic nervous system.

CN: Physiological integrity; CNS: Pharmacological and parenteral therapies; CL: Application

34. A 20-year-old client with myasthenia gravis will undergo plasmapheresis. Which action describes the purpose of this procedure?

1. Preventing exacerbations during pregnancy
2. Removing T and B lymphocytes that attack acetylcholine receptors
3. Delivering acetylcholinesterase inhibitor directly into the bloodstream
4. Separating and removing acetylcholine receptor antibodies from the blood

34. 4. The purpose of plasmapheresis in myasthenia gravis is to separate and remove circulating acetylcholine receptor antibodies from the blood of clients refractory to the usual therapies or clients in crisis. Although stress, including pregnancy, may precipitate crisis, this isn't the purpose of the procedure. Plasmapheresis doesn't remove T and B lymphocytes, nor does it deliver acetylcholinesterase inhibitor directly into the bloodstream.

CN: Physiological integrity; CNS: Pharmacological and parenteral therapies; CL: Application

35. When assessing a client with glaucoma, a nurse expects which finding?

1. Complaints of double vision
2. Complaints of halos around lights
3. Intraocular pressure of 15 mm Hg
4. Soft globe on palpation

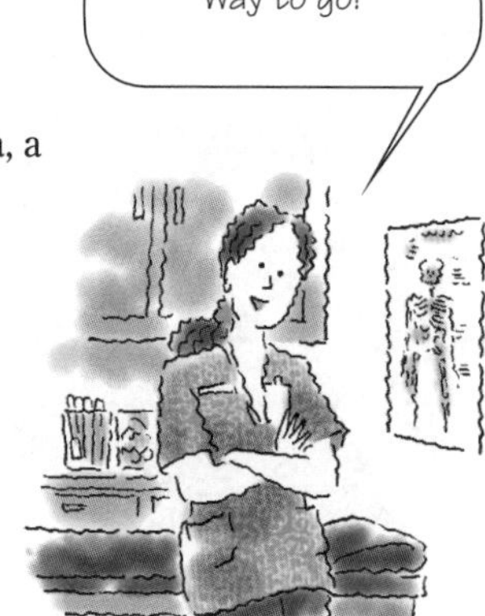

35. 2. Complaints of halos around lights is a common finding in a client with glaucoma. Symptoms of glaucoma don't include double vision but can include loss of peripheral vision or blind spots, reddened sclera, firm globe, decreased accommodation, halos around lights, and occasional eye pain, but clients may be asymptomatic. Normal intraocular pressure is 10 to 21 mm Hg.

CN: Physiological integrity; CNS: Physiological adaptation; CL: Application

36. A client at the eye clinic is newly diagnosed with glaucoma. Client teaching includes the need to take his medication because noncompliance may lead to which condition?

1. Diplopia
2. Permanent vision loss
3. Progressive loss of peripheral vision
4. Pupillary constriction

36. 2. Without treatment, glaucoma may progress to irreversible blindness. Treatment won't restore visual damage, but will halt disease progression. Blurred or foggy vision, not diplopia, is typical in glaucoma. Central vision loss is typical in glaucoma. Miotics, which constrict the pupil, are used in the treatment of glaucoma to permit outflow of the aqueous humor.

CN: Physiological integrity; CNS: Pharmacological and parenteral therapies; CL: Application

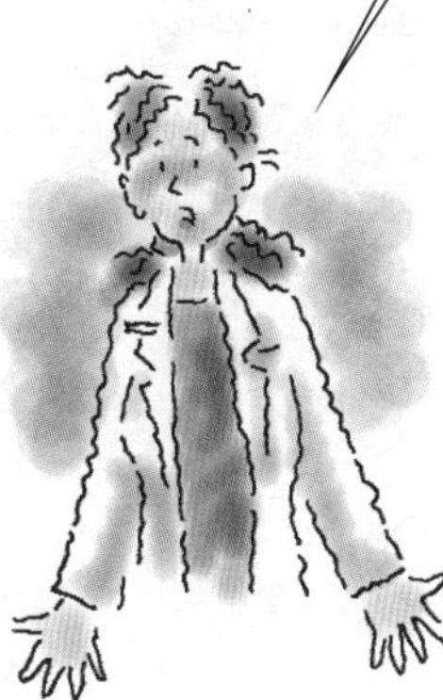

Don't get all discombobulated, now. Remember the abbreviations?

37. Pilocarpine, 2 gtt both eyes q.i.d., should be instilled according to which procedure?

1. Two drops of the drug in both eyes four times daily
2. Two drops on the sclera of both eyes two times daily
3. Two drops over the lacrimal duct of both eyes four times daily
4. Two drops of the drug toward the nasal side of each conjunctival sac three times daily

37. 1. *Q.i.d.* means four times daily and *gtt* means drops. Medications placed on the nasal side near the lacrimal duct will enter the nose and be ineffective.

CN: Physiological integrity; CNS: Pharmacological and parenteral therapies; CL: Application

38. When evaluating the extent of Parkinson's disease, a nurse observes for which condition?

1. Bulging eyeballs
2. Diminished distal sensation
3. Increased dopamine levels
4. Muscle rigidity

38. 4. Parkinson's disease is characterized by the slowing of voluntary muscle movement, muscular rigidity, and resting tremor. Bulging eyeballs (exophthalmos) occur in Graves' disease. Diminished distal sensation doesn't occur in Parkinson's disease. Dopamine is deficient in this disorder.

CN: Physiological integrity; CNS: Physiological adaptation; CL: Application

39. A client is admitted with Parkinson's disease. The client's face is expressionless and their speech is monotone. Which of the following observations by the nurse is <u>most accurate</u>?

1. The client is most likely depressed and should be left alone.
2. These are common symptoms of Parkinson's disease that produce an undesired façade of an alert and responsive individual.
3. The client's antipsychotic medication may need to be adjusted.
4. The client probably has dementia.

39. 2. The nurse should recognize that these are common symptoms of Parkinson's disease. The symptoms do not indicate depression or dementia, although these are common in Parkinson's disease. Antipsychotic medication will often mimic Parkinson's disease extrapyramidal symptoms and is not indicated. Parkinson's disease is caused by degeneration of the substantia nigra in the basal ganglia of the brain, where dopamine is produced and stored. This degeneration results in motor dysfunction.

CN: Physiological integrity; CNS: Physiological adaptation; CL: Application

40. Which client would be most at risk for secondary Parkinson's disease caused by pharmacotherapy?

1. A 30-year-old client with schizophrenia taking chlorpromazine (Thorazine)
2. A 50-year-old client taking nitroglycerin tablets for angina
3. A 60-year-old client taking prednisone for chronic obstructive pulmonary disease
4. A 75-year-old client using naproxen for rheumatoid arthritis

40. 1. Phenothiazines such as chlorpromazine deplete dopamine, which may lead to tremor rigidity (extrapyramidal effects). The other drugs don't place the client at a greater risk for developing Parkinson's disease.

CN: Physiological integrity; CNS: Pharmacological and parenteral therapies; CL: Application

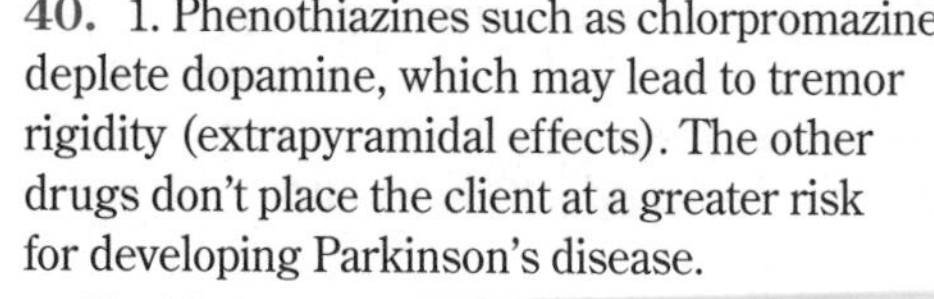

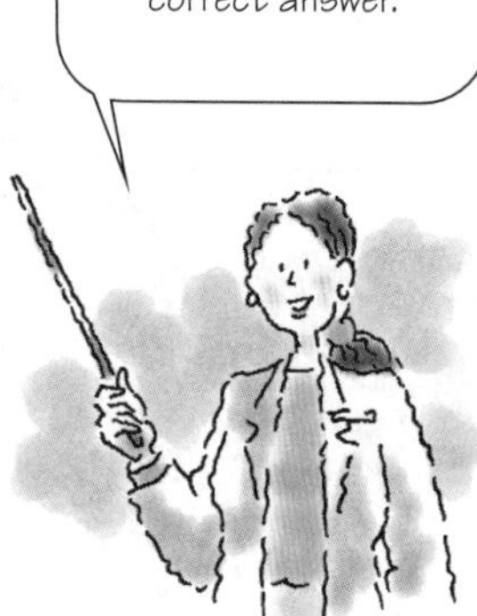

Read question 41 carefully to get the correct answer.

41. Which symptom occurs initially in Parkinson's disease?

1. Akinesia
2. Aspiration of food
3. Dementia
4. Pill rolling movements of the hand

41. 4. Early symptoms of Parkinson's disease include coarse resting tremors of the fingers and thumb. Akinesia and aspiration are late signs of Parkinson's disease. Dementia occurs in only 20% of the clients with Parkinson's disease.

CN: Health promotion and maintenance; CNS: None; CL: Application

42. To evaluate the effectiveness of levodopa-carbidopa (Sinemet), a nurse should watch for which result?

1. Improved visual acuity
2. Decreased dyskinesia
3. Reduction in short-term memory
4. Lessened rigidity and tremor

42. 4. Levodopa-carbidopa increases the amount of dopamine in the central nervous system, allowing for more smooth, purposeful movements. The drug doesn't affect visual acuity and should improve dyskinesia and short-term memory.

CN: Physiological integrity; CNS: Pharmacological and parenteral therapies; CL: Application

43. Two days after starting therapy with trihexyphenidyl, a client complains of a dry mouth. Which nursing intervention would best relieve the client's dry mouth?

1. Offer the client ice chips and frequent sips of water.
2. Withhold the drug and notify the physician.
3. Change the client's diet to clear liquid until the symptoms subside.
4. Encourage the use of supplemental puddings and shakes to maintain weight.

43. 1. Trihexyphenidyl is an anticholinergic agent that causes blurred vision, dry mouth, constipation, and urine retention. There's no need to withhold the drug unless hypotension or tachyarrhythmia occurs. A clear liquid diet doesn't provide adequate nutrition and may be more difficult to swallow than thickened liquids if dysphagia is present; it isn't indicated at this time. Weight loss may occur with Parkinson's disease; however, the question relates to effects of trihexyphenidyl.

CN: Physiological integrity; CNS: Pharmacological and parenteral therapies; CL: Analysis

44. Which antiparkinsonian drug can cause drug tolerance or toxicity if taken for too long at one time?

1. Amantadine (Symmetrel)
2. Levodopa-carbidopa (Sinemet)
3. Pergolide
4. Selegiline (Eldepryl)

44. 2. Long-term therapy with levodopa-carbidopa can result in drug tolerance or toxicity, shown by confusion, hallucinations, or decreased drug effectiveness. The other drugs don't require that the client take a drug holiday.

CN: Physiological integrity; CNS: Pharmacological and parenteral therapies; CL: Application

45. A young female client has been recently diagnosed with multiple sclerosis (MS) and wants more information on the disease. In teaching the client, which statement by the nurse is most accurate?

1. MS is an autoimmune disease.
2. MS is more common in men than women.
3. MS is characterized by remyelination.
4. MS is an acute and curable disease.

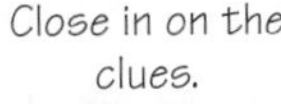

Close in on the clues.

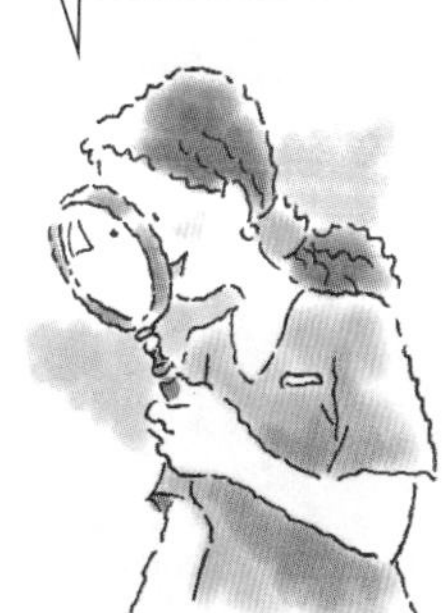

45. 1. MS is a chronic autoimmune disease that is more common in women than in men. It is characterized by multiple areas of demyelination and scarring (sclerosis) of the underlying nerve fibers. There are no known cures for MS, although treatment can help promote remissions and prevent exacerbations.

CN: Physiological integrity; CNS: Physiological adaptation; CL: Application

46. A client with multiple sclerosis (MS) is started on 20 mg of glatiramer (Copaxone) subcutaneously daily. Immediately after the injection, the client experiences flushing and chest pain. Which of the following would be the most appropriate nursing intervention?

1. Call a code.
2. Call the physician to inform him of the client's adverse reaction.
3. Administer oxygen.
4. Monitor the client to see if the symptoms quickly dissipate.

46. 4. Glatiramer helps to decrease the number of relapses in the MS client. Flushing, chest pain, palpitations, anxiety, shortness of breath, and itching occur in some clients following administration of the medication. They typically are transient and self-limiting and don't need specific treatment.

CN: Physiological integrity; CNS: Pharmacological and parenteral therapies; CL: Analysis

47. Which symptom usually occurs early in multiple sclerosis (MS)?

1. Diplopia
2. Grief
3. Paralysis
4. Dementia

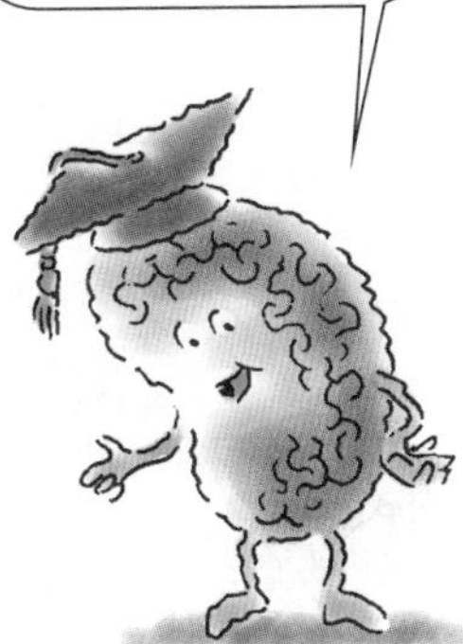

Client teaching is very important.

47. 1. Early symptoms of MS include slurred speech and diplopia. Grief isn't a clinical manifestation. Paralysis is a late symptom of MS. Although depression and a short attention span may occur, dementia is rarely associated with MS.

CN: Physiological integrity; CNS: Physiological adaptation; CL: Application

48. Which measure would be included in teaching the client with multiple sclerosis (MS) to avoid exacerbation of the disease?

1. Patching the affected eye
2. Sleeping 8 hours each night
3. Taking hot baths for relaxation
4. Drinking 1½ to 2 qt (1.5 to 2 L) of fluid daily

48. 2. MS is exacerbated by exposure to stress, fatigue, and heat. Clients should balance activity with rest. Patching the affected eye may result in improvement in vision and balance but won't prevent exacerbation of the disease. Adequate hydration will help prevent urinary tract infections secondary to a neurogenic bladder.

CN: Physiological integrity; CNS: Reduction of risk potential; CL: Application

49. Which condition or activity may exacerbate multiple sclerosis (MS)?

1. Pregnancy
2. Range-of-motion (ROM) exercises
3. Swimming
4. Urine retention

49. 1. Pregnancy, stress, fatigue, and heat may exacerbate MS. Exercise to maintain ROM is encouraged; swimming is particularly effective due to weightlessness and the cooling of nerves. Urine retention is common due to neurogenic bladder but doesn't lead to the exacerbation of symptoms.

CN: Physiological integrity; CNS: Reduction of risk potential; CL: Application

50. A client with suspected multiple sclerosis (MS) undergoes a lumbar puncture. Which abnormality is typically found in the cerebrospinal fluid (CSF) of clients with MS?

1. Blood or increased red blood cells
2. Elevated white blood cells (WBCs) or pus
3. Increased glucose concentrations
4. Increased protein levels

50. 4. Elevated gamma globulin fraction in CSF without an elevated level in the blood occurs in MS. WBCs or pus indicates infection. Blood may be found with trauma or subarachnoid hemorrhage. Increased glucose concentration is a nonspecific finding indicating infection or subarachnoid hemorrhage.

CN: Physiological integrity; CNS: Physiological adaptation; CL: Analysis

51. Which term describes involuntary, jerking, rhythmic movements of the eyes?

1. Diplopia
2. Exophthalmos
3. Nystagmus
4. Oculogyric crisis

51. 3. *Nystagmus* refers to jerking movements of the eye. *Diplopia* means double vision. *Exophthalmos* refers to bulging eyeballs, as seen in Graves' disease. Oculogyric crisis involves deviation of the eyes.

CN: Health promotion and maintenance; CNS: None; CL: Application

52. Which nursing intervention takes priority for the client having a tonic-clonic seizure?

1. Maintaining a patent airway
2. Timing the duration of the seizure
3. Noting the origin of seizure activity
4. Inserting a padded tongue blade to prevent the client from biting his tongue

52. 1. The priority during and after a seizure is to maintain a patent airway. Timing the seizure activity and noting the origin of motor dysfunction are done, but not first. Nothing should be placed in the client's mouth during a seizure because teeth may be dislodged or the tongue pushed back, further obstructing the airway.

CN: Safe, effective care environment; CNS: Management of care; CL: Application

53. A client recalls smelling an unpleasant odor before his seizure. Which term describes this symptom?

1. Atonic seizure
2. Aura
3. Icterus
4. Postictal experience

53. 2. An aura occurs in some clients as a warning before a seizure. The client may experience a certain smell, a vision such as flashing lights, or a sensation. *Atonic seizure* or *drop attack* refers to an abrupt loss of muscle tone. Icterus refers to jaundice. Postictal experience occurs after a seizure, during which the client may be confused, somnolent, and fatigued.

CN: Physiological integrity; CNS: Physiological adaptation; CL: Application

54. A client with new-onset seizures of unknown cause is started on phenytoin (Dilantin), 750 mg I.V. now and 100 mg P.O. t.i.d. Which statement best describes the purpose of the loading dose?

1. To ensure that the drug reaches the cerebrospinal fluid
2. To prevent the need for surgical excision of the epileptic focus
3. To reduce secretions in case another seizure occurs
4. To more quickly attain therapeutic levels

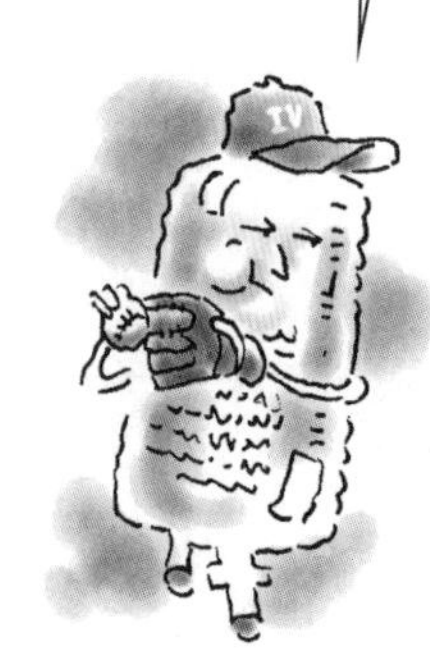

The question said "loading" dose, not "loaded bases."
IV

54. 4. A loading dose of phenytoin and other drugs is given to reach therapeutic levels more quickly; maintenance dosing follows. A loading dose of phenytoin can be oral or parenteral. Surgical excision of an epileptic focus is considered when seizures aren't controlled with anticonvulsant therapy. Phenytoin doesn't reduce secretions.

CN: Physiological integrity; CNS: Pharmacological and parenteral therapies; CL: Application

55. Which adverse effect may occur during phenytoin (Dilantin) therapy?
1. Dry mouth
2. Furry tongue
3. Somnolence
4. Tachycardia

56. Which symptom may occur with a phenytoin level of 32 mg/dl?
1. Ataxia and confusion
2. Sodium depletion
3. Tonic-clonic seizure
4. Urinary incontinence

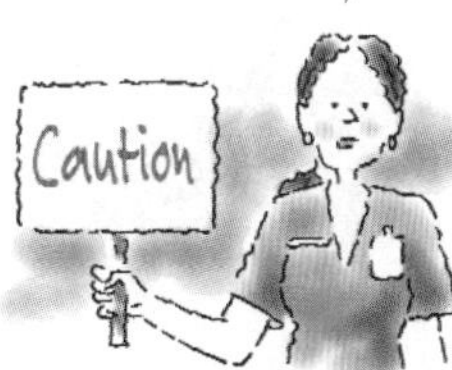

Caution! Can you find the clues here?
Caution

57. Which precaution must be taken when giving phenytoin (Dilantin) to a client with a nasogastric (NG) tube for feeding?
1. Check the phenytoin level after giving the drug to check for toxicity.
2. Elevate the head of the bed before giving phenytoin through the NG tube.
3. Give phenytoin 1 hour before or 2 hours after NG tube feedings to ensure absorption.
4. Verify proper placement of the NG tube by placing the end of the tube in a glass of water and observing for bubbles.

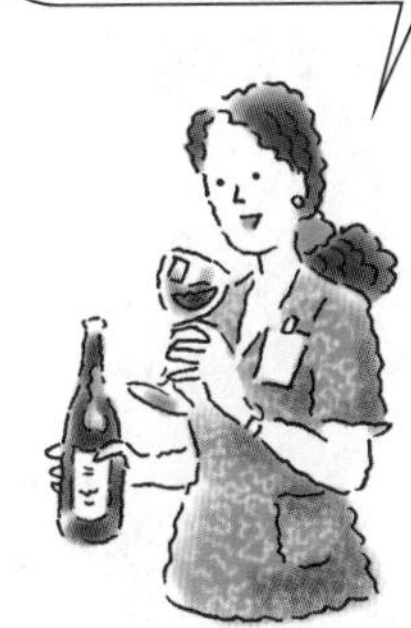

So, why doesn't alcohol get along with phenytoin?

58. What's the most important concern for clients who drink alcohol while taking phenytoin?
1. Alcohol increases phenytoin activity.
2. Alcohol raises the seizure threshold.
3. Alcohol impairs judgment and coordination.
4. Alcohol decreases the effectiveness of phenytoin.

59. When assessing vital signs in a client with a seizure disorder, which measure is used?
1. Checking for a pulse deficit
2. Checking for pulsus paradoxus
3. Taking axillary instead of oral temperatures
4. Checking the blood pressure for an auscultatory gap

55. 3. Adverse effects of phenytoin include sedation, somnolence, gingival hyperplasia, blood dyscrasia, and toxicity. The other symptoms aren't adverse effects of phenytoin.
CN: Physiological integrity; CNS: Pharmacological and parenteral therapies; CL: Application

56. 1. A therapeutic phenytoin level is 10 to 20 mg/dl. A level of 32 mg/dl indicates phenytoin toxicity. Symptoms of toxicity include confusion and ataxia. Phenytoin doesn't cause hyponatremia, seizure, or urinary incontinence. Incontinence may occur during or after a seizure.
CN: Physiological integrity; CNS: Pharmacological and parenteral therapies; CL: Analysis

57. 3. Nutritional supplements and milk interfere with the absorption of phenytoin, decreasing its effectiveness. Phenytoin levels are checked before giving the drug and the drug is withheld for elevated levels to avoid compounding toxicity. The head of the bed is elevated when giving all drugs or solutions and isn't specific to phenytoin administration. The nurse verifies NG tube placement by checking for stomach contents before giving drugs and feedings.
CN: Physiological integrity; CNS: Pharmacological and parenteral therapies; CL: Application

58. 4. Alcohol decreases phenytoin activity, diminishing its effectiveness. Although alcohol also reduces the seizure threshold and impairs judgement and coordination, these effects aren't the primary concern.
CN: Physiological integrity; CNS: Pharmacological and parenteral therapies; CL: Application

59. 3. To reduce the risk of injury, the nurse should take an axillary temperature or use a metal thermometer when taking an oral temperature to prevent injury if a seizure occurs. Pulse deficit occurs in an arrhythmia. Pulsus paradoxus may occur with cardiac tamponade. An auscultatory gap occurs in hypertension.
CN: Physiological integrity; CNS: Reduction of risk potential; CL: Application

60. A client in status epilepticus arrives at the emergency department. His family is interviewed to determine the cause of this problem. Which event may have predisposed the client to this condition?

1. Abruptly stopping anticonvulsant therapy
2. Airplane travel
3. Exposure to sunlight
4. Recent upper respiratory infection

60. 1. Status epilepticus (seizures not responsive to usual therapies) occurs with the abrupt cessation of anticonvulsant drugs or ethanol intake. The other options don't cause status epilepticus.

CN: Physiological integrity; CNS: Pharmacological and parenteral therapies; CL: Analysis

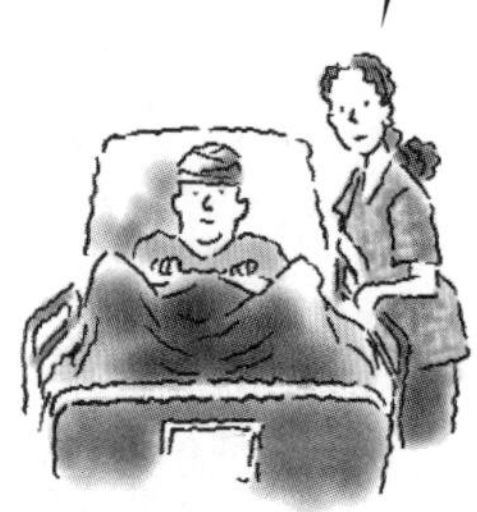

61. A client comes to the emergency department after hitting his head in a motor vehicle collision. He's alert and oriented. Which nursing intervention should be done first?

1. Assess full range of motion (ROM) to determine the extent of injuries.
2. Call for an immediate chest X-ray.
3. Immobilize the client's head and neck.
4. Open the airway with the head-tilt, chin-lift maneuver.

61. 3. All clients with a head injury are treated as if a cervical spine injury is present until X-rays confirm their absence. ROM would be contraindicated at this time. There is no indication the client needs a chest X-ray. The airway doesn't need to be opened since the client appears alert and not in respiratory distress. The head-tilt, chin-lift maneuver wouldn't be used until cervical spine injury is ruled out.

CN: Safe, effective care environment; CNS: Management of care; CL: Application

62. A client with a C6 spinal injury would most likely have which symptom?

1. Aphasia
2. Hemiparesis
3. Paraplegia
4. Quadriplegia

62. 4. Quadriplegia occurs as a result of cervical spine injuries. Aphasia refers to difficulty expressing or understanding spoken words. Hemiparesis describes weakness of one side of the body. Paraplegia occurs as a result of injury to the thoracic cord and below.

CN: Physiological integrity; CNS: Physiological adaptation; CL: Application

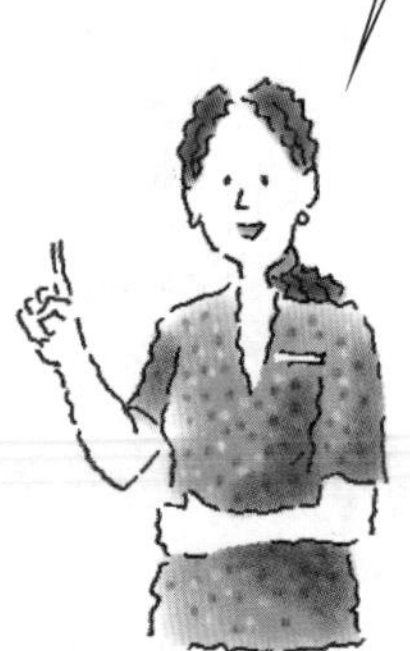

Let's see, what do all three of these brain areas have in common?

63. Nursing care of a client with damage to the hippocampus, amygdala, and fornix should focus on which of the following?

1. Frequent monitoring of vital signs
2. Coordination
3. Memory and emotion
4. Pain control

63. 1. The hippocampus, amygdala, and fornix make up the limbic system, which regulates emotions. The hippocampus and associated structures are also important for short-term memory. Coordination is a function of the cerebellum. The midbrain, pons, medulla oblongata, and reticular formation regulate vital functions.

CN: Safe, effective care environment; CNS: Management of care; CL: Application

64. A 30-year-old client is admitted to the progressive care unit with a C5 fracture from a motorcycle collision. Which assessment would take priority?

1. Bladder distention
2. Neurologic deficit
3. Pulse oximetry readings
4. The client's feelings about the injury

64. 3. After a spinal cord injury, ascending cord edema may cause a higher level of injury. The diaphragm is innervated at the level of C4, so assessment of adequate oxygenation and ventilation is necessary. Although the other options would be necessary at a later time, observation for respiratory failure is the priority.

CN: Safe, effective care environment; CNS: Management of care; CL: Application

CN: Client needs category CNS: Client needs subcategory CL: Cognitive level

65. While in the emergency department, a client with C8 quadriplegia develops a blood pressure of 80/44 mm Hg, pulse of 48 beats/minute, and respiratory rate of 18 breaths/minute. The nurse suspects which condition?

1. Autonomic dysreflexia
2. Hemorrhagic shock
3. Neurogenic shock
4. Pulmonary embolism

65. 3. Symptoms of neurogenic shock include hypotension, bradycardia, and warm, dry skin due to loss of adrenergic stimulation below the level of the lesion. Hypertension, bradycardia, flushing, and sweating of the skin are seen with autonomic dysreflexia. Hemorrhagic shock presents with anxiety, tachycardia, and hypotension; this wouldn't be suspected without an injury. Pulmonary embolism presents with chest pain, hypotension, hypoxemia, tachycardia, and hemoptysis; this may be a later complication of spinal cord injury due to immobility.

CN: Physiological integrity; CNS: Physiological adaptation; CL: Analysis

66. A client is admitted with a spinal cord injury at the level of T12. He has limited movement of his upper extremities. Which medication should be used to control edema of the spinal cord?

1. Acetazolamide (Diamox)
2. Furosemide (Lasix)
3. Methylprednisolone (Solu-Medrol)
4. Sodium bicarbonate

66. 3. High doses of methylprednisolone are used within 8 hours of spinal cord injury to reduce cord swelling and limit neurologic deficit. The other drugs aren't indicated in this circumstance.

CN: Physiological integrity; CNS: Pharmacological and parenteral therapies; CL: Application

67. A 22-year-old client with quadriplegia is apprehensive and flushed, with a blood pressure of 210/100 mm Hg and heart rate of 50 beats/minute. Which nursing intervention should be done <u>first</u>?

1. Place the client flat in bed.
2. Assess patency of the indwelling urinary catheter.
3. Give one sublingual nitroglycerin tablet.
4. Raise the head of the bed immediately to 90 degrees.

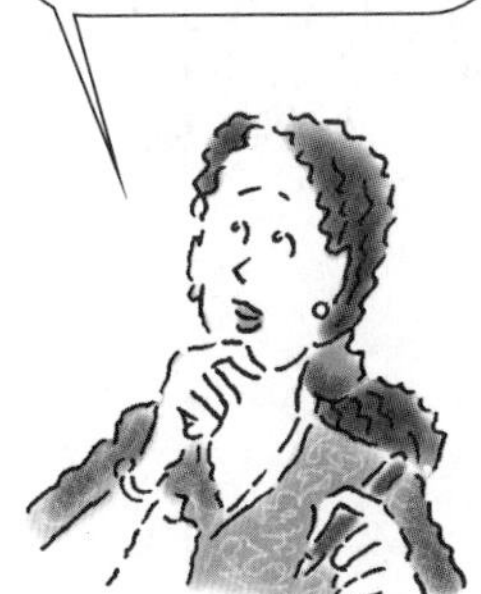

Which nursing intervention comes first?

67. 4. Anxiety, flushing above the level of the lesion, piloerection, hypertension, and bradycardia are symptoms of autonomic dysreflexia, typically caused by such noxious stimuli as a full bladder, fecal impaction, or pressure ulcer. Putting the client flat will cause the blood pressure to increase more. The indwelling urinary catheter should be assessed immediately after the head of the bed is raised. Nitroglycerin is given to relieve chest pain and reduce preload; it isn't used for hypertension or dysreflexia.

CN: Safe, effective care environment; CNS: Management of care; CL: Analysis

68. A client with paraplegia from a T10 injury is getting ready to transfer to a rehabilitation hospital. When the nurse offers to assist him, the client throws his suitcase on the floor and says, "You don't want to help me." Which response would be the <u>most appropriate</u> for the nurse to give?

1. "You know I want to help you. I offered."
2. "I'll pick these things up for you and come back later."
3. "You seem angry today. Going to rehab may be scary."
4. "When you get to rehab, they won't let you behave like a spoiled brat."

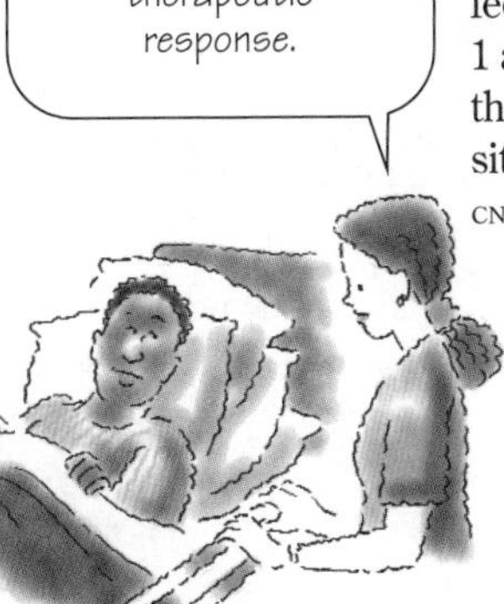

Choose the most therapeutic response.

68. 3. The nurse should always focus on the feelings underlying a particular action. Options 1 and 4 are confrontational. Offering to pick up the client's belongings doesn't deal with the situation and assumes he can't do it alone.

CN: Psychosocial integrity; CNS: None; CL: Application

69. A client with a cervical spine injury is placed in a Minerva body vest. The client is uncomfortable and would like to try a different device. The nurse should explain which of the following to the client?

1. The vest protects the neck against excessive motion.
2. The vest will provide for immobilization of the mid-cervical segments.
3. The vest will provide significant immobilization including lateral flexion.
4. There are other soft type collars that can be used.

69. 3. The Minerva vest will provide significant immobilization including lateral flexion. Most soft collars do not limit cervical motion, but act as a reminder against excessive motion. More rigid devices such as the Philadelphia collar provide reasonable immobilization of the mid-cervical segments for flexion and extension, but not for lateral flexion.

CN: Physiological integrity; CNS: Physiological adaptation; CL: Application

70. When a client with a halo vest is discharged from the hospital, which instruction should the nurse give the client and family?

1. "Don't use the wheelchair while the halo vest is in place."
2. "Clean the pin sites with peroxide."
3. "Keep the wrench that opens the vest attached to the client at all times."
4. "Perform range-of-motion (ROM) exercises to the neck and shoulders four times daily."

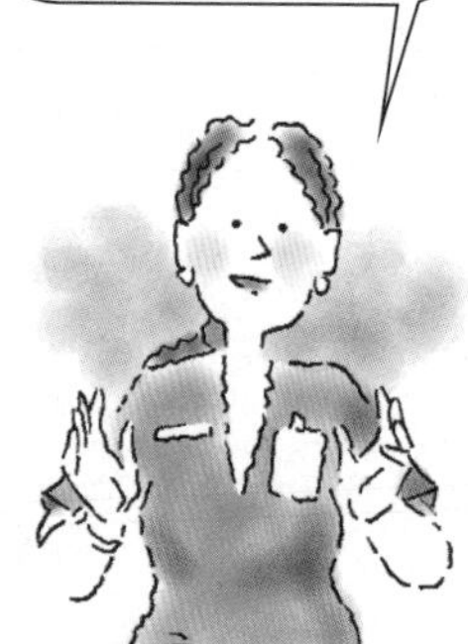
Teaching is second nature to a nurse.

70. 3. The wrench must be attached at all times to remove the vest in case the client needs cardiopulmonary resuscitation. The vest is designed to improve mobility; the client may use a wheelchair. Peroxide, especially full-strength, can disrupt the healing process and normal flora. The purpose of the vest is to immobilize the neck; ROM exercises to the neck are prohibited but should be performed to other areas.

CN: Physiological integrity; CNS: Reduction of risk potential; CL: Application

71. A client is admitted with intervertebral disk prolapse and now shows new symptoms of loss of bladder control and paralysis of both legs. Which of the following nursing interventions should be the priority?

1. Obtaining an order for a urinary drainage device.
2. Notifying the physician immediately.
3. Increasing the frequency of vital signs.
4. Administering medication to decrease inflammation.

71. 2. Cauda equina syndrome occurs when there is compression on the nerve roots. It affects areas below the level of these nerve roots. It is an emergency that requires surgical intervention; if not treated, it may lead to permanent loss of bladder and bowel control and paralysis of the legs. Inserting a urinary drainage device, increasing the frequency of vital signs, and administering anti-inflammatory medication may be interventions that are needed; however, they are not the priority.

CN: Safe, effective care environment; CNS: Management of care; CL: Analysis

72. Which intervention describes an appropriate bladder program for a client in rehabilitation for spinal cord injury?

1. Insert an indwelling urinary catheter.
2. Schedule intermittent catheterization every 2 to 4 hours.
3. Perform a straight catheterization every 8 hours while the client is awake.
4. Perform Credé's maneuver to the lower abdomen before the client voids.

72. 2. Intermittent catheterization should begin every 2 to 4 hours early in treatment. When residual volume is less than 400 ml, the schedule may advance to every 4 to 6 hours. Indwelling catheters may predispose the client to infection and are removed as soon as possible. Credé's maneuver is applied after voiding to enhance bladder emptying.

CN: Physiological integrity; CNS: Basic care and comfort; CL: Application

73. A 46-year-old client with breast cancer complains of back pain and difficulty moving her legs. Which nursing intervention is the most appropriate?

1. Notify the physician.
2. Position the client on her side, and prop her with a foam wedge.
3. Ask the physician for a physical therapy consultation.
4. Give acetaminophen, and reassure the client that the pain will disappear soon.

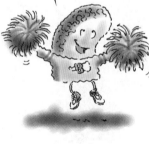

73. 1. Symptoms of back pain and neurologic deficits may be symptoms of metastasis. The physician should be notified. Repositioning the client, physical therapy, or giving acetaminophen may help the pain but may delay evaluation and treatment.

CN: Health promotion and maintenance; CNS: None; CL: Analysis

74. A client was admitted to the hospital because of a transient ischemic attack secondary to atrial fibrillation. He should be given which medication to prevent further neurologic deficit?

1. Digoxin (Lanoxin)
2. Diltiazem (Cardizem)
3. Heparin
4. Quinidine gluconate

74. 3. Atrial fibrillation may lead to the formation of mural thrombi, which may embolize to the brain. Heparin will prevent further clot formation and prevent clot enlargement. The other drugs are used in the treatment and control of atrial fibrillation but won't affect clot formation.

CN: Physiological integrity; CNS: Pharmacological and parenteral therapies; CL: Application

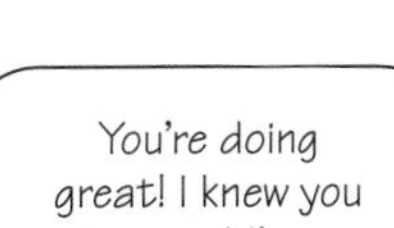

You're doing great! I knew you would!

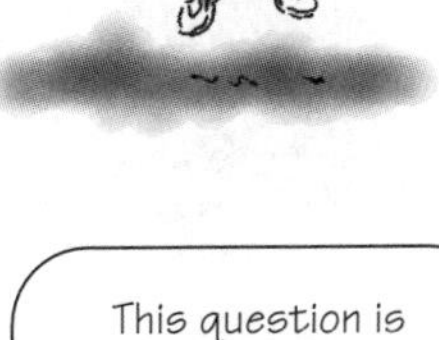

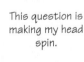

75. A client is diagnosed with Ménière's disease. Which nursing diagnosis would take priority for this client?

1. *Risk for ineffective cerebral tissue perfusion*
2. *Imbalanced nutrition: More than body requirements*
3. *Impaired social interaction*
4. *Risk for injury*

75. 4. Ménière's disease results in dizziness, so the client should be protected from falling. Ménière's disease doesn't alter cerebral tissue perfusion or directly affect nutrition. Although hearing loss may occur, causing impaired social interaction, this isn't a priority.

CN: Safe, effective care environment; CNS: Management of care; CL: Application

76. Which position would be the most appropriate for a client who has undergone stapedectomy?

1. On the affected side
2. On the unaffected side
3. Prone
4. Sims'

76. 2. The client should be positioned with the operative ear up, on the unaffected side. Although Sims' position is a side-lying position, it doesn't consider which side is best for after ear surgery.

CN: Physiological integrity; CNS: Physiological adaptation; CL: Application

77. Which symptom should the nurse expect to find when assessing a client with Ménière's disease?

1. Epistaxis
2. Facial pain
3. Ptosis
4. Tinnitus

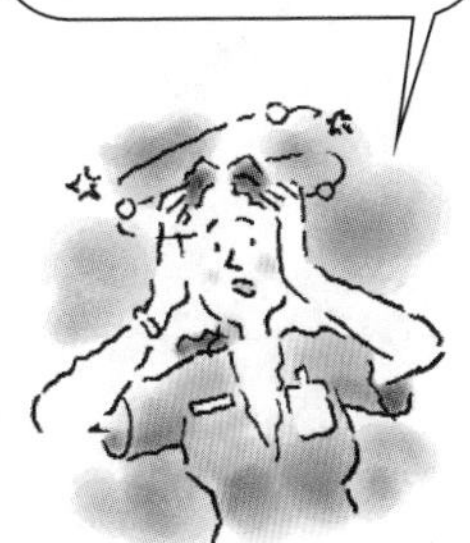

This question is making my head spin.

77. 4. Tinnitus, dizziness, and vertigo occur in Ménière's disease. Epistaxis may occur with a variety of blood dyscrasias or local lesions. Facial pain may occur with trigeminal neuralgia. Ptosis occurs with a variety of conditions, including myasthenia gravis.

CN: Physiological integrity; CNS: Physiological adaptation; CL: Application

78. Which nursing intervention has priority for an occupational nurse treating a client with a foreign body protruding from the eye?

1. Irrigate the eye with sterile saline.
2. Assess visual acuity with a Snellen chart.
3. Remove the foreign body with sterile forceps.
4. Patch both eyes until seen by the ophthalmologist.

78. 4. One or both eyes may be patched to prevent pain with extraocular movement or accommodation. Chemicals or small foreign bodies may be irrigated. Assessment of visual acuity isn't a priority, although it may be done after treatment. Protruding objects aren't removed by the nurse because the vitreous body may rupture.

CN: Safe, effective care environment; CNS: Management of care; CL: Application

79. A client with severe eye pain requests a prescription for the topical anesthetic the ophthalmologist instilled. A nurse explains these drugs shouldn't be used on an ongoing basis for which reason?

1. They are a way for pathogens to enter.
2. They cause dependence and rebound pain.
3. Damage could occur to the cornea due to lack of sensation.
4. The resulting blurred vision from mydriasis makes activity hazardous.

79. 3. Corneal damage may occur with the prolonged use of topical anesthetics. If the bottle isn't touched to the eye or lashes, the entry of pathogens should be limited. Dependence and rebound don't occur from topical anesthetics. Anesthetics don't cause mydriasis.

CN: Physiological integrity; CNS: Reduction of risk potential; CL: Application

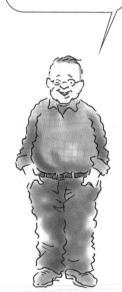

80. An 86-year-old client admitted to the hospital with chest pain is hearing-impaired. Which method should be used when assessing the client?

1. Obtain an ear wick.
2. Shout into the better ear.
3. Lower your voice pitch while facing the client.
4. Ask the family to go home and get the client's hearing aid.

80. 3. Hearing loss in an elderly client typically involves the upper ranges; lowering the pitch of your voice and facing the client is essential for the client to use other means of understanding, such as lip reading, mood, and so on. An ear wick is used to allow medications to enter the ear canal. Shouting is typically in the upper ranges and could cause anxiety to an already anxious client. Alternative means of communication such as writing may also be used to assess chest pain while waiting for the family to bring the hearing aid from home.

CN: Physiological integrity; CNS: Basic care and comfort; CL: Application

81. A client is scheduled for magnetic resonance imaging (MRI) of the head. Which area is essential to assess before the procedure?

1. Food or drink intake within the past 8 hours
2. Metal fillings, prostheses, or a pacemaker
3. The presence of carotid artery disease
4. Voiding before the procedure

81. 2. Strong magnetic waves may dislodge metal in the client's body, causing tissue injury. Although the client may be told to restrict food for 8 hours, particularly if contrast is used, metal is an absolute contraindication for this procedure. Voiding beforehand would make the client more comfortable and better able to remain still during the procedure, but isn't essential for the test. Having carotid artery disease isn't a contraindication to having an MRI.

CN: Safe, effective care environment; CNS: Safety and infection control; CL: Application

82. The nurse is providing teaching for a client being discharged with a prescription reading 1 gtt both ears t.i.d. Which of the following statements by the nurse would be most accurate?

1. Place one drop into each ear three times daily.
2. Place one drop into each ear two times daily.
3. Place one drop into each ear four times daily.
4. Place three drops into both ears once daily.

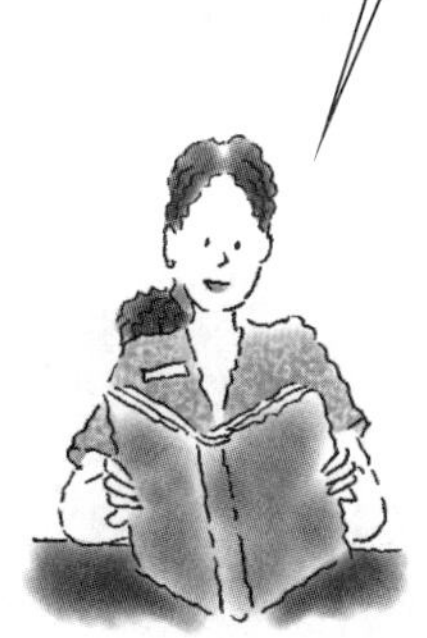

Prevent errors. Know your abbreviations.

82. 1. The nurse would instruct the client that *t.i.d.* means three times daily and that *gtt* means drop.

CN: Physiological integrity; CNS: Pharmacological and parenteral therapies; CL: Application

83. To properly instill eardrops in a 28-year-old client with otitis externa, which method is correct?

1. Pulling the pinna down and back
2. Pulling the pinna up and back
3. Pulling the tragus up and back
4. Separating the palpebral fissures with a clean gauze pad

83. 2. To straighten the ear canal of an adult, the pinna is pulled up and back. Options 1 and 3 aren't appropriate methods for preparing the ear to receive eardrops. The palpebral fissures are in the eye.

CN: Physiological integrity; CNS: Pharmacological and parenteral therapies; CL: Application

84. Which instruction given to a client after cataract surgery is inappropriate?

1. "Avoid bending and straining."
2. "Avoid high-sodium foods to reduce intraocular pressure."
3. "Don't drive or sleep on the affected side."
4. "Don't use makeup on the affected eye."

Check out the in before appropriate.

84. 2. After cataract surgery, there's no need to restrict sodium. Using makeup, bending, straining, lifting, vomiting, and sleeping on the affected side may increase intraocular pressure and put strain on the sutures.

CN: Physiological integrity; CNS: Reduction of risk potential; CL: Application

85. Which sign or symptom of increased intracranial pressure (ICP) after head trauma would appear first?

1. Bradycardia
2. Large amounts of very dilute urine
3. Restlessness and confusion
4. Widened pulse pressure

85. 3. The earliest symptom of increased ICP is a change in mental status. Bradycardia, widened pulse pressure, and bradypnea occur later. The client may void large amounts of very dilute urine if there's damage to the posterior pituitary.

CN: Physiological integrity; CNS: Physiological adaptation; CL: Analysis

86. A client admitted to the emergency department for head trauma is diagnosed with an epidural hematoma. Which of the following would most likely cause this condition?

1. Laceration of the middle meningeal artery
2. Rupture of the carotid artery
3. Thromboembolism from a carotid artery
4. Venous bleeding from the arachnoid space

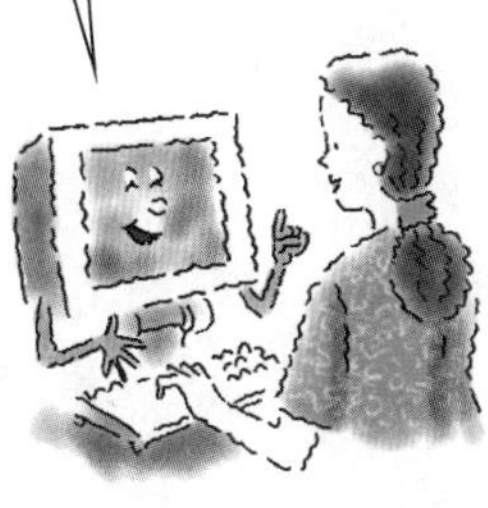

The words "most likely" help you choose the correct answer.

86. 1. Epidural hematoma or extradural hematoma is usually caused by laceration of the middle meningeal artery. An embolic stroke is a thromboembolism from a carotid artery that ruptures. Venous bleeding from the arachnoid space is usually observed with subdural hematoma.

CN: Physiological integrity; CNS: Physiological adaptation; CL: Application

87. A 23-year-old client has been hit on the head with a baseball bat. The nurse notes clear fluid draining from his ears and nose. Which nursing intervention should be done first?

1. Position the client flat in bed.
2. Check the fluid for glucose with a dipstick.
3. Suction the nose to maintain airway patency.
4. Insert nasal and ear packing with sterile gauze.

87. 2. Clear liquid from the nose (rhinorrhea) or ear (otorrhea) can be determined to be cerebral spinal fluid or mucus by the presence of glucose. Placing the client flat in bed may increase intracranial pressure and promote pulmonary aspiration. The nose wouldn't be suctioned because of the risk of suctioning brain tissue through the sinuses. Nothing is inserted into the ears or nose of a client with a skull fracture because of the risk of infection.
CN: Physiological integrity; CNS: Physiological adaptation; CL: Analysis

88. When discharging a client from the emergency department after a head trauma, the nurse teaches the guardian to observe for a lucid interval. Which statement by the nurse is most accurate?

1. An interval when the client's speech is garbled
2. An interval when the client is alert but can't recall recent events
3. An interval when the client is oriented but then becomes somnolent
4. An interval when the client has a "warning" symptom, such as an odor or visual disturbance

88. 3. A *lucid interval* is described as a brief period of unconsciousness followed by alertness; after several hours, the client again loses consciousness. Garbled speech is known as *dysarthria.* An interval in which the client is alert but can't recall recent events is known as *amnesia.* Warning symptoms or auras typically occur before seizures.
CN: Physiological integrity; CNS: Reduction of risk potential; CL: Application

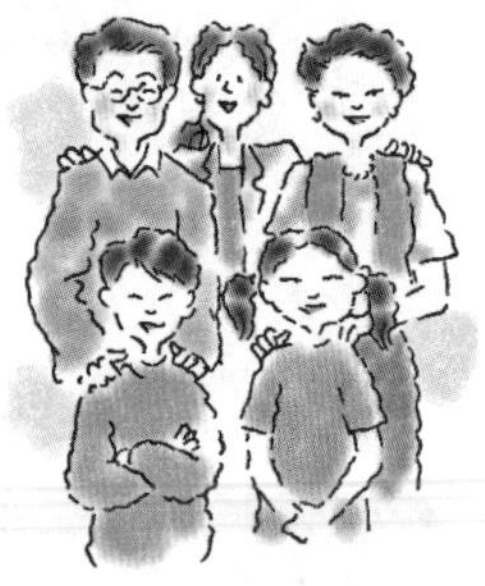

Teaching the family is as important as teaching the client.

89. When teaching the family of a client with C4 quadriplegia how to suction his tracheostomy, the nurse includes which instruction?

1. Suction for 10 to 15 seconds at a time.
2. Regulate the suction machine to –300 cm suction.
3. Apply suction to the catheter during insertion only.
4. Pass the suction catheter into the opening of the tracheostomy tube ¾″ to 1¼″ (2 to 3 cm).

89. 1. Suction should be applied for 10 to 15 seconds at a time. Suction is regulated to 80 to 120 cm. Suction should be applied only during withdrawal of the catheter. When suctioning the trachea, the catheter is inserted 4″ to 6″ (10 to 15 cm) or until resistance is felt.
CN: Physiological integrity; CNS: Reduction of risk potential; CL: Application

90. Which condition is the leading risk factor for hemorrhagic stroke?

1. Coronary artery disease
2. Diabetes
3. Hypertension
4. Recent viral infection

90. 3. Uncontrolled hypertension is the major cause of hemorrhagic stroke. Both diabetes and heart disease increase the probability of stroke by hastening atherosclerosis. A recent viral infection is not directly linked to this problem.
CN: Physiological integrity; CNS: Reduction of risk potential; CL: Application

91. An 86-year-old client with a stroke in evolution and a history of coronary artery disease is brought to the medical-surgical floor. His medications include heparin and isosorbide (Isordil). Which condition should be avoided in a client with a stroke?

1. Dehydration
2. Hypocarbia
3. Hypotension
4. Tube feeding

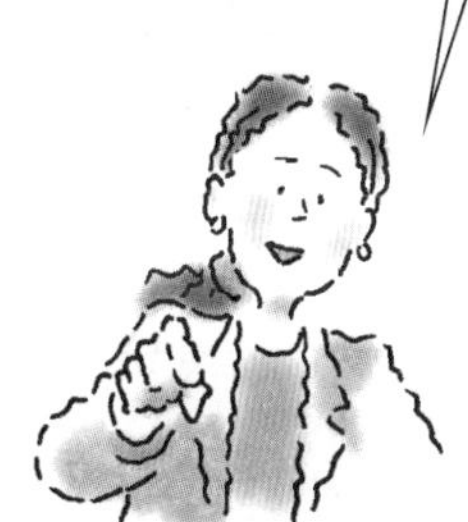

91. 3. Isosorbide can cause hypotension, which reduces brain perfusion and should be avoided in a client with a stroke. Dehydration would be inappropriate in this instance. Hypocarbia is used to reduce intracranial pressure through cerebral vasoconstriction. Nutrition may be delivered by tube when dysphagia exists.

CN: Physiological integrity; CNS: Physiological adaptation; CL: Application

92. Which client on the rehabilitation unit is most likely to develop autonomic dysreflexia?

1. A client with brain injury
2. A client with herniated nucleus pulposus
3. A client with a high cervical spine injury
4. A client with a stroke

92. 3. *Autonomic dysreflexia* refers to uninhibited sympathetic outflow in clients with spinal cord injuries most commonly above the level of T6. The other clients aren't prone to dysreflexia.

CN: Safe, effective care environment; CNS: Management of care; CL: Application

93. Which condition indicates that spinal shock is <u>resolving</u> in a client with C7 quadriplegia?

1. Absence of pain sensation in the chest
2. Spasticity
3. Spontaneous respirations
4. Urinary continence

93. 2. Spasticity, the return of reflexes, is a sign of resolving shock. Spinal or neurogenic shock is characterized by hypotension, bradycardia, dry skin, flaccid paralysis, or the absence of reflexes below the level of injury. The absence of pain sensation in the chest doesn't apply to spinal shock. Spinal shock descends from the injury, and respiratory difficulties occur at C4 and above. Slight muscle contraction at the bulbocavernosus reflex occurs, but not enough for urinary continence.

CN: Physiological integrity; CNS: Physiological adaptation; CL: Analysis

94. When discharging a client from the hospital after a laminectomy, the nurse recognizes that the client needs further teaching when he makes which statement?

1. "I'll sleep on a firm mattress."
2. "I won't drive for 2 to 4 weeks."
3. "When I pick things up, I'll bend my knees."
4. "I can't wait to pick up my 1-year-old-granddaughter."

94. 4. Lifting more than 10 lb (4.5 kg) for several weeks after surgery is contraindicated. The other responses are appropriate.

CN: Physiological integrity; CNS: Reduction of risk potential; CL: Analysis

95. When assessing a client with herniated nucleus pulposus of L4–L5, the nurse should expect to find which sign or symptom of spinal cord compression?

1. Lower back pain
2. Pain radiating across the buttocks
3. Positive Kernig's sign
4. Urinary incontinence

95. 4. Progressive neurologic deficits at L4–L5, including worsening muscle weakness, paresthesia, and loss of bowel and bladder control, are symptoms of spinal cord compression. The other symptoms usually occur in clients with herniated nucleus pulposus without spinal cord compression.

CN: Physiological integrity; CNS: Physiological adaptation; CL: Analysis

96. A nurse assesses a client who has episodes of autonomic dysreflexia. Which condition can cause autonomic dysreflexia?

1. Headache
2. Lumbar spinal cord injury
3. Neurogenic shock
4. Noxious stimuli

96. 4. Noxious stimuli, such as a full bladder, fecal impaction, or a decubitus ulcer, may cause autonomic dysreflexia. A headache is a symptom of autonomic dysreflexia, not a cause. Autonomic dysreflexia is most commonly seen with injuries at T6 or above. Neurogenic shock isn't a cause of dysreflexia.

CN: Physiological integrity; CNS: Physiological adaptation; CL: Application

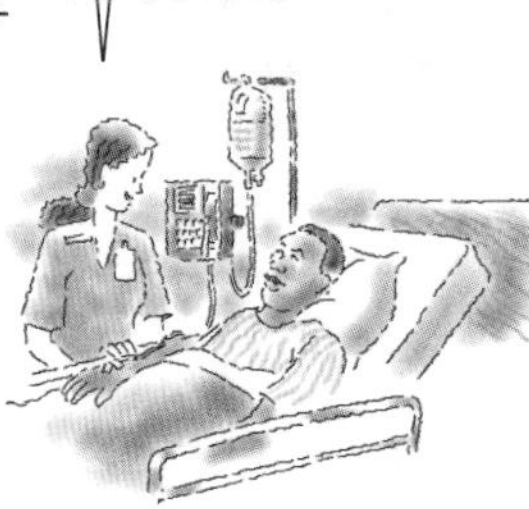

Correct positioning will help relieve your client's symptoms.

97. During an episode of autonomic dysreflexia in which a client becomes hypertensive, the nurse should perform which intervention?

1. Elevate the client's legs.
2. Put the client flat in bed.
3. Put the bed in Trendelenburg's position.
4. Put the client in high Fowler's position.

97. 4. Putting the client in high Fowler's position will decrease cerebral blood flow, decreasing hypertension. Elevating the client's legs, putting the client flat in bed, or putting the bed in Trendelenburg's position places the client in positions that improve cerebral blood flow, worsening hypertension.

CN: Physiological integrity; CNS: Reduction of risk potential; CL: Application

98. A client recovering from a spinal cord injury has a great deal of spasticity. Which medication may be used to control spasticity?

1. Hydralazine
2. Baclofen (Lioresal)
3. Lidocaine (Xylocaine)
4. Methylprednisolone (Medrol)

98. 2. Baclofen is a skeletal muscle relaxant used to decrease spasms. Hydralazine is an antihypertensive and afterload reducing agent. Lidocaine is an antiarrhythmic and a local anesthetic agent. Methylprednisolone, an anti-inflammatory drug, is used to decrease spinal cord edema.

CN: Physiological integrity; CNS: Pharmacological and parenteral therapies; CL: Application

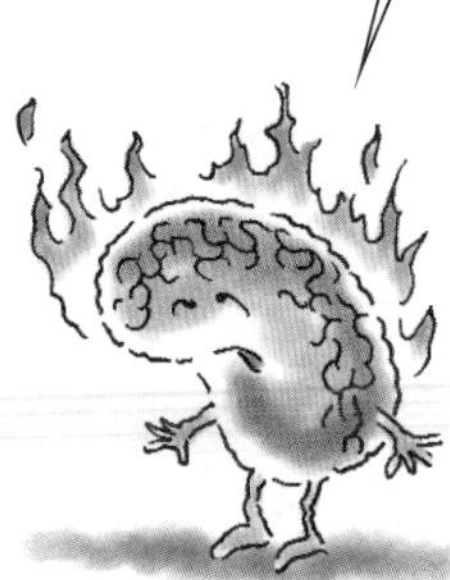

I know you're feeling fried at this point, but keep going!

99. Client teaching for a client with Gardner-Wells tongs should include which reason for their use?

1. To reduce intracranial pressure (ICP)
2. To reduce dislocations and pain
3. To prevent deep vein thrombosis (DVT)
4. To improve neurologic outcome

99. 2. Gardner-Wells tongs are used to reduce dislocations, subluxations, pain, and spasm in cervical spinal cord injuries. They aren't used to reduce ICP, prevent DVT, or improve neurologic outcome.

CN: Physiological integrity; CNS: Reduction of risk potential; CL: Application

100. A client with a T1 spinal cord injury arrives at the emergency department with a blood pressure of 82/40 mm Hg; pulse, 34 beats/minute; dry skin, and flaccid paralysis of the lower extremities. Which condition should be suspected?

1. Autonomic dysreflexia
2. Hypervolemia
3. Neurogenic shock
4. Sepsis

100. 3. Loss of sympathetic control and unopposed vagal stimulation below the level of the injury typically cause hypotension, bradycardia, pallor, flaccid paralysis, and warm, dry skin in the client in neurogenic shock. Hypervolemia is indicated by a rapid and bounding pulse and edema. Autonomic dysreflexia occurs after neurogenic shock abates. Signs of sepsis would include elevated temperature, increased heart rate, and increased respiratory rate.

CN: Physiological integrity; CNS: Physiological adaptation; CL: Analysis

101. A client has a cervical spine injury at the level of C5. Which condition should the nurse anticipate during the acute phase?

1. Absent corneal reflex
2. Decerebrate posturing
3. Movement of only the right or left half of the body
4. The need for mechanical ventilation

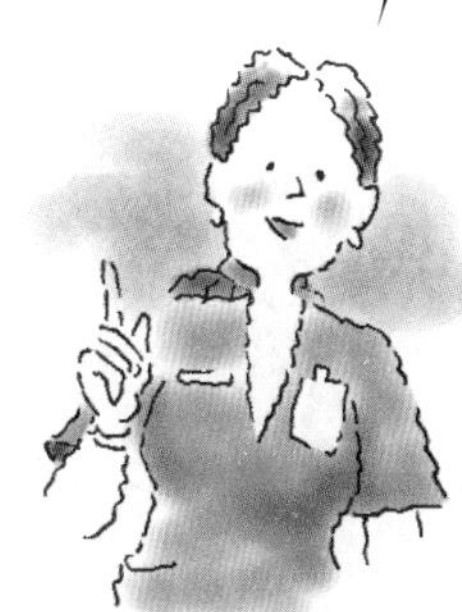

Pay close attention to the word acute.

102. When caring for a client with quadriplegia, which nursing intervention takes priority?

1. Forcing fluids to prevent renal calculi
2. Maintaining skin integrity
3. Obtaining adaptive devices for more independence
4. Preventing atelectasis

103. A client with C7 quadriplegia is flushed and anxious and complains of a pounding headache. Which symptoms should also be anticipated?

1. Decreased urine output or oliguria
2. Hypertension and bradycardia
3. Respiratory depression
4. Symptoms of shock

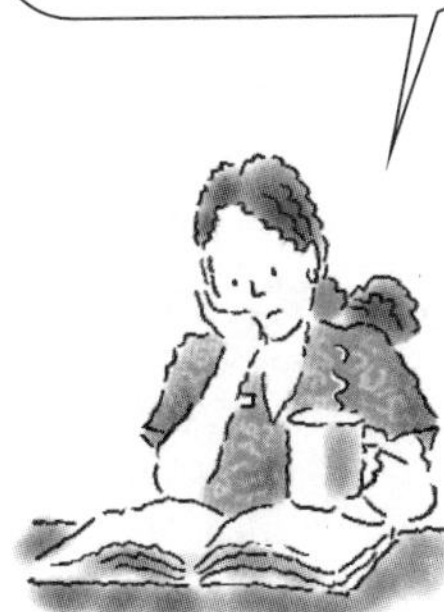

Keep alert! You've got 44 questions to go!

104. The nurse is teaching a client who has a diagnosis of a stroke versus a transient ischemic attack (TIA). Which statement by the nurse describing to the client the difference between stroke and TIA would be the most accurate?

1. TIAs resolve in less than 24 hours.
2. TIAs may be hemorrhagic in origin.
3. TIAs may cause a permanent motor deficit.
4. TIAs may predispose the client to a myocardial infarction (MI).

105. A client with a right stroke has a flaccid left side. Which intervention would best prevent shoulder subluxation?

1. Splint the wrist.
2. Use an air splint.
3. Put the affected arm in a sling.
4. Perform range-of-motion exercises on the affected side.

101. 4. The diaphragm is stimulated by nerves at the level of C4. Initially, this client may need mechanical ventilation due to cord edema. This may resolve in time. Absent corneal reflexes, decerebrate posturing, and hemiplegia occur with brain injuries, not spinal cord injuries.

CN: Physiological integrity; CNS: Physiological adaptation; CL: Application

102. 4. Clients with quadriplegia have paralysis or weakness of the diaphragm, abdominal, or intercostal muscles. Maintenance of airway and breathing take top priority. Although forcing fluids, maintaining skin integrity, and obtaining adaptive devices for more independence are all important interventions, preventing atelectasis has more priority.

CN: Physiological integrity; CNS: Reduction of risk potential; CL: Application

103. 2. Hypertension, bradycardia, anxiety, blurred vision, and flushing above the lesion occur with autonomic dysreflexia due to uninhibited sympathetic nervous system discharge. The other options are incorrect.

CN: Physiological integrity; CNS: Physiological adaptation; CL: Analysis

104. 1. Symptoms of a TIA result from a transient lack of oxygen to the brain and usually resolve within 24 hours, and the average time is less than 30 minutes. Hemorrhage into the brain has the worst neurologic outcome and isn't associated with a TIA. A permanent motor deficit doesn't result from a TIA. Unstable angina, not a TIA, may predispose the client to a future MI.

CN: Physiological integrity; CNS: Physiological adaptation; CL: Analysis

105. 3. Due to the weight of the flaccid extremity, the shoulder may disarticulate. A sling will support the extremity. The other options won't support the shoulder.

CN: Physiological integrity; CNS: Basic care and comfort; CL: Application

106. A 40-year-old paraplegic client must perform intermittent catheterization of the bladder. Which instruction should be given?

1. "Clean the meatus from back to front."
2. "Measure the quantity of urine."
3. "Gently rotate the catheter during removal."
4. "Clean the meatus with soap and water."

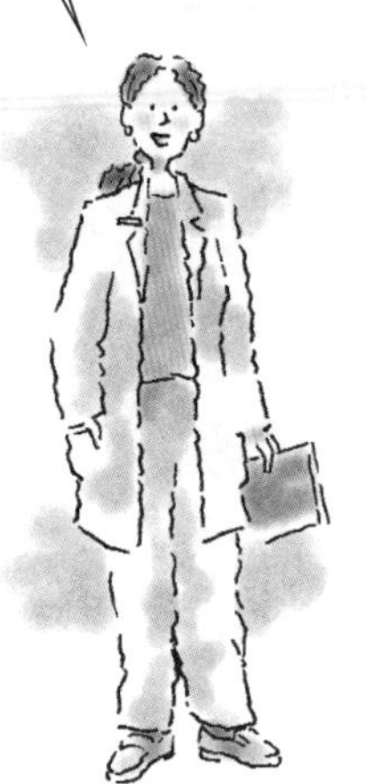
Which instruction should be given?

106. 4. Intermittent catheterization may be performed chronically with clean technique, using soap and water to clean the urinary meatus. The meatus is always cleaned from front to back in a woman, or in expanding circles working outward from the meatus in a man. It isn't necessary to measure the urine. The catheter doesn't need to be rotated during removal.

CN: Physiological integrity; CNS: Basic care and comfort; CL: Application

107. Which method should be used to assess pupil accommodation?

1. Assessing for peripheral vision
2. Touching the cornea lightly with a wisp of cotton
3. Having the client follow an object upward, downward, obliquely, and horizontally
4. Observing for pupil constriction and convergence while focusing on an object coming toward the client

107. 4. Accommodation refers to convergence and constriction of the pupil while following a near object. Assessing for peripheral vision refers to visual fields. Touching the cornea lightly with a wisp of cotton describes assessment of the corneal reflex. Having the client follow an object upward, downward, obliquely, and horizontally refers to cardinal fields of gaze.

CN: Physiological integrity; CNS: Reduction of risk potential; CL: Application

108. A client at the eye clinic reports difficulty seeing at night. This may result from which nutritional deficiency?

1. Vitamin A
2. Vitamin B_6
3. Vitamin C
4. Vitamin K

108. 1. Night blindness (nyctalopia) may be caused by a vitamin A deficiency or dysfunctional rod receptors. None of the other deficiencies lead to nyctalopia.

CN: Health promotion and maintenance; CNS: None; CL: Application

109. A client with a spinal cord injury has a neurogenic bladder. When planning for discharge, the nurse anticipates the client will need which procedure or program?

1. Intermittent catheterization program
2. Kock pouch
3. Transurethral prostatectomy
4. Ureterostomy

109. 1. Intermittent catheterization, starting with 2-hour intervals and increasing to 4- to 6-hour intervals, is used to manage neurogenic bladder. A Kock pouch is a type of urinary diversion. Transurethral prostatectomy is indicated for obstruction to urinary outflow by benign prostatic hyperplasia or for the treatment of cancer. An ileostomy or ureterostomy isn't necessary.

CN: Physiological integrity; CNS: Basic care and comfort; CL: Application

110. When using a Snellen alphabet chart, a nurse records a client's vision as 20/40. Which statement best describes 20/40 vision?

1. The client has alterations in near vision and is legally blind.
2. The client can see at 20 feet what the person with normal vision sees at 40 feet.
3. The client can see at 40 feet what the person with normal vision sees at 20 feet.
4. The client has a 20% decrease in acuity in one eye, and 40% decrease in the other eye.

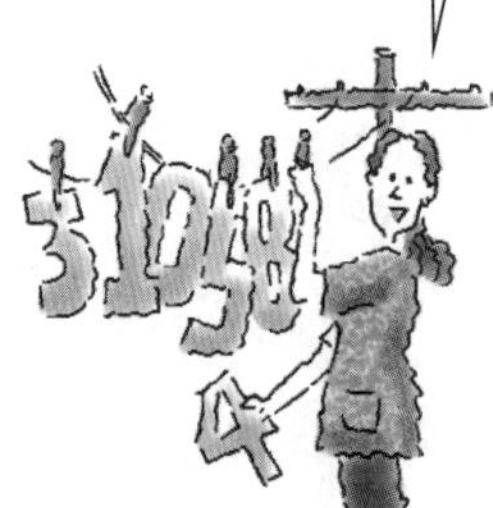
Keep those numbers straight!

110. 2. The numerator refers to the client's vision while comparing the normal vision in the denominator. Legal blindness refers to 20/150 or less. Alterations in near vision may be due to loss of accommodation caused by the aging process (presbyopia) or farsightedness.

CN: Physiological integrity; CNS: Reduction of risk potential; CL: Analysis

111. Which instrument is used to record intraocular pressure?

1. Goniometer
2. Ophthalmoscope
3. Slit lamp
4. Tonometer

111. 4. A tonometer is a device used in glaucoma screening to record intraocular pressure. A goniometer measures joint movement and angles. An ophthalmoscope examines the interior of the eye, especially the retina. A slit lamp evaluates structures in the anterior chamber of the eye.

CN: Physiological integrity; CNS: Reduction of risk potential; CL: Comprehension

112. After a nurse instills atropine drops into both eyes for a client undergoing an ophthalmic examination, which instruction should be given to the client?

1. "Be careful because the blink reflex is paralyzed."
2. "Avoid wearing your regular glasses when driving."
3. "Be aware that the pupils may be unusually small."
4. "Wear dark glasses in bright light because the pupils are dilated."

112. 4. Atropine, an anticholinergic drug, has mydriatic effects causing pupil dilation. This allows more light onto the retina and may cause photophobia and blurred vision. Atropine doesn't paralyze the blink reflex or cause miosis (pupil constriction). Driving may be contraindicated due to blurred vision.

CN: Physiological integrity; CNS: Pharmacological and parenteral therapies; CL: Application

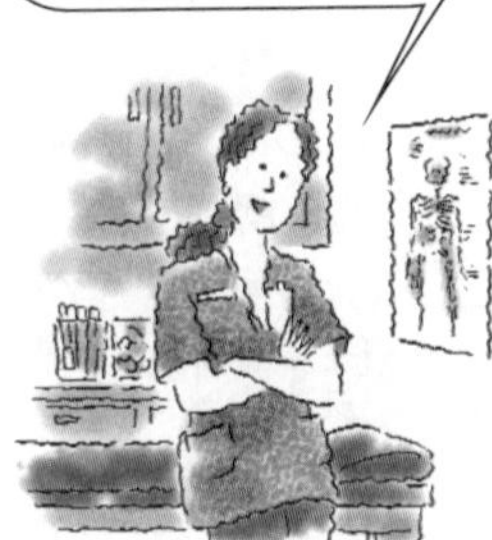

113. Which procedure or assessment must a nurse perform when preparing a client for eye surgery?

1. Clipping the client's eyelashes
2. Verifying the affected eye has been patched for 24 hours before surgery
3. Verifying the client has had nothing by mouth since midnight or at least 8 hours before surgery
4. Obtaining informed consent

113. 3. Maintaining nothing-by-mouth status for at least 8 hours before surgical procedures prevents vomiting and aspiration. There's no need to patch an eye before most surgeries or to clip the eyelashes unless specifically ordered by the physician. The physician is responsible for obtaining informed consent; the nurse validates that the consent is obtained.

CN: Physiological integrity; CNS: Reduction of risk potential; CL: Application

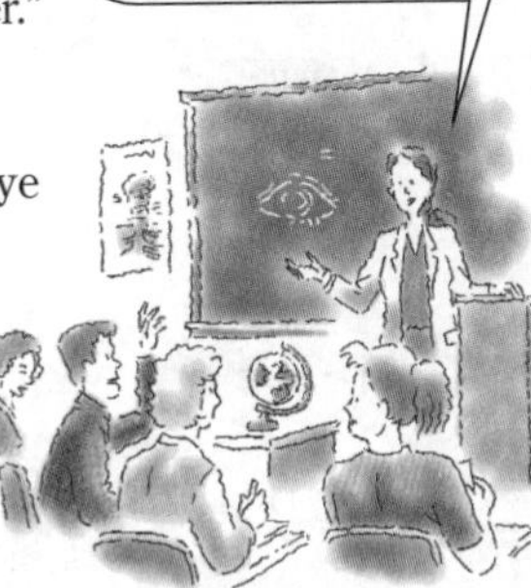

Teaching isn't complete if your client doesn't understand.

114. Which statement indicates that a client needs additional teaching after cataract surgery?

1. "I'll avoid eating until the nausea subsides."
2. "I can't wait to pick up my granddaughter."
3. "I'll avoid bending over to tie my shoelaces."
4. "I'll avoid touching the dropper to my eye when using my eyedrops."

114. 2. Lifting, usually involving the Valsalva maneuver, increases intraocular pressure (IOP) and strain on the surgical site. Preventing nausea and subsequent vomiting will prevent increased IOP, as will avoiding bending or placing the head in a dependent position. Touching the eye dropper to the eye will contaminate the dropper and thus the entire bottle of medication.

CN: Physiological integrity; CNS: Reduction of risk potential; CL: Analysis

115. Cataract surgery results in aphakia. Which statement best describes this term?

1. Absence of the crystalline lens
2. A "keyhole" pupil
3. Loss of accommodation
4. Retinal detachment

115. 1. *Aphakia* means without lens. A keyhole pupil results from iridectomy. Loss of accommodation is a normal response to aging. A retinal detachment is usually associated with retinal holes created by vitreous traction.

CN: Physiological integrity; CNS: Physiological adaptation; CL: Comprehension

116. When developing a teaching session on glaucoma for the community, which statement should the nurse stress?

1. Glaucoma is easily corrected with eyeglasses.
2. White and Asian individuals are at the highest risk for glaucoma.
3. Yearly screening for people ages 20 to 40 is recommended.
4. Glaucoma can be painless and vision may be lost before the person is aware of a problem.

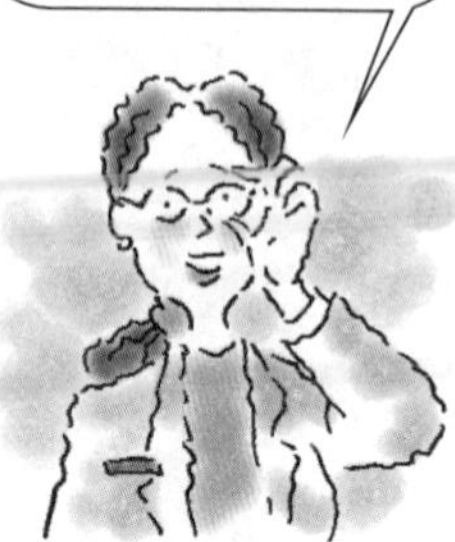

This question should be painless.

116. 4. Open-angle glaucoma causes a painless increase in intraocular pressure (IOP) with loss of peripheral vision. A variety of miotics and agents to decrease IOP and occasionally surgery are used to treat glaucoma. Blacks have a threefold greater chance of developing glaucoma with an increased chance of blindness than other groups. Individuals older than age 40 should be screened.
CN: Health promotion and maintenance; CNS: None; CL: Application

117. For a client having an episode of acute angle-closure glaucoma, the nurse expects to give which medication?

1. Acetazolamide (Diamox)
2. Atropine
3. Furosemide (Lasix)
4. Urokinase

117. 1. Acetazolamide, a carbonic anhydrase inhibitor, decreases intraocular pressure (IOP) by decreasing the secretion of aqueous humor. Atropine dilates the pupil and decreases outflow of aqueous humor, causing a further increase in IOP. Furosemide is a loop diuretic, and urokinase is a thrombolytic agent; they aren't used in the treatment of glaucoma.
CN: Physiological integrity; CNS: Pharmacological and parenteral therapies; CL: Application

118. Which symptom would occur in a client with a detached retina?

1. Flashing lights and floaters
2. Homonymous hemianopia
3. Loss of central vision
4. Ptosis

118. 1. Signs and symptoms of retinal detachment include abrupt flashing lights, floaters, loss of peripheral vision, or a sudden shadow or curtain in the vision. Occasionally, vision loss is gradual.
CN: Physiological integrity; CNS: Physiological adaptation; CL: Application

119. A client underwent an enucleation of the right eye for a malignancy. Which intervention will the nurse perform?

1. Instilling miotics as ordered to the affected eye
2. Teaching the client to clean the prosthesis in soap and water
3. Assessing reactivity of the pupils to light and accommodation
4. Teaching the client to prevent straining at stool leading to increased intraocular pressure

119. 2. *Enucleation of the eye* refers to surgical removal of the entire eye; therefore, the client needs instructions about the prosthesis. There are no activity restrictions or need for eyedrops; however, prophylactic antibiotics may be used in the immediate postoperative period.
CN: Physiological integrity; CNS: Physiological adaptation; CL: Application

120. A nurse should question an order to irrigate the ear canal in which circumstance?

1. Ear pain
2. Hearing loss
3. Otitis externa
4. Perforated tympanic membrane

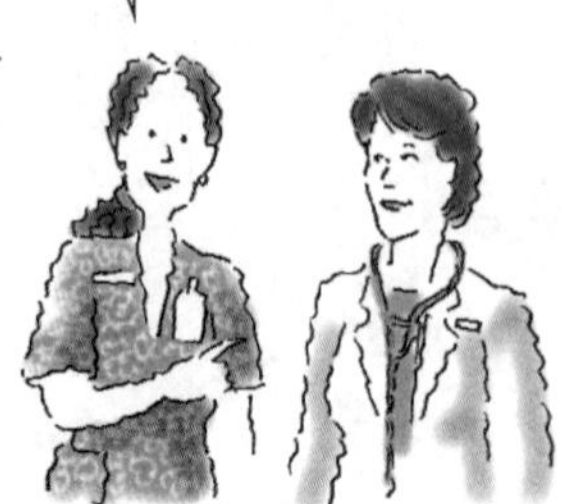

If you're unsure about an order, ask.

120. 4. Irrigation of the ear canal is contraindicated with perforation of the tympanic membrane because solution entering the inner ear may cause dizziness, nausea, vomiting, and infection. The other conditions aren't contraindications to irrigation of the ear canal.
CN: Physiological integrity; CNS: Reduction of risk potential; CL: Application

121. Which intervention is essential when instilling Cortisporin suspension, 2 gtt right ear?

1. Verifying the proper client and route
2. Warming the solution to prevent dizziness
3. Holding an emesis basin under the client's ear
4. Positioning the client in the semi-Fowler's position

121. 1. When giving medications, a nurse follows the five R's of medication administration: right client, right drug, right dose, right route, and right time. The drops may be warmed to prevent pain or dizziness, but this action isn't essential. An emesis basin would be used for irrigation of the ear. The client should be placed in the lateral position, not semi-Fowler's position, to prevent the drops from draining out for 5 minutes.

CN: Physiological integrity; CNS: Pharmacological and parenteral therapies; CL: Application

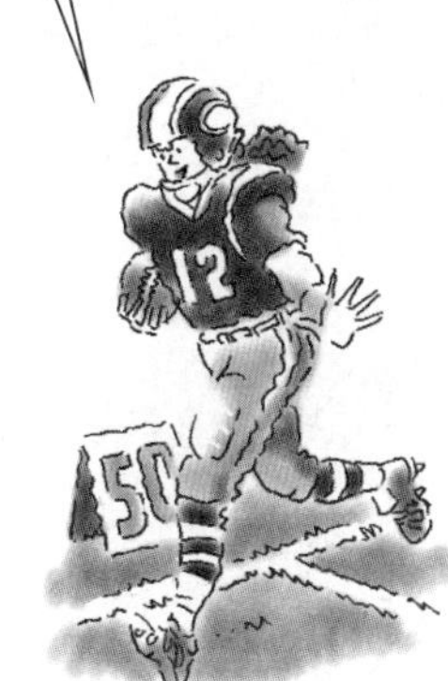

Giving I.V. drugs isn't a game. Know the right way to do it.
12
50

122. When teaching the client with Ménière's disease, which instruction should the nurse give about vertigo?

1. "Report dizziness at once."
2. "Drive in daylight hours only."
3. "Get up slowly, turning the entire body."
4. "Change your position using the logroll technique."

122. 3. Turning the entire body, not the head, will prevent vertigo. Dizziness is expected but can be prevented with Ménière's disease. The client shouldn't drive because he may reflexively turn the wheel to correct for vertigo. Turning the client in bed slowly and smoothly will be helpful; logrolling isn't needed.

CN: Physiological integrity; CNS: Reduction of risk potential; CL: Application

123. When giving I.V. phenytoin (Dilantin), which method should be used?

1. Administering rapidly
2. Withholding other anticonvulsants
3. Mixing the drug with saline solution only
4. Flushing the I.V. catheter with dextrose solution

123. 3. Phenytoin is compatible only with saline solutions; dextrose causes an insoluble precipitate to form. Phenytoin should be administered slowly (50 mg/minute). There's no need to withhold additional anticonvulsants.

CN: Physiological integrity; CNS: Pharmacological and parenteral therapies; CL: Application

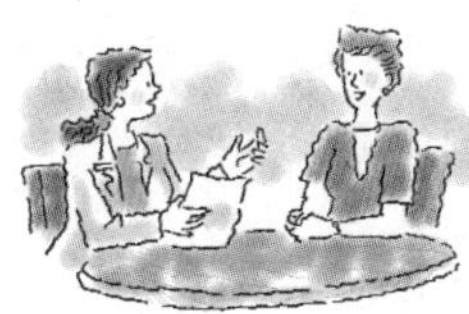

Instruct the client's mother about the care for her son's injury.

124. An 18-year-old client was hit in the head with a baseball during practice. When discharging him to the care of his mother, the nurse gives which instruction?

1. "Watch him for keyhole pupil for the next 24 hours."
2. "Expect profuse vomiting for 24 hours after the injury."
3. "Wake him every hour and assess his orientation to person, time, and place."
4. "Notify the physician immediately if he has a headache."

124. 3. Changes in level of consciousness (LOC) may indicate expanding lesions such as subdural hematoma; orientation and LOC are assessed frequently for 24 hours. A keyhole pupil is found after iridectomy. Profuse or projectile vomiting is a symptom of increased intracranial pressure and should be reported immediately. A slight headache may last for several days after concussion; severe or worsening headaches should be reported.

CN: Physiological integrity; CNS: Physiological adaptation; CL: Application

125. A client is taking carbamazepine (Tegretol). For which of the following potential complications should the nurse be monitoring the client?

1. Acute respiratory distress syndrome (ARDS)
2. Diplopia
3. Elevated levels of phenytoin (Dilantin)
4. Leukocytosis

125. 2. Complications of carbamazepine include diplopia, dizziness, ataxia, and rash. ARDS isn't a complication of carbamazepine. Carbamazepine decreases blood levels of phenytoin and hormonal contraceptives; it also causes agranulocytosis because of the reduction in leukocytes.

CN: Physiological integrity; CNS: Pharmacological and parenteral therapies; CL: Application

126. For a client with damage to the caudate nucleus, putamen, and globus pallidus, which condition should be monitored?

1. Eye movement
2. Modulation of sounds
3. Motor movement
4. Muscle synergy

126. 3. Motor movement is regulated by the basal ganglia, which consists of the caudate nucleus, putamen, and globus pallidus. Eye movement is too vague because there are several cranial nerves responsible for various forms of eye movement. Modulation of sounds occurs from the occipital lobe. The cerebellum regulates muscle synergy.

CN: Safe, effective care environment; CNS: Management of care; CL: Application

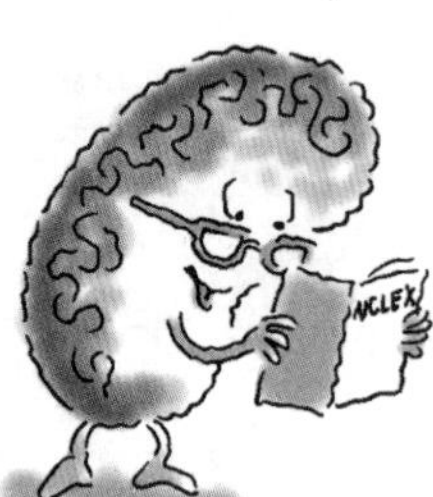
Different areas of the brain (Hey, that's me!) regulate different functions.
NCLEX

127. Which of the following should the nurse anticipate in a client with injury to the thalamus, such as in a thalamic stroke?

1. Burning or aching sensation over one half of the body
2. Seizures
3. Problems initiating movement
4. Memory lapses

127. 1. Damage to the thalamus may result in thalamic syndrome, which is characterized by pain, burning, or an aching sensation over one half of the body. It is often accompanied by mood swings. Problems initiating movement are associated with the basal ganglia and memory problems with the hippocampus. Seizures are not specific to thalamic injury.

CN: Physiological integrity; CNS: Physiological adaptation; CL: Application

128. A client is admitted with second stage Alzheimer's disease. In communicating with the client, which of the following techniques will be the most successful?

1. Listening carefully and deciphering word substitutions
2. Avoiding repeated messages, as this may agitate the client
3. Avoiding yes or no questions
4. Avoiding the subject-verb-object format

128. 1. Listening and deciphering word substitutions are the most helpful, as the client may have difficulty expressing their thoughts. Sentences should be repeated as often as needed. In questioning the client, yes-no or multiple-choice questions are very helpful. Sentences should be short and literal, following the subject-verb-object format.

CN: Psychosocial integrity; CNS: None; CL: Application

129. The family of a client recently admitted to the hospital is describing to the nurse how the client was cooking and was slightly burned because he could not feel the hot temperature of the oven. Which of the following areas of the brain would the nurse suspect to be dysfunctional?

1. Frontal lobe
2. Occipital lobe
3. Parietal lobe
4. Temporal lobe

129. 3. The parietal lobe regulates sensory function, which would include the ability to sense hot or cold objects. The frontal lobe regulates thinking, planning, and judgment, and the occipital lobe is primarily responsible for vision function. The temporal lobe regulates memory.

CN: Physiological integrity; CNS: Physiological adaptation; CL: Application

130. When assessing the ability of a client's pupil to constrict, which cranial nerve (CN) is being tested?

1. II
2. III
3. IV
4. V

130. 2. CN III, the oculomotor nerve, controls pupil constriction. CN II is the optic nerve, which controls vision. CN IV is the trochlear nerve, which coordinates eye movement. CN V is the trigeminal nerve, which innervates the muscles of chewing.

CN: Physiological integrity; CNS: Physiological adaptation; CL: Application

131. A nurse is discussing the purpose of an EEG with the family of a client with massive cerebral hemorrhage and loss of consciousness. Which of the following responses by the nurse would be the most accurate in describing what the test measures?

1. Extent of intracranial bleeding
2. Sites of brain injury
3. Activity of the brain
4. Percent of functional brain tissue

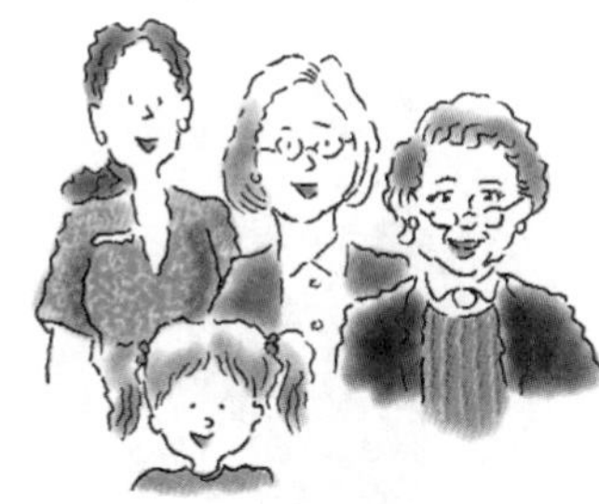
What should I be telling the family of a client about an EEG?

131. 3. An EEG measures the electrical activity of the brain. Extent of intracranial bleeding and location of the injury site would be determined by computerized tomography or magnetic resonance imaging. Percent of functional brain tissue would be determined by a series of tests.

CN: Physiological integrity; CNS: Reduction of risk potential; CL: Application

132. A nurse is teaching a client and his family about dietary practices related to Parkinson's disease. Which signs and symptoms would be <u>most important</u> for the nurse to address?

1. Fluid overload and drooling
2. Aspiration and anorexia
3. Choking and diarrhea
4. Dysphagia and constipation

132. 4. The eating problems associated with Parkinson's disease include dysphagia, risk of choking, drooling, aspiration, and constipation. Fluid overload, anorexia, and diarrhea aren't problems specifically related to Parkinson's disease.

CN: Physiological integrity; CNS: Reduction of risk potential; CL: Analysis

133. In some clients with multiple sclerosis (MS), plasmapheresis diminishes symptoms. Plasmapheresis achieves this effect by removing which blood component?

1. Catecholamines
2. Antibodies
3. Plasma proteins
4. Lymphocytes

133. 2. In plasmapheresis, antibodies are removed from the client's plasma. Antibodies attack the myelin sheath of the neuron causing the manifestations of MS. The treatment of MS with plasmapheresis isn't for the purpose of removing catecholamines, plasma proteins, or lymphocytes.

CN: Physiological integrity; CNS: Physiological adaptation; CL: Comprehension

134. A nurse performs a neurologic assessment on a client complaining of headache and dizziness. Which assessment technique helps assess the motor function of cranial nerve VII?

1. Asking the client to clench his jaw
2. Testing the gag reflex by placing an applicator against the pharynx
3. Asking the client to frown, smile, and raise his eyebrows
4. Asking the client to swallow

134. 3. To assess the motor function of cranial nerve VII, the nurse should ask the client to frown, smile, and raise his eyebrows. If these facial expressions are symmetrical, motor function is intact. Jaw clenching is a test for cranial nerve V function. Testing the gag reflex by placing an applicator against the pharynx, and assessing swallowing ability are ways to evaluate cranial nerve IX function. Testing the gag reflex also helps assess cranial nerve X function.

CN: Health promotion and maintenance; CNS: None; CL: Application

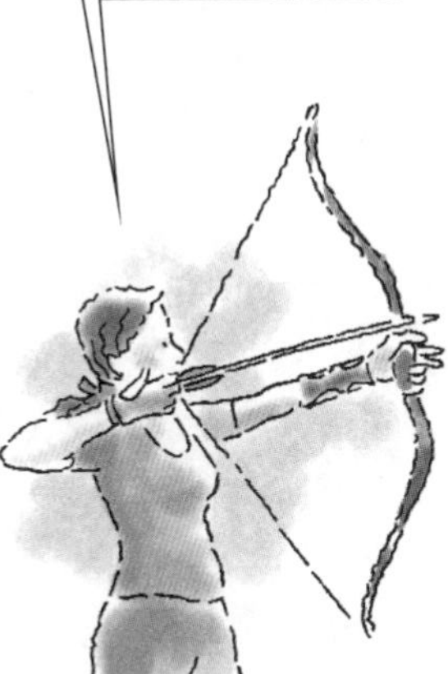
Prioritizing hits the mark on this question.

135. An unconscious client is receiving mechanical ventilation. Which nursing diagnosis takes <u>priority</u>?

1. *Ineffective airway clearance related to the inability to expectorate*
2. *Risk for impaired skin integrity related to immobility*
3. *Imbalanced nutrition: Less than body requirements related to inability to swallow*
4. *Dressing self-care deficit related to unconsciousness*

135. 1. *Ineffective airway clearance related to the inability to expectorate* takes priority in an unconscious client. The other nursing diagnoses are appropriate but are less important than airway, breathing, and circulation.

CN: Physiological integrity; CNS: Physiological adaptation; CL: Analysis

136. An 18-year-old client is admitted with a closed head injury sustained in a motor vehicle collision. His intracranial pressure (ICP) shows an upward trend. Which intervention should the nurse perform first?

1. Reposition the client to avoid neck flexion.
2. Administer 1 g of mannitol (Osmitrol) I.V. as ordered.
3. Increase the ventilator's respiratory rate to 20 breaths/minute.
4. Administer 100 mg of pentobarbital I.V. as ordered.

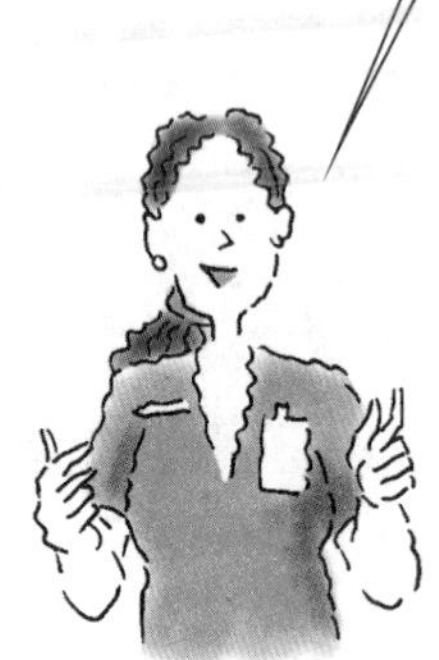

In this case, save the best for first.

136. 1. The nurse should first attempt a nursing intervention, such as repositioning the client to avoid neck flexion, which increases venous return and lowers ICP. If nursing measures prove ineffective, notify the physician, who may prescribe mannitol, pentobarbital, or hyperventilation therapy.

CN: Safe, effective care environment; CNS: Management of care; CL: Application

137. A client arrives at the emergency department after slipping on a patch of ice and hitting his head. A computed tomography scan of the head shows a collection of blood between the skull and dura mater. Which type of head injury does this finding suggest?

1. Subdural hematoma
2. Subarachnoid hemorrhage
3. Epidural hematoma
4. Contusion

137. 3. An epidural hematoma occurs when blood collects between the skull and dura mater. In a subdural hematoma, venous blood collects between the dura mater and arachnoid mater. In a subarachnoid hemorrhage, blood collects between the pia mater and arachnoid membrane. A contusion is a bruise on the brain's surface.

CN: Physiological integrity; CNS: Physiological adaptation; CL: Application

138. After falling 20′ (6 m), a 36-year-old construction worker sustains a C6 fracture with spinal cord transection. Which other findings should the nurse expect?

1. Quadriplegia with gross arm movement and diaphragmatic breathing
2. Quadriplegia and loss of respiratory function
3. Paraplegia with intercostal muscle loss
4. Loss of bowel and bladder control

138. 1. A client with a spinal cord injury at levels C5 to C6 has quadriplegia with gross arm movement and diaphragmatic breathing. Injuries at levels C1 to C4 lead to quadriplegia with total loss of respiratory function. Paraplegia with intercostal muscle loss occurs with injuries at T1 to L2. Injuries below L2 cause paraplegia and loss of bowel and bladder control.

CN: Physiological integrity; CNS: Physiological adaptation; CL: Application

139. A client with a subarachnoid hemorrhage is prescribed a 1,000-mg loading dose of phenytoin (Dilantin) I.V. Which consideration is most important when administering this dose?

1. Therapeutic drug levels should be maintained between 20 and 30 mg/ml.
2. Rapid phenytoin administration can cause cardiac arrhythmias.
3. Phenytoin should be mixed in dextrose in water before administration.
4. Phenytoin should be administered through an I.V. catheter in the client's hand.

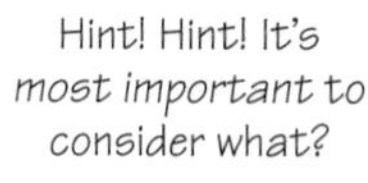

Hint! Hint! It's most important to consider what?

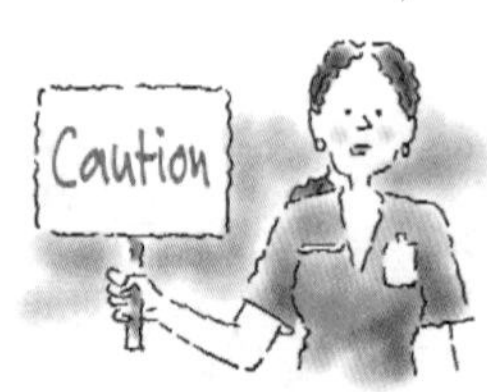

Caution

139. 2. Phenytoin I.V. shouldn't be given at a rate exceeding 50 mg/minute; rapid administration can depress the myocardium, causing arrhythmias. Therapeutic drug levels range from 10 to 20 mg/ml. Phenytoin shouldn't be mixed in solution for administration. However, because it's compatible with normal saline solution, it can be injected through an I.V. line containing normal saline solution. When given through an I.V. catheter in the hand, phenytoin may cause purple glove syndrome.

CN: Physiological integrity; CNS: Pharmacological and parenteral therapies; CL: Application

140. A nurse is developing a discharge teaching plan for a client who has been prescribed phenytoin (Dilantin). Which instruction should the plan include?

1. "Take the drug on an empty stomach."
2. "You can consume alcoholic beverages in moderation."
3. "You can take any phenytoin brand because all brands are the same."
4. "Don't stop taking the drug except with medical supervision."

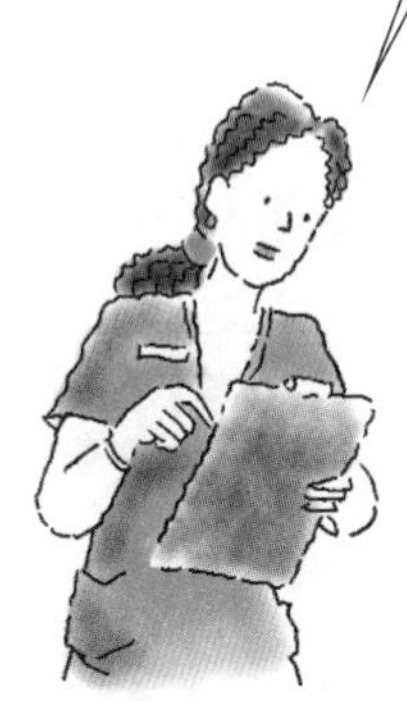

Which instruction shall I include in the teaching plan?

140. 4. Abrupt phenytoin withdrawal may trigger status epilepticus, so the client should be warned not to stop taking the drug unless the physician approves. Taking phenytoin with food minimizes GI distress. Alcoholic beverages can decrease the drug's effectiveness. Changing phenytoin brands may alter the therapeutic effect.

CN: Physiological integrity; CNS: Pharmacological and parenteral therapies; CL: Application

141. A 20-year-old client who fell approximately 30′ (9 m) is unresponsive and breathless. A cervical spine injury is suspected. How should the first-responder open the client's airway for rescue breathing?

1. By inserting a nasopharyngeal airway
2. By inserting an oropharyngeal airway
3. By performing the jaw-thrust maneuver
4. By performing the head-tilt, chin-lift maneuver

141. 3. If the client has a suspected cervical spine injury, the jaw-thrust maneuver should be used to open the airway. If the tongue or relaxed throat muscles are obstructing the airway, a nasopharyngeal or oropharyngeal airway can be inserted; however, the client must have spontaneous respirations when the airway is open. The head-tilt, chin-lift maneuver requires neck hyperextension, which can worsen a cervical spine injury.

CN: Physiological integrity; CNS: Physiological adaptation; CL: Analysis

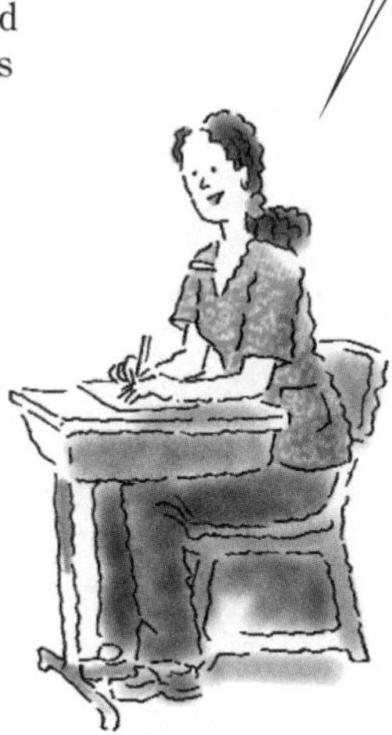

Documentation is key. Remember to always write it down!

142. An 87-year-old client is admitted with a stroke. During the admission interview and assessment, his speech is slow, nonfluent, and labored. How should the nurse document this finding?

1. Receptive aphasia
2. Wernicke's aphasia
3. Expressive aphasia
4. Global aphasia

142. 3. Expressive (Broca's) aphasia results from damage to Broca's area, located in the frontal lobe of the brain's dominant hemisphere. Typically, the client with expressive aphasia has difficulty expressing himself and his speech is slow, nonfluent, and labored; however, comprehension of written and verbal communication is intact. With receptive (Wernicke's) aphasia (which results from injury to Wernicke's area, located in the temporal lobe of the dominant hemisphere), the client can't comprehend written or verbal communication; his speech is normal but he conveys information poorly. With global aphasia—a combination of receptive and expressive aphasia—most of the brain's communication system is damaged. Global aphasia results from extensive damage to Broca's and Wernicke's areas.

CN: Physiological integrity; CNS: Physiological adaptation; CL: Application

143. A nurse is developing a teaching plan for a client who will undergo a stapedectomy for treatment of otosclerosis. Which point should the plan include?

1. Ringing in the ears is common after surgery.
2. Vertigo and dizziness are common after surgery.
3. Hearing should return immediately after surgery.
4. Excessive drainage is common after surgery.

143. 2. Vertigo is the most frequent complication of stapedectomy. The client should move slowly to avoid triggering or worsening vertigo and should ask for assistance with ambulation. Ringing in the ears (tinnitus) rarely follows this surgery and should be reported to the physician. Hearing typically decreases after surgery because of ear packing and tissue swelling, but commonly returns over the next 2 to 6 weeks. Usually, postoperative drainage and pain are minimal; excessive drainage should be reported.

CN: Physiological integrity; CNS: Reduction of risk potential; CL: Application

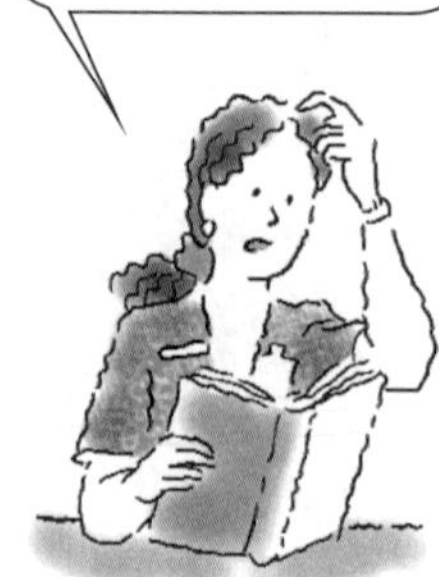
Hmmm. My priority is to answer the last five questions of this test.

144. A client has just been diagnosed with primary open-angle glaucoma and requires teaching about the disease. Which nursing diagnosis takes priority?

1. *Risk for injury related to peripheral vision loss*
2. *Chronic pain related to increased intraocular pressure*
3. *Ineffective health maintenance related to medication adverse effects*
4. *Deficient knowledge related to new diagnosis of glaucoma*

144. 1. *Risk for injury related to peripheral vision loss* takes priority because open-angle glaucoma limits peripheral vision; the client risks injury from stumbling over peripheral objects that he can't see. Angle-closure glaucoma—not open-angle glaucoma—commonly causes acute pain. Primary open-angle glaucoma is an incurable disease that requires life-long treatment; adverse effects of medications are common. Although *Ineffective health maintenance* is an appropriate diagnosis for this client, safety takes priority. *Deficient knowledge* is appropriate for any client with a new diagnosis, but it takes lower priority than safety.

CN: Physiological integrity; CNS: Reduction of risk potential; CL: Analysis

145. When teaching a client how to administer mydriatic agents, which instruction should the nurse provide?

1. "Your pupils will be small and your night vision will be diminished."
2. "Blurred vision is an adverse effect and you should report it to the physician immediately."
3. "Eye pain is common after administration."
4. "Compress the lacrimal sac for 1 minute after instillation."

145. 4. To prevent systemic absorption, the client should compress the lacrimal sac for 1 minute after instilling a mydriatic agent. The drug makes the pupils large and causes light sensitivity. Blurred vision is an expected effect of mydriatics and need not be reported immediately. The client should discontinue the drug if eye pain occurs.

CN: Physiological integrity; CNS: Pharmacological and parenteral therapies; CL: Application

CN: Client needs category CNS: Client needs subcategory CL: Cognitive level

146. A nurse is performing a neurologic assessment on a client during a routine physical examination. To assess the Babinski reflex, indicate the point where the nurse should place the tongue blade to begin the stroke of the foot.

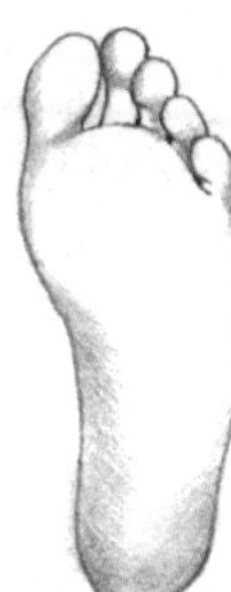

146. To test for the Babinski reflex, use a tongue blade to slowly stroke the lateral side of the underside of the foot. Start at the heel and move toward the great toe. The normal response in an adult is plantar flexion of the toes. Upward movement of the great toe and fanning of the little toes, called the Babinski reflex, is abnormal.

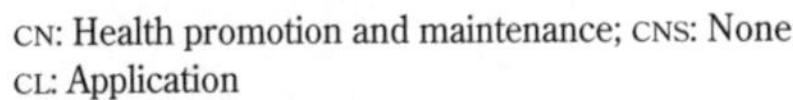

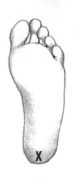

CN: Health promotion and maintenance; CNS: None; CL: Application

147. The nurse is assessing a client's deep tendon reflexes. Which graphic shows assessing the biceps reflex?

1. 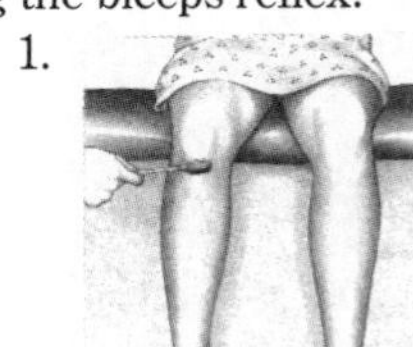
2. 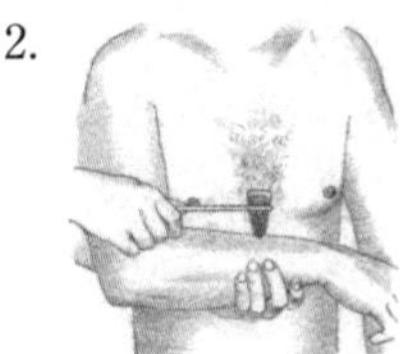
3. 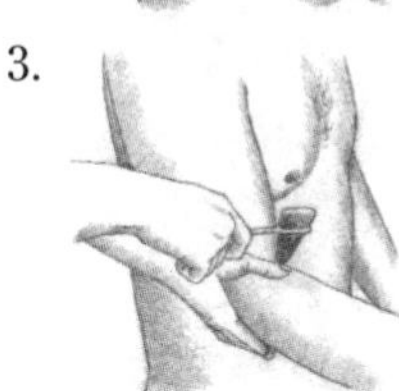
4. 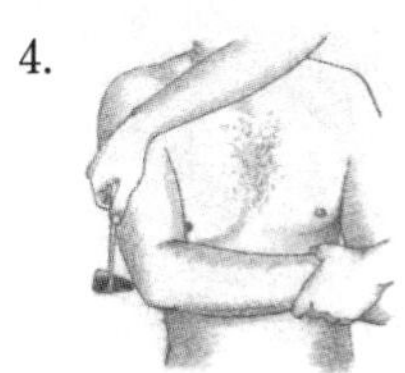

147. 3. To test the biceps reflex, the client's elbow is flexed at a 45-degree angle. The nurse places her thumb or index finger over the biceps tendon and strikes the digit with the pointed end of the reflex hammer, watching and feeling for the contraction of the biceps muscle and flexion of the forearm. Option 1 shows assessment of the patellar reflex. Option 2 shows assessment of the brachioradialis reflex. Option 4 shows assessment of the triceps reflex.

CN: Physiological integrity; CNS: Reduction of risk potential; CL: Analysis

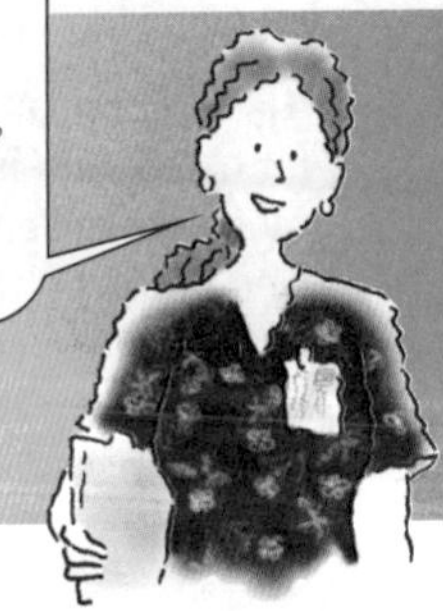

Here's a test that covers nursing care for clients with a disorder of the musculoskeletal system. So get moving! (Get it? Moving? Hmmm. I must be losing my touch.)

Chapter 7 Musculoskeletal disorders

1. A 70-year-old female client complains of pain in her lower back. She has a markedly aged appearance and says she doesn't eat well. She's diagnosed with osteoporosis. The nurse teaches the client about injury prevention because the nurse is concerned about preventing which condition that is the primary complication of osteoporosis?

1. Pain
2. Fracture
3. Hardening of the bones
4. Increased bone matrix and remineralization

1. 2. The primary complication of osteoporosis is fractures. With osteoporosis, bones soften, and there's a decrease in bone matrix and remineralization. Pain may occur, but fractures can be life-threatening.
CN: Physiological integrity; CNS: Physiological adaptation; CL: Application

2. A nurse admits a 76-year-old woman with a history of osteoporosis who has experienced a right wrist fracture. Which nursing diagnosis has the highest priority?

1. *Acute pain*
2. *Dressing self-care deficit*
3. *Imbalanced nutrition: Less than body requirements*
4. *Risk for impaired skin integrity*

2. 1. Relieving pain and making the client more comfortable should have the highest priority. All the other nursing diagnoses would be lower priorities.
CN: Physiological integrity; CNS: Physiological adaptation; CL: Analysis

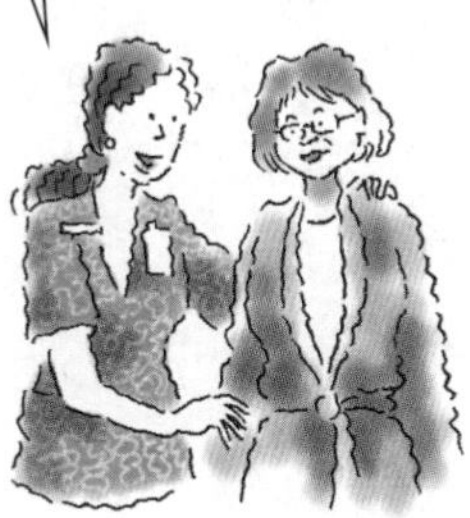

A client may have different postoperative risk factors.

3. The nurse is teaching a client about the cause of osteoporosis. Which statement by the nurse would be the most accurate in stating the primary cause?

1. Alcoholism
2. Hormonal imbalance
3. Malnutrition
4. Osteogenesis imperfecta

3. 2. Hormonal imbalance, faulty metabolism, and poor dietary intake of calcium cause primary osteoporosis. Alcoholism, malnutrition, osteogenesis imperfecta, rheumatoid arthritis, liver disease, scurvy, lactose intolerance, hyperthyroidism, and trauma cause secondary osteoporosis.
CN: Physiological integrity; CNS: Physiological adaptation; CL: Application

4. A 42-year-old client recently had a total hysterectomy and bilateral oopherectomy. Which response by the client indicates that the nurse's teaching about osteoporosis has been effective?
1. "My risk for osteoporosis is low because I still have my thyroid gland."
2. "Osteoporosis affects only women over 65-years old."
3. "I'm still producing hormones, so I don't have to worry about osteoporosis."
4. "I need to take precautions to protect myself from osteoporosis because I've had surgically-induced menopause."

4. 4. Menopause at any age puts women at risk for osteoporosis because of the associated hormonal imbalance. This client's thyroid gland won't protect her from osteoporosis. With her ovaries removed, she's no longer producing hormones.

CN: Physiological integrity; CNS: Physiological adaptation; CL: Analysis

5. <u>Primary</u> prevention of osteoporosis includes which measure?
1. Place items within reach of the client.
2. Install bars in the bathroom to prevent falls.
3. Maintain the optimal calcium intake.
4. Use a professional alert system in the home in case a fall occurs when the client is alone.

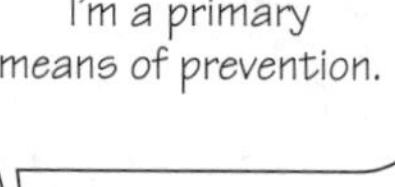
I'm a primary means of prevention.

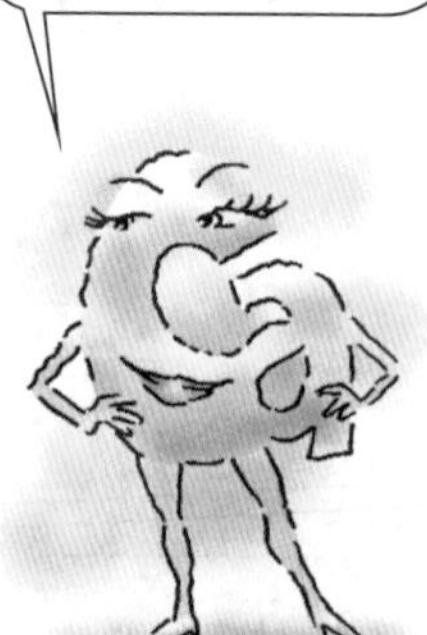

5. 3. Primary prevention of osteoporosis includes maintaining optimal calcium intake. Placing items within reach of the client, using a professional alert system in the home, and installing bars in bathrooms are all secondary and tertiary prevention methods to prevent falls.

CN: Health promotion and maintenance; CNS: None; CL: Application

6. A nurse is providing nutritional consulting to a client with a diagnosis of gout. Which of the client's favorite foods should she instruct him to limit?
1. Blackberries
2. Tofu
3. Liver
4. Tomatoes

6. 3. A client with gout should reduce his intake of purine rich food, such as liver. Blackberries, tofu, and tomatoes aren't rich in purine.

CN: Physiological integrity; CNS: Basic care and comfort; CL: Application

7. A nurse is providing care to a client with an acute gout attack. Which action should the nurse plan to take first?
1. Force fluids.
2. Instruct the client on relaxation techniques.
3. Encourage bed rest.
4. Administer analgesics.

7. 4. Administering analgesics to relieve pain should be the priority. The other actions are appropriate measures to institute but aren't the priority.

CN: Physiological integrity; CNS: Physiological adaptation; CL: Analysis

8. Which phrase best explains the usual pattern of nonchronic gout?
1. Frequent painful attacks
2. Generally painful joints at all times
3. Painful attacks with pain-free periods
4. Painful attacks with less painful periods, but pain never subsides

8. 3. The usual pattern of gout involves painful attacks with pain-free periods. Chronic gout may lead to frequent attacks with persistently painful joints.

CN: Physiological integrity; CNS: Physiological adaptation; CL: Application

9. A client has been prescribed a diet that limits purine-rich foods. Which foods should the nurse teach him to avoid eating?
1. Bananas and dried fruits
2. Milk, ice cream, and yogurt
3. Wine, cheese, preserved fruits, meats, and vegetables
4. Anchovies, sardines, kidneys, sweetbreads, and lentils

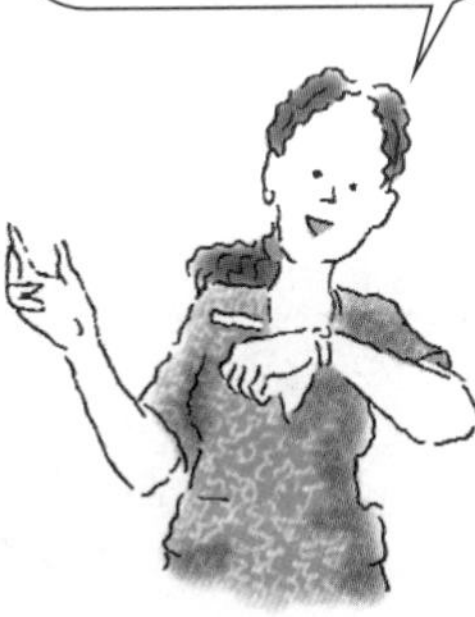

You'll answer these questions in no time!

9. 4. Anchovies, sardines, kidneys, sweetbreads, and lentils are high in purines. Bananas and dried fruits are high in potassium. Milk, ice cream, and yogurt are rich in calcium. Wine, cheese, preserved fruits, meats, and vegetables contain tyramine.

CN: Physiological integrity; CNS: Basic care and comfort; CL: Application

10. A client is recovering from an attack of gout. Client teaching should include the need to lose weight for which reason?
1. Weight loss will decrease purine levels.
2. Weight loss will decrease inflammation.
3. Weight loss will increase uric acid levels and decrease stress on joints.
4. Weight loss will decrease uric acid levels and decrease stress on joints.

10. 4. Weight loss will decrease uric acid levels and decrease stress on joints. Weight loss won't decrease purine levels, increase uric acid levels, or decrease inflammation.

CN: Health promotion and maintenance; CNS: None; CL: Application

11. A physician tells a client diagnosed with gout that his X-rays are normal. Which response would be the <u>most appropriate</u> when the client asks if he still has gout?
1. "No, you're cured."
2. "Yes, X-rays are unreliable."
3. "Yes, X-rays are normal in the early stages of gout."
4. "Yes, X-ray changes are only seen with acute attacks."

Question 11 asks you to choose the most appropriate answer. That means more than one may be suitable.

11. 3. X-rays are normal in the early stages of gout and can be very valuable in the diagnosis of gout. Telling the client that he's cured would be incorrect, because he may be in the early stages of gout when X-rays appear normal. With chronic gout, X-rays show damage to cartilage and bone. When X-ray changes occur, they're present during attacks and remissions.

CN: Physiological integrity; CNS: Physiological adaptation; CL: : Application

12. A client who has recently been diagnosed with gout asks the nurse to explain why he needs to take colchicine. The nurse plans her response based on the understanding that colchicine:
1. increases estrogen levels in the blood stream.
2. decreases the risk of infection.
3. decreases inflammation.
4. decreases bone demineralization.

12. 3. The action of colchicine is to decrease inflammation by reducing the migration of leukocytes to synovial fluid. Colchicine doesn't replace estrogen, decrease infection, or decrease bone demineralization.

CN: Physiological integrity; CNS: Pharmacological and parenteral therapies; CL: Application

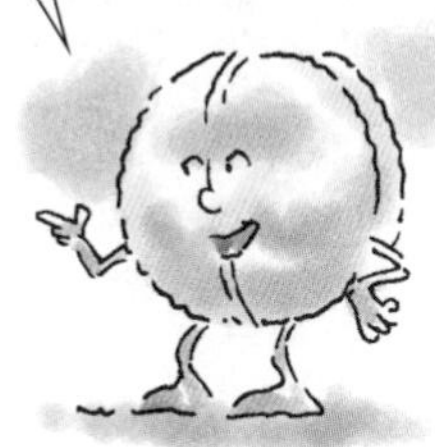

I'm just a little guy, but I'm ready to take action.

13. Which statement by a client diagnosed with gout indicates that he understands his discharge instructions?
1. "I'll increase my fluids so that the inflammation will be reduced."
2. "Increasing fluid intake will increase the calcium my body absorbs."
3. "Increasing fluid intake will cause my body to excrete more uric acid."
4. "Increasing fluids will help provide a cushion for my bones."

13. 3. Fluids promote the excretion of uric acid. Fluids don't decrease inflammation, increase calcium absorption, or provide a cushion for weakened bones.

CN: Physiological integrity; CNS: Physiological adaptation; CL: Application

14. A nurse is performing an admission assessment on a client with osteoarthritis. Which finding should she expect to note?

1. Joint pain after exercise relieved by rest
2. Symmetrical swelling of the joints of both hands
3. Morning stiffness lasting longer than 30 minutes
4. Fever

14. 1. The most common symptom of osteoarthritis is joint pain after exercise or weight-bearing, usually relieved by rest. The other options are all symptoms of rheumatoid arthritis.

CN: Physiological integrity; CNS: Physiological adaptation; CL: Application

15. A client with gout is receiving indomethacin for pain. Which statement should be included in teaching a client who's taking nonsteroidal anti-inflammatory drugs (NSAIDs)?

1. "Bleeding isn't a problem with NSAIDs."
2. "Take NSAIDs with food to avoid an upset stomach."
3. "Take NSAIDs on an empty stomach to increase absorption."
4. "Don't take NSAIDs at bedtime because they may cause excitement."

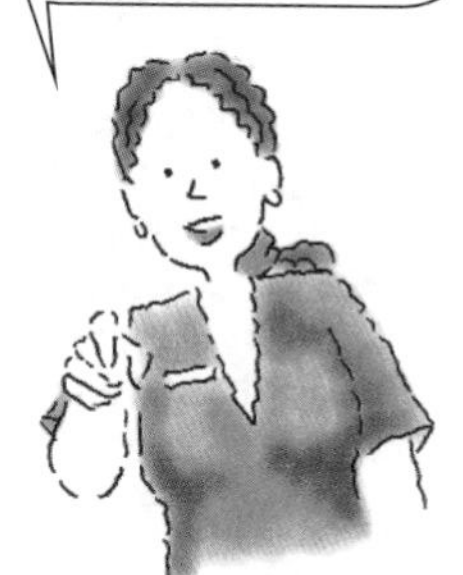

Your client depends on you for information.

15. 2. Indomethacin, like other NSAIDs, should be taken with food because it can be irritating to the GI mucosa and lead to GI bleeding. It can cause drowsiness, not excitement, and potential bleeding complications.

CN: Physiological integrity; CNS: Pharmacological and parenteral therapies; CL: Application

16. A client asks for information about osteoarthritis. Which statement should you include in teaching the client about this condition?

1. Osteoarthritis is rarely debilitating.
2. Osteoarthritis is a rare form of arthritis.
3. Osteoarthritis is the most common form of arthritis.
4. Osteoarthritis afflicts people over age 60.

16. 3. Osteoarthritis is the most common form of arthritis and can be extremely debilitating. It can afflict people of any age, although most are elderly.

CN: Physiological integrity; CNS: Physiological adaptation; CL: Application

17. Which condition or actions can cause primary osteoarthritis?

1. Overuse of joints, aging, obesity
2. Obesity, diabetes mellitus, aging
3. Congenital abnormality, aging, overuse of joints
4. Diabetes mellitus, congenital abnormality, aging

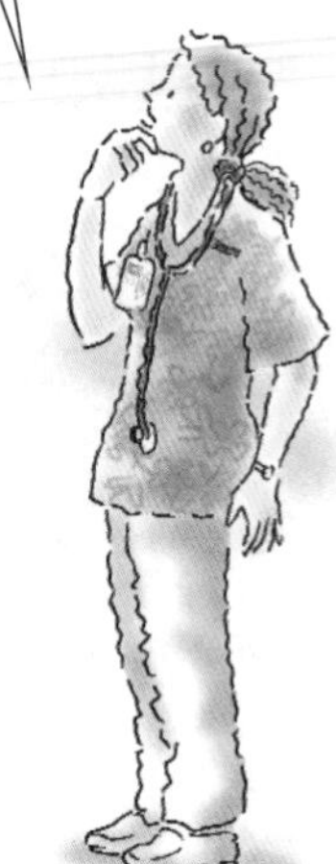

Don't be fooled. What does primary mean in this question?

17. 1. Primary osteoarthritis may be caused by the overuse of joints, aging, or obesity. Congenital abnormalities and diabetes mellitus can cause secondary osteoarthritis.

CN: Physiological integrity; CNS: Physiological adaptation; CL: Application

18. The nurse knows that a client with osteoarthritis of the knee understands the discharge instructions when the client makes which statement?

1. "I'll take my ibuprofen (Motrin) on an empty stomach."
2. "I'll try taking a warm shower in the morning."
3. "I'll wear my knee splint every night."
4. "I'll jog at least a mile every morning."

18. 2. A client with osteoarthritis has joint stiffness that may be partially relieved with a warm shower on arising in the morning. Ibuprofen should be taken with food, as should all nonsteroidal anti-inflammatory medications. Splints are usually used by clients with rheumatoid arthritis. Because the problem is continued stress on the joint, the client may want to try to an exercise that puts less strain on the joint, such as swimming.

CN: Physiological integrity; CNS: Basic care and comfort; CL: Application

CN: Client needs category CNS: Client needs subcategory CL: Cognitive level

19. A client is taking salicylates for osteoarthritis. The presence of which of the following indicates that further assessment is needed?

1. Hearing loss
2. Increased pain in joints
3. Decreased calcium absorption
4. Increased bone demineralization

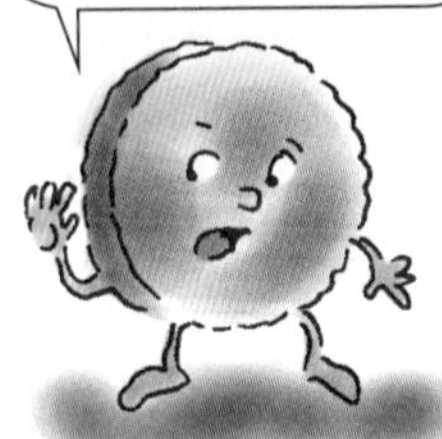

What did you say?

19. 1. Many elderly people already have diminished hearing, and salicylate use can lead to further or total hearing loss. Salicylates don't increase pain in joints, decrease calcium absorption, or increase bone demineralization.

CN: Physiological integrity; CNS: Pharmacological and parenteral therapies; CL: Application

20. Clients with osteoarthritis may be on bed rest for prolonged periods. Which nursing intervention would be appropriate for these clients?

1. Encourage coughing and deep breathing, and limit fluid intake.
2. Provide only passive range of motion (ROM), and decrease stimulation.
3. Have the client lie as still as possible, and give adequate pain medicine.
4. Turn the client every 2 hours, and encourage coughing and deep breathing.

20. 4. A bedridden client needs to be turned every 2 hours, have adequate nutrition, and cough and deep breathe. Hydration, active and passive ROM, and adequate pain medication are also appropriate nursing measures. To prevent contractures, the client shouldn't limit his fluid intake or lie as still as possible.

CN: Physiological integrity; CNS: Basic care and comfort; CL: Application

21. A client asks the nurse, "What's the difference between rheumatoid arthritis and osteoarthritis?" Which statement in response is the most correct?

1. Osteoarthritis is gender-specific; rheumatoid arthritis isn't.
2. Osteoarthritis is a localized disease; rheumatoid arthritis is systemic.
3. Osteoarthritis is a systemic disease; rheumatoid arthritis is localized.
4. Osteoarthritis has dislocations and subluxations; rheumatoid arthritis doesn't.

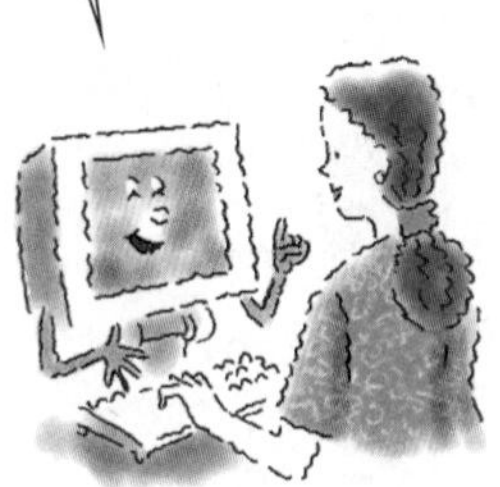

It's important to know the difference between these two common diseases.

21. 2. Osteoarthritis is a localized disease, rheumatoid arthritis is systemic. Osteoarthritis isn't gender-specific, but rheumatoid arthritis is. Clients have dislocations and subluxations in both disorders.

CN: Physiological integrity; CNS: Physiological adaptation; CL: Application

22. The nurse is assessing a client with a diagnosis of osteoarthritis. Which of the following signs would the nurse most likely assess?

1. Elevated sedimentation rate
2. Multiple subcutaneous nodules
3. Asymmetrical joint involvement
4. Signs and symptoms of inflammation, such as heat, fever, and malaise

22. 3. Asymmetrical joint involvement is present in osteoarthritis. Elevated sedimentation rate, multiple subcutaneous nodules, and such signs and symptoms of inflammation as heat, fever, and malaise are all present in rheumatoid arthritis.

CN: Physiological integrity; CNS: Physiological adaptation; CL: Analysis

23. Which instruction would be considered primary prevention of injury from osteoarthritis?

1. "Stay on bed rest."
2. "Avoid physical activity."
3. "Perform only repetitive tasks."
4. "Warm up before exercise and avoid repetitive tasks."

23. 4. Primary prevention of injury from osteoarthritis includes warming up before exercise and avoiding repetitive tasks. Bed rest would contribute to many other systemic complications. Physical activity is important to remain fit and healthy and to maintain joint function.

CN: Health promotion and maintenance; CNS: None; CL: Application

24. A client with osteoarthritis wants to know what it is. Client teaching would include which description for osteoarthritis?

1. A systemic inflammatory joint disease
2. A disease involving fusion of the joints in the hands
3. An inflammatory joint disease, with degeneration and loss of articular cartilage in synovial joints
4. A noninflammatory joint disease, with degeneration and loss of articular cartilage in synovial joints

24. 4. Osteoarthritis is a noninflammatory joint disease, with degeneration and loss of articular cartilage in synovial joints. Rheumatoid arthritis is a systemic inflammatory joint disease. Arthrodesis is fusion of the joints.
CN: Physiological integrity; CNS: Physiological adaptation; CL: Application

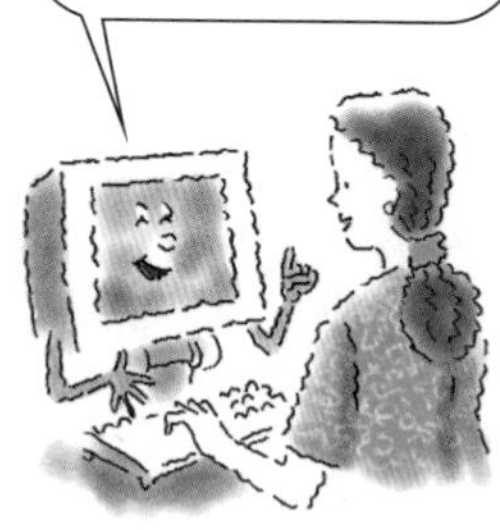

You've finished 25 questions already!

25. Use of which articles or types of clothing would help a client with osteoarthritis perform activities of daily living at home?

1. Zippered clothing
2. Tied shoes to promote stability
3. Velcro clothing, slip-on shoes, and rubber grippers
4. Buttoned clothing, slip-on shoes, and rubber grippers

25. 3. Velcro clothing, slip-on shoes, and rubber grippers make it easier for the client to dress and grip objects. Zippers, ties, and buttons may be difficult for the client to use.
CN: Physiological integrity; CNS: Basic care and comfort; CL: Application

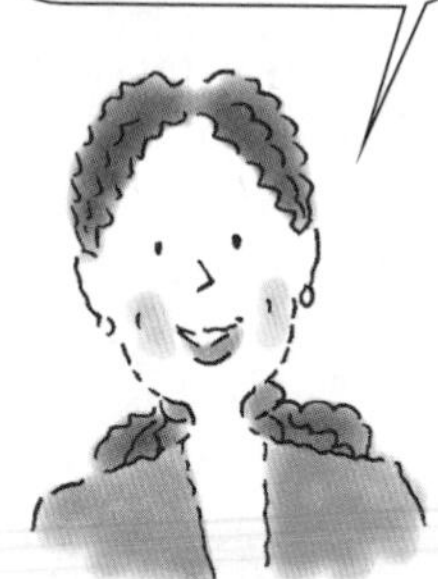

What would be the best way to help the client?

26. A client with osteoarthritis is refusing to perform his own daily care. Which approach would be most appropriate to use with this client?

1. Perform the care for the client.
2. Explain that he needs to maintain complete independence.
3. Encourage him to perform as much care as his pain will allow.
4. Tell him that once he's completed his care, he'll receive his pain medication.

26. 3. A client with osteoarthritis should be encouraged to perform as much of his care as he's able to. The nurse's goal should be to allow him to maintain his self-care abilities with help as needed but not to perform the care for him. It's never appropriate to use pain medication as a bargaining tool.
CN: Psychosocial integrity; CNS: None; CL: Analysis

27. Which of the following terms would a client in the late stages of osteoarthritis most likely use to describe his joint pain?

1. Grating
2. Dull ache
3. Deep aching pain
4. Deep aching, relieved with rest

27. 1. In the late stages of osteoarthritis, the client often describes joint pain as grating. As the disease progresses, the cartilage covering the ends of bones is destroyed and bones rub against each other. Osteophytes, or bone spurs, may also form on the ends of bones. A dull ache and deep aching pain with or without relief with rest is often seen in the earlier stages of osteoarthritis.
CN: Physiological integrity; CNS: Physiological adaptation; CL: Application

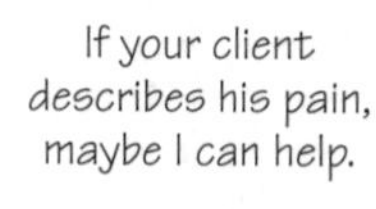

If your client describes his pain, maybe I can help.

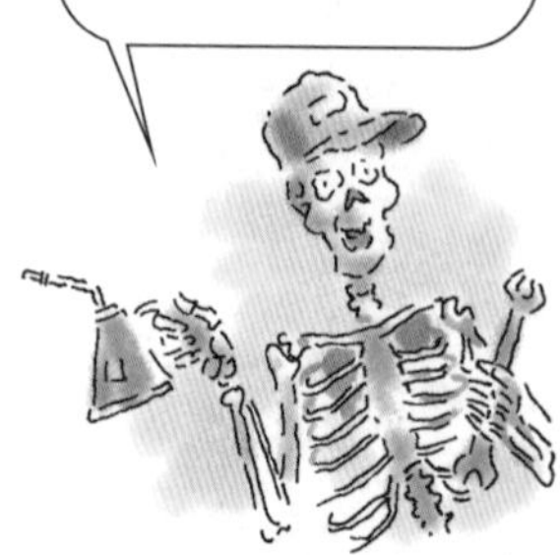

CN: Client needs category CNS: Client needs subcategory CL: Cognitive level

28. A client uses a cane for assistance in walking. Which statement is true about a cane or other assistive devices?
1. A walker is a better choice than a cane.
2. The cane should be used on the affected side.
3. The cane should be used on the unaffected side.
4. A client with osteoarthritis should be encouraged to ambulate without the cane.

28. 3. A cane should be used on the unaffected side. A client with osteoarthritis should be encouraged to ambulate with a cane, walker, or other assistive device as needed; their use takes weight and stress off of joints.
CN: Physiological integrity; CNS: Basic care and comfort; CL: Application

29. Which instruction about activity should be given to a client with osteoarthritis after he returns home?
1. "Learn to pace activity."
2. "Remain as sedentary as possible."
3. "Return to a normal level of activity."
4. "Include vigorous exercise in your daily routine."

29. 1. A client with osteoarthritis should pace his activities and avoid overexertion. Overexertion can increase degeneration and cause pain. The client shouldn't become sedentary because he'll have a high risk of pneumonia and contractures.
CN: Physiological integrity; CNS: Basic care and comfort; CL: Application

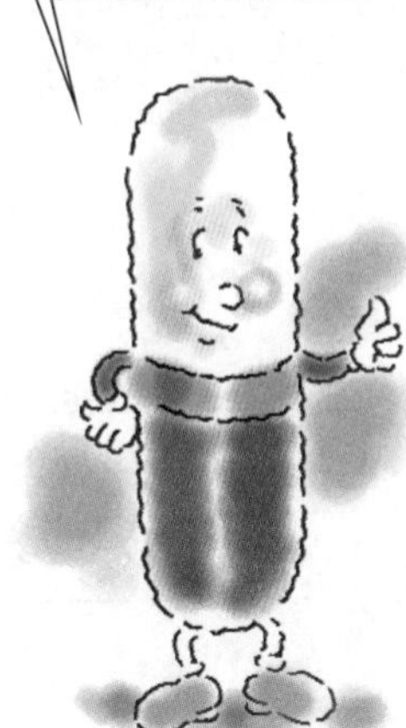

You might have to stick with me for a while so I can do my job.

30. A client was prescribed an anti-inflammatory drug for osteoarthritis 5 days ago. He says the pain has decreased some but not completely. Which nursing intervention would be the most appropriate?
1. Continue the present dose and offer other pain relief measures.
2. Notify the physician and suggest increasing the dose.
3. Notify the physician and suggest stopping the medication.
4. Notify the physician and suggest adding another medication.

30. 1. Anti-inflammatory medications may take 2 to 3 weeks to provide full benefits. If the client can tolerate the pain, continue on the medication and offer other pain measures, such as rest, massage, heat, or cold. Increasing, stopping, or adding another medication aren't appropriate because the medication hasn't been taken long enough to provide full benefit.
CN: Physiological integrity; CNS: Pharmacological and parenteral therapies; CL: Application

31. A client is diagnosed with a herniated nucleus pulposus, or herniated disk. Which statement should the nurse include in her teaching about a herniated disk?
1. The disk slips out of alignment.
2. The disk shatters, and fragments place pressure on nerve roots.
3. The nucleus tissue itself remains centralized, and the surrounding tissue is displaced.
4. The nucleus of the disk puts pressure on the annulus, causing pressure on the nerve root.

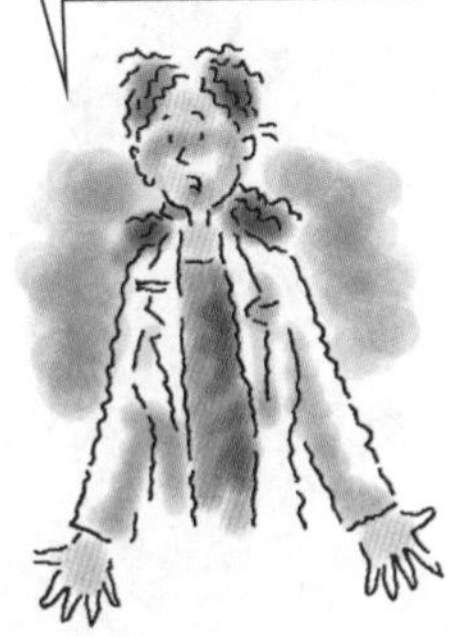

Why am I feeling so much pressure?

31. 4. With a herniated nucleus pulposus, or herniated disk, the nucleus of the disk puts pressure on the annulus, causing pressure on the nerve root. The disk itself doesn't slip, rupture, or shatter. The nucleus tissue usually moves from the center of the disk.
CN: Physiological integrity; CNS: Physiological adaptation; CL: Application

32. A client complains of low back pain that radiates down the right leg, with numbness and weakness of the right leg. The nurse recognizes these complaints as related to which disorder?

1. Herniated nucleus pulposus
2. Muscular dystrophy
3. Parkinson's disease
4. Osteoarthritis

32. 1. Compression of nerves by the herniated nucleus pulposus causes back pain that radiates into the leg, with numbness and weakness of the leg. Muscular dystrophy causes wasting of skeletal muscles. Parkinson's disease is characterized by progressive muscle rigidity and tremors. Osteoarthritis causes deep, aching joint pain.

CN: Physiological integrity; CNS: Physiological adaptation; CL: Analysis

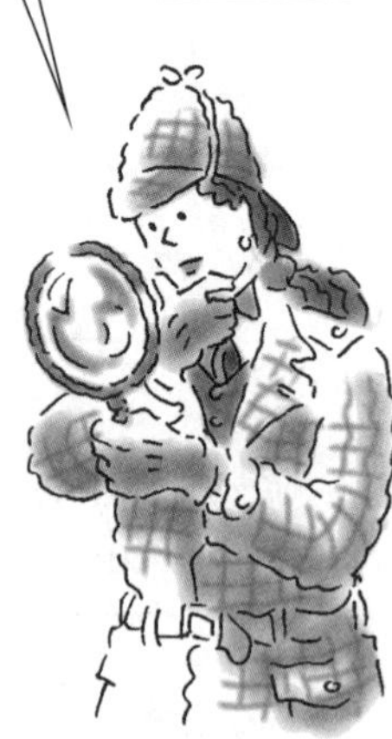

The word conservative is a clue to the right answer.

33. Conservative treatment of a herniated nucleus pulposus would include which measures?

1. Surgery
2. Bone fusion
3. Bed rest, pain medication, physiotherapy
4. Strenuous exercise, pain medication, physiotherapy

33. 3. Conservative treatment of a herniated nucleus pulposus may include bed rest, pain medication, and physiotherapy. Aggressive treatment may include surgery such as a bone fusion.

CN: Physiological integrity; CNS: Reduction of risk potential; CL: Application

34. Which instruction should a nurse include in her preoperative teaching for a client scheduled for closed spine surgery?

1. "There is a greater associated risk with closed spine surgery."
2. "Intense physical therapy is needed after the procedure."
3. "An endoscope is used to perform the surgery."
4. "Recovery time is twice as long as with open spine surgery."

34. 3. Closed spine surgery uses endoscopy to fix a herniated disk. It's less risky than open surgery and has a shorter recovery time; it's commonly done as a same-day surgical procedure. Physical therapy may be less intensive or not needed at all.

CN: Physiological integrity; CNS: Reduction of risk potential; CL: Application

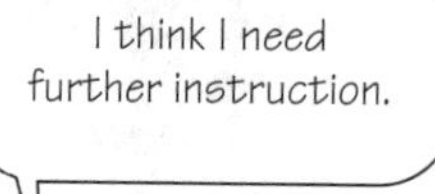

I think I need further instruction.

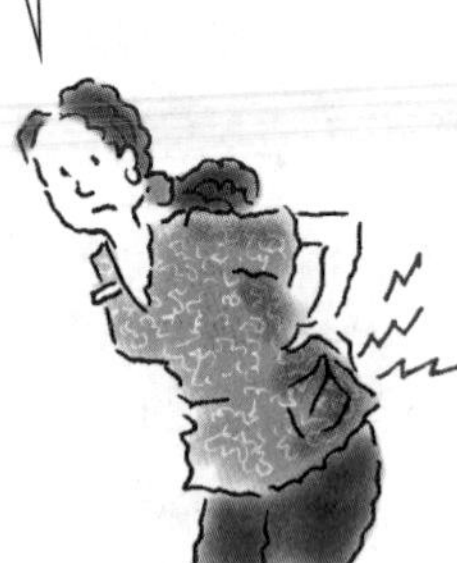

35. A nurse provided teaching to a client with a herniated lumbar disk. Which statement indicates the client needs further instruction?

1. "I can strengthen my back muscles by doing pelvic tilt exercises."
2. "I should increase my fiber and fluid intake."
3. "I should bend at the waist when picking up objects."
4. "I need to maintain a healthy weight to limit back strain."

35. 3. The client should bend at the knees, not the waist, to maintain proper body mechanics. Pelvic tilt exercises are recommended to strengthen back muscles. Increasing fiber and fluid intake helps soften stool, thereby preventing straining which increases intraspinal pressure. Any extra weight carried by the client increases back strain.

CN: Physiological integrity; CNS: Physiological adaptation; CL: Application

36. A client asks the nurse why she has applied a cold pack to a sprained ankle. Which response by the nurse would be the most appropriate?

1. "It decreases pain and increases circulation."
2. "It numbs the nerves and dilates the blood vessels."
3. "It promotes circulation and reduces muscle spasm."
4. "It constricts local blood vessels and decreases swelling."

36. 4. Application of a cold pack causes the blood vessels to constrict, which reduces the leakage of fluid into the tissues and prevents swelling. It may have an effect on muscle spasms. Cold therapy may reduce pain by numbing the nerves and tissues. Cold therapy doesn't promote circulation or dilate the blood vessels.

CN: Physiological integrity; CNS: Basic care and comfort; CL: Application

37. The nurse is teaching a community class about back injuries. Which of the following statements by the nurse would be the most accurate concerning the area that is common for vertebral herniation?

1. It is the L1–L2, L4–L5 vertebra.
2. It is the L1–L2, L5–S1 vertebra.
3. It is the L4–L5, L5–S1 vertebra.
4. It is the L5–S1, S2–S3 vertebra.

37. 3. The most common areas of herniation are L4–L5, L5–S1.

CN: Health promotion and maintenance; CNS: None; CL: Application

38. A 50-year-old client is admitted to the emergency department with severe lower back pain, weakness, and atrophy of her leg muscles. Suspecting a herniated disk, which diagnostic test would the nurse expect a physician to order?

1. Chest X-ray, magnetic resonance imaging (MRI), computed tomography (CT) scan
2. Lumbar puncture, chest X-ray, MRI, CT scan
3. Lumbar puncture, chest X-ray, myelography
4. Myelography, MRI, CT scan

38. 4. Tests used to diagnose a herniated nucleus pulposus include myelography, MRI, and CT scan. Chest X-ray and lumbar puncture aren't conclusive for a herniated disk.

CN: Physiological integrity; CNS: Physiological adaptation; CL: Application

39. Which instructions should be included when teaching a client how to protect his back?

1. "Sleep on your side, and carry objects at arm's length."
2. "Sleep on your back, and carry objects at arm's length."
3. "Sleep on your side, and carry objects close to your body."
4. "Sleep on your back, and carry objects close to your body."

39. 3. By sleeping on the side and carrying objects close to the body, there's less strain on the back. Sleeping on the back and carrying objects at arm's length adds pressure to the back.

CN: Health promotion and maintenance; CNS: None; CL: Application

40. Skeletal muscle relaxants may be used in the acute treatment of a herniated nucleus pulposus. Which instruction should be included in client teaching?

1. "Change your position quickly to avoid dizziness."
2. "Double a missed dose to ensure proper muscle relaxation."
3. "Cough and cold medications are appropriate to take, if needed."
4. "Avoid activities that require alertness; muscle relaxants can cause drowsiness."

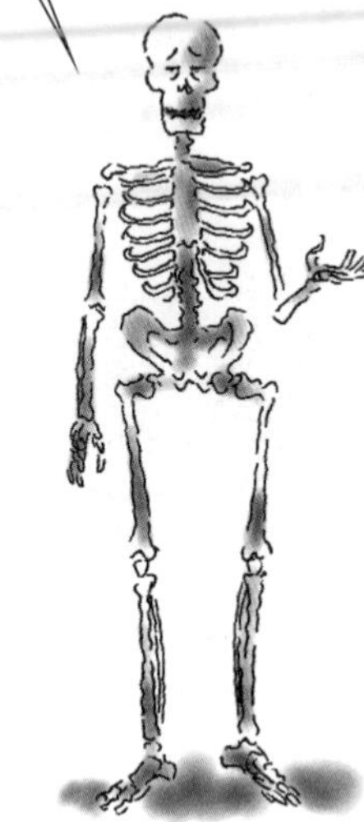
Now I know why
they call them
relaxants.

40. 4. Client teaching should include avoiding activities that require alertness; muscle relaxants can cause drowsiness. Tell the client to change position slowly to avoid dizziness. The client shouldn't double a missed dose or take cough and cold medications because this will increase the likelihood of adverse effects.

CN: Physiological integrity; CNS: Pharmacological and parenteral therapies; CL: Application

41. A client with a recent fracture is suspected of having compartment syndrome. Assessment findings may include which symptom?

1. Body-wide decrease in bone mass
2. A growth in and around the bone tissue
3. Inability to perform active movement; pain with passive movement
4. Inability to perform passive movement; pain with active movement

41. 3. With compartment syndrome, the client can't perform active movement, and pain occurs with passive movement. Osteoporosis brings a body-wide decrease in bone mass. A bone tumor shows growth in and around the bone tissue.

CN: Physiological integrity; CNS: Physiological adaptation; CL: Application

42. A client who was casted for a recent fracture of the right ulna complains of severe pain, numbness, and tingling of the right arm. What would be the nurse's most appropriate response?

1. Administer acetaminophen (Tylenol) as prescribed.
2. Lower the arm below the level of the heart.
3. Immediately report the client's symptoms.
4. Apply a heating pad.

42. 3. Severe pain, numbness, and tingling are symptoms of impaired circulation due to compartment syndrome, which is a medical emergency. Don't give analgesics until the client has been assessed and treated. Lowering the arm below the level of the heart and applying heat will decrease venous outflow and impair the circulation even more.

CN: Physiological integrity; CNS: Physiological adaptation; CL: Application

43. The nurse is assessing a client with a hemorrhage from compartment syndrome. Which of the following symptoms would the nurse expect to find?

1. Edema
2. Decreased venous pressure
3. Increased venous circulation
4. Increased arterial circulation

43. 1. The hemorrhage in compartment syndrome causes edema, increased venous pressure, and decreased venous and arterial circulation.

CN: Physiological integrity; CNS: Physiological adaptation; CL: Application

44. A client has developed compartment syndrome following application of a cast to a fractured tibia. Which of the following responses is the most accurate for prompt action in treating compartment syndrome?

1. Decrease the level of pain.
2. Prevent tissue death, which can occur within 2 to 4 hours.
3. Prevent further complications.
4. Decrease the swelling in the extremity.

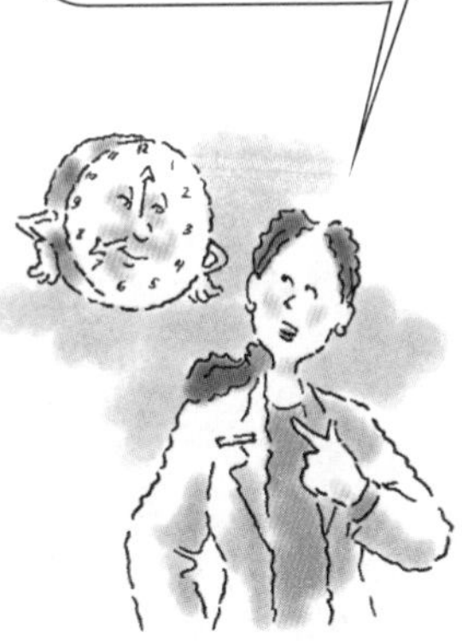

You'll have this
answer in no time.

44. 2. Following development of compartment syndrome, there is an increase in pressure within the affected compartment that compromises circulation to the muscle tissue and to nerves. This may lead to death of these tissues and can occur within 2 to 4 hours. Decreasing pain levels, preventing further complication, and decreasing the swelling in the affected extremity are important goals of treatment, but they are not the priority of treatment.
CN: Physiological integrity; CNS: Physiological adaptation; CL: Application

45. Treatment of compartment syndrome includes which measure?

1. Amputation
2. Casting
3. Fasciotomy
4. Observation; no treatment necessary

45. 3. Treatment of compartment syndrome includes fasciotomy, which involves cutting the fascia over the affected area to permit muscle expansion. Amputation and casting aren't treatments for compartment syndrome.
CN: Physiological integrity; CNS: Physiological adaptation; CL: Application

46. A client is admitted to the emergency department with a foot fracture. The nurse is teaching the client about the brace that will be applied. The teaching has been effective when the client states which of the following responses regarding the reason for the brace?

1. "It acts as a splint."
2. "It prevents infection."
3. "It allows for movement."
4. "It encourages direct contact."

46. 1. The purpose of the brace is to act as a splint, maintain immobility, and prevent direct contact. A brace doesn't prevent infection.
CN: Physiological integrity; CNS: Reduction of risk potential; CL: Application

47. Which of the following symptoms are considered signs of paresthesia?

1. Fever and chills
2. Change in range of motion (ROM)
3. Pain and blanching
4. Numbness and tingling

47. 4. Paresthesia is described as numbness and tingling. It isn't associated with fever and chills or change in ROM nor is it described as pain or blanching.
CN: Physiological integrity; CNS: Physiological adaptation; CL: Application

48. A client has been treated for compartment syndrome by undergoing a fasciotomy. Which nursing diagnosis is the most appropriate?

1. *Risk for infection*
2. *Chronic pain*
3. *Impaired gas exchange*
4. *Decreased cardiac output*

48. 1. *Risk for infection* is the most appropriate diagnosis following a fasciotomy. A fasciotomy involves the excision of the fascia and leaving the wound unsutured. The wound is covered with dressings that are moistened with sterile saline. The client may develop infection in this open wound. Although there is pain involved, the pain should decrease due to the surgical decompression of the fascia. Gas exchange and cardiac output should not be affected by the fasciotomy.
CN: Physiological integrity; CNS: Physiological adaptation; CL: Analysis

49. The community health nurse found an elderly female client lying in the snow, unable to move her right leg because of a fracture. What's the nurse's first priority?

1. Realign the fracture ends.
2. Reduce the fracture.
3. Immobilize the fracture in its present position.
4. Elevate the leg on whatever is available.

49. 3. Initial treatment of obvious and suspected fractures includes immobilizing and splinting the limb. Any attempt to realign or rest the fracture at the stem may cause further injury and complications. The leg may be elevated only after immobilization.

CN: Safe, effective care environment; CNS: Management of care; CL: Analysis

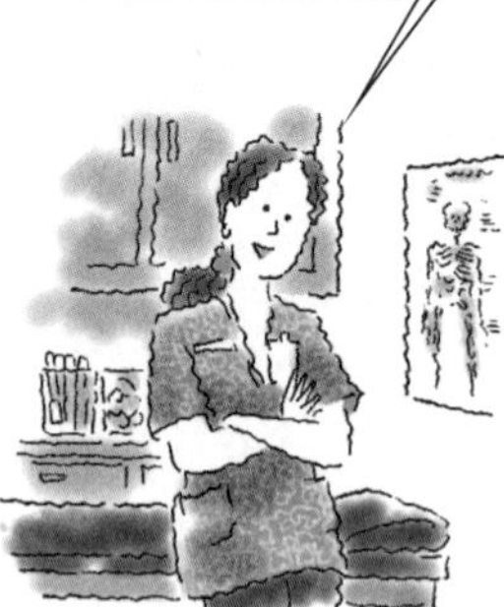

Knowing normal signs will alert you to what is wrong.

50. A nurse determines a client understands the teaching regarding compartment syndrome if he reports which early symptom?

1. Heat
2. Paresthesia
3. Skin pallor
4. Swelling

50. 2. Paresthesia is the earliest sign of compartment syndrome. Pain, heat, and swelling are also signs but occur after paresthesia. Skin pallor isn't a sign of compartment syndrome.

CN: Physiological integrity; CNS: Physiological adaptation; CL: Analysis

51. Which symptoms are considered signs of a fracture?

1. Tingling, coolness, loss of pulses
2. Loss of sensation, redness, coolness
3. Coolness, redness, new site of pain
4. Redness, warmth, pain at the site of injury

51. 4. Signs of a fracture may include redness, warmth, numbness or loss of sensation, and new site of pain. Coolness, tingling, and loss of pulses are signs of a vascular problem.

CN: Physiological integrity; CNS: Physiological adaptation; CL: Application

52. Which areas should be included in a neurovascular assessment?

1. Orientation, movement, pulses, warmth
2. Capillary refill, movement, pulses, warmth
3. Orientation, pupillary response, temperature, pulses
4. Respiratory pattern, orientation, pulses, temperature

52. 2. A correct neurovascular assessment should include capillary refill, movement, pulses, and warmth. Neurovascular assessment involves nerve and blood supply to an area. Respiratory pattern, orientation, temperature, and pupillary response aren't part of a neurovascular examination.

CN: Physiological integrity; CNS: Reduction of risk potential; CL: Application

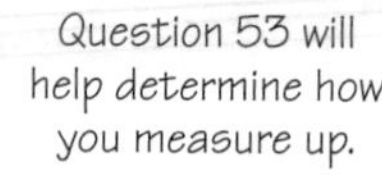

Question 53 will help determine how you measure up.

53. A nurse has instructed a client to accurately measure the circumference of both calves each morning and to report any increase in circumference. Which statement by the client indicates that the teaching has been effective?

1. "I'll use a measuring tape to check circumference."
2. "I only have to call if one leg is significantly larger than the other."
3. "I can measure my calves either near the knee or closer to the ankle."
4. "I'll use the standardized chart for limb circumference."

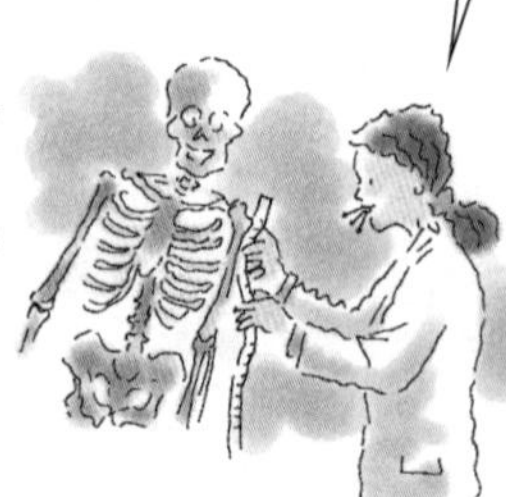

53. 1. The correct method for measuring calf circumference is to use a measuring tape: place the tape at the level where the calf circumference is largest and measure at the same place each time. The client was instructed to report any increase in circumference. A significant increase in calf circumference size might be unilateral or bilateral. There's no standardized chart for limb circumference.

CN: Health promotion and maintenance; CNS: None; CL: Application

54. If pulses aren't palpable, which intervention should be performed <u>first</u>?

1. Check again in 1 hour.
2. Alert the nurse in charge immediately.
3. Verify the findings with Doppler ultrasonography.
4. Alert the physician immediately.

54. 3. If pulses aren't palpable, verify the assessment with Doppler ultrasonography. If pulses can't be found with Doppler ultrasonography, immediately notify the physician.

CN: Safe, effective care environment; CNS: Management of care; CL: Application

55. A client describes a foul odor from his cast. Which response or intervention would be the <u>most appropriate</u>?

1. Assess further because this may be a sign of infection.
2. Teach him proper cast care, including hygiene measures.
3. This is normal, especially when a cast is in place for a few weeks.
4. Assess further because this may be a sign of neurovascular compromise.

55. 1. A foul odor from a cast may be a sign of infection. The nurse needs to assess for fever, malaise and, possibly, an elevation in white blood cells. Odor from a cast is never normal, and it isn't a sign of neurovascular compromise, which would include decreased pulses, coolness, and paresthesia.

CN: Physiological integrity; CNS: Reduction of risk potential; CL: Analysis

56. To reduce the roughness of a cast, which measure should be used?

1. Petal the edges.
2. Elevate the limb.
3. Break off the rough area.
4. Distribute pressure evenly.

56. 1. To reduce the roughness of the cast, petal the edges. Elevating the limb will prevent swelling. Never break a rough area off the cast. Distributing pressure evenly will prevent pressure ulcers.

CN: Physiological integrity; CNS: Basic care and comfort; CL: Application

57. Elevating a limb with a cast will prevent swelling. Which action best describes how this is done?

1. Place the limb with the cast close to the body.
2. Place the limb with the cast at the level of the heart.
3. Place the limb with the cast below the level of the heart.
4. Place the limb with the cast above the level of the heart.

57. 4. To reduce swelling, place the limb with the cast above the level of the heart. To elevate a cast, the limb may need to be extended from the body. Placing it below or at the level of the heart won't reduce swelling.

CN: Physiological integrity; CNS: Basic care and comfort; CL: Application

58. A client asks why a plaster cast can't get wet. Which response would be the most <u>appropriate</u>?

1. A wet cast can cause a foul odor.
2. A wet cast will weaken or be destroyed.
3. A wet cast is heavy and difficult to maneuver.
4. It's all right to get the cast wet, just use a hair dryer to dry it off.

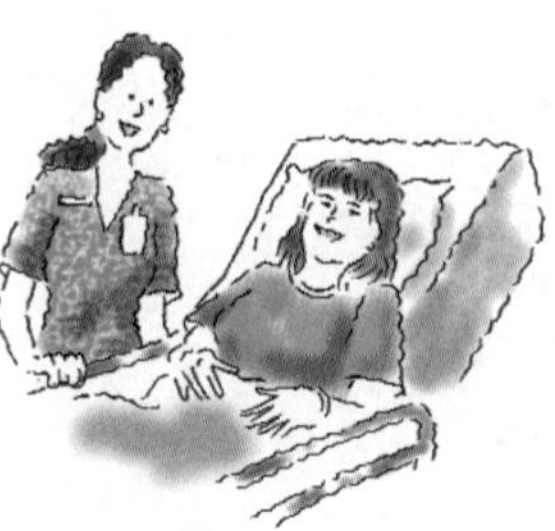

Your client depends on you to know the answers.

58. 2. A wet cast will weaken or be destroyed. A foul odor is a sign of infection. It's never all right to get a cast wet. Fiberglass casts do not lose integrity or strength when wet or damp.

CN: Physiological integrity; CNS: Reduction of risk potential; CL: Application

59. A client comes to the emergency department complaining of dull, deep bone pain unrelated to movement. Which statement is correct to help decide if the bone pain is caused by a fracture?

1. These are classic symptoms of a fracture.
2. Fracture pain is sharp and related to movement.
3. Fracture pain is sharp and unrelated to movement.
4. Fracture pain is dull and deep and related to movement.

59. 2. Fracture pain is sharp and related to movement. Pain that's dull and deep and unrelated to movement isn't typical of a fracture.
CN: Health promotion and maintenance; CNS: None; CL: Analysis

60. A client with skeletal traction to his right leg complains of severe right leg pain. Which action should the nurse take first?

1. Call the physician.
2. Check the client's alignment in bed.
3. Remove the weights from the traction.
4. Perform pin care.

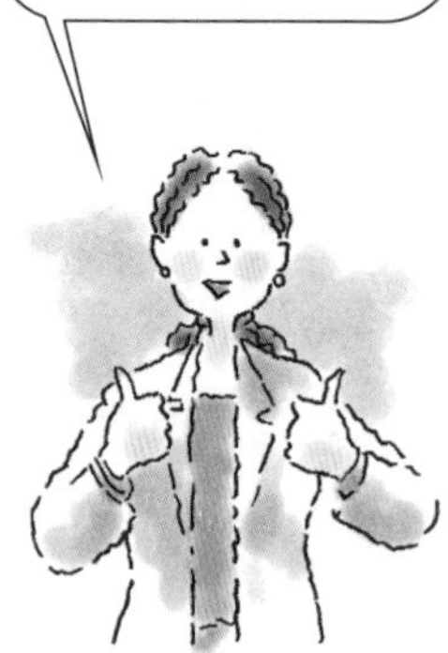

60. 2. A client who complains of severe leg pain may need realignment to ease some pressure on the fracture site. If this is ineffective, then the physician may need to be notified. The weights ordered may be too heavy but the nurse can't remove them without a physician's order. Performing pin care isn't appropriate at this time.
CN: Safe, effective care environment; CNS: Management of care; CL: Application

61. A male client with a fractured femur is in Russell's traction. He asks the nurse to help him with back care. Which nursing action is the most appropriate?

1. Telling the client that he can't have back care while he's in traction.
2. Removing the weight to give the client more slack to move.
3. Supporting the weight to give the client more slack to move.
4. Telling the client to use the trapeze to lift his back off the bed.

61. 4. The traction must not be disturbed, to maintain correct alignment. Therefore, the client should use the trapeze to lift his back off of the bed. The client can have back care as long as he uses the trapeze and doesn't disturb the alignment. The weight shouldn't be moved without a physician's order; it should hang freely without touching anything.
CN: Physiological integrity; CNS: Basic care and comfort; CL: Application

62. A client is involved in an automobile accident and is being sent to a trauma center. For which classic fractures that typically occur from trauma should the staff be prepared to assess?

1. Brachial and clavicle
2. Brachial and humerus
3. Humerus and clavicle
4. Occipital and humerus

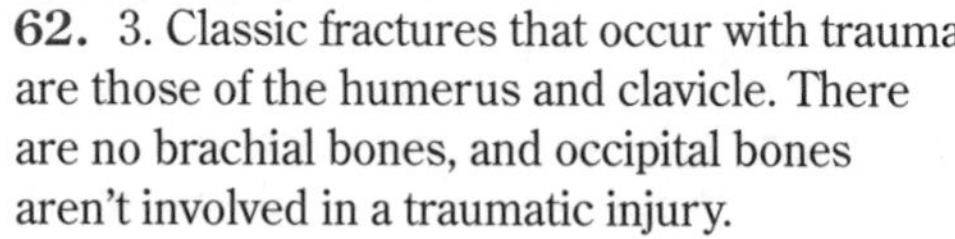

62. 3. Classic fractures that occur with trauma are those of the humerus and clavicle. There are no brachial bones, and occipital bones aren't involved in a traumatic injury.
CN: Physiological integrity; CNS: Physiological adaptation; CL: Analysis

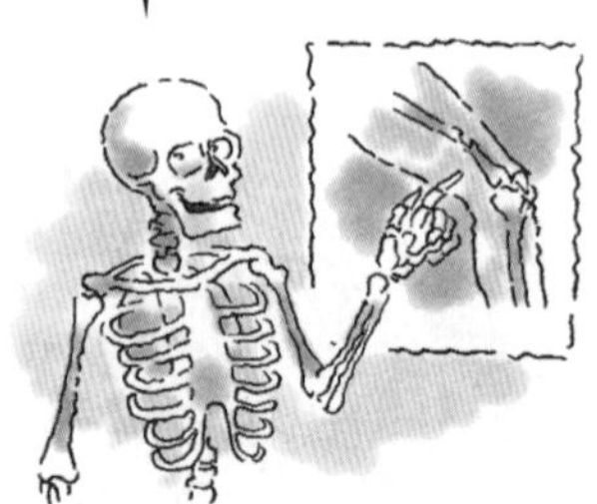

It's important to understand the different types of fractures.

63. A client asks why he's being placed in traction prior to surgery. Which response by the nurse is the most appropriate?

1. Traction will help prevent skin breakdown.
2. Traction helps with repositioning while in bed.
3. Traction allows for more activity.
4. Traction helps to prevent trauma and overcome muscle spasms.

63. 4. Traction prevents trauma and overcomes muscle spasms. Traction doesn't help in preventing skin breakdown, repositioning the client, or allowing the client to become active.
CN: Physiological integrity; CNS: Basic care and comfort; CL: Application

64. A 75-year-old client with Paget's disease is undergoing tests for a suspected fracture. The nurse should expect to see which type of fracture?

1. Linear
2. Longitudinal
3. Oblique
4. Transverse

64. 4. A transverse fracture commonly occurs with such bone diseases as osteomalacia and Paget's disease. Linear, longitudinal, and oblique fractures generally occur with trauma.
CN: Physiological integrity; CNS: Physiological adaptation; CL: Application

65. A 20-year-old female client is complaining of severe pain in her right upper arm. If the nurse suspects domestic abuse, which X-ray finding would indicate the need for further investigation?

1. Longitudinal
2. Oblique
3. Spiral
4. Transverse

65. 3. Spiral fractures are commonly seen in the upper extremities and are related to physical abuse. Longitudinal and oblique fractures generally occur with trauma. A transverse fracture commonly occurs with such bone diseases as osteomalacia and Paget's disease.
CN: Physiological integrity; CNS: Physiological adaptation; CL: Application

66. A 25-year-old male client has just had a plaster cast applied to his right forearm following the reduction of a closed radius fracture due to an in-line skating accident. It's most important for the nurse to check which of the following?

1. Whether the cast is completely dry
2. Sensation and movement of the fingers
3. Whether the client is having any pain
4. Whether the cast needs petaling

66. 2. Neurovascular checks are most important because they're used to determine if any impairment exists after cast application and reduction of the fracture. Checking to see if the cast is completely dry isn't the nurse's highest priority. Petaling to smooth the cast edge is done when the cast is completely dry.
CN: Physiological integrity; CNS: Reduction of risk potential; CL: Application

67. A nurse is caring for a client with a femoral shaft fracture. Which serious complication is seen with this condition?

1. Constipation
2. Decreased urine output
3. Hemorrhage
4. Pain

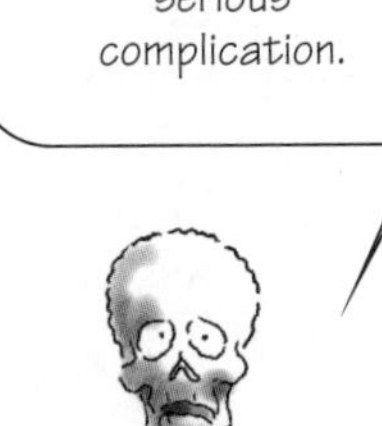
Wow! This is a serious complication.

67. 3. Femoral shaft fractures may cause hemorrhage, with as much as 1,000 to 1,500 ml of blood loss. Constipation and decreased urine output aren't direct complications of a fracture. Pain may occur, but it can be controlled with analgesia.
CN: Physiological integrity; CNS: Physiological adaptation; CL: Analysis

68. Which serious complication is most frequently seen with long bone fractures?
1. Bone emboli
2. Fat emboli
3. Platelet emboli
4. Serous emboli

68. 2. A serious complication of long bone fractures is the development of fat emboli. Bone or platelet emboli are rare occurrences and infrequently associated with long bone fractures. There aren't emboli known as serous emboli.
CN: Physiological integrity; CNS: Physiological adaptation; CL: Analysis

69. A client is diagnosed with fat emboli. Which signs and symptoms would the nurse expect to find when assessing his client?
1. Tachypnea, tachycardia, shortness of breath, paresthesia
2. Paresthesia, bradypnea, bradycardia, petechial rash on chest and neck
3. Bradypnea, bradycardia, shortness of breath, petechial rash on chest and neck
4. Tachypnea, tachycardia, shortness of breath, petechial rash on chest and neck

69. 4. Signs and symptoms of fat emboli include tachypnea, tachycardia, shortness of breath, and a petechial rash on the chest and neck. The fat molecules enter the venous circulation and travel to the lung, obstructing pulmonary circulation. Bradycardia, bradypnea, and paresthesia aren't usual symptoms.
CN: Health promotion and maintenance; CNS: None; CL: Analysis

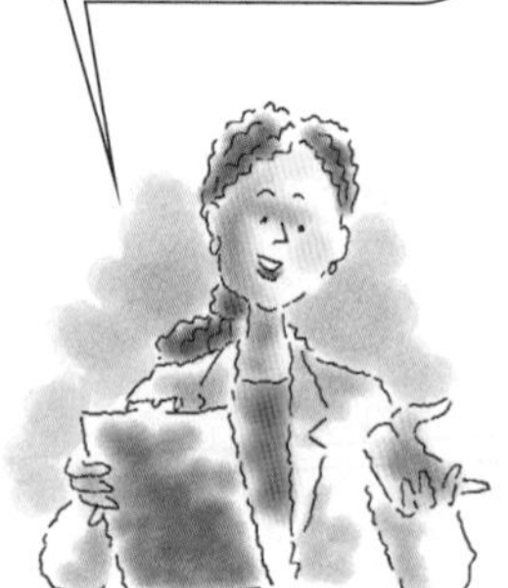

Assessment is a key skill for nurses in every field.

70. Treatment of a fat embolus may include which therapies?
1. Albuterol, oxygen, I.V. fluids, steroids
2. Oxygen, I.V. fluids, steroids, antibiotics
3. Morphine, oxygen, I.V. fluids, antibiotics
4. Theophylline, morphine, oxygen, I.V. fluids

70. 2. Treatment of a fat embolus may include oxygen, I.V. fluids, steroids to counteract inflammation in the lungs and correct cerebral edema, and antibiotics to prevent infection. Albuterol, morphine, and theophylline aren't commonly used to treat fat emboli.
CN: Physiological integrity; CNS: Physiological adaptation; CL: Analysis

71. A high-protein diet is ordered for a client recovering from a fracture. High protein is ordered for which reason?
1. Protein promotes gluconeogenesis.
2. Protein has anti-inflammatory properties.
3. Protein promotes cell growth and bone union.
4. Protein decreases pain medication requirements.

71. 3. High-protein intake promotes cell growth and bone union. Protein doesn't promote gluconeogenesis, exert anti-inflammatory properties, or decrease pain medication requirements.
CN: Physiological integrity; CNS: Basic care and comfort; CL: Application

72. The nurse is instructing a nursing assistant on the proper car of a client in Buck's extension traction following a fracture of his left fibula. Which observation indicates that the teaching was effective?
1. The weights are allowed to hang freely over the end of the bed.
2. The nursing assistant lifts the weights when assisting the client to move up in bed.
3. The leg in traction is kept externally rotated.
4. The nursing assistant instructs the client to perform ankle rotation exercises.

72. 1. In Buck's traction, the weights should hang freely without touching the bed or floor. Lifting the weights would break the traction. The client should be moved up in bed, allowing the weight to move freely along with the client. The leg should be kept in straight alignment. Performing ankle rotation exercises could cause the leg to go out of alignment.
CN: Physiological integrity; CNS: Basic care and comfort; CL: Application

73. A 61-year-old client has undergone a total hip replacement on her right side. After surgery, how often should the nurse turn the client?
1. Every 1 to 2 hours, from the unaffected side to the back
2. Every 1 to 2 hours, from the affected side to the back
3. Every 4 to 6 hours, from the unaffected side to the back
4. Every 4 to 6 hours, from the affected side to the back

73. 1. The client should be turned at least every 2 hours and always from the unaffected side to the back. The client should never be placed on the affected side. Turning the client every 4 to 6 hours places her at greater risk for skin breakdown.

CN: Physiological integrity; CNS: Reduction of risk potential; CL: Application

74. A client is receiving nutritional counseling following application of a plaster cast for a fracture. Vitamin D intake is emphasized to promote the:
1. excretion of calcium and phosphorus.
2. excretion of potassium and calcium.
3. absorption and use of potassium and phosphorus.
4. absorption and use of calcium and phosphorus.

74. 4. Vitamin D increases the absorption and use of calcium and phosphorus. It doesn't affect potassium, nor does it reduce the absorption or affect the excretion of calcium and phosphorus.

CN: Physiological integrity; CNS: Pharmacological and parenteral therapies; CL: Application

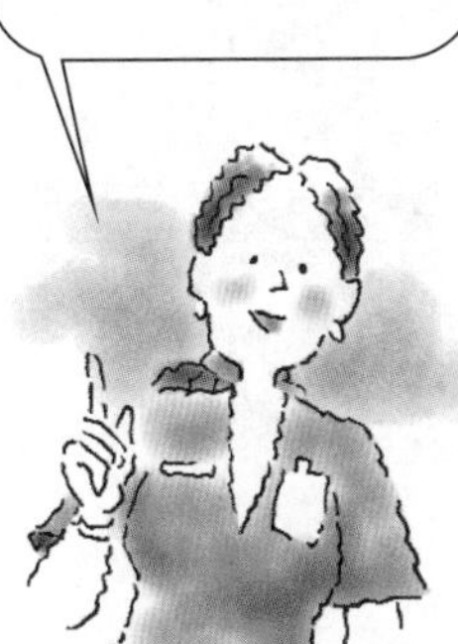

Placing the client in the correct position after hip surgery is critical.

75. After surgical repair of a hip, which position is best for a client's legs and hips?
1. Abduction
2. Adduction
3. Prone
4. Subluxated

75. 1. After surgical repair of the hip, the desired position of the legs and hips is abduction. Adduction, prone, or subluxated positions don't keep the prosthesis within the acetabulum.

CN: Physiological integrity; CNS: Reduction of risk potential; CL: Application

76. A nurse is reviewing discharge instructions for a client after a left hip replacement. Which statement indicates that the client understands the activity instructions?
1. "I must remain on bed rest."
2. "I have no activity restrictions."
3. "I can't bear any weight for 2 months."
4. "I am allowed limited weight bearing."

76. 4. After a hip replacement, the client's activity is usually ordered as limited weight bearing. The client is allowed to move with restrictions for approximately 2 to 3 months. The hip shouldn't be flexed more than 90 degrees. Abduction past the midline of the body is prohibited. Progressive weight bearing reduces the complications of immobility.

CN: Physiological integrity; CNS: Basic care and comfort; CL: Application

77. Which intervention would help prevent deep vein thrombosis (DVT) after hip surgery?
1. Bed rest
2. Egg crate mattress
3. Vigorous pulmonary care
4. Subcutaneous heparin and pneumatic compression boots

77. 4. To prevent DVT after hip surgery, subcutaneous heparin and pneumatic compression boots are used. Bed rest can cause DVT. Egg crate mattresses and pulmonary care don't prevent DVT.

CN: Physiological integrity; CNS: Reduction of risk potential; CL: Application

78. Which discharge instructions should be given to a client after surgery for repair of a hip fracture?

1. "Don't flex the hip more than 30 degrees, don't cross your legs, and get help putting on your shoes."
2. "Don't flex the hip more than 60 degrees, don't cross your legs, and get help putting on your shoes."
3. "Don't flex the hip more than 90 degrees, don't cross your legs, and get help putting on your shoes."
4. "Don't flex the hip more than 120 degrees, don't cross your legs, and get help putting on your shoes."

78. 3. Discharge instructions should include not flexing the hip more than 90 degrees, not crossing the legs, and getting help to put on shoes. These restrictions prevent dislocation of the new prosthesis.
CN: Physiological integrity; CNS: Reduction of risk potential; CL: Application

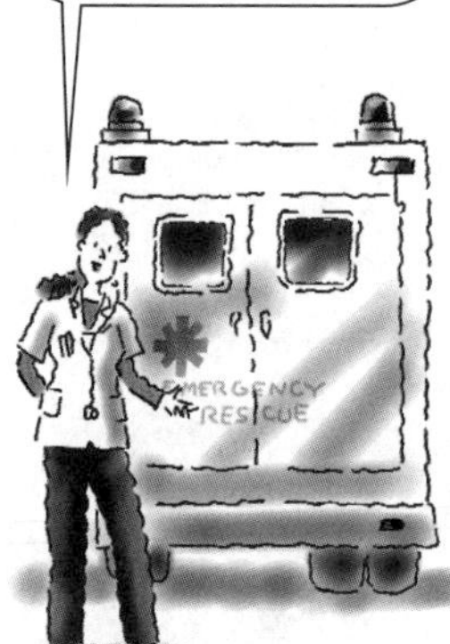
Make sure your initial intervention is the correct one.
EMERGENCY RESCUE

79. At the scene of an accident, which intervention applies to a client with a suspected fracture?

1. Don't move the client.
2. Move the client to safety immediately.
3. Sit the client up to facilitate his airway.
4. Immobilize the extremity, and move the client to safety.

79. 4. At the scene of an accident, a client with a suspected fracture should have the extremity immobilized and be moved to safety. If the client is in a safe place, don't try to move him. Never try to sit the client up; this could make the fracture worse.
CN: Safe, effective care environment; CNS: Safety and infection control; CL: Application

80. After instructing a client on a 3-point gait using crutches, the client demonstrates an understanding when he places weight on the:

1. feet.
2. axillary areas.
3. palms of the hands.
4. palms and axillary areas.

80. 3. To avoid damage to the brachial plexus nerves in the axilla, the palms of the hands should bear the client's weight. Minimal weight should be placed on the affected leg.
CN: Physiological integrity; CNS: Basic care and comfort; CL: Application

81. A client with a right hip fracture is complaining of left-sided leg pain and edema and has a positive Homans' sign. Which condition would show those symptoms?

1. Deep vein thrombosis (DVT)
2. Fat emboli
3. Infection
4. Pulmonary embolism

81. 1. Unilateral leg pain and edema with a positive Homans' sign (not always present) might be symptoms of DVT. Symptoms of fat emboli include restlessness, tachypnea, and tachycardia and are more common in long-bone injuries. It's unlikely an infection would occur on the opposite side of the fracture without cause. Tachycardia, chest pain, and shortness of breath may be symptoms of a pulmonary embolism.
CN: Physiological integrity; CNS: Reduction of risk potential; CL: Application

82. Which nursing intervention is appropriate for a client in traction?

1. Assess the pin sites every shift and as needed.
2. Add and remove weights as the client wants.
3. Make sure the knots in the rope catch on the pulley.
4. Give range of motion (ROM) to all joints, including those immediately proximal and distal to the fracture, every shift.

82. 1. Nursing care for a client in traction may include assessing pin sites every shift and as needed and making sure the knots in the rope don't catch on the pulley. Add and remove weights as the physician orders, and give ROM to all joints except those immediately proximal and distal to the fracture every shift.
CN: Physiological integrity; CNS: Basic care and comfort; CL: Application

83. After helping a physician apply a cast, which nursing intervention is included in the immediate cast care?

1. Rest the cast on the bedside table.
2. Dispose of the plaster water in the sink.
3. Support the cast with the palms of the hands.
4. Wait until the cast dries before cleaning the surrounding skin.

83. 3. After helping the physician apply a cast, support it with the palms of the hands; don't rest the cast on a hard or sharp surface. Dispose of the plaster water in a sink with a plaster trap or in a garbage bag. Clean the surrounding skin before the cast dries.

CN: Safe, effective care environment; CNS: Management of care; CL: Application

84. The physician has just removed the cast from a 20-year-old male client's lower leg. During the removal, a small superficial abrasion occurred over the ankle. Which statement by the client indicates the need for additional client teaching?

1. "I must use a moisturizing lotion on the dry areas."
2. "The dry, peeling skin will go away by itself."
3. "I can wash the abrasion on my ankle with soap and water."
4. "I'll wait until the abrasion is healed before I go swimming."

84. 1. The dry, peeling skin will heal in a few days with normal cleaning; therefore, lotions are unnecessary. Vigorous scrubbing isn't necessary. Washing the abrasion and delaying swimming until healing are correct procedures to follow after removal of a cast.

CN: Physiological integrity; CNS: Reduction of risk potential; CL: Application

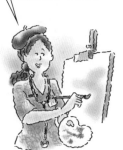

So, when can I sign your cast?

85. Which statement by a client who recently had a cast applied indicates that the nurse's teaching has been effective?

1. "The cast will need to be removed if I feel any heat."
2. "Heat is a normal sensation as a cast dries."
3. "The heat I feel is most likely caused by an infection."
4. "I'll call my physician if I feel any heat."

85. 2. Normally, as the cast dries, a client may complain of heat from the cast. Offer reassurance. The cast won't need to be removed and the physician doesn't need to be notified. Heat from the cast isn't a sign of infection.

CN: Physiological integrity; CNS: Reduction of risk potential; CL: Application

The word *prevent* is a hint. Look for a preventive measure, not a treatment.

86. A nurse is providing care for a client with a leg cast. To help prevent footdrop, which action by the nurse is the most appropriate?

1. Encouraging bed rest.
2. Supporting the foot with 45 degrees of flexion.
3. Supporting the foot with 90 degrees of flexion.
4. Placing a stocking on the foot to provide warmth.

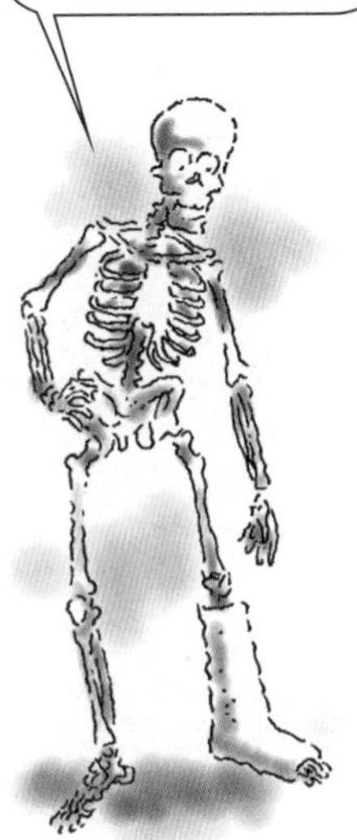

86. 3. To prevent foot drop in a leg with a cast, the foot should be supported with 90 degrees of flexion. Bed rest can cause foot drop. Keeping the extremity warm won't prevent foot drop.

CN: Health promotion and maintenance; CNS: None; CL: Application

87. A client with a hip-spica cast should avoid gas-forming foods. Which rationale best explains why?

1. To prevent flatus
2. To prevent diarrhea
3. To prevent constipation
4. To prevent abdominal distention

87. 4. A client with a hip-spica cast should avoid gas-forming foods to prevent abdominal distention. Gas-forming foods may cause flatus, but that isn't a reason to avoid them. Gas-forming foods generally don't cause diarrhea or constipation.
CN: Physiological integrity; CNS: Reduction of risk potential; CL: Application

88. A client is demonstrating his understanding of touchdown weight bearing prior to discharge. The nurse is satisfied with:

1. full weight bearing on the affected extremity.
2. 30% to 50% weight bearing on the affected extremity.
3. no weight on the extremity, but may touch the floor with it.
4. no weight on the extremity, and keep it elevated at all times.

88. 3. Touchdown weight bearing involves no weight on the extremity, but the client may touch the floor with the affected extremity. Full weight bearing allows for full weight to be put on the affected extremity. Partial weight bearing allows for 30% to 50% weight bearing on affected extremity. Non-weight bearing is no weight on the extremity.
CN: Physiological integrity; CNS: Basic care and comfort; CL: Application

89. A client has attended the Sports Medicine Clinic to reduce his risk of experiencing a sports-related injury. Which activity indicates his understanding?

1. Warming up
2. Pacing the activity
3. Building strength
4. Working with moderate intensity

89. 1. The best way to prevent sports-related injuries is to warm up. Pacing the activity, building strength, and using moderate intensity are also prevention measures, but warming up is the most effective.
CN: Physiological integrity; CNS: Reduction of risk potential; CL: Application

90. A client has just returned from the post anesthesia care unit after undergoing internal fixation of a left femoral neck fracture. The nurse should place the client in which position?

1. On his left side with his right knee bent
2. On his back with two pillows between his legs
3. On his right side with his left knee bent
4. Sitting at a 90-degree angle

90. 2. The operative leg must be kept abducted to prevent dislocation of the hip. Placing the client on the left or right side with knee bent doesn't promote abduction. Acute flexion of the operated hip may cause dislocation. The head of the bed may be raised 35 to 49 degrees.
CN: Physiological integrity; CNS: Reduction of risk potential; CL: Application

91. Which symptom would lead the nurse to suspect a fat embolus in a client who has a fracture of his left femur?

1. Dyspnea
2. Sudden headache
3. Muscle spasm in the left thigh
4. Numbness in the left leg

91. 1. A fat embolism usually presents as an acute respiratory distress. Symptoms include chest pain, cyanosis, dyspnea, tachypnea, and apprehension. A sudden headache isn't a symptom of a fat embolism. Muscle spasms in the left thigh are a neuromuscular response of the local muscle around the femoral fracture. Numbness would be a neurovascular response.
CN: Physiological integrity; CNS: Physiological adaptation; CL: Application

92. Which statement explains an open reduction of a fractured femur?

1. Traction will be used.
2. A cast will be applied.
3. Crutches will be used after surgery.
4. Some form of screw, plate, nail, or wire is usually used to maintain alignment.

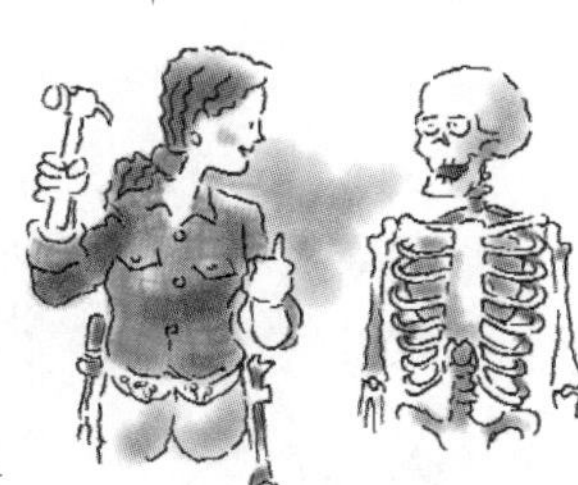

"Screws, nails, wires—who knew open reduction was so much like home repair?"

92. 4. Open reduction means that the tissue must be surgically opened and the fractured bones realigned. To maintain proper alignment, a screw, plate, nail, or wire is inserted to prevent the bones from separating. Although traction may have been used before surgery, it won't be needed any longer once the fracture is reduced. A cast or crutches may be used after surgery, but the question asks specifically about the surgical procedure.

CN: Physiological integrity; CNS: Physiological adaptation; CL: Application

93. Dislocation of the hip includes which symptoms?

1. Pain relieved with pressure
2. Pain in the inguinal area, abnormal gait
3. Internal rotation of the knee, abduction of the leg
4. Pain in the hip, the thigh appears longer than the unaffected leg

93. 2. A dislocated hip will create problems with walking, and pain is often due to a pinched nerve in the joint. Pressure shouldn't be applied to a painful joint or fracture unless there's hemorrhage. The leg is usually adducted and shortened.

CN: Physiological integrity; CNS: Physiological adaptation; CL: Analysis

94. A 20-year-old client developed osteomyelitis 2 weeks after a fishhook was removed from his foot. Which rationale best explains the expected long-term antibiotic therapy needed?

1. Bone has poor circulation.
2. Tissue trauma requires antibiotics.
3. Feet are normally more difficult to treat.
4. Fishhook injuries are highly contaminated.

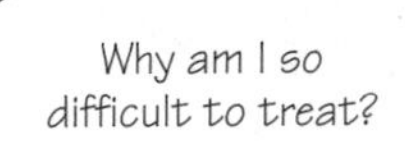

Why am I so difficult to treat?

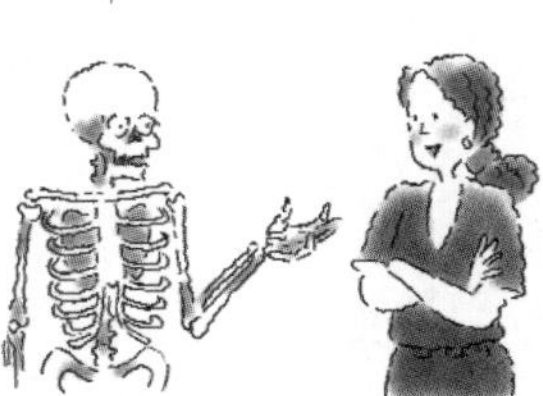

94. 1. Bone has very poor blood circulation, making it difficult to treat an infection in the bone. This requires the long-term use of I.V. antibiotics to make sure the infection is cleared. Tissue trauma doesn't always require antibiotics, at least not long term. Feet aren't more difficult to treat than other parts of the body unless the client has a circulatory problem or diabetes mellitus. Fishhooks may not be any more contaminated than another instrument that caused an injury.

CN: Physiological integrity; CNS: Pharmacological and parenteral therapies; CL: Application

95. The nurse is teaching a client with degenerative joint disease, also commonly known as osteoarthritis. The teaching has been effective when the client states the following about the condition?

1. "It is a noninflammatory joint disease."
2. "It is an immune-mediated joint disease."
3. "It is a joint inflammation after a viral infection."
4. "It is a joint inflammation related to systemic infections."

95. 1. Degenerative joint disease is joint disease due to the noninflammatory wear and tear on joints and is often seen in athletes. It isn't immune-mediated, or inflammatory, or caused by systemic infections.

CN: Physiological integrity; CNS: Physiological adaptation; CL: Application

96. Client education about gout includes which information?

1. Good foot care will reduce complications.
2. Increased dietary intake of purine is needed.
3. Production of uric acid in the kidney affects joints.
4. Uric acid crystals cause inflammatory destruction of the joint.

96. 4. The client needs to know that uric acid crystals collect in the joint of the great toe and cause inflammation. The kidney excretes uric acid, an end product of metabolism. A diet low in purines would be indicated. Good foot care doesn't affect the development of complications, but increasing water intake may help prevent urinary stone formation.
CN: Physiological integrity; CNS: Reduction of risk potential; CL: Application

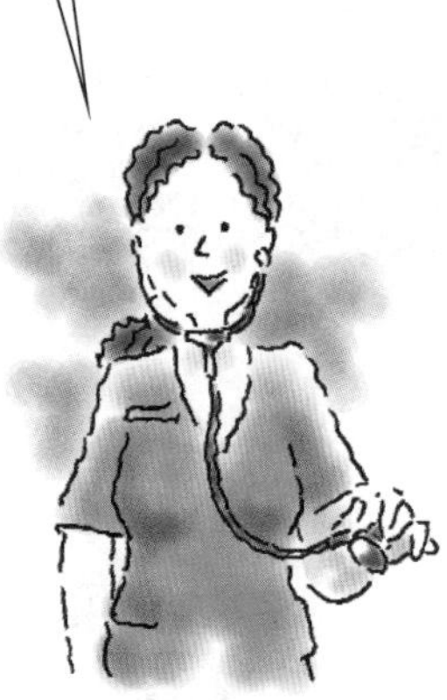

The words "most appropriate" in question 97 are a clue to the answer.

97. A client has been treated with IV antibiotics for osteomyelitis. The treatment has not been effective. Which intervention would be the most appropriate for this client?

1. Bone grafts
2. Hyperbaric oxygen therapy
3. Amputation of the extremity
4. Debridement of necrotic tissue

97. 4. The tissues may need to be debrided to eliminate necrotic tissue and allow new tissue to form. A bone graft would be done after debridement. Hyperbaric oxygen therapy is a new treatment modality that has been used in the successful treatment of osteomyelitis, but it isn't universally available. Amputation isn't indicated in the treatment of acute osteomyelitis.
CN: Physiological integrity; CNS: Physiological adaptation; CL: Application

98. A high-protein diet is ordered for a client recovering from a fracture. High protein is ordered for which reason?

1. Protein promotes gluconeogenesis.
2. Protein has anti-inflammatory properties.
3. Protein promotes cell growth and bone union.
4. Protein decrease pain medication requirements.

98. 3. High-protein intake promotes cell growth and bone union. Protein doesn't decrease pain medication requirements, exert anti-inflammatory properties; or promote gluconeogenesis.
CN: Physiological integrity; CNS: Basic care and comfort; CL: Application

99. Nursing interventions to treat a musculoskeletal injury may include cold or heat therapy. Cold therapy is ordered for which reason?

1. Promotes analgesia and circulation
2. Numbs the nerves and dilates the vessels
3. Promotes circulation and reduces muscle spasms
4. Causes local vasoconstriction and prevents edema or muscle spasm

99. 4. Cold causes the blood vessels to constrict, which reduces the leakage of fluid into the tissues and prevents swelling and muscle spasms. Cold therapy may reduce pain by numbing the nerves and tissues. Heat therapy promotes circulation, enhances flexibility, reduces muscle spasms, and also provides analgesia.
CN: Physiological integrity; CNS: Basic care and comfort; CL: Application

100. What discharge information should be given to a client with a cast?

1. "Use powder under the cast as needed."
2. "Itching under the cast indicates infection."
3. "Keep the extremity in a dependent position."
4. "Report fever and foul odors around the cast."

101. Which diagnosis would place a client at risk for traction-related complications?

1. Coronary artery disease
2. Diabetes mellitus
3. Hip fracture
4. Hypertension

102. A client complains that he experiences pain and numbness in his fingers when he types on a computer keyboard. Which action will help the nurse assess for Phalen's sign?

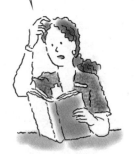

1. Having the client hold both hands above his head with his arms straight for 30 seconds
2. Having the client hold both wrists in acute flexion with the dorsal surfaces touching for 60 seconds
3. Tapping gently over the median nerve in the wrist
4. Having the client extend his wrists while the nurse provides resistance

Which action will help the nurse assess for Phalen's sign?

103. A client has a knee-high cast removed 6 weeks after suffering an ankle fracture. Palpation reveals a hard, nontender lump at the fracture site. How should the nurse interpret this finding?

1. Abnormal; the bone may have healed in misalignment, possibly from the short leg cast.
2. Abnormal; remodeling should have occurred by now, so the findings suggest malunion.
3. Normal; swelling and bruising may persist after a traumatic fracture.
4. Normal; callus formation normally occurs at this stage and may feel like a lump on the bone.

100. 4. Fever, foul odor, and warmth over a specific area of the cast after it's dry may be signs of infection. Itchy skin results from dry skin, and powder shouldn't be used. The extremity should be elevated for 24 to 48 hours.

CN: Health promotion and maintenance; CNS: None; CL: Application

101. 2. Because people with diabetes commonly have microvascular compromise and delayed wound healing, they need careful monitoring for early signs of skin breakdown. The other conditions don't increase the risk of traction-related complications.

CN: Physiological integrity; CNS: Reduction of risk potential; CL: Analysis

102. 2. Acute wrist flexion places pressure on the inflamed median nerve, causing the pain and numbness of carpal tunnel syndrome (Phalen's sign). Holding the hands above the head with arms straight for 30 seconds isn't an assessment technique. Tapping gently over the median nerve tests for Tinel's sign, another sign of carpal tunnel syndrome. Placing the wrists in extension against resistance tests strength.

CN: Physiological integrity; CNS: Physiological adaptation; CL: Application

103. 4. Callus formation is a normal stage of bone repair. It's characterized by an overgrowth of bone that's reabsorbed gradually during the remodeling stage. This deformity is painless, whereas misalignment and malunion typically cause pain. Swelling and bruising should have disappeared by this time.

CN: Physiological integrity; CNS: Physiological adaptation; CL: Analysis

104. A client is being discharged from the emergency department after cast application for a tibial fracture. A serious complication of this injury is identified with the nursing diagnosis *Impaired gas exchange: Fat embolus related to long bone fracture.* Based on this diagnosis, which instruction should the nurse provide?

1. "Cough and deep breathe at least every 2 hours."
2. "Keep the leg elevated and apply ice for the first 24 to 48 hours."
3. "Call the physician at once if you experience apprehensiveness, shortness of breath, fever, or palpitations."
4. "Restrict your fluid intake to 1 L per day."

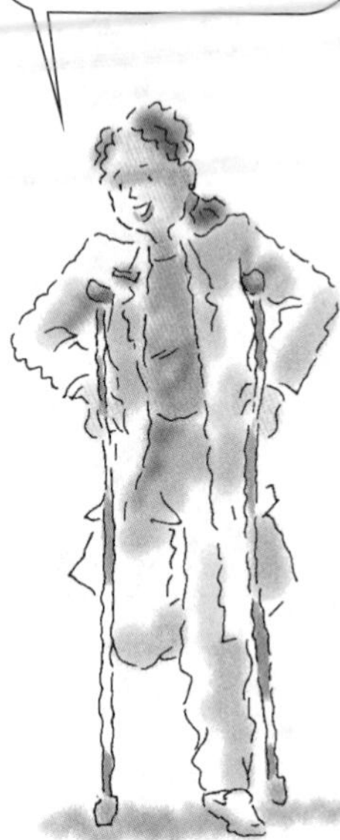
Which instruction should the nurse provide?

104. 3. Fat embolism is a complication of a long bone fracture. Signs and symptoms include apprehension, altered mental status, respiratory distress, tachycardia, tachypnea, fever, and petechiae over the neck, upper arms, and chest. Coughing and deep-breathing exercises as well as leg elevations with ice applications can help prevent other complications of a long bone fracture but have no effect on fat emboli. The client should also be instructed that drinking plenty of fluids to stay well hydrated will help him avoid embolic complications.

CN: Physiological integrity; CNS: Reduction of risk potential; CL: Application

105. A client who's receiving acetaminophen for osteoarthritis complains of continuing pain. The physician prescribes celecoxib (Celebrex). Which medication instruction should the nurse provide?

1. "Don't take the medication with dairy products."
2. "Report black, tarry stools to the physician."
3. "If you miss a dose, take a double dose the next day."
4. "Use a stool softener or fiber laxative daily to prevent constipation."

105. 2. Black, tarry stools are a sign of GI bleeding and may necessitate a medication change. Dairy products help reduce GI irritation. The celecoxib dose should never be doubled. Constipation isn't an adverse effect of this drug.

CN: Physiological integrity; CNS: Pharmacological and parenteral therapies; CL: Application

106. A client has an above-the-knee amputation 4 days after a traumatic injury. Which nursing diagnosis is most appropriate?

1. *Risk for impaired skin integrity related to decreased peripheral circulation*
2. *Impaired gas exchange related to fat embolism caused by surgical removal of bone and tissue*
3. *Acute pain related to phantom limb pain caused by surgical removal of leg after traumatic injury*
4. *Decreased cardiac output related to shock caused by decreased fluid volume*

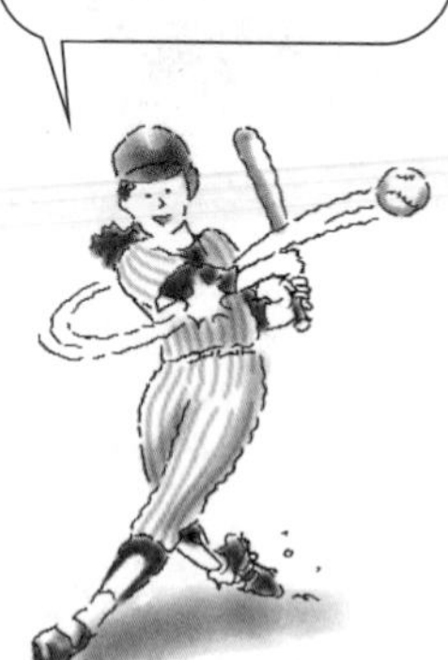
This question is a double-hinter.

106. 3. Phantom limb pain is common after limb amputation and may be more severe with traumatic injury. Because the limb was severed traumatically rather than removed because of poor circulation, peripheral circulation should be adequate. Fat embolism is more typical with long bone fractures. The risk of shock is relatively low on the 4th postoperative day.

CN: Psychosocial integrity; CNS: None; CL: Analysis

107. A nurse is assigned to care for a 70-year-old client with acute rheumatoid arthritis. Which assessment finding should the nurse expect to find during the physical examination?

1. Tender, painful, stiff joints
2. Radial deviation of the distal phalanges
3. Heberden's nodes
4. Bouchard's nodes

107. 1. Tender, painful, stiff joints characterize acute rheumatoid arthritis. The other assessment findings characterize osteoarthritis, including nodules on the dorsolateral aspects of the distal interphalangeal joints (Herbeden's nodules), flexion and deviation deformities, like radial deviation of the distal phalanges, and nodules on the proximal interphalangeal joints (Bouchard's nodes).

CN: Physiological integrity; CNS: Physiological adaptation; CL: Application

108. A client with lactose intolerance requires dietary teaching. Which foods should the nurse advise him to eat to ensure adequate calcium intake?

1. Bananas and avocados
2. Beef liver and broccoli
3. Cheese and yogurt
4. Collard greens and spinach

108. 4. Dark green, leafy vegetables are the best nondairy sources of calcium. Bananas and avocados are good sources of vitamin K. Beef liver and broccoli supply iron. Cheese and yogurt are dairy products, which this client should avoid because of the lactose intolerance.

CN: Physiological integrity; CNS: Basic care and comfort; CL: Application

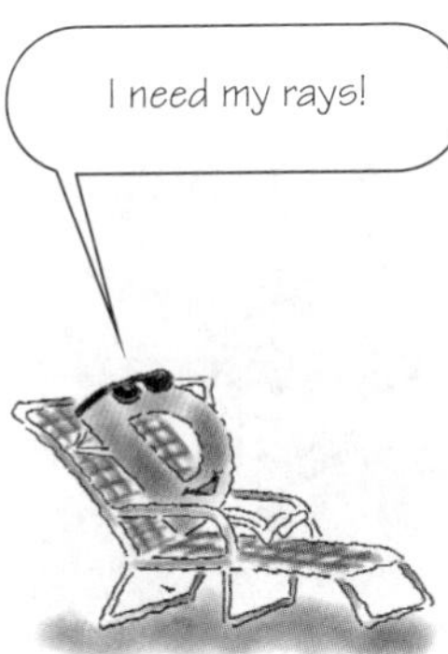
I need my rays!

109. An elderly client in a nursing home is particularly susceptible to bone loss. Which factor can contribute to bone loss?

1. Calcium channel blockers
2. Chronic use of stool softeners
3. Decreased mobility
4. Lack of sunlight exposure

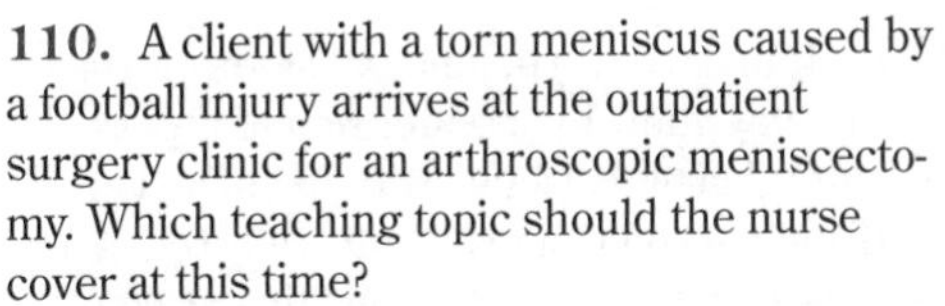

109. 4. Lack of sunlight exposure decreases absorption of vitamin D, which must be present for calcium to be absorbed from the small intestine. Calcium channel blockers don't affect serum calcium levels. Stool softeners don't increase peristalsis, so they don't impair calcium absorption. Decreased mobility is a result, not a cause, of bone loss. Immobility results in a loss of bone density.

CN: Health promotion and maintenance; CNS: None; CL: Analysis

110. A client with a torn meniscus caused by a football injury arrives at the outpatient surgery clinic for an arthroscopic meniscectomy. Which teaching topic should the nurse cover at this time?

1. Exactly how the procedure will be performed
2. Avoidance of weight bearing for 2 weeks after the surgery
3. Postoperative exercises, such as straight-leg raising and quadriceps setting
4. The possibility of severe postoperative pain for 24 to 48 hours after surgery

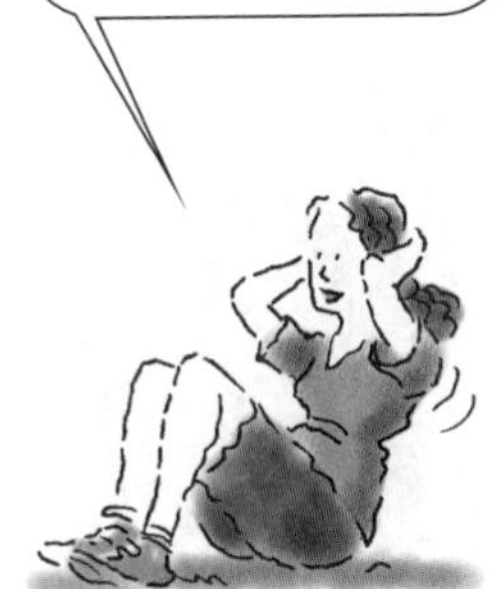
Exercise your
knowledge by
teaching your client.

110. 3. The best time to teach about postoperative care is preoperatively. Straight-leg raising and quadriceps setting exercises help maintain the strength of the affected extremity. The physician, not the nurse, should explain the surgical procedure. Weight bearing may begin as soon as the day of surgery. Usually, pain is mild to moderate after arthroscopic surgery.

CN: Physiological integrity; CNS: Basic care and comfort; CL: Application

111. A client is ready to be discharged after arthroscopic knee surgery. Which instruction should the nurse expect the physician to write on the discharge instructions?

1. "Ice and elevate the extremity for 12 hours after discharge."
2. "Infection isn't a potential problem because of the small incision size."
3. "Swelling and coolness of the joint and limb are normal right after surgery."
4. "Take acetaminophen with codeine every 4 hours as necessary for pain relief."

111. 4. Mild to moderate pain is normal after this type of surgery and can be relieved by oral narcotic analgesics. To minimize swelling, the client should ice and elevate the extremity for at least 24 hours after surgery. Infection is a potential problem after an invasive procedure. Swelling and coolness of the joint and limb may indicate complications from tourniquet use during surgery.

CN: Physiological integrity; CNS: Basic care and comfort; CL: Application

112. A perimenopausal client, age 50, is at high risk for osteoporosis because of her family history, lactose intolerance, and small body frame. She asks the nurse how to prevent osteoporosis. Which information should the nurse provide?

1. Increase the amount of calcium and vitamin D in your diet.
2. Have a bone density test yearly.
3. It's not necessary to stop smoking.
4. Hormone replacement therapy (HRT) is recommended.

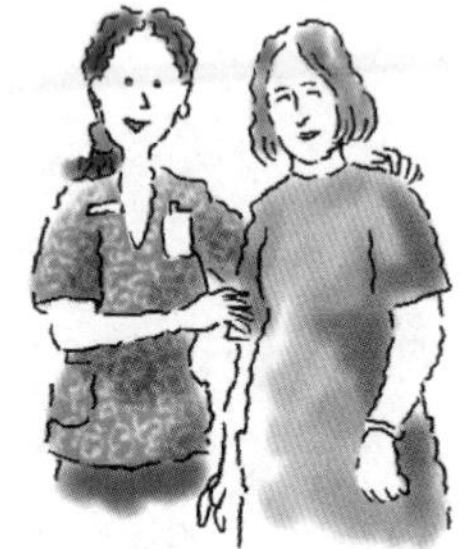

Counsel your client about health history risk factors.

112. 1. Adequate calcium and vitamin D intake are an important part of an overall prevention program. Bone density tests can evaluate the risk for osteoporosis but don't need to be done yearly. Smoking is a risk factor for developing osteoporosis. Studies show that estrogen in HRT may influence the development of breast and uterine cancers.

CN: Physiological integrity; CNS: Pharmacological and parenteral therapies; CL: Analysis

113. For a client diagnosed with Ewing's sarcoma, which test is <u>most</u> useful in determining the extent of metastasis?

1. Bone scan
2. Computed tomography (CT) scan
3. Magnetic resonance imaging (MRI)
4. Positron emission tomography (PET)

113. 1. A bone scan views the entire skeletal structure, indicating areas of possible metastases. CT scan, MRI, and PET scan visualize only one body area at a time.

CN: Physiological integrity; CNS: Reduction of risk potential; CL: Application

114. An 80-year-old client with pneumonia is admitted to the hospital. His past medical history includes <u>chronic</u> rheumatoid arthritis. Which assessment finding should the nurse expect during the physical examination?

1. Flattened thenar eminence
2. Thickened plaque overlying the flexor tendon of the ring finger
3. Cystic swelling on the dorsum of the wrist
4. Swan neck deformity

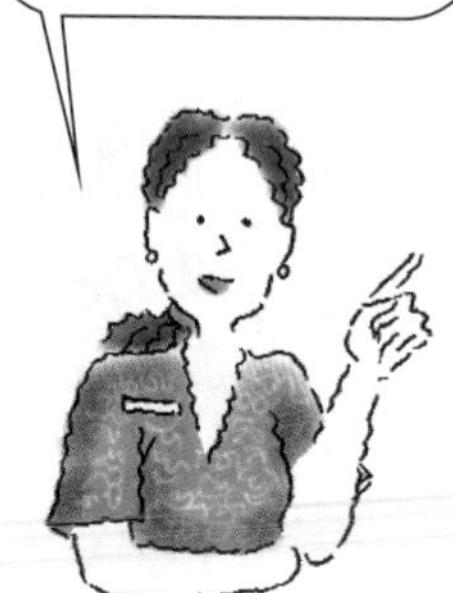

Pay close attention to the word chronic and what it implies.

114. 4. In chronic rheumatoid arthritis, the fingers may show hyperextension of the proximal interphalangeal joints with fixed flexion of the distal interphalangeal joints, referred to as *swan neck deformities.* Flattened thenar eminence characterizes thenar atrophy, a condition which suggests an ulnar nerve disorder. The first sign of a Dupuytren's contracture is a thickened plaque overlying the flexor tendon of the ring finger and possibly the little finger at the level of the distal palmar crease. Ganglia are cystic, round, usually nontender swellings located along tendon sheaths or joint capsules; ganglia frequently involve the dorsum of the wrist.

CN: Physiological integrity; CNS: Physiological adaptation; CL: Application

115. A 64-year-old client with complications related to metastatic cancer and complaints of back pain is admitted to the hospital. Which assessment finding should the nurse expect during the physical examination?

1. A rounded thoracic convexity
2. A gibbous
3. Gentle concavities in the cervical and lumbar regions and a convexity in the thorax
4. An accentuation of the normal lumbar curve

115. 2. Gibbous is an angular deformity of collapsed vertebra and is frequently caused by metastatic cancer or tuberculosis of the spine. A rounded thoracic convexity, kyphosis, is common in aging, especially in women. Gentle curves of the normal spine include concavities in the cervical and lumbar regions and a convexity of the thorax. An accentuation of the normal lumbar curve, called *lordosis,* frequently develops to compensate for the protuberant abdomen of pregnancy or marked obesity.

CN: Physiological integrity; CNS: Physiological adaptation; CL: Application

116. An elderly client with rheumatoid arthritis is being treated with prednisone (Deltasone). Which conditions can occur with long-term prednisone therapy?

1. Breast and uterine cancer
2. Osteoporosis and diabetes mellitus
3. Deep vein thrombosis (DVT), pulmonary embolus, and stroke
4. Weight loss and lactose intolerance

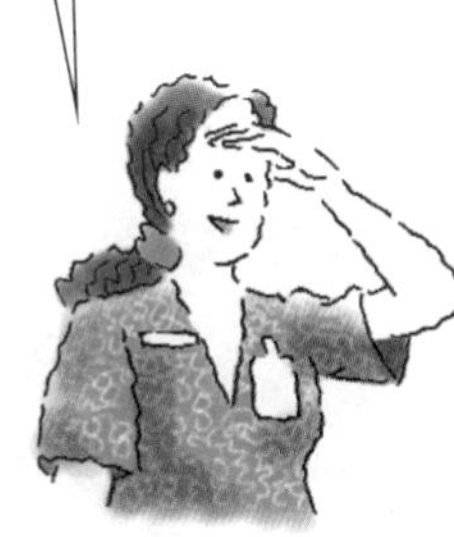

116. 2. Long-term prednisone therapy can increase the loss of calcium from bones, slow down the formation of new bone tissue (resulting in osteoporosis), and alter glucose metabolism (resulting in diabetes mellitus). Breast and uterine cancer, DVT, pulmonary embolus, stroke, weight loss, and lactose intolerance aren't common adverse effects of prednisone.

CN: Physiological integrity; CNS: Pharmacological and parenteral therapies; CL: Analysis

117. A client with a femoral fracture is in skeletal traction. During the initial shift assessment, the nurse finds that the weight used in traction is heavier than specified by the nursing care plan. Which action should the nurse take first?

1. Ask the physician during rounds if the order for the weight was changed.
2. Assume that if the weight was changed, the physician ordered it.
3. Check the physician's orders to see if they include a weight change.
4. Remove the weight and replace it with the weight specified in the plan.

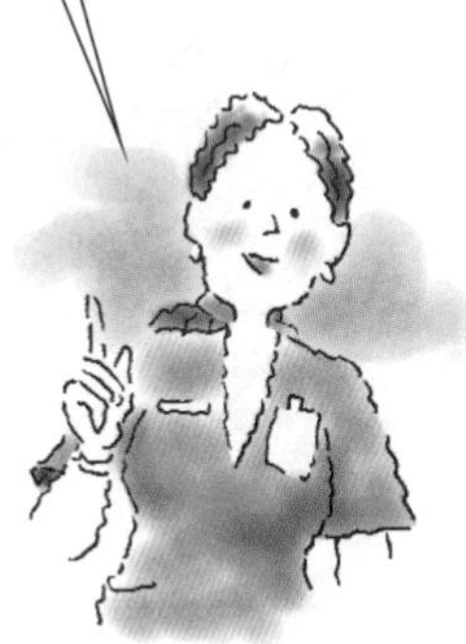
What's the first thing you would do?

117. 3. First, the nurse should check the physician's orders to see if a weight change was ordered. If it was, the nurse responsible for ensuring implementation of the care plan should investigate why the change wasn't incorporated in the plan.

CN: Safe, effective care environment; CNS: Management of care; CL: Analysis

118. The nurse is assessing a client's response to skeletal traction applied to the lower extremity. Which finding would be considered normal?

1. Coolness and pallor below the fracture level
2. Erythema and swelling immediately around the pin insertion site
3. Moderate to severe muscle spasms around the fracture area
4. Serous drainage and crust formation at the pin insertion site

118. 4. Serous drainage around the pin insertion site is a normal finding; some institutions don't recommend crust removal because of its protective nature. A pale extremity may indicate arterial compromise. Erythema and swelling signal infection. Severe muscle spasms may indicate improper alignment of the body or traction.

CN: Physiological integrity; CNS: Reduction of risk potential; CL: Analysis

119. Which nursing diagnosis is appropriate for a client with diabetes who is placed in skeletal traction after a motor vehicle collision?

1. *Imbalanced nutrition: Less than body requirements related to malabsorption of nutrients*
2. *Risk for infection related to the skeletal pin*
3. *Risk for injury related to subluxation of the joint above the pin insertion site*
4. *Risk for autonomic dysreflexia*

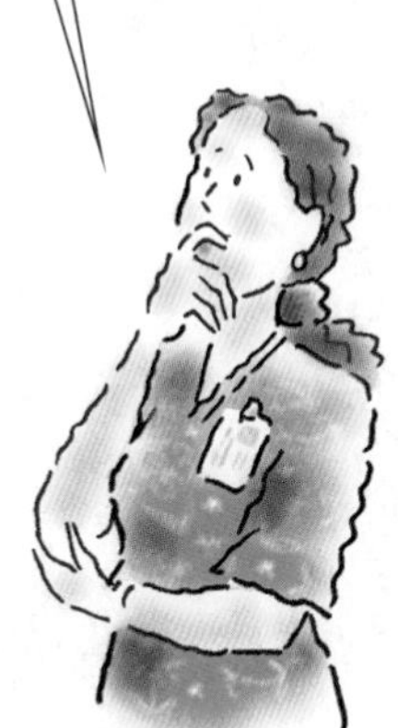
Which nursing diagnosis is appropriate?

119. 2. This client has a significant risk of osteomyelitis secondary to the skeletal pin. A dangerous bone infection that's hard to eradicate, osteomyelitis should be prevented at all costs—especially in a client with diabetes, who is already prone to infection. Based on the information provided, the other nursing diagnoses aren't appropriate.

CN: Physiological integrity; CNS: Reduction of risk potential; CL: Analysis

120. A client in skeletal traction complains of pain even though he received an analgesic 1 hour ago. The nurse wants to offer an alternative pain-management measure. Which measure can she implement within her scope of practice?

1. Acupressure and shiatsu
2. Hypnosis and therapeutic touch
3. Relaxation and imagery
4. Swedish massage and the Feldenkrais method

120. 3. Relaxation and imagery are effective adjuncts to pharmacologic pain management that the nurse can implement without a physician's order. Although the other therapies may promote pain management, they require special training or certification.

CN: Physiological integrity; CNS: Basic care and comfort; CL: Application

121. While examining the hands of a client with osteoarthritis, the nurse notes Heberden's nodes on the second (pointer) finger. Identify the area on the finger where the nurse observed the node.

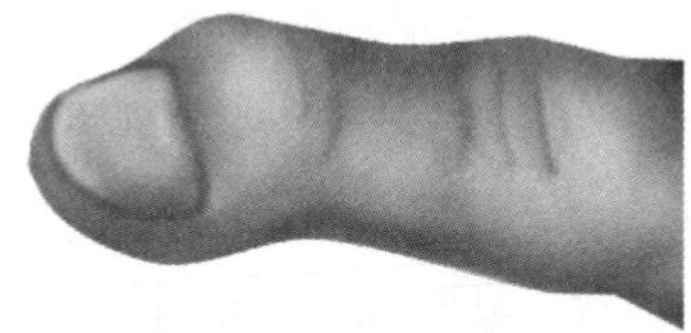

121. Heberden's nodes appear on the distal interphalangeal joints. These bony and cartilaginous enlargements are usually hard and painless and typically occur in middle-aged and elderly clients with osteoarthritis.

CN: Physiological integrity; CNS: Physiological adaptation: CL: Application

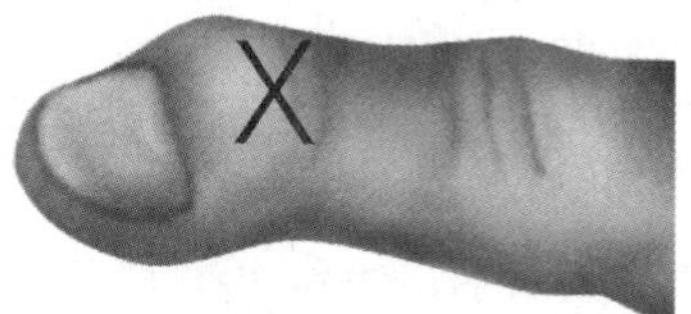

122. A client is diagnosed with gout. Which foods should the nurse instruct the client to avoid? Select all that apply:

1. Green, leafy vegetables
2. Liver
3. Cod
4. Chocolate
5. Sardines
6. Eggs

122. 2, 3, 5. Clients with gout should avoid foods that are high in purines, such as liver, cod, and sardines. They should also avoid anchovies, sweetbreads, lentils, and alcoholic beverages, especially beer and wine. Green, leafy vegetables, chocolate, and eggs aren't high in purines.

CN: Physiological integrity; CNS: Basic care and comfort; CL: Application

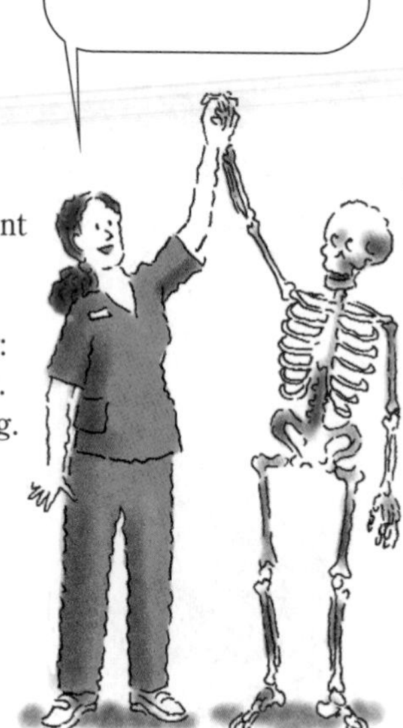

123. A client is in the emergency department with a suspected fracture of the right hip. Which assessment findings of the right leg should the nurse expect? Select all that apply:

1. The right leg is longer than the left leg.
2. The right leg is shorter than the left leg.
3. The right leg is abducted.
4. The right leg is adducted.
5. The right leg is externally rotated.
6. The right leg is internally rotated.

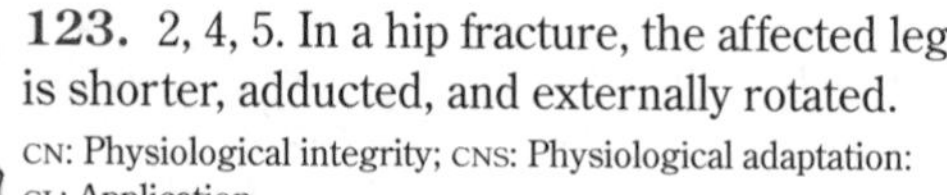

123. 2, 4, 5. In a hip fracture, the affected leg is shorter, adducted, and externally rotated.

CN: Physiological integrity; CNS: Physiological adaptation: CL: Application

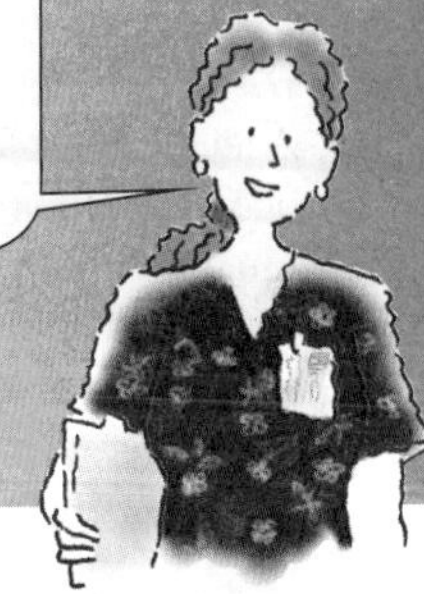

From hiatal hernias to diverticulitis to pancreatitis, this chapter covers all the GI disorders you could ask for, in one handy package. Gotta love it!

Chapter 8 Gastrointestinal disorders

1. Which condition can cause a hiatal hernia?
1. Increased intrathoracic pressure
2. Weakness of the esophageal muscle
3. Increased esophageal muscle pressure
4. Weakness of the diaphragmatic muscle

1. 4. A hiatal hernia is caused by weakness of the diaphragmatic muscle and increased intra-abdominal—not intrathoracic—pressure. This weakness allows the stomach to slide into the esophagus. The esophageal supports weaken, but esophageal muscle weakness or increased esophageal muscle pressure isn't a factor in hiatal hernia.
CN: Physiological integrity; CNS: Physiological adaptation; CL: Application

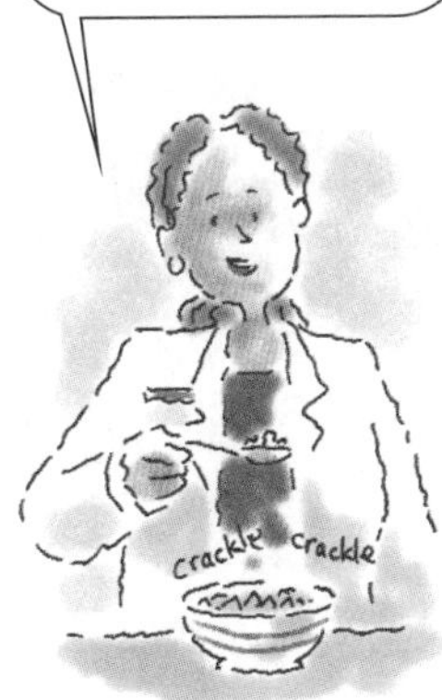

You know what they say, "You are what you eat."

2. Risk factors for the development of hiatal hernias are those that lead to increased abdominal pressure. Which complication is most likely to <u>cause</u> increased abdominal pressure?
1. Obesity
2. Volvulus
3. Constipation
4. Intestinal obstruction

2. 1. Obesity may cause increased abdominal pressure that pushes the lower portion of the stomach into the thorax. A volvulus is a type of intestinal obstruction. Constipation has no effect on a hiatal hernia. Obstructions may complicate a rolling hiatal hernia, but they don't cause the hernia.
CN: Physiological integrity; CNS: Physiological adaptation; CL: Application

3. A client is admitted with a hiatal hernia. The nurse should assess the client for which symptom?
1. Left arm pain
2. Lower back pain
3. Esophageal reflux
4. Abdominal cramping

3. 3. Esophageal reflux is a common symptom of hiatal hernia. This seems to be associated with chronic exposure of the lower esophageal sphincter to the lower pressure of the thorax, making it less effective. Left arm pain is a common symptom of heart attack. Lower back pain can be caused by lumbar strain. Abdominal cramping can be caused by intestinal infection.
CN: Physiological integrity; CNS: Physiological adaptation; CL: Application

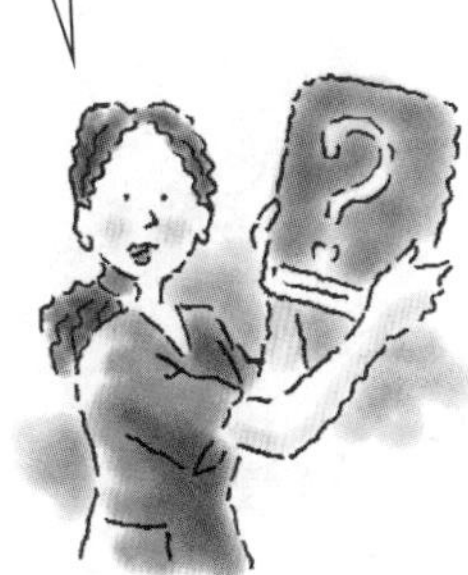

4. A nurse is preparing to teach a client with a hiatal hernia. The nurse should provide instruction on which test?
1. Colonoscopy
2. Lower GI series
3. Barium swallow
4. Abdominal X-ray series

4. 3. A barium swallow with fluoroscopy shows the position of the stomach in relation to the diaphragm. A colonoscopy and a lower GI series show disorders of the intestine. An abdominal X-ray series will show structural defects but not necessarily a hiatal hernia, unless it's sliding or rolling at the time of the X-ray.
CN: Health promotion and maintenance; CNS: None; CL: Application

CN: Client needs category   CNS: Client needs subcategory   CL: Cognitive level

5. A client is admitted with right lower quadrant pain, anorexia, nausea, low-grade fever, and elevated white blood cell count. Which complication is most likely the cause?

1. A fecalith
2. Bowel kinking
3. Internal bowel occlusion
4. Abdominal wall swelling

5. 1. The client is experiencing appendicitis. A fecalith is a fecal calculus, or stone, that occludes the lumen of the appendix and is the most common cause of appendicitis. Bowel wall swelling, kinking of the appendix, and external occlusion, not internal occlusion, of the bowel by adhesions can also be causes of appendicitis.
CN: Physiological integrity; CNS: Physiological adaptation; CL: Analysis

6. The nurse is assessing a client with suspected appendicitis. The nurse would expect the client to use which of the following terms to describe their pain?

1. Aching
2. Fleeting
3. Intermittent
4. Steady

6. 4. The pain begins in the epigastrium or periumbilical region, then shifts to the right lower quadrant and becomes steady. The pain may be moderate to severe.
CN: Physiological integrity; CNS: Physiological adaptation; CL: Application

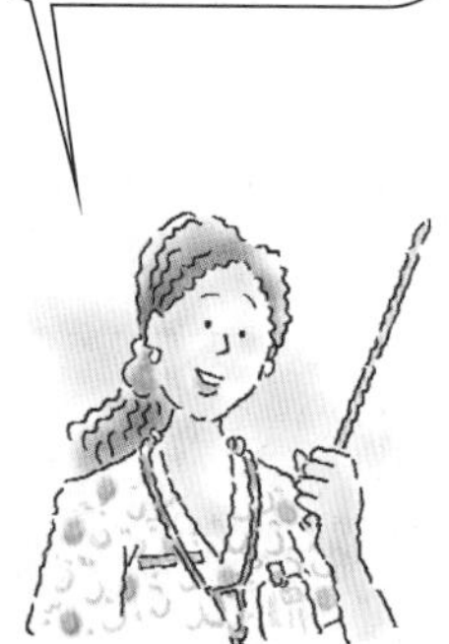

Evaluate each position to determine which one will ease your client's pain.

7. Which position should a nurse direct a client with appendicitis to assume to help relieve the pain?

1. Prone
2. Sitting
3. Supine, stretched out
4. Lying with legs drawn up

7. 4. Lying still with the legs drawn up toward the chest helps relieve tension on the abdominal muscles, which helps to reduce the amount of discomfort felt. Lying flat or sitting may increase the amount of pain experienced.
CN: Physiological integrity; CNS: Physiological adaptation; CL: Application

8. Which nursing intervention should be the priority when caring for a client with appendicitis?

1. Assessing for pain
2. Encouraging oral intake of clear fluids
3. Providing discharge teaching
4. Assessing for symptoms of peritonitis

8. 4. The focus of care is to assess for peritonitis, or inflammation of the peritoneal cavity. Peritonitis is most commonly caused by appendix rupture and invasion of bacteria, which could be lethal. The client with appendicitis will have pain that should be controlled with analgesia. The nurse should discourage oral intake in preparation for surgery. Discharge teaching is important; however, in the acute phase, management should focus on minimizing preoperative complications and recognizing when such may be occurring.
CN: Safe, effective care environment; CNS: Management of care; CL: Application

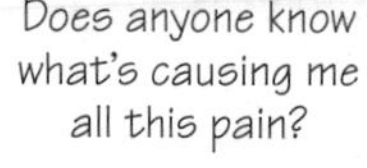

Does anyone know what's causing me all this pain?

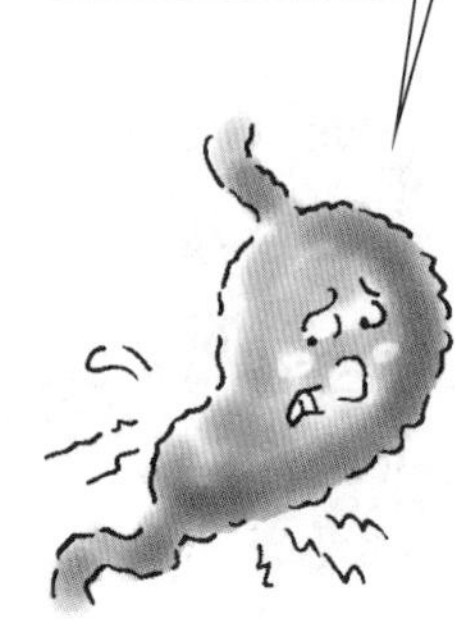

9. The nurse is teaching the client about gastritis. Which of the following statements by the nurse would be the most accurate in describing gastritis?

1. Erosion of the gastric mucosa
2. Inflammation of a diverticulum
3. Inflammation of the gastric mucosa
4. Reflux of stomach acid into the esophagus

9. 3. Gastritis is an inflammation of the gastric mucosa that may be acute (often resulting from exposure to local irritants) or chronic (associated with autoimmune infections or atrophic disorders of the stomach). Erosion of the mucosa results in ulceration. Inflammation of a diverticulum is called diverticulitis; reflux of stomach acid is known as gastroesophageal reflux disease.
CN: Physiological integrity; CNS: Physiological adaptation; CL: Analysis

CN: Client needs category CNS: Client needs subcategory CL: Cognitive level

10. A 30-year-old client is complaining of reflux in his esophagus 1 to 2 hours after eating or when lying down for the last 2 weeks. The nurse recognizes that this symptom is related to which disorder?

1. Myocardial infarction (MI)
2. Lumbar strain
3. Hiatal hernia
4. Intestinal infection

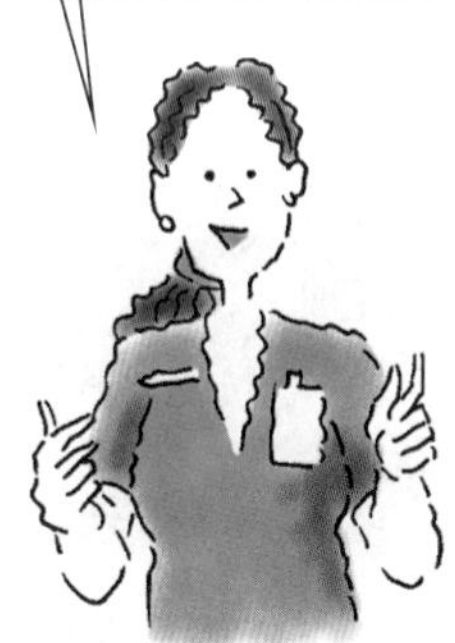

You'll most likely know this answer if you just give it some thought.

10. 3. Esophageal reflux is a common symptom of hiatal hernia. This condition seems to be associated with chronic exposure of the lower esophageal sphincter to the lower pressure of the thorax, making it less effective. MI may present with indigestion but not reflux. This symptom isn't associated with the other conditions.

CN: Physiological integrity; CNS: physiological adaptation; CL: Analysis

11. Which nursing intervention should be included in the <u>immediate</u> postoperative management of a client who has undergone gastric resection?

1. Monitoring gastric pH to detect complications
2. Assessing for bowel sounds
3. Providing nutritional support
4. Monitoring for symptoms of hemorrhage

11. 4. The client should be monitored closely for signs and symptoms of hemorrhage, such as bright red blood in the nasogastric tube suction, tachycardia, or a drop in blood pressure. Gastric pH may be monitored to evaluate the need for histamine-2 receptor antagonists. Bowel sounds may not return for up to 72 hours postoperatively. Nutritional needs should be addressed soon after surgery.

CN: Physiological integrity; CNS: Reduction of risk potential; CL: Analysis

12. Which treatment should be included in the immediate management of acute gastritis?

1. Reducing work stress
2. Completing gastric resection
3. Treating the underlying cause
4. Administering enteral tube feedings

12. 3. Discovering and treating the cause of gastritis is the most beneficial approach. Reducing the amount of stress and reducing or eliminating oral intake until the symptoms are gone are important in the recovery phase. A gastric resection is only an option when serious erosion has occurred.

CN: Safe, effective care environment; CNS: Safety and infection control; CL: Analysis

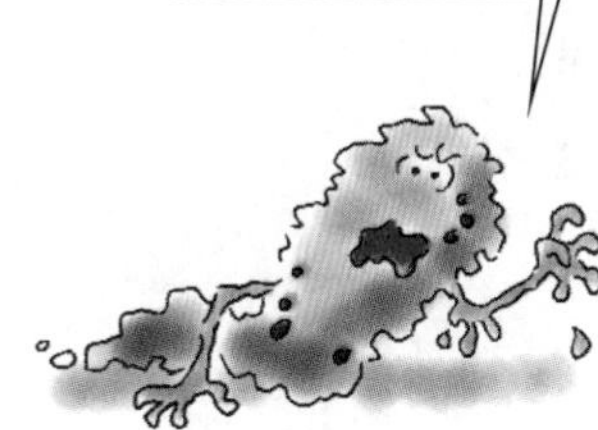

I can cause a stomach to writhe in pain!

13. Which risk factor can lead to chronic gastritis?

1. Young age
2. Antibiotic usage
3. Gallbladder disease
4. *Helicobacter pylori* infection

13. 4. *H. pylori* infection can lead to chronic atrophic gastritis. Chronic gastritis can occur at any age but is more common in older adults. It may be caused by conditions that allow reflux of bile acids into the stomach. Drugs such as nonsteroidal anti-inflammatory agents, not antibiotics, may cause gastritis. Chronic gastritis isn't related to gallbladder disease.

CN: Health promotion and maintenance; CNS: None; CL: Analysis

14. Which factor associates chronic gastritis with pernicious anemia?

1. Chronic blood loss
2. Inability to absorb vitamin B_{12}
3. Overproduction of stomach acid
4. Overproduction of vitamin B_{12}

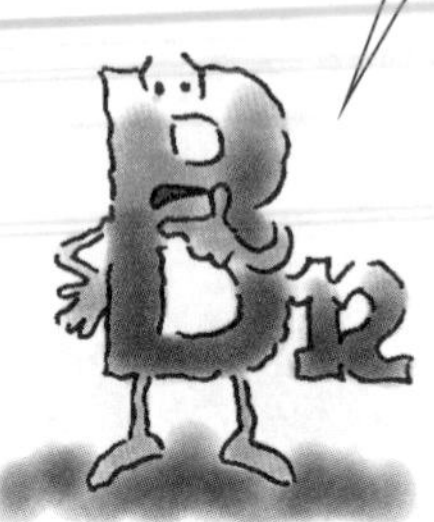

14. 2. With gastritis, the stomach lining becomes thin and atrophic, decreasing stomach acid secretion (the source of intrinsic factor). This causes a reduction in the absorption of vitamin B_{12}, leading to pernicious anemia.

CN: Physiological integrity; CNS: Physiological adaptation; CL: Analysis

15. In which developmental stage would the nurse note that a client is at risk of developing diverticulosis?

1. Infant
2. School age
3. Young adult
4. Older adult

15. 4. As clients age, the incidence of diverticulosis increases. Almost two-thirds of the population is diagnosed with diverticulosis by age 85.

CN: Health promotion and maintenance; CNS: None; CL: Application

16. Which type of diet is implicated in the development of diverticulosis?

1. Low-fiber diet
2. High-fiber diet
3. High-protein diet
4. Low-carbohydrate diet

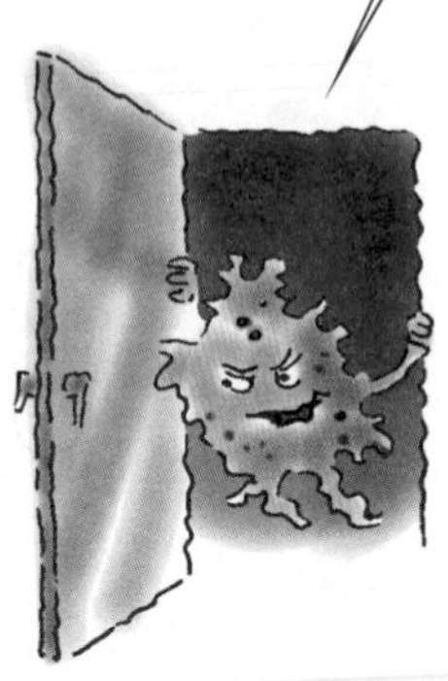

Looks like the door is wide open for my entrance!

16. 1. Low-fiber diets have been implicated in the development of diverticula because these diets decrease the bulk in the stool and predispose the person to the development of constipation. A high-fiber diet is recommended to help prevent diverticulosis. A high-protein or low-carbohydrate diet has no effect on the development of diverticulosis.

CN: Physiological integrity; CNS: Basic care and comfort; CL: Analysis

17. Which mechanism can facilitate the development of diverticulosis into diverticulitis?

1. Treating constipation with chronic laxative use, leading to dependence on the laxatives
2. Chronic constipation causing an obstruction, reducing forward flow of intestinal contents
3. Herniation of the intestinal mucosa, rupturing the wall of the intestine
4. Undigested food blocking the diverticulum, predisposing the area to bacterial invasion

17. 4. Undigested food can block the diverticulum, decreasing blood supply to the area and predisposing the area to the invasion of bacteria. Chronic laxative use is a common problem in elderly clients, but it doesn't cause diverticulitis. Chronic constipation can cause an obstruction—not diverticulitis. Herniation of the intestinal mucosa causes an intestinal perforation.

CN: Physiological integrity; CNS: Physiological adaptation; CL: Analysis

18. Which symptoms indicate diverticulosis?

1. No symptoms exist
2. Change in bowel habits
3. Anorexia and low-grade fever
4. Episodic, dull or steady midabdominal pain

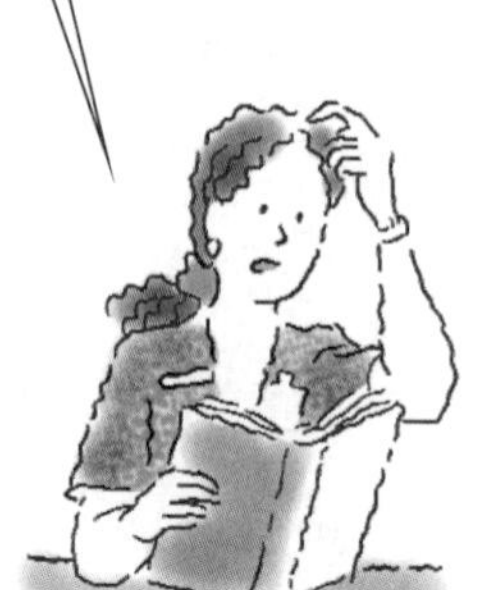

Sometimes you have to read between the lines.

18. 1. Diverticulosis is an asymptomatic condition. The other choices are signs and symptoms of diverticulitis.

CN: Physiological integrity; CNS: Physiological adaptation; CL: Application

19. Which test should the nurse expect to be ordered for a client suspected of having diverticulosis?

1. Abdominal ultrasound
2. Barium enema
3. Barium swallow
4. Gastroscopy

19. 2. A barium enema will cause diverticula to fill with barium and be easily seen on an X-ray. An abdominal ultrasound can tell more about structures, such as the gallbladder, liver, and spleen, than the intestine. A barium swallow and gastroscopy view upper GI structures.
CN: Health promotion and maintenance; CNS: None; CL: Application

20. A client was hospitalized and treated for acute diverticulitis. The nurse has provided discharge teaching. Which statement by the client indicates that he understands his discharge instructions?

1. "I'll reduce my fluid intake."
2. "I'll decrease the fiber in my diet."
3. "I'll take all of my antibiotics."
4. "I'll exercise to increase my intra-abdominal pressure."

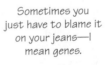

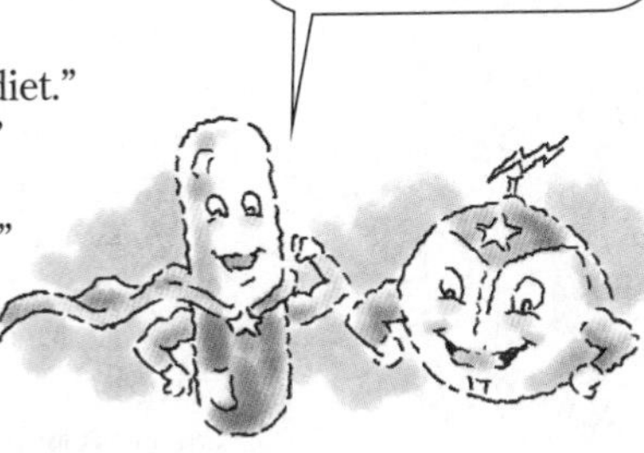

It's time for us to get to work.

20. 3. Antibiotics are used to reduce the inflammation. The client typically isn't allowed anything orally until the acute episode subsides. Parenteral fluids are given until the client feels better; then it's recommended that the client drink 8-oz glasses of water per day and gradually increase fiber in the diet to improve intestinal motility. During the acute phase, activities that increase intra-abdominal pressure should be avoided to decrease pain and the chance of intestinal obstruction.
CN: Physiological integrity; CNS: Physiological adaptation; CL: Analysis

21. Crohn's disease can be described as a chronic relapsing disease. Which area of the GI system may be involved with this disease?

1. The entire length of the large colon
2. Only the sigmoid area
3. The entire large colon through the layers of mucosa and submucosa
4. The small intestine and colon, affecting the entire thickness of the bowel

21. 4. Crohn's disease more commonly involves any segment of the small intestine, the colon, or both, affecting the entire thickness of the bowel. However, it can also affect the digestive system anywhere from the mouth to the anus. Options 1 and 3 describe ulcerative colitis. Option 2 is too specific and, therefore, not likely.
CN: Physiological integrity; CNS: Physiological adaptation; CL: Application

22. A client presents with a recurrence of Crohn's disease. Which area of the alimentary canal does the nurse suspect is involved?

1. Ascending colon
2. Descending colon
3. Sigmoid colon
4. Terminal ileum

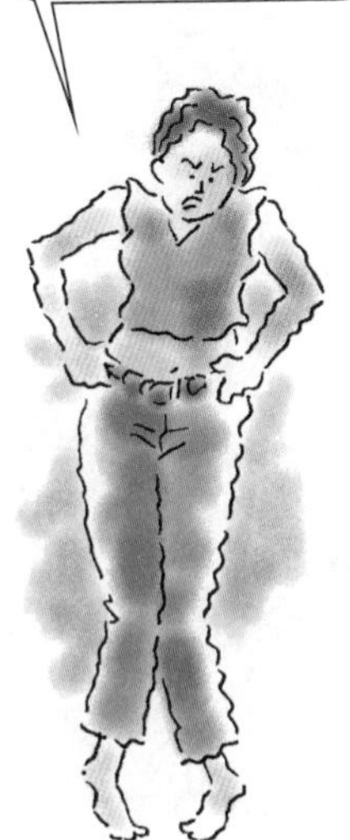

Sometimes you just have to blame it on your jeans—I mean genes.

22. 4. Studies have shown that the terminal ileum is the most common site for recurrence in clients with Crohn's disease. The other areas may be involved but aren't as common.
CN: Physiological integrity; CNS: Physiological adaptation; CL: Application

23. A nurse is preparing the teaching plan for a client with Crohn's disease. Which factor should the nurse include as a possible link to the development of this disease?

1. Constipation
2. Diet
3. Heredity
4. Lack of exercise

23. 3. Although the definitive cause of Crohn's disease is unknown, it's thought to be associated with infectious, immune, or psychological factors. Because it has a higher incidence in siblings, it may have a genetic cause.
CN: Health promotion and maintenance; CNS: None; CL: Analysis

24. A nurse is reviewing the causes of ulcerative colitis with a client. Which factor is believed to cause ulcerative colitis?

1. Acidic diet
2. Altered immunity
3. Chronic constipation
4. Emotional stress

24. 2. Several theories exist regarding the cause of ulcerative colitis. One suggests altered immunity as the cause based on the extraintestinal characteristics of the disease, such as peripheral arthritis and cholangitis. Diet and constipation have no effect on the development of ulcerative colitis. Emotional stress may exacerbate the attacks but isn't believed to be the primary cause.

CN: Health promotion and maintenance; CNS: None; CL: Analysis

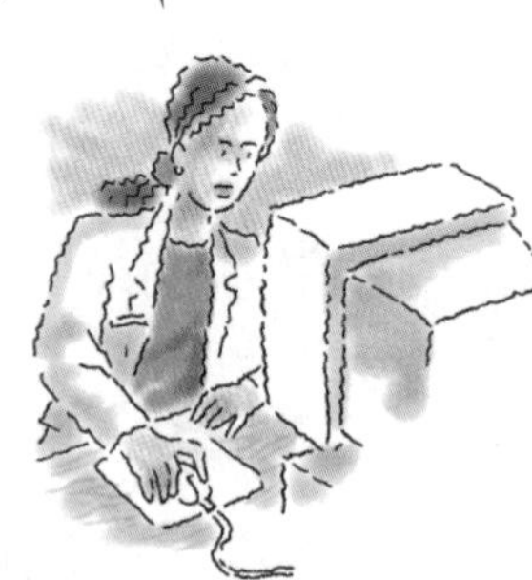

NCLEX questions sure can be a fistula full of trouble!

25. A client is admitted with an anorectal fistula. Which underlying disorder does the client most likely have?

1. Crohn's disease
2. Diverticulitis
3. Diverticulosis
4. Ulcerative colitis

25. 1. As the disease progresses, the lesions of Crohn's disease become *transmural;* that is, they involve all thicknesses of the bowel. These lesions may perforate the bowel wall, forming fistulas with adjacent structures. Fistulas don't develop in diverticulitis or diverticulosis. The ulcers that occur in the submucosal and mucosal layers of the intestine in ulcerative colitis usually don't progress to fistula formation as in Crohn's disease.

CN: Physiological integrity; CNS: Physiological adaptation; CL: Analysis

26. A client with Crohn's disease experiences 20 watery stools per day. Which sign would indicate dehydration?

1. Poor skin turgor
2. Decreased heart rate
3. Dilute urine
4. Elevated blood pressure

26. 1. Signs and symptoms of dehydration include poor skin turgor, increased heart rate, concentrated urine, and decreased blood pressure. Other signs are dry skin and mouth, sunken eyes, and lethargy.

CN: Physiological integrity; CNS: Physiological adaptation; CL: Analysis

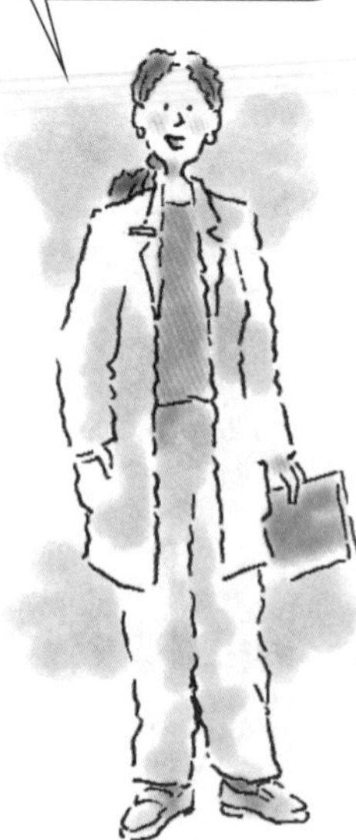

Many GI disorders have similar symptoms. Pay attention to which one the question is asking about.

27. Which associated disorder might a client with ulcerative colitis exhibit?

1. Gallstones
2. Hydronephrosis
3. Nephrolithiasis
4. Toxic megacolon

27. 4. Toxic megacolon is extreme dilation of a segment of the diseased colon caused by paralysis of the colon, resulting in complete obstruction. This disorder is associated with both Crohn's disease *and* ulcerative colitis. The other disorders are more commonly associated with Crohn's disease.

CN: Physiological integrity; CNS: Physiological adaptation; CL: Analysis

28. Which associated disorder might a client with Crohn's disease exhibit most often?

1. Ankylosing spondylitis
2. Colon cancer
3. Malabsorption
4. Lactase deficiency

28. 3. Because of the transmural nature of Crohn's disease lesions, malabsorption may occur with Crohn's disease. Although ankylosing spondylitis and colon cancer are more commonly associated with ulcerative colitis, they may be seen in clients with Crohn's disease. Lactase deficiency is caused by a congenital defect in which an enzyme isn't present.

CN: Physiological integrity; CNS: Physiological adaptation; CL: Analysis

CN: Client needs category CNS: Client needs subcategory CL: Cognitive level

29. A client with Crohn's disease is admitted with fever, weight loss, leg cramping, diarrhea, frequent premature ventricular contractions, and abdominal pain. Which laboratory finding should be treated first?

1. Hypoalbuminemia
2. Leukocytosis
3. Increased erythrocyte sedimentation rate
4. Hypokalemia

29. 4. A low potassium level can lead to cardiac arrest. The client is already having leg cramps and arrhythmias, so this finding is the priority.

CN: Physiological integrity; CNS: Physiological adaptation; CL: Analysis

30. Which diet would be most appropriate for a client with ulcerative colitis?

1. Low-fat, low-protein
2. Low-residue, high-protein
3. High-calorie, low-fiber
4. High-residue, high-fiber

30. 2. Clients with ulcerative colitis should follow a low-residue, high-protein diet. More protein is needed for tissue healing. High residue food, such as grains and nuts, should be avoided. There is no need for clients with ulcerative colitis to follow a low-fat diet.

CN: Physiological integrity; CNS: Basic care and comfort; CL: Application

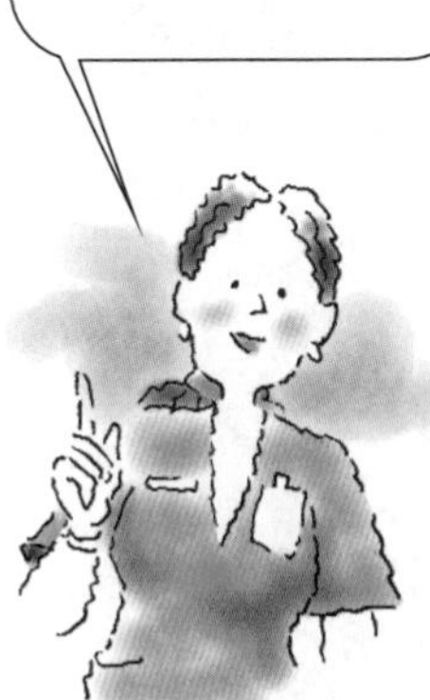

One of these tests can help you distinguish between two GI disorders.

31. If a client had irritable bowel syndrome, which diagnostic test would determine if the diagnosis is Crohn's disease or ulcerative colitis?

1. Abdominal computed tomography (CT) scan
2. Abdominal X-ray
3. Barium swallow
4. Colonoscopy with biopsy

31. 4. A colonoscopy with biopsy can be performed to determine the state of the colon's mucosal layers, presence of ulcerations, and level of cytologic involvement. An abdominal X-ray or a CT scan wouldn't provide the cytologic information necessary to diagnose which disease it is. A barium swallow doesn't involve the intestine.

CN: Physiological integrity; CNS: Physiological adaptation; CL: Analysis

32. Which intervention should be included in the medical management of Crohn's disease?

1. Increasing oral intake of fiber
2. Administering laxatives
3. Using long-term steroid therapy
4. Increasing physical activity

32. 3. Management of Crohn's disease may include long-term steroid therapy to reduce the extensive inflammation associated with the deeper layers of the bowel wall. Other management focuses on bowel rest (not increasing oral intake) and reducing diarrhea with medications (not giving laxatives). The pain associated with Crohn's disease may require bed rest, not an increase in physical activity.

CN: Physiological integrity; CNS: Basic care and comfort; CL: Application

33. A client with Crohn's disease is experiencing an exacerbation. Which instruction would be a priority in planning his care?

1. Increasing current weight
2. Encourage ambulation
3. Promoting bowel rest
4. Controlling rectal bleeding

33. 3. Promoting bowel rest is the priority during an acute exacerbation. This is accomplished by decreasing activity and initially putting the client on nothing-by-mouth status. Weight loss may occur, but the priority is bowel rest. Rectal bleeding usually isn't expected in Crohn's disease.

CN: Safe, effective care environment; CNS: Management of care; CL: Analysis

34. A nurse would expect to prepare a client with ulcerative colitis for surgery if the client develops which condition?

1. Gastritis
2. Bowel herniation
3. Bowel outpouching
4. Bowel perforation

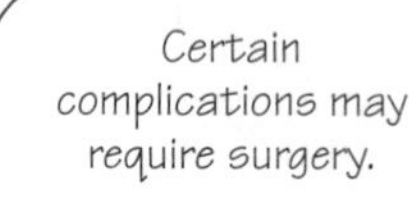
Certain complications may require surgery.

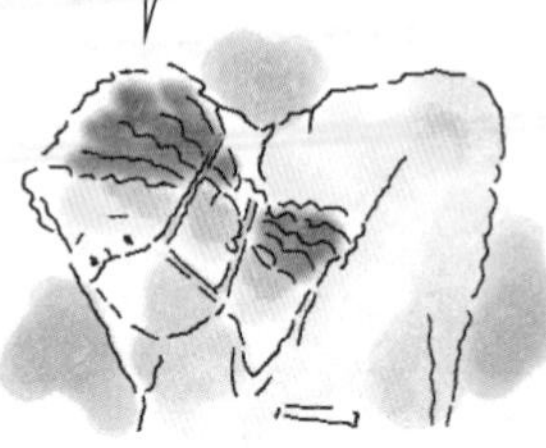

34. 4. Bowel perforation, obstruction, hemorrhage, and toxic megacolon are common complications of ulcerative colitis that may require surgery. Gastritis and herniation aren't associated with irritable bowel diseases, and outpouching of the bowel wall is diverticulosis.
CN: Physiological integrity; CNS: Physiological adaptation; CL: Application

35. Which medication is most effective for treating the pain associated with irritable bowel disease?

1. Acetaminophen
2. Opiates
3. Steroids
4. Stool softeners

35. 3. The pain of irritable bowel disease is caused by inflammation, which steroids can reduce. Acetaminophen has little effect on the pain, and opiates won't treat its underlying cause. Stool softeners aren't necessary.
CN: Physiological integrity; CNS: Pharmacological and parenteral therapies; CL: Analysis

36. During the first few days of recovery from ostomy surgery for ulcerative colitis, which aspect should be the <u>first priority</u> of client care?

1. Body image
2. Ostomy care
3. Sexual concerns
4. Skin care

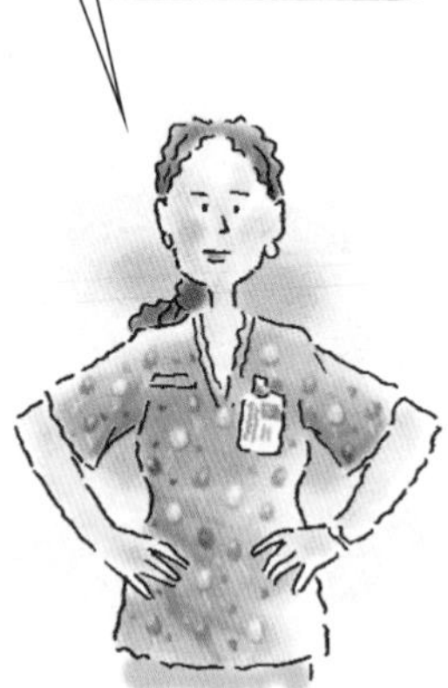
Question 36 is asking you to prioritize.

36. 2. Although all of these are concerns the nurse should address, being able to safely manage the ostomy is crucial for the client before discharge.
CN: Safe, effective care environment; CNS: Management of care; CL: Analysis

37. The nursing assessment of a client with colon cancer may also include a past medical history of which condition?

1. Appendicitis
2. Hemorrhoids
3. Hiatal hernia
4. Ulcerative colitis

37. 4. Chronic ulcerative colitis, granulomas, and familial polyposis seem to increase a person's chance of developing colon cancer. The other conditions listed have no known effect on colon cancer risk.
CN: Health promotion and maintenance; CNS: None; CL: Application

38. A nurse is providing nutritional teaching for a client with a family history of colon cancer. Which dietary choice by the client demonstrates that he understands the correct diet to follow?

1. Vegetarian chili
2. Hot dogs and sauerkraut
3. Egg salad on rye bread
4. Spaghetti and meat sauce

38. 1. A high-fiber, low-fat food, such as vegetarian chili, increases motility and decreases the chance of constipation and is recommended to help avoid colon cancer. The other choices don't represent a high-fiber, low-fat diet.
CN: Physiological integrity; CNS: Basic care and comfort; CL: Application

39. Which diagnostic test should be performed annually after age 50 to screen for colon cancer?
1. Abdominal computed tomography (CT) scan
2. Abdominal X-ray
3. Colonoscopy
4. Fecal occult blood test

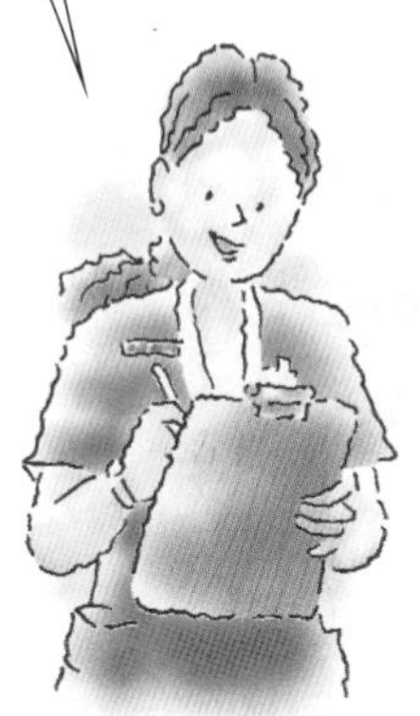

Screening for colon cancer should be on the "to do" list of anyone over age 50.

39. 4. Surface blood vessels of polyps and cancers are fragile and often bleed with the passage of stools, so a fecal occult blood test should be performed annually. Abdominal X-ray and CT scan can help establish tumor size and metastasis. A colonoscopy can help to locate a tumor as well as polyps, but is only recommended every 10 years.
CN: Health promotion and maintenance; CNS: None; CL: Application

40. A client with colon cancer is scheduled to receive radiation therapy prior to surgery. What should the nurse include in her teaching about the use of radiation therapy?
1. It helps reduce the size of the tumor.
2. It eliminates the malignant cells.
3. It may cure the cancer.
4. It helps heal the bowel after surgery.

40. 1. Radiation therapy is used before surgery to reduce the size of the tumor, making it easier to be resected. Radiation therapy isn't curative, can't eliminate the malignant cells (though it helps to define tumor margins), and could slow postoperative healing.
CN: Physiological integrity; CNS: Physiological adaptation; CL: Application

41. Which symptom is a client with colon cancer most likely to exhibit?
1. A change in appetite
2. A change in bowel habits
3. An increase in body weight
4. An increase in body temperature

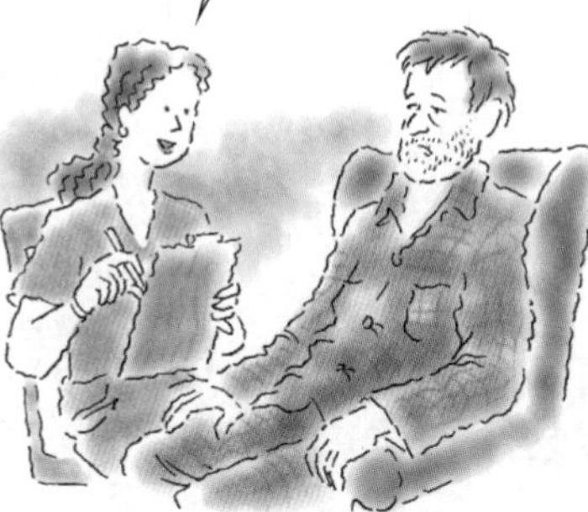

It's important to ask the client about his symptoms.

41. 2. The most common complaint of the client with colon cancer is a change in bowel habits. The client may have anorexia, secondary abdominal distention, or weight loss. Fever isn't related to colon cancer.
CN: Physiological integrity; CNS: Physiological adaptation; CL: Application

42. A client has just had surgery for colon cancer. The nurse would observe the client for symptoms that might indicate the development of which complication?
1. Peritonitis
2. Diverticulosis
3. Partial bowel obstruction
4. Complete bowel obstruction

42. 1. Bowel spillage could occur during surgery, resulting in peritonitis. Diverticulosis doesn't result from surgery for colon cancer. Complete or partial intestinal obstruction may occur *before* bowel resection.
CN: Physiological integrity; CNS: Physiological adaptation; CL: Application

43. Which symptom, if reported by a client, would lead the nurse to suspect gastric cancer?
1. Abdominal cramping
2. Constant hunger
3. Feeling of fullness
4. Weight gain

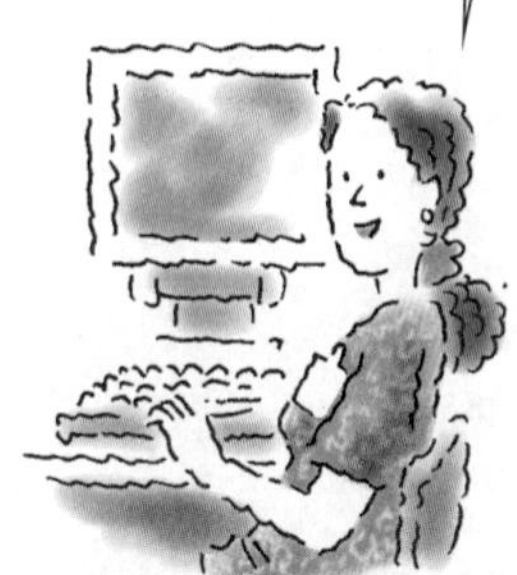

Read the question carefully and know what disorder is being addressed.

43. 3. The client with gastric cancer may report a feeling of fullness in the stomach, but not enough to cause him to seek medical care. Abdominal cramping isn't associated with gastric cancer. Anorexia and weight loss (not increased hunger or weight gain) are common symptoms of gastric cancer.
CN: Physiological integrity; CNS: Physiological adaptation; CL: Application

44. Which diagnostic test may be performed to determine if a client has gastric cancer?
1. Barium enema
2. Colonoscopy
3. Endoscopy
4. Serum chemistry levels

44. 3. An endoscopy will allow direct visualization of the tumor. A colonoscopy or a barium enema would help to diagnose colon cancer, not gastric cancer. Serum chemistry levels don't contribute data useful to the assessment of gastric cancer.
CN: Health promotion and maintenance; CNS: None; CL: Application

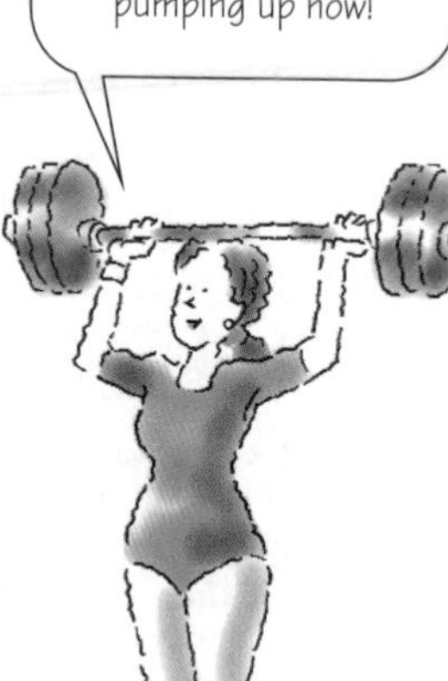

You're really pumping up now!

45. A client with gastric cancer can expect to have surgery for resection. Which intervention should be the nursing management priority for the preoperative client with gastric cancer?
1. Discharge planning
2. Correction of nutritional deficits
3. Prevention of deep vein thrombosis (DVT)
4. Instruction regarding radiation treatment

45. 2. Clients with gastric cancer commonly have nutritional deficits and may be cachectic. Discharge planning before surgery is important, but correcting the nutritional deficit is a higher priority. Prevention of DVT also isn't a high priority prior to surgery, though it assumes greater importance after surgery. At present, radiation therapy hasn't been proven effective for gastric cancer, and teaching about it preoperatively wouldn't be appropriate.
CN: Safe, effective care environment; CNS: Management of care; CL: Application

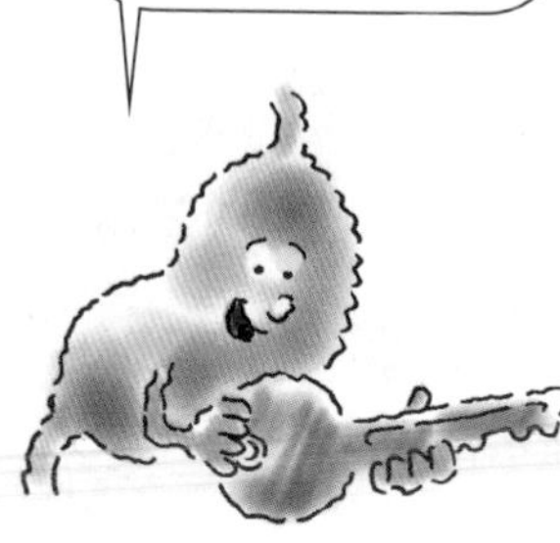

Do you know the key to the treatment of GI disorders in general?

46. Which factor is the priority postoperative care need of the client after gastric resection?
1. Body image
2. Nutritional needs
3. Skin care
4. Spiritual needs

46. 2. After gastric resection, a client may require total parenteral nutrition or jejunostomy tube feedings to maintain adequate nutritional status which promotes healing. Body image isn't much of a problem for this client at this point because clothing can cover the incision site. Wound care of the incision site is necessary to prevent infection; otherwise the skin shouldn't be affected. Spiritual needs may be a concern, depending on the client, and should be addressed as the client demonstrates readiness to share concerns.
CN: Safe, effective care environment; CNS: Management of care; CL: Analysis

47. Which complication of gastric resection should a nurse teach the client to watch for?
1. Constipation
2. Dumping syndrome
3. Gastric spasm
4. Intestinal spasms

47. 2. Dumping syndrome is a problem that occurs postprandially after gastric resection because ingested food rapidly enters the jejunum without proper mixing and without the normal duodenal digestive processing. Diarrhea, not constipation, may also be a symptom. Gastric or intestinal spasms don't occur, but antispasmodics may be given to slow gastric emptying.
CN: Physiological integrity; CNS: Reduction of risk potential; CL: Application

48. A client reports having several episodes of rectal bleeding, ribbon-shaped stools, and abdominal cramping. The nurse recognizes these signs and symptoms as related to which disorder?

1. Hemorrhoids
2. Irritable bowel syndrome
3. Colorectal cancer
4. Liver cancer

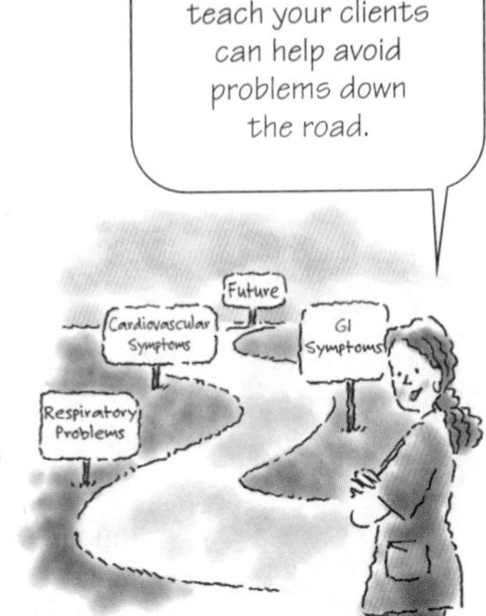
Knowing what to teach your clients can help avoid problems down the road.
Future
Cardiovascular Symptoms
GI Symptoms
Respiratory Problems

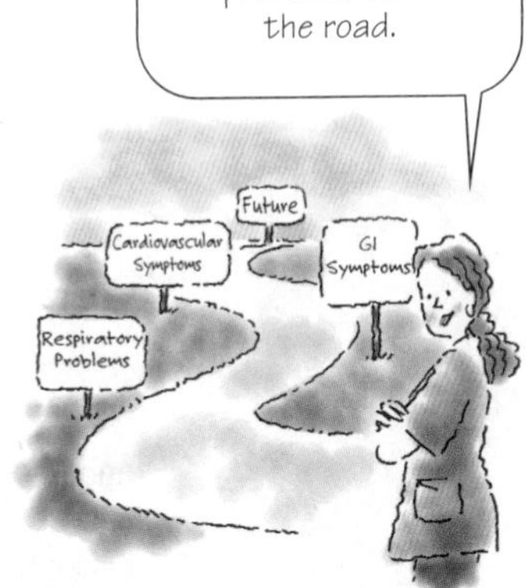

48. 3. Rectal bleeding, ribbon-shaped stool, and abdominal cramping are all associated with colorectal cancer but these signs and symptoms aren't all associated with the other conditions. IBS can produce abdominal cramping but not rectal bleeding. Hemorrhoids can cause rectal bleeding. Liver cancer isn't related to these symptoms.

CN: Physiological integrity; CNS: Physiological adaptation; CL: Analysis

49. A client with which condition may be likely to develop rectal cancer?

1. Adenomatous polyps
2. Diverticulitis
3. Hemorrhoids
4. Peptic ulcer disease

49. 1. A client with adenomatous polyps has a higher risk for developing rectal cancer than others do. Clients with diverticulitis are more likely to develop colon cancer. Hemorrhoids don't increase the chance of any type of cancer. Clients with peptic ulcer disease have a higher incidence of gastric cancer.

CN: Health promotion and maintenance; CNS: None; CL: Analysis

50. A client recently diagnosed with colon cancer tells the nurse that he's been having trouble sleeping and is preoccupied with thoughts of how his life will change after surgery. Which is the most appropriate nursing diagnosis?

1. *Anxiety related to upcoming surgery*
2. *Powerlessness related to illness*
3. *Disturbed sleep pattern related to fear of the unknown*
4. *Ineffective coping related to the diagnosis of colon cancer*

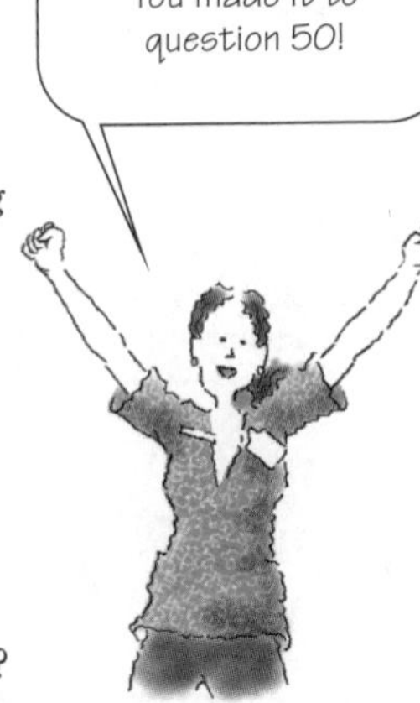
You made it to question 50!

50. 3. The client is having trouble sleeping because of his concerns about life changes. Although he may be experiencing anxiety and powerlessness, the information supports a diagnosis of insomnia. There is no evidence of ineffective coping.

CN: Safe, Physiological integrity; CNS: Basic care and comfort; CL: Analysis

51. Which condition may lead to hemorrhoids?

1. Diarrhea
2. Diverticulosis
3. Portal hypertension
4. Rectal bleeding

51. 3. Portal hypertension and other conditions associated with persistently high intra-abdominal pressure such as pregnancy can lead to hemorrhoids. The passing of hard stool, not diarrhea, can aggravate hemorrhoids. Diverticulosis has no relationship to hemorrhoids. Rectal bleeding can be a symptom of hemorrhoids.

CN: Physiological integrity; CNS: Physiological adaptation; CL: Analysis

52. Which assessment is most relevant with the diagnosis of hemorrhoids?
1. Abdominal assessment
2. Diet history
3. Digital rectal examination
4. Sexual history

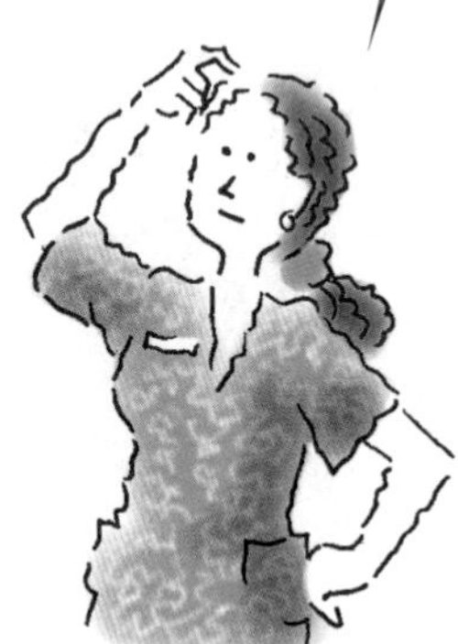
Now let me think. Which treatment would be appropriate?

52. 3. Digital rectal examination is important to assess for internal hemorrhoids and to determine if other causes of the pain and bleeding are present. Abdominal assessment isn't necessary for hemorrhoids. Diet history is relevant because constipation can worsen hemorrhoids, but it isn't as important to diagnosis as a digital rectal examination. Sexual history may also be relevant, but again, the history isn't as important as a digital rectal examination.
CN: Physiological integrity; CNS: Physiological adaptation; CL: Analysis

53. Which of the following should be part of the teaching plan for a client with hemorrhoids?
1. Recommending a high-fiber diet
2. Applying cold to reduce swelling
3. Using astringent lotions to reduce swelling
4. Elevating the buttocks to reduce engorgement

53. 1. A high-fiber diet will add bulk to the stool and ease its passage through the rectum. Application of cold isn't recommended because it can cause injury to the tissue. Astringent lotions can be used to reduce pain, but they aren't a treatment. The buttocks should be elevated only when prolapsed hemorrhoids are present.
CN: Physiological integrity; CNS: Physiological adaptation; CL: Application

54. Which response should a nurse offer to a client who asks why he's having a vagotomy to treat his ulcer?
1. To repair a hole in the stomach
2. To reduce the ability of the stomach to produce acid
3. To prevent the stomach from sliding into the chest
4. To remove a potentially malignant lesion in the stomach

Client education is an important tool for obtaining compliance.

54. 2. A vagotomy is performed to eliminate the acid-secreting stimulus to gastric cells. A perforation would be repaired with a gastric resection. Repair of hiatal hernia (fundoplication) prevents the stomach from sliding through the diaphragm. Removal of a potentially malignant tumor wouldn't reduce the entire acid-producing mechanism.
CN: Physiological integrity; CNS: Reduction of risk potential; CL: Application

55. Which condition is most likely to directly cause peritonitis?
1. Cholelithiasis
2. Gastritis
3. Perforated ulcer
4. Incarcerated hernia

55. 3. The most common cause of peritonitis is a perforated ulcer, which can pour contaminants into the peritoneal cavity, causing inflammation and infection within the cavity. The other conditions—cholelithiasis, gastritis, and incarcerated hernia—don't by themselves cause peritonitis. However, if cholelithiasis leads to rupture of the gall bladder, gastritis leads to erosion of the stomach wall, or an incarcerated hernia leads to rupture of the intestines, peritonitis may develop.
CN: Physiological integrity; CNS: Physiological adaptation; CL: Application

CN: Client needs category CNS: Client needs subcategory CL: Cognitive level

56. Which symptom would a client in the early stages of peritonitis exhibit?

1. Abdominal distention
2. Abdominal pain and rigidity
3. Hyperactive bowel sounds
4. Right upper quadrant pain

56. 2. Abdominal pain causing rigidity of the abdominal muscles is characteristic of peritonitis. Abdominal distention may occur as a late sign but not early on. Bowel sounds may be normal or decreased but not increased. Right upper quadrant pain is characteristic of cholecystitis or hepatitis.

CN: Health promotion and maintenance; CNS: None; CL: Application

57. Which laboratory result would be expected in a client with peritonitis?

1. Partial thromboplastin time above 100 seconds
2. Hemoglobin level below 10 mg/dl
3. Potassium level above 5.5 mEq/L
4. White blood cell (WBC) count above 15,000/µl

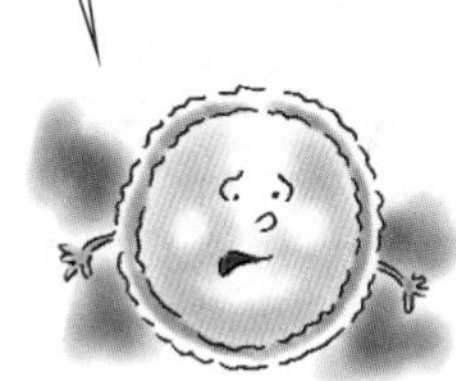

In my case, more is not necessarily better.

57. 4. Because of infection, the client's WBC count will be elevated. A partial thromboplastin time longer than 100 seconds may suggest disseminated intravascular coagulation, a serious complication of septic shock. A hemoglobin level below 10 mg/dl may occur from hemorrhage. A potassium level above 5.5 mEq/L may suggest renal failure.

CN: Physiological integrity; CNS: Reduction of risk potential; CL: Application

58. A recently admitted client is suspected of having peritonitis. He's requesting a glass of water to drink. Which would be the nurse's best response to the client?

1. "I can give you small amounts of water frequently."
2. "You're getting your fluids intravenously."
3. "I'll check with the physician."
4. "Until your diagnosis is confirmed and bowel function returns, it wouldn't be safe to give you anything to drink."

58. 4. The client with peritonitis commonly isn't allowed anything orally until the source of the peritonitis is confirmed and treated. I.V. fluids are given to maintain hydration and hemodynamic stability and to replace electrolytes. However, saying to a client that, "You're getting your fluids intravenously," doesn't explain to the client why he can't have fluids orally. Checking with the physician isn't necessary.

CN: Physiological integrity; CNS: Physiological adaptation; CL: Application

59. Which aspect is the priority focus of nursing care for a client with peritonitis?

1. Fluid and electrolyte balance
2. Gastric irrigation
3. Pain management
4. Psychosocial issues

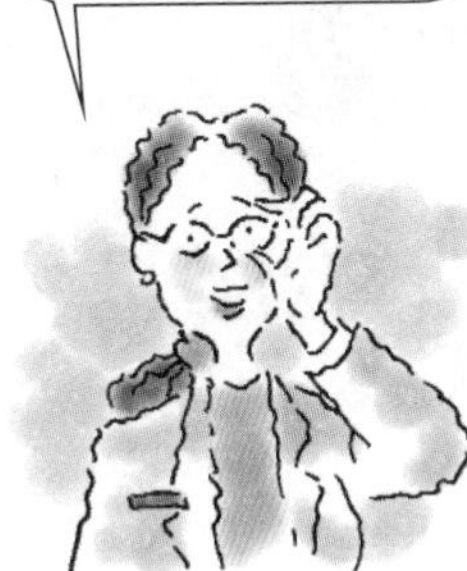

59. 1. Peritonitis can advance to shock and circulatory failure, so fluid and electrolyte balance is the priority focus of nursing management. Gastric irrigation may be needed periodically to ensure patency of the nasogastric tube. Although pain management is important for comfort and psychosocial care will address concerns such as anxiety, focusing on fluid and electrolyte balance will maintain hemodynamic stability.

CN: Safe, effective care environment; CNS: Management of care; CL: Analysis

60. Which factor is most commonly associated with the development of pancreatitis?

1. Alcohol abuse
2. Hypercalcemia
3. Hyperlipidemia
4. Pancreatic duct obstruction

60. 1. Alcohol abuse is the major cause of acute pancreatitis in males, although gallbladder disease is more commonly implicated in women. Hypercalcemia, hyperlipidemia, and pancreatic duct obstruction are also causes of pancreatitis but occur less frequently.

CN: Physiological integrity; CNS: Reduction of risk potential; CL: Application

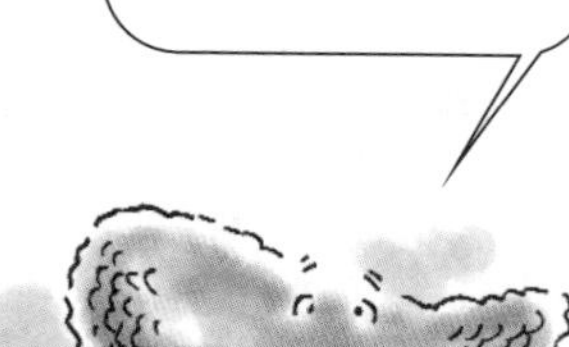

Read question 61 carefully before you answer. Make sure you know what it's asking.

61. Which action of pancreatic enzymes can cause pancreatic damage?

1. Utilization by the intestine
2. Autodigestion of the pancreas
3. Reflux into the pancreas
4. Clogging of the pancreatic duct

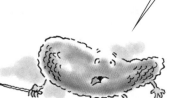

61. 2. In pancreatitis, pancreatic enzymes become activated and begin to autodigest the pancreas. The enzymes are activated but aren't used properly by the intestine. Reflux of bile into the pancreatic duct and clogging of the pancreatic duct may occur before autodigestion of the pancreas occurs.

CN: Physiological integrity; CNS: Physiological adaptation; CL: Analysis

62. Which laboratory test is used to diagnose pancreatitis?

1. Amylase level
2. Hemoglobin level
3. Blood glucose level
4. White blood cell (WBC) count

62. 1. Amylase is an enzyme secreted by the pancreas; when elevated, it's useful in diagnosing pancreatitis. Hemoglobin level can be low in pancreatitis, but there are other causes for this. The blood glucose level may be elevated with pancreatitis, but this factor isn't diagnostic. The WBC count may also be elevated in pancreatitis, but this symptom can be due to infection.

CN: Health promotion and maintenance; CNS: None; CL: Analysis

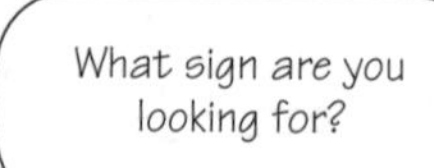

What sign are you looking for?

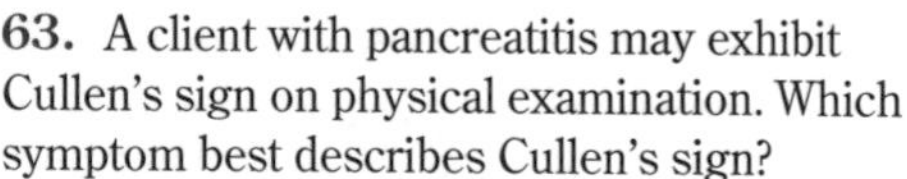

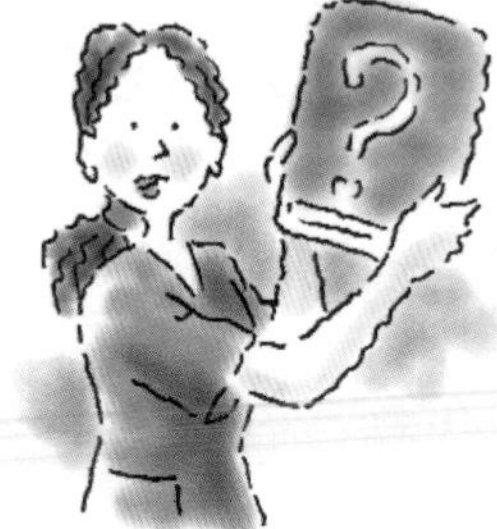

63. A client with pancreatitis may exhibit Cullen's sign on physical examination. Which symptom best describes Cullen's sign?

1. Jaundiced sclera
2. Pain that occurs with movement
3. Bluish discoloration of the left flank area
4. Bluish discoloration of the periumbilical area

63. 4. Cullen's sign is bluish discoloration of the periumbilical area from subcutaneous intraperitoneal hemorrhagic pancreatitis. Jaundiced sclera occurs with hepatitis. Pain with movement is a common finding with peritonitis. Turner's sign is the bluish discoloration of the left flank area, which can be present in peritonitis.

CN: Health promotion and maintenance; CNS: None; CL: Analysis

64. Which factor should be the initial focus of nursing management in a client with acute pancreatitis?

1. Dietary management
2. Prevention of skin breakdown
3. Management of hypoglycemia
4. Pain control

64. 4. The priority is to provide adequate pain control. This is essential to minimize discomfort and restlessness, which may stimulate pancreatic secretion further. Initially, the client with acute pancreatitis isn't permitted food and oral intake. Although prevention of skin breakdown is important, it isn't the initial focus. Clients are at risk for hyperglycemia, not hypoglycemia.

CN: Physiological integrity; CNS: Physiological adaptation; CL: Analysis

CN: Client needs category CNS: Client needs subcategory CL: Cognitive level

65. When admitting a client to the hospital with suspected acute pancreatitis, which electrolyte disorder would be expected?

1. Hypoglycemia
2. Hypernatremia
3. Hypocalcemia
4. Hyperkalemia

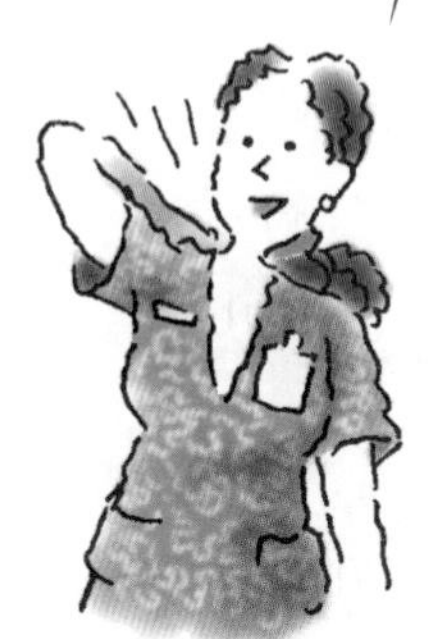

Give yourself a pat on the back: You're doing great!

65. 3. The client with acute pancreatitis may exhibit hypocalcemia due to the deposit of calcium in areas of fat necrosis. Hyperglycemia, not hypoglycemia, may occur due to reduced insulin production caused by islet of Langerhans involvement. Hypokalemia and hyponatremia may occur because potassium is lost in emesis, but hypernatremia is unlikely.

CN: Physiological integrity; CNS: Physiological adaptation; CL: Analysis

66. If a gastric ulcer perforates, which action should be included in the management of the client?

1. Removal of the nasogastric (NG) tube
2. Antacid administration
3. H_2-receptor antagonist administration
4. Fluid and electrolyte replacement

66. 4. The client should be treated with antibiotics as well as fluid, electrolyte, and blood replacement. NG tube suction should also be performed to prevent further spillage of stomach contents into the perineal cavity. Antacids and H_2-receptor antagonists aren't helpful in this situation.

CN: Physiological integrity; CNS: Physiological adaptation; CL: Application

67. A client presents to the emergency department with abdominal pain, weight loss, steatorrhea, and a random glucose of 417 mg/dl. The nurse should expect which diagnostic test to be ordered?

1. Upper GI series
2. Lower GI series
3. Ultrasound of the abdomen
4. Colonoscopy

67. 3. The symptoms described correlate with chronic pancreatitis. An abdominal ultrasound could reveal pancreatic changes. The other tests are of no value in evaluating the pancreas.

CN: Physiological integrity; CNS: Physiological adaptation; CL: Analysis

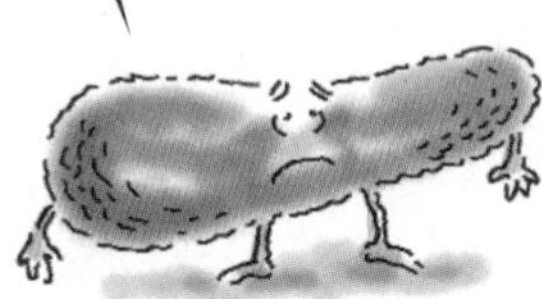

I'm really feeling under the influence.

68. In alcohol-related pancreatitis, which intervention is the best way to reduce the exacerbation of pain?

1. Lying in a supine position
2. Taking aspirin
3. Eating a low-fat diet
4. Abstaining from alcohol

68. 4. Abstaining from alcohol is imperative to reduce the injury to the pancreas; in fact, it may be enough to completely control pain. Lying in a supine position usually aggravates the pain because it stretches the abdominal muscles. Taking aspirin can cause bleeding in hemorrhagic pancreatitis. During an attack of acute pancreatitis, the client usually isn't allowed to ingest anything orally.

CN: Physiological integrity; CNS: Reduction of risk potential; CL: Application

69. A client with cirrhosis complains that his skin always feels itchy. The nurse recognizes that the itching is a result of which abnormality associated with cirrhosis?

1. Prolonged prothrombin time
2. Decreased protein level
3. Increased bilirubin level
4. Increased aspartate aminotransferase level

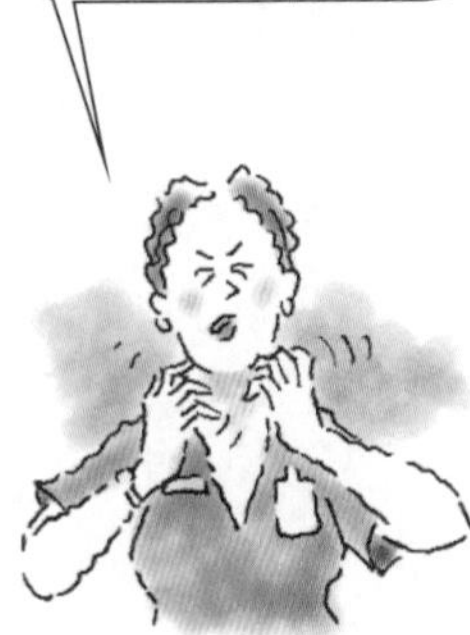

I'm itching to be done with this question.

69. 3. High bilirubin levels irritate peripheral nerves, causing an intense itching sensation. Itching isn't a symptom of prolonged prothrombin time, decreased protein levels, or increased aspartate aminotransferase levels.

CN: Physiological integrity; CNS: Physiological adaptation; CL: Analysis

70. Which factor causes biliary cirrhosis?
1. Acute viral hepatitis
2. Alcohol hepatotoxicity
3. Chronic biliary inflammation or obstruction
4. Heart failure with prolonged venous hepatic congestion

70. 3. Chronic biliary inflammation or obstruction causes biliary cirrhosis. Acute viral hepatitis can cause postnecrotic cirrhosis. Alcohol hepatotoxicity is Laënnec's cirrhosis. Heart failure with prolonged venous hepatic congestion will cause cardiac cirrhosis.
CN: Physiological integrity; CNS: Physiological adaptation; CL: Application

71. Which finding would strongly indicate the possibility of cirrhosis?
1. Dry skin
2. Hepatomegaly
3. Peripheral edema
4. Pruritus

One of these findings is a red flag for cirrhosis.
STOP

71. 2. The client with cirrhosis has a liver that is enlarged (hepatomegaly), fibrotic, and nodular, which makes it palpable. The client may develop dry skin, pruritus, and peripheral edema, but these symptoms may have other causes.
CN: Physiological integrity; CNS: Physiological adaptation; CL: Analysis

72. For a definitive diagnosis of cirrhosis, the nurse will assist with which diagnostic test?
1. Albumin level
2. Bromsulfophthalein dye excretion
3. Liver biopsy
4. Liver enzyme levels

72. 3. A liver biopsy can reveal the exact cause of the hepatomegaly. The albumin level will be low, but that can be caused by poor nutritional states. Bromsulfophthalein dye excretion may be reduced, but other hepatocirculatory disorders could also cause this. Liver enzymes may be elevated, but other liver conditions may cause these elevations.
CN: Physiological integrity; CNS: Physiological adaptation; CL: Application

73. Which of the following assessment findings would be consistent with a client's diagnosis of cirrhosis?
1. Increased carbon dioxide level
2. Increased pH level
3. Increased prothrombin time
4. Increased white blood cell (WBC) count

73. 3. Clotting factors may not be produced normally when a client has cirrhosis, increasing the potential for bleeding. There's no associated change in carbon dioxide level or pH unless the client is developing other comorbidities, such as metabolic alkalosis. The WBC count can be elevated in acute cirrhosis but isn't always altered.
CN: Physiological integrity; CNS: Physiological adaptation; CL: Application

74. Which measure should the nurse focus on for a client with esophageal varices?
1. Recognizing hemorrhage
2. Controlling blood pressure
3. Encouraging nutritional intake
4. Teaching the client about varices

74. 1. Recognizing the rupture of esophageal varices, or hemorrhage, is the focus of nursing care because the client could succumb to this quickly. Controlling blood pressure is also important because it helps reduce the risk of variceal rupture. It's also important to teach the client what foods he should avoid, such as spicy foods, and what varices are.
CN: Physiological integrity; CNS: Physiological adaptation; CL: Application

75. Several children at a daycare center have been infected with hepatitis A virus. Which instruction by the nurse would reduce the risk of hepatitis A to other children and staff members?

1. Hand washing after diaper changes
2. Isolation of the sick children
3. Use of masks during contact with the children
4. Sterilization of all eating utensils

75. 1. Children in day care centers are at risk of hepatitis A infection which is transmitted via fecal-oral route due to poor hand hygiene practices and poor sanitation. Isolation of sick children, use of mask during contact, and sterilization of all eating utensils would not be useful in breaking the chain of infection.

CN: Safe, effective care environment; CNS: Safety & Infection control; CL: Application

76. A client is being evaluated for hepatitis A. Which activity places him at the highest risk for contracting hepatitis A?

1. Helping his roommate with an epistaxis episode
2. Receiving an elective blood transfusion after surgery
3. Eating a shrimp platter at a local restaurant
4. Having sexual intercourse with his fianceé

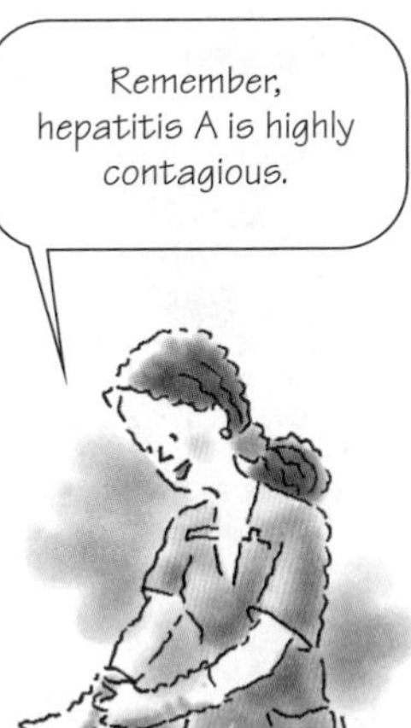
Remember, hepatitis A is highly contagious.

76. 3. Hepatitis A can be caused by contact with contaminated feces and may be transmitted through infected water, milk, or food, especially shellfish from contaminated waters. Hepatitis B is caused by blood contact and sexual contact. Hepatitis C is usually caused by contact with infected blood, including blood transfusions.

CN: Health promotion and maintenance; CNS: None; CL: Application

77. The nurse is teaching a client with a peptic ulcer about discharge instructions. The client asks the nurse which type of analgesic he may take. Which of the following responses by the nurse would be the most accurate?

1. Aspirin
2. Acetaminophen
3. Naproxen
4. Ibuprofen

77. 2. Acetaminophen is recommended for pain relief because it does not promote irritation of the mucosa. Aspirin, and nonsteroidal anti-inflammatory drugs such as naproxen and ibuprofen, may cause irritation of the mucosa and subsequent bleeding.

CN: Physiological integrity; CNS: Pharmacological and parenteral therapies; CL: Application

78. The nurse is performing an assessment on a client being evaluated for viral hepatitis. Which symptom will the nurse most likely assess on this client?

1. Arthralgia
2. Excitability
3. Headache
4. Polyphagia

78. 1. Arthralgia is common in clients with viral hepatitis. Other symptoms of viral hepatitis include lethargy, flulike symptoms, anorexia, nausea and vomiting, abdominal pain, diarrhea, constipation, and fever. Excitability, headache, and polyphagia are *not* symptoms of viral hepatitis.

CN: Physiological integrity; CNS: Physiological adaptation; CL: Application

79. A client is admitted with a diagnosis of hepatic encephalopathy. The nurse's assessment documentation will include which of the following?

1. Asterixis
2. Good concentration
3. Increased energy
4. Talkativeness

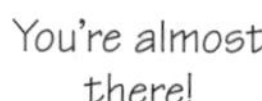

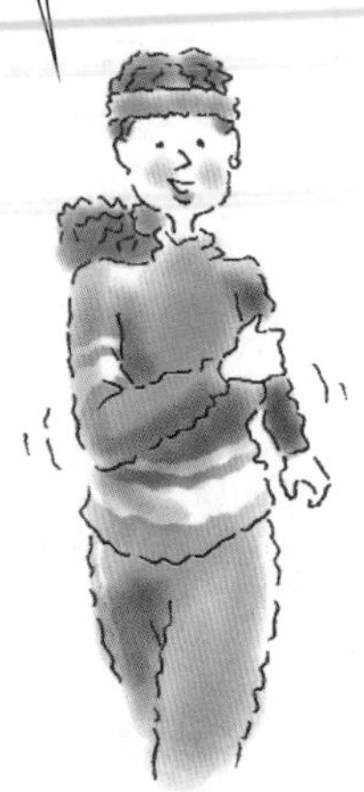

79. 1. Asterixis, also known as *liver flap,* is commonly present in clients with hepatic encephalopathy. It can be easily elicited by applying a blood pressure cuff and noting if the flapping is present when the cuff is released. Lack of concentration, fatigue, and introversion are also symptoms of encephalopathy.

CN: Physiological integrity; CNS: Physiological adaptation; CL: Application

80. Which dietary instructions should the nurse give to a client with toxic hepatitis?

1. No foods or drinks allowed.
2. Eat low-calorie foods.
3. Consume only low-residue foods.
4. Eat high-calorie foods.

80. 4. Instructions to a client with toxic hepatitis should include consuming a high-calorie diet. The client is allowed to eat and drink and does not need to consume low-calorie or low-residue foods.

CN: Physiological integrity; CNS: Basic care and comfort; CL: Application

81. Which test is the most accurate for diagnosing liver cancer?

1. Abdominal ultrasound
2. Abdominal flat plate X-ray
3. Cholangiogram
4. Computed tomography (CT) scan

81. 4. A client with suspected liver cancer will likely undergo CT imaging to identify tumors. The results of a CT scan are much more definitive than the findings of an ultrasound or X-ray. A cholangiogram evaluates the gallbladder, not the liver.

CN: Health promotion and maintenance; CNS: None; CL: Analysis

Closely monitor a client for complications following surgery.

Caution

82. Immediately after a liver biopsy, which complication should a client be closely monitored for?

1. Abdominal cramping
2. Hemorrhage
3. Nausea and vomiting
4. Potential infection

82. 2. The liver is very vascular, and taking a biopsy could cause the client to hemorrhage. The client may experience some discomfort but typically not cramping. Nausea and vomiting may be present, and infection may occur but not immediately after the procedure.

CN: Physiological integrity; CNS: Reduction of risk potential; CL: Application

83. When a client who has a liver disorder is having an invasive procedure, the nurse helps assure safety by assessing the results of which test?

1. Coagulation studies
2. Liver enzyme levels
3. Serum chemistries
4. White blood cell count

83. 1. The liver produces coagulation factors. If the liver is affected negatively, production of these factors may be altered, placing the client at risk for hemorrhage. The other laboratory tests should also be monitored, but the results may not necessarily relate to the safety of the procedure.

CN: Physiological integrity; CNS: Reduction of risk potential; CL: Analysis

84. A nurse is giving preoperative and postoperative instructions to a client who will undergo a liver biopsy the next morning. In this situation, client-teaching information for which problem is the most critical?

1. Paralytic ileus
2. Hemorrhage
3. Renal shutdown
4. Constipation

What to do, what to do. I hope someone knows what to do.

84. 2. Because the most common adverse effect of a liver biopsy is bleeding, the nurse should provide relevant information regarding the potential for hemorrhage. There's no reason to provide the client with information about paralytic ileus. Renal shutdown isn't an expected complication after a liver biopsy. The nurse would have no reason to suspect that the client will have a problem with constipation after a liver biopsy.

CN: Physiological integrity; CNS: Reduction of risk potential; CL: Application

85. Which procedure is likely to be most necessary for a client with a small tumor confined to one liver segment or lobe?

1. Chemotherapy only
2. Cryoablation or liver resection
3. Liver transplant
4. Radiation therapy only

85. 2. If the tumor is confined and small, the best treatment would be cryoablation of the tumor or liver resection, removing the segment involved. Chemotherapy and radiation therapy may also be used to reduce the chance of cancerous hepatocytes from regrowing. Liver transplantation usually isn't indicated for liver cancer.

CN: Physiological integrity; CNS: Physiological adaptation; CL: Application

86. When counseling a client in the ways to prevent cholecystitis, which guideline is most important?

1. Eat a low-protein diet.
2. Eat a low-fat, low-cholesterol diet.
3. Limit exercise to 10 minutes a day.
4. Keep weight proportional to height.

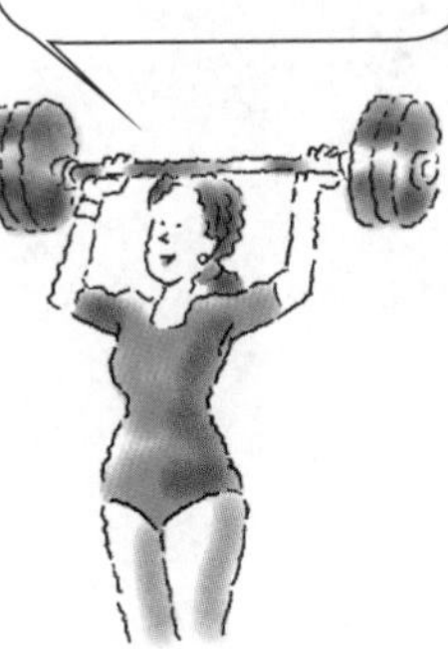

The correct answer carries a lot of weight towards preventing cholecystitis.

86. 4. Obesity is a known cause of cholecystitis, and maintaining a recommended weight will help to protect against cholecystitis. Excessive dietary intake of cholesterol is associated with the development of gallstones in many people. Dietary protein isn't implicated in cholecystitis. Liquid protein and low-calorie diets (with rapid weight loss of more than 5 lb [2.3 kg] per week) *are* implicated as the cause of some cases of cholecystitis. Regular exercise (30 minutes/three times a week) may help to reduce weight and improve fat metabolism. Reducing stress may reduce bile production, which may also indirectly decrease the chances of developing cholecystitis.

CN: Health promotion and maintenance; CNS: None; CL: Application

87. Which symptom best describes Murphy's sign?

1. Periumbilical ecchymosis exists.
2. On deep palpation and release, pain is elicited.
3. On palpation and deep inspiration, pain is elicited and the client stops breathing in.
4. Abdominal muscles are tightened in anticipation of palpation.

87. 3. Murphy's sign is elicited when the client reacts to pain and stops breathing in. It's a common finding in clients with cholecystitis. Periumbilical ecchymosis (Cullen's sign) is present in peritonitis. Pain on deep palpation and release is rebound tenderness. Tightening up abdominal muscles in anticipation of palpation is guarding, not Murphy's sign.

CN: Physiological integrity; CNS: Physiological adaptation; CL: Application

88. A client is suspected of having cholecystitis. The nurse will prepare the client for which of the following diagnostic tests?

1. Abdominal computed tomography (CT) scan
2. Abdominal ultrasound
3. Barium swallow
4. Endoscopy

88. 2. An abdominal ultrasound can show if the gallbladder is enlarged, if gallstones are present, if the gallbladder wall is thickened, or if distention of the gallbladder lumen is present. An abdominal CT scan can be used to diagnose cholecystitis, but it usually isn't necessary. A barium swallow looks at the stomach and the duodenum. Endoscopy looks at the esophagus, stomach, and duodenum.

CN: Health promotion and maintenance; CNS: None; CL: Application

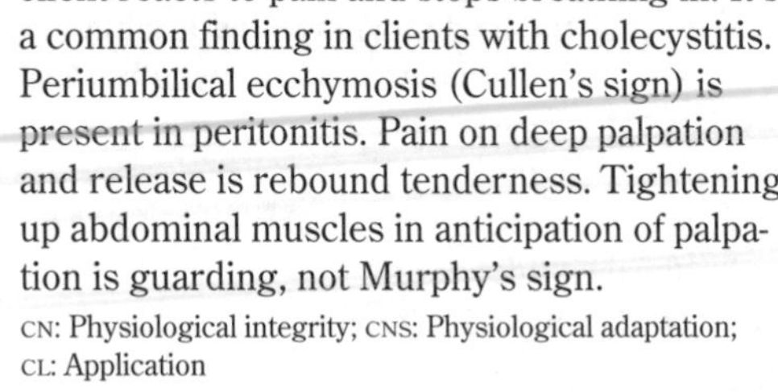

Question 89 is asking you to prioritize again.

89. Which factor should be the main focus of nursing management for a client hospitalized for acute cholecystitis?

1. Administration of antibiotics
2. Assessment for complications
3. Preparation for lithotripsy
4. Preparation for surgery

89. 2. The client with acute cholecystitis should *first* be monitored for such complications as perforation, fever, abscess, fistula, and sepsis. After assessment, antibiotics will be administered to reduce the infection. Lithotripsy is used for only a small percentage of clients. Surgery is usually done after the acute infection has subsided.

CN: Safe, effective care environment; CNS: Management of care; CL: Application

90. A nurse has given discharge instructions to a client with chronic cholecystitis. Which response by the client indicates the teaching has been effective?

1. "I need to rest more."
2. "I should avoid taking antacids."
3. "I should increase the fat in my diet."
4. "I will take my anticholinergic medications as prescribed."

90. 4. Conservative therapy for chronic cholecystitis includes weight reduction by increasing physical activity, a low-fat diet (not low-protein), antacid use to treat dyspepsia, and anticholinergic use to relax smooth muscles and reduce ductal tone and spasm, thereby reducing pain.

CN: Physiological integrity; CNS: Reduction of risk potential; CL: Application

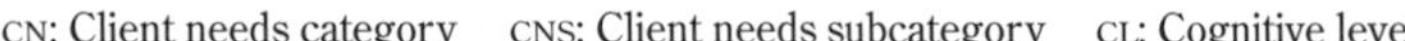

CN: Client needs category CNS: Client needs subcategory CL: Cognitive level

91. Documentation of assessment by the nurse for a client with duodenal ulcer will most likely reveal which of the following findings?

1. Hematemesis
2. Malnourishment
3. Melena
4. Pain with eating

91. 3. The client with a duodenal ulcer may have bleeding at the ulcer site, which shows up as melena. The other findings are consistent with a gastric ulcer.

CN: Physiological integrity; CNS: Physiological adaptation; CL: Application

92. To reduce occurrences of the dumping syndrome, the nurse should instruct a client to do which of the following?

1. Sip fluids with meals
2. Eat three meals daily
3. Rest after meals for 30 minutes
4. Diet should be high-carbohydrate, low-fat, and low-protein

92. 3. To reduce the occurrences of the dumping syndrome, clients should be taught to lie down after eating for 30 minutes; take fluids only between meals, none with meals; eat smaller amounts more frequently in a semi-recumbent position; and eat a low-carbohydrate diet, with high-protein and moderate-fat foods, and avoid sweets.

CN: Physiological integrity; CNS: Reduction of risk potential; CL: Application

I know some food
will relieve this pain.

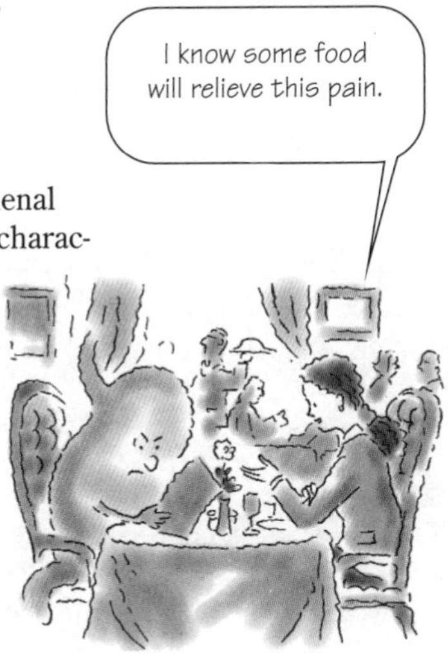

93. Assessment of a client with a duodenal ulcer will reveal which of the following characteristics?

1. Early satiety
2. Pain on eating
3. Dull upper epigastric pain
4. Pain on an empty stomach

93. 4. Pain of a duodenal ulcer on an empty stomach is relieved by taking food or antacids. The other symptoms are those of a gastric ulcer.

CN: Physiological integrity; CNS: Physiological adaptation; CL: Application

94. Which is the major diagnostic test for peptic ulcers?

1. Abdominal X-ray
2. Barium swallow
3. Computed tomography (CT) scan of the abdomen
4. Esophagogastroduodenoscopy (EGD)

94. 4. The EGD can visualize the entire upper GI tract as well as allow for tissue specimens and electrocautery if needed. The barium swallow could locate a gastric ulcer and may be an initial test performed. A CT scan and an abdominal X-ray aren't useful in the diagnosis of an ulcer.

CN: Health promotion and maintenance; CNS: None; CL: Application

95. Which process best describes the method of action of medications, such as ranitidine (Zantac), which are used in the treatment of peptic ulcer disease?

1. Neutralize acid
2. Reduce acid secretions
3. Stimulate gastrin release
4. Protect the mucosal barrier

95. 2. Ranitidine is a histamine-2 receptor antagonist that reduces acid secretion by inhibiting gastrin secretion. Antacids neutralize acid, and mucosal barrier fortifiers protect the mucosal barrier.

CN: Physiological integrity; CNS: Pharmacological and parenteral therapies; CL: Application

96. Which laboratory values will a nurse interpret as confirming a client's diagnosis of pancreatitis?

1. Elevated amylase, elevated lipase, elevated serum glucose, and decreased serum calcium levels
2. Elevated amylase, elevated lipase, decreased serum glucose, and decreased serum calcium levels
3. Decreased amylase, decreased lipase, elevated serum glucose, and increased serum calcium levels
4. Decreased amylase, decreased lipase, decreased serum glucose, and increased serum calcium levels

96. 1. Inflammation of the pancreas causes it to excrete pancreatic enzymes. The inflammation also causes a blockage of the ducts from the pancreas to the GI tract; therefore, the pancreatic enzymes are released into the blood, resulting in an elevation of amylase and lipase levels. Carbohydrate metabolism is impaired secondary to damage to pancreatic beta cells. This impairment causes the client to become hyperglycemic. As in many other disease processes, serum calcium level decreases because of the saponification of calcium by fatty acids in the area of the inflamed pancreas.

CN: Physiological integrity; CNS: Physiological adaptation; CL: Analysis

97. Which instruction should a nurse give a client with pancreatitis during discharge teaching?

1. Consume high-fat meals
2. Consume low-calorie meals
3. Limit daily intake of alcohol
4. Avoid beverages that contain caffeine

It's irritating to give up my cup of joe.

97. 4. A client with pancreatitis must avoid foods or beverages that can cause a relapse of the disease. Caffeine must be avoided because it's a stimulant that will further irritate the pancreas. The client with pancreatitis must avoid all alcohol because chronic alcohol use is one of the causes of pancreatitis. The diet should be low in fats and high in calories, especially carbohydrates.

CN: Physiological integrity; CNS: Reduction of risk potential; CL: Application

98. After a liver biopsy, a nurse should place a client in which position?

1. Left side-lying position, with the bed flat
2. Right side-lying position, with the bed flat
3. Left side-lying position, with the bed in semi-Fowler's position
4. Right side-lying position, with the bed in semi-Fowler's position

98. 2. Lying the client on his right side with the bed flat will splint the biopsy site and minimize bleeding. The other positions won't do this and may cause increased bleeding at the site or internally.

CN: Physiological integrity; CNS: Reduction of risk potential; CL: Application

99. A client with irritable bowel syndrome is being prepared for discharge. Which meal plan should the nurse give the client?

1. Low-fiber, low-fat
2. High-fiber, low-fat
3. Low-fiber, high-fat
4. High-fiber, high-fat

99. 2. The client with irritable bowel syndrome needs to be on a diet that contains at least 25 grams of fiber per day. Fatty foods are to be avoided because they may precipitate symptoms.

CN: Physiological integrity; CNS: Basic care and comfort; CL: Application

100. A client presents to the emergency department, reporting that he has been vomiting every 30 to 40 minutes for the past 8 hours. Frequent vomiting puts him at risk for which condition?

1. Metabolic acidosis and hyperkalemia
2. Metabolic acidosis and hypokalemia
3. Metabolic alkalosis and hyperkalemia
4. Metabolic alkalosis and hypokalemia

100. 4. Gastric acid contains large amounts of potassium, chloride, and hydrogen ions. Excessive loss of these substances, such as from vomiting, can lead to metabolic alkalosis and hypokalemia. It doesn't cause metabolic acidosis or hyperkalemia.

CN: Physiological integrity; CNS: Reduction of risk potential; CL: Application

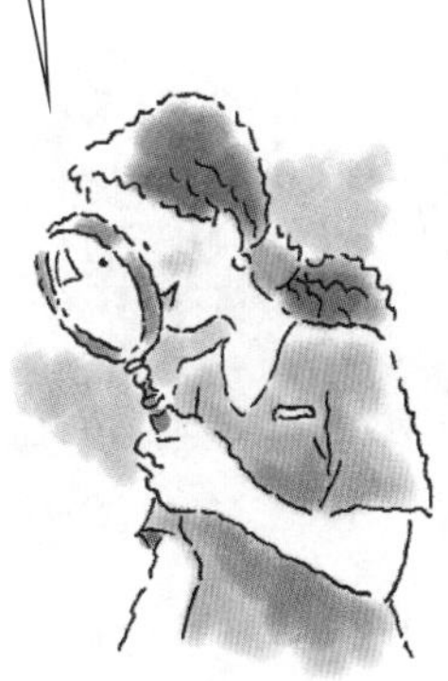

Closely examine the answers to question 100; it's easy to confuse them.

101. Five days after undergoing surgery, a client develops a small-bowel obstruction. A Miller-Abbott tube is inserted for bowel decompression. Which nursing diagnosis takes priority?

1. *Imbalanced nutrition: Less than body requirements*
2. *Acute pain*
3. *Deficient fluid volume*
4. *Excess fluid volume*

101. 3. Fluid shifts to the site of the bowel obstruction, causing a fluid deficit in the intravascular spaces. If the obstruction isn't resolved immediately, the client may experience *Imbalanced nutrition: Less than body requirements;* however, *Deficient fluid volume* takes priority. The client also may experience pain, but that nursing diagnosis is also of lower priority than *Deficient fluid volume.*

CN: Safe, effective care environment; CNS: Management of care; CL: Analysis

102. A client presents to the clinic for a follow-up appointment after diagnostic tests show he has gastroesophageal reflux disease. Which instruction should the nurse provide?

1. "Lie down and rest after each meal."
2. "Avoid alcohol and caffeine."
3. "Drink 16 ounces of water with each meal."
4. "Eat three well-balanced meals every day."

102. 2. A client with gastroesophageal reflux disease should avoid alcohol, caffeine, and foods that increase acidity, all of which can cause epigastric pain. To further prevent reflux, the client should remain upright for 2 to 3 hours after eating; avoid eating for 2 to 3 hours before bedtime; avoid bending and wearing tight clothing; avoid drinking large fluid volumes with meals; and eat small, frequent meals to help reduce gastric acid secretion.

CN: Physiological integrity; CNS: Reduction of risk potential; CL: Application

103. When teaching an elderly client how to prevent constipation, which instruction should the nurse include?

1. "Drink six glasses of fluid each day."
2. "Avoid grain products and nuts."
3. "Add at least 4 grams of bran to your cereal each morning."
4. "Be sure to get regular exercise."

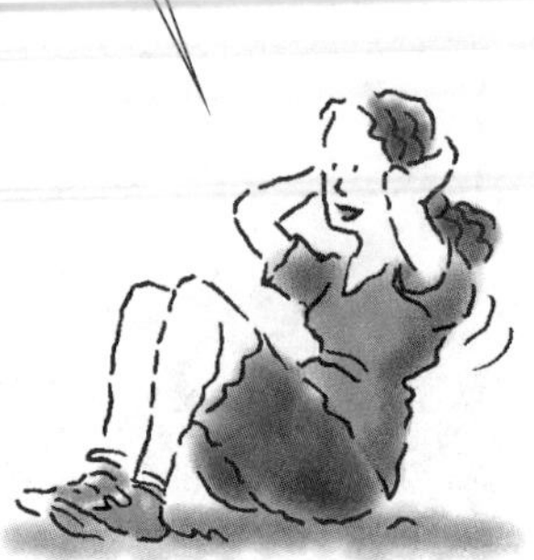

If you keep moving, you'll keep moving.

103. 4. Exercise helps prevent constipation. Fluids and dietary fiber promote normal bowel function. The client should drink eight to ten glasses of fluid per day. Although adding bran to cereal helps prevent constipation by increasing dietary fiber, the client should start with a small amount of bran and gradually increase the amount as tolerated to a maximum of 2 grams daily.

CN: Health promotion and maintenance; CNS: None; CL: Application

104. In a client with diarrhea, which outcome indicates that fluid resuscitation is successful?

1. The client passes formed stools at regular intervals.
2. The client reports a decrease in stool frequency and liquidity.
3. The client exhibits firm skin turgor.
4. The client no longer experiences perianal burning.

104. 3. Firm skin turgor would be one indication of successful fluid resuscitation. Other indications would include moist mucous membranes and urine output of at least 30 ml/hour. Passage of formed stools at regular intervals and a decrease in stool frequency and liquidity indicate successful resolution of diarrhea. The absence of perianal burning indicates that the irritation from the diarrhea is gone.

CN: Physiological integrity; CNS: Basic care and comfort; CL: Analysis

105. When teaching a community group about measures to prevent colon cancer, which instruction should a nurse include?

1. "Limit fat intake to 20% to 25% of your total daily calories."
2. "Include 15 to 20 grams of fiber in your daily diet."
3. "Get an annual rectal examination after age 35."
4. "Undergo sigmoidoscopy annually after age 50."

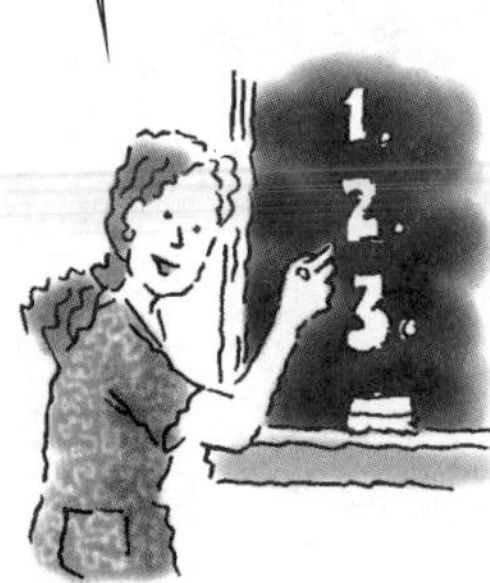

Eliminating the wrong answers can be as important as selecting the right one.
1.
2.
3.

105. 1. To help prevent colon cancer, fats should account for no more than 20% to 25% of total daily calories and the diet should include 25 to 30 grams of fiber per day. A digital rectal examination isn't recommended as a stand-alone test for colorectal cancer. For colorectal cancer screening, the American Cancer Society advises clients over age 50 to have a flexible sigmoidoscopy every 5 years, yearly fecal occult blood tests, a double-contrast barium enema every 5 years, or a colonoscopy every 10 years.

CN: Health promotion and maintenance; CNS: None; CL: Application

106. A 30-year-old client experiences weight loss, abdominal distention, crampy abdominal pain, and intermittent diarrhea after the birth of her second child. Diagnostic tests reveal gluten-induced enteropathy. Which foods must she eliminate from her diet permanently?

1. Milk and dairy products
2. Protein-containing foods
3. Cereal grains (except rice and corn)
4. Carbohydrates

106. 3. To manage gluten-induced enteropathy, the client must eliminate gluten, which means avoiding all cereal grains except rice and corn. In initial disease management, clients eat a high-calorie, high-protein diet with mineral and vitamin supplements to help normalize the nutritional status. Lactose intolerance is sometimes an associated problem, so milk and dairy products are limited until improvement occurs. Cereal grains are the only carbohydrates this client must eliminate.

CN: Physiological integrity; CNS: Basic care and comfort; CL: Application

CN: Client needs category CNS: Client needs subcategory CL: Cognitive level

107. After a right hemicolectomy for treatment of colon cancer, a 57-year-old client is reluctant to turn while on bed rest. Which action by the nurse would be appropriate?

1. Asking a coworker to help turn the client
2. Explaining to the client why turning is important
3. Allowing the client to turn when he's ready to do so
4. Telling the client that the physician's order states he must turn every 2 hours

107. 2. The appropriate action is to explain the importance of turning to avoid postoperative complications. Asking a coworker to help turn the client against his will would infringe on his rights. Allowing him to turn when he's ready would increase his risk for postoperative complications. Telling him he must turn because of the physician's orders would put him on the defensive and exclude him from participating in care decisions.

CN: Physiological integrity; CNS: Reduction of risk potential CL: Application

108. A nurse assists a physician during paracentesis. When documenting the procedure, which information should the nurse include?

1. Exactly what the nurse did during the procedure
2. The reason for the procedure
3. The physician's name and the client's response to the procedure
4. Diagnostic tests performed before obtaining the specimen

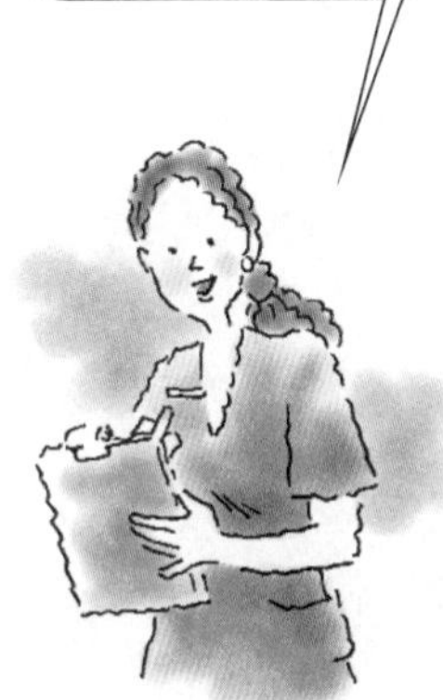
Good record
keeping is a key
factor in client care.

108. 3. The nurse should document the date and time of the procedure, the physician's name, pertinent information about the procedure (including tests done on the specimen obtained), the client's response, and client teaching. Documentation should include response to her interventions during the procedure. The reason for the procedure doesn't need to be documented.

CN: Physiological integrity; CNS: Reduction of risk potential; CL: Analysis

109. A client has a percutaneous endoscopic gastrostomy tube inserted for tube feedings. Before starting a continuous feeding, the nurse should place the client in which position?

1. Semi-Fowler's
2. Supine
3. Reverse Trendelenburg
4. High Fowler's

109. 1. To prevent aspiration of stomach contents, the nurse should place the client in semi-Fowler's position. The supine and reverse Trendelenburg positions may cause aspiration. High-Fowler's position isn't necessary and may not be tolerated as well as semi-Fowler's.

CN: Physiological integrity; CNS: Reduction of risk potential; CL: Application

110. An enema is prescribed for a client with suspected appendicitis. Which action should the nurse take?

1. Prepare 750 ml of irrigating solution warmed to 100° F (37.8° C).
2. Question the physician about the order.
3. Provide privacy and explain the procedure to the client.
4. Assist the client to left lateral Sims' position.

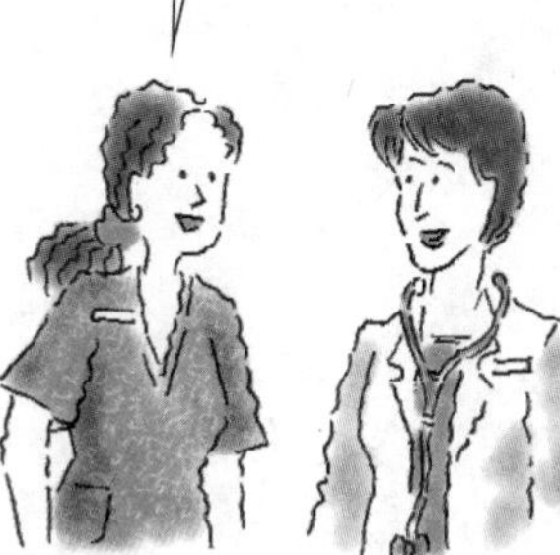
When in doubt ...
always ask!

110. 2. Enemas are contraindicated in an acute abdominal condition of unknown origin (such as suspected appendicitis) as well as after recent colon or rectal surgery or myocardial infarction, so questioning the physician about the order would be the correct thing to do. The other answers are correct only when enema administration is appropriate.

CN: Safe, effective care environment; CNS: Safety and infection control; CL: Application

111. A 75-year-old client is admitted to the hospital with lower GI bleeding. His hemoglobin on admission to the emergency department is 7.3 g/dl. The physician prescribes 2 units of packed red blood cells (RBCs) to infuse over 1 hour each. Each unit of packed RBCs contains 250 ml. The blood administration set has a drip factor of 10 gtt/ml. What is the flow rate in drops per minute? Record your answer using a whole number.

______________________ gtt/minute

111. 42. Each unit of packed RBCs contains 250 ml. Each unit is to infuse over 1 hour (60 minutes). Use the following equation:
250 ml/60 minutes = 4.16 ml.
Multiply by the drip factor:
4.16 ml × 10 gtt = 41.6 gtt/minute
(42 gtt/minute).

CN: Physiological integrity; CNS: Pharmacological and parenteral therapies; CL: Analysis

112. A nurse is assessing a client's abdomen. Identify the area where the nurse's hand should be placed to palpate the liver.

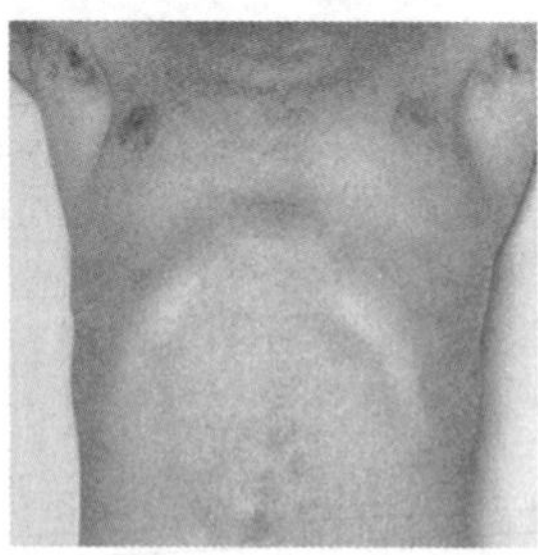

112. The nurse can palpate the liver by standing at the client's right side and placing her right hand on the client's abdomen, to the right of midline. The nurse should point the fingers of her right hand toward the client's head, just under the right rib margin.

CN: Health promotion and maintenance; CNS: None; CL: Application

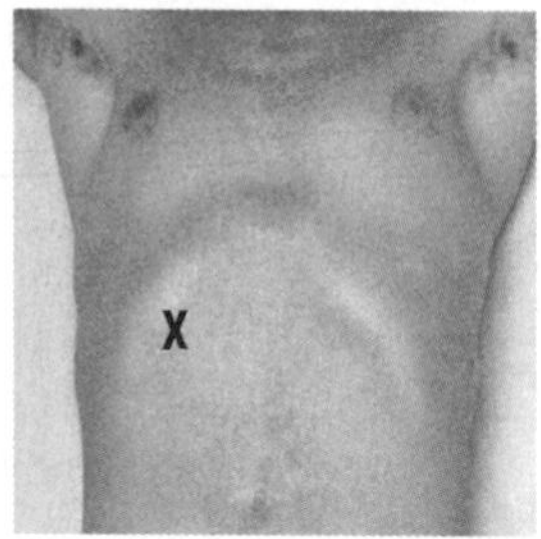

113. A nurse is caring for a client who has had extensive abdominal surgery and is in critical condition. Dextrose 5% in half-normal saline solution is infusing through a triple-lumen central catheter at 125 ml/hour. The physician's orders include: gentamicin 80 mg I.V. piggyback in 50 ml D_5W over 30 minutes; Ranitidine (Zantac) 50 mg I.V. in 50 ml D_5W over 30 minutes; one unit of 250 ml of packed red blood cells (RBCs) over 3 hours; and a nasogastric tube flush with 30 ml normal saline solution every 2 hours. How many milliliters should the nurse document as the intake for the 8-hour shift? Record your answer using a whole number.

______________________ milliliters

113. 1,470. The regular I.V. at 125 ml × 8 hours = 1,000 ml; gentamicin piggyback = 50 ml; ranitidine (Zantac) piggyback = 50 ml; packed RBCs = 250 ml; and nasogastric flushes of 30 ml × 4 = 120 ml. Totalled together, this equals 1,470 ml.

CN: Physiological integrity; CNS: Pharmacological and parenteral therapies; CL: Application

This chapter covers diabetes mellitus and other endocrine disorders, typically a difficult area for nursing students. Don't worry, though, I'll help you through all the tough spots.

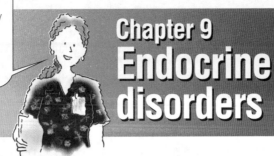

Chapter 9 Endocrine disorders

1. A client who is started on metformin and glyburide would have initially presented with which symptoms?

1. Polydipsia, polyuria, and weight loss
2. Weight gain, tiredness, and bradycardia
3. Irritability, diaphoresis, and tachycardia
4. Diarrhea, abdominal pain, and weight loss

1. 1. Symptoms of hyperglycemia include polydipsia, polyuria, and weight loss. Metformin and sulfonylureas are commonly ordered medications. Weight gain, tiredness, and bradycardia are symptoms of hypothyroidism. Irritability, diaphoresis, and tachycardia are symptoms of hypoglycemia. Symptoms of Crohn's disease include diarrhea, abdominal pain, and weight loss.

CN: Physiological integrity; CNS: Reduction of risk potential; CL: Analysis

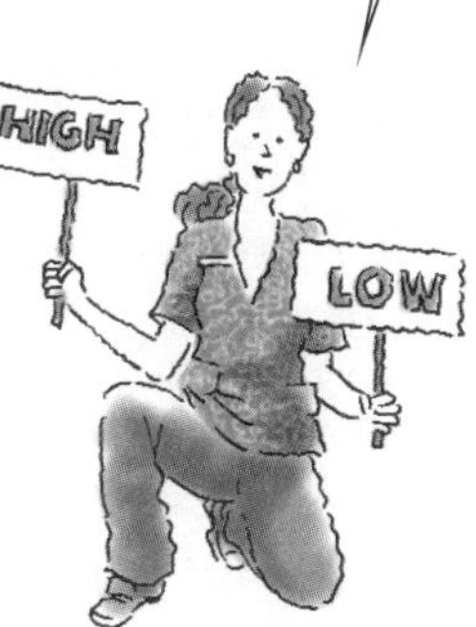

Make sure you don't confuse hyper and hypo!
HIGH
LOW

2. A client presents with diaphoresis, palpitations, jitters, and tachycardia approximately 1½ hours after taking his regular morning insulin. Which treatment is appropriate for this client?

1. Check blood glucose level and administer carbohydrates.
2. Give nitroglycerin and perform an electrocardiogram (ECG).
3. Check pulse oximetry and administer oxygen therapy.
4. Restrict salt, administer diuretics, and perform a paracentesis.

2. 1. The client is experiencing symptoms of hypoglycemia. Checking the blood glucose level and administering carbohydrates will elevate blood glucose. ECG and nitroglycerin are treatments for myocardial infarction. Administering oxygen won't help correct the low blood glucose level. Restricting salt, administering diuretics, and performing a paracentesis are treatments for ascites.

CN: Physiological integrity; CNS: Physiological adaptation; CL: Application

3. Which nursing consideration must be taken into account for a client with type 1 diabetes mellitus on the morning of surgery?

1. The client should take one-half of his usual daily dose of intermediate-acting insulin.
2. The client should receive an oral antidiabetic agent.
3. The client should receive an I.V. insulin infusion.
4. The client should take his full daily insulin dose with no dextrose infusion.

3. 1. If the client takes his full daily dose of intermediate-acting insulin when he isn't allowed anything orally before surgery, he'll become hypoglycemic. One-half of the insulin dose will provide all that is needed. Clients with type 1 diabetes don't take oral antidiabetic agents. I.V. insulin infusions aren't standard for routine surgery; they're used in the management of clients undergoing stressful procedures, such as transplants or coronary artery bypass surgery.

CN: Physiological integrity; CNS: Physiological adaptation; CL: Application

CN: Client needs category CNS: Client needs subcategory CL: Cognitive level

4. Which type of diabetes is controlled primarily through diet, exercise, and oral antidiabetic agents?

1. Diabetes insipidus
2. Diabetic ketoacidosis
3. Type 1 diabetes mellitus
4. Type 2 diabetes mellitus

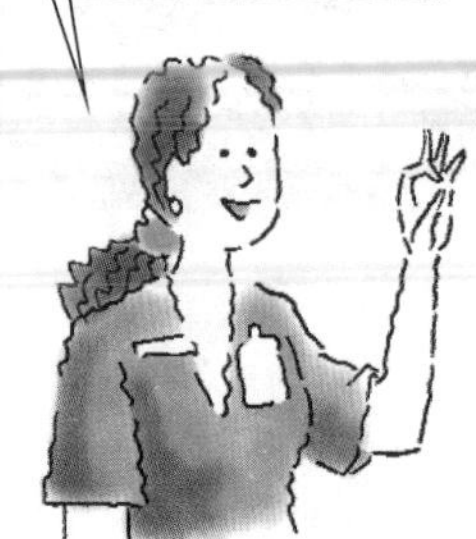

Okay. You've got this question under control.

4. 4. Type 2 diabetes mellitus is controlled primarily through diet, exercise, and oral antidiabetic agents. Desmopressin acetate, a long-acting vasopressin given intranasally, is the treatment of choice for diabetes insipidus. Treament for diabetic ketoacidosis includes restoration of fluid volume, electrolyte management, reversal of acidosis, and control of blood glucose. Diet and exercise are important in type 1 diabetes mellitus, but blood glucose levels are controlled by insulin injections in that disorder.

CN: Physiological integrity; CNS: Reduction of risk potential; CL: Analysis

5. Which nursing intervention should be taken for a client who complains of nausea and vomits 1 hour after taking his morning glyburide (DiaBeta)?

1. Give glyburide again.
2. Give subcutaneous insulin and monitor blood glucose.
3. Monitor blood glucose closely, and look for signs of hypoglycemia.
4. Monitor blood glucose, and assess for symptoms of hyperglycemia.

5. 3. When a client who has taken an oral antidiabetic agent vomits, the nurse should monitor glucose and assess him frequently for signs of hypoglycemia. Most of the medication has probably been absorbed. Therefore, repeating the dose would further lower glucose levels later in the day. Giving insulin also will lower glucose levels, causing hypoglycemia. The client wouldn't have hyperglycemia if the glyburide was absorbed.

CN: Physiological integrity; CNS: Pharmacological and parenteral therapies; CL: Analysis

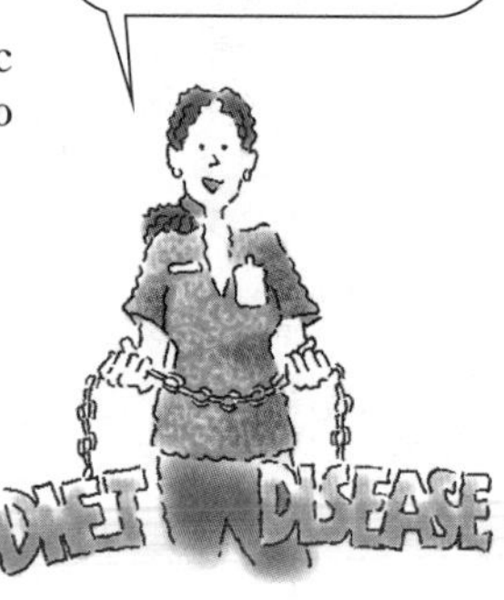

Teach your client about the link between diet and diabetes.
DIET
DISEASE

6. When teaching a newly diagnosed diabetic client about diet and exercise, it's important to include which directive?

1. Use of fiber laxatives and bulk-forming agents
2. Management of fluid, protein, and electrolytes
3. Reduction of calorie intake before exercising
4. Caloric goals, food consistency, and physical activity

6. 4. Diabetic clients must be taught the relationship among caloric goals, consistency of food composition, and physical activity. Fiber laxatives and bulk-forming agents are treatments for constipation. Management of fluids, proteins, and electrolytes is important for a client with acute renal failure. The diabetic client may need to intake additional calories before exercising.

CN: Health promotion and maintenance; CNS: None; CL: Application

7. A nurse is teaching a client with diabetes mellitus about chronic complications associated with the disease. Which information should she include in her teaching?

1. Buy shoes that are a half size larger.
2. Annual eye examinations are recommended.
3. Excessive exercise increases insulin resistance.
4. Podiatry visits are necessary every 5 years.

7. 2. Retinopathy is a chronic complication of diabetes mellitus. Therefore, yearly eye examinations are recommended. Because of the risk of serious foot injuries, shoes should fit properly and be the correct size. Exercise decreases insulin resistance. A podiatrist should be seen on a yearly basis.

CN: Physiological integrity; CNS: Reduction of risk potential; CL: Application

8. Rotating injection sites when administering insulin prevents which complication?
 1. Insulin edema
 2. Insulin lipodystrophy
 3. Insulin resistance
 4. Systemic allergic reactions

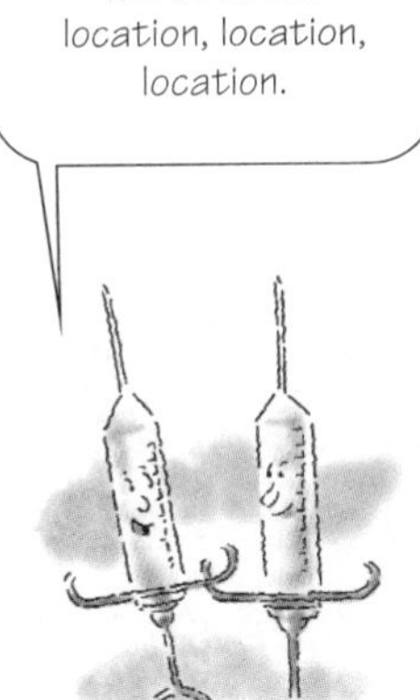

It's all about location, location, location.

8. 2. Insulin lipodystrophy produces fatty masses at the injection sites, causing unpredictable absorption of insulin injected into these sites. Insulin edema is generalized retention of fluid, sometimes seen after normal blood glucose levels are established in a client with prolonged hyperglycemia. Insulin resistance occurs mostly in overweight clients and is due to insulin binding with antibodies, decreasing the amount of absorption. Systemic allergic reactions range from hives to anaphylaxis; rotating injection sites won't prevent these.
CN: Physiological integrity; CNS: Pharmacological and parenteral therapies; CL: Application

9. Which of the following laboratory results would be most important for a nurse to monitor in a client who is on a regimen of twice daily NPH insulin and premeal insulin lispro (Humalog)?
 1. Capillary blood glucose test
 2. Serum ketone test
 3. Serum T_4 test
 4. Urine glucose test

9. 1. A capillary blood glucose test is a rapid test used to show blood glucose levels, which are necessary to give the correct insulin dose. A serum ketone test is used to document diabetic ketoacidosis by titration and may allow determination of serum ketone concentration. A serum T_4 test is used to diagnosis thyroid disorders. Most of the time, however, neither serum ketone levels nor T_4 levels are useful in determining blood glucose levels. A urine glucose test monitors glucose levels in urine and is influenced by both glucose and water excretion. Therefore, results correlate poorly with blood glucose levels.
CN: Physiological integrity; CNS: Reduction of risk potential; CL: Comprehension

10. A client is scheduled to start an insulin regimen. Based on an understanding of peak effect times, which of the following insulin is prescribed to provide basal coverage?
 1. Insulin lispro (Humalog)
 2. Insulin aspart (Novolog)
 3. Novolin NPH
 4. Humalin R

10. 3. Novolin NPH is an intermediate-acting insulin with a peak effect of 6–16 hours. It is used to provide basal coverage. Humalog and Novolog are rapid-acting types of insulin with a peak effect of 2–6 hours. Humalin R is a short-acting insulin with a peak of 2–4 hours.
CN: Physiological integrity; CNS: Pharmacological and parenteral therapies; CL: Application

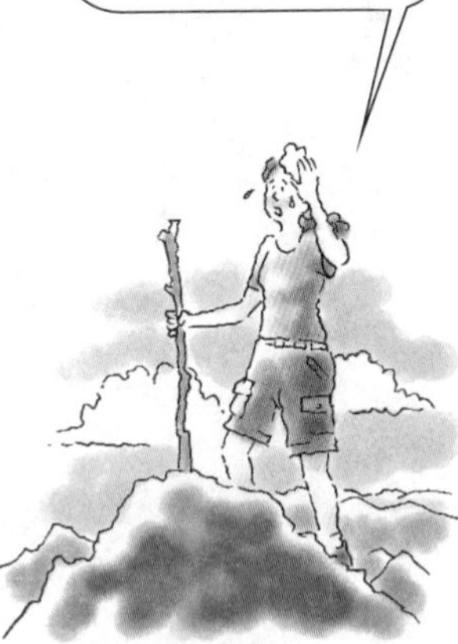

I wonder how long this "peak effect" lasts?

11. A 52-year-old client reports weight gain and tiredness. On assessment, her vital signs are blood pressure 120/74 mm Hg, pulse rate 52 beats/minute, respiratory rate 20 breaths/minute, and temperature 98° F. Laboratory results show low thyroxine (T_4) and triiodothyronine (T_3) levels. The nurse knows these symptoms are associated with which condition?
 1. Tetany
 2. Hypothyroidism
 3. Hyperthyroidism
 4. Hypokalemia

11. 2. Weight gain, lethargy, and slow pulse rate along with decreased T_3 and T_4 levels indicate hypothyroidism. T_3 and T_4 are thyroid hormones that affect growth and development as well as metabolic rate. Tetany is related to low calcium levels. Hypokalemia is a low potassium level.
CN: Physiological integrity; CNS: Physiological adaptation; CL: Analysis

12. The nurse should anticipate administration of which medication to a client with hypothyroidism?

1. Dexamethasone
2. Lactulose
3. Levothyroxine
4. Lidocaine

12. 3. Levothyroxine, a synthetic form of the thyroid hormone T_4, is the medication of choice for treating hypothyroidism. Dexamethasone is a steroid and an antithyroid medication. Lactulose is used to produce an osmotic diarrhea, resulting in an acidic diarrhea. Lidocaine is used to treat ventricular arrhythmias.
CN: Physiological integrity; CNS: Pharmacological and parenteral therapies; CL: Application

13. The thyroid gland is properly palpated by which action?

1. Have the client flex his neck onto his chest and cough while the nurse palpates the anterior neck with her fingertips.
2. Place hands around the client's neck, with the thumbs in the front of the neck, and gently massage the anterior neck.
3. Encircle the client's neck with both hands, have the client slightly extend his neck, and ask him to swallow.
4. Have the client hyperextend his neck and take slow, deep inhalations while the nurse palpates the neck with her fingertips.

13. 3. This approach is the correct method for palpating the thyroid gland. As the client swallows, the gland is palpated for enlargement as the tissue rises and falls. Having the client flex his neck wouldn't allow for palpation. Massaging the area or checking during inhalation doesn't allow for the movement of tissue that swallowing provides.
CN: Physiological integrity; CNS: Reduction of risk potential; CL: Analysis

14. A client with hypothyroidism who experiences trauma, emergency surgery, or severe infection is at risk for developing which condition?

1. Hepatitis B
2. Malignant hyperthermia
3. Myxedema coma
4. Thyroid storm

14. 3. Myxedema coma can be precipitated by opioids, stress (such as surgery), trauma, and infections. It represents the most severe form of hypothyroidism. Hepatitis B is a virus and isn't caused by thyroid disorders. The client would be hypothermic, not hyperthermic. Thyroid storm is a complication of hyperthyroidism.
CN: Physiological integrity; CNS: Pharmacological and parenteral therapies; CL: Application

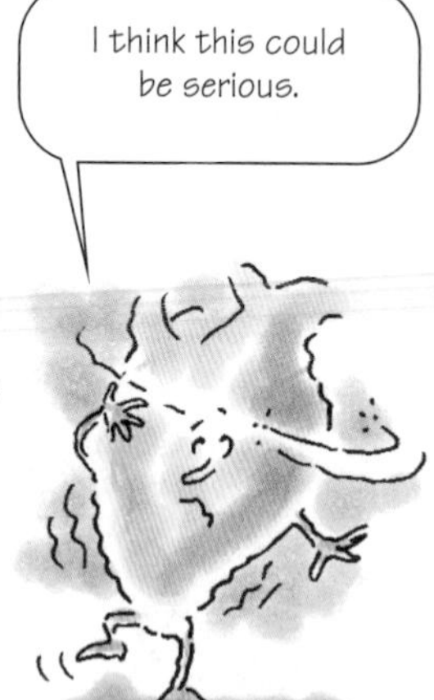
I think this could be serious.

15. When assessing a client who is being treated for hypothyroidism, which of these findings would indicate a potentially serious complication?

1. Chills, fever, and hypotension
2. Palpitations and chest pain
3. Decreased visual acuity
4. Low platelet counts

15. 2. Palpitations and chest pain are cardiac symptoms, which can be precipitated with thyroid replacement therapy, especially in clients with preexisting heart disease. Chills, fever, and hypotension could indicate several complications, such as sepsis related to infection, or transfusion reactions, which are not related to hypothyroid therapy. Decreased visual acuity and low platelet count are not related to hypothyroidism.
CN: Physiological integrity; CNS: Physiological adaptation; CL: Application

16. A client presents with weight gain, intolerance to cold, constipation, and lethargy. Which test should the nurse expect to be ordered?

1. Liver function tests
2. Hemoglobin A_{1C}
3. T_4 and thyroid-stimulating hormone
4. 24-hour urine free cortisol measurement

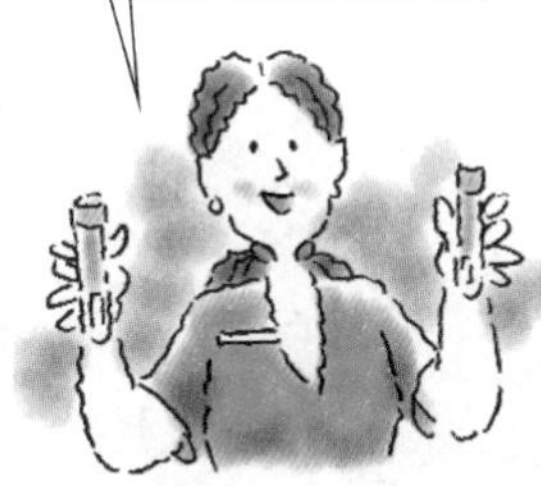

Know which test to order to ensure a proper diagnosis.

16. 3. The client's symptoms suggest hypothyroidism. Levels of thyroid-stimulating hormone and T_4 should be measured if hypothyroidism is suspected. Liver function tests are used to determine liver disease. Hemoglobin A_{1C} measurement is used to assess hyperglycemia. As part of the screening process for Cushing's syndrome, a 24-hour urine free cortisol measurement is completed.

CN: Physiological integrity; CNS: Physiological adaptation; CL: Application

17. A client with hypothyroidism may present with which symptom?

1. Polyuria, polydipsia, and weight loss
2. Heat intolerance, nervousness, weight loss, and hair loss
3. Coarsening of facial features and extremity enlargement
4. Tiredness, cold intolerance, weight gain, and constipation

17. 4. Tiredness, cold intolerance, weight gain, and constipation are symptoms of hypothyroidism, secondary to a decrease in cellular metabolism. Polyuria, polydipsia, and weight loss are symptoms of type 1 diabetes mellitus. Hyperthyroidism has symptoms of heat intolerance, nervousness, weight loss, and hair loss. Coarsening of facial features and extremity enlargement are symptoms of acromegaly.

CN: Physiological integrity; CNS: Physiological adaptation; CL: Application

18. After a client is admitted with an adrenal malfunction, the nurse demonstrates an understanding of the function of the adrenal gland by identifying which hormones as being released by the adrenal medulla?

1. Epinephrine and norepinephrine
2. Glucocorticoids, mineralocorticoids, and androgens
3. Thyroxine, triiodothryonine, and calcitonin
4. Insulin, glucagon, and somatostatin

18. 1. The medulla of the adrenal gland causes the release of epinephrine and norepinephrine. Glucocorticoids, mineralocorticoids, and androgens are released from the adrenal cortex. Thyroxine, triiodothyronine, and calcitonin are secreted by the thyroid gland. The islet cells of the pancreas secrete insulin, glucagon, and somatostatin.

CN: Physiological integrity; CNS: Physiological adaptation; CL: Analysis

19. A client is scheduled for several tests. Which test should be performed after the thyroid function tests?

1. Ultrasound of the carotid arteries
2. EEG
3. Chest X-ray
4. Computed tomography scan of the head with contrast

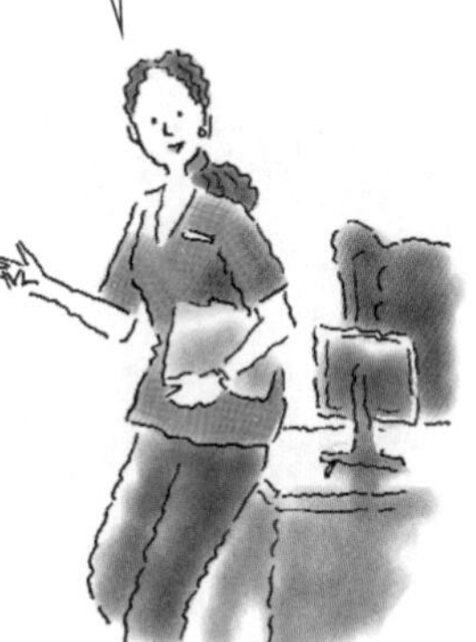

Sometimes the order of the tests performed is as important as the results.

19. 4. Contrast media contains iodine and can alter thyroid function test results. The other studies don't require contrast media and don't need to be performed after the thyroid function tests.

CN: Physiological integrity; CNS: Reduction of risk potential; CL: Application

20. Which disorder can cause a client to retain fluid and develop hyponatremia secondary to the inability to excrete dilute urine?
1. Thyrotoxic crisis
2. Diabetes insipidus
3. Primary adrenocortical insufficiency
4. Syndrome of inappropriate antidiuretic hormone (SIADH)

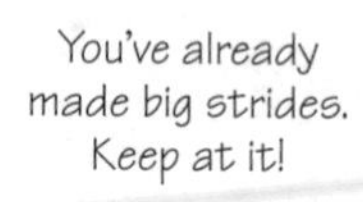

You've already made big strides. Keep at it!

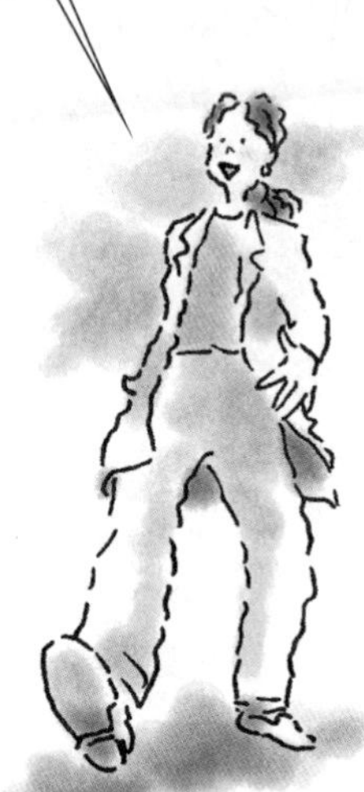

20. 4. SIADH is a condition in which the client has excessive levels of antidiuretic hormone (ADH) and can't excrete the dilute urine. Therefore, the client retains fluids. This disorder causes a dilutional hyponatremia. Thyrotoxic crisis occurs with severe hyperthyroidism. Diabetes insipidus creates an ADH deficiency, causing dilute urine and hypernatremia. Primary adrenocortical insufficiency (Addison's disease) is caused by deficiency of a cortical hormone.
CN: Physiological integrity; CNS: Reduction of risk potential; CL: Application

21. Adrenal insufficiency develops secondary to inadequate secretion of which pituitary hormone?
1. Corticotropin
2. Antidiuretic hormone (ADH)
3. Follicle-stimulating hormone (FSH)
4. Thyroid-stimulating hormone (TSH)

21. 1. Inadequate secretion of corticotropin from the pituitary gland results in adrenal insufficiency. ADH is secreted by the pituitary gland but doesn't affect the adrenal gland. FSH is also secreted by the pituitary gland but doesn't affect the adrenal gland; it stimulates the gonads. TSH is also secreted by the pituitary gland and stimulates the thyroid gland.
CN: Physiological integrity; CNS: Reduction of risk potential; CL: Application

22. A nurse is caring for a client with syndrome of inappropriate antidiuretic hormone (SIADH). Which laboratory value is most important for the nurse to monitor?
1. Glucose
2. Hemoglobin
3. Creatinine
4. Sodium

22. 4. SIADH occurs as a result of excessive release of antidiuretic hormone which disturbs fluid and electrolyte balance, especially sodium. Clients need to be closely monitored for hyponatremia.
CN: Physiological integrity; CNS: Reduction of risk potential; CL: Analysis

23. A 37-year-old client complains of muscle weakness, anorexia, and darkening of his skin. The nurse reviews his laboratory data and notes findings of low serum sodium and high serum potassium levels. The nurse recognizes these signs and symptoms are associated with which condition?
1. Addison's disease
2. Cushing's disease
3. Diabetes insipidus
4. Thyrotoxic crisis

23. 1. The clinical picture of Addison's disease includes muscle weakness, anorexia, darkening of the skin's pigmentation, low sodium level, and high potassium level. Cushing's syndrome presents with obesity, "buffalo hump," "moonface," and thin extremities. Symptoms of diabetes insipidus include excretion of large volumes of dilute urine, leading to hypernatremia and dehydration. Thyrotoxic crisis can occur with severe hyperthyroidism.
CN: Physiological integrity; CNS: Physiological adaptation; CL: Application

24. A nurse is caring for a client following surgical ablation of the pituitary gland. Which condition must she be alert for?

1. Addison's disease
2. Cushing's syndrome
3. Diabetes insipidus
4. Hypothyroidism

24. 3. The cause of diabetes insipidus is unknown, but it may be secondary to head trauma, brain tumors, or surgical ablation of the pituitary gland. Addison's disease is caused by a deficiency of cortical hormones, whereas Cushing's syndrome is an excess of cortical hormones. Hypothyroidism occurs when the thyroid gland secretes low levels of thyroid hormone.

CN: Physiological integrity; CNS: Physiological adaptation; CL: Analysis

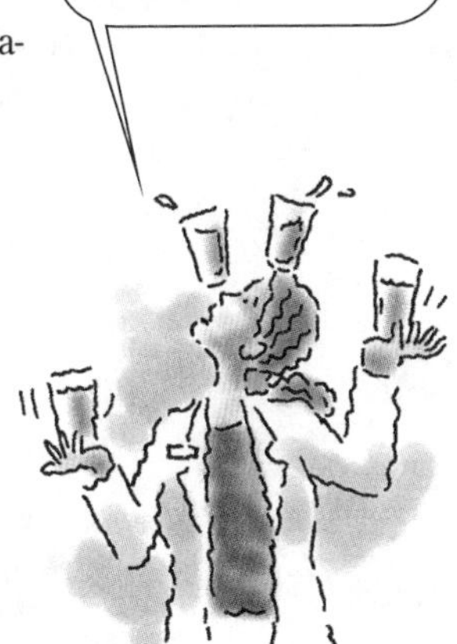

Knowing how much water a client should have can be a real juggling act.

25. If fluid intake is limited in a client with diabetes insipidus, which complication will he be at risk for developing?

1. Hypertension and bradycardia
2. Glucosuria and weight gain
3. Peripheral edema and hyperglycemia
4. Severe dehydration and hypernatremia

25. 4. A client with diabetes insipidus has high volumes of urine, even without fluid replacement. Therefore, limiting fluid intake will cause severe dehydration and hypernatremia. A client undergoing a fluid deprivation test may experience tachycardia and hypotension. A client with diabetes insipidus will usually experience weight loss, and his urine doesn't contain glucose. Diabetes insipidus has no effect on blood glucose. Therefore, the client wouldn't suffer from hyperglycemia. Peripheral edema isn't a symptom of diabetes insipidus.

CN: Physiological integrity; CNS: Physiological adaptation; CL: Analysis

26. When caring for a client with a diagnosis of diabetes insipidus, which nursing intervention should be the priority?

1. Watching for signs and symptoms of septic shock.
2. Maintain adequate fluid intake.
3. Check weight every 3 days.
4. Monitor urine for specific gravity greater than 1.030.

26. 2. In a client with diabetes insipidus, maintaining fluid intake is essential to prevent severe dehydration. The client is at risk for developing hypovolemic shock because of increased urine output. Weight should be measured on a daily basis to check for adequate fluid balance. Urine specific gravity should be monitored for low osmolality, generally less than 1.005, due to the body's inability to concentrate urine.

CN: Safe, effective care environment; CNS: Management of care; CL: Application

27. Which disorder is suggested by polydipsia and large amounts of waterlike urine with a specific gravity of 1.003?

1. Diabetes mellitus
2. Diabetes insipidus
3. Diabetic ketoacidosis
4. Syndrome of inappropriate antidiuretic hormone (SIADH)

27. 2. Diabetes insipidus is characterized by a great thirst (polydipsia) and large amounts of waterlike urine, which has a specific gravity of 1.001 to 1.005. Diabetes mellitus presents with polydipsia, polyuria, and polyphagia, but the client also has hyperglycemia. Diabetic ketoacidosis presents with weight loss, polyuria, and polydipsia, and the client has a severe acidosis. A client with SIADH can't excrete a dilute urine; he retains fluid and develops a sodium deficiency.

CN: Physiological integrity; CNS: Physiological adaptation; CL: Analysis

28. A client with diabetes insipidus is receiving desmopressin (DDAVP). Which adverse effect associated with DDAVP administration should be immediately reported to the physician?

1. Rash and difficulty breathing
2. Abdominal cramping
3. Burning at the injection site
4. Headache

28. 1. Rash and difficulty breathing may indicate an allergic reaction to the medication which requires immediate intervention. The other symptoms may occur but aren't life-threatening.

CN: Physiological integrity; CNS: Pharmacological and parenteral therapies; CL: Application

29. The nurse is caring for a client with a low vasopressin level. In teaching the client about the illness, which of the following areas of the body would the nurse describe as the area where the deficiency originates?

1. Adrenal gland
2. Parathyroid gland
3. Pituitary gland
4. Thyroid gland

29. 3. Low vasopressin level is a deficiency of antidiuretic hormone, which is a disorder of the posterior pituitary gland. The adrenal, parathyroid, and thyroid glands aren't involved.

CN: Physiological integrity; CNS: Physiological adaptation; CL: Application

30. A client is diagnosed with diabetes insipidus. The nurse develops a care plan based on the understanding that which hormone is deficient?

1. Androgen
2. Epinephrine
3. Norepinephrine
4. Vasopressin

30. 4. Clients with diabetes insipidus have a deficiency of vasopressin, the antidiuretic hormone. Androgen, epinephrine, and norepinephrine are hormones secreted by the adrenal gland and aren't related to diabetes insipidus.

CN: Physiological integrity; CNS: Physiological adaptation; CL: Knowledge

31. Which test is used to diagnose diabetes insipidus?

1. Capillary blood glucose test
2. Fluid deprivation test
3. Serum ketone test
4. Urine glucose test

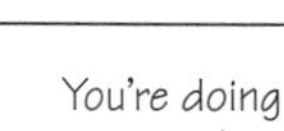

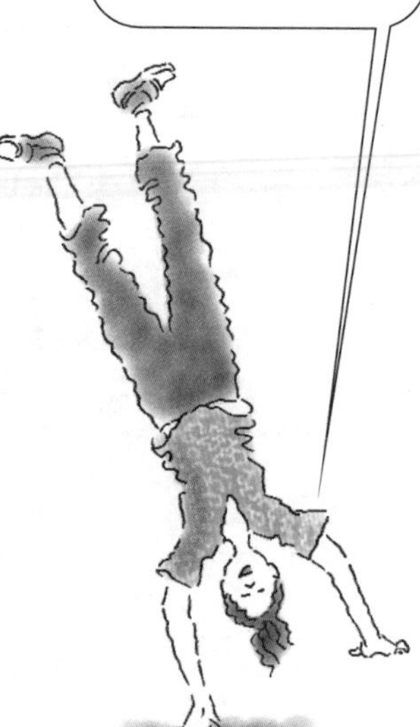

31. 2. The fluid deprivation test involves withholding water for 4 to 18 hours and checking urine osmolarity periodically. Plasma osmolarity is also checked. A client with diabetes insipidus will have an increased serum osmolarity (of less than 300 mOsm/kg). Urine osmolarity won't increase. The capillary blood glucose test allows a rapid measurement of glucose in whole blood. The serum ketone test documents diabetic ketoacidosis. The urine glucose test monitors glucose levels in urine, but diabetes insipidus doesn't affect urine glucose levels.

CN: Physiological integrity; CNS: Reduction of risk potential; CL: Analysis

32. Which medical emergency may occur when a client with Addison's disease develops acute hypotension secondary to hypoadrenocorticism?
1. Addisonian crisis
2. Diabetic ketoacidosis
3. Myxedema
4. Thyrotoxic crisis

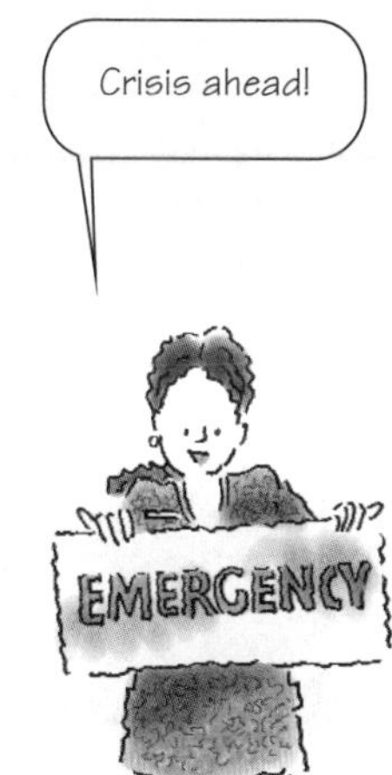
Crisis ahead!
EMERGENCY

32. 1. As Addison's disease progresses, the client moves into an addisonian crisis, a medical emergency marked by cyanosis, fever, and signs of shock. Diabetic ketoacidosis is a form of hyperglycemia. Myxedema is a form of severe hypothyroidism. Thyrotoxic crisis is a form of severe hyperthyroidism.
CN: Physiological integrity; CNS: Physiological adaptation; CL: Analysis

33. A client with Addison's disease would exhibit which sign or symptoms?
1. Hunger
2. Muscle spasm
3. Weight gain
4. Lethargy

33. 4. Lethargy and depression are early symptoms of Addison's disease. Most clients experience loss of appetite and weight loss. Muscles become weak not spastic.
CN: Physiological integrity; CNS: Physiological adaptation; CL: Application

34. What's the best indicator for determining if a client with Addison's disease is receiving the correct amount of glucocorticoid replacement?
1. Daily weight
2. Temperature
3. Skin turgor
4. Blood pressure

34. 1. Daily weight is an objective way to monitor fluid balance. Rapid variations in weight reflect changes in fluid volume and the need for more glucocorticoids. Temperature and blood pressure aren't direct measurements of fluid balance. Skin turgor isn't as reliable as daily weight.
CN: Physiological integrity; CNS: Physiological adaptation; CL: Application

35. Which intervention is the priority for a client with addisonian crisis?
1. Preventing irreversible shock
2. Preventing infection
3. Relieving anxiety
4. Lowering blood pressure

35. 1. In addisonian crisis there's an uncontrolled loss of sodium in the urine and impaired mineralocorticoid function resulting in loss of extracellular fluid and low blood volume and possible irreversible shock. Preventing infection isn't an appropriate goal in this life-threatening situation. Relieving anxiety is appropriate after the client is stabilized. The client in addisonian crisis is hypotensive so blood pressure should be raised not lowered.
CN: Safe, effective care environment; CNS: Management of care; CL: Analysis

36. A nurse reviews the laboratory data of a 60-year-old client. The data reveals increased blood and urine levels of triiodothyronine (T_3) and thyroxine (T_4). The nurse knows these values are associated with which condition?
1. Addison's disease
2. Cushing's syndrome
3. Hyperthyroidism
4. Hypopituitarism

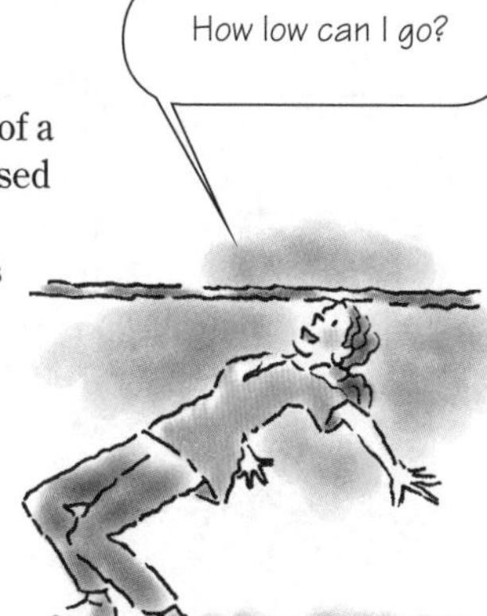
How low can I go?

36. 3. With hyperthyroidism, the client has high levels of T_3 and T_4. A definitive diagnosis of Addison's disease must reflect low levels of adrenocortical hormones. A client with Cushing's syndrome would have excessive amounts of adrenocortical hormones. Lower pituitary hormone secretion levels are consistent with hypopituitarism.
CN: Physiological integrity; CNS: Physiological adaptation; CL: Analysis

37. An appropriate nursing diagnosis for a client with Addison's disease would include which assessment?
1. *Fatigue*
2. *Excess fluid volume*
3. *Ineffective thermoregulation*
4. *Impaired gas exchange*

37. 1. Clients with Addison's disease experience fatigue related to decreased metabolic energy production and altered body chemistry. Clients with Addison's disease experience fluid volume deficit, secondary to decreased mineralocorticoid secretion. Heat intolerance is a symptom of hyperthyroidism. The respiratory system isn't directly affected, and gas exchange shouldn't be affected.

CN: Health promotion and maintenance; CNS: None; CL: Analysis

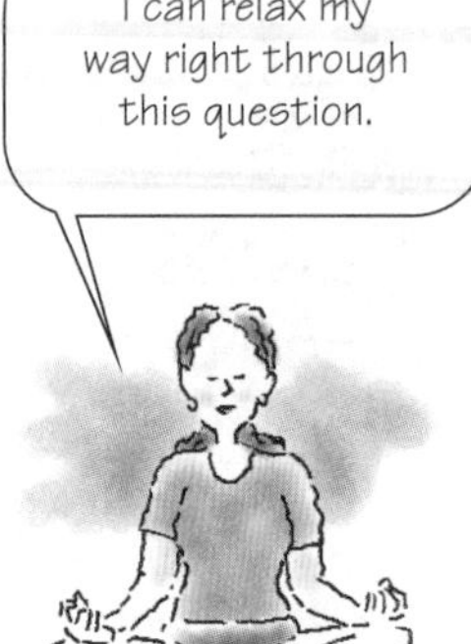

I can relax my way right through this question.

38. Nursing care for a client with Addison's disease may include which goal?
1. Limiting fluid intake to 100 ml/day
2. Participating in relaxation techniques
3. Ambulating in the hall five to six times per day
4. Knowing which high-sodium foods to avoid

38. 2. Stress can precipitate a hypotensive crisis in clients with Addison's disease. These clients need to learn ways to identify and cope with stressors. Fluids shouldn't be restricted; fluid intake should be 3 qt (3 L) or more per day. Activity should be monitored closely for fatigue and weakness. Sodium shouldn't be restricted.

CN: Physiological integrity; CNS: Physiological adaptation; CL: Analysis

39. Which outcome is expected for a client being treated for Addison's disease?
1. Avoiding alcohol to decrease abdominal girth
2. Avoiding hot and uncomfortable environments
3. Reporting absence of postural hypotension symptoms
4. Selecting and eating foods high in protein, calcium, and vitamin D

39. 3. Clients with Addison's disease may experience postural hypotension if the hormone replacement dose is too low. Clients with pancreatitis may have an increase in abdominal girth with alcohol consumption. A large abdomen isn't a typical finding with Addison's disease. Clients with hyperthyroidism should avoid hot and uncomfortable environments because the disorder causes heat intolerance. A diet high in protein, calcium, and vitamin D would be beneficial for clients with Cushing's syndrome. Clients with Addison's disease must monitor salt intake.

CN: Physiological integrity; CNS: Physiological adaptation; CL: Analysis

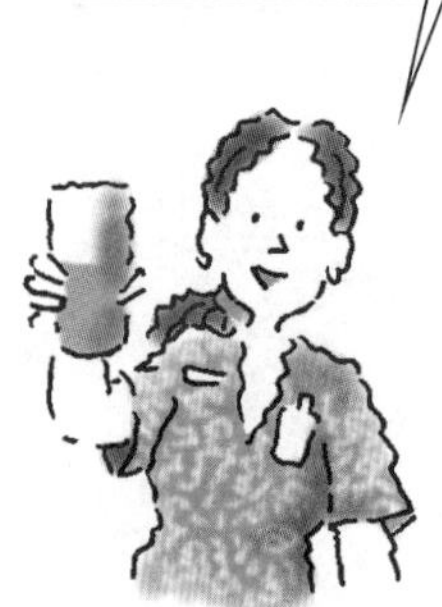

Here's to you! You've finished 40 questions already! That's excellent!

40. A nurse can expect to see which signs and symptoms when a client overproduces adrenocortical hormone?
1. Arrested growth and obesity
2. Weight loss and heat intolerance
3. Changes in skin texture and low body temperature
4. Polyuria and dehydration

40. 1. Overproduction of adrenocortical hormone results in growth arrest and obesity. Weight loss and heat intolerance indicate thyroid hormone overproduction. Changes in skin texture and low body temperature indicate thyroid hormone underproduction. Polyuria and dehydration indicate diabetic ketoacidosis.

CN: Physiological integrity; CNS: Physiological adaptation; CL: Application

41. A client has thin extremities but an obese truncal area and a "buffalo hump" at the shoulder area. The client also complains of weakness and disturbed sleep. What long-term complication can develop from this disorder?

1. Pathologic fractures
2. Diabetes mellitus
3. Ataxia
4. Mèniére's disease

41. 2. The symptoms describe Cushing's syndrome. One of the long-term complications may be diabetes mellitus. The other choices do not relate to Cushing's syndrome.

CN: Physiological integrity; CNS: Physiological adaptation; CL: Analysis

42. Sodium and water retention in a client with Cushing's syndrome contribute to which commonly seen disorders?

1. Hypoglycemia and dehydration
2. Hypotension and hyperglycemia
3. Pulmonary edema and dehydration
4. Hypertension and heart failure

42. 4. Increased mineralocorticoid activity resulting in sodium and water retention in a client with Cushing's syndrome commonly contributes to hypertension and heart failure. Hypoglycemia and dehydration are uncommon in a client with Cushing's syndrome. Diabetes mellitus and hyperglycemia may develop, but hypotension is *not* part of the disease process. Pulmonary edema and dehydration also aren't complications of Cushing's syndrome.

CN: Physiological integrity; CNS: Physiological adaptation; CL: Analysis

43. High serum sodium and glucose levels, low potassium level and eosinophil count, and disappearance of lymphoid tissue are associated with which disease process?

1. Addison's disease
2. Cushing's syndrome
3. Graves' disease
4. Myxedema

43. 2. Test results in Cushing's syndrome include high serum sodium and glucose levels, low potassium level, reduction of eosinophils, and disappearance of lymphoid tissue. Addison's disease is the opposite of Cushing's syndrome, with low serum sodium and glucose levels and a high potassium level. Graves' disease would have increased thyroid hormone levels. Myxedema would have low levels of thyroid hormones.

CN: Physiological integrity; CNS: Physiological adaptation; CL: Analysis

44. A client presents with a "buffalo hump" at the shoulder area and an obese truncal area with thin extremities. Which test should the nurse anticipate?

1. Fluid deprivation test
2. Glucose tolerance test
3. Low-dose dexamethasone suppression test
4. Thallium stress test

44. 3. A low-dose dexamethasone suppression test is used to detect changes in plasma cortisol levels and to diagnose Cushing's syndrome. A fluid deprivation test is used to diagnose diabetes insipidus. The glucose tolerance test is used to determine gestational diabetes in pregnant women. A thallium stress test is used to monitor heart function under stress.

CN: Physiological integrity; CNS: Physiological adaptation; CL: Analysis

45. Treatment for Cushing's syndrome may involve removal of one of the adrenal glands, which could cause a temporary state of which condition?

1. Hyperkalemia
2. Adrenal insufficiency
3. Excessive adrenal hormone
4. Syndrome of inappropriate antidiuretic hormone (SIADH)

45. 2. Removing a major source of adrenal hormones may cause a state of temporary adrenal insufficiency, requiring short-term replacement therapy. When both adrenal glands are removed, the client requires lifelong hormone replacement. A client with Cushing's syndrome would have a low—not high—potassium level. The client wouldn't have excessive adrenal hormone if all or part of the adrenal glands were removed. SIADH doesn't involve the adrenal gland; it involves the pituitary gland.
CN: Physiological integrity; CNS: Physiological adaptation; CL: Analysis

46. Which nursing diagnosis is appropriate for a client with Cushing's syndrome?

1. *Risk for infection*
2. *Deficient fluid volume*
3. *Acute pain*
4. *Functional urinary incontinence*

46. 1. Clients with Cushing's syndrome have an increased susceptibility to injury or infection, secondary to the immunosuppression caused by excessive cortisol. Fluid volume deficit, related to inadequate adrenal hormones, is common in clients with Addison's disease. Pain and functional incontinence aren't common in Cushing's syndrome.
CN: Physiological integrity; CNS: Reduction of risk potential; CL: Application

47. Which nursing intervention should be performed for a client with Cushing's syndrome?

1. Suggest clothing or bedding that is cool and comfortable.
2. Suggest consumption of high-carbohydrate and low-protein foods.
3. Explain that physical changes are a result of excessive corticosteroids.
4. Explain the rationale for increasing salt and fluid intake in times of illness, increased stress, and very hot weather.

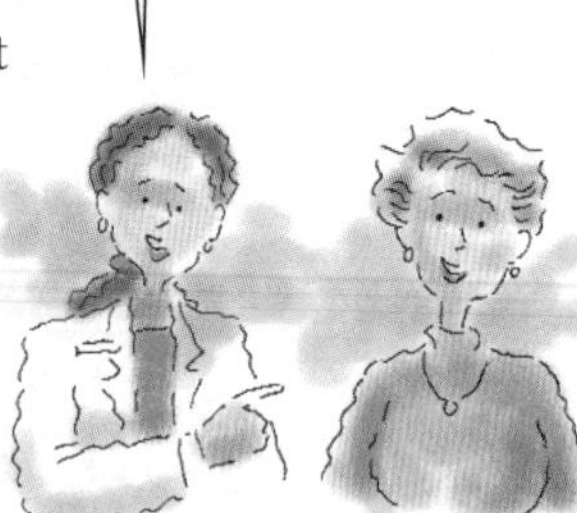

Explaining physical changes that may result from corticosteroid use can help ease your client's mind.

47. 3. Clients with Cushing's syndrome have physical changes related to excessive corticosteroids. Clients with hyperthyroidism are heat intolerant and must have comfortable, cool clothing and bedding. Clients with Cushing's syndrome should have a high-protein, not low-protein, diet. Clients with Addison's disease must increase sodium intake and fluid intake in times of stress to prevent hypotension.
CN: Physiological integrity; CNS: Physiological adaptation; CL: Application

48. Which disease process is caused by an absence of insulin or inadequate amount of insulin, resulting in hyperglycemia and leading to a series of biochemical disorders?

1. Diabetes insipidus
2. Hyperaldosteronism
3. Diabetic ketoacidosis
4. Hyperosmolar hyperglycemic nonketotic syndrome (HHNS)

48. 3. Diabetic ketoacidosis is caused by inadequate amounts of insulin or absence of insulin, and leads to a series of biochemical disorders. Diabetes insipidus is caused by a deficiency of vasopressin. Hyperaldosteronism is an excess in aldosterone production, causing sodium and fluid excesses and hypertension. HHNS is a coma state in which hyperglycemia and hyperosmolarity dominate.
CN: Physiological integrity; CNS: Physiological adaptation; CL: Analysis

49. A client who is insulin-dependent fails to take insulin regularly; he is at risk for which complication?

1. Diabetic ketoacidosis
2. Hypoglycemia
3. Pancreatitis
4. Respiratory failure

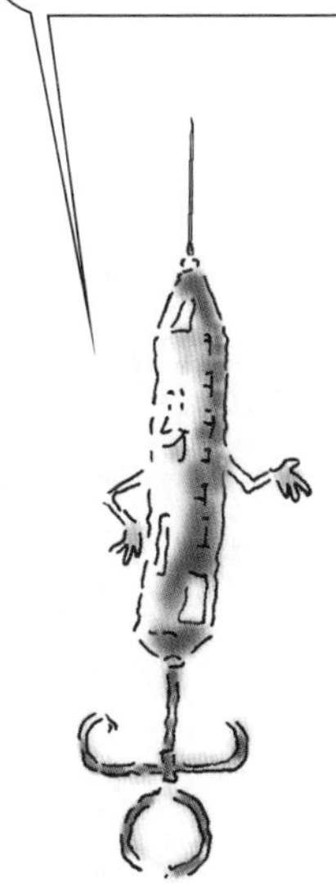

I'm a real shot in the arm towards your client's good health.

49. 1. A client who fails to regularly take his insulin is at risk for hyperglycemia, which could lead to diabetic ketoacidosis. Hypoglycemia wouldn't occur because the lack of insulin would lead to increased levels of sugar in the blood. A client with chronic pancreatitis may develop diabetes (secondary to the pancreatitis), but insulin-dependent diabetes mellitus doesn't lead to pancreatitis. Respiratory failure isn't related to insulin levels.

CN: Physiological integrity; CNS: Physiological adaptation; CL: Application

50. A client with diabetes presents with polyphagia, polydipsia, and oliguria; he also complains of headache, malaise, and some visual changes. Assessment shows signs of dehydration. Which diagnosis could be made?

1. Diabetes insipidus
2. Diabetic ketoacidosis
3. Hypoglycemia
4. Syndrome of inappropriate antidiuretic hormone (SIADH)

50. 2. Early manifestations of diabetic ketoacidosis include polydipsia, polyphagia, and polyuria. As the client dehydrates and loses electrolytes, this condition often leads to oliguria, malaise, and visual changes. Diabetes insipidus may result in dehydration but not polyphagia and polydipsia. Symptoms of hypoglycemia include diaphoresis, tachycardia, and nervousness. A client with SIADH is unable to excrete a dilute urine, causing hyponatremia.

CN: Physiological integrity; CNS: Physiological adaptation; CL: Application

51. The nurse is completing a physical assessment of the thyroid gland on a client. This is most commonly done as the nurse is also assessing which part of the body?

1. Head and neck
2. Lungs
3. Abdomen
4. Genitalia

51. 1. The thyroid gland is located in the lower neck near the trachea. The thyroid gland is not located in any of the other body areas listed.

CN: Health promotions and maintenance; CNS: None; CL: Application

52. A client exhibiting exophthalmus, weight loss, and tachycardia would be evaluated by checking the levels of which hormones?

1. Amylase, lipase, and trypsin
2. Triiodothyronine (T_3), thyroxine (T_4), and thyroid-stimulating hormone (TSH)
3. Glucocorticoids, mineralocorticoids, and androgens
4. Vasopressin and oxytocin

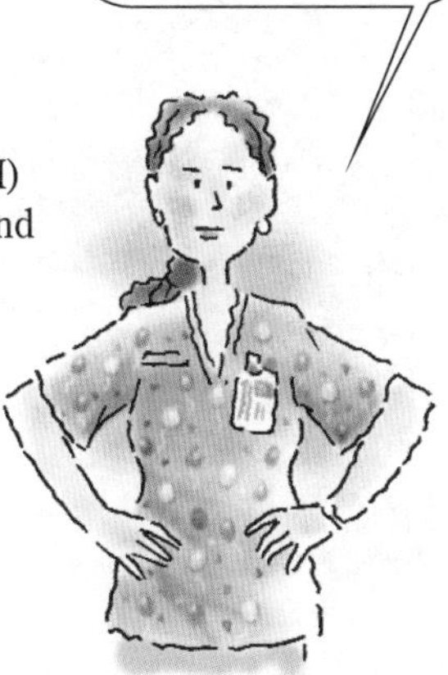

Do you know which glands produce which hormones? Here's a chance to test your knowledge.

52. 2. The symptoms reflect a potential dysfunction of the thyroid gland. T_3, T_4, and TSH are all secreted by the thyroid gland. Amylase, lipase, and trypsin are enzymes produced by the pancreas that aid in digestion. Glucocorticoids, mineralocorticoids, and androgens are produced by the adrenal gland. The pituitary gland secretes vasopressin and oxytocin.

CN: Health promotion and maintenance; CNS: None; CL: Application

53. The nurse is teaching a client with hypothyroidism about the thyroid gland. Which of the following statements by the nurse would be the most accurate about which gland controls the secretion of thyroid hormone?

1. Adrenal gland
2. Parathyroid gland
3. Pituitary gland
4. Thyroid gland

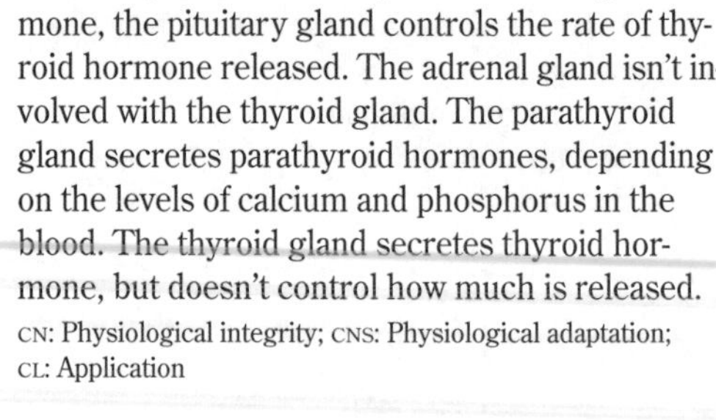

53. 3. By secretion of thyroid-stimulating hormone, the pituitary gland controls the rate of thyroid hormone released. The adrenal gland isn't involved with the thyroid gland. The parathyroid gland secretes parathyroid hormones, depending on the levels of calcium and phosphorus in the blood. The thyroid gland secretes thyroid hormone, but doesn't control how much is released.

CN: Physiological integrity; CNS: Physiological adaptation; CL: Application

54. Which treatment can be used for hyperthyroidism?

1. Cholelithotomy
2. Irradiation of the thyroid
3. Administration of oral thyroid hormones
4. Whipple procedure

54. 2. Irradiation, involving administration of the ^{131}I, destroys the thyroid gland and thereby treats hyperthyroidism. Cholelithotomy is used to treat gallstones. Oral thyroid hormones are the treatment for hypothyroidism. The Whipple procedure is a surgical treatment for pancreatic cancer.

CN: Physiological integrity; CNS: Pharmacological and parenteral therapies; CL: Analysis

55. Which group of symptoms of hyperthyroidism is <u>most commonly</u> found in elderly clients?

1. Depression, apathy, and weight loss
2. Palpitations, irritability, and heat intolerance
3. Cold intolerance, weight gain, and thinning hair
4. Numbness, tingling, and cramping of extremities

55. 1. Most elderly clients present with depression, apathy, and weight loss, which are typical signs and symptoms of hyperthyroidism. Palpitations, irritability, and heat intolerance can be present with hyperthyroidism, but these aren't typical symptoms in elderly clients. Cold intolerance, weight gain, and thinning hair are some of the signs of hypothyroidism. Numbness, tingling, and cramping of extremities are symptoms of hypocalcemia, which may be a symptom of hypoparathyroidism.

CN: Physiological integrity; CNS: Physiological adaptation; CL: Application

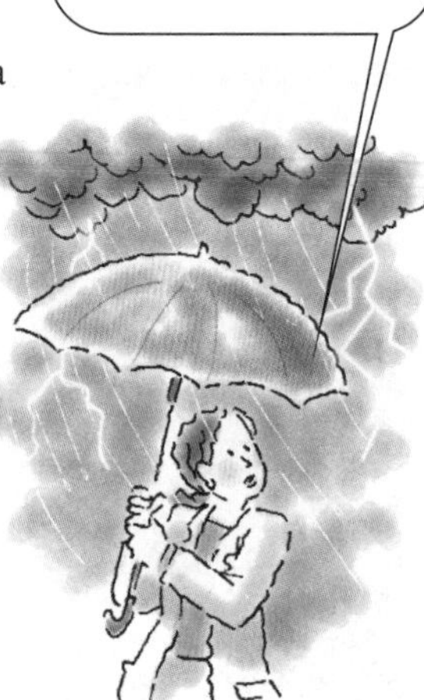
I think there's a storm on the way.

56. A client with hyperthyroidism develops a high fever, extreme tachycardia, and altered mental status. The nurse suspects which of the following?

1. Hepatic coma
2. Thyroid storm
3. Myxedema coma
4. Hyperosmolar hyperglycemic nonketotic syndrome (HHNS)

56. 2. Thyroid storm is a form of severe hyperthyroidism that can be precipitated by stress, injury, or infection. Hepatic coma occurs in clients with profound liver failure. Myxedema coma is a rare disorder characterized by hypoventilation, hypotension, hypoglycemia, and hypothyroidism. HHNS occurs in clients with type 2 diabetes mellitus who are dehydrated and have severe hyperglycemia.

CN: Physiological integrity; CNS: Physiological adaptation; CL: Analysis

57. A client is admitted with Graves' disease. Which laboratory test should the nurse expect to be ordered?

1. Serum glucose
2. Serum calcium
3. Lipid panel
4. Thyroid panel

57. 4. Hyperthyroidism is known as Graves' disease. Therefore the nurse should expect a thyroid panel to be ordered.
CN: Physiological integrity; CNS: Physiological adaptation; CL: Application

58. A client is admitted with a diagnosis of hyperparathyroidism. Which of the following characteristics would the nurse anticipate the client to present?

1. Bulging eyes
2. Renal calculi
3. Weight gain
4. Weight loss

58. 2. Hyperparathyroidism is overproduction of parathyroid hormone, characterized by bone calcification or renal calculi. Bulging eyes and weight loss are signs of hyperthyroidism and weight gain is a sign of hypothyroidism.
CN: Physiological integrity; CNS: Physiological adaptation; CL: Application

59. A client presents with flushed skin, bulging eyes, and perspiration, and states that he has been "irritable" and having palpitations. This client is presenting with symptoms of which disorder?

1. Hyperthyroidism
2. Hyperparathyroidism
3. Hypothyroidism
4. Type 1 diabetes mellitus

59. 1. Signs and symptoms of hyperthyroidism include nervousness, palpitations, irritability, bulging eyes, heat intolerance, weight loss, and weakness. Hyperparathyroidism is characterized by weakness and anorexia. Signs and symptoms of hypothyroidism include fatigue, cool skin, and sensitivity to cold. Type 1 diabetes mellitus presents with polyuria, polydipsia, and weight loss.
CN: Physiological integrity; CNS: Physiological adaptation; CL: Analysis

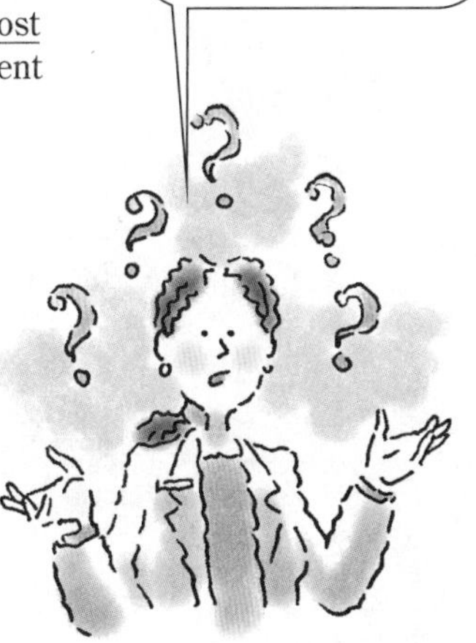
The words most important are a clue to how to answer question 60.

60. Which of the following would be most important for the nurse to assess in a client with anterior pituitary hypofunction?

1. Date of least menstrual period
2. Weight gain
3. Changes in urinary output
4. Chest pain

60. 1. Amenorrhea is a sign of decreased follicle-stimulation hormone, which is one of the anterior pituitary hormones. Weight gain is associated with Cushing's syndrome, which is associated with the adrenal cortex. Urinary output is related to posterior pituitary function and chest pain is not related to hormone levels.
CN: Health promotion and maintenance; CNS: None; CL: Application

61. A client is brought into the emergency department with a brain stem contusion. Two days after admission, the client has a large amount of urine and a serum sodium level of 155 mEq/dl. Which condition may be developing?

1. Myxedema coma
2. Diabetes insipidus
3. Type 1 diabetes mellitus
4. Syndrome of inappropriate antidiuretic hormone (SIADH)

61. 2. Two leading causes of diabetes insipidus are hypothalamic or pituitary tumors and closed head injuries. Myxedema coma is a form of hypothyroidism. Type 1 diabetes mellitus isn't caused by a brain injury. A client with SIADH would have hyponatremia; this client's sodium level was 155 mEq/dl, which is above normal levels of 135 to 145 mEq/dl.

CN: Physiological integrity; CNS: Reduction of risk potential; CL: Application

62. A client is exhibiting Kussmaul's respirations, abdominal discomfort, and lethargy. If a random serum glucose is 325 mg/dl, which additional test should be conducted?

1. Complete blood count (CBC)
2. Serum ketones
3. Blood urea nitrogen (BUN)/creatinine
4. Liver enzymes

62. 2. Clients with Kussmaul's respirations, abdominal discomfort, lethargy, and serum glucose levels above 300 mg/dl could be diagnosed with diabetic ketoacidosis. Serum ketones would aid in confirming the diagnosis. CBC, BUN/creatinine, and liver enzymes are not indicated in a diabetic ketoacidosis workup.

CN: Physiological integrity; CNS: Reduction of risk potential; CL: Application

Make sure you know which disorder the question is asking you to treat.

63. Objectives for treating diabetic ketoacidosis (DKA) include administration of which treatment?

1. Glucagon
2. Blood products
3. Glucocorticoids
4. Insulin and I.V. fluids

63. 4. A client with DKA would receive insulin to lower glucose and I.V. fluids to correct hypotension. Glucagon is given to treat hypoglycemia; DKA involves hyperglycemia. Blood products aren't needed to correct DKA. Glucocorticoids aren't needed because the adrenal glands aren't involved.

CN: Physiological integrity; CNS: Pharmacological and parenteral therapies; CL: Application

64. Which method of insulin administration would be used in the initial treatment of hyperglycemia in a client with diabetic ketoacidosis?

1. Subcutaneous
2. I.M.
3. I.V. bolus only
4. I.V. bolus, followed by continuous infusion

64. 4. An I.V. bolus of insulin is given initially to control the hyperglycemia, followed by a continuous infusion that's titrated to control blood glucose. After the client is stabilized, subcutaneous insulin is given. Insulin is never given I.M.

CN: Physiological integrity; CNS: Pharmacological and parenteral therapies; CL: Application

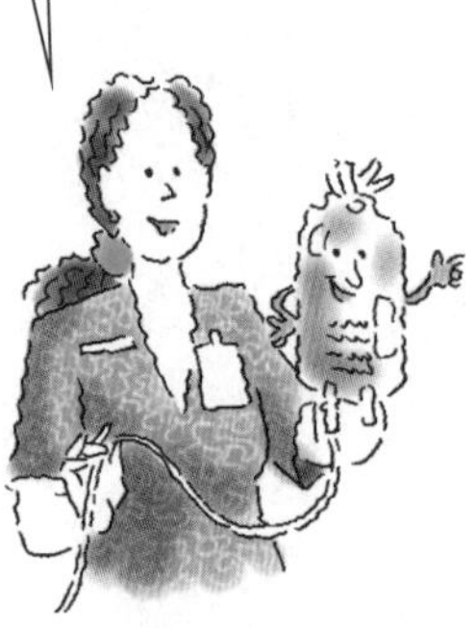

This question calls for a concentrated effort.

65. Which electrolyte imbalance should a nurse be alert for in a client started on an insulin drip?

1. Hypercalcemia
2. Hypermagnesemia
3. Hypophosphatemia
4. Hypokalemia

65. 4. Insulin forces potassium out of the plasma, back into the cells, causing hypokalemia. Calcium, magnesium, and phosphorus aren't affected by insulin.

CN: Physiological integrity; CNS: Physiological adaptation; CL: Application

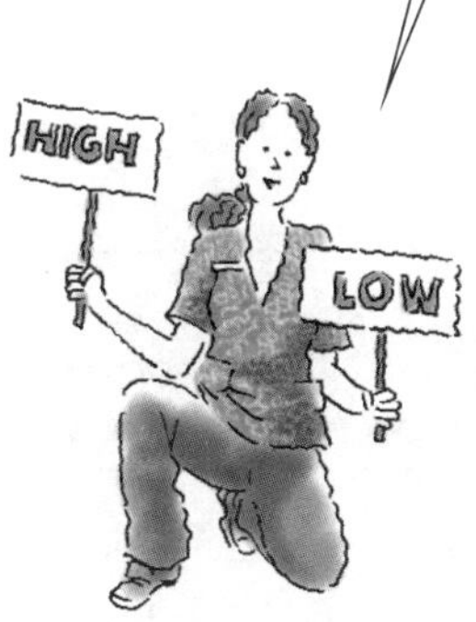

Keep your eyes open for the highs and lows.
HIGH
LOW

66. Which combination of adverse effects must be carefully monitored when administering I.V. insulin to a client diagnosed with diabetic ketoacidosis?

1. Hypokalemia and hypoglycemia
2. Hypocalcemia and hyperkalemia
3. Hyperkalemia and hyperglycemia
4. Hypernatremia and hypercalcemia

66. 1. Blood glucose needs to be monitored because there's a chance for hyperglycemia or hypoglycemia. Hypoglycemia might occur if too much insulin is administered. Hypokalemia might occur because I.V. insulin forces potassium into cells, thereby lowering the plasma levels of potassium. The client would *not* have hyperkalemia. Calcium and sodium levels aren't affected.

CN: Physiological integrity; CNS: Pharmacological and parenteral therapies; CL: Application

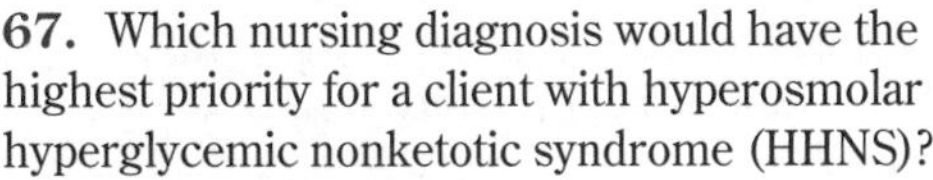

67. Which nursing diagnosis would have the highest priority for a client with hyperosmolar hyperglycemic nonketotic syndrome (HHNS)?

1. *Risk for infection*
2. *Risk for acute confusion*
3. *Deficient fluid volume*
4. *Impaired skin integrity*

67. 3. A client with HHNS has severe dehydration which requires immediate intervention. The other nursing diagnoses are all appropriate but aren't the priority.

CN: Physiological integrity; CNS: Physiological adaptation; CL: Analysis

68. Which disease process releases enough insulin to prevent ketosis but not enough to prevent hyperglycemia?

1. Diabetes insipidus
2. Diabetic ketoacidosis
3. Type 2 diabetes mellitus
4. Hyperosmolar hyperglycemic nonketotic syndrome (HHNS)

68. 4. In HHNS, enough insulin is released to prevent ketosis but not enough to prevent hyperglycemia. Diabetes insipidus doesn't involve hyperglycemia. Diabetic ketoacidosis involves hyperglycemia and ketosis. In type 2 diabetes mellitus, the body produces insulin, but hyperglycemia results from insulin resistance or insufficiency.

CN: Physiological integrity; CNS: Physiological adaptation; CL: Analysis

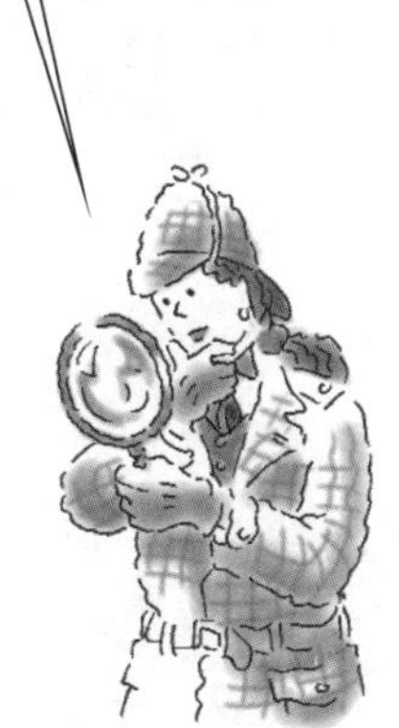

Don't let this one trip you up. The most obvious answer may not be the correct one.

69. In a client with hyperosmolar hyperglycemic nonketotic syndrome (HHNS) due to hyperosmolarity, which condition causes cellular dehydration?

1. Diuresis
2. Hyperglycemia
3. Polyphagia
4. Pulmonary edema

69. 1. Hyperosmolarity causes cellular dehydration and diuresis. The client has hyperglycemia, but it isn't related to hyperosmolarity. Polyphagia and pulmonary edema aren't symptoms of HHNS.

CN: Physiological integrity; CNS: Physiological adaptation; CL: Analysis

70. A client presents to the emergency department with weakness, thirst, warmth and an inability to concentrate. His laboratory results are serum glucose 712 mg/dl, urine negative for ketones, and minimal electrolyte imbalance. Which complication should the client be evaluated for?

1. Hypoglycemia
2. Diabetes insipidus
3. Diabetic ketoacidosis (DKA)
4. Hyperosmolar hyperglycemic nonketotic syndrome (HHNS)

70. 4. A serum glucose level over 600 mg/dl and no ketones in the urine suggest HHNS. Excessive insulin will lead to hypoglycemia. Dysfunctions in antidiuretic hormone secretion lead to diabetes insipidus. The absence of ketones suggests that DKA isn't present.

CN: Physiological integrity; CNS: Physiological adaptation; CL: Application

71. A client presents with a temperature of 103° F (39.4° C), hypotension, dry mucus membranes, and a blood glucose level of 590 mg/dl. Which of the following conditions would the nurse suspect for this client?

1. Diabetes mellitus
2. Diabetes insipidus
3. Diabetic ketoacidosis
4. Hyperosmolar hyperglycemic nonketotic syndrome (HHNS)

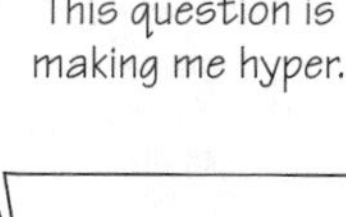
This question is making me hyper.

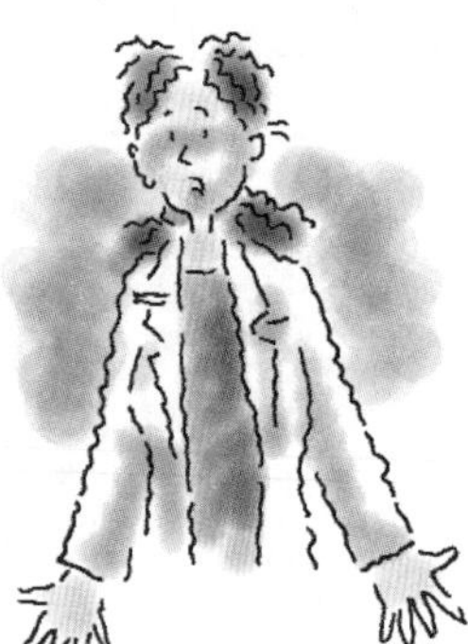

71. 4. HHNS usually presents with hypotension, dehydration, fever, and tachycardia. Diabetes mellitus presents with polyuria, polyphagia, polydipsia, and blood glucose levels above normal. Diabetes insipidus presents with large amounts of dilute urine. Diabetic ketoacidosis presents with polyuria, polydipsia, and possibly oliguria secondary to dehydration.

CN: Physiological integrity; CNS: Physiological adaptation; CL: Analysis

72. A diabetic client suddenly develops hypoglycemia. What should the nurse do first?

1. Give the client a glass of orange juice to drink.
2. Administer 5 more units of regular insulin.
3. Check the client's blood glucose level.
4. Call the client's physician.

72. 1. Drinking a glass of orange juice should raise the client's blood glucose level, thus correcting hypoglycemia. Receiving additional insulin would lower the client's blood glucose level even further, causing hypoglycemia to worsen. The nurse shouldn't check the blood glucose level or call the physician at this time because the client needs immediate attention to prevent loss of consciousness.

CN: Safe, effective care environment; CNS: Management of care; CL: Application

73. A diabetic client who has had a stroke has right-sided paralysis and incontinence and is in the rehabilitation center. Which action should be the nurse's priority in caring for the client?

1. Apply body powder every 4 hours to keep the client dry.
2. To conserve energy, maintain bed rest when the client isn't in therapy.
3. Insert an indwelling urinary catheter to keep the client continent.
4. Wash the client's skin with soap and water, gently patting it dry.

73. 4. The skin of a diabetic client should be kept dry to prevent breakdown and infection. The nurse should avoid excessive use of powder, which can cake with perspiration and cause irritation. Clients undergoing rehabilitation should be upright in a chair, except for short rest periods during the day, to promote optimal recovery. Diabetic clients are especially prone to infections. Urinary tract infections are commonly caused by the use of indwelling catheters. Other methods should be used to encourage continence.

CN: Safe, effective care environment; CNS: Management of care; CL: Application

74. Which laboratory results support a diagnosis of primary hyperparathyroidism?
1. High parathyroid hormone and high calcium levels
2. High magnesium and high thyroid hormone levels
3. Low parathyroid hormone and low potassium levels
4. Low thyroid-stimulating hormone (TSH) and high phosphorus levels

74. 1. A diagnosis of primary hyperparathyroidism is established based on increased serum calcium levels and elevated parathyroid hormone levels. Potassium, magnesium, TSH, and thyroid hormone levels aren't used to diagnose hyperparathyroidism.
CN: Physiological integrity; CNS: Physiological adaptation; CL: Application

75. Which type of medication is <u>contraindicated</u> in the treatment of clients with hyperparathyroidism?
1. Acetaminophen
2. Aspirin
3. Potassium-wasting diuretics
4. Thiazide diuretics

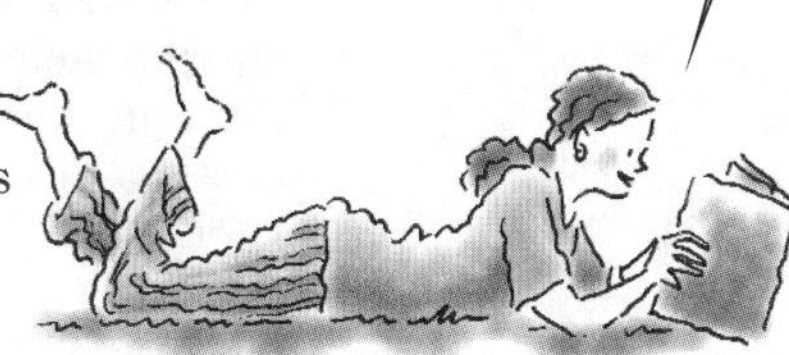
The word contraindicated makes this a tricky question.

75. 4. Thiazide diuretics shouldn't be used because they decrease renal excretion of calcium, thereby raising serum calcium levels even higher. There are no contraindications to acetaminophen or aspirin for clients with hyperparathyroidism. Potassium loss isn't an issue for clients with hyperparathyroidism.
CN: Physiological integrity; CNS: Pharmacological and parenteral therapies; CL: Application

76. The serum calcium level of a client with hyperthyroidism is 14.6 mg/dl. Which treatment should the nurse anticipate?
1. Withholding fluids
2. Starting oral calcium supplements
3. Giving vitamin D supplements
4. Administering I.V. fluids at 200 ml/hour

76. 4. Normal calcium levels are 8.5 to 10.5 mg/dl, so a level of 14.6 mg/dl is dangerously high. To decrease the calcium level, intake of calcium should be reduced, and calcium excretion should be promoted by administering I.V. and oral fluids and diuretics. Vitamin D increases the calcium level.
CN: Physiological integrity; CNS: Physiological adaptation; CL: Analysis

77. Hyperphosphatemia and hypocalcemia are indicative of which disorder?
1. Cushing's syndrome
2. Graves' disease
3. Hypoparathyroidism
4. Hypothyroidism

77. 3. Symptoms of hypoparathyroidism include hyperphosphatemia and hypocalcemia. Excessive adrenocortical activity indicates Cushing's syndrome. Excessive thyroid hormone levels indicate Graves' disease (hyperthyroidism). Low thyroid hormone levels indicate hypothyroidism.
CN: Physiological integrity; CNS: Physiological adaptation; CL: Analysis

78. A 55-year-old client is admitted with hyperthyroidism. Which nursing intervention should be the priority to decrease the client's anxiety?
1. Keeping the client warm
2. Encouraging the client to increase activity
3. Providing a calm, restful environment
4. Placing the client in semi-Fowler's position

78. 3. Clients with hyperthyroidism are typically anxious, diaphoretic, nervous, and fatigued; they need a calm, restful environment in which to relax and get adequate rest. Clients with hyperthyroidism are usually warm and diaphoretic, and need a cool environment. Activity shouldn't be increased. If a client is exhibiting dyspnea, he would benefit from high Fowler's position.
CN: Safe, effective care environment; CNS: Management of care; CK: Application

79. A nurse is providing teaching to a client with hypoparathyroidism. Which vitamin therapy should she include in her teaching?
1. Vitamin A
2. Vitamin C
3. Vitamin D
4. Vitamin E

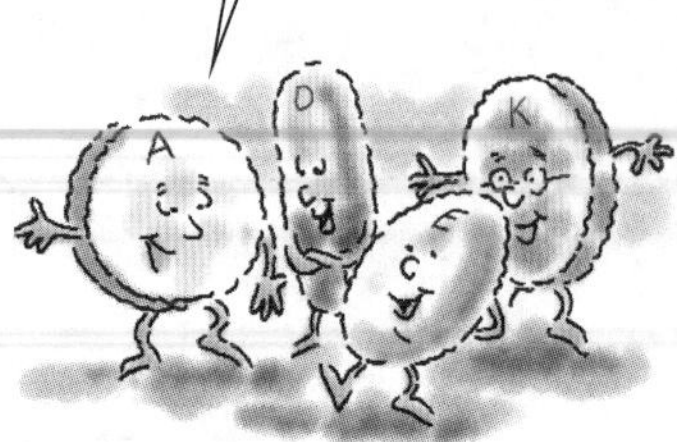

One of us needs to get involved.
A
D
K

79. 3. A client with hypoparathyroidism has a decreased calcium level. Variable doses of vitamin D preparations enhance the absorption of calcium from the GI tract. Vitamins A, C, and E aren't involved with this process.

CN: Physiological integrity; CNS: Pharmacological and parenteral therapies; CL: Analysis

80. Coarsening of facial features and soft tissue swelling of the hands and feet are early clinical manifestations of which condition?
1. Acromegaly
2. Cushing's syndrome
3. Graves' disease
4. Pheochromocytoma

80. 1. Acromegaly is marked by coarsening of facial features and soft tissue swelling of the hands and feet. Cushing's syndrome causes thin extremities, truncal obesity, and a "moonface." Graves' disease causes bulging of the eyes, weight loss, and heat intolerance. Pheochromocytoma is a tumor of the adrenal gland that causes hypertension.

CN: Physiological integrity; CNS: Physiological adaptation; CL: Application

81. A nurse is teaching a client about insulin. The physician has ordered, "Regular insulin 6 units U100." Which statement by the client indicates that teaching has been effective?
1. "The insulin is cloudy."
2. "The insulin vial should be shaken vigorously before I draw the insulin into the syringe."
3. "U100 means there are 100 units in each milliliter of the insulin and that 6 units are to be administered."
4. "The insulin should be drawn up in a tuberculin syringe."

81. 3. There are 100 units of insulin in each milliliter of U100 insulin, and it should be drawn up in a U100 syringe (orange needle cap). Regular insulin is clear. Cloudy insulin has a zinc precipitate that must be evenly distributed in the solution. Insulin syringes are the only type of syringe used for drawing up insulin.

CN: Physiological integrity; CNS: Pharmacological and parenteral therapies; CL: Application

82. A client is diagnosed with a somatotrophin-secreting tumor that could lead to development of acromegaly, Cushing's syndrome, and hypopituitarism. Which gland is related to this tumor?
1. Adrenal gland
2. Hypothalamus
3. Pituitary gland
4. Thyroid gland

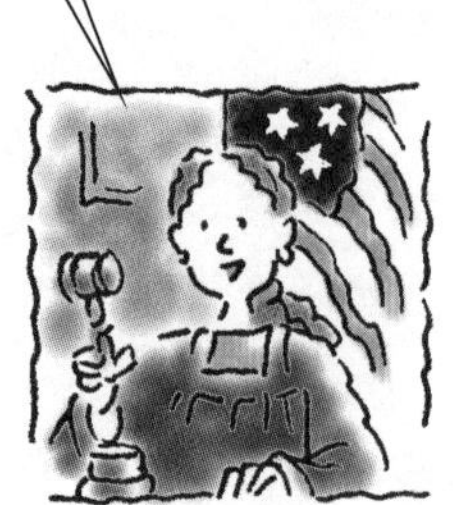

Here's a case for knowing your hormones cold.

82. 3. Tumors that affect the pituitary gland would lead to acromegaly, Cushing's syndrome, and hypopituitarism. Tumors of the adrenal gland would cause symptoms such as hypertension. The hypothalamus secretes corticotropin-releasing factor, which stimulates the anterior pituitary to secrete corticotropin. Tumors affecting the thyroid gland would involve thyroid hormones.

CN: Physiological integrity; CNS: Physiological adaptation; CL: Application

83. The nurse is reviewing a client's chart and notes that the client developed a carpopedal spasm when the blood flow in his arm was occluded for 3 minutes with a blood pressure cuff. Which of the following terms correctly describes this sign?

1. Negative Chvostek's sign
2. Positive Chvostek's sign
3. Negative Trousseau's sign
4. Positive Trousseau's sign

83. 4. A Trousseau's sign is positive when a carpopedal spasm is induced by occluding the blood flow of an arm for 3 minutes using a blood pressure cuff. Chvostek's sign is positive when a sharp tapping over the facial nerve, in front of the parotid gland and anterior to the ear, causes the mouth, nose, and eye to twitch.
CN: Physiological integrity; CNS: Reduction of risk potential; CL: Application

84. After undergoing a thyroidectomy, a client develops hypocalcemia and tetany. Which medication should the nurse anticipate administering?

1. Calcium gluconate
2. Potassium chloride
3. Sodium bicarbonate
4. Sodium phosphorus

84. 1. Immediate treatment for a client who develops hypocalcemia and tetany after thyroidectomy is calcium gluconate. Potassium chloride and sodium bicarbonate aren't indicated. Sodium phosphorus wouldn't be given because phosphorus levels are already elevated.
CN: Physiological integrity; CNS: Pharmacological and parenteral therapies; CL: Application

85. A client is diagnosed with acute pancreatitis. The nurse is teaching the client about the causes. Which of the following responses is most correct?

1. Gallstones
2. Crohn's disease
3. High gastric acid levels
4. Low thyroid hormone level

85. 1. Gallstones may cause obstruction and swelling at the ampulla of Vater, preventing flow of pancreatic juices into the duodenum and leading to pancreatitis. Gallbladder obstruction and alcoholism are the major causes of acute pancreatitis. Crohn's disease usually involves the terminal ileum and wouldn't affect the pancreas. High gastric acid levels and low thyroid hormone levels aren't related to an acute pancreatitis attack.
CN: Physiological integrity; CNS: Physiological adaptation; CL: Application

86. Which test should a nurse expect to be ordered for a client with severe abdominal pain in the midepigastric region, back tenderness, nausea, and vomiting?

1. Amylase
2. C-peptide
3. Stool culture
4. Colonoscopy

86. 1. Severe abdominal pain in the midepigastric region, back tenderness, nausea, and vomiting may be due to irritation of the pancreas. Therefore an amylase level test should be ordered. C-peptide, a stool culture, and a colonoscopy wouldn't be ordered for the presenting symptoms.
CN: Physiological integrity; CNS: Physiological adaptation; CL: Analysis

87. A 48-year-old client has been admitted with complaints of acute abdominal pain in the midepigastric region, back tenderness, nausea, and vomiting. The nurse recognizes these findings to be associated with which condition?

1. Acute pancreatitis
2. Crohn's disease
3. Hypophysectomy
4. Pheochromocytoma

87. 1. Signs and symptoms of acute pancreatitis include midepigastric abdominal pain, back pain, nausea, and vomiting. Crohn's disease is associated with right lower quadrant abdominal pain (in acute disease) and cramping abdominal pain (in chronic disease). Hypophysectomy is the surgical removal of the pituitary gland. Pheochromocytoma is a tumor of the adrenal gland and doesn't cause abdominal or back symptoms.
CN: Physiological integrity; CNS: Physiological adaptation; CL: Application

88. The nurse is modifying the plan of care for a client who is recovering form acute pancreatitis. Which of these measures would be the most appropriate to include in the care plan?

1. Eat small, frequent meals that are bland, high-carbohydrate, high-protein, and low-fat.
2. Consume no more than one alcoholic drink per day, and limit coffee to three cups per day.
3. Include fruits and vegetables that are high in vitamin C and K, and increase fiber.
4. Maintain a diet that is low-residue, low-protein, and high in calcium.

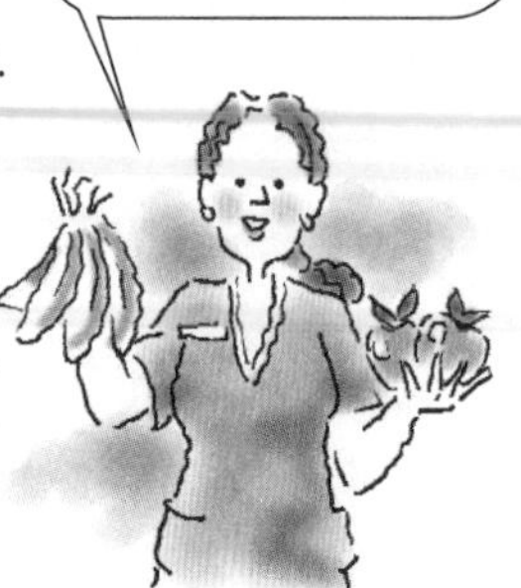

Teach your client the importance of making healthy food choices.

88. 1. In order to restore energy and nutrients, small frequent meals that are high-carbohydrate, high-protein, and low-fat are advised. Spicy foods, caffeine, and alcohol should be avoided. The other instructions do not relate to pancreatitis.

CN: Physiological integrity; CNS: Basic care and comfort; CL: Application

89. If a pancreatitis attack has been brought on by gallstones or gallbladder disease, a client may require reinforcement about the need to follow which type of diet?

1. High-calorie, high-protein diet
2. High-fiber diet, encouraging fluid intake
3. Low-fat diet, avoiding heavy meals
4. Diet high in protein, calcium, and vitamin D

89. 3. A client who survives an acute pancreatitis attack caused by gallstones or gallbladder disease requires reinforcement to maintain a low-fat diet and to avoid heavy meals. A high-calorie, high-protein diet is appropriate for clients with hyperthyroidism. A diet high in fiber, encouraging fluid intake, is recommended for constipation. A client with Cushing's syndrome should follow a diet high in protein, calcium, and vitamin D.

CN: Physiological integrity; CNS: Reduction of risk potential; CL: Application

90. A client with diabetes mellitus and a hearing impairment is admitted. For this client, the nurse is developing a care plan that includes daily self-administration of insulin. Which intervention should the nurse include in this plan?

1. Use facial expressions as needed.
2. Chew gum while giving instructions.
3. Shine a light on the client's face.
4. Raise an arm or hand to get attention.

90. 4. To get the client's attention, the nurse should raise an arm or hand before presenting instructions. The nurse should avoid relying on facial expressions because they may be misinterpreted as signs of annoyance or other feelings by a client who depends on visual cues. The nurse shouldn't chew gum when teaching a client with limited hearing because it can distort the sounds that the client can hear.

CN: Health promotion and maintenance; CNS: None; CL: Application

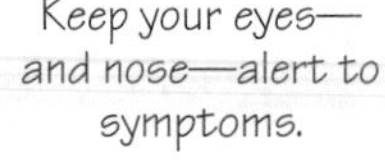

Keep your eyes—and nose—alert to symptoms.

91. A client is in diabetic ketoacidosis, secondary to infection. As the condition progresses, which symptoms might the nurse see?

1. Kussmaul's respirations and a fruity odor on the breath
2. Shallow respirations and severe abdominal pain
3. Decreased respirations and increased urine output
4. Cheyne-Stokes respirations and foul-smelling urine

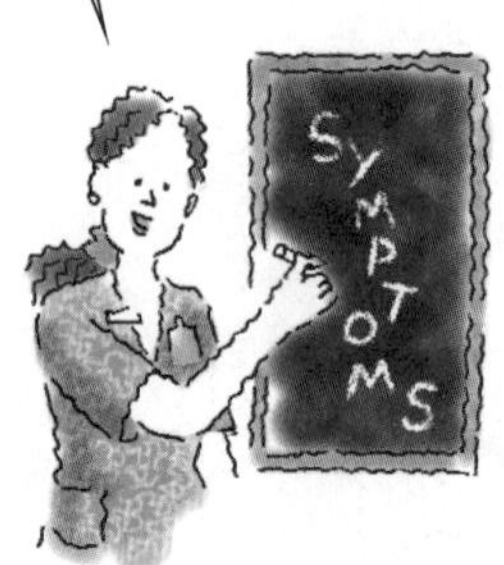

91. 1. Coma and severe acidosis are ushered in with Kussmaul's respirations (very deep but not labored respirations) and a fruity odor on the breath (acidemia). Shallow respirations and severe abdominal pain may be symptoms of pancreatitis. Decreased respirations and increased urine output aren't symptoms related to acidemia. Cheyne-Stokes respirations and foul-smelling urine don't result from diabetic ketoacidosis.

CN: Physiological integrity; CNS: Physiological adaptation; CL: Application

92. A nurse is preparing to administer "Regular insulin 4 units subcutaneously" to a client with type 1 diabetes mellitus. Which equipment does the nurse need to perform the injection?

1. 27-guage, ½″ needle
2. 22-guage, ½″ needle
3. 27-guage, 1″ needle
4. 22-guage, 1″ needle

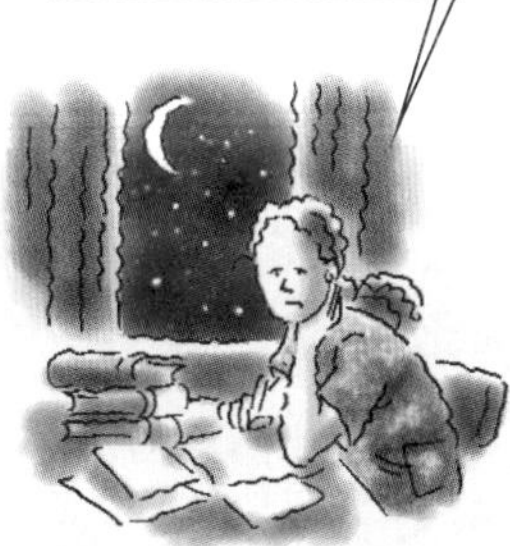
Don't give up now.
You're doing great!

92. 1. To administer medication, the nurse will be using a subcutaneous injection, which should be administered with a 25-guage to 27-guage, ⅝″ to ½″ needle. A 22-guage needle is too large for a subcutaneous injection. A 1″ needle will deliver the medication into the muscle rather than subcutaneous tissue.

CN: Physiological integrity; CNS: Pharmacological and parenteral therapies; CL: Application

93. Clients with insulin-dependent diabetes mellitus may require which change to their daily routine during periods of infection?

1. No changes
2. Less insulin
3. More insulin
4. Oral antidiabetic agents

93. 3. During periods of infection or illness, insulin-dependent clients may need even more insulin to compensate for increased blood glucose levels. Since the client has insulin-dependent diabetes, oral antidiabetic agents wouldn't be indicated.

CN: Physiological integrity; CNS: Pharmacological and parenteral therapies; CL: Application

94. A physician prescribes an oral antidiabetic medication and weekly glucose monitoring for a 42-year-old male client recently diagnosed with type 2 diabetes. The client is moderately overweight and has a poor diet and a stressful job. He asks how his diagnosis will affect his life. Which response is the most appropriate?

1. "The medication will help maintain a steady glucose level, but you need to cut back on snacking."
2. "Type 2 diabetes is common and easily treated. You don't have to make changes."
3. "I'll refer you to a diabetes nurse specialist. She'll help you develop a plan."
4. "You may want to change careers because your job takes so much of your energy."

94. 3. A referral to a nurse specialist who can develop an ongoing relationship and spend time assessing the client's personal needs and developing a workable plan with him would be the most appropriate. Although the medication does help to maintain steady glucose levels, this response ignores the other factors contributing to the client's poor health habits. Telling the client that he won't have to make any lifestyle changes is inappropriate, as is suggesting he change careers.

CN: Health promotion and maintenance; CNS: None; CL: Application

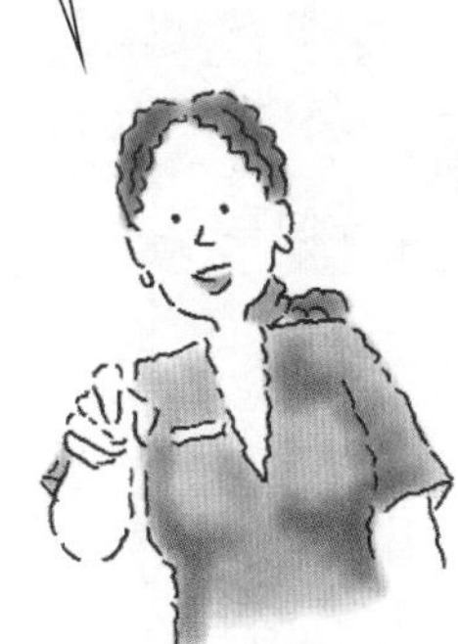
Make sure you
know the standard
guidelines of
common disorders.

95. A nonpregnant client tells the nurse that two recent fasting blood glucose results were 132 mg/dl and 146 mg/dl. The nurse should expect which of the following actions to occur?

1. These are normal results; no further action is needed.
2. These results indicate diabetes mellitus; further follow-up is needed.
3. The fasting blood glucose tests should be repeated two more times.
4. The client should be scheduled for an HbA_{1C} test.

95. 2. Based on the American Diabetes Association guidelines, fasting blood glucose of 126 mg/dl or more, on at least two occasions, is indicative of diabetes mellitus. These are not normal results. Further tests to make a definitive diagnosis of diabetes mellitus should be random blood glucose or glucose tolerance tests, not a fasting blood glucose of HbA_{1C} test.

CN: Physiological integrity; CNS: Reduction of risk potential; CL: Analysis

96. Which condition is associated with the adrenal gland and causes hypertension and paroxysmal tachycardia?
1. Apical aneurysm
2. Endemic goiter
3. Pheochromocytoma
4. Ulcerogenic tumor

96. 3. A pheochromocytoma is usually a benign tumor of the adrenal medulla that secretes epinephrine and nonepinephrine, resulting in hypertension and paroxysmal tachycardia. An apical aneurysm is located in the heart. An endemic goiter is an iodine-deficient enlargement of the thyroid gland. Ulcerogenic tumors are located in the islets of Langerhans (part of the pancreas).
CN: Physiological integrity; CNS: Physiological adaptation; CL: Application

97. The nurse is caring for a client with an adrenal medulla tumor. Which of the following symptoms would the nurse expect to assess?
1. Carpopedal spasm
2. Hyperglycemia
3. Hypertension
4. "Moonface"

97. 3. Tumors of the adrenal medulla usually produce hypertension because they release excessive amounts of epinephrine and norepinephrine. Carpopedal spasm occurs as a result of hypocalcemia. Hyperglycemia is a result of low insulin levels. Clients with Cushing's syndrome usually have a "moonface."
CN: Physiological integrity; CNS: Physiological adaptation; CL: Application

98. The nurse is administering corticosteroid therapy to a client. The nurse should be alert for which of the following adverse effects of this therapy?
1. Hyponatremia
2. Hypoglycemia
3. Change in metabolism
4. Change in pituitary secretions

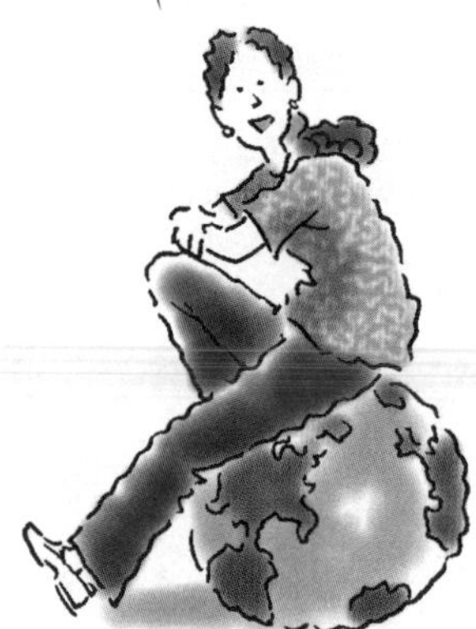

You should feel on top of the world! You're almost finished.

98. 3. A major adverse effect of corticosteroid therapy is a slowing of metabolism. This therapy also produces hyperglycemia and hypernatremia. Changes in pituitary secretions aren't affected by corticosteroid therapy.
CN: Physiological integrity; CNS: Pharmacological and parenteral therapies; CL: Analysis

99. Which condition contributes to hyperparathyroidism?
1. Chronic renal failure
2. Thyroidectomy
3. Elevated serum calcium level
4. Steroid use

99. 1. Because failing kidneys can't convert vitamin D, the serum calcium level declines, causing hyperparathyroidism from increased release of parathyroid hormones. Thyroidectomy may lead to hypoparathyroidism if the parathyroid is also removed during surgery. Hyperparathyroidism may cause serum calcium levels to rise. Steroid use induces calcium to leave bone, suppressing parathyroid hormone.
CN: Physiological integrity; CNS: Physiological adaptation; CL: Analysis

100. A previously healthy 70-year-old male client has a serum glucose level of 1,200 mg/dl, a normal serum bicarbonate level, and urine free from acetone. The nurse should suspect which condition?

1. Diabetic ketoacidosis (DKA)
2. Diabetes insipidus
3. Hyperglycemic hyperosmolar nonketotic coma
4. Syndrome of inappropriate antidiuretic hormone (SIADH)

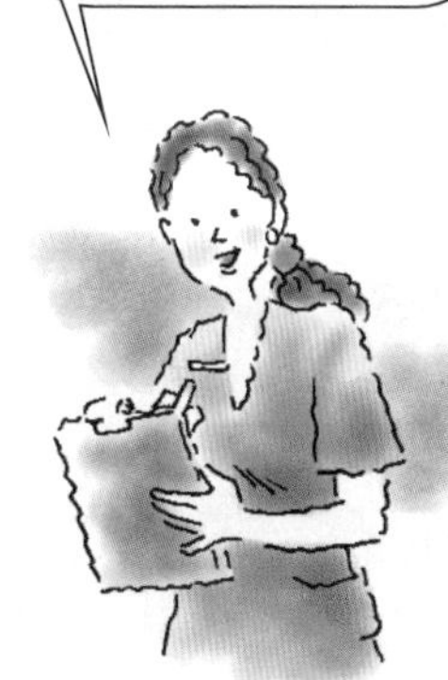

Always note the stated age. It can influence the answer.

100. 3. Elderly clients are at risk for developing a hyperosmolar state as their taste preferences shift to softer, higher-carbohydrate foods. The urine free from acetone indicates that the client isn't experiencing breakdown of fats and proteins, so the nurse shouldn't suspect DKA. The client's laboratory values don't indicate a disturbance in the production, secretion, or use of antidiuretic hormone, which would result in diabetes insipidus or SIADH.

CN: Physiological integrity; CNS: Physiological adaptation; CL: Analysis

101. A client with Addison's disease is receiving a maintenance dose of steroids. Which topic should the nurse include in discharge teaching?

1. Importance of restricting fluids
2. Watching for signs of hypoglycemia
3. Taking steroids exactly as prescribed
4. Adjusting steroid doses based on dietary intake and exercise

101. 3. A client with Addison's disease needs more steroids than the body produces. Taking a lower dose may trigger an addisonian crisis; taking a higher dose increases the effects of potassium depletion, hyperglycemia, and fluid retention, leading to a life-threatening situation. Fluid restriction isn't desirable and could cause dehydration. Steroids tend to increase, not decrease, blood sugar. Steroid doses aren't adjusted for diet and exercise, although the client may need to administer insulin and adjust insulin doses.

CN: Physiological integrity; CNS: Pharmacological and parenteral therapies; CL: Application

102. A client is being treated for adrenal crisis (addisonian crisis). Which laboratory values are <u>most</u> important to monitor?

1. Serum bicarbonate and sodium
2. Serum glucose and ketones
3. Serum sodium and potassium
4. Serum calcium and magnesium

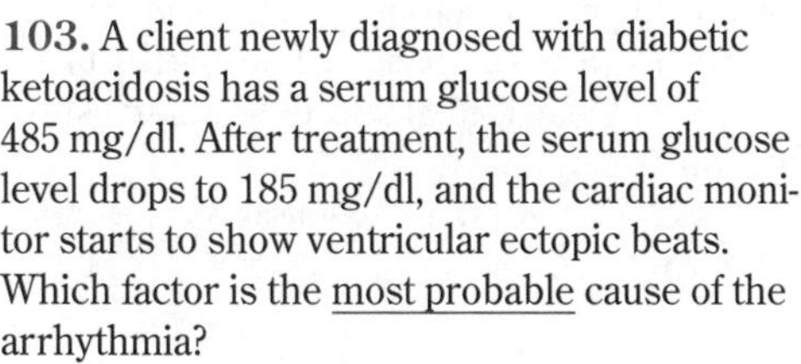

Be careful!
Combo answers can be tricky!

102. 3. If steroid replacement therapy is inadequate, sodium loss and potassium retention persist. If the steroid dose is too high, sodium and water are retained, and large amounts of potassium are excreted. Steroid replacement can affect glucose, but the replacement doesn't have as great an impact on ketones, bicarbonate, calcium, or magnesium as it does on sodium and potassium.

CN: Physiological integrity; CNS: Reduction of risk potential; CL: Analysis

103. A client newly diagnosed with diabetic ketoacidosis has a serum glucose level of 485 mg/dl. After treatment, the serum glucose level drops to 185 mg/dl, and the cardiac monitor starts to show ventricular ectopic beats. Which factor is the <u>most probable</u> cause of the arrhythmia?

1. Decreased serum chloride level
2. Decreased serum potassium level
3. Elevated serum glucose level
4. Elevated serum sodium level

103. 2. Correction of an elevated serum glucose level may alter the serum potassium level, predisposing the client to arrhythmias. Serum chloride and sodium changes are more likely to contribute to an altered level of consciousness, whereas elevated serum glucose contributes to long-term effects of diabetes mellitus, such as coronary artery disease, hypertension, and peripheral vascular disease.

CN: Physiological integrity; CNS: Physiological adaptation; CL: Analysis

104. When teaching a diabetic client about nutritional planning, which food selection would be considered one healthy serving of carbohydrate?

1. One small orange
2. ½ cup of vanilla ice cream
3. 2 slices of white bread
4. 2 cups of whole grain rice

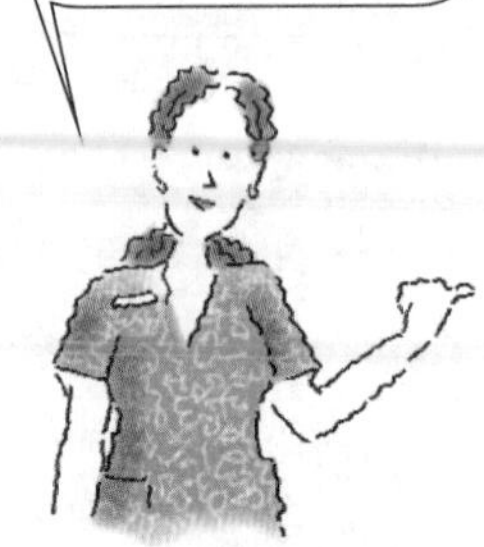

Teaching is crucial for clients with diabetes.

104. 1. One small orange is one serving of a healthy carbohydrate. Besides providing vitamins and water content, an orange contains fiber. Vanilla ice cream contains both carbohydrate and saturated fat. Two slices of white bread are two servings of carbohydrate. Two cups of whole grain rice is approximately 3 to 4 servings of a carbohydrate.

CN: Physiological integrity; CNS: Basic care and comfort; CL: Application

105. An unemployed client with no health insurance hasn't filled his prescriptions for some time. According to his roommate, the client has been "getting sicker by the day." Which problem suggests the client isn't taking his prescribed levothyroxine (Synthroid)?

1. Diarrhea and vomiting
2. Rapid heart rate
3. Warm, dry, flushed skin
4. Temperature of 94° F (34.4° C)

105. 4. Levothyroxine is prescribed for hypothyroidism, which causes a hypodynamic state; failure to maintain levothyroxine therapy can lead to a low body temperature. The other problems indicate a hypermetabolic state; although the client may also experience these symptoms, they stem from infection and dehydration.

CN: Physiological integrity; CNS: Physiological adaptation; CL: Application

106. A client with newly diagnosed diabetes mellitus is ready for discharge. Discharge teaching must include instruction on which topic?

1. Foot care and the need for a high-calorie diet
2. How to balance diet, exercise, and medication
3. Fasting before health care maintenance visits
4. Avoiding all carbohydrates and drinking 2 qt (2 L) of water daily

106. 2. With type 1, type 2, or gestational diabetes mellitus, balancing diet, exercise, and medication is essential to diabetes control. High-calorie and non-carbohydrate diets are contraindicated in diabetes. While fasting may reduce the serum glucose level temporarily, glycosylated hemoglobin tests show the effectiveness of long-term diabetes control.

CN: Physiological integrity; CNS: Physiological adaptation; CL: Application

107. Which statement indicates that a client with diabetes understands proper foot care?

1. "I'll call for a physician's appointment if my feet start to ache."
2. "I'll rotate insulin injection sites from my left foot to my right foot."
3. "I'll go barefoot around the house to avoid pressure areas on my feet."
4. "I'll wear cotton socks with well-fitting shoes."

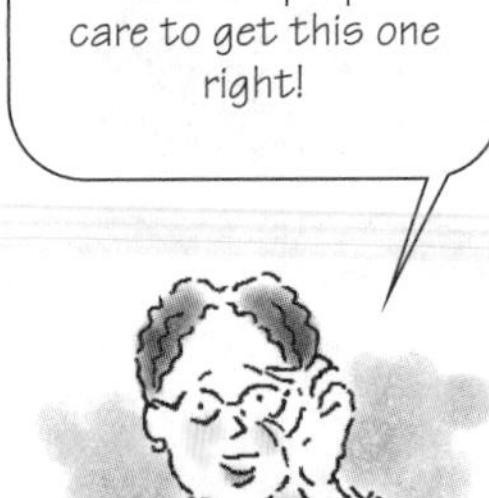

Focus on proper care to get this one right!

107. 4. Cotton socks wisk moisture away from the skin, helping to prevent fungal infections; proper shoe fit helps avoid pressure areas. Aching isn't a common sign of foot problems; however, a tingling sensation in the feet indicates neurovascular changes. Injecting insulin into the foot may lead to infection. Going barefoot can cause injury.

CN: Physiological integrity; CNS: Reduction of risk potential; CL: Analysis

108. A 17-year-old client with diabetes has a decreased level of consciousness, with a finger-stick glucose level of 39. Her family reports that she has been skipping meals in an effort to lose weight. Which nursing intervention is most appropriate?

1. Placing a Salem sump tube and providing tube feedings
2. Administering a 500-ml bolus of normal saline solution
3. Administering 1 ampule of 50% dextrose solution
4. Calling the physician for orders

108. 3. Administering 50% dextrose solution helps preserve and restore the client's physiologic integrity. Providing a feeding tube is appropriate only in a less urgent situation; during the time it takes to insert a nasogastric tube, administer a feeding, and wait for digestion to occur, the client may suffer permanent brain damage and seizures from severe hypoglycemia. A blood pressure drop wasn't mentioned; a bolus of normal saline solution would correct only the client fluid status, not his glucose level. Calling the physician would delay treatment at a time when rapid intervention is crucial.

CN: Physiological integrity; CNS: Physiological adaptation; CL: Application

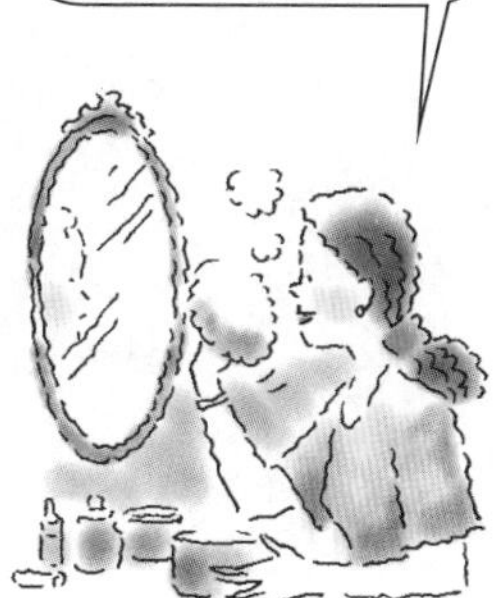

Lookin' good. Only 5 questions to go!

109. A client is admitted to the telemetry floor with a diagnosis of pancreatitis. Which nursing intervention is appropriate?

1. Providing generous servings at mealtime
2. Reserving one antecubital site for a peripherally inserted central catheter (PICC)
3. Providing a glass of wine with each meal because the client wasn't admitted to treat alcoholism
4. Serving coffee with breakfast to help clear the client's mind

109. 2. Pancreatitis treatment commonly involves resting the GI tract; use of a PICC enables the client to receive long-term total parenteral nutrition. Alcohol and caffeine stimulate the pancreas, increase pain, and may lead to a pseudocyst, with eventual rupture resulting in peritonitis.

CN: Physiological integrity; CNS: Physiological adaptation; CL: Application

110. A client is diagnosed with Cushing's disease. Which statement indicates that he understands his disease?

1. "My blood sugar is high only because I produce too much cortisone, so I don't need to watch my diet."
2. "I don't like fruits and vegetables, and potassium isn't that important to me."
3. "Because I'm susceptible to infection and heal poorly, I should get a Pneumovax (pneumococcal vaccine)."
4. "I'll continue to teach ice skating when I get out of the hospital."

110. 3. The client's concern about preventing disease shows an understanding of the body's response to elevated steroid levels. Elevated serum glucose or decreased serum potassium levels could lead to life-threatening health crises. With elevated steroid levels, minerals leave the bones, making the bones more fragile; a minor spill when walking or skating could cause long-bone or compression fractures.

CN: Health promotion and maintenance; CNS: None; CL: Application

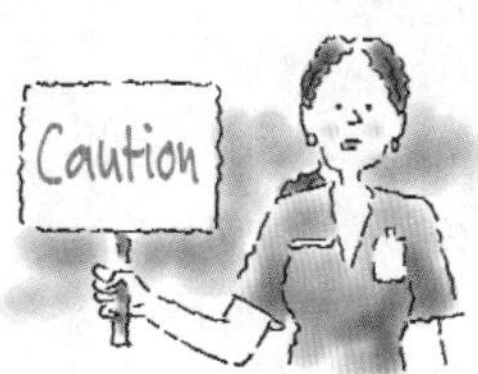

Read series answers carefully to be certain all are correct.
Caution

111. The most common signs and symptoms of hypothyroidism include:

1. increased body temperature, tachycardia, and fatigue.
2. tachycardia, pitting, and facial edema.
3. facial edema, weight gain, and diarrhea.
4. cold intolerance, swollen hands and feet, and mental sluggishness.

111. 4. Hypothyroidism slows the metabolic rate and mental responses, causing edema, decreased body temperature, and slower respiratory and heart rates. Hyperthyroidism causes increased body temperature, tachycardia, and fatigue. Tachycardia, pitting, and facial edema suggest a cardiac problem. Diarrhea and facial edema suggest hyperthyroidism.

CN: Physiological integrity; CNS: Physiological adaptation; CL: Analysis

112. A client is admitted with a diagnosis of diabetic ketoacidosis. An insulin drip is initiated with 50 units of insulin in 100 ml of normal saline solution. The I.V. is being infused via an infusion pump and the pump is currently set at 10 ml/hour. The nurse determines that the client is receiving how many units of insulin each hour? Record your answer using a whole number.

____________________units

112. 5. To determine the number of insulin units the client is receiving per hour, the nurse must first calculate the number of units in each ml of fluid (50 units ÷ 100 ml = 0.5 units/ml). Next, she should multiply the units/ml by the rate of ml/hour (0.5 units × 10 ml/hour = 5 units).

CN: Physiological integrity; CNS: Pharmacological and parenteral therapies; CL: Application

113. A client with Addison's disease is scheduled for discharge after being hospitalized for an adrenal crisis. Which statements by the client would indicate that the nurse's teaching has been effective? Select all that apply:

1. "I have to take my steroids for 10 days."
2. "I need to weigh myself daily to be sure I don't eat too many calories."
3. "I need to call my physician to discuss my steroid needs before I have dental work."
4. "I will call the physician if I suddenly feel profoundly weak or dizzy."
5. "If I feel like I have the flu, I'll carry on as usual because this is an expected response."
6. "I need to obtain and wear a medical alert bracelet."

113. 3, 4, 6. Dental work can be a cause of physical stress; therefore, the client's physician needs to be informed and may need to adjust the steroid dosage. Fatigue, weakness, and dizziness are symptoms of inadequate dosing; the physician should be notified if these symptoms occur. A medical alert bracelet allows health care providers to access the client's history of Addison's disease if she can't communicate this information. For this client, routine administration of steroids is a lifetime treatment. Daily weight is monitored for changes in fluid balance, not caloric intake. Influenza is an added physical stressor; the client shouldn't "carry on as usual."

CN: Physiological integrity; CNS: Reduction of risk potential; CL: Analysis

114. A client who suffered a brain injury after falling off a ladder has recently developed syndrome of inappropriate antidiuretic hormone (SIADH). What findings indicate that the treatment he's receiving for SIADH is effective? Select all that apply:

1. Decrease in body weight
2. Rise in blood pressure; drop in heart rate
3. Absence of wheezes in the lungs
4. Increase in urine output
5. Decrease in urine osmolarity

114. 1, 4, 5. SIADH is an abnormality involving an excessive release of antidiuretic hormone. The predominant feature is water retention with oliguria, edema, and weight gain. Successful treatment should result in a reduction of weight, increased urine output, and a decrease in urine concentration (osmolarity).

CN: Physiological integrity; CNS: Physiological adaptation; CL: Analysis

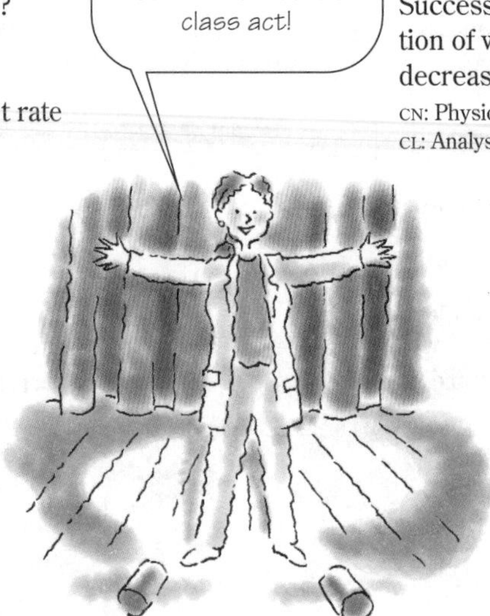
Congratulations! You finished! You're a class act!

CN: Client needs category CNS: Client needs subcategory CL: Cognitive level

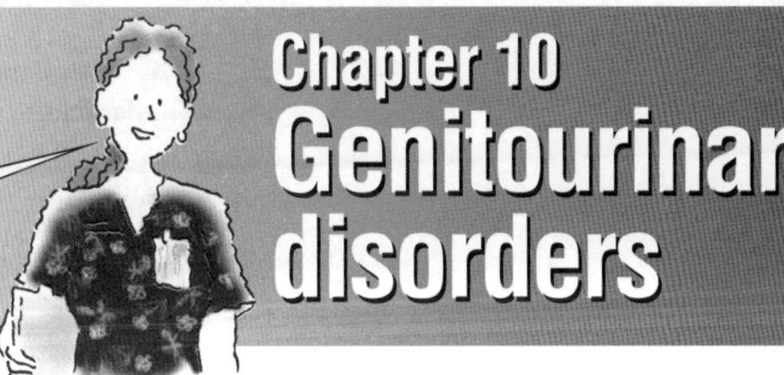

For more information about genitourinary system disorders, visit the Web site of the National Institute of Diabetes and Digestive and Kidney Diseases at www.niddk.nih.gov.

Chapter 10 Genitourinary disorders

1. Which statement best explains why it's important to empty the bowel before treatment with intracavitary radiation for cancer of the cervix?

1. Feces in the bowel increase the risk for ileus.
2. An empty bowel allows the applicator to be positioned with little or no discomfort.
3. Bowel movements increase the risk of inadvertent contamination of the vagina and urethra.
4. Pressure changes in the pelvis associated with bowel movements can alter the position of the applicator and the radiation source.

1. 4. A position change of the radioactive implant could deliver more radiation to healthy tissue and less to the malignant lesion. This increases the risk of injury to healthy tissue and decreases the effectiveness of treatment on the cancer. Feces in the bowel increase the likelihood of a bowel movement, which can change the position of the applicator and radiation source. Feces in the bowel don't increase the risk of ileus or inadvertent contamination of the vagina and urethra from a bowel movement. Applicators are usually inserted under anesthesia in the operating room.

CN: Physiological integrity; CNS: Reduction of risk potential; CL: Analysis

2. A physician tells a client to return 1 week after treatment to have a repeat culture done to verify the cure. This order would be appropriate for a woman with which condition?

1. Genital warts
2. Genital herpes
3. Gonorrhea
4. Syphilis

2. 3. Gonococcal infections can be completely eliminated by drug therapy. This is documented by a negative culture 4 to 7 days after therapy is finished. Genital warts aren't curable and are identified by appearance, not culture. Genital herpes isn't curable and is identified by the appearance of the lesions or by cytologic studies. The diagnosis of syphilis is by darkfield microscopy or serologic tests.

CN: Physiological integrity; CNS: Physiological adaptation; CL: Application

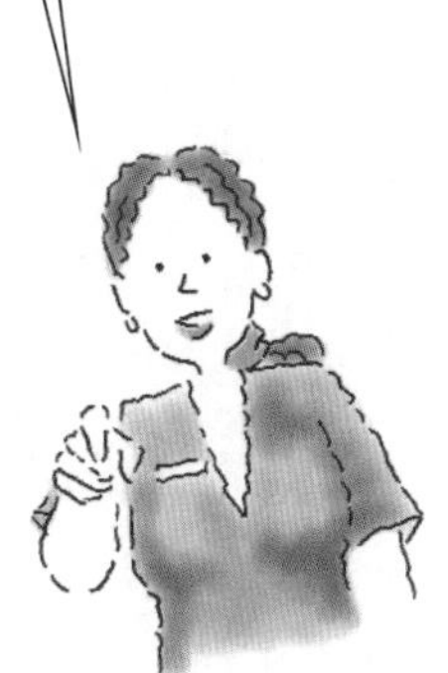

You're the greatest at choosing the correct answer.

3. Which client is at <u>greatest</u> risk for having a false-positive Venereal Disease Research Laboratory (VDRL) result?

1. An alcoholic
2. A narcotics addict
3. A transfusion recipient
4. A breast-feeding mother

3. 2. The VDRL test is a nontreponemal test used to check for the presence of reagins in the client's serum. It isn't specific for syphilis, so false-positive results occur for a variety of reasons, most commonly in clients with chronic infection, autoimmune disease, and narcotics addiction. History of alcoholism, transfusion, or breast-feeding alone doesn't constitute a risk of a false-positive VDRL result.

CN: Physiological integrity; CNS: Physiological adaptation; CL: Analysis

CN: Client needs category CNS: Client needs subcategory CL: Cognitive level

4. Which statement made by a client with a chlamydial infection indicates an understanding of the potential complications?

1. "I'm glad I'm not pregnant; I'd hate to have a malformed baby from this disease."
2. "I hope this medicine works before this disease gets into my urine and destroys my kidneys."
3. "If I had known a diaphragm would put me at risk for this, I would've taken birth control pills."
4. "I need to treat this infection so it doesn't spread into my pelvis because I want to have children some day."

4. 4. Chlamydia is a common cause of pelvic inflammatory disease and infertility. It doesn't cause birth defects or affect the kidneys. It can cause conjunctivitis and respiratory infection in neonates exposed to infected cervicovaginal secretions during delivery. Use of a diaphragm isn't a risk factor.

CN: Physiological integrity; CNS: Reduction of risk potential; CL: Application

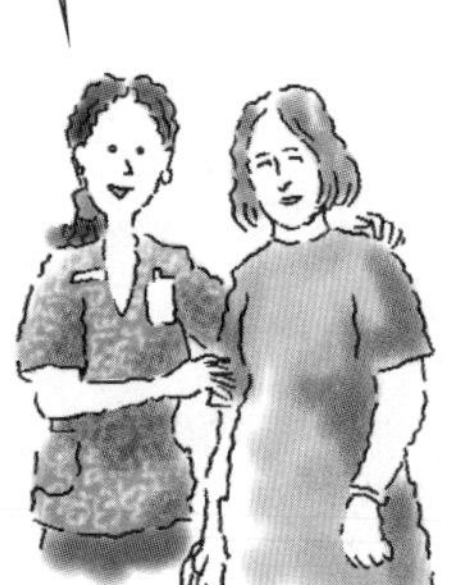

Your client relies on you for accurate instruction.

5. Which comfort measure can be recommended to a client with genital herpes?

1. Wear loose cotton underwear.
2. Apply a water-based lubricant to the lesions.
3. Rub rather than scratch in response to an itch.
4. Pour hydrogen peroxide and water over the lesions.

5. 1. Wearing loose cotton underwear promotes drying and helps avoid irritation of the lesions. The use of lubricants is contraindicated because they can prolong healing time and increase the risk of secondary infection. Lesions shouldn't be rubbed or scratched because of the risk of tissue damage and additional infection. Cool, wet compresses can be used to soothe the itch. The use of hydrogen peroxide and water on lesions isn't recommended.

CN: Physiological integrity; CNS: Basic care and comfort; CL: Application

6. Giving instructions for breast self-examination is particularly important for clients with which medical problem?

1. Cervical dysplasia
2. A dermoid cyst
3. Endometrial polyps
4. Ovarian cancer

6. 4. Clients with ovarian cancer are at increased risk for breast cancer. Breast self-examination supports early detection and treatment and is very important. There isn't a known relationship between breast cancer and cervical dysplasia, or endometrial polyps, or dermoid cysts, so breast self-examination is no more or less important for these clients.

CN: Health promotion and maintenance; CNS: None; CL: Application

7. On a follow-up visit after having a vaginal hysterectomy, a 32-year-old client has an elevated temperature and decreased hematocrit. Which complication does this suggest?

1. Hematoma
2. Hypovolemia
3. Infection
4. Thromboembolism

7. 1. An elevated temperature and decreased hematocrit are signs of hematoma, a delayed complication of abdominal and vaginal hysterectomy. Symptoms of hypovolemia include increased hematocrit and hemoglobin values. Temperature is a classic sign of infection, but a decreased hematocrit isn't. Abrupt onset of fever is a symptom of thromboembolism, but other symptoms include dyspnea, chest pain, cough, hemoptysis, restlessness, and signs of shock.

CN: Physiological integrity; CNS: Reduction of risk potential; CL: Application

CN: Client needs category CNS: Client needs subcategory CL: Cognitive level

8. Which client is at greatest risk for dehydration?
1. A 48-year-old having intracavitary radiation for cancer of the cervix
2. A 59-year-old 1 week after a radical vulvectomy
3. A 67-year-old receiving adjuvant tamoxifen therapy for breast cancer
4. A 72-year-old with a vesicovaginal fistula

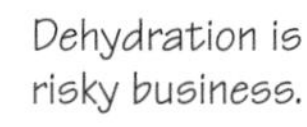

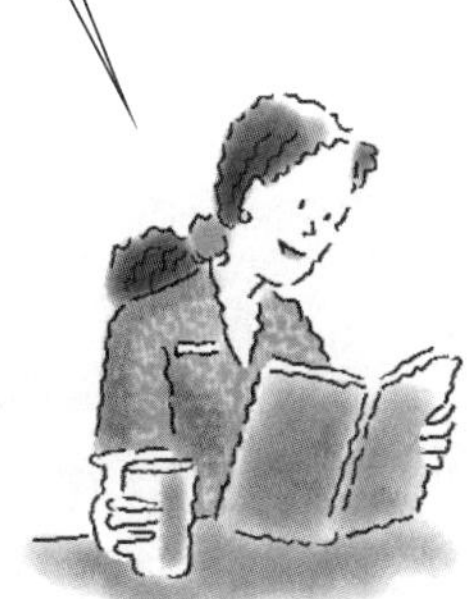

8. 1. Regardless of age, dehydration is a risk caused by fluid loss secondary to tissue destruction at the site of irradiation. After radical vulvectomy, wound drains are generally removed by postoperative day 4 or 5 and don't create a significant risk of dehydration. Tamoxifen therapy is unrelated to dehydration. Although urine may escape through the vagina as a result of a vesicovaginal fistula, it doesn't cause an unusual amount of urine or other fluid to be lost.

CN: Physiological integrity; CNS: Physiological adaptation; CL: Analysis

9. In which group is it most important for a client to understand the importance of an annual Papanicolaou test?
1. Clients with a history of recurrent candidiasis
2. Clients with a pregnancy before age 20
3. Clients infected with the human papillomavirus (HPV)
4. Clients with a long history of oral contraceptive use

9. 3. HPV causes genital warts, which are associated with an increased incidence of cervical cancer. Recurrent candidiasis, pregnancy before age 20, and use of oral contraceptives don't increase the risk of cervical cancer.

CN: Health promotion and maintenance; CNS: None; CL: Analysis

10. Which factor in a client's history indicates she's at risk for candidiasis?
1. Nulliparity
2. Menopause
3. Use of corticosteroids
4. Use of spermicidal jelly

10. 3. Small numbers of the fungus *Candida albicans* commonly are found in the vagina. Because corticosteroids decrease host defense, they increase the risk of candidiasis. Pregnancy, not nulliparity, increases the risk of candidiasis. Candidiasis is rare before menarche and after menopause. The use of oral contraceptives, not spermicidal jelly, increases the risk of candidiasis.

CN: Health promotion and maintenance; CNS: None; CL: Application

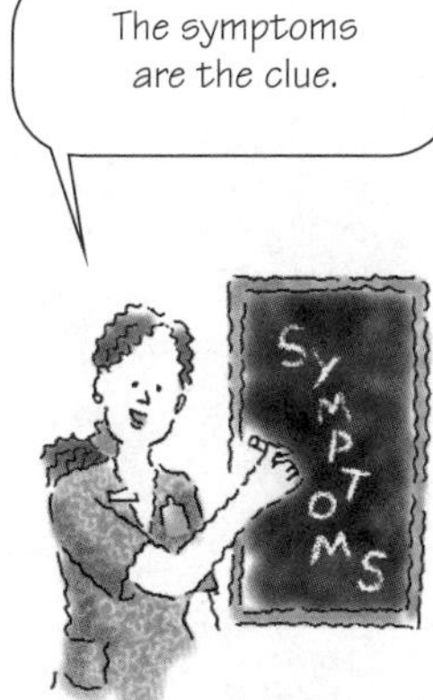

11. Copious amounts of frothy, greenish vaginal discharge would be a symptom with which infection?
1. Candidiasis
2. *Gardnerella vaginalis* vaginitis
3. Gonorrhea
4. Trichomoniasis

11. 4. The discharge associated with infection caused by *Trichomonas* organisms is homogenous, greenish gray, watery, and frothy or purulent. The discharge associated with candidiasis is thick and white and resembles cottage cheese in appearance, while that associated with infection due to *Gardnerella vaginalis* is thin and grayish white, with a marked fishy odor. With gonorrhea, vaginal discharge is purulent when present but, in many women, gonorrhea is asymptomatic.

CN: Physiological integrity; CNS: Physiological adaptation; CL: Application

12. A 19-year-old woman reports an intermittent milky vaginal discharge. She isn't sexually active and denies itching or burning. Which factor is the most likely cause of the milky-appearing discharge?

1. Inadequate cleaning of the perineal area
2. Sensitivity to a feminine hygiene product
3. Normal fluctuation in estrogen and progesterone levels
4. Reaction to heat and moisture from wearing tight clothing

12. 3. Vaginal fluid is clear, milky, or cloudy, depending on the fluctuating levels of estrogen and progesterone. A milky-appearing vaginal discharge is normal and isn't associated with inadequate cleaning, sensitivity, or reaction to heat or moisture.

CN: Health promotion and maintenance; CNS: None; CL: Application

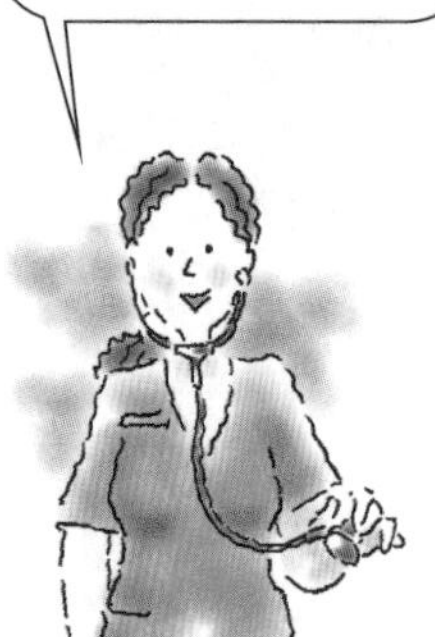

Postoperative care depends on the type of surgery.

13. Which nursing intervention is appropriate for a client who had breast reconstruction surgery?

1. Prevent hypothermia.
2. Maintain even pressure on the wound.
3. Position the client on the operative side.
4. Raise the client's arms over her head four times daily.

13. 1. Hypothermia causes a decrease in surface circulation. This can lead to ischemia of the skin or muscle graft and ultimately to tissue necrosis in clients who had breast reconstruction surgery. Because of the importance of maintaining good circulation, pressure on the breast wound must be avoided, so the client is positioned on the back or nonoperative side. Arms shouldn't be lifted above shoulder level for 4 to 6 weeks.

CN: Physiological integrity; CNS: Reduction of risk potential; CL: Application

14. A client who had intracavitary radiation treatment for cancer of the cervix 1 month earlier reports small amounts of vaginal bleeding. This most likely represents which condition?

1. Recurrence of the carcinoma
2. Development of a rectovaginal fistula
3. Expected effect of the radiation therapy
4. Infection secondary to a change in vaginal flora

14. 3. After intracavitary radiation, some vaginal bleeding occurs for 1 to 3 months. Intermittent painless vaginal bleeding is a classic symptom of cervical cancer, but given the client's history, bleeding is more likely a result of the radiation than recurrent cancer. The passage of feces through the vagina, not vaginal bleeding, is a sign of rectovaginal fistula. Vaginal infections show various types of vaginal discharge but not vaginal bleeding.

CN: Physiological integrity; CNS: Physiological adaptation; CL: Application

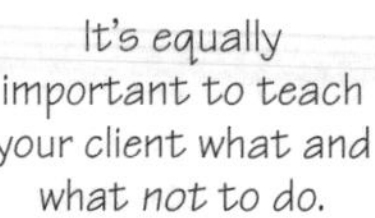

It's equally important to teach your client what and what not to do.

15. A nurse enters the room of a client who had a left modified mastectomy 8 hours earlier. Which observation indicates that the nursing assistant assigned to the client needs further instruction and guidance?

1. The client is squeezing a ball in her left hand.
2. The client is wearing a robe with elastic cuffs.
3. The client's affected arm is elevated on a pillow.
4. A blood pressure cuff is on the client's right arm.

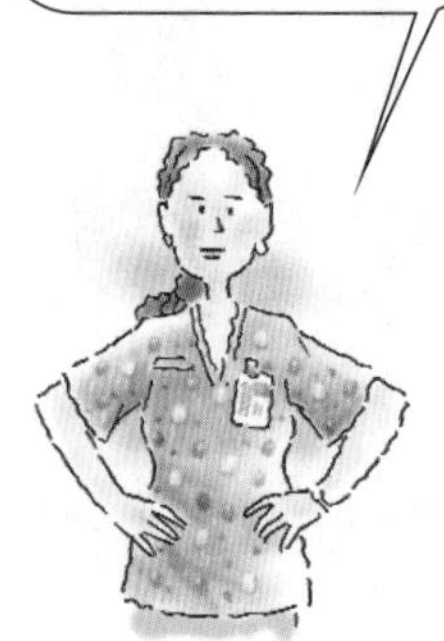

15. 2. Elastic cuffs can contribute to the development of lymphedema and should be avoided. Simple exercises, such as squeezing a ball, help promote circulation and should be started as soon as possible after surgery. Elevation of the affected arm promotes venous and lymphatic return from the extremity. Blood pressure measurements in the affected arm also should be avoided.

CN: Safe, effective care environment; CNS: Management of care; CL: Analysis

16. For which symptom should a client at risk for evisceration be monitored after an abdominal hysterectomy?

1. Tachycardia accompanied by a weak, thready pulse
2. Hypotension with a decreased level of consciousness (LOC)
3. Shallow, rapid respirations and increasing vaginal drainage
4. Low-grade fever with increasing serosanguineous incisional drainage

16. 4. Signs of impending evisceration are low-grade fever and increasing serosanguineous drainage. Tachycardia; weak, thready pulse; hypotension; decreased LOC; shallow, rapid respirations; and vaginal drainage after abdominal hysterectomy are all unrelated to impending evisceration, although they may be associated with other serious problems such as shock.

CN: Physiological integrity; CNS: Reduction of risk potential; CL: Application

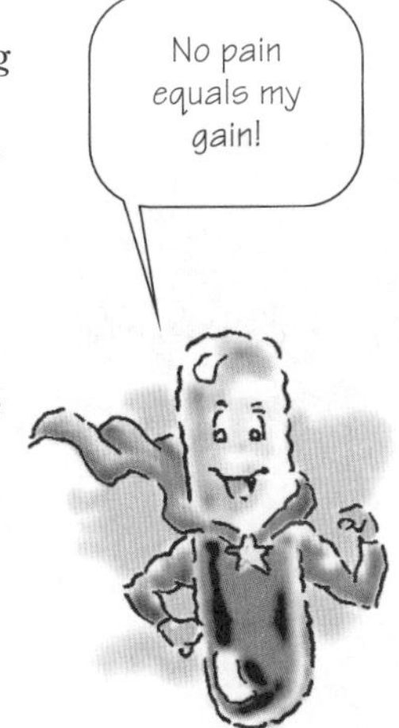
No pain equals my gain!

17. Which finding indicates that oxycodone (OxyContin) given to a client with breast cancer metastasized to the bone is exerting the desired effect?

1. Bone density is increased.
2. Pain is 0 to 2 on a 10-point scale.
3. Alpha-fetoprotein level is decreased.
4. Serum calcium level is within normal range.

17. 2. Oxycodone is an opioid analgesic used for alleviating severe pain, especially in terminal illness. If a client's pain has decreased to 0 to 2 on a 10-point scale (0 is no pain and 10 is the worst pain), the medication is working as desired. The drug doesn't directly affect bone density, alpha-fetoprotein level, or serum calcium level.

CN: Physiological integrity; CNS: Pharmacological and parenteral therapies; CL: Analysis

18. Which instruction should be given to a client with prostatitis who's receiving co-trimoxazole double strength (Bactrim DS)?

1. Don't expect improvement of symptoms for 7 to 10 days.
2. Drink six to eight glasses of fluid daily while taking this medication.
3. If a sore mouth or throat develops, take the medication with milk or an antacid.
4. Use a sunscreen of at least SPF-15 with para-aminobenzoic acid (PABA) to protect against drug-induced photosensitivity.

18. 2. Six to eight glasses of fluid daily are needed to prevent renal problems, such as crystalluria and stone formation. The symptoms should improve in a few days if the drug is effective. Sore throat and sore mouth are adverse effects that should be reported right away. The drug causes photosensitivity, but a PABA-free sunscreen should be used because PABA can interfere with the drug's action.

CN: Physiological integrity; CNS: Pharmacological and parenteral therapies; CL: Application

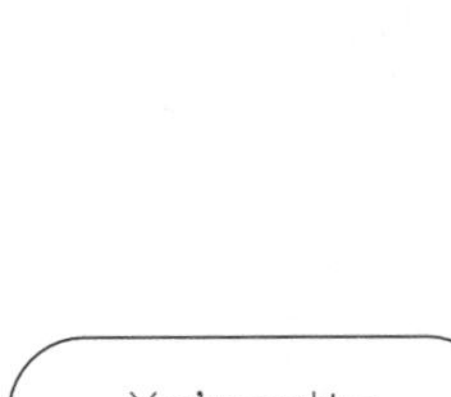
You're making great strides. Keep going!

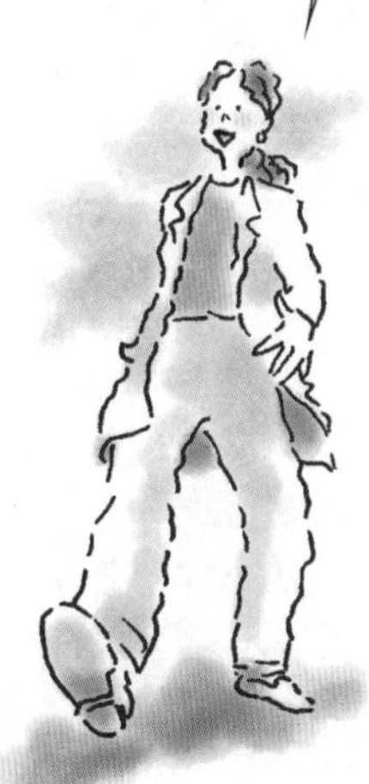

19. Which factor should be checked when evaluating the effectiveness of an alpha-adrenergic blocker given to a client with benign prostatic hyperplasia (BPH)?

1. Voiding pattern
2. Size of the prostate
3. Creatinine clearance
4. Serum testosterone level

19. 1. Alpha-adrenergic blockers relax the smooth muscle of the bladder neck and prostate, so the urinary voiding symptoms (frequency, urgency, hesitancy) of BPH are reduced in many clients. These drugs don't affect the size of the prostate, renal function, or production or metabolism of testosterone.

CN: Physiological integrity; CNS: Pharmacological and parenteral therapies; CL: Application

20. A nursing diagnosis addressing *Risk for impaired tissue integrity* would be most appropriate for which client?

1. A client with endometriosis
2. A client taking oral contraceptives
3. A client with a vaginal packing in place
4. A client having reconstructive breast surgery

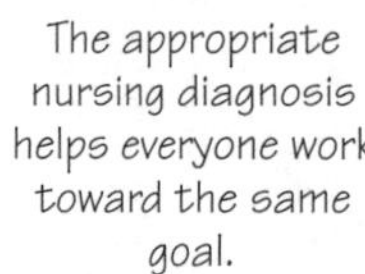

The appropriate nursing diagnosis helps everyone work toward the same goal.

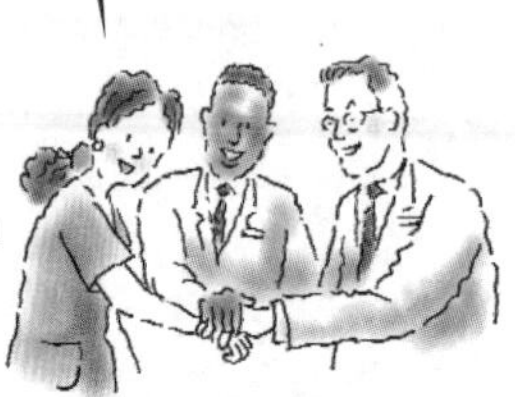

20. 4. Reconstructive breast surgery places the client at risk for insufficient blood supply to the muscle graft and skin, which can lead to tissue necrosis. Endometriosis or oral contraceptives aren't generally associated with altered tissue perfusion. Pressure from vaginal packing can sometimes put pressure on the bladder neck and interfere with voiding.

CN: Physiological integrity; CNS: Reduction of risk potential; CL: Analysis

21. A 27-year-old man arrives at the clinic with priapism. The nurse arranges for an immediate urologic consult because of the risk of which condition?

1. Disseminated intravascular coagulation (DIC)
2. Hydronephrosis
3. Penile gangrene
4. Testicular atrophy

21. 3. Priapism is a condition in which the penis is persistently erect and painful. It's a urologic emergency because gangrene secondary to ischemia can result if venous drainage of the corpora cavernosa doesn't occur. Priapism doesn't cause DIC, hydronephrosis, or testicular atrophy.

CN: Physiological integrity; CNS: Reduction of risk potential; CL: Application

22. Which instruction is the most important to give women to decrease the risk of toxic shock syndrome?

1. Avoid douching.
2. Wear loose cotton underwear.
3. Use pads, not tampons, overnight.
4. Avoid sexual intercourse during menses.

22. 3. The cause of toxic shock syndrome is a toxin produced by *Staphylococcus aureus* bacteria. It occurs most commonly in menstruating women using tampons. Tampons, particularly when left in place for more than 8 hours (such as overnight), are believed to provide a good environment for growth of the bacteria, which then enter the bloodstream through breaks in the vaginal mucosa. Douching, use of loose cotton underwear, and sexual intercourse during menstruation have no direct association with toxic shock syndrome.

CN: Health promotion and maintenance; CNS: None; CL: Analysis

23. Which response is the most appropriate when a client asks what activity limitations are necessary after a dilatation and curettage procedure?

1. Tampons may be used during exercise.
2. Avoid strenuous work and sexual intercourse for at least 2 weeks.
3. Stay on bed rest for 3 days; then gradually resume normal activity.
4. Take a soaking tub bath each day to promote relaxation.

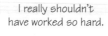

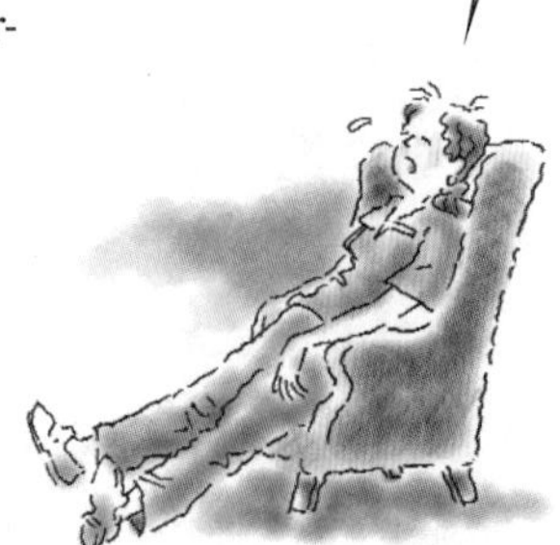

I really shouldn't have worked so hard.

23. 2. Strenuous work, which can result in increased bleeding, should be avoided for 2 weeks to allow time for healing. Sexual intercourse should also be avoided for 2 weeks to allow healing and thus decrease the risk of infection. Tampons and tub baths should be avoided for 1 week. Overall activity should be gradually resumed, reaching preoperative levels in the 2-week period, but bed rest isn't necessary. No other restrictions are routinely necessary.

CN: Physiological integrity; CNS: Reduction of risk potential; CL: Application

24. Which assessment finding is expected in a client receiving bicalutamide (Casodex) and leuprolide (Lupron) for advanced prostate cancer?

1. Abdominal distention
2. Acromegaly
3. Colicky pain
4. Hot flashes

24. 4. Bicalutamide, a nonsteroidal antiandrogen, and leuprolide, a gonadotropin-releasing hormone agonist, decrease the production of testosterone. This helps to decrease the production of cancer cells involved in the prostate cancer. Because androgens are responsible for the development of the male genitalia and secondary male sex characteristics, low androgen levels can cause genital atrophy, breast enlargement, and hot flashes. Abdominal distention, acromegaly, and colicky pain aren't caused by bicalutamide and leuprolide therapy.

CN: Physiological integrity; CNS: Pharmacological and parenteral therapies; CL: Analysis

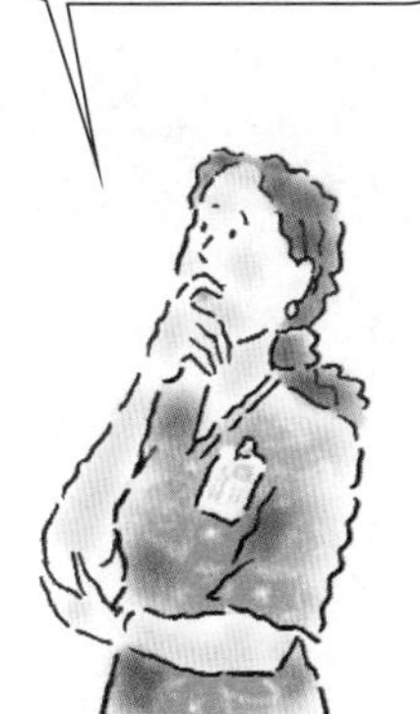

What is abnormal about this client's findings?

25. Which assessment finding is abnormal in a 72-year-old male client?

1. Decreased sperm count
2. Small, firm testes on palpation
3. History of slowed sexual response
4. Decreased plasma testosterone level

25. 1. Sperm continues to be produced despite the age-related degenerative changes that occur in the male reproductive system. Among the normal age-related changes are decreased size and increased firmness of the testes, a decrease in sexual potency, and decreased production of testosterone and progesterone.

CN: Physiological integrity; CNS: Physiological adaptation; CL: Application

26. Which comment made by a client being treated for chronic prostatitis indicates that self-care instructions need to be clarified?

1. "I miss not being able to have sex."
2. "I enjoy frequent soaking in a hot tub of water."
3. "Cutting down on coffee hasn't been as hard as I expected."
4. "I'm used to getting up and moving, not just sitting for long periods."

26. 1. Ejaculation can aid in the treatment of chronic prostatitis by decreasing the retention of prostatic fluid. Coffee should be eliminated from the diet because it can increase prostate secretion. Warm sitz baths and not sitting for too long at a time promote comfort.

CN: Physiological integrity; CNS: Physiological adaptation; CL: Application

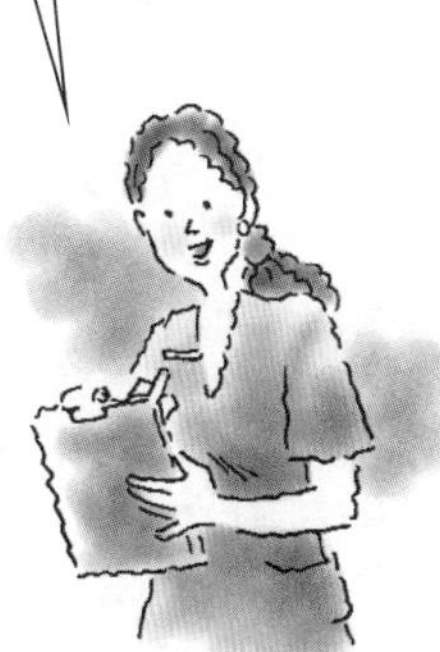

Client teaching includes making sure your client understands your instructions.

27. Perineal pain in the absence of any observable cause is suggestive of which condition?

1. Endometriosis
2. Internal hemorrhoids
3. Prostatitis
4. Renal calculus

27. 3. Prostatitis can cause prostate pain, which is felt as perineal discomfort. Endometriosis can cause pain low in the abdomen, deep in the pelvis, or in the rectal or sacrococcygeal area, depending on the location of the ectopic tissue. Hemorrhoids cause rectal pain and pressure. Renal calculi typically produce flank pain.

CN: Health promotion and maintenance; CNS: None; CL: Analysis

28. Which assessment finding would be a cause for alarm in a client taking finasteride (Proscar)?

1. Azotemia
2. Breast enlargement
3. Decreased prostate size
4. Flushing

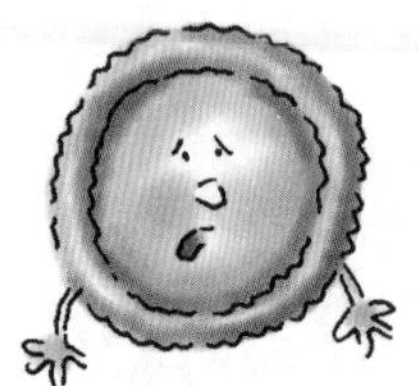
Which assessment finding is cause for alarm? Here's a hint: I think it's a waste.

28. 1. Azotemia, a buildup of nitrogenous waste products in the blood, indicates impaired renal function. Finasteride, an antiandrogenic agent, is prescribed for chronic urinary retention with large residual volumes secondary to benign prostatic hypertrophy. Azotemia in a client on finasteride therapy can indicate the drug isn't effective in relieving the urinary symptoms associated with benign prostatic hypertrophy or that an unrelated renal problem has occurred. Breast enlargement, decrease in prostate size, and flushing are expected effects of finasteride.

CN: Physiological integrity; CNS: Pharmacological and parenteral therapies; CL: Application

29. Which treatment is appropriate for a client with cervical polyps who has been treated with cryosurgery?

1. Daily douche
2. Oral antibiotics
3. Intravaginal antibiotic cream
4. Use of tampons for 72 hours

29. 3. Intravaginal antibiotic cream is commonly used to aid healing and prevent infection. Oral antibiotics are used for clients with acute cervicitis or perimetritis. Douching is generally avoided for 2 weeks, as is the use of tampons.

CN: Physiological integrity; CNS: Reduction of risk potential; CL: Application

30. Which intervention would be correct for a woman having intracavitary radiation for cancer of the cervix?

1. High-residue diet
2. Fowler's position when in bed
3. Intermittent urinary catheterization
4. Bed rest

30. 4. Clients having intracavitary radiation therapy are on strict bed rest, with the head of the bed elevated no more than 10 to 15 degrees to avoid displacing the radiation source. A low- residue diet is used to prevent diarrhea during treatment. An order for Fowler's position when in bed is incorrect. An indwelling urinary catheter, not intermittent urinary catheterization, is used to prevent urine from distending the bladder and changing the position of tissues relative to the radiation source.

CN: Physiological integrity; CNS: Physiological adaptation; CL: Analysis

31. Which condition of the female reproductive system generally requires the identification and treatment of sexual partners?

1. Bartholinitis
2. Candidiasis
3. Chlamydia
4. Endometriosis

31. 3. Chlamydia is a common sexually transmitted disease requiring the treatment of all current sexual partners to prevent reinfection. Bartholinitis results from obstruction of a duct. Sexual partners may become infected, although men can usually be treated with over-the-counter products. Candidiasis is a yeast infection that typically occurs as a result of antibiotic use. Endometriosis occurs when endometrial cells are seeded throughout the pelvis and isn't a sexually transmitted disease.

CN: Health promotion and maintenance; CNS: None; CL: Application

32. Which information should be given to a client taking metronidazole (Flagyl)?

1. Breathlessness and cough are common adverse effects.
2. Urine may develop a greenish tinge while the client is taking this drug.
3. Mixing this drug with alcohol causes severe nausea and vomiting.
4. Heart palpitations may occur and should be immediately reported.

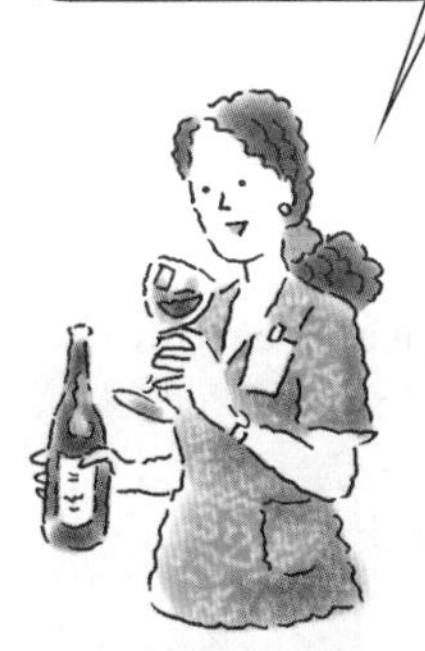

Drugs and alcohol typically don't mix.

32. 3. When mixed with alcohol, metronidazole causes a disulfiram-like effect involving nausea, vomiting, and other unpleasant symptoms. Urine may turn reddish brown, not greenish, from the drug. Cardiovascular or respiratory effects aren't associated with use of this drug.

CN: Physiological integrity; CNS: Pharmacological and parenteral therapies; CL: Application

33. Which symptom is an adverse reaction of hydrocodone with acetaminophen that a client with metastatic prostate cancer should be instructed to report to the physician?

1. Blurred vision
2. Diarrhea
3. Unusual dreams
4. Vomiting

33. 4. Vomiting is an adverse reaction to the drug that should be reported because it impairs the client's quality of life and places the client at risk for dehydration. Taking the medication with food may prevent vomiting. If not, other opiate analgesics may be better tolerated. Blurred vision and diarrhea aren't associated with the use of hydrocodone with acetaminophen. Unusual dreams are a common adverse effect but don't need to be reported unless they're bothersome to the client.

CN: Physiological integrity; CNS: Pharmacological and parenteral therapies; CL: Application

34. Which intervention is appropriate for a client having hysterosalpingography?

1. Give the client a perineal pad to wear after the procedure.
2. Give the client nothing by mouth after midnight the night before the procedure.
3. Position the client in the knee-chest position during the procedure.
4. Keep the client in a dorsal recumbent position for 4 hours after the procedure.

34. 1. A perineal pad is needed after hysterosalpingography because the contrast medium may leak from the vagina for several hours and stain the clothing. The bowel needs to be cleaned before the procedure, but the client doesn't have to refrain from having anything by mouth after midnight. The procedure is performed with the client in the lithotomy position, and no special positioning is required after the procedure.

CN: Physiological integrity; CNS: Basic care and comfort; CL: Application

35. The nurse is instructing a client with vulvovaginal candidiasis on the use of the prescribed Nystatin vaginal tablets. Which of the following statements indicates the client needs additional teaching?

1. "I will need to refrigerate the Nystatin tablets."
2. "I can get up to do other activities after inserting the medicine."
3. "I will finish all the tablets even if I am feeling better."
4. "I should report any increased skin irritation to my doctor."

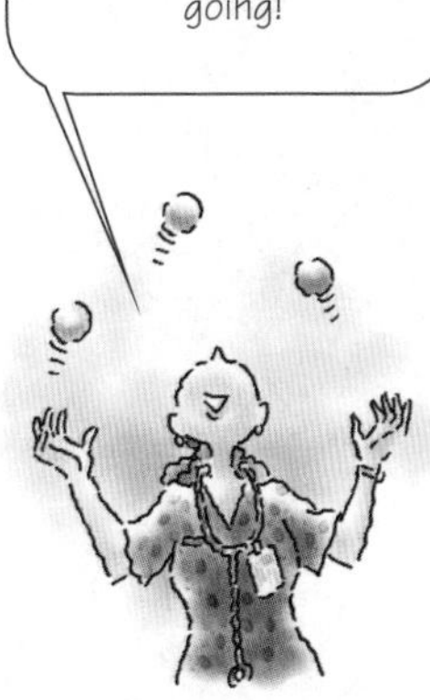

You've got it all under control. Keep going!

35. 2. The client needs to continue lying down for at least 30 minutes after insertion of the vaginal tablets. Refrigerating Nystatin tablets, finishing all the tablets, and reporting any increased skin irritation to the doctor are all important interventions concerning this medication.

CN: Physiological integrity; CNS: Pharmacological and parenteral therapies; CL: Application

36. A 36-year-old client who has never had mumps reports that he was just notified that an 8-year-old child of a family with whom he stayed recently has been diagnosed with mumps. Which treatment should the client receive?

1. I.V. antibiotics
2. Ice packs to the scrotum
3. Application of a scrotal support
4. Administration of gamma globulin

36. 4. Gamma globulin provides passive immunity to mumps. Antibiotic therapy is used in the treatment of bacterial orchitis. Ice and the use of a scrotal support are used as comfort measures in the treatment of orchitis.

CN: Health promotion and maintenance; CNS: None; CL: Application

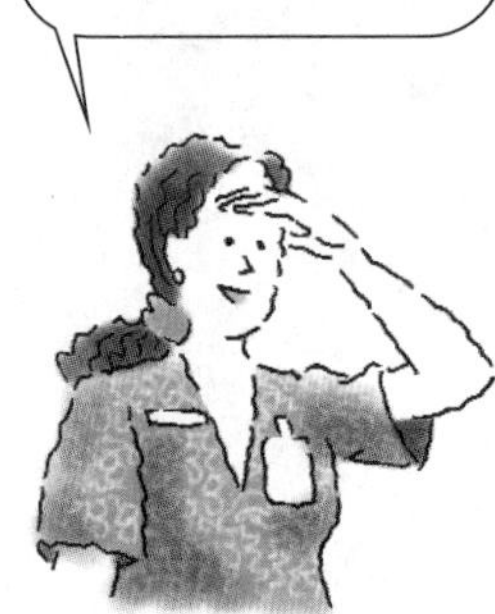

Look for signs that your client doesn't understand the information.

37. Which statement by a client scheduled for a vasectomy indicates he needs further teaching about the procedure?

1. "I'm glad I won't have to worry about contraception as soon as this procedure is done."
2. "I'll need to place an ice pack over the incision several times a day when I first go home."
3. "I know this procedure can be reversed, but the success rate is low."
4. "I'll have to limit my usual activities for about 1 week."

37. 1. After vasectomy, the client remains fertile for several weeks until sperm stored distal to the severed vas are evacuated. After this occurs, sperm are still produced but they don't enter the ejaculate and are absorbed by the body. The other statements are accurate.

CN: Physiological integrity; CNS: Physiological adaptation; CL: Analysis

38. Which area of client teaching should be stressed when the goal is preventing the development of phimosis in a 20-year-old uncircumcised client?

1. Proper cleaning of the prepuce
2. Importance of regular ejaculation
3. Technique of testicular self-examination
4. Proper hand washing before touching the genitals

38. 1. Proper cleaning of the preputial area to remove secretions is critical to the prevention of noncongenital phimosis. Regular ejaculation can decrease the symptoms of chronic prostatitis, but it has no effect on the development of phimosis. Testicular self-examination is important in the early detection and treatment of testicular cancer. Hand washing is important in preventing the spread of infection.

CN: Health promotion and maintenance; CNS: None; CL: Application

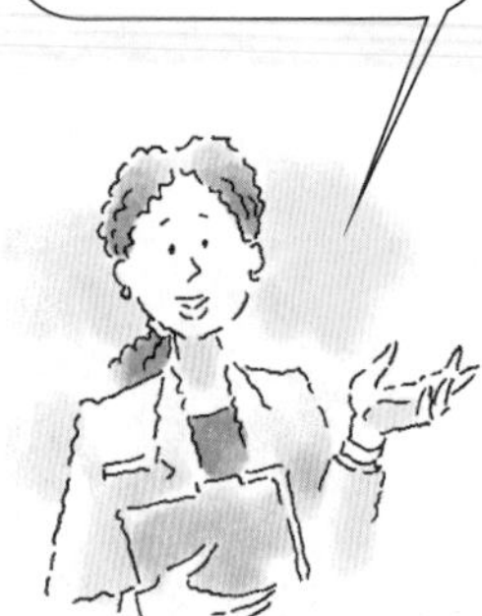

You can ease your client's worries through effective teaching efforts.

39. Which statement should be included when teaching a client newly diagnosed with testicular cancer?

1. Testicular cancer isn't responsive to chemotherapy, but it's highly curative with surgery.
2. Radiation therapy is never used, so the unaffected testicle remains healthy.
3. Testicular self-examination is still important because there's increased risk for a second tumor.
4. Taking testosterone after orchiectomy prevents changes in appearance and sexual function.

39. 3. A history of a testicular malignancy puts the client at increased risk for a second tumor. Testicular self-examination allows for early detection and treatment and is critical. Chemotherapy is added for clients who have evidence of metastasis after irradiation. Radiation therapy is used on the retroperitoneal lymph nodes. Testosterone usually isn't needed because the unaffected testis usually produces sufficient hormone.

CN: Physiological integrity; CNS: Reduction of risk potential; CL: Application

CN: Client needs category CNS: Client needs subcategory CL: Cognitive level

40. Which instruction should be given when teaching penile hygiene?
1. Use warm water without soap.
2. Dry all areas of the penis thoroughly.
3. Wash from the base of the shaft to the tip.
4. Avoid retracting the foreskin if not circumcised.

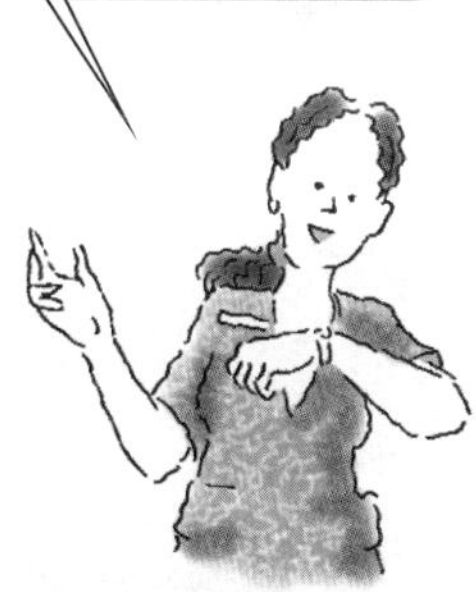

You've made it through 40 questions in no time!

40. 2. Careful drying is essential to avoid maceration of the penis. To decrease the risk of genitourinary infection, wash the penis from the tip to the base to reduce the risk for introducing pathogens into the urethral meatus. Effective cleaning requires soap and thorough rinsing. It's also essential to remove secretions that accumulate under the foreskin because they can lead to inflammation and are associated with the development of penile cancer. The foreskin in uncircumcised men must be retracted for cleaning, then replaced to prevent paraphimosis.
CN: Health promotion and maintenance; CNS: None; CL: Application

41. Which statement shows the significance of a persistent elevation in alpha-fetoprotein level after orchiectomy for testicular cancer?
1. Fertility is maintained.
2. The cancer has recurred.
3. There's metastatic disease.
4. Testosterone levels are low.

41. 3. Alpha-fetoprotein is a tumor marker elevated in nonseminomatous malignancies of the testicle. After the tumor is removed, the level should decrease. A persistent elevation after orchiectomy indicates a tumor is present someplace outside the testicle that was removed. The level of alpha-fetoprotein isn't related to fertility or testosterone level. A recurrence of the cancer is indicated by a postsurgical decrease in alpha-fetoprotein level followed by an elevation as a new tumor starts to grow.
CN: Physiological integrity; CNS: Physiological adaptation; CL: Analysis

42. Which discharge instruction should be given to a client after a prostatectomy?
1. Avoid straining at stool.
2. Report clots in the urine right away.
3. Soak in a warm tub daily for comfort.
4. Return to your usual activities in 3 weeks.

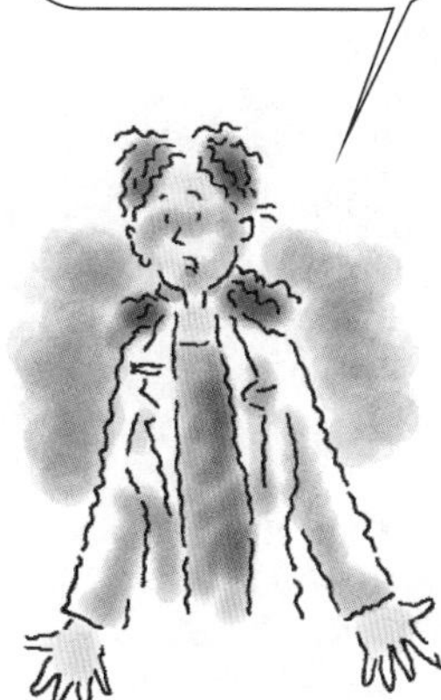

This test has been a real strain on my brain.

42. 1. Straining at stool after prostatectomy can cause bleeding. Small blood clots or pieces of tissue commonly are passed in the urine for up to 2 weeks postoperatively. Tub baths are prohibited because they cause dilation of pelvic blood vessels. Other activities are resumed based on the guidance of the physician. Sexual intercourse and driving are usually prohibited for about 3 weeks. Exercising and returning to work are usually prohibited for about 6 weeks.
CN: Physiological integrity; CNS: Reduction of risk potential; CL: Application

43. After a biopsy of the prostate, which symptom should a nurse instruct a client to report?
1. Pain on the following day
2. Discolored semen
3. Difficulty urinating
4. Temperature greater than 99°F (37.2° C)

43. 3. Difficulty urinating suggests urethral obstruction. Mild pain is expected for 1 to 3 days after the biopsy. Semen may be discolored for up to a month after the biopsy. Temperature higher than 101°F (38.3° C) should be reported because it suggests infection.
CN: Physiological integrity; CNS: Reduction of risk potential; CL: Analysis

44. Two days after a transrectal biopsy of the prostate, a client calls the clinic to report that his stool is streaked with blood. Which response is appropriate?

1. Tell the client to take a laxative.
2. Tell the client to come in for examination.
3. Reassure the client that this is an expected occurrence.
4. Ask the client to collect a stool specimen for testing.

44. 3. After a transrectal prostatic biopsy, blood in the stool is expected for a number of days. Because blood in the stool is expected, testing the stool or examining the client isn't necessary. Stool softeners are prescribed if the client complains of constipation; straining at stool can precipitate bleeding, but laxatives generally aren't necessary.
CN: Physiological integrity; CNS: Reduction of risk potential; CL: Application

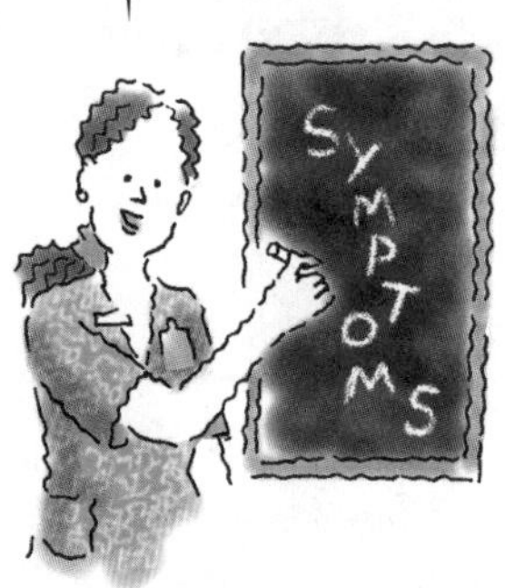
Teach your client the prodromal symptoms of an outbreak of genital herpes.
SYMPTOMS

45. A nurse is caring for clients who have a history of genital herpes infection. Which client is most at risk for an outbreak of genital herpes?

1. A client who complains of a headache and fever
2. A client who complains of vaginal and urethral discharge
3. A client who complains of dysuria and lymphadenopathy
4. A client who complains of genital pruritus and paresthesia

45. 4. Pruritus and paresthesia as well as redness of the genital area are prodromal symptoms of recurrent herpes infection. These symptoms occur 30 minutes to 48 hours before the lesions appear. Headache and fever are symptoms of viremia associated with the primary infection. Vaginal and urethral discharge is also a local sign of primary infection. Dysuria and lymphadenopathy are local symptoms of primary infection that may also occur with recurrent infection.
CN: Physiological integrity; CNS: Physiological adaptation; CL: Analysis

46. Which instruction should be given to a female client newly diagnosed with genital herpes?

1. Obtain a Papanicolaou (Pap) test every year.
2. Have your partner use a condom when lesions are present.
3. Use a water-soluble lubricant for relief of pruritus.
4. Limit stress and emotional upset as much as possible.

46. 4. Stress, anxiety, and emotional upset seem to predispose to recurrent outbreaks of genital herpes. Because a relationship has been found between genital herpes and cervical cancer, a Pap test is recommended every 6 months. Sexual intercourse should be avoided during outbreaks, and a condom should be used between outbreaks; it isn't known if the virus can be transmitted at this time. During an outbreak, creams and lubricants should be avoided because they may prolong healing.
CN: Physiological integrity; CNS: Physiological adaptation; CL: Application

47. A client newly diagnosed with genital herpes is crying and wringing her hands as the nurse approaches her. Which nursing diagnosis is the most appropriate to this situation?

1. *Acute pain*
2. *Impaired tissue integrity*
3. *Anxiety*
4. *Deficient knowledge*

47. 3. The client is demonstrating *Anxiety*; this problem needs to be incorporated into the plan of care. *Acute pain* and *Impaired tissue integrity* are not nursing diagnoses for the client. The client may have *Deficient knowledge* concerning the new diagnosis; however, that is not being demonstrated at this time.
CN: Psychosocial integrity; CNS: None; CL: Application

CN: Client needs category CNS: Client needs subcategory CL: Cognitive level

48. A client is describing how she palpates her breasts for breast self-examination. Which statement indicates the need for further teaching?

1. "I put lotion on my breasts before I begin to palpate them."
2. "I palpate both breasts standing up and then lying on my back."
3. "I'm careful to palpate under each arm and up to 2 inches below my collarbone."
4. "I start at the outer edge of the breast and work in to the nipple in smaller and smaller circles."

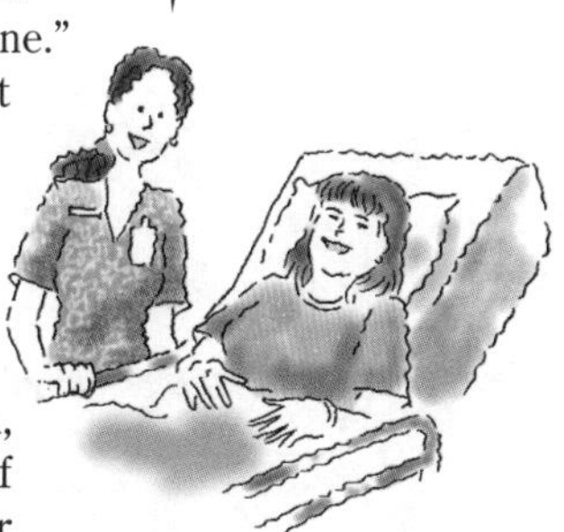
Make sure your client understands the proper technique for breast self-examination.

48. 3. Breast self-examination requires palpation of all breast tissue. This includes checking the area above the breast up to the collarbone and all the way over to the shoulder as well as the area between the breast and the underarm, including the underarm itself. Lotion or powder helps the fingers glide over the skin and facilitates palpation. Breasts need to be palpated in both erect and lying positions. Any pattern of palpation may be used in performing breast self-examination as long as each quadrant of the breast, tail, and axilla are examined.

CN: Health promotion and maintenance; CNS: None; CL: Application

49. During a routine physical examination, a firm mass is palpated in the right breast of a 35-year-old female client. Which finding or client history would suggest cancer of the breast as opposed to fibrocystic disease?

1. Mass located in upper, outer quadrant
2. Cyclic change in mass size
3. History of anovulatory cycles
4. Increased vascularity of the breast

49. 4. Increase in breast size or vascularity is consistent with cancer of the breast. Masses associated with fibrocystic disease of the breast are firm, most commonly located in the upper outer quadrant of the breast, and increase in size prior to menstruation. They may be bilateral in a mirror image and are typically well demarcated and freely moveable.

CN: Health promotion and maintenance; CNS: None; CL: Application

50. After which procedure is a postoperative wound infection most likely?

1. Radical prostatectomy
2. Perineal prostatectomy
3. Suprapubic prostatectomy
4. Transurethral resection of the prostate (TURP)

50. 2. The incision in a perineal prostatectomy is close to the rectum, which normally contains gram-negative organisms that can cause infection if introduced into other areas of the body. Therefore, a perineal incision will become contaminated more often than either no external incision, as with TURP, or abdominal incisions, as with radical or suprapubic prostatectomy.

CN: Physiological integrity; CNS: Reduction of risk potential; CL: Analysis

Read this question carefully.

51. A client with pneumonia is transfered to the intensive care unit for mechanical ventilation. His blood pressure is 70/40, his heart rate is 115 beats/minute, and his respiratory rate is 32 breaths/minute with accessory muscle use. I.V.s are infusing at 150 ml/hour. Urine output is 50 ml for the past 4 hours. This client is most at risk for which of the following?

1. Postrenal failure
2. Prerenal failure
3. Intrarenal failure
4. Chronic renal failure

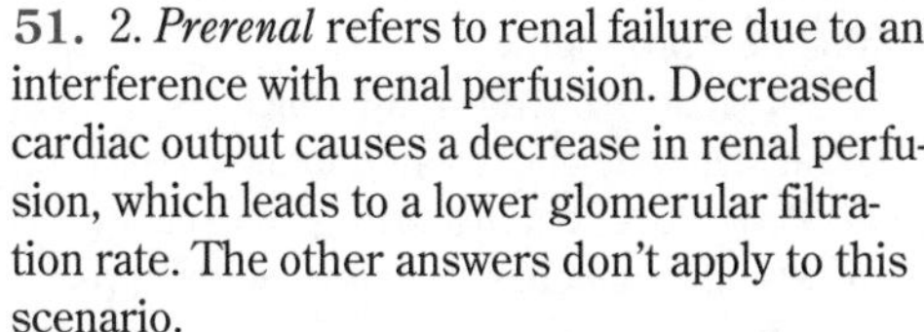

51. 2. *Prerenal* refers to renal failure due to an interference with renal perfusion. Decreased cardiac output causes a decrease in renal perfusion, which leads to a lower glomerular filtration rate. The other answers don't apply to this scenario.

CN: Physiological integrity; CNS: Physiological adaptation; CL: Analysis

52. A client admitted for acute pyelonephritis is about to start antibiotic therapy. Which symptom would be expected in this client?
1. Hypertension
2. Flank pain on the affected side
3. Pain that radiates toward the unaffected side
4. No tenderness with deep palpation over the costovertebral angle

52. 2. The client may complain of pain on the affected side because the kidney is enlarged and might have formed an abscess. Hypertension is associated with chronic pyelonephritis. Pain may radiate down the ureters or to the epigastrium. The client would have tenderness with deep palpation over the costovertebral angle.
CN: Physiological integrity; CNS: Physiological adaptation; CL: Application

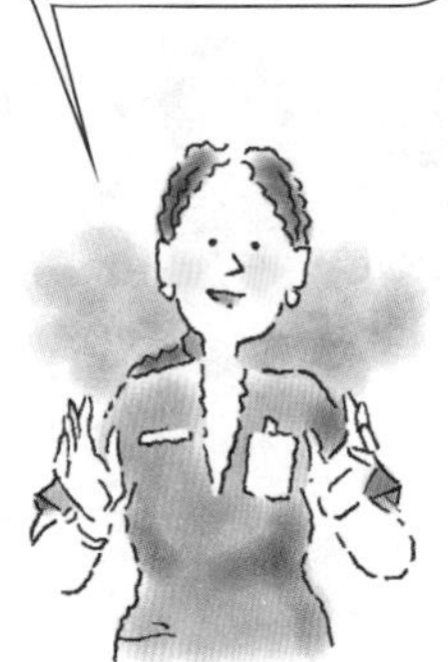

Here's another question about client teaching, an essential topic on NCLEX examinations.

53. Discharge instructions for a client treated for acute pyelonephritis should include which statement?
1. Avoid taking any dairy products.
2. Return for follow-up urine cultures.
3. Stop taking the prescribed antibiotics when the symptoms subside.
4. Recurrence is unlikely because you've been treated with antibiotics.

53. 2. The client needs to return for follow-up urine cultures because bacteriuria may be present but asymptomatic. Intake of dairy products won't contribute to pyelonephritis. Antibiotics need to be taken for the full course of therapy regardless of symptoms. Pyelonephritis typically recurs as a relapse or new infection and frequently recurs within 2 weeks of completing therapy.
CN: Health promotion and maintenance; CNS: None; CL: Application

54. A client is complaining of severe flank and abdominal pain. A flat plate of the abdomen shows urolithiasis. Which intervention is important?
1. Strain all urine.
2. Limit fluid intake.
3. Enforce strict bed rest.
4. Encourage a high-calcium diet.

54. 1. Urine should be strained for calculi and sent to the laboratory for analysis. Fluid intake of 3 to 4 qt (3 to 4 L)/day is encouraged to flush the urinary tract and prevent further calculi formation. Ambulation is encouraged to help pass the calculi through gravity. A low-calcium diet is recommended to help prevent the formation of calcium calculi.
CN: Physiological integrity; CNS: Reduction of risk potential; CL: Application

55. A client is receiving a radiation implant for the treatment of bladder cancer. Which intervention is appropriate?
1. Flush all urine down the toilet.
2. Restrict the client's fluid intake.
3. Place the client in a semiprivate room.
4. Monitor the client for signs and symptoms of cystitis.

55. 4. Cystitis is the most common adverse reaction of clients undergoing radiation therapy; symptoms include dysuria, frequency, urgency, and nocturia. Urine of clients with radiation implants for bladder cancer should be sent to the radioisotopes laboratory for monitoring. It's recommended that fluid intake be increased. Clients with radiation implants require a private room.
CN: Physiological integrity; CNS: Physiological adaptation; CL: Application

56. A client has undergone a radical cystectomy and has an ileal conduit for the treatment of bladder cancer. Which postoperative assessment finding must be reported to the physician immediately?

1. A red, moist stoma
2. A dusky colored stoma
3. Urine output more than 30 ml/hour
4. Slight bleeding from the stoma when changing the appliance

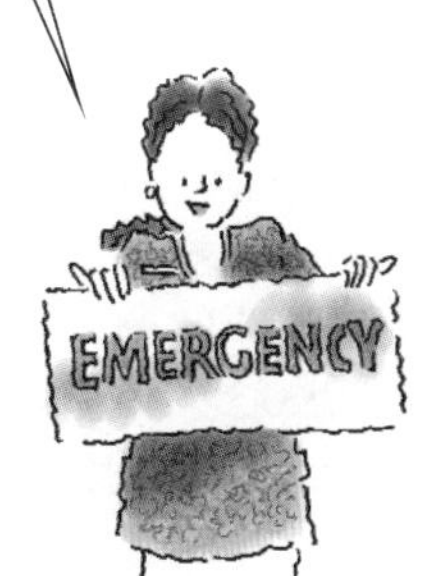

Question 56 asks you to prioritize responses according to which is most urgent.
EMERGENCY

56. 2. The stoma should be red and moist, indicating adequate blood flow. A dusky or cyanotic stoma indicates insufficient blood supply and is an emergency needing prompt intervention. Urine output less than 30 ml/hour or no urine output for more than 15 minutes should be reported. Slight bleeding from the stoma when changing the appliance may occur because the intestinal mucosa is fragile.

CN: Physiological integrity; CNS: Reduction of risk potential; CL: Application

57. Which instruction about skin care at the stoma site should be given to a client with an ileal conduit?

1. Change the appliance at bedtime.
2. Leave the stoma open to air while changing the appliance.
3. Clean the skin around the stoma with mild soap and water, and dry it thoroughly.
4. Cut the faceplate or wafer of the appliance no more than 4 mm larger than the stoma.

57. 3. Cleaning the skin around the stoma with mild soap and water and drying it thoroughly helps keep the area clean from urine, which can irritate the skin. Change the appliance in the early morning when urine output is less to decrease the amount of urine in contact with the skin. The stoma should be covered with a gauze pad when changing the appliance to prevent seepage of urine onto the skin. The faceplate or wafer of the appliance shouldn't be more than 3 mm larger than the stoma to reduce the skin area in contact with urine.

CN: Physiological integrity; CNS: Basic care and comfort; CL: Application

58. A client is diagnosed with cystitis. Client teaching aimed at preventing a recurrence should include which instruction?

1. Bathe in a tub.
2. Wear cotton underwear.
3. Use a feminine hygiene spray.
4. Limit your intake of cranberry juice.

58. 2. Cotton underwear prevents infection because it allows for air to flow to the perineum. Women should shower instead of taking a tub bath to prevent infection. Feminine hygiene spray can act as an irritant. Cranberry juice helps prevent cystitis because it increases urine acidity; alkaline urine supports bacterial growth, so cranberry juice intake should be increased, not limited.

CN: Health promotion and maintenance; CNS: None; CL: Application

59. When performing a physical assessment, the nurse discovers a client's urinary drainage bag lying next to him. Based on this finding, the nurse identifies which priority nursing diagnosis?

1. *Risk for infection*
2. *Reflex urinary incontinence*
3. *Impaired comfort*
4. *Risk for compromised human dignity*

59. 1. The drainage bag shouldn't be placed alongside the client or on the floor because of the increased risk of infection caused by microorganisms. It should hang on the bed in a dependent position. The other nursing diagnoses are not appropriate for this assessment finding.

CN: Safe, effective care environment; CNS: Management of care; CL: Application

60. Which method should be used to collect a specimen for urine culture?

1. Have the client void in a clean container.
2. Clean the foreskin of the penis of uncircumcised men before specimen collection.
3. Have the client void into a urinal, and then pour the urine into the specimen container.
4. Have the client begin the stream of urine in the toilet and catch the urine in a sterile container midstream.

60. 4. Catching urine midstream reduces the amount of contamination by microorganisms at the meatus. Voiding in a clean container is done for a random specimen, not a clean-catch specimen for urine culture. When cleaning an uncircumcised male, the foreskin should be retracted and the glans penis should be cleaned to prevent specimen contamination. Voiding in a urinal doesn't allow for an uncontaminated specimen because the urinal isn't sterile.

CN: Physiological integrity; CNS: Reduction of risk potential; CL: Application

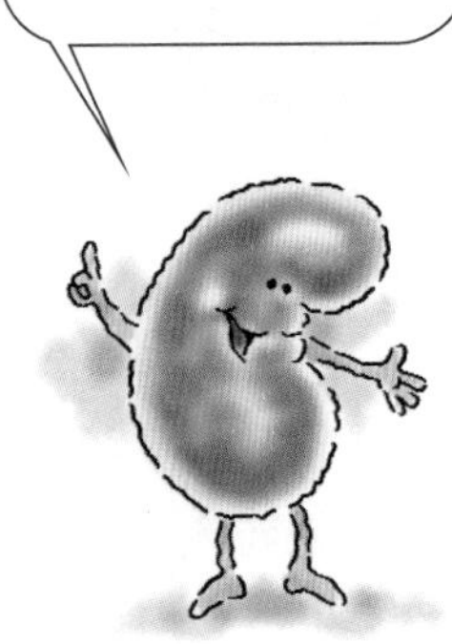

If I can't do my job properly, I get a little hyper.

61. A client with a history of chronic renal failure is admitted to the unit with pulmonary edema after missing his dialysis treatment yesterday. His laboratory result levels are serum potassium 6.0 mEq/L, serum sodium 130mEq/l, and serum bicarbonate 18mEq/L. The nurse interprets that the client has which of the following conditions?

1. Alkalemia
2. Hyperkalemia
3. Hypernatremia
4. Hypokalemia

61. 2. The kidneys are responsible for excreting potassium. In renal failure, the kidneys are no longer able to excrete potassium, resulting in hyperkalemia. The kidneys are responsible for regulating the acid-base balance; in renal failure, acidemia would be seen. Generally, hyponatremia would be seen because of the dilutional effect of water retention. Hypokalemia is generally seen in clients undergoing diuresis.

CN: Physiological integrity; CNS: Physiological adaptation; CL: Analysis

62. A client with acute renal failure has a serum potassium level of 7.0 mEq/L. The nurse's priority for this client is to assess which of the following?

1. Urine specific gravity
2. Electrocardiogram (ECG) results
3. Mental status
4. Blood pressure

62. 2. Acute renal failure can result in hyperkalemia, which can manifest in widening of the PR and QRS intervals on the ECG. Urine specific gravity, mental status, and blood pressure are not a priority with this client.

CN: Safe, effective care environment; CNS: Management of care; CL: Application

63. A client has just received a renal transplant and has started cyclosporine therapy to prevent graft rejection. Which discharge instruction should be emphasized?

1. Report any signs of depression or a decreased appetite.
2. Report any dizziness and bleeding from the incision.
3. Report any fever, a flushed feeling, or lethargy.
4. Report any stomach discomfort or dyspepsia.

63. 3. Fever, a flushed feeling, or lethargy suggests infection, which is the major complication to watch for in clients on cyclosporine therapy because it's an immunosuppressive drug. The other symptoms aren't indicative of cyclosporine therapy.

CN: Physiological integrity; CNS: Pharmacological and parental therapies; CL: Application

CN: Client needs category CNS: Client needs subcategory CL: Cognitive level

64. A client received a kidney transplant 2 months ago. He's admitted to the hospital with the diagnosis of acute rejection. Which assessment finding should be expected?

1. Hypotension
2. Normal body temperature
3. Decreased white blood cell (WBC) counts
4. Elevated blood urea nitrogen (BUN) and creatinine levels

64. 4. In a client with acute renal graft rejection, evidence of deteriorating renal function (elevated BUN and creatinine levels) is expected. The client would most likely have acute hypertension. The nurse would see fever and elevated WBC counts because the body is recognizing the graft as foreign and is attempting to fight it.

CN: Physiological integrity; CNS: Reduction of risk potential; CL: Analysis

65. A client is diagnosed with chronic renal failure and is told he must start hemodialysis. Client teaching should include which instruction?

1. Follow a high-potassium diet.
2. Strictly follow the hemodialysis schedule.
3. There will be few changes in your lifestyle.
4. Use alcohol on the skin to clean it because of integumentary changes.

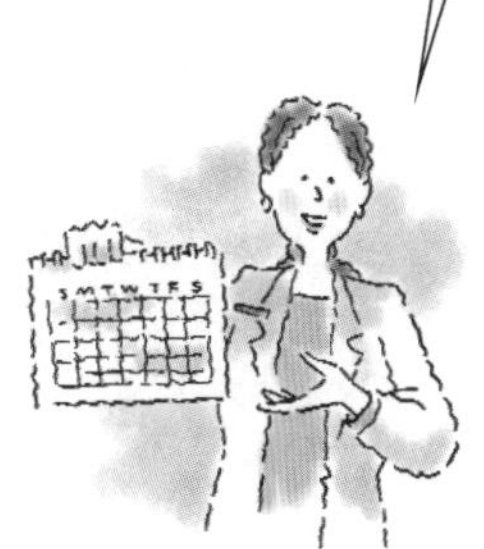

It's important that your client follow scheduled treatment.

65. 2. To prevent life-threatening complications, the client must follow the dialysis schedule. The client should follow a low-potassium diet because potassium levels increase in chronic renal failure. The client should know that hemodialysis is time-consuming and will definitely cause a change in current lifestyle. Alcohol would further dry the client's skin more than it already is.

CN: Physiological integrity; CNS: Reduction of risk potential; CL: Application

66. A client is to undergo a kidney transplantation with a living donor. Which preoperative assessment is the most important?

1. Urine output
2. Signs of graft rejection
3. Signs and symptoms of infection
4. Client's support system and understanding of lifestyle changes

66. 4. The client undergoing a renal transplantation will need vigilant follow-up care and must adhere to the medical regimen. The client is most likely anuric or oliguric preoperatively but postoperatively will require close monitoring of urine output to make sure the transplanted kidney is functioning optimally. Rejection can occur postoperatively. Although the client will always need to be monitored for signs and symptoms of infection, it's most important postoperatively because of the initiation of immunosuppressive therapy.

CN: Psychosocial integrity; CNS: None; CL: Application

67. A client is undergoing peritoneal dialysis. The dialysate dwell time is completed, and the clamp is opened to allow the dialysate to drain. The nurse notes that drainage has stopped and that only 500 ml has drained; the amount of dialysate instilled was 1,500 ml. Which intervention should be done first?

1. Change the client's position.
2. Call the physician.
3. Check the catheter for kinks or obstruction.
4. Clamp the catheter and instill more dialysate at the next exchange time.

This question is asking for the first thing you should do.

67. 3. The first intervention should be to check for kinks and obstructions because that could be preventing drainage. After checking for kinks, have the client change position to promote drainage. Don't give the next scheduled exchange until the dialysate is drained because abdominal distention will occur, unless the output is within the parameters set by the physician. If unable to get more output despite checking for kinks and changing the client's position, the nurse should then call the physician to determine the proper intervention.

CN: Physiological integrity; CNS: Reduction of risk potential; CL: Analysis

68. A client receiving hemodialysis treatments arrives at the hospital with a blood pressure of 200/100 mm Hg, a heart rate of 110 beats/minute, and a respiratory rate of 36 breaths/minute. Oxygen saturation on room air is 89%. He complains of shortness of breath, and +2 pedal edema is noted. His last hemodialysis treatment was yesterday. Which intervention should be done first?

1. Administer oxygen.
2. Elevate the foot of the bed.
3. Restrict the client's fluids.
4. Prepare the client for hemodialysis.

68. 1. Airway and oxygenation are always the first priority. Because the client is complaining of shortness of breath and his oxygen saturation is only 89%, the nurse needs to try to increase the partial pressure of arterial oxygen by administering oxygen. The foot of the bed may be elevated to reduce edema, but this isn't a priority. The client is in pulmonary edema from fluid overload and will need to be dialyzed and have his fluids restricted, but the first intervention should be aimed at the immediate treatment of hypoxia.

CN: Physiological integrity; CNS: Physiological adaptation; CL: Analysis

69. A client with renal insufficiency is admitted with a diagnosis of pneumonia. He's being treated with I.V. antibiotics, which can be nephrotoxic. Which laboratory value(s) should be monitored closely?

1. Blood urea nitrogen (BUN) and creatinine levels
2. Arterial blood gas (ABG) levels
3. Platelet count
4. Potassium level

69. 1. BUN and creatinine levels should be monitored closely to detect elevations due to nephrotoxicity. ABG determinations are inappropriate for this situation. Platelets and potassium levels should be monitored according to routine.

CN: Physiological integrity; CNS: Reduction of risk potential; CL: Analysis

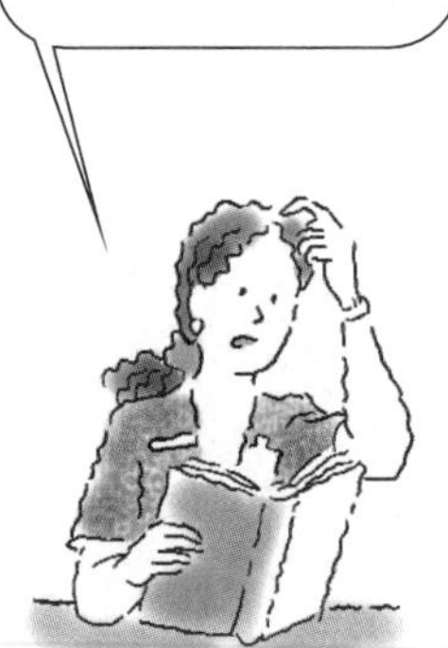

Lots to do, but what's the most important?

70. A client had transurethral prostatectomy for benign prostatic hypertrophy and is currently being treated with a continuous bladder irrigation. He's complaining of an increase in severity of bladder spasms. Which intervention should be done <u>first</u>?

1. Administer an oral analgesic.
2. Stop the irrigation and call the physician.
3. Administer a belladonna and opium suppository as ordered by the physician.
4. Check for the presence of clots, and make sure the catheter is draining properly.

70. 4. Blood clots and blocked outflow of the urine can increase spasms. The irrigation shouldn't be stopped as long as the catheter is draining because clots will form. A belladonna and opium suppository should be given to relieve spasms but only *after* assessment of the drainage. Oral analgesics should be given if the spasms are unrelieved by the belladonna and opium suppository.

CN: Physiological integrity; CNS: Physiological adaptation; CL: Analysis

71. Proper maintenance of a continuous bladder irrigation system includes which intervention?

1. Regulate irrigant flow to maintain red urine.
2. Regulate irrigant flow to maintain pink urine.
3. Maintain a slow flow rate of irrigant to prevent bladder distention.
4. Stop the irrigation if there's leakage of large amounts of urine around the catheter.

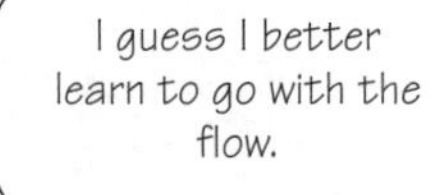

I guess I better learn to go with the flow.

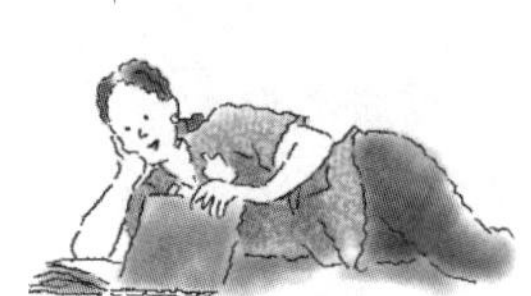

71. 2. The irrigant should be infused at a rate fast enough to maintain pink urine. Red urine indicates inadequate irrigation and possible clot formation. Bladder distention shouldn't occur as long as the system is draining properly and no clots are obstructing the outflow of urine. Leakage of urine around the catheter indicates clot formation on the catheter tip, needing manual irrigation. The irrigation shouldn't be stopped because of the potential for clot formation.

CN: Physiological integrity; CNS: Physiological adaptation; CL: Application

CN: Client needs category CNS: Client needs subcategory CL: Cognitive level

72. A client has an indwelling urinary catheter, and urine is leaking from a hole in the collection bag. Which nursing intervention would be most appropriate?

1. Cover the hole with tape.
2. Remove the catheter, and insert a new one using sterile technique.
3. Disconnect the drainage bag from the catheter, and replace it with a new bag.
4. Place a towel under the bag to prevent spillage of urine on the floor, which could cause the client to slip and fall.

72. 2. The system is no longer a closed system, and bacteria might have been introduced into the system, so a new sterile catheter should be inserted. Taping up the hole and placing a towel under the bag leave the system open, which increases the risk of infection. Replacing the drainage bag by disconnecting the old one from the catheter opens up the entire system and isn't recommended because of the increased risk of infection.

CN: Safe, effective care environment; CNS: Safety and infection control; CL: Analysis

73. A client is admitted with a diagnosis of hydronephrosis secondary to calculi. The calculi have been removed, and postobstructive diuresis is occurring. Which intervention should be performed?

1. Take vital signs every 8 hours.
2. Weigh the client every other day.
3. Assess the urine output every shift.
4. Monitor the client's electrolyte levels.

73. 4. Postobstructive diuresis seen in hydronephrosis can cause electrolyte imbalances; laboratory values must be checked so electrolytes can be replaced as needed. Vital signs should initially be taken every 30 minutes for the first 4 hours and then every 2 hours. Urine output needs to be assessed hourly. The client's weight should be taken daily to assess fluid status more closely.

CN: Physiological integrity; CNS: Reduction of risk potential; CL: Analysis

74. A client is admitted with severe nausea, vomiting, and diarrhea. He is hypotensive and is noted to have severe oliguria with elevated blood urea nitrogen (BUN) and creatinine levels. The physician will most likely write an order for which treatment?

1. Force oral fluids.
2. Give furosemide 20 mg I.V.
3. Start hemodialysis after a temporary access is obtained.
4. Start I.V. fluid of normal saline solution bolus followed by a maintenance dose.

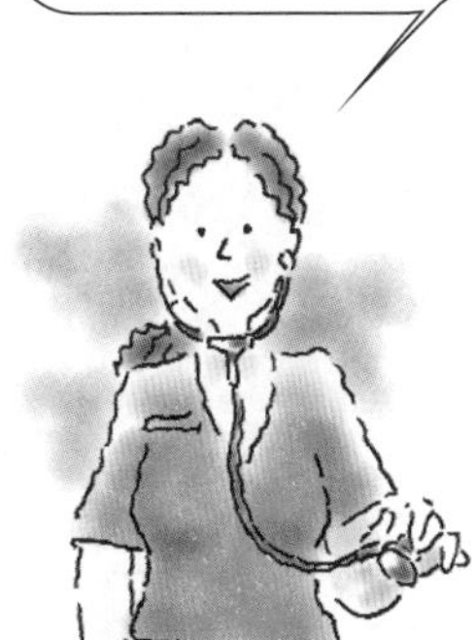

Which answer is most likely to be correct?

74. 4. The client is prerenal secondary to hypovolemia. I.V. fluids should be given to rehydrate the client, urine output should increase, and the BUN and creatinine levels will normalize. The client wouldn't be able to tolerate oral fluids because of the nausea, vomiting, and diarrhea. The client isn't fluid overloaded, and her urine output won't increase with furosemide. The client won't need dialysis because the oliguria and increased BUN and creatinine levels are due to dehydration.

CN: Physiological integrity; CNS: Physiological adaptation; CL: Analysis

75. A client has a history of chronic renal failure and receives hemodialysis treatments three times a week through an arteriovenous (AV) fistula in the left arm. Which intervention is included in this client's care?

1. Keep the AV fistula site dry.
2. Keep the AV fistula wrapped in gauze.
3. Take the blood pressure in the left arm.
4. Assess the AV fistula for a bruit and thrill.

75. 4. Assessment of the AV fistula for a bruit and thrill is important because, if not present, it indicates a nonfunctioning fistula. When not being dialyzed, the AV fistula site may get wet. Immediately after a dialysis treatment, the access site is covered with adhesive bandages. No blood pressures or venipunctures should be taken in the arm with the AV fistula.

CN: Physiological integrity; CNS: Physiological adaptation; CL: Application

76. During a health history, which statement by a client indicates a risk of renal calculi?

1. "I've been drinking a lot of cola soft drinks lately."
2. "I've been jogging more than usual."
3. "I've had more stress since we adopted a child last year."
4. "I'm a vegetarian and eat cheese two or three times each day."

76. 4. Renal calculi are commonly composed of calcium. Diets high in calcium may predispose a person to renal calculi. Milk and milk products are high in calcium. Cola soft drinks don't contain ingredients that would increase the risk of renal calculi. Jogging and increased stress aren't considered risk factors for renal calculi formation.

CN: Health promotion and maintenance; CNS: None; CL: Analysis

77. The nurse is assessing a client who reports painful urination during and after voiding. The nurse suspects the client may have a problem with which area of the client's urinary system?

1. Bladder
2. Kidneys
3. Ureters
4. Urethra

77. 1. Pain during or after voiding indicates a bladder problem, usually infection. Kidney and ureter pain would be in the flank area, and problems of the urethra would cause pain at the external orifice that's commonly felt at the start of voiding.

CN: Health promotion and maintenance; CNS: None; CL: Application

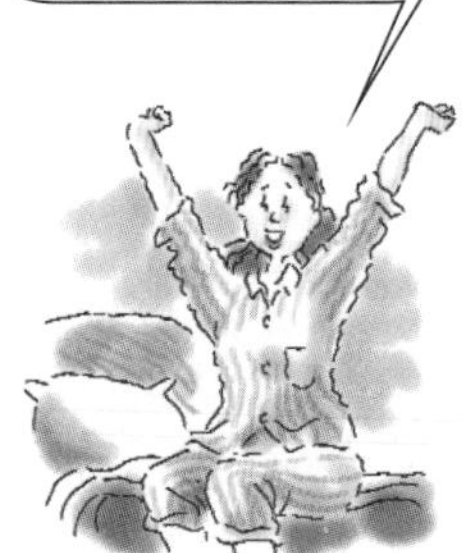
This is the best time of day.

78. A client is ordered diuretics. Which of the following would be the best time of day for the nurse to schedule this medication?

1. Anytime
2. Nighttime
3. Morning
4. Noon

78. 3. A diuretic given in the morning has time to work throughout the day. Diuretics given at nighttime will cause the client to get up to go to the bathroom frequently, interrupting sleep.

CN: Physiological integrity; CNS: Pharmacological and parenteral therapies; CL: Application

79. Which intervention would be the most appropriate for a client with postoperative urinary retention?

1. Give a diuretic.
2. Pour warm water over the perineum.
3. Consider inserting a bladder catheter.
4. Lay the client flat in bed.

79. 2. Urinary retention reflects bladder distention from urine. Sitting the client upright and pouring warm water over the perineum may help the client void. A diuretic isn't necessary. If these measures aren't successful, the nurse should consider inserting a bladder catheter to drain the bladder. This procedure needs an order from the primary healthcare provider.

CN: Physiological integrity; CNS: Basic care and comfort; CL: Application

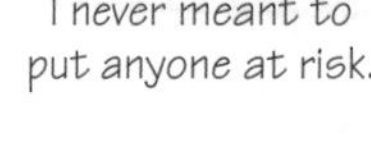
I never meant to put anyone at risk.

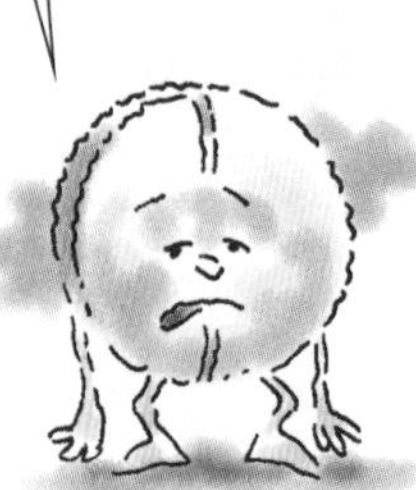

80. A client has not voided 10 hours following an inguinal hernia repair. The nurse determines that the nursing diagnosis for this client would be *Urinary retention related to* which of the following?

1. *Dehydration*
2. *History of smoking*
3. *Duration of surgery*
4. *Preoperative atropine*

80. 4. Anticholinergic medications, such as atropine, may cause urinary retention, particularly for the client who has surgery in the pelvic area (inguinal hernia, hysterectomy). Dehydration, smoking, and duration of surgery aren't risk factors for retention, although opiate analgesics are risk factors.

CN: Physiological integrity; CNS: Reduction of risk potential; CL: Application

81. The nurse is caring for a client with urine retention. The physician has ordered the client to be catheterized. Which of the following catheters would be the most appropriate for the nurse to select to perform the procedure?

1. Coudé
2. Indwelling urinary
3. Straight
4. Three-way

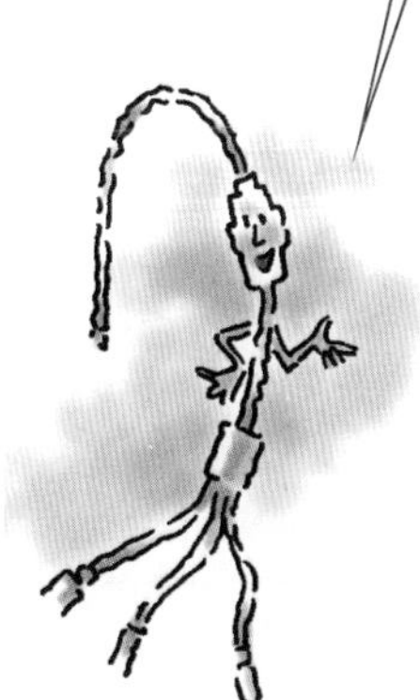

All catheters are not created equal.

81. 3. Urine retention is usually a temporary problem that requires insertion of a straight catheter. An indwelling urinary catheter is used for longer-term bladder problems. A catheter coudé is used only when it's difficult to insert a standard catheter, usually because of an enlarged prostate. A three-way catheter is used for clients who need bladder irrigation such as after a prostate resection.

CN: Physiological integrity; CNS: Basic care and comfort; CL: Application

82. An 80-year-old male client reports urine retention. Which factor may contribute to this client's problem?

1. Benign prostatic hyperplasia (BPH)
2. Diabetes
3. Diet
4. Hypertension

82. 1. BPH is common among elderly men and typically results in urine retention, frequency, dribbling, and difficulty starting the urine stream. Diabetes, diet, and hypertension usually don't affect urine retention.

CN: Physiological integrity; CNS: Reduction of risk potential; CL: Application

83. A 75-year-old client is admitted with dehydration. The client's laboratory results are serum sodium 145 mg/dl, serum potassium 5.0 mEq/L, blood urea nitrogen 23 mg/dl, and serum creatinine 3.0 mg/dl. Based on these results, the nurse determines that the client is at risk for developing which of the following conditions?

1. Acute confusion
2. Urinary retention
3. Acute renal failure
4. Cardiac arrhythmias

83. 3. The laboratory results indicate an elevated serum creatinine (normal ranges are from 0.7 to 1.5 mg/dl), which is reflective of dehydration. Volume depletion or dehydration is a risk factor for developing acute renal failure due to decreased perfusion of the kidneys.

CN: Physiological integrity; CNS: Reduction of risk potential; CL: Application

84. A client with an overactive neurogenic bladder is complaining of a dry mouth from his medication oxybutynin (Ditropan). The nurse is aware that this adverse effect is commonly found with which of the flowing drug classifications?

1. Anti-infective
2. Corticosteroid
3. Urinary antiseptic
4. Spasmolytic

84. 4. Oxybutynin belongs to the spasmolytic drug classification. A common side effect is dry mouth. The other drug classifications do not commonly have an adverse effect of dry mouth.

CN: Physiological integrity; CNS: Pharmacological and parenteral therapies; CL: Application

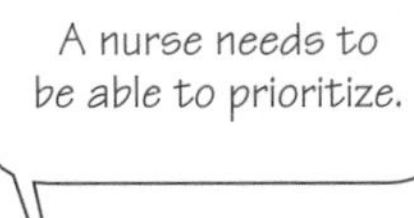

A nurse needs to be able to prioritize.

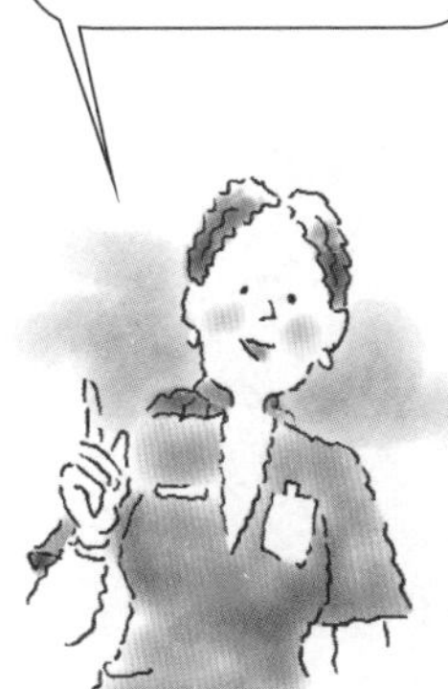

85. A client is injected with radiographic contrast medium and immediately shows signs of dyspnea, flushing, and pruritis. Which intervention should take <u>priority</u>?

1. Check vital signs.
2. Make sure the airway is patent.
3. Apply a cold pack to the I.V. site.
4. Call the physician.

85. 2. The client is showing symptoms of an allergy to the iodine in the contrast medium. The first action is to make sure the client's airway is patent. If compromised, call a cardiac arrest code. Checking vital signs and calling for the physician are important nursing actions but should follow making sure the airway is patent. A cold pack isn't indicated.

CN: Physiological integrity; CNS: Physiological adaptation; CL: Analysis

86. An 80-year-old man is admitted for a cystoscopy with biopsy of the bladder. After obtaining a history, surgery is postponed. Which reason would be cause to postpone this client's surgery?

1. The client stopped taking his anticoagulant 3 days ago.
2. The client has a urinary tract infection.
3. The client has previously been treated for carcinoma of the bladder.
4. The client took an antibiotic prior to the procedure.

86. 2. Bladder biopsies shouldn't be done when an active urinary tract infection is present because sepsis may result. Anticoagulants should be discontinued for 3 to 5 days before the procedure. The client who has been treated for bladder cancer may still require the producedure to check effectiveness of treatment. Antibiotics are sometimes given prophylactically prior to the procedure.

CN: Physiological integrity; CNS: Reduction of risk potential; CL: Analysis

87. Unless there are postoperative complications, a cystoscopy client is discharged to home within 24 hours. Which instruction is given at discharge?

1. Expect bloody urine for about a week.
2. Drink 8 to 10 glasses of water every 8 hours.
3. Try to urinate frequently, and measure your output.
4. Check the color, consistency, and amount of urine in the indwelling urinary catheter bag every 4 to 8 hours.

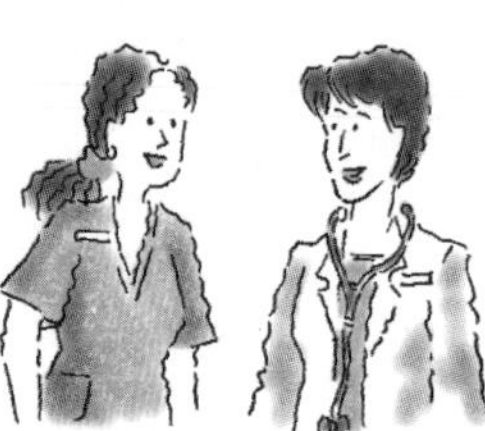

It's important to share vital client information.

87. 3. The bladder needs to be emptied frequently, and output should be measured to make sure the bladder is emptying. Blood in the urine isn't normal except for small amounts during the first 24 hours after the procedure. Large amounts of fluids help flush microorganisms out of the body, but 8 to 10 glasses every 8 hours may not be reasonable. Also, clients don't tend to think in time periods, so instructions should be given per day. The client may not have an indwelling urinary catheter.

CN: Physiological integrity; CNS: Reduction of risk potential; CL: Application

88. Before a renal biopsy, which information is most important to tell the physician?

1. The client signed a consent form.
2. The client understands the procedure.
3. The client has normal urinary elimination.
4. The client regularly takes aspirin or nonsteroidal anti-inflammatory drugs (NSAIDs).

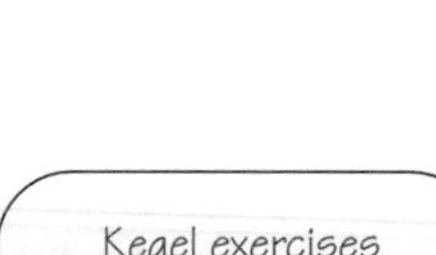

88. 4. Aspirin and NSAIDs cause increased bleeding times and commonly result in hemorrhaging when biopsies are performed. It's the physician's responsibility to make sure the client understands the procedure, which is needed for informed consent. It isn't necessary to report that the client has normal urinary elimination.

CN: Physiological integrity; CNS: Reduction of risk potential; CL: Application

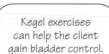

89. Kegel exercises are used to gain control of bladder function in women with stress incontinence and in some men after prostate surgery. Which instruction would help the client perform these exercises?

1. Completely empty the bladder.
2. Do the exercise 200 times per day.
3. Sit or stand with your legs together.
4. Drink small amounts of fluid frequently.

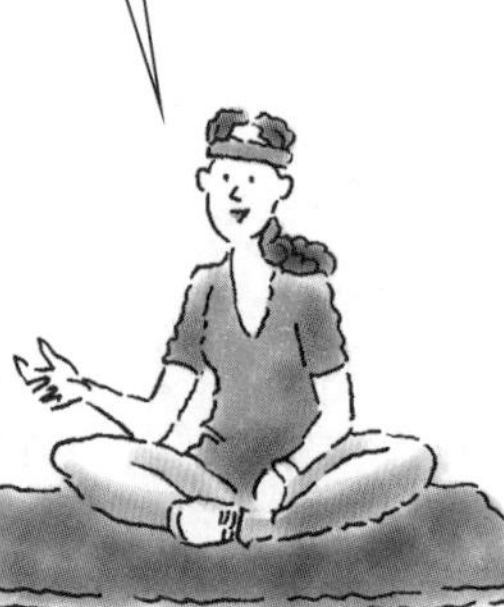

Kegel exercises can help the client gain bladder control.

89. 2. Exercises begin with tightening and relaxing the vagina, rectum, and urethra four or five times during each session and gradually increasing to 25 times for each session. The client stops the flow of urine during urination to practice holding the flow. Standing or sitting with the legs apart facilitates the exercise. Clients should drink plenty of fluids to prevent urinary problems.

CN: Physiological integrity; CNS: Physiological adaptation; CL: Application

90. Which instruction is given to clients with chronic pyelonephritis?
1. Stay on bed rest for up to 2 weeks.
2. Use analgesia on a regular basis for up to 6 months.
3. Have a urine culture every 2 weeks for up to 6 months.
4. Antibiotic treatment may be needed for several weeks or months.

90. 4. Chronic pyelonephritis can be a long-term condition requiring antibiotic treatment for several weeks or months as well as close monitoring to prevent permanent damage to the kidneys. Bed rest and analgesia may be used during the acute stage but usually aren't required long-term. A urine culture is done 2 weeks after stopping antibiotics to make sure the infection has been eradicated.
CN: Physiological integrity; CNS: Reduction of risk control; CL: Application

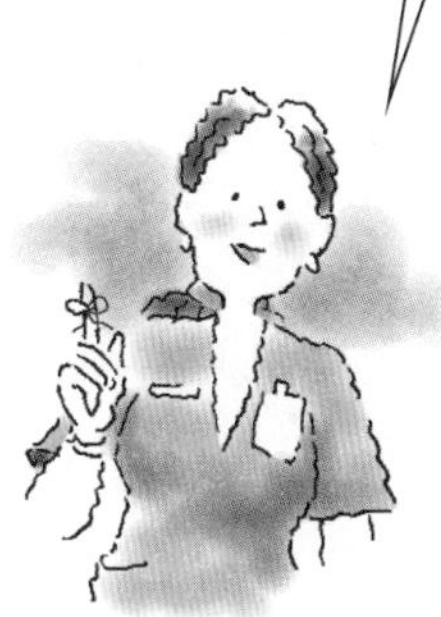

Remember, it's what you should do first that's important.

91. A client had transurethral prostatectomy for benign prostatic hypertrophy. He's currently being treated with continuous bladder irrigation and is complaining of an increase in severity of bladder spasms. What should the nurse do first for this client?
1. Administer an oral analgesic.
2. Stop the irrigation and call the physician.
3. Administer a belladonna and opium suppository as ordered by the physician.
4. Check for the presence of clots, and make sure that the catheter is draining properly.

91. 4. Blood clots and blocked outflow of urine can increase spasms. The irrigation shouldn't be stopped as long as the catheter is draining because clots will form. A belladonna and opium suppository should be given to relieve spasm only *after* assessment of the drainage. Oral analgesics should be given if the spasms are unrelieved by the belladonna and opium suppository.
CN: Physiological integrity; CNS: Reduction of risk potential; CL: Analysis

92. Which client is at greatest risk for developing acute renal failure?
1. A dialysis client who gets influenza
2. A teenager who has an appendectomy
3. A pregnant woman who has a fractured femur
4. A client with diabetes who has a heart catheterization

92. 4. Clients with diabetes are prone to renal insufficiency and renal failure. The contrast used for heart catheterization must be eliminated by the kidneys, which further stresses them and may produce acute renal failure. A dialysis client already has end-stage renal disease and wouldn't develop acute renal failure. A teenager who has an appendectomy and a pregnant woman who fractures a femur aren't at increased risk for renal failure.
CN: Health promotion and maintenance; CNS: None; CL: Analysis

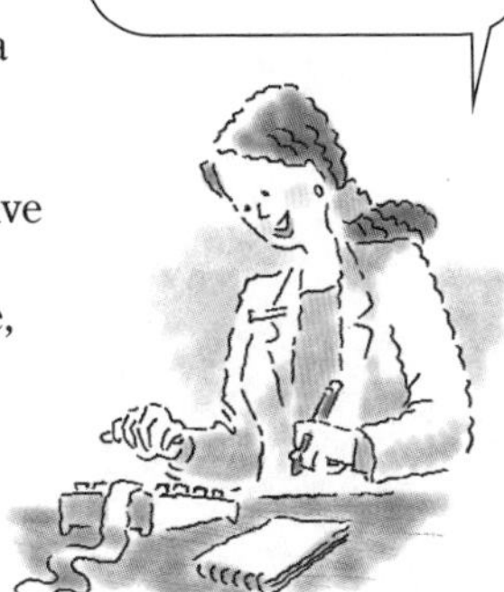

I never did understand calculus.

93. Which intervention should be done for a client with urinary calculus?
1. Save any calculi larger than 0.25 cm.
2. Strain the urine, limit oral fluids, and give pain medications.
3. Encourage fluid intake, strain the urine, and give pain medications.
4. Insert an indwelling urinary catheter, check intake and output, and give pain medications.

93. 3. Encourage fluid intake and strain all urine, saving all calculi, including "flecks." Give pain medications because renal calculi are painful. Indwelling urinary catheters aren't usually needed.
CN: Physiological integrity; CNS: Physiological adaptation; CL: Application

94. The nurse is caring for a client who is receiving hemodialysis treatments. Which of the following interventions would be the most appropriate for this client?

1. Palpate for a thrill on the arm with the fistula.
2. Palpate for a thrill on the arm without the fistula.
3. Document the absence of a bruit as a normal finding.
4. Take the blood pressure on the arm with the fistula.

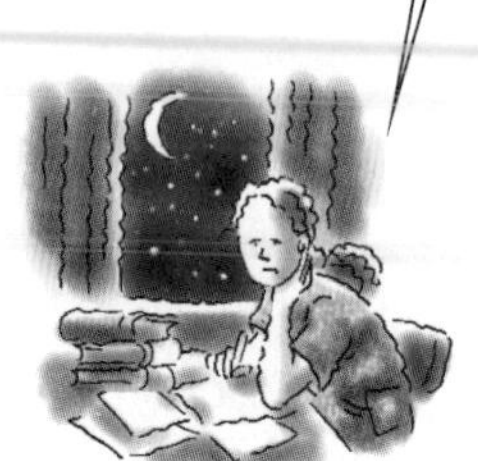

94. 1. The nurse would palpate for a thrill and auscultate for a bruit on the arm with a fistula but no procedures (blood pressure, I.V. access, or blood draw) should be done on the arm with a fistulae because it could damage the fistula. The absence of a thrill or bruit should be reported promptly to the physician because it indicates an occlusion and is not a normal finding.

CN: Physiological integrity; CNS: Reduction of risk potential; CL: Application

95. A client has passed a renal calculus. The nurse sends the specimen to the laboratory so it can be analyzed for which factor?

1. Antibodies
2. Type of infection
3. Composition of calculus
4. Size and number of calculi

95. 3. The calculus should be analyzed for composition to determine appropriate interventions such as dietary restrictions. Calculi don't result from infections. The size and number of calculi aren't relevant, and they don't contain antibodies.

CN: Physiological integrity; CNS: Reduction of risk potential; CL: Application

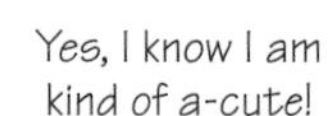

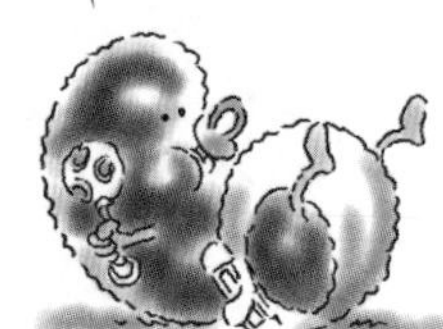

96. Which symptom may indicate <u>acute</u> rejection of a transplanted kidney?

1. Increased urine output
2. Hypotension
3. Pain at the graft site
4. Decreased white blood cell (WBC) count

96. 3. Signs and symptoms of acute rejection of a transplanted kidney include pain at the graft site, decreased (not increased) urine output, hypertension (not hypotension), elevated (not decreased) WBC count, fever, and elevated creatinine level.

CN: Physiological integrity; CNS: Physiological adaptation; CL: Analysis

97. Adverse reactions of prednisone therapy include which conditions?

1. Acne and bleeding gums
2. Sodium retention and constipation
3. Mood swings and increased temperature
4. Increased blood glucose levels and decreased wound healing

97. 4. Steroid use tends to increase blood glucose levels, particularly in clients with diabetes and borderline diabetes. Steroids also contribute to poor wound healing and may cause acne, mood swings, and sodium and water retention. Steroids don't affect bleeding tendencies, constipation, or thermoregulation.

CN: Physiological integrity; CNS: Pharmacological and parenteral therapies; CL: Analysis

98. Steroids, such as prednisone and methylprednisolone, are used to suppress the inflammatory immune response following a kidney transplant. Which information should be given to a client with a transplant?

1. Alopecia may occur.
2. Weight loss is common.
3. Cholesterol levels may become elevated.
4. Hypokalemia may result.

98. 4. Steroids may decrease serum potassium levels but don't increase cholesterol levels. Hirsutism may occur, but not alopecia. Weight gain is commonly reported, not weight loss.

CN: Physiological integrity; CNS: Pharmacological and parenteral therapies; CL: Analysis

99. A nurse suspects that a client with polyuria is experiencing water diuresis. Which laboratory value suggests water diuresis?

1. High urine specific gravity
2. High urine osmolarity
3. Normal to low urine specific gravity
4. Elevated urine pH

99. 3. Water diuresis causes low urine specific gravity, low urine osmolarity, and a normal to elevated serum sodium level. High urine specific gravity indicates dehydration. Elevated urine pH can result from potassium deficiency, a high-protein diet, or uncontrolled diabetes.

CN: Physiological integrity; CNS: Physiological adaptation; CL: Application

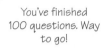

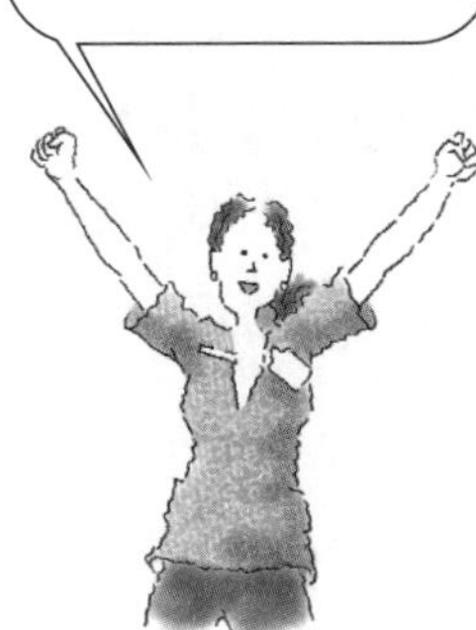

You've finished 100 questions. Way to go!

100. A client with bladder cancer has had his bladder removed and an ileal conduit created for urine diversion. While changing this client's pouch, the nurse observes that the area around the stoma is red, weeping, and painful. What should the nurse conclude?

1. The skin wasn't lubricated before the pouch was applied.
2. The pouch faceplate doesn't fit the stoma.
3. A skin barrier was applied properly.
4. Stoma dilation wasn't performed.

100. 2. If the pouch faceplate doesn't fit the stoma properly, the skin around the stoma will be exposed to continuous urine flow from the stoma, causing excoriation and red, weeping, painful skin. A lubricant shouldn't be used because it would prevent the pouch from adhering to the skin. When properly applied, a skin barrier prevents skin excoriation. Stoma dilation isn't performed with an ileal conduit, although it may be done with a colostomy, if ordered.

CN: Physiological integrity; CNS: Basic, care and comfort; CL: Analysis

101. A client is diagnosed with prostate cancer. The physician is most likely to order which test to monitor the client's progress?

1. Serum creatinine
2. Complete blood count (CBC)
3. Prostate specific antigen (PSA)
4. Serum potassium

101. 3. The PSA test is used to monitor prostate cancer progression; higher PSA levels indicate a greater tumor burden. Serum creatinine levels may suggest blockage from an enlarged prostate. CBC is used to diagnose anemia and polycythemia. Serum potassium levels identify hypokalemia and hyperkalemia.

CN: Physiological integrity; CNS: Physiological adaptation; CL: Application

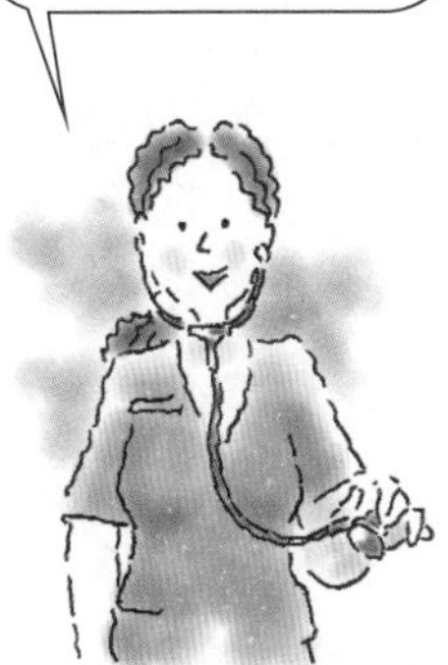

Location. It's a hint to help you answer question 102.

102. When teaching a client about cystitis, a nurse explains that females are more prone to the disorder than males. Which factor explains a female's increased susceptibility?

1. Higher estrogen levels
2. Inadequate fluid intake
3. Urethral proximity to the rectum
4. Continuous nature of the mucosa

102. 3. In females, the urethra and rectum are in close proximity, posing a greater risk for urethral contamination with feces after a bowel movement. Decreased estrogen levels may reduce vaginal and urethral lubrication, increasing the chance of irritation during coitus. Males and females can have equivalent fluid intake. The mucosa is continuous in both males and females.

CN: Physiological integrity; CNS: Physiological adaptation; CL: Application

103. A client presents with a possible urinary tract infection. Which urine characteristic should the nurse assess <u>first</u>?

1. Urine clarity
2. Urine specific gravity
3. Urine acetone
4. Urine protein

103. 1. First, the nurse should assess urine clarity; cloudy urine usually indicates drainage, which may reflect infection. Urine specific gravity yields information about fluid balance. Neither urine acetone nor urine protein indicates infection.

CN: Health promotion and maintenance; CNS: None; CL: Analysis

104. A 70-year-old male client is diagnosed with syphilis in the secondary stage. Which finding should the nurse expect during assessment?

1. Chronic bone and joint irritation
2. Tender lymphadenopathy
3. Generalized rash on the palms and soles
4. Personality changes and mental confusion

104. 3. In secondary syphilis, a maculopapular nonpruritic rash appears on the palms and soles. Chronic bone and joint irritation aren't related to secondary syphilis. During the second stage of syphilis, nontender lymphadenopathy occurs. Personality changes occur during the late stage of syphilis.

CN: Physiological integrity; CNS: Basic care and comfort; CL: Application

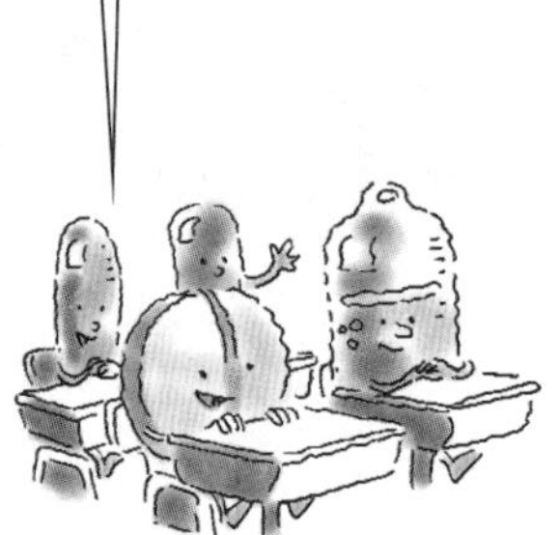

The question is, which one of us can help?

105. Which medication is most likely to be prescribed for a client with gonorrhea?

1. Penicillin (Penicillin G)
2. Azithromycin (Zithromax)
3. Ceftriaxone (Rocephin)
4. Trichloroacetic acid

105. 3. According to the Centers for Disease Control guidelines, ceftriaxone (Rocephin) or cefixime (Suprax) are the drugs of choice for treating gonorrhea. Penicillin is used to treat syphilis. Azithromycin is used for chlamydial infection. Topical trichloroacetic acid is used for human papilloma virus.

CN: Physiological integrity; CNS: Pharmacological and parenteral therapies; CL: Application

106. In a client with renal failure, which assessment finding may indicate hypocalcemia?

1. Headache
2. Serum calcium level of 10 mg/dl
3. Increased blood coagulation
4. Diarrhea

106. 4. In renal failure, calcium absorption from the intestine declines, leading to increased smooth-muscle contractions, causing diarrhea. Central nervous system changes in renal failure rarely cause headache. A serum calcium level of 9 to 10.5 mg/dl is a normal calcium level. As renal failure progresses, bleeding tendencies increase.

CN: Health promotion and maintenance; CNS: None; CL: Application

107. A 27-year-old client, who became paraplegic after a swimming accident, is experiencing autonomic dysreflexia. Which condition is the most common cause of autonomic dysreflexia?

1. Upper respiratory infection
2. Incontinence
3. Bladder distention
4. Diarrhea

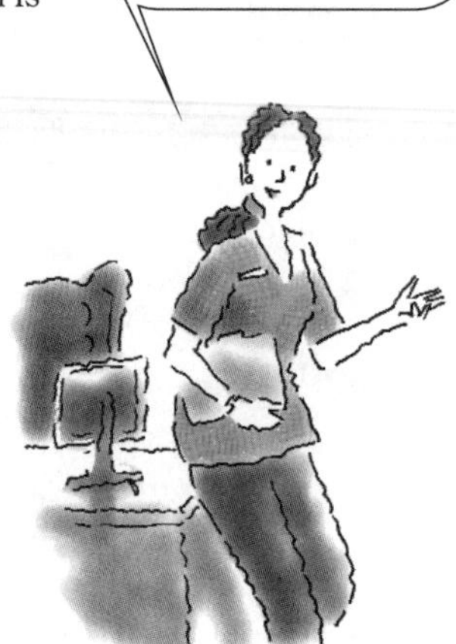

There may be many causes, but which is *most common*?

107. 3. Autonomic dysreflexia is a potentially life-threatening complication of spinal cord injury, occuring from obstruction of the urinary system or bowel. An upper respiratory infection could obstruct the respiratory system but not the urinary or bowel system. Incontinence and diarrhea don't result in obstruction of the urinary system or bowel, respectively.

CN: Physiological integrity; CNS: Physiological adaptation; CL: Analysis

108. When teaching a client how to prevent recurrences of acute glomerulonephritis, which instruction should the nurse include?

1. "Avoid physical activity."
2. "Strain all urine."
3. "Seek early treatment for respiratory infection."
4. "Monitor urine specific gravity every day."

108. 3. Hemolytic streptococci are common in throat infections and can cause an immune reaction that causes glomerular damage. Therefore, the client should seek early treatment for respiratory infection. Avoiding physical activity may promote urination but doesn't prevent recurrence of glomerulonephritis. Straining all urine helps identify renal calculi that have passed through the urine. Daily monitoring of urine specific gravity helps assess hydration status but doesn't aid in glomerulonephritis prevention.

CN: Physiological integrity; CNS: Reduction of risk potential; CL: Analysis

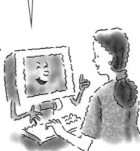

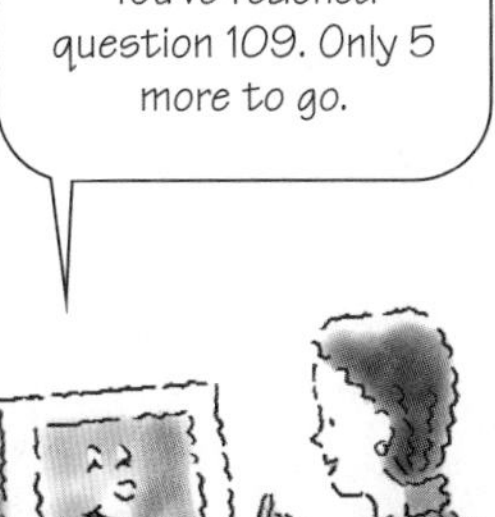

You've reached question 109. Only 5 more to go.

109. After radical prostatectomy for prostate cancer, a client has an indwelling catheter removed. He then begins to have periods of incontinence. During the postoperative period, which intervention should be implemented first?

1. Kegel exercises
2. Fluid restriction
3. Artificial sphincter use
4. Self-catheterization

109. 1. Kegel exercises are noninvasive and are recommended as the initial intervention for incontinence. Fluid restriction is useful for a client with increased detrusor contraction related to acidic urine. Artificial sphincter use isn't a primary intervention for postprostatectomy incontinence. Self-catheterization may be used as a temporary measure but isn't a primary intervention.

CN: Physiological integrity; CNS: Physiological adaptation; CL: Application

110. When providing discharge teaching for a client with uric acid calculi, the nurse should include an instruction to avoid which type of food?

1. Cottage cheese
2. Beets
3. Spinach
4. Organ meats

110. 4. To control uric acid calculi, the client should avoid high purine foods such as organ meats. Beets and spinach are high in oxalate. Cottage cheese is high in calcium.

CN: Physiological integrity; CNS: Reduction of risk potential; CL: Application

111. When a client with nephrotic syndrome manifests anasarca, the nurse relates this assessment finding to which abnormally low laboratory value?

1. Cholesterol
2. Prothrombin time
3. Albumin
4. Calcium

111. 3. When the glomeruli are damaged, as in nephrotic syndrome, the kidneys are excessively permeable to plasma protein, causing proteinuria and hypoalbuminemia. This leads to a decreased oncotic pressure, which results in anasarca (massive generalized edema).

CN: Physiological integrity; CNS: Physiological adaptation; CL: Application

112. After a retropubic prostatectomy, a client needs continuous bladder irrigation. The client has an I.V. of dextrose 5% in water infusing at 40 ml/hour and a triple-lumen urinary catheter with normal saline solution infusing at 200 ml/hour. The nurse empties the urinary catheter drainage bag three times during an 8-hour period for a total of 2,780 ml. How many milliliters does the nurse calculate as urine? Record your answer using a whole number.

____________________ milliliters

112. 1,180. During 8 hours, 1,600 ml of bladder irrigation has been infused (200 ml × 8 hours = 1,600 ml/8 hours). The nurse then subtracts this amount of infused bladder irrigation from the total volume in the drainage bag (2,780 ml − 1,600 ml = 1,180 ml) to determine urine output.

CN: Physiological integrity; CNS: Basic care and comfort; CL: Analysis

113. A nurse is caring for a client with chronic renal failure. The laboratory results indicate hypocalcemia and hyperphosphatemia. When assessing the client, the nurse should be alert for which symptom? Select all that apply:

1. Trousseau's sign
2. Cardiac arrhythmias
3. Constipation
4. Decreased clotting time
5. Drowsiness and lethargy
6. Fractures

113. 1, 2, 6. Hypocalcemia is a calcium deficit that causes nerve fiber irritability and repetitive muscle spasms. Signs and symptoms of hypocalcemia include Trousseau's sign, cardiac arrhythmias, diarrhea, increased clotting, anxiety, and irritability. The calcium–phosphorus imbalance leads to brittle bones and pathologic fractures.

CN: Physiological integrity; CNS: Reduction of risk potential; CL: Application

114. A 26-year-old client with chronic renal failure plans to receive a kidney transplant. Recently, the physician told the client that he's a poor candidate for transplant because of chronic uncontrolled hypertension and diabetes mellitus. Now the client tells the nurse, "I want to go off dialysis. I'd rather not live than be on this treatment for the rest of my life." Which response is appropriate? Select all that apply:

1. Take a seat next to the client and sit quietly.
2. Say to the client, "We all have days when we don't feel like going on."
3. Leave the room to allow the client to collect his thoughts.
4. Say to the client, "You're feeling upset about the news you got about the transplant."
5. Say to the client, "The treatments are only 3 days a week. You can live with that."

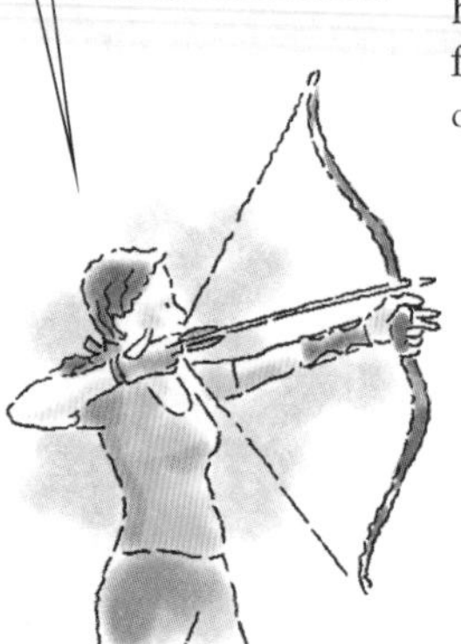

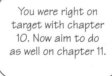

You were right on target with chapter 10. Now aim to do as well on chapter 11.

114. 1, 4. Silence is a therapeutic communication technique that allows the nurse and client to reflect on what has taken place or been said. By waiting quietly and attentively, the nurse encourages the client to initiate and maintain conversation. By reflecting the client's implied feelings, the nurse also promotes communication. Using such platitudes as "We all have days when we don't feel like going on" fails to address the client's needs. The nurse shouldn't leave the client alone because he may harm himself. Reminding the client of the treatment frequency doesn't address his feelings.

CN: Psychosocial integrity; CNS: None; CL: Analysis

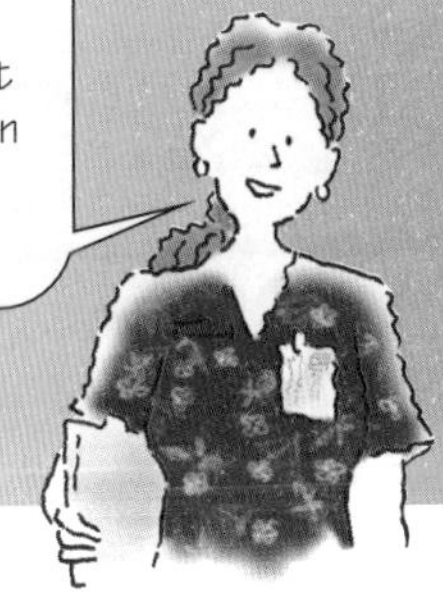

So, you think the care of the client with a skin disorder isn't your strong suit, eh? Maybe you'd like to check out this Web site before taking on this chapter: www.aad.org. Enjoy!

Chapter 11 Integumentary disorders

1. Adequate nutrition is essential for a burn client. Which statement is correct about the nutritional needs of a burn client?

1. The client needs 100 cal/kg throughout hospitalization.
2. The hypermetabolic state after a burn injury contributes to poor healing.
3. A cool environment decreases caloric demand.
4. Maintaining a hypermetabolic rate decreases the client's risk of infection.

1. 2. A burn injury causes a hypermetabolic state resulting in protein and lipid catabolism that affects wound healing. Calories need to be 1½ to 2 times the basal metabolic rate, with at least 1.5 to 2 g/kg of body weight of protein daily. An environmental temperature within normal range lets the body function efficiently and devote caloric expenditure to healing and normal physiologic processes. If the temperature is too warm or too cold, the body gives energy to warming or cooling, which takes away from energy used for tissue repair. High metabolic rates increase the risk of infection.

CN: Physiological integrity; CNS: Basic care and comfort; CL: Application

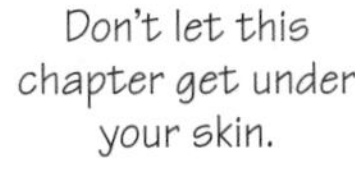

Don't let this chapter get under your skin.

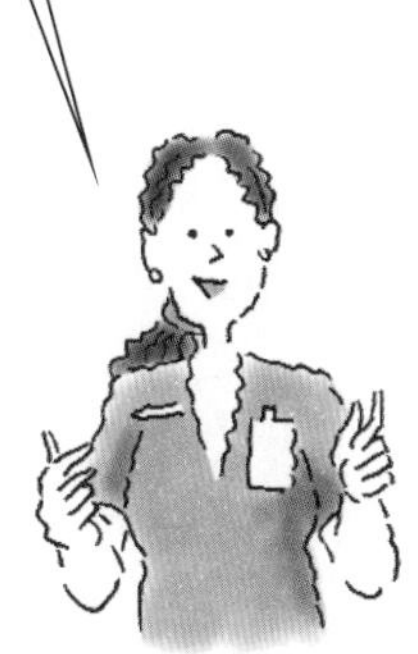

2. A 30-year-old client is admitted to the emergency department with a deep partial-thickness burn on his arm after a fire in the workplace. Which signs and symptoms should the nurse expect to see?

1. Pain and redness
2. Minimal damage to the epidermis
3. Necrotic tissue through all layers of skin
4. Necrotic tissue through most of the dermis

2. 4. A deep partial-thickness burn causes necrosis of the epidermal and dermal layers. Redness and pain are characteristics of a superficial injury. Superficial burns cause slight epidermal damage. Necrosis through all skin layers is seen with full-thickness injuries.

CN: Physiological integrity; CNS: Physiological adaptation; CL: Application

3. A client comes to the emergency department after being bitten by a brown recluse spider. Which characteristic should the nurse expect to find during the assessment?

1. Bull's-eye rash
2. Painful rash around a necrotic lesion
3. Herald patch of oval lesions
4. Line of papules and vesicles that appear 1 to 3 days after exposure

3. 2. Necrotic, painful rashes are associated with the bite of a brown recluse spider. A bull's-eye rash located primarily at the site of the bite is a classic sign of Lyme disease. A herald patch — a slightly raised, oval lesion about 2 to 6 cm in diameter and appearing anywhere on the body — is indicative of pityriasis rosea. A linear, papular, vesicular rash is characteristic of exposure to poison ivy.

CN: Physiological integrity; CNS: Physiological adaptation; CL: Application

CN: Client needs category CNS: Client needs subcategory CL: Cognitive level

4. Which instruction should be observed when administering a Mantoux test?
1. Use the deltoid muscle.
2. Rub the site to help absorption.
3. Read the results within 72 hours.
4. Read the results by checking for a rash.

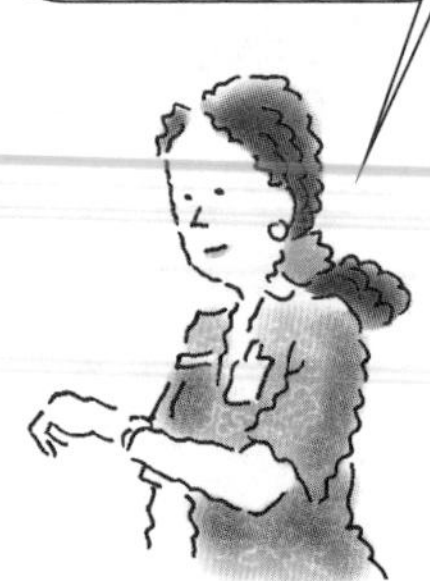
Sometimes timing is everything.

4. 3. The test results should be read 48 to 72 hours after placement by measuring the diameter of the induration that develops at the site. The Mantoux test is injected intradermally on the volar surface of the forearm, not I.M. Rubbing the site could cause leakage from the injection site. An induration develops, not a rash.
CN: Physiological integrity; CNS: Reduction of risk potential; CL: Application

5. A woman is worried she might have lice. Which assessment finding is associated with this infestation?
1. Diffuse pruritic wheals
2. Oval, white dots stuck to the hair shafts
3. Pain, redness, and edema with an embedded stinger
4. Pruritic papules, pustules, and linear burrows of the finger and toe webs

5. 2. Nits, the eggs of lice, are seen as white oval dots. Diffuse pruritic wheals are associated with an allergic reaction. Bites from honeybees are associated with a stinger, pain, and redness. Pruritic papules, vesicles, and linear burrows are diagnostic for scabies.
CN: Physiological integrity; CNS: Physiological adaptation; CL: Application

6. Which type of injury will most likely result from the bite of a large dog?
1. Abrasion
2. Crush injury
3. Fracture
4. Puncture wound

6. 2. The bite of a large dog can exert between 150 to 400 psi of pressure, causing a crush injury, not a fracture. An abrasion is caused by friction. A bite from a small animal such as a cat will cause puncture wounds.
CN : Physiological integrity; CNS: Physiological adaptation; CL: Application

7. A 19-year-old client comes to the clinic with dark red lesions on her hands, wrist, and waistline. She has scratched several of the lesions so that they're open and bleeding. The nurse instructs the client to try pressing on the itchy lesions. What's the rationale for this intervention?
1. Pressing the skin spreads the beneficial microorganisms.
2. Pressing is suggested before scratching.
3. Pressing the skin promotes breaks in the skin.
4. Pressing the skin stimulates nerve endings.

7. 4. Pressing the skin stimulates nerve endings and can reduce the sensation of itching. Scratching (not pressing) the skin spreads microorganisms and opens portals of entry for bacteria. Scratching isn't recommended at all. Pressing the skin doesn't promote breaks in the skin.
CN : Physiological integrity; CNS: Physiological adaptation; CL: Application

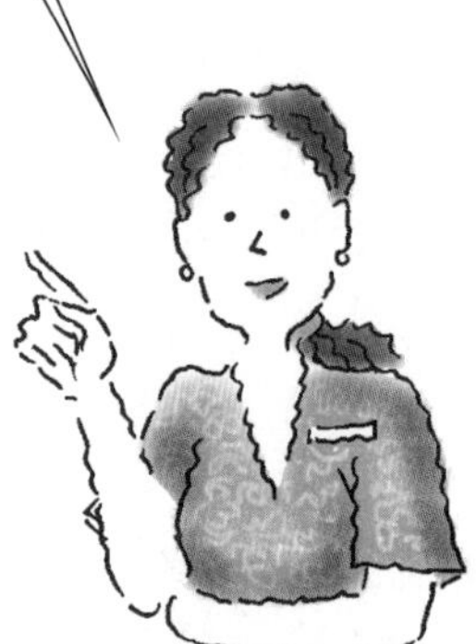
Your most important skill is assessment.

8. A client arrives at the office of his physician complaining of a rash. The nurse assesses the client and notes several palpable, elevated masses, each about 0.5 cm. Which term would the nurse use to accurately describe these masses?
1. Erosions
2. Macules
3. Papules
4. Vesicles

8. 3. Papules are masses elevated up to 0.5 cm, and nodules and tumors are masses elevated more than 0.5 cm. Erosions are characterized as loss of the epidermis layer. Macules and patches are nonpalpable, flat changes in skin color. Fluid-filled lesions are vesicles and pustules.
CN: Health promotion and maintenance; CNS: None; CL: Application

CN: Client needs category CNS: Client needs subcategory CL: Cognitive level

9. A nurse is teaching a female client about the use of isotretinoin (Accutane). She should include the need to take:
   1. contraceptive precautions.
   2. antiemetics.
   3. analgesics.
   4. antidiarrheals.

9. 1. Even small amounts of isotretinoin are associated with severe birth defects. Most female clients are also prescribed oral contraceptives. The other medications aren't necessary for a client on isotretinoin.
CN: Physiological integrity; CNS: Pharmacological and parenteral therapies; CL: Application

10. A client complains of small, red, pruritic dots between his fingers and toes. Which condition is the most likely diagnosis?
   1. Contusion
   2. Herpes zoster
   3. Scabies
   4. Varicella

10. 3. Scabies are seen as linear burrows between the fingers and toes caused by a mite. Contusions don't have small pruritic dots. The varicella zoster virus causes herpes zoster, characterized by papulovesicular lesions that erupt along a dermatome, usually with hyperesthesia, pain, and tenderness. The papulovesicular lesions of varicella are distributed over the trunk, face, and scalp and don't follow a dermatome.
CN: Physiological integrity; CNS: Physiological adaptation; CL: Application

11. Which instruction is given to a client taking nystatin (Mycostatin) oral solution?
   1. Take the drug right after meals.
   2. Take the drug right before meals.
   3. Mix the drug with small amounts of food.
   4. Take half the dose before and half after meals.

11. 1. Nystatin oral solution should be swished around the mouth after eating for the best contact with mucous membranes. Taking the drug before or with meals doesn't allow for the best contact with the mucous membranes.
CN: Physiological integrity; CNS: Pharmacological and parenteral therapies; CL: Application

12. A client is examined and found to have pinpoint, pink-to-purple, nonblanching macular lesions 1 to 3 mm in diameter. Which term best describes these lesions?
   1. Ecchymosis
   2. Hematoma
   3. Petechiae
   4. Purpura

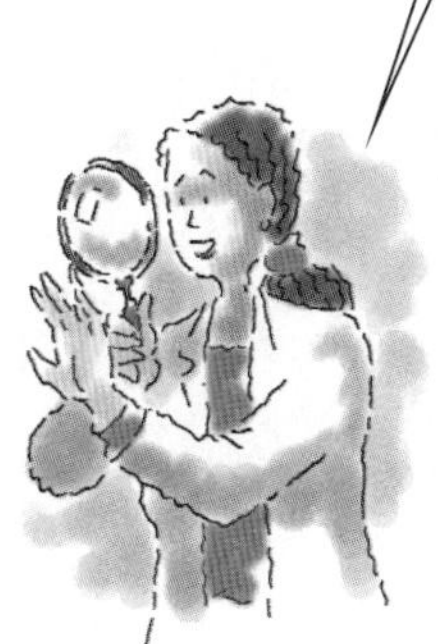
What type of rash is this lesion suggesting?

12. 3. Petechiae are small macular lesions 1 to 3 mm in diameter. Ecchymosis is a purple-to-brown bruise, macular or papular, and varied in size. A hematoma is a collection of blood from ruptured blood vessels more than 1 cm in diameter. Purpura are purple macular lesions larger than 1 cm.
CN: Physiological integrity; CNS: Physiological adaptation; CL: Application

13. A client has a rash consisting of scattered lesions on various parts of the body. Which type of rash is this?
   1. Annular
   2. Confluent
   3. Diffuse
   4. Linear

13. 3. A diffuse rash usually has widely distributed scattered lesions. An annular rash is ring shaped. Confluent lesions are touching or adjacent to each other. Linear rashes are lesions arranged in a line.
CN: Physiological integrity; CNS: Physiological adaptation; CL: Application

14. A nurse is assessing a client recently admitted to the hospital and observes hair loss in small round circles on the client's scalp. Which of the following would most accurately describe this condition?

1. Alopecia
2. Amblyopia
3. Exotropia
4. Seborrhea

14. 1. Alopecia is the correct term for thinning hair loss. Exotropia and amblyopia are eye disorders. Seborrhea is a chronic inflammatory dermatitis.
CN: Physiological integrity; CNS: Physiological adaptation; CL: Application

15. A client is diagnosed with atopic dermatitis. He is upset and asks how to avoid another outbreak. The nurse understands that the client needs information about:

1. avoiding bacterial infections.
2. avoiding fungal infections.
3. hereditary factors.
4. avoiding viral infections.

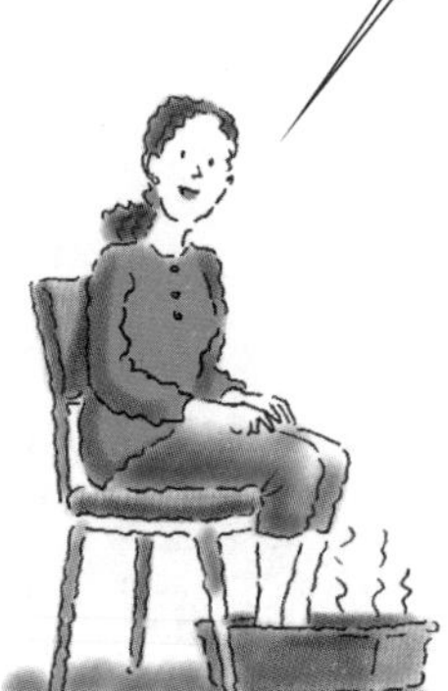

I wish I knew the sole cause of my aching feet.

15. 3. Atopic dermatitis is a hereditary disorder associated with a family history of asthma, allergic rhinitis, or atopic dermatitis. Atopic dermatitis isn't a bacterial, fungal, or viral infection.
CN: Physiological integrity; CNS: Physiological adaptation; CL: Application

16. A client has rough papules on the soles of his feet that are sometimes painful when he walks. The nurse suspects that the client has a:

1. filiform wart.
2. flat wart.
3. plantar wart.
4. venereal wart.

16. 3. Plantar warts are rough papules commonly found on the soles of the feet. Filiform warts are long, spiny projections from the skin surface. Flat warts are flat-topped, smooth-surfaced lesions. Venereal warts appear on the genital mucosa and are confluent papules with rough surfaces.
CN: Physiological integrity; CNS: Physiological adaptation; CL: Application

17. What should the nurse expect to observe on the client who has been recently diagnosed with tinea corporis?

1. A fungal infection of the skin
2. A group of small, red papule lesions
3. A flat, scaling popular lesion with raised borders
4. Itching and sweating of the feet accompanied by a foul odor

17. 3. Tinea corporis, or ringworm, is a flat, scaling papular lesion with raised borders. Candidiasis is a fungal infection of the skin or mucous membranes commonly found in the oral, vaginal, and intestinal mucosal tissue. Molluscum contagiosum is a viral skin infection with small, red, papular lesions. Tinea pedis is a superficial fungal infection on the feet, commonly called athletes' foot, that causes itching and sweating and a foul odor.
CN: Physiological integrity; CNS: Physiological adaptation; CL: Application

18. A client has thick, discolored nails with splintered hemorrhages, easily separated from the nail bed. There are also "ice pick" pits and ridges. The nurse should explain that these findings are most closely associated with:

1. paronychia.
2. psoriasis.
3. seborrhea.
4. scabies.

18. 2. Psoriasis, a chronic skin disorder with an unknown cause, shows these characteristic skin changes. A paronychia is a bacterial infection of the nail bed. Seborrhea is a chronic inflammatory dermatitis known as cradle cap. Scabies are mites that burrow under the skin, generally between the webbing of the fingers and toes.
CN: Physiological integrity; CNS: Physiological adaptation; CL: Application

19. A client found unconscious at home is brought to the emergency department. Physical examination shows cherry-red mucous membranes, nail beds, and skin. Which factor is the most likely cause of his condition?

1. Spider bite
2. Aspirin ingestion
3. Hydrocarbon ingestion
4. Carbon monoxide poisoning

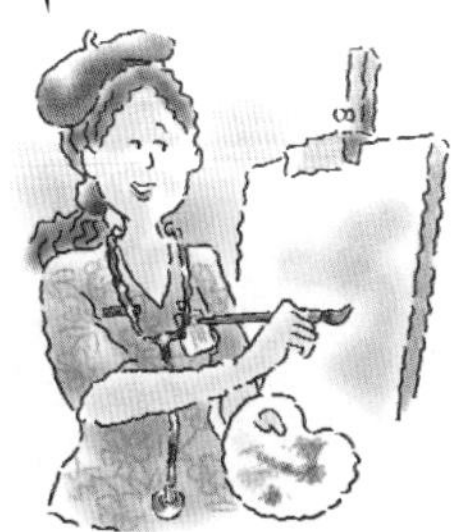

Color can be a classic sign of some conditions.

19. 4. Cherry-red skin indicates exposure to high levels of carbon monoxide. Spider bite reactions are usually localized to the area of the bite. Nausea and vomiting and pale skin are symptoms of aspirin ingestion. Hydrocarbon or petroleum ingestion usually causes respiratory symptoms and tachycardia.

CN: Physiological integrity; CNS: Physiological adaptation; CL: Analysis

20. A client is diagnosed with a fungal infection of the scalp. The nurse documents this as:

1. tinea capitis.
2. tinea corporis.
3. tinea cruris.
4. tinea pedis.

20. 1. Tinea capitis is a fungal infection of the scalp. Tinea corporis describes fungal infections of the body. Tinea cruris describes fungal infections of the inner thigh and inguinal creases, and tinea pedis is the term for fungal infections of the foot.

CN: Physiological integrity; CNS: Physiological adaptation; CL: Application

21. What should the nurse expect to observe upon assessment of a client with secondary syphilis?

1. Chancre ulcers
2. No significant symptoms
3. Nodular, pustular, annular lesions
4. Destructive lesions involving many organs and tissues

21. 3. Nodular, pustular, annular lesions and generalized lymphadenopathy occur in secondary syphilis. The chancre, a painless, shallow ulcer, develops in primary syphilis and appears 3 weeks after exposure. The latent phase occurs between the secondary and tertiary stages. Tertiary syphilis has destructive lesions involving many organs and tissues.

CN: Physiological integrity; CNS: Physiological adaptation; CL: Application

22. An intubated client with full-thickness, circumferential burns to the chest is experiencing pressure from edema that's inhibiting chest wall expansion. Which intervention should correct this condition?

1. Cricothyrotomy
2. Escharotomy
3. Needle thoracentesis
4. Insertion of a chest tube

22. 2. Escharotomy is a surgical incision used to relieve pressure from edema. It's needed with circumferential burns that prevent chest expansion or circulatory compromise. Cricothyrotomy is an emergency procedure that involves puncturing the trachea through the cricothyroid membrane to create an airway. This client is already intubated. Needle thoracentesis and insertion of a chest tube are performed to relieve a pneumothorax.

CN: Physiological integrity; CNS: Physiological adaptation; CL: Analysis

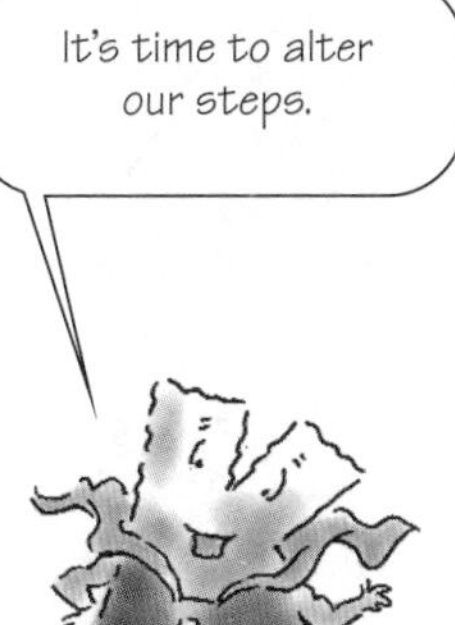

It's time to alter our steps.

23. A client has just arrived at the emergency department after sustaining a major burn injury. Which metabolic alterations are expected during the first 8 hours postburn?

1. Hyponatremia and hypokalemia
2. Hyponatremia and hyperkalemia
3. Hypernatremia and hypokalemia
4. Hypernatremia and hyperkalemia

23. 2. During the first 48 hours after a burn, capillary permeability increases, allowing fluids to shift from the plasma to the interstitial spaces. This fluid is high in sodium, causing a decrease in serum sodium levels. Potassium also leaks from the cells into the plasma, causing hyperkalemia.

CN: Physiological integrity; CNS: Physiological adaptation; CL: Analysis

24. A client has partial-thickness burns to both lower extremities and portions of the trunk. Which I.V. fluid is given first?

1. Albumin
2. Dextrose 5% in water
3. Lactated Ringer's solution
4. Normal saline solution with 2 mEq of potassium per 100 ml

24. 3. Lactated Ringer's solution replaces lost sodium and corrects metabolic acidosis, both of which commonly occur following a burn. Albumin is used as adjunct therapy, not primary fluid replacement. Dextrose isn't given to burn clients during the first 24 hours because it can cause pseudodiabetes. The client is hyperkalemic from the potassium shift from the intracellular space to the plasma, so potassium would be detrimental.

CN: Physiological integrity; CNS: Pharmacological and parenteral therapies; CL: Application

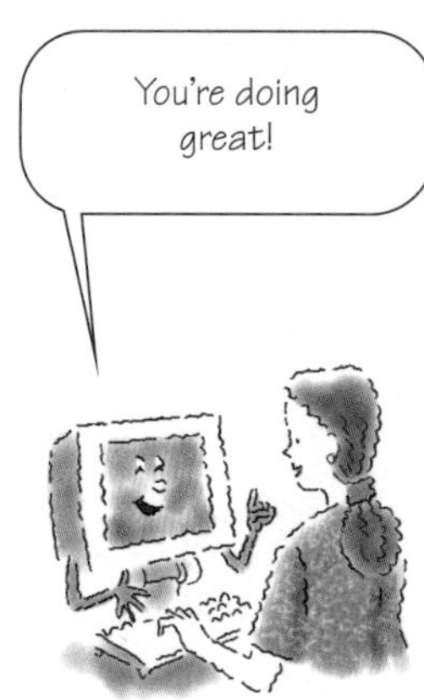
You're doing great!

25. Which method is best for making sure a client receives an ordered dressing change each shift?

1. Write the order in the client's care plan.
2. Put a sign above the head of the client's bed.
3. Tell the nurse about the treatment in the report.
4. Document the dressing change in the narrative note.

25. 1. Writing the order in the client's care plan notifies everyone of the treatment. Posting a sign above the head of the bed is a good reminder but doesn't ensure that the treatment will be performed. Verbally reporting to the nurse on the upcoming shift doesn't ensure the dressing change will be done. Although the intervention should be documented in the narrative note, this doesn't guarantee that the next nurse will do the treatment.

CN: Safe, effective care environment; CNS: Management of care; CL: Application

26. Which nursing diagnosis is correct for a client with a reddened sacrum unrelieved by position change?

1. *Sedentary lifestyle*
2. *Risk for impaired skin integrity*
3. *Noncompliance*
4. *Impaired skin integrity*

26. 4. This client has an actual—not potential—skin impairment. There isn't enough information to indicate a sedentary lifestyle or noncompliance.

CN: Physiological integrity; CNS: Basic care and comfort; CL: Application

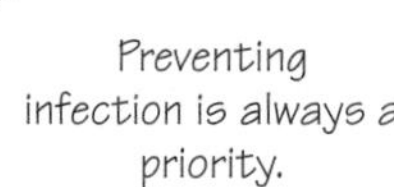
Preventing infection is always a priority.

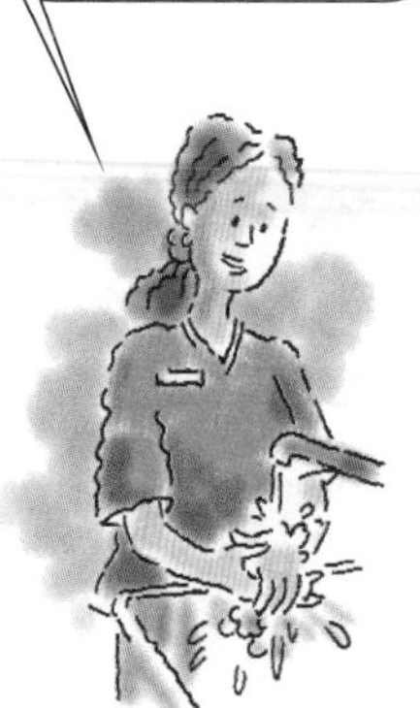

27. After the initial phase of a burn injury, the primary focus of a client's cure is:

1. enhancing self-esteem.
2. promoting hygiene.
3. reducing anxiety.
4. preventing infection.

27. 4. Because the body's protective barrier is damaged and the immune system is compromised, preventing infection is the primary goal. Enhancing self-esteem, promoting hygiene, and reducing anxiety are important but aren't the primary focus.

CN: Physiological integrity; CNS: Physiological adaptation; CL: Application

28. Which client is at greatest risk for impaired wound healing after surgery?

1. A 65-year-old client with hypertension
2. A 60-year-old client who's slightly overweight
3. An 78-year-old client in general good health
4. A 75-year-old client with poorly controlled diabetes mellitus

28. 4. Poorly controlled diabetes is a serious risk factor for impaired wound healing. Other factors that delay wound healing include advanced age, inadequate blood supply, nutritional deficiencies, and obesity.

CN: Physiological integrity; CNS: Physiological adaptation; CL: Analysis

29. A client has a possible postoperative wound infection. Which technique should the nurse use to obtain a wound culture from the surgical site?

1. Thoroughly irrigate the wound before collecting the culture.
2. Use a sterile swab to wipe the crusty area around the outside of the wound.
3. Gently roll a sterile swab from the center of the wound outward to collect drainage.
4. Use one sterile swab to collect drainage from several possible infected sites along the incision.

29. 3. Rolling a swab from the center outward is the right way to culture a wound. Irrigating the wound washes away drainage, debris, and many of the microorganisms colonizing or infecting the wound. The outside of the wound may be colonized with microorganisms from this wound, another wound, or the normal microorganisms on the client's skin. These may grow in culture and confuse the interpretation of results. All sources of drainage in an incision or surgical wound may not be infected or may be infected with different microorganisms, so each swab should be used on only one site.

CN: Safe, effective care environment; CNS: Safety and infection control; CL: Application

30. The nurse who is assessing a client with an abdominal incision suspects there is a potential for delayed wound healing. Which one of the following observations would most likely support this finding?

1. Sutures dry and intact
2. Wound edges in close approximation
3. Purulent drainage on soiled wound dressing
4. Sanguineous drainage in wound collection drainage bag

30. 3. Purulent drainage contains white blood cells, which fight infection, and indicates possible delay in wound healing. The sutures from a wound draining purulent secretions would pull away with an infection. Wound edges can't approximate with an infection in the wound. Sanguineous drainage indicates bleeding, not infection.

CN: Physiological integrity; CNS: Physiological adaptation; CL: Analysis

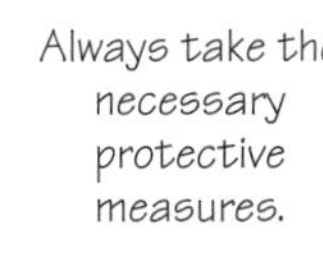
Always take the necessary protective measures.

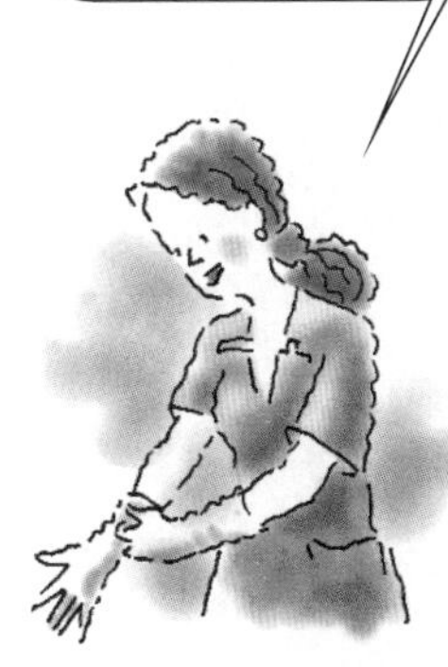

31. A nursing assistant will be changing the soiled bed linens of a client with a draining pressure ulcer. Which protective equipment should the nursing assistant wear?

1. Mask
2. Clean gloves
3. Sterile gloves
4. Shoe protectors

31. 2. Clean gloves protect the hands and wrists from microorganisms in the linens. Sterile gloves allow one to touch a sterile object or area without contaminating it. A mask protects the wearer and client from droplet nuclei and large particle aerosols. Shoe protectors prevent static and microorganism transmission from the floor of one room to another.

CN: Safe, effective care environment; CNS: Safety and infection control; CL: Analysis

32. Which intervention is most appropriate for preventing pressure ulcers in a bedridden elderly client?

1. Slide instead of lift the client when turning.
2. Turn and reposition the client at least every 8 hours.
3. Apply lotion after bathing the client, and vigorously massage the skin.
4. Post a turning schedule at the client's bedside, and adapt position changes to the client's situation.

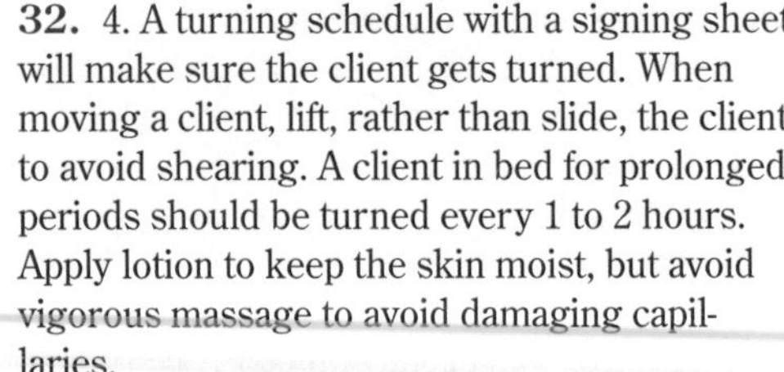

32. 4. A turning schedule with a signing sheet will make sure the client gets turned. When moving a client, lift, rather than slide, the client to avoid shearing. A client in bed for prolonged periods should be turned every 1 to 2 hours. Apply lotion to keep the skin moist, but avoid vigorous massage to avoid damaging capillaries.

CN: Physiological integrity; CNS: Basic care and comfort; CL: Analysis

33. Which instruction is the most important to give a client who has recently had a skin graft?

1. Continue physical therapy.
2. Protect the graft from direct sunlight.
3. Use cosmetic camouflage techniques.
4. Apply lubricating lotion to the graft site.

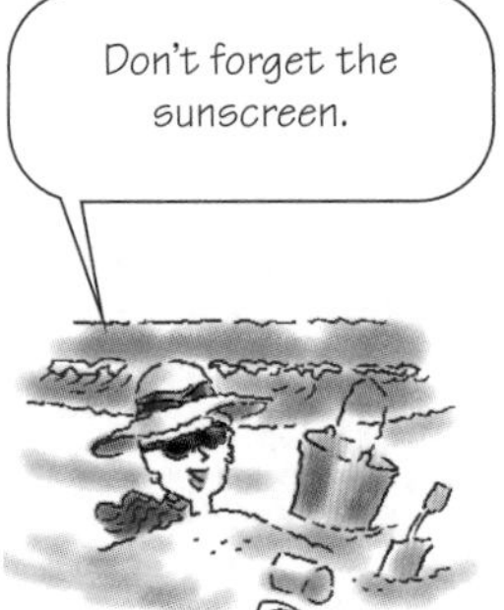
Don't forget the sunscreen.

33. 2. To avoid burning and sloughing, the client must protect the graft from direct sunlight. The other three interventions are all helpful to the client and his recovery.

CN: Physiological integrity; CNS: Physiological adaptation; CL: Analysis

34. The nurse is teaching the client how to prevent development of basal cell epithelioma. Which of the following statements is the most important when the nurse instructs the client?

1. Avoid burns.
2. Avoid exposure to the sun.
3. Avoid immnosuppression.
4. Avoid exposure to radiation.

34. 2. The sun is the best-known and most common cause of basal cell epithelioma. Burns, immunosuppression, and radiation are less common causes.

CN: Physiological integrity; CNS: Reduction of risk potential; CL: Application

35. The nurse is assessing an older client's skin turgor and finds inelasticity present. What is the nurse's most accurate interpretation of this finding?

1. The client is overhydrated.
2. The skin is considered to be normal skin turgor.
3. The skin is considered to be a normal part of the aging process.
4. The client is dehydrated.

35. 3. Inelastic skin turgor is a normal part of aging. Overhydration causes the skin to appear edematous and spongy. Normal skin turgor is dry and firm. Dehydration causes inelastic skin with tenting.

CN: Health promotion and maintenance; CNS: None; CL: Application

36. A client has a stage II sacral pressure ulcer that's receiving a transparent film dressing. Which statement is correct for this type of dressing?

1. The dressing will maintain a moist environment for the wound.
2. The dressing should be allowed to dry out before removal.
3. A gauze dressing should cover the transparent film dressing.
4. The transparent film dressing should be tightly packed into the wound.

36. 1. A transparent film dressing keeps the wound moist and enhances autolysis of necrotic tissue. There's no need to cover the transparent film dressing with a gauze dressing. The dressing should never be allowed to dry or be packed into the wound.

CN: Physiological integrity; CNS: Physiological adaptation; CL: Analysis

37. A 19-year-old client presents with second-degree sunburn on her face and both arms. Which intervention should the nurse implement first?

1. Administer analgesic medication as ordered.
2. Apply cold, moist towels to the burns.
3. Apply sterile, dry towels to the burns.
4. Apply vitamin A, D, and E ointment to the burns.

37. 2. Cold, moist towels help stop the burning process. Analgesics should be administered as ordered after the burning process has been controlled. Dry towels would retain the heat and aren't used. Ointments are applied during the healing phase, but not initially.
CN: Physiological integrity; CNS: Basic care and comfort; CL: Application

38. A client received burns to his entire back and left arm. Using the Rule of Nines, the nurse calculates that he has sustained burns to which percentage of his body?

1. 9%
2. 18%
3. 27%
4. 36%

One back and one arm equal…

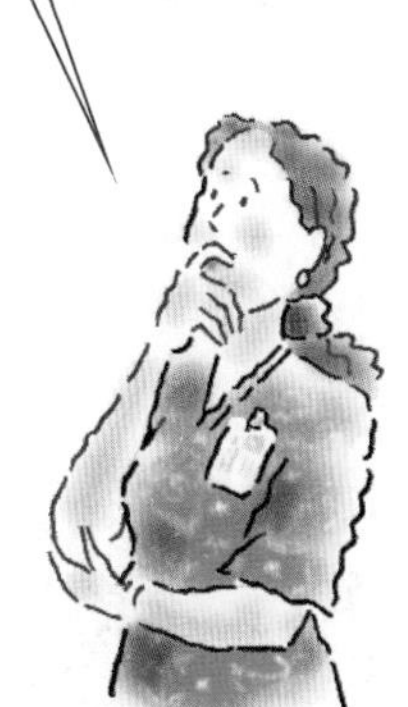

38. 3. According to the Rule of Nines, the posterior trunk, anterior trunk, and legs are each 18% of the total body surface. The head, neck, and arms are each 9% of total body surface, and the perineum is 1%. In this case, the client received burns to his back (18%) and one arm (9%), totaling 27% of his body.
CN: Physiological integrity; CNS: Reduction of risk potential; CL: Application

39. Which technique will maintain surgical asepsis?

1. Change the sterile field after sterile water is spilled on it.
2. Put on sterile gloves; then open a container of sterile saline.
3. Place a sterile dressing ½″ (1.3 cm) from the edge of the sterile field.
4. Clean the wound with a circular motion, moving from outer circles toward the center.

39. 1. A sterile field is considered contaminated when it becomes wet. Moisture can act as a wick, allowing microorganisms to contaminate the field. The outside of containers such as sterile saline bottles aren't sterile. The containers should be opened before sterile gloves are put on, and the solution poured over the sterile dressings placed in a sterile basin. The outer inch of a sterile field isn't considered sterile. Wounds should be cleaned from the most contaminated area to the least contaminated area, for example, from the center outward.
CN: Safe, effective care environment; CNS: Safety and infection control; CL: Application

40. For a client with a burn wound, which intervention decreases the chance of hypertrophied scarring during later stages of healing?

1. Removing all tissue in the wound area
2. Applying continuous pressure using elastic wraps
3. Wearing clothing to protect the burn from the sun
4. Maintaining wound dressing changes

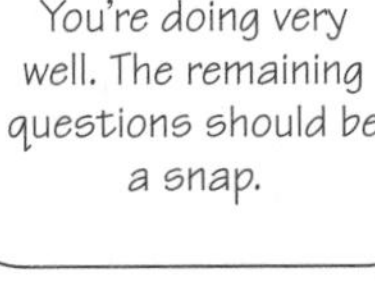

You're doing very well. The remaining questions should be a snap.

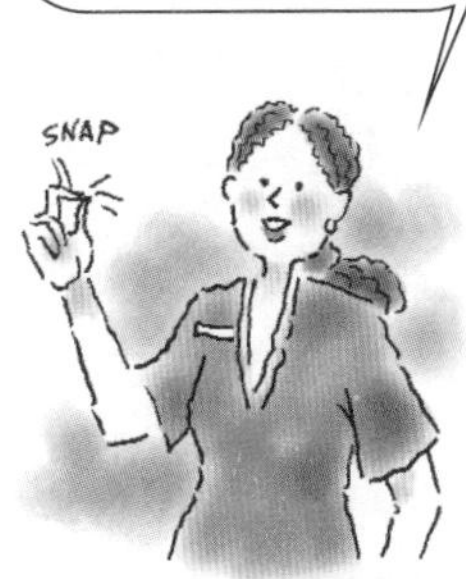

SNAP

40. 2. Using elastic wraps and bandages to apply continuous pressure during the early stages of wound healing can help prevent keloid scar formation. Removing tissue, especially eschar, promotes wound healing as do dressing changes, but neither directly decreases scar formation. Wearing clothing prevents sunburn but doesn't decrease scar formation.
CN: Physiological integrity; CNS: Physiological adaptation; CL: Application

41. Which piece of equipment for the wheelchair- or bed-bound client impedes circulation to the area it's meant to protect?

1. Waterbed
2. Ring or donut
3. Gel flotation pad
4. Polyurethane foam mattress

41. 2. Rings or donuts shouldn't be used because they restrict circulation. The waterbed distributes pressure over the entire surface. Gel pads give with weight. Foam mattresses distribute pressure evenly.
CN: Physiological integrity; CNS: Reduction of risk potential; CL: Application

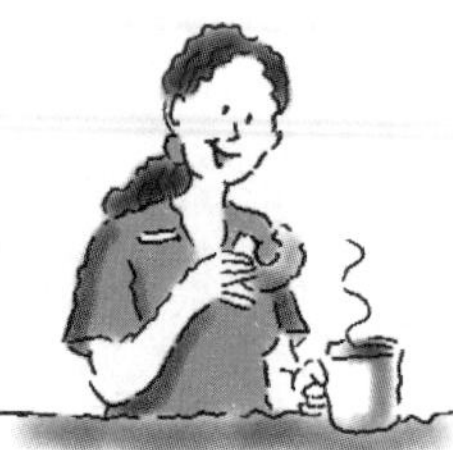
I should know better than to indulge.

42. Which intervention is the priority in treating postoperative wound evisceration?

1. Give prophylactic antibiotics as ordered.
2. Place the client on nothing-by-mouth (NPO) status.
3. Explain to the client what's happening, and give support.
4. Cover the protruding internal organs with sterile gauze moistened with sterile saline.

42. 4. Covering the wound with moistened gauze is the priority to prevent the organs from drying. Both the gauze and the saline must be sterile to reduce the risk of infection. Because evisceration usually requires emergency surgery, the nurse should place the client on NPO status. Evisceration is a frightening situation for any client. While the nurse works quickly to get the client treated, she can provide support to reduce the client's anxiety. Antibiotics will usually be ordered and should be started as soon as possible.
CN: Physiological integrity; CNS: Physiological adaptation; CL: Analysis

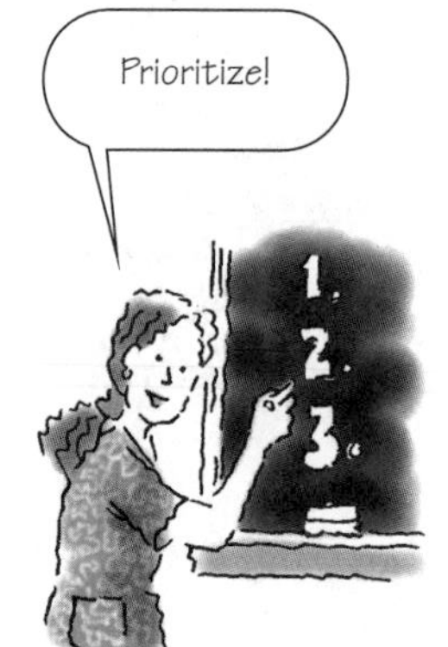
Prioritize!
1.
2.
3.

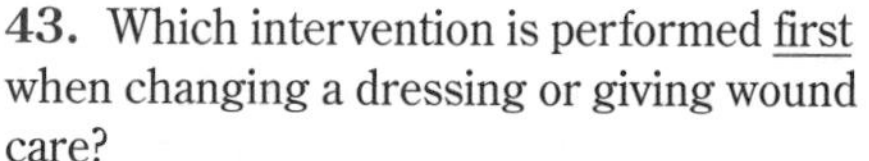

43. Which intervention is performed <u>first</u> when changing a dressing or giving wound care?

1. Put on gloves.
2. Wash hands thoroughly.
3. Slowly remove the soiled dressing.
4. Observe the dressing for the amount, type, and odor of drainage.

43. 2. The first thing the nurse must do is wash her hands. Putting on gloves, removing the dressing, and observing the drainage are all parts of the procedure for a dressing change.
CN: Safe, effective care environment; CNS: Management of care; CL: Application

44. When caring for a client who spends all or most of the time in bed, a turning schedule prevents the development of complications. Which schedule is best for most clients?

1. Turn every half hour.
2. Turn every 1 to 2 hours.
3. Turn once every 8 hours.
4. Keep the client on his back as much as possible.

44. 2. Turning the client every 1 to 2 hours will prevent pressure areas from developing and help prevent atelectasis and other pulmonary complications. Turning every half hour is too frequent, and turning every 8 hours would make the client vulnerable to the development of complications. The client should spend time on his back according to the turning schedule. During that period, the head of the bed should be raised to prevent the client from aspirating.
CN: Physiological integrity; CNS: Basic care and comfort; CL: Application

CN: Client needs category CNS: Client needs subcategory CL: Cognitive level

45. Which instruction is most important when teaching a client about hypersensitivity skin test results?
1. Wash the sites daily with a mild soap.
2. Have the sites read on the correct date.
3. Keep the skin test areas moist with a mild lotion.
4. Stay out of direct sunlight until the tests are read.

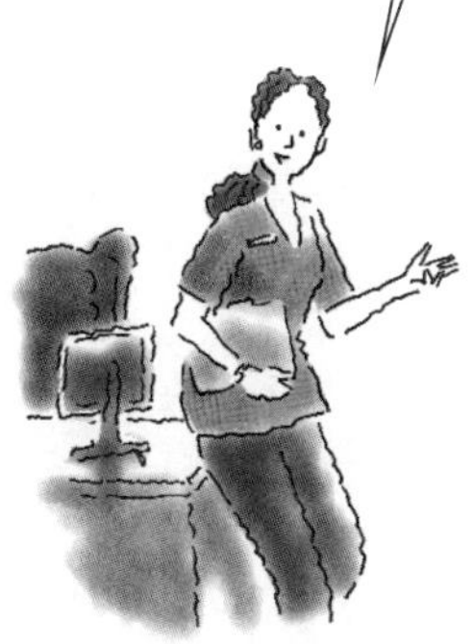

It's most important that you read this question carefully.

45. 2. An important facet of evaluating skin tests is to read the skin test results at the proper time. Evaluating the skin test too late or too early will give inaccurate and unreliable results. Both the gauze and the saline must be sterile to reduce the risk of infection. There's no need to wash the sites with soap. The sites should be kept dry. Direct sunlight isn't prohibited.

CN: Health promotion and maintenance; CNS: None; CL: Application

46. A client with disseminated herpes zoster is given I.V. hydrocortisone (Solu-Cortef). Which laboratory value should the nurse expect to be elevated as a result of this therapy?
1. Calcium
2. Glucose
3. Magnesium
4. Potassium

46. 2. Corticosteroids increase blood sugar and tend to lower serum potassium and calcium levels. Their effect on magnesium isn't substantial.

CN: Physiological integrity; CNS: Pharmacological and parenteral therapies; CL: Analysis

47. A client has been admitted to the burn unit with extensive full-thickness burns. Which consideration has priority?
1. Fluid status
2. Body image
3. Level of pain
4. Risk of infection

47. 1. In early burn care, the client's greatest need is fluid resuscitation because of large-volume fluid loss through the damaged skin. Body image, pain, and infection are important concerns in the nursing care of a burn client but don't take precedence over fluid management in the early phase of burn care.

CN: Safe, effective care environment; CNS: Management of care; CL: Analysis

48. A nurse is performing a skin assessment on a recently admitted client. Which factor is the most important in planning care for the client?
1. Family history of pressure ulcers
2. Presence of existing pressure ulcers
3. Overall risk of developing pressure ulcers
4. Potential areas of pressure ulcer development

48. 2. Areas of existing pressure ulcers need immediate treatment, and therefore are the most important. Family history of pressure ulcers isn't a risk factor for the development of pressure ulcers. Overall risk and potential areas of pressure development are important in planning care but don't take priority.

CN: Safe, effective care environment; CNS: Management of care; CL: Analysis

49. A client with extensive burns has a new donor site. Which consideration is important in positioning the client?
1. Make the site dependent.
2. Avoid pressure on the site.
3. Keep the site fully covered.
4. Allow ventilation of the site.

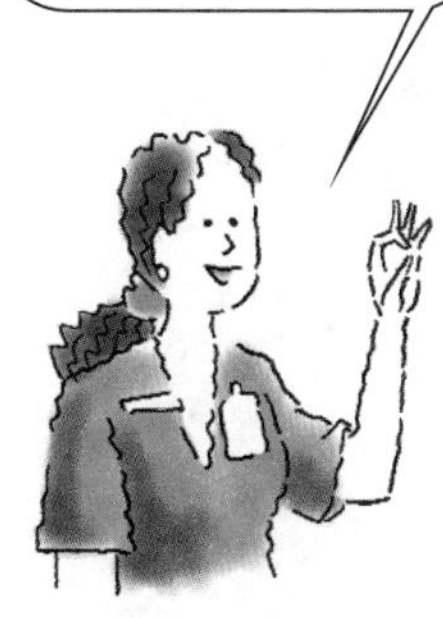

You're almost at question 50, and you're doing OK. Does that take some of the pressure off?

49. 2. A universal concern in the care of donor sites for burn care is to keep the site away from sources of pressure. Placing the site in a position of dependence isn't a justified aspect of donor site care. Ventilation of the site and keeping the site fully covered are practices in some institutions but aren't hallmarks of donor site care.

CN: Physiological integrity; CNS: Physiological adaptation; CL: Application

50. A client has been diagnosed with late stage Lyme disease. Upon assessment, which complication should the nurse expect to observe in the client?

1. Arthritis
2. Lung abscess
3. Renal failure
4. Sterility

50. 1. If Lyme disease goes untreated, arthritis, neurologic problems, and cardiac abnormalities may arise as late complications. Lung abscess, renal failure, and sterility aren't complications of Lyme disease.

CN: Physiological integrity; CNS: Physiological adaptation; CL: Application

51. A client is admitted with suspected malignant melanoma on his left shoulder. When performing the physical assessment, the nurse should expect to observe which sign?

1. Brown birthmark that has lightened in color
2. Brown or black mole with red, white, or blue areas
3. Petechiae
4. Red birthmark that has recently become darker

51. 2. Melanomas have an irregular shape and lack uniformity in color. They may appear brown or black with red, white, or blue areas. Melanoma lesions don't appear as petechiae or as birthmarks that have changed color.

CN: Health promotion and maintenance; CNS: None; CL: Application

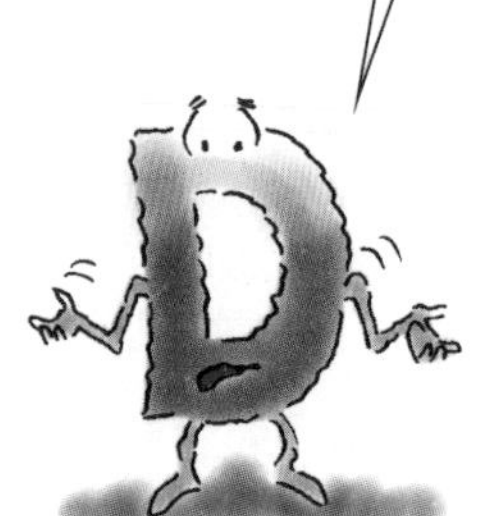

Why is everyone always trying to change me?

52. A nurse educator is presenting a hygiene class to nursing students. Which statement by a student indicates the need for further teaching?

1. "The skin absorbs fluids."
2. "The skin serves as the body's first line of defense."
3. "The skin excretes waste products."
4. "The skin changes vitamin D to a form the body can use."

52. 4. The skin doesn't change vitamin D to a form the body can use. (The sun helps to convert vitamin D.) The skin absorbs fluids, serves as the body's first line of defense, and excretes waste products.

CN: Physiological integrity; CNS: Physiological adaptation; CL: Analysis

53. The nurse is teaching a client how to care for his skin. What should the nurse instruct the client regarding sebum?

1. "It is the most superficial layer of the skin."
2. "It is the oil secreted by the skin."
3. "It is a pouchlike depression from which a hair grows."
4. "It is the deepest layer of the skin."

53. 2. Sebum is the oil secreted by the skin. The epidermis and dermis are skin layers. A follicle is a pouchlike depression from which a hair grows.

CN: Physiological integrity; CNS: Physiological adaptation; CL: Application

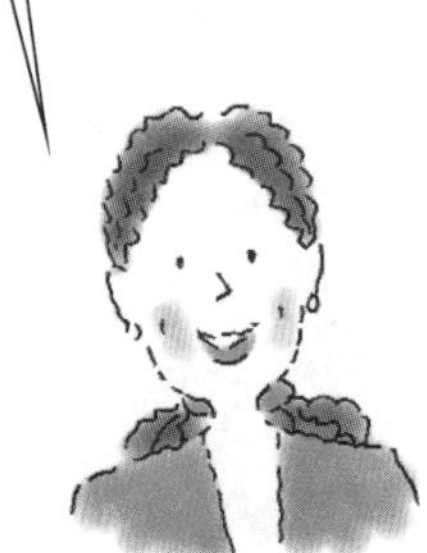

With your knowledge of burns, this question should take minimal effort.

54. During the late stages of healing, which intervention helps a burn wound to heal with minimal scarring?

1. Removing eschar from the skin
2. Applying continuous-compression wraps
3. Wearing clothing to protect the burn from the sun
4. Maintaining wound care irrigation

54. 2. Applying continuous-compression wraps aids skin healing and prevents hypertrophied tissue from forming. The other interventions are appropriate for the client with a burn wound but don't necessarily help minimize scarring.

CN: Physiological integrity; CNS: Reduction of risk potential; CL: Application

55. A client has an inflamed area on the right forearm that's causing considerable discomfort. The nurse should expect the physician to order which treatment?
1. Warm, moist compresses
2. An elastic bandage
3. Hydrocortisone cream
4. Nonadherent dressing

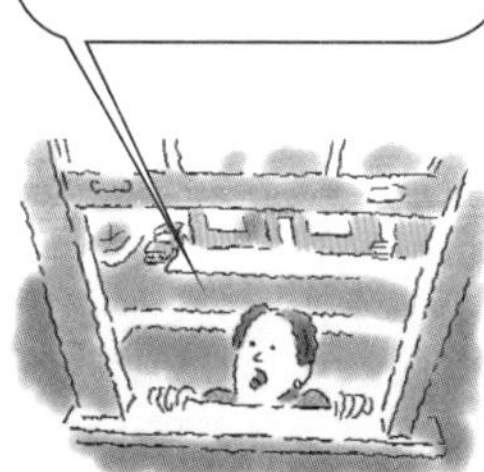

You've answered 55 questions! Hang in there!

56. An elderly client has a sore on the inside of his ankle that he says won't heal. After noting varicosities and coarse discoloration around the sore, the nurse should suspect which finding?
1. Acute venous insufficiency
2. Chronic venous insufficiency
3. Acute arterial occlusive disease
4. Chronic arterial occlusive disease

57. A nurse prepares a client for a shave biopsy of a skin lesion. Which point should be the priority in the teaching plan?
1. How to care for the suture line
2. The need for a skin graft
3. The need for sedation
4. How to care for the dressing

58. The physician orders a wet-to-dry dressing for a client who has a pressure ulcer with infected, necrotic tissue. What's the rationale for this treatment?
1. To prevent extension of the infection
2. To debride the wound
3. To keep the wound moist
4. To reduce pain

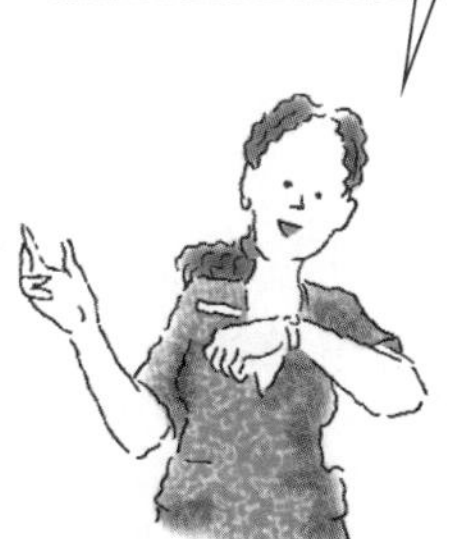

Observe the time in a question of this type.

59. A client has moist saline dressings applied to an open ulcer of the foot. Ten days after ulcer development, the wound should have which appearance?
1. Red, swollen tissue
2. Dry, crusted scab
3. Deep, wide keloid
4. Warm, painful tissue

55. 1. Warm, moist compresses increase circulation to the area, reducing discomfort and redness. An elastic bandage decompresses the area but doesn't ease inflammation. Hydrocortisone cream is useful on an inflamed area that itches. A nonadherent dressing doesn't relieve inflammation or pain.

CN: Physiological integrity; CNS: Basic care and comfort; CL: Application

56. 2. Classic signs of chronic venous insufficiency include skin discoloration (from blood extravasation in subcutaneous tissue) and stasis ulcers, usually found on the ankle's medial aspect. Asymmestric moderate edema, normal pulses, and deep muscle pain relieved by elevation are signs of acute venous insufficiency. Acute or chronic arterial occlusive disease usually causes intermittent claudication and severe burning pain.

CN: Physiological integrity; CNS: Physiological adaptation; CL: Application

57. 4. Dressing care should be included in the teaching plan. A shave biopsy removes only the first or second layer of skin, causing a superficial wound with no suture line and minimal scarring. There's no need for a skin graft or sedation with a shave biopsy.

CN: Physiological integrity; CNS: Physiological adaptation; CL: Application

58. 2. A wet-to-dry dressing placed over a necrotic area adheres to dead tissue and is debrided as the dressing is removed. Antibiotics, not dressings, help prevent extension of the infection. Keeping the wound moist would prevent the necessary debridement. The dressing has no analgesic effect.

CN: Physiological integrity; CNS: Physiological adaptation; CL: Application

59. 2. Ten days into healing, an ulcer should be at the end of the lag phase of healing, as indicated by a dry, crusted scab. Tissue is red, swollen, warm, or painful during the inflammatory phase, which occurs 2 to 7 days after the ulcer develops. A deep, wide keloid may appear 3 weeks to 2 years after ulcer development.

CN: Physiological integrity; CN: Physiological adaptation; CL: Application

60. When changing a dressing on a pressure ulcer, a nurse notes necrotic wound tissue. Which treatment should the nurse expect the physician to order?

1. Wound incision and drainage
2. Wound culturing
3. Wound debridement
4. Wound irrigation with an antiseptic

60. 3. For healing to occur, necrotic (dead) tissue must be removed from the wound; usually, this is done by debridement. Wound incision and drainage and wound culturing are done when infection is present or suspected. Wound irrigation with an antiseptic may damage sensitive tissue and prevent healing.

CN: Physiological integrity; CNS: Physiological adaptation; CL: Application

61. After a traumatic injury, a client's wound heals and a smooth, pink, thickened, rubbery lesion forms over the wound. Which cause should the nurse suspect?

1. Erosion
2. Fissure
3. Keloid
4. Abscess

61. 3. A keloid results from a defect in the healing process in which excess collagen develops at the healing site. Erosion refers to loss of part or all of the skin surface, usually from infection or pressure. A fissure is a slit in the wound. Abscess, which results from accumulation of purulent drainage, causes the wound to appear red, swollen, and tender.

CN: Physiological integrity; CNS: Physiological adaptation; CL: Analysis

62. A client is diagnosed with urticaria. Which statement describes the wheal that commonly accompanies urticaria?

1. Elevated, firm circumscribed lesion in the dermis, 1 to 2 cm in diameter
2. Flat, nonpalpable, irregularly shaped lesion, more than 1 cm in diameter
3. Transient, elevated, solid, firm, irregularly shaped area of cutaneous edema, with a variable diameter
4. Elevated, circumscribed lesion in the dermis or subcutaneous layer, filled with liquid or semisolid material

These questions aren't easy, but you've got a good hand-le on it.

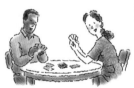

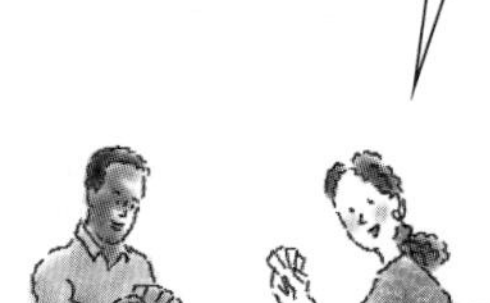

62. 3. A wheal is a transient, elevated, firm lesion of irregular shape and size. A nodule is an elevated lesion in the dermis with a diameter of 1 to 2 cm. A patch is a flat lesion with a diameter exceeding 1 cm. A cyst is an elevated, circumscribed lesion filled with liquid or semisolid material.

CN: Physiological integrity; CNS: Physiological adaptation; CL: Application

63. A 70-year-old client who spilled hot coffee on his lap 3 days ago has multiple blisters. As the nurse provides care, two of the blisters break. Which action should the nurse take?

1. Remove the raised skin, because the blister has been compromised.
2. Wash the area vigorously with soap and water.
3. Apply alcohol to the area.
4. Clean the area with normal saline solution, and cover it with a dressing.

63. 4. To maintain asepsis, the nurse should clean the area with normal saline solution and cover it with a dressing. Removing the raised skin would cause further skin damage. Washing the area vigorously with soap and water would damage the tissue and cause drying. Alcohol would dry out the tissue.

CN: Safe, effective care environment; CNS: Safety and infection control; CL: Application

64. A client undergoes cryosurgery to remove a cancerous skin lesion. When assessing the wound a few days later, the nurse should expect to find:

1. dry, itchy patches.
2. oozing and pain.
3. dryness, tenderness, and sutures.
4. swelling, blistering, and tenderness.

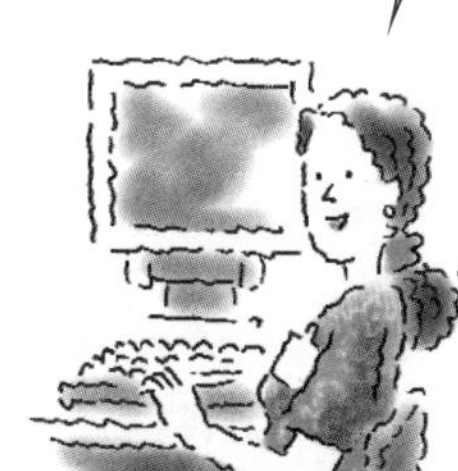

Know your assessment facts; they're critical in nursing and on the NCLEX.

64. 4. Cryosurgery leaves a wound resembling a burn, with swelling, blistering, and tenderness. Oozing and pain suggest an infection. The wound wouldn't be dry or itchy and wouldn't have sutures.

CN: Physiological integrity; CNS: Physiological adaptation; CL: Analysis

65. A client with facial lacerations requires hospitalization for 1 week. During assessment, the nurse notes scabs on the wounds. This finding corresponds to which phase of wound healing?

1. Contraction phase
2. Inflammatory phase
3. Proliferative phase
4. Remodeling phase

65. 3. During the proliferative phase of wound healing, which lasts from the 4th to 21st day after injury, granulation tissue appears (scabs form) and the wound edges start to pull together. Contraction, the third phase of wound healing, may begin around the 7th day and involves a significant decrease in the wound surface. The inflammatory phase, the first healing phase, immediately follows the injury and lasts 4 to 6 days; it involves control of bleeding and release of chemicals needed for healing. The remodeling phase, the final phase, may lead to scar flattening and correction of any deformities that occurred during the third phase.

CN: Physiological integrity; CNS: Basic care and comfort; CL: Analysis

66. An 85-year-old female client who has spent a great deal of time outdoors tells the home health nurse that her skin is dry and itchy. Which instruction should the nurse provide?

1. "Soak in a bubble bath once per day."
2. "Bathe with antimicrobial soap once per day."
3. "Bathe with mild soap and water or with water only."
4. "Scrub the skin vigorously to remove dead skin cells."

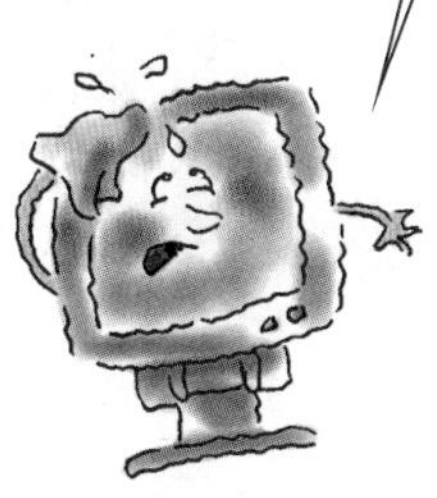

Only four more questions to go. Whew!

66. 3. Bathing with mild soap and water or with water only can relieve skin itching and dryness. Bubble baths and antimicrobial soap can be very drying to an elderly person's sensitive skin. Scrubbing vigorously may worsen skin dryness.

CN: Physiological integrity; CNS: Basic care and comfort; CL: Application

67. A client has a maculopapular rash on his trunk, which follows skin cleavage lines in a Christmas tree pattern. He reports that the rash started as a small lesion 4 days ago. What is the <u>most likely</u> cause of the rash?

1. Tinea corporis
2. Pityriasis rosea
3. Allergic reaction to a drug
4. Eczema

67. 2. Pityriasis rosea starts with a "herald patch" and then erupts in a Christmas tree pattern on the trunk. Tinea corporis is a skin infestation, usually seen as fine lines under the skin. Allergic reactions to drugs typically affect the entire body. Eczema is an erythematous papular rash typically affecting the antecubital and popliteal fossae.

CN: Physiological integrity; CNS: Physiological adaptation; CL: Analysis

68. At an outpatient clinic, a medical assistant interviews a client and documents her findings as follows:

Progress notes

12/13/10	Client very anxious because new
0900	black mole with shades of brown
	noted on upper outer right
	thigh. Asymmetrical in shape
	with an irregular border.
	——— M. Rosenfeld, MA

After reading the chart note, a nurse begins planning based on which nursing diagnosis?

1. *Deficient knowledge related to potential diagnosis of basal cell carcinoma*
2. *Fear related to potential diagnosis of malignant melanoma*
3. *Risk for impaired skin integrity related to potential squamous cell carcinoma*
4. *Readiness for enhanced knowlege: Skin care precautions related to benign mole*

69. The nurse is examining the back of a client and notes a rash with a discrete lesion configuration. Which graphic shows a discrete lesion configuration?

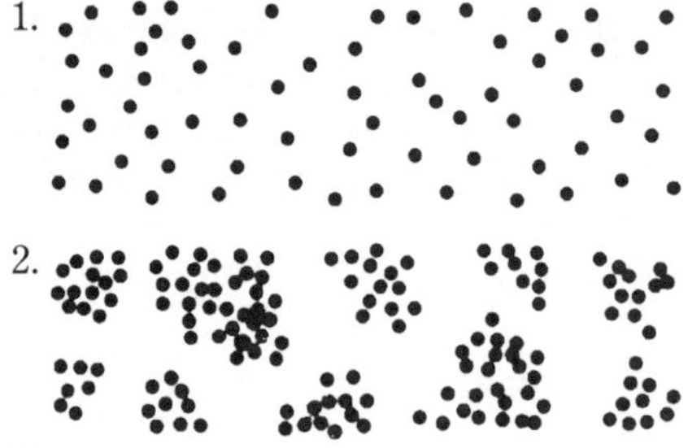

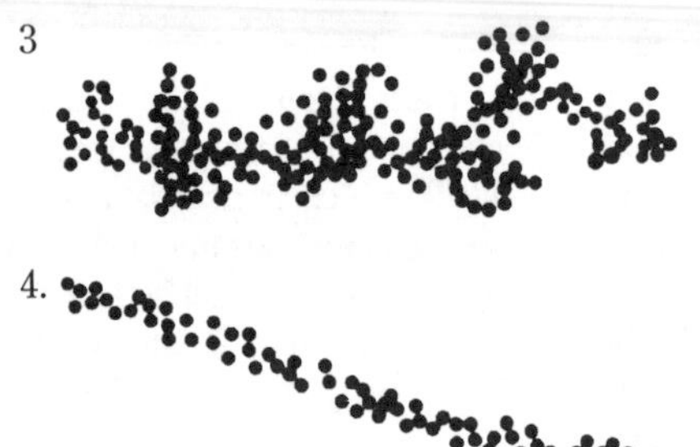

68. 2. Documentation reveals that the client is anxious about her symptoms. These symptoms (asymmetry, variable color, and border irregularity) most closely resemble malignant melanoma. The nursing note contains no indication that the client currently has deficient knowledge. The characteristics of the lesion aren't consistent with basal or squamous cell carcinoma or a benign nevus (mole).

CN: Physiological integrity; CNS: Physiological adaptation; CL: Analysis

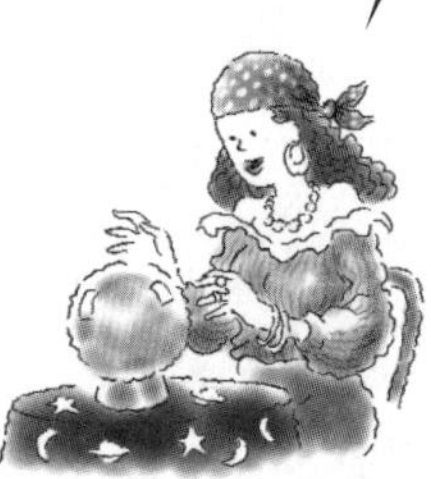

Hooray! You've finished Part II. I see your future success in Part III.

69. 1. In a discrete pattern, individual lesions are separate and distinct. Option 2 shows a grouped pattern, in which lesions are clustered together. Option 3 is a confluent pattern. In this configuration, lesions merge so that individual lesions aren't visible or palpable. Option 4 is a linear pattern, in which lesions form a line.

CN: Physiological integrity; CNS: Physiological adaptation; CL: Analysis

Part III Care of the psychiatric client

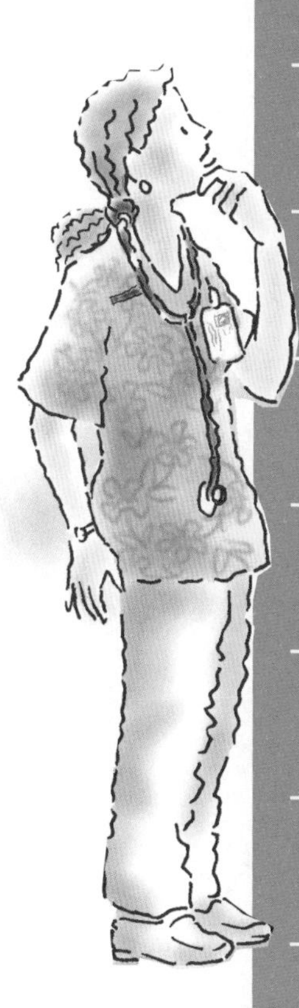

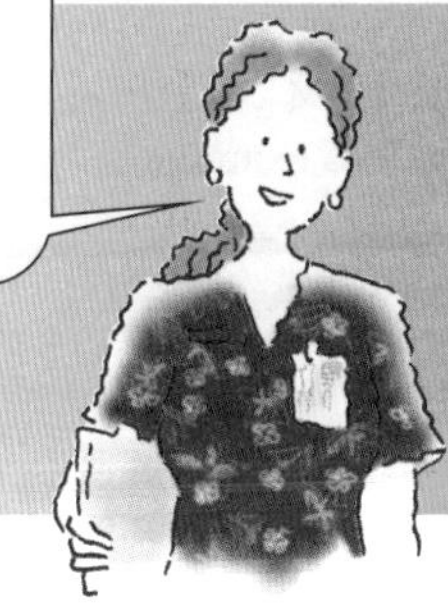

Before you take the
tests relating to
psychiatric care, take
this test relating to
tests (and treatments,
too) in psychiatric care.

Chapter 12 Essentials of psychiatric care

1. A 50-year-old client is scheduled for electroconvulsive therapy (ECT). ECT is most commonly prescribed for which condition?
1. Major depression
2. Antisocial personality disorder
3. Chronic schizophrenia
4. Somatoform disorder

1. 1. ECT is most commonly used for the treatment of major depression in clients who haven't responded to antidepressants or who have medical problems that contraindicate the use of antidepressants. ECT isn't commonly used for treatment of personality disorders. ECT doesn't appear to be of value to individuals with chronic schizophrenia and isn't the treatment of choice for clients with somatoform disorders.
CN: Psychosocial integrity; CNS: None; CL: Application

2. A patient with bipolar disorder becomes verbally aggressive in a group therapy session. Which response by the nurse would be best?
1. "You're behaving in an unacceptable manner, and you need to control yourself."
2. "If you continue to talk like that, no one will want to be around you."
3. "You're frightening everyone in the group. Leave the room immediately."
4. "Other people are disturbed by your profanity. I'll walk with you down the hall to help release some of that energy."

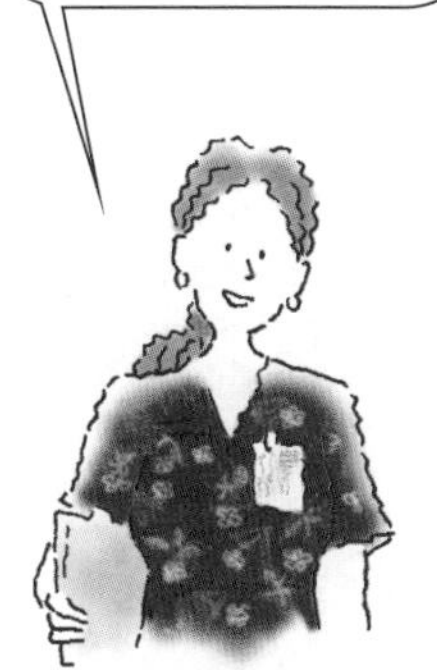

options might be

which is *best?*

2. 4. This response informs the client that, although the behavior is unacceptable, the client is still worthy of help. The other responses are nontherapeutic and blaming.
CN: Safe, effective care environment; CNS: Management of care; CL: Application

3. A newly admitted client is extremely hostile toward a staff member he has just met, without apparent reason. According to Freudian theory, the nurse should suspect that the client is exhibiting which phenomena?
1. Intellectualization
2. Transference
3. Triangulation
4. Splitting

3. 2. Transference is the unconscious assignment of negative or positive feelings evoked by a significant person in the client's past to another person. Intellectualization is a defense mechanism in which the client avoids dealing with emotions by focusing on facts. Triangulation refers to conflicts involving three family members. Splitting is a defense mechanism commonly seen in clients with personality disorders in which the world is perceived as all good or all bad.
CN: Psychosocial integrity; CNS: None; CL: Analysis

CN: Client needs category CNS: Client needs subcategory CL: Cognitive level

4. Which intervention would be typical of a nurse using a cognitive-behavioral approach to a client experiencing low self-esteem?

1. Use of unconditional positive regard
2. Analysis of free associations
3. Classical conditioning
4. Examination of negative thought patterns

4. 4. Popular cognitive-behavioral approaches examine the validity of habitual patterns of thinking and belief systems that influence feelings and behaviors. "Unconditional positive regard" is a phrase from Carl Rogers's client-centered therapy and describes a supportive, nonjudgmental, neutral approach by a therapist. Analysis of free associations is characteristic of Freudian psychoanalysis. Classical conditioning is characteristic of a pure behavioral intervention.
CN: Psychosocial integrity; CNS: None; CL: Application

5. During group therapy, a client listening to another client's description of an abusive incident that occurred during childhood says, "I didn't think anyone else felt like I did as a child." The nurse recognizes this statement as a reflection of which curative factor of group therapy, as identified by Yalom?

1. Altruism
2. Universality
3. Catharsis
4. Existential factors

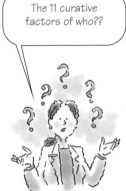

5. 2. One of the 11 curative factors of group therapy identified by Yalom is universality, which assists group participants in recognizing common experiences and responses. This action helps reduce anxiety and allows other group members to provide support and understanding. Altruism, catharsis, and existential factors are other curative factors Yalom described, but they don't describe this particular incident. Altruism refers to finding meaning through helping others; catharsis is an open expression of previously suppressed feelings; and existential factors describe the recognition that one has control over the quality of one's life.
CN: Psychosocial integrity; CNS: None; CL: Application

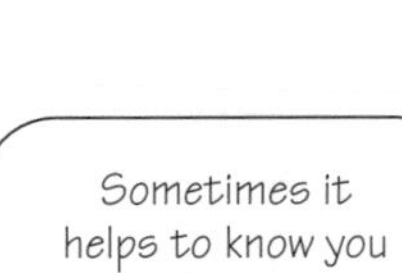

Sometimes it helps to know you aren't alone.

6. Which statement best describes the key advantage of using groups in psychotherapy?

1. Decreases the focus on the individual
2. Fosters the physician–client relationship
3. Confronts individuals with their shortcomings
4. Fosters a new learning environment

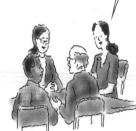

6. 4. In a group, the individual has the opportunity to learn that others have the same problems and needs. The group can also provide an arena where new methods of relating to others can be tried. Decreasing focus on the individual isn't a key advantage (and sometimes isn't an advantage at all). Groups don't, by themselves, foster the physician–client relationship, and they aren't always used to confront individuals.
CN: Psychosocial integrity; CNS: None; CL: Analysis

7. A client who has recently lost his wife and children in a car collision is being treated at the outpatient psychiatric clinic. Which therapy should be most effective with this client?

1. Electroconvulsive therapy (ECT)
2. Group therapy
3. Hypnotherapy
4. Individual therapy

7. 2. The client history strongly suggests post-traumatic stress disorder. Group therapy has been especially effective with this diagnosis. ECT, hypnotherapy, and individual therapy may be useful to this client, but these therapies aren't as strongly advocated as group therapy.
CN: Psychosocial integrity; CNS: None; CL: Analysis

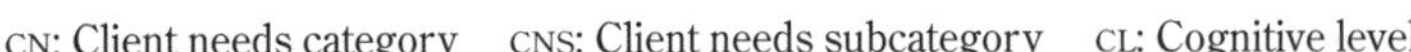
CN: Client needs category CNS: Client needs subcategory CL: Cognitive level

8. During a group therapy session, a teenage girl says that she's fat and ugly and that everybody makes fun of her. This statement reflects which common adolescent fear or anxiety?
1. Fear of the unknown
2. Fear of loss of respect, love, and emerging self-esteem
3. Anxiety related to guilt
4. Anxiety about body image and changes in physical appearance

8. 4. Anxiety about body image and changes in physical appearance is a common fear of adolescents. Fear of the unknown is associated with toddlerhood. Fear of loss of respect, love, and emerging self-esteem is associated with the school-age developmental phase. Anxiety related to guilt is also associated with the school-age developmental phase.
CN: Psychosocial integrity; CNS: None; CL: Application

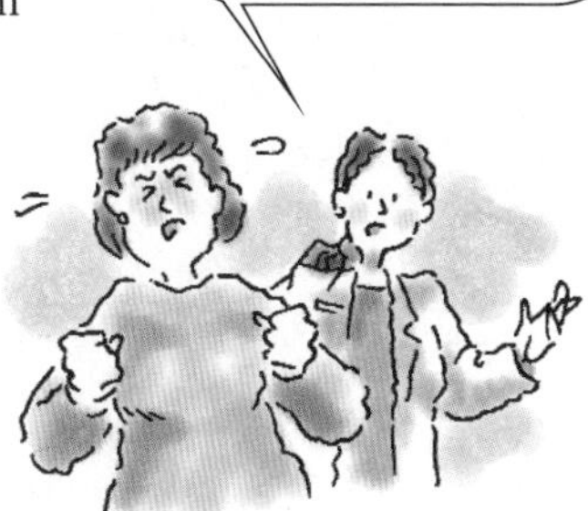
In psychiatric care, the nurse needs to recognize verbal as well as physical clues.

9. After telling a nurse to "pray for me," a client gives away personal possessions and shows a sudden calmness. The nurse recognizes that this behavior may signal which condition?
1. Major depression
2. Panic attack
3. Suicidal ideation
4. Severe anxiety

9. 3. Verbal clues to suicidal ideation include such statements as "Pray for me," and "I won't be here when you get back." Nonverbal clues include giving away personal possessions, a sudden calmness, and risk-taking behaviors. The nurse should recognize the combination of these signs as indicating suicidal ideation—not depression, panic, or anxiety. Clients with major depression generally don't exhibit suicidal behavior until their outlook on their problems begins to improve (an improvement in behavior should raise suspicion, especially if accompanied by sudden calmness).
CN: Psychosocial integrity; CNS: None; CL: Application

10. A client recently lost his spouse. Which of the following behaviors indicates that the client is going through a normal stage of grieving?
1. The client starts using chemicals.
2. The client becomes an overachiever.
3. The client shows signs of hyperactivity.
4. The client shows a loss of warmth when interacting with others.

10. 4. Hostile reactions, such as loss of warmth when interacting with others, occur during normal grieving. Chemical use, overachieving, and hyperactivity commonly correlate with complicated grieving.
CN: Psychosocial integrity; CNS: None; CL: Application

11. Two 16-year-old clients are being treated in an adolescent unit. During a recreational activity, they begin to physically fight. How should the nurse intervene?
1. Remove the teenagers to separate areas and set limits.
2. Remind the teenagers of the unit rules.
3. Obtain an order to place the teenagers in seclusion.
4. Obtain an order to place the teenagers in restrains.

11. 1. Setting limits and removing the clients from the situation is the best way to handle aggression. Reminders of appropriate behavior aren't likely to be effective at this time and seclusion and restraints are reserved for more serious situations.
CN: Psychosocial integrity; CNS: None; CL: Application

12. A client is prescribed sertraline (Zoloft), a selective serotonin reuptake inhibitor. Which information about this drug's adverse effects should the nurse include when creating a medication teaching plan? Select all that apply:

1. Agitation
2. Agranulocytosis
3. Sleep disturbance
4. Intermittent tachycardia
5. Dry mouth
6. Seizures

12. 1, 3, 5. Common adverse effects of sertraline include agitation, sleep disturbance, and dry mouth. Agranulocytosis, intermittent tachycardia, and seizures are adverse effects of clozapine (Clozaril).

CN: Physiological integrity; CNS: Pharmacological and parenteral therapies; CL: Application

13. A physician prescribes lithium for a client diagnosed with bipolar disorder. The nurse needs to provide appropriate education for the client on this drug. Which topics should the nurse cover? Select all that apply:

1. The potential for addiction
2. Signs and symptoms of drug toxicity
3. The potential for tardive dyskinesia
4. A low-tyramine diet
5. The need to consistently monitor blood levels
6. The expected time frame for noticing improvements in mood

13. 2, 5, 6. Client education should cover the signs and symptoms of drug toxicity as well as the need to report them to the physician. The client should be instructed to monitor his lithium levels on a regular basis to avoid toxicity. The nurse should explain that 7 to 21 days may pass before the client notes a change in his mood. Lithium doesn't have addictive properties. Tardive dyskinesia isn't associated with lithium. Tyramine is a potential concern for clients taking monoamine-oxidase inhibitors.

CN: Physiological integrity; CNS: Pharmacological and parenteral therapies; CL: Application

14. A physician starts a client on the antipsychotic medication haloperidol (Haldol). The nurse is aware that this medication has extrapyramidal adverse effects. Which measures should the nurse take during haloperidol administration? Select all that apply:

1. Review subcutaneous injection technique.
2. Closely monitor vital signs, especially temperature.
3. Provide the client with the opportunity to pace.
4. Monitor blood glucose levels.
5. Provide the client with hard candy.
6. Monitor for signs and symptoms of urticaria.

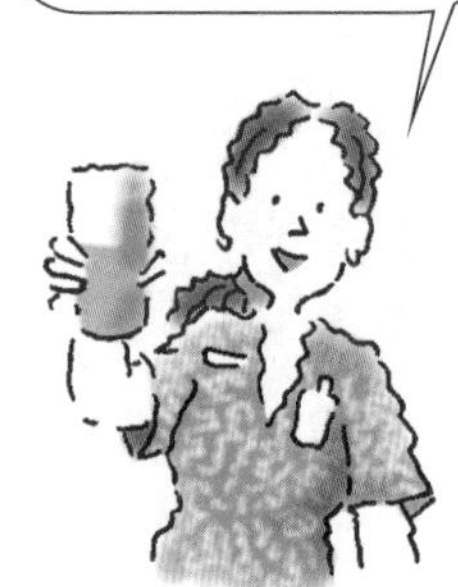

Here's to you! You've just zipped through another important NCLEX topic.

14. 2, 3, 5. Neuroleptic malignant syndrome is a life-threatening adverse effect of antipsychotic medications such as haloperidol. It's associated with a rapid increase in temperature. The most common extrapyramidal adverse effect, akathisia, is a form of psychomotor restlessness that can typically be relieved by pacing. Haloperidol and the anticholinergic medications that are provided to alleviate its extrapyramidal effects can result in a dry mouth. Providing the client with hard candy to suck on can help with this problem. Haloperidol isn't given subcutaneously and doesn't affect blood glucose levels. Urticaria isn't usually associated with haloperidol administration.

CN: Physiological integrity; CNS: Pharmacological and parenteral therapies; CL: Analysis

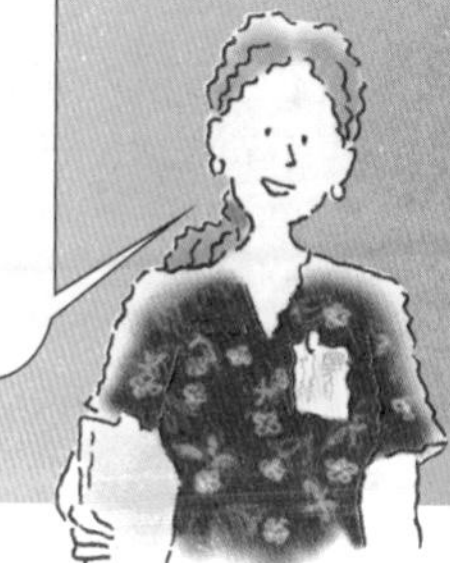

Can't remember much
about a particular

Type this address into
your Web browser:
www.emedicine.com.
Then search for the

Chapter 13 Somatoform & sleep disorders

1. The nurse is teaching a student nurse about somatoform disorders. Which of the following statements by the nurse would be the most accurate in describing somatoform disorders?

1. They usually seek medical attention.
2. They have organic pathologic disorders.
3. They regularly attend psychotherapy sessions without encouragement.
4. They're eager to discover the true reasons for their physical symptoms.

1. 1. A client with a somatization disorder usually seeks medical attention. These clients have a history of multiple physiologic complaints without associated demonstrable organic pathologic causes. The expected behavior for this type of disorder is to seek treatment from several medical physicians for somatic complaints, not psychiatric evaluation.

CN: Health promotion and maintenance; CNS: None; CL: Application

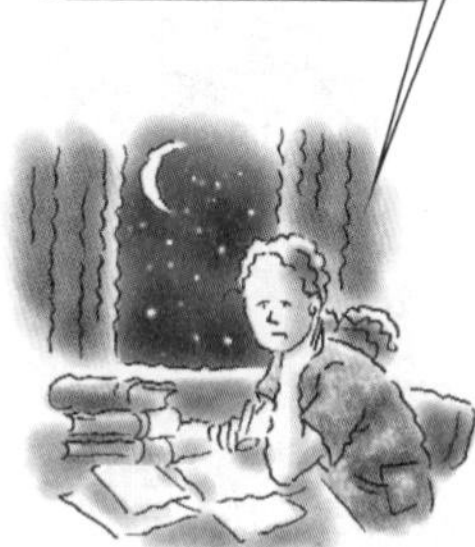

I hope I stay
awake long enough
to finish these
questions.

2. A nurse is caring for a client with a somatoform disorder. In providing education to the family, the nurse discusses that these disorders:

1. are limited to one organ system.
2. occur with a recent physical illness.
3. are physical conditions with organic pathologic causes.
4. occur in the absence of organic findings.

2. 4. The essential feature of somatoform disorders is a physical or somatic complaint without any demonstrable organic findings to account for the complaint. Somatic complaints aren't limited to one organ system. There are no known physiologic mechanisms to explain the findings. The diagnostic criteria for somatoform disorders state that the client has a history of many physical complaints beginning before age 30 that occur over several years.

CN: Psychosocial integrity; CNS: None; CL: Application

3. Which rationale best explains the physical symptoms experienced by a client with a somatoform disorder?

1. The client complains of physical symptoms that can be explained by a known physiologic cause.
2. The client complains of physical symptoms to gain attention.
3. The client experiences physical symptoms in response to anxiety.
4. The client complains of physical symptoms to cope with delusional thinking.

3. 3. In a client with a somatoform disorder, physical symptoms are manifestations of psychological distress, such as anxiety and depression, that have no apparent physiologic cause. The physical symptoms enable the client to avoid unpleasant emotions, not seek individual attention intentionally. The attention received, if any, is a secondary gain that stems from the primary gain of anxiety relief. Somatic delusions are characteristic of schizophrenia.

CN: Psychosocial integrity; CNS: None; CL: Analysis

4. A nurse is caring for a client who's demonstrating an ego defense mechanism. Which finding supports the nurse's observations?

1. Repression of anger
2. Suppression of grief
3. Denial of depression
4. Preoccupation with pain

Remember, you're looking for a defense mechanism.

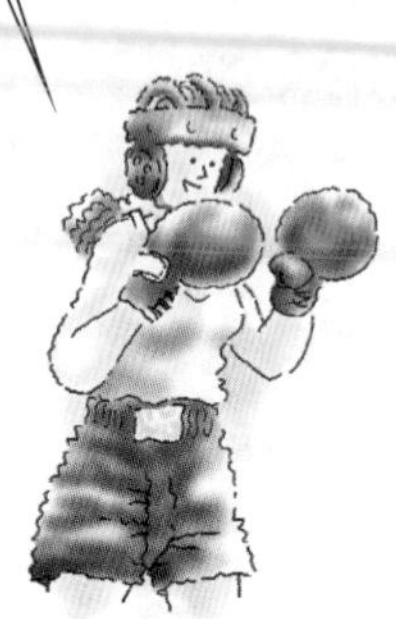

4. 1. One psychodynamic theory states that somatization is the transformation of aggressive and hostile wishes toward others into physical complaints. Repressed anger originating from past disappointments and unfilled needs for nurturing and caring are expressed by soliciting other people's concern and rejecting them as ineffective. Denial, suppression, and preoccupation aren't the defense mechanisms underlying the dynamics of somatization disorders.
CN: Psychosocial integrity; CNS: None; CL: Application

5. An 86-year-old client in an extended care facility is anxious most of the time and frequently complains of a number of vague symptoms that interfere with his ability to eat. These symptoms indicate which disorder?

1. Conversion disorder
2. Hypochondriasis
3. Severe anxiety
4. Sublimation

5. 2. Complaints of vague physical symptoms that have no apparent medical causes are characteristic of clients with hypochondriasis. In many cases, the GI system is affected. Conversion disorders are characterized by one or more neurologic symptoms. The client's symptoms don't suggest severe anxiety. A client experiencing sublimation channels maladaptive feelings or impulses into socially acceptable behavior.
CN: Psychosocial integrity; CNS: None; CL: Analysis

Accurate nursing diagnoses make sure all staff are working toward the same goal!

6. Which nursing diagnosis is most appropriate for the disorder known as hypochondriasis?

1. *Risk for injury*
2. *Grieving*
3. *Risk for situational low self-esteem*
4. *Deficient diversional activity*

6. 3. Hypochondriasis is a disorder manifested by fear, risk for situational low self-esteem, and feelings of worthlessness. *Risk for injury, Grieving,* and *Deficient diversional activity* have no correlation to the disorder.
CN: Safe, effective care environment; CNS: Management of care; CL: Application

7. A college student frequently visited the health center during the past year with multiple vague complaints of GI symptoms before course examinations. Although physical causes have been eliminated, the student continues to express her belief that she has a serious illness. These symptoms are typical of which disorder?

1. Conversion disorder
2. Depersonalization
3. Hypochondriasis
4. Somatization disorder

7. 3. Hypochondriasis in this case is shown by the client's belief that she has a serious illness, although pathologic causes have been eliminated. The disturbance usually lasts at least 6 months, and the GI system is commonly affected. Exacerbations are usually associated with identifiable life stressors such as, in this case, course examinations. Conversion disorders are characterized by one or more neurologic symptoms. Depersonalization refers to persistent, recurrent episodes of feeling detached from one's self or body. Somatoform disorders generally have a chronic course with few remissions.
CN: Psychosocial integrity; CNS: None; CL: Analysis

8. A nursing goal for a client diagnosed with hypochondriasis should focus on which area?

1. Determining the cause of the sleep disturbance
2. Relieving the fear of serious illness
3. Recovering the lost or altered function
4. Giving positive reinforcement for accomplishments related to physical appearance

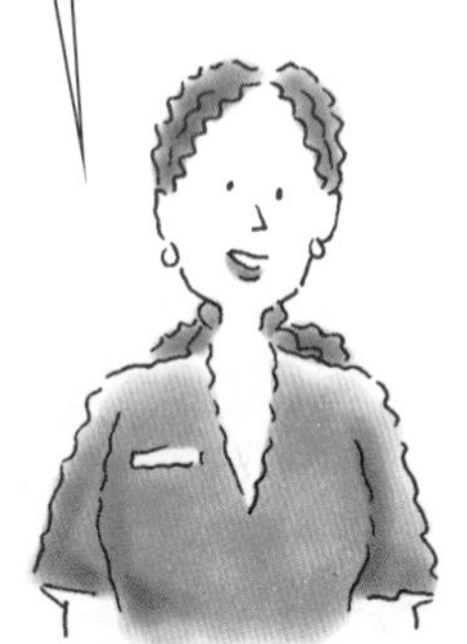
Nursing goals target emotional outcomes as well as physical ones.

8. 2. The nursing goal for hypochondriasis is relief of fear. For insomnia, the goal is focused on determining the cause of the sleep disturbance. The nursing goal for a conversion disorder focuses on the recovery of the lost or altered function. An appropriate goal for body dysmorphic disorder focuses on positive reinforcement for accomplishments related to physical appearance.

CN: Psychosocial integrity; CNS: None; CL: Application

9. Which nursing intervention is appropriate for a client diagnosed with hypochondriasis?

1. Teach the client adaptive coping strategies.
2. Help the client eliminate the stress in her life.
3. Confront the client with the statement, "It's all in your head."
4. Encourage the client to focus on identification of physical symptoms.

9. 1. Because of weak ego strength, a client with hypochondriasis is unable to use coping mechanisms effectively. The nursing focus is to teach adaptive coping mechanisms. It isn't realistic to eliminate all stress. A client should never be confronted with the statement, "It's all in your head," because this wouldn't facilitate a long-term therapeutic relationship, which is necessary to offer reassurance that no physical disease is present. Calling attention to physical symptoms is counterproductive to treatment.

CN: Psychosocial integrity; CNS: None; CL: Application

10. After repeated office visits, physical examinations, and diagnostic tests for assorted complaints, a client is referred to a psychiatrist. The client later tells a friend, "I can't imagine why my doctor wants me to see a psychiatrist." Which statement is the most likely explanation for the client's statement?

1. The client probably believes psychiatrists are only for "crazy" people.
2. The client probably doesn't understand the correlation of symptoms and stress.
3. The client probably believes his physician has made an error in diagnosis.
4. The client probably believes his physician wants to get rid of him as a client.

10. 3. The preoccupation in hypochondriasis is related to bodily functions or physical sensations. Repeated physical examinations, diagnostic tests, and reassurance from the physician don't allay the concerns about bodily disease. There's a belief that a health care professional has poor insight if he sees the concern about having a serious illness as excessive or unreasonable. The other responses aren't valid.

CN: Psychosocial integrity; CNS: None; CL: Analysis

11. Which therapeutic strategy is used to reduce anxiety in a client diagnosed with hypochondriasis?

1. Suicide precautions
2. Relaxation exercises
3. Electroconvulsive therapy (ECT)
4. Aversion therapy

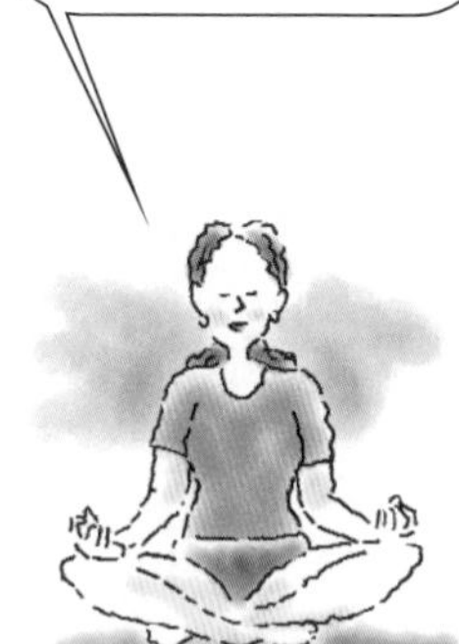
Meditating is so therapeutic.

11. 2. Relaxation exercises help to decrease anxiety in a client with hypochondriasis. In a hypochondriasis disorder, no threat of suicide exists. ECT and aversion therapy aren't therapeutic strategies for hypochondriasis.

CN: Psychosocial integrity; CNS: None; CL: Application

12. A client is given triazolam (Halcion) for a sleep disorder. The nurse is reinforcing some teaching precautions concerning the medication. The nurse determines that the client understands the precautions when the client states:

1. "I take the medication with citrus juice."
2. "I shouldn't confuse this medication with Haldol."
3. "It's okay to take a short drive after taking the medication."
4. It's okay to smoke while I take this medication."

12. 2. Haldol is an antipsychotic that has a spelling similar to Halcion and is used for clients with psychoses, Tourette's syndrome, severe behavioral problems in children, and emergency sedation of severely agitated psychotic clients. Halcion is one of a group of sedative-hypnotic medications that can be used only for a limited time because of the risk of dependence. Grapefruit and grapefruit juices can alter the absorption of Halcion. The client should avoid driving and other tasks that require alertness or motor skills because the medication may cause drowsiness. Smoking reduces drug effectiveness.

CN: Physiological integrity; CNS: Pharmacological and parenteral therapies; CL: Analysis

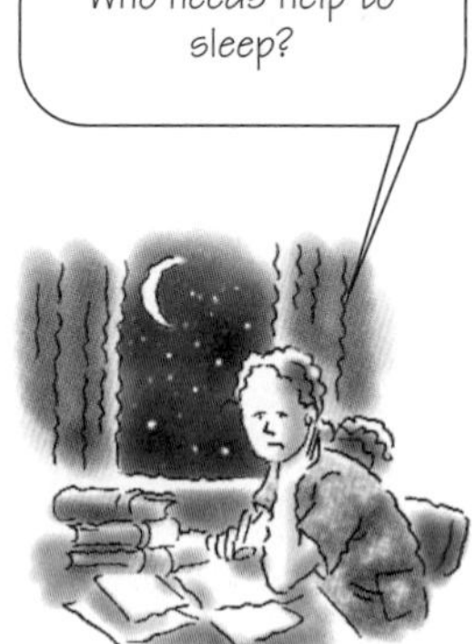

13. Which measure should be included when teaching a client strategies to help sleep?

1. Keep the room warm.
2. Eat a large meal before bedtime.
3. Schedule bedtime when you feel tired.
4. Avoid caffeine, excessive fluid intake, alcohol, and stimulating drugs before bedtime.

13. 4. Caffeine, excessive fluid intake, alcohol, and stimulating drugs act as stimulants; avoiding them should promote sleep. Maintaining a cool temperature in the room will better facilitate sleeping. Excessive fullness or hunger may interfere with sleep. Setting a regular bedtime and wake-up time facilitates physiologic patterns.

CN: Health promotion and maintenance; CNS: None; CL: Application

14. A nurse is interviewing a client newly admitted to the unit. While stating a list of medications, the client falls asleep. The nurse understands that the client is most likely exhibiting which sleep disorder?

1. Hypersomnia
2. Insomnia
3. Narcolepsy
4. Parasomnia

14. 3. Narcolepsy is also known as sleep attacks. Hypersomnia, or somnolence, refers to excessive sleepiness or seeking excessive amounts of sleep. Insomnia is a sleep disorder in which an individual has difficulty initiating or maintaining sleep. Parasomnia refers to unusual or undesired behavior that occurs during sleep, such as nightmares and sleepwalking.

CN: Physiological integrity; CNS: Physiological adaptation; CL: Analysis

15. Treatments for sleep disorders include which method?

1. Behavior therapy
2. Biofeedback
3. Group therapy
4. Insight-oriented psychotherapy

15. 2. Biofeedback, relaxation therapy, and psychopharmacology are appropriate treatments for sleep disorders. Behavior therapy, group therapy, and insight-oriented psychotherapy are treatments related to somatoform disorders.

CN: Physiological integrity; CNS: Basic care and comfort; CL: Application

16. Which nursing intervention would be the most appropriate for a depressed client with a nursing diagnosis of *Disturbed sleep pattern related to external factors*?

1. Consult the physician about prescribing a bedtime sleep medication.
2. Allow the client to sit at the nurses' station for comfort.
3. Allow the client to watch television until he's sleepy.
4. Encourage the client to take a warm bath before retiring.

16. 4. Sleep-inducing activities, such as a warm bath, help promote relaxation and sleep. Although consulting a physician about prescribing a bedtime sleep medication is possible, it wouldn't be the best nursing intervention for this client. Encouraging the client to watch television or sit at the nurses' station wouldn't necessarily promote sleep. In fact, these activities may provide too much stimulation, further preventing sleep.

CN: Physiological integrity; CNS: Basic care and comfort; CL: Application

17. Which condition characterizes rapid eye movement (REM) sleep?

1. Disorientation and disorganized thinking
2. Jerky limb movements and position changes
3. Pulse rate slowed by 5 to 10 beats/minute
4. Highly active brain and physiologic activity levels

17. 4. Highly active brain and physiologic activity levels characterize REM stage. Stages 3 and 4 of non-REM sleep are characterized by disorientation and disorganization. During REM sleep, body movement ceases except for the eyes. The pulse rate slows by 5 or 10 beats/minute during non-REM sleep, not REM sleep.

CN: Physiological integrity; CNS: Physiological adaptation; CL: Analysis

18. A client with sleep terror disorder might have autonomic signs of intense anxiety. Which autonomic sign or symptom should the nurse monitor?

1. Tachycardia
2. Pupil constriction
3. Cool, clammy skin
4. Decreased muscle tone

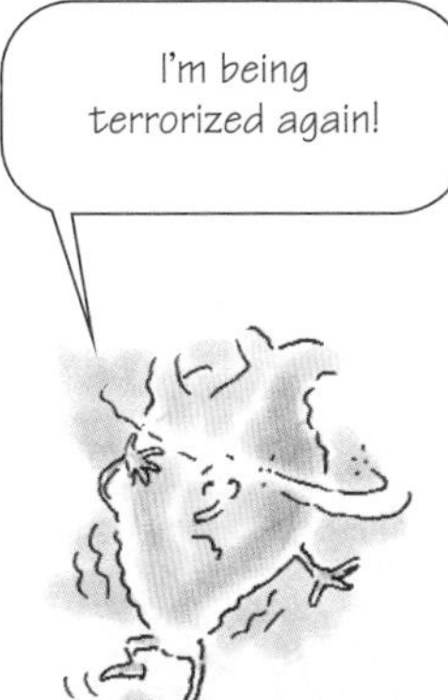
I'm being terrorized again!

18. 1. Autonomic arousal includes tachycardia, which should be closely monitored by the nurse to prevent the occurrence of further complications such as arrhythmia. Sweating, increased muscle tone, and pupillary dilation are responses that may also occur but aren't considered life-threatening.

CN: Physiological integrity; CNS: Physiological adaptation; CL: Application

19. Which consideration is important in planning care for a client experiencing sleep deprivation?

1. Sleep is influenced by biological rhythms.
2. The natural body clock follows a 24-hour cycle.
3. Long sleepers have more rapid eye movement periods.
4. Prolonged periods of sleep deprivation can lead to ego disorganization, hallucinations, and delusions.

19. 4. Sleep deprivation can lead to hallucinations and delusions. Uninterrupted sleep is an important nursing consideration in planning care. All other data are expected and shouldn't cause sleep deprivation.

CN: Physiological integrity; CNS: Physiological adaptation; CL: Application

20. A nurse is instructing a 38-year-old male client undergoing treatment for anxiety and insomnia. The practitioner has prescribed lorazepam (Ativan) 1 mg by mouth three times per day. The nurse determines that the teaching regarding the client's medication has been effective when the client gives which of the following responses?

1. "I'll avoid caffeine."
2. "I'll avoid aged cheese."
3. "I'll avoid sunlight."
4. "I'll maintain adequate salt intake."

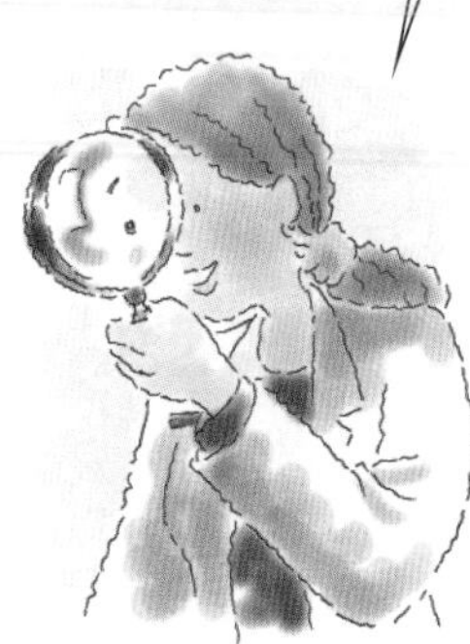

In question 20, you're looking for what could exacerbate the client's symptoms.

20. 1. Lorazepam is a benzodiazepine used to treat various forms of anxiety and insomnia. Caffeine is contraindicated because it's a stimulant and increases anxiety. A client on a monoamine oxidase inhibitor should avoid aged cheeses. Clients taking certain antipsychotic medications should avoid sunlight. Salt intake has no effect on lorazepam.

CN: Physiological integrity CNS: Pharmacological and parenteral therapies; CL: Analysis

21. A client diagnosed with a sleep disorder awakens abruptly with a piercing scream. Which disorder best explains this behavior?

1. Hypersomnia
2. Nightmare disorder
3. Sleep terror disorder
4. Sleepwalking

21. 3. Sleep terror disorder refers to an abrupt arousal from sleep with a piercing scream or cry. Hypersomnia is excessive sleepiness or seeking excessive amounts of sleep. Nightmares are frightening dreams that lead to awakenings from sleep and are severe enough to interfere with social or occupational functioning. Sleepwalking refers to motor activity initiated during sleep in which the individual may leave the bed and walk around.

CN: Psychosocial integrity; CNS: None; CL: Analysis

22. Which nursing diagnosis is appropriate for a client with a sleep disorder?

1. *Fear*
2. *Risk for injury*
3. *Risk for situational low self-esteem*
4. *Disturbed sensory perception (auditory)*

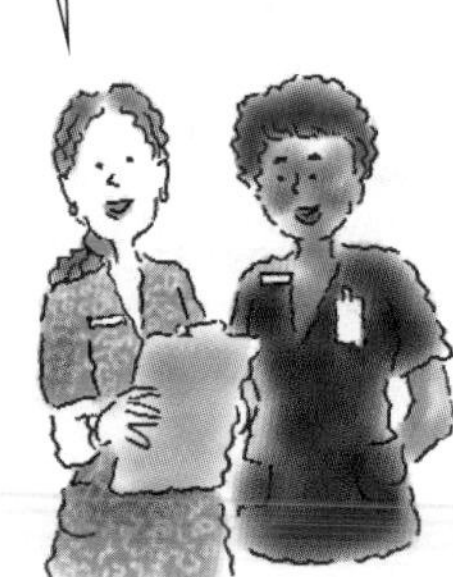

Nursing diagnoses are the professional language of nursing.

22. 2. A client with a sleep disorder may be at *Risk for injury* due to drowsiness and decreased concentration. *Fear* may be applicable to hypochondriasis. *Risk for situational low self-esteem* may be related to an alteration in self-concept or self-esteem. No evidence of a *Disturbed sensory perception (auditory)* problem exists.

CN: Safe, effective care environment; CNS: Management of care; CL: Analysis

23. A 35-year-old female client is diagnosed with conversion disorder with paralysis of the legs. What's the best nursing intervention for the nurse to use?

1. Discuss with the client ways to live with the paralysis.
2. Focus interactions on results of medical tests.
3. Encourage the client to move her legs as much as possible.
4. Avoid focusing on the client's physical limitations.

23. 4. The paralysis is used as an unhealthy way of expressing unmet psychological needs. The nurse should avoid speaking about the paralysis to shift the client's attention to the mental aspect of the disorder. The other options focus too much on the paralysis, which doesn't allow for recognition of the underlying psychological motivations.

CN: Psychological integrity; CNS: None; CL: Application

24. Which statement is correct about conversion disorders?

1. The symptoms can be controlled.
2. The psychological conflict is repressed.
3. The client is aware of the psychological conflict.
4. The client shouldn't be made aware of the conflicts underlying the symptoms.

24. 2. In conversion disorder, physical symptoms are manifestations of a repressed psychological conflict. The client isn't able to control or produce symptoms and is unaware of the psychological conflict. Understanding the principles and conflicts behind the symptoms can prove helpful during a client's therapy.
CN: Psychosocial integrity; CNS: None; CL: Analysis

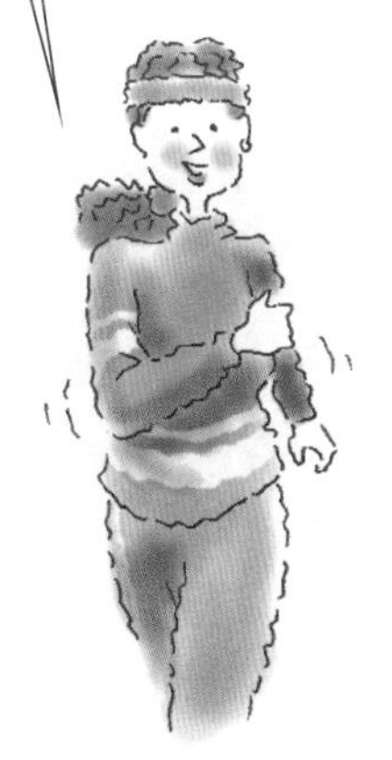

You've run through 24 questions. You're almost there.

25. A client is admitted for abrupt onset of paralysis in his left arm. Although no physiologic cause has been found, the symptoms are exacerbated when he speaks of losing custody of his children in a recent divorce. These assessment findings are characteristic of which of the following disorders?

1. Body dysmorphic disorder
2. Conversion disorder
3. Delusional disorder
4. Malingering

25. 2. Conversion disorders are characterized by one or more neurologic symptoms associated with psychological conflict. Body dysmorphic disorder is an imagined belief that there's a defect in the appearance of all or part of the body. The client doesn't have a delusion; this is the sole manifestation of a delusional disorder. Malingering is the intentional production of symptoms to avoid obligations or obtain rewards.
CN: Psychosocial integrity; CNS: None; CL: Analysis

26. A client has been hospitalized with a diagnosis of conversion-disorder blindness. Which statement best explains this manifestation?

1. The client is suppressing her true feelings.
2. The client's anxiety has been relieved through her physical symptoms.
3. The client is acting indifferent because she doesn't want to show her actual fear.
4. The client's needs are being met, so she doesn't need to be anxious.

26. 2. Conversion accomplishes anxiety reduction through the production of a physical symptom symbolically linked to an underlying conflict. The client isn't aware of the internal conflict. Hospitalization doesn't remove the source of the conflict.
CN: Psychosocial integrity; CNS: None; CL: Analysis

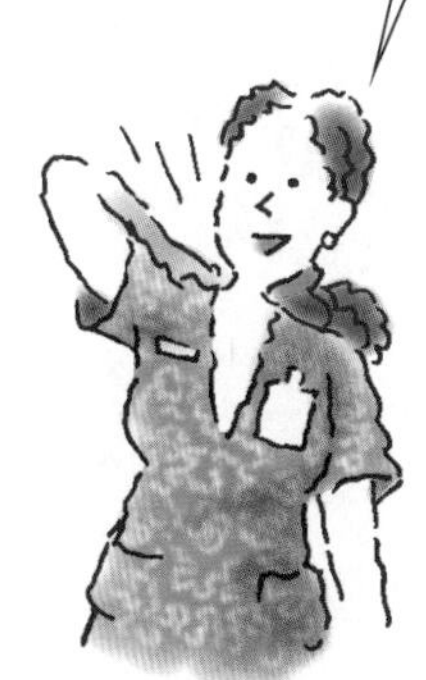

You deserve a pat on the back for answering these questions.

27. A client with hypochondriasis complains of pain in his right side that he hasn't had before. Which response is the most appropriate?

1. "It's time for group therapy now."
2. "Tell me about this new pain you're having. You'll miss group therapy today."
3. "I'll report this pain to your physician. In the meantime, group therapy starts in 5 minutes. You must leave now to be on time."
4. "I'll call your physician and see whether he'll order a new pain medication. Why don't you get some rest for now?"

27. 3. The amount of time focused on discussing physical symptoms should be decreased. Lack of positive reinforcement may help stop the maladaptive behavior. However, avoiding the statement altogether demeans the client and doesn't address the underlying problem. Asking the client to further explain the pain emphasizes physical symptoms and prevents the client from attending group therapy. All physical complaints need to be evaluated for physiologic causes by the physician.
CN: Psychosocial integrity; CNS: None; CL: Application

28. Which intervention would help a client with conversion-disorder blindness to eat?

1. Direct the client to independently locate items on the tray and feed himself.
2. See to the needs of the other clients in the dining room; then feed this client last.
3. Establish a "buddy" system with other clients who can feed the client at each meal.
4. Expect the client to feed himself after explaining the location of food on the tray.

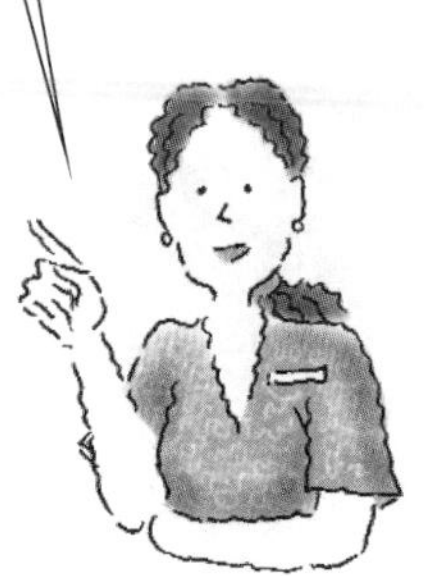

A client with a disorder of psychologic origin may need the same interventions as one with a disorder of physical origin.

28. 4. The client is expected to maintain some level of independence by feeding himself, while at the same time the nurse provides some direction and is supportive in a matter-of-fact way. Feeding the client leads to dependence.

CN: Psychosocial integrity; CNS: None; CL: Application

29. A client diagnosed with conversion disorder who's experiencing left-sided paralysis tells the nurse that he has received a lot of attention in the hospital and that it's unfortunate that others outside the hospital don't find him interesting. Which nursing diagnosis is appropriate for this client?

1. *Interrupted family processes*
2. *Ineffective health maintenance*
3. *Ineffective coping*
4. *Social isolation*

29. 3. The client can't express his internal conflicts in appropriate ways. There are no defining characteristics to support the other nursing diagnoses.

CN: Psychosocial integrity; CNS: None; CL: Application

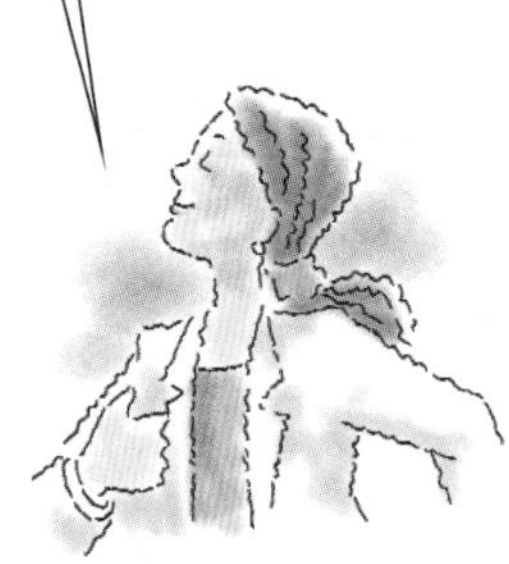

It's nice to feel special.

30. To help a client with conversion disorder increase self-esteem, which nursing intervention is appropriate?

1. Set large goals so the client can see positive gains.
2. Focus attention on the client as a person rather than on the symptom.
3. Discuss the client's childhood to link present behaviors with past traumas.
4. Encourage the client to use avoidant-interactional patterns rather than assertive patterns.

30. 2. Focusing on the client directs attention away from the symptom. This approach eventually reduces the client's need to gain attention through physical symptoms. Small goals ensure success and reinforce self-esteem. Discussion of childhood has no correlation with self-esteem. Avoiding interactional situations doesn't foster self-esteem.

CN: Psychosocial integrity; CNS: None; CL: Application

31. A nurse is caring for a client with a conversion disorder. What sign or symptom should she expect to observe or have the client report?

1. Delusions
2. Feelings of depression or euphoria
3. A feeling of dread accompanied by somatic signs
4. One or more neurologic symptoms associated with psychological conflict or need

31. 4. Symptoms of conversion disorders are neurologic in nature (paralysis, blindness). Delusional disorders are characterized by delusions. Mood disorders are characterized by abnormal feelings of depression or euphoria. Anxiety is characterized by a feeling of dread.

CN: Health promotion and maintenance; CNS: None; CL: Application

32. Which nursing diagnosis is appropriate for a client with conversion disorder who has little energy to expend on activities or interactions with friends?
1. *Powerlessness*
2. *Hopelessness*
3. *Impaired social interaction*
4. *Compromised family coping*

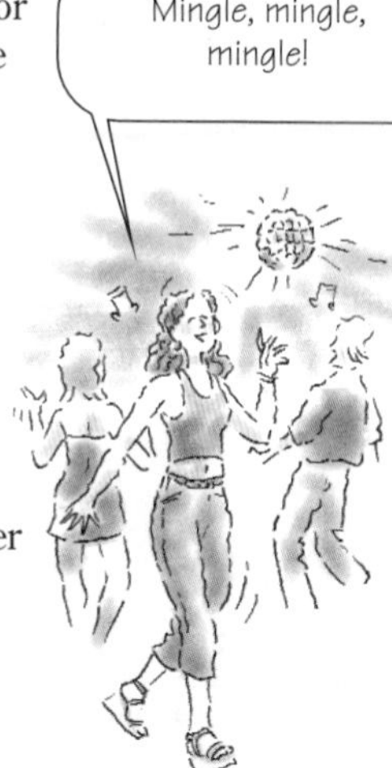

32. 3. When clients focus their mental and physical energy on somatic symptoms, they have little energy to expend on social or diversional activities. Such a client needs nursing assistance to become involved in social interactions. Although the other diagnoses are common for a client with conversion disorder, the information given in the question doesn't support them.
CN: Psychosocial integrity; CNS: None; CL: Application

33. A client diagnosed with conversion disorder has a nursing diagnosis of *Interrupted family processes related to the client's disability.* Which goal is appropriate for this client?
1. The client will resume former roles and tasks.
2. The client will take over roles of other family members.
3. The client will rely on family members to meet all client needs.
4. The client will focus energy on problems occurring in the family.

33. 1. The client who uses somatization has typically adopted a sick role in the family, characterized by dependence. Increasing independence and resumption of former roles are necessary to change this pattern. The client shouldn't be expected to take on the roles or responsibilities of other family members. Focusing energy on problems occuring in the family doesn't address the nursing diagnosis and related factors.
CN: Psychosocial integrity; CNS: None; CL: Application

34. A new client admitted to a psychiatric unit is diagnosed with conversion disorder. The client shows a lack of concern for his sudden paralysis, although his athletic abilities have always been a source of pride to him. The nurse understands that the client is demonstrating:
1. acute dystonia.
2. la belle indifference.
3. malingering.
4. secondary gain.

34. 2. La belle indifference is a lack of concern about the present illness. Acute dystonia refers to muscle spasms. Malingering is voluntary production of symptoms. Secondary gain refers to the benefits of illness.
CN: Psychosocial integrity; CNS: None; CL: Application

35. Which nursing intervention is the <u>most appropriate</u> for a client who had pseudoseizures and is diagnosed with conversion disorder?
1. Explain that the pseudoseizures are imaginary.
2. Promote dependence so that unfilled dependency needs are met.
3. Encourage the client to discuss his feelings about the pseudoseizures.
4. Promote independence, and withdraw attention from the pseudoseizures.

35. 4. Successful performance of independent activities enhances self-esteem. Telling the client that the symptoms are imaginary may jeopardize the nurse-client relationship. Positive reinforcement encourages the use of maladaptive responses. Focus shouldn't be on the disability because it may provide positive gains for the client.
CN: Psychosocial integrity; CNS: None; CL: Application

36. Which therapeutic approach would enable a client to cope effectively with life stress without using conversion?

1. Focus on the symptoms.
2. Ask for clarification of the symptoms.
3. Listen to the client's symptoms in a matter-of-fact manner.
4. Point out that the client's symptoms are an escape from dealing with conflict.

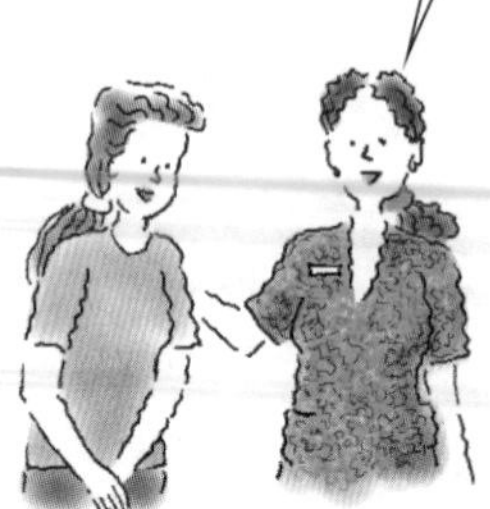
Focus on what
the client is saying.

36. 3. Listening in a matter-of-fact manner doesn't focus on the client's symptoms. All other interventions focus on the client's symptoms, which draw attention to the physical symptoms, not the underlying cause.

CN: Health promotion and maintenance; CNS: None; CL: Application

37. Which statement made by a client with a pain disorder shows the nurse that the goal of stress management was attained?

1. "My arm hurts."
2. "I enjoy being dependent on others."
3. "I don't really understand why I'm here."
4. "My muscles feel relaxed after that progressive relaxation exercise."

37. 4. The client is experiencing positive results from the relaxation exercise. All other responses alert the nurse that the client needs further interventions.

CN: Physiological integrity; CNS: Basic care and comfort; CL: Analysis

38. Which nursing diagnosis is appropriate for a client with hypochondriasis disorder?

1. *Disturbed sensory perception (visual)*
2. *Hopelessness*
3. *Imbalanced nutrition: Less than body requirements*
4. *Risk for other-directed violence*

38. 3. A client with hypochondriasis has a preoccupying fear of having a serious disease and is at risk for not getting adequate nutrition. Delusions are not a symptom of hypochondriasis. Although hopelessness may be present, it is not the primary focus. Clients with hypochondriasis are not prone to violence toward themselves or others.

CN: Safe, effective care environment; CNS: Management of care; CL: Application

39. A nurse is teaching the family of a client diagnosed with a somatoform pain disorder. Which of the following statements by the nurse most accurately describes this disorder?

1. A preoccupation with pain in the absence of physical disease
2. A physical or somatic complaint without any demonstrable organic findings
3. A morbid fear or belief that one has a serious disease where none exists
4. One or more neurologic symptoms associated with psychological conflict or need

39. 1. Somatoform pain disorder is a preoccupation with pain in the absence of physical disease. A physical or somatic complaint refers to somatoform disorders in general. A morbid fear of serious illness is hypochondriasis. Neurologic symptoms are associated with conversion disorders.

CN: Psychosocial integrity; CNS: None; CL: Application

40. By which process does a client conceal the true motivations for his thoughts, actions, or feelings?
1. Displacement
2. Rationalization
3. Regression
4. Substitution

40. 2. Rationalization is a process by which an individual deals with emotional conflict or internal or external stressors by concealing the true motivations for his thoughts, actions, and feelings through the elaboration of reassuring or self-serving, but incorrect, explanations. This process isn't a defense mechanism related to pain disorders. Displacement, substitution, and regression are defense mechanisms that would be expected from a client with a pain disorder.
CN: Psychosocial integrity; CNS: None; CL: Application

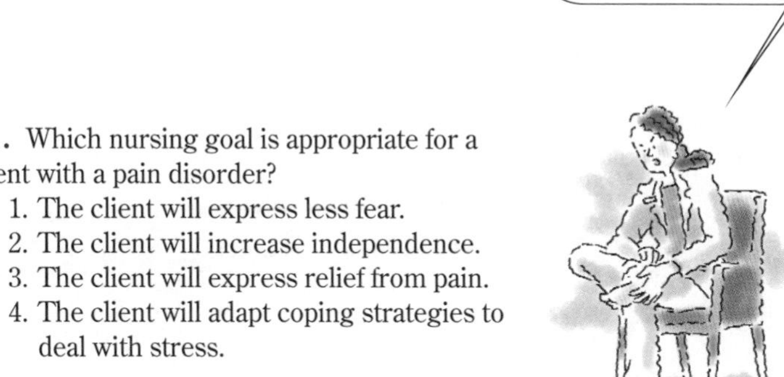

41. Which nursing goal is appropriate for a client with a pain disorder?
1. The client will express less fear.
2. The client will increase independence.
3. The client will express relief from pain.
4. The client will adapt coping strategies to deal with stress.

41. 3. Relief of pain should be a priority for clients experiencing pain. Expression of less fear applies to a client with hypochondriasis. A focus on independence is appropriate for a client diagnosed with conversion disorder. The development of coping strategies would be beneficial for a client with a somatization disorder.
CN: Physiological integrity; CNS: Physiological adaptation; CL: Application

42. Which conditions or situations are most likely to result in difficulty sleeping? Select all that apply:
1. Shift work
2. Sleep apnea
3. Reduction of external stimuli
4. Caffeine intake in the evening
5. Consistent bedtime routine
6. Excessive worry or anxiety

42. 1, 2, 4, 6. Shift work can disrupt the circadian rhythm. Sleep apnea can cause a reduction in oxygen to the brain, which can reduce the quality of rest. Caffeine is a stimulant and, if taken too close to bedtime, can interfere with falling asleep. Excessive worry or anxiety causes an increase in adrenaline, which enhances alertness and reduces sleepiness. A consistent bedtime routine and reduction of external stimuli promote good sleep.
CN: Health promotion and maintenance; CNS: None; CL: Analysis

43. Based on a nursing diagnosis of *Ineffective coping* for a client with somatoform pain disorder, which nursing goal is most realistic?
1. The client will be free from injury.
2. The client will recognize sensory impairment.
3. The client will discuss beliefs about spiritual issues.
4. The client will verbalize the absence or significant reduction of physical symptoms.

43. 4. Expression of feelings enables the client to ventilate emotions, which decreases anxiety and draws attention away from the physical symptoms. The client isn't experiencing a safety issue. There's no apparent correlation with any sensory-perceptual alterations. Spiritual issues are related to spiritual distress, and no evidence exists to support that the client is having spiritual distress.
CN: Physiological integrity; CNS: Basic care and comfort; CL: Analysis

44. Which statement made by a client best meets the diagnostic criteria for pain disorder?
1. "I can't move my right leg."
2. "I'm having severe stomach and leg pain."
3. "I'm so afraid I might have human immunodeficiency virus."
4. "I'm having chest pain and pain radiating down my left arm that began more than 1 hour ago."

44. 2. The diagnostic criteria for pain disorders state that pain in one or more anatomic sites is the predominant focus of the clinical presentation and is of sufficient severity to warrant clinical attention. A client with a conversion disorder can experience a motor neurologic symptom such as paralysis. Hypochondriasis is a morbid fear or belief that one has a serious disease where none exists. Unremitting chest pain with radiation of pain down the left arm is symptomatic of a myocardial infarction.
CN: Psychosocial integrity; CNS: None; CL: Application

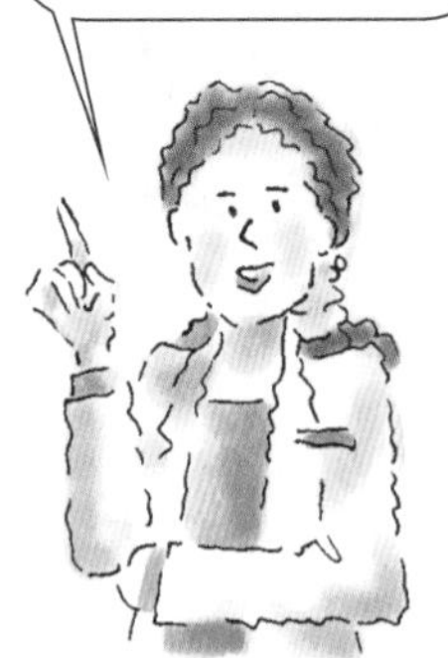

Remember, diagnostic criteria for psychologic problems come from the latest edition of the *Diagnostic and Statistical Manual of Mental Disorders,* currently known as DSM-IV-TR.

45. Which nursing diagnosis is appropriate for a client with somatoform pain disorder?
1. *Interrupted family processes*
2. *Disturbed body image*
3. *Ineffective denial*
4. *Ineffective coping*

45. 4. A somatoform pain disorder is closely associated with the client's inability to handle stress and conflict. Although *Interrupted family processes* and *Ineffective denial* may be present, they aren't the primary focus. *Disturbed body image* isn't directly correlated with this disorder.
CN: Safe, effective care environment; CNS: Management of care; CL: Application

46. Which statement made by a nurse will help a client diagnosed with somatoform pain disorder become independent in self-care?
1. "I'll call you for all the group activities."
2. "I'll help you on a daily basis with your care."
3. "The staff will help you with your basic needs for today."
4. "We'll wait until you have no more pain before you participate in activities."

46. 3. Limited time in assisting a client will help the client develop independence. All other options would promote dependence on the staff.
CN: Safe, effective care environment; CNS: Management of care; CL: Application

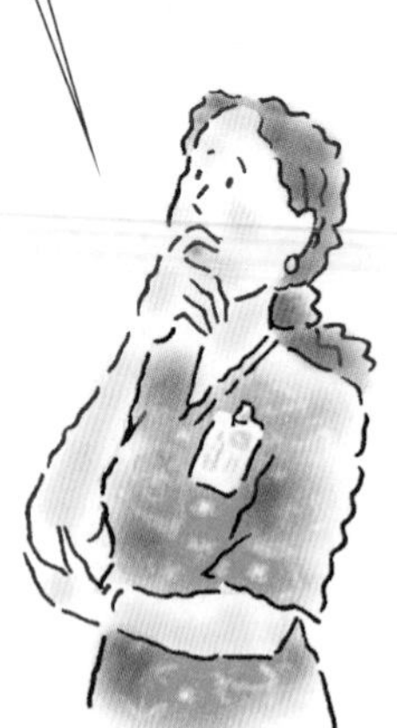

What is the *initial* intervention?

47. Which initial therapeutic intervention is the most appropriate for a client diagnosed with ineffective coping related to a pain disorder?
1. Make an accurate assessment.
2. Promote expression of feelings.
3. Promote insight into the disorder.
4. Help the client develop alternative coping strategies.

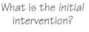

47. 1. It's essential to accurately assess the client first before any interventions. Promoting expression of feelings and insight and helping the client develop coping strategies are appropriate interventions that can be implemented after the initial assessment.
CN: Psychosocial integrity; CNS: None; CL: Application

48. A client with a somatoform pain disorder may obtain secondary gain. Which statement refers to a secondary gain?
1. It brings some stability to the family.
2. It decreases the preoccupation with the physical illness.
3. It enables the client to avoid some unpleasant activity.
4. It promotes emotional support or attention for the client.

48. 4. Secondary gain refers to the benefits of the illness that allow the client to receive emotional support or attention. A dysfunctional family may disregard the real issue, although some conflict is relieved. Somatoform pain disorder is a preoccupation with pain in the absence of physical disease. Primary gain enables the client to avoid some unpleasant activity.
CN: Psychosocial integrity; CNS: None; CL: Analysis

49. Which nursing intervention is appropriate for a client diagnosed with a somatoform pain disorder?

1. Reinforce the client's behavior when it isn't focused on pain.
2. Allow the client to verbalize anxieties related to body image.
3. Allow the client to verbalize relief of fear related to the illness.
4. Assist the client in recovery of the lost or altered function of a body part.

49. 1. Help the client get attention and see himself as valuable without using pain. Verbalization of anxieties related to body image may be beneficial in a client with body dysmorphic disorder. Fear of illness is related to hypochondriasis. The recovery of a lost or altered function of a part is related to conversion disorders.
CN: Psychosocial integrity; CNS: None; CL: Application

50. A client has primary insomnia and requires pharmaceutical assistance to sleep. The physician orders secobarbital sodium (Seconal) 75 mg by mouth at bedtime. The nurse has secobarbital sodium 25-mg tablets on hand. How many tablets should the nurse administer to the client? Record your answer using a whole number.

___________ tablets

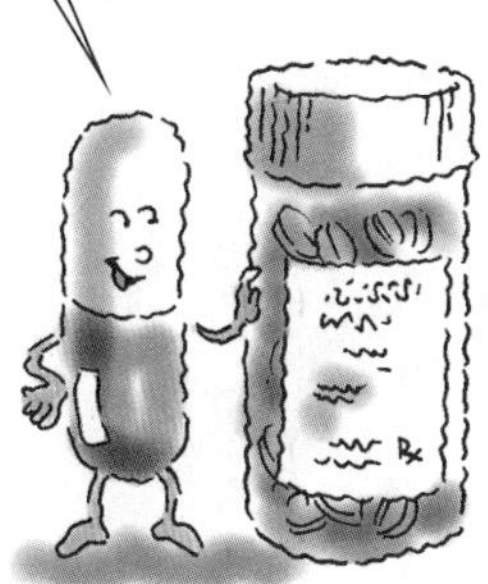

Remember to use the correct formula when calculating the appropriate drug dose.

50. 3. Each tablet contains 25 mg of the medication. The correct formula to calculate this drug dose is:

Dose of each tablet × X = Prescribed dose
25 mg × X (# of tablets) = 75 mg
25X = 75
X = 75/25
X = 3

CN: Physiological integrity; CNS: Pharmacological and parenteral therapies; CL: Analysis

51. A home health nurse is caring for a client diagnosed with a conversion disorder manifested by paralysis in the left arm. An organic cause for the deficit has been ruled out. Which nursing intervention is the <u>most appropriate</u> for this client?

1. Perform all physical tasks for the client to foster dependence.
2. Allot an hour each day to discuss the paralysis and its cause.
3. Identify primary or secondary gains that the physical symptom provides.
4. Allow the client to withdraw from all physical activities.

51. 3. Primary or secondary gains should be identified because they're etiological factors that can be used in problem resolution. The nurse should encourage the client to be as independent as possible and should intervene only when the client requires assistance. The nurse shouldn't focus on the disability. The nurse should encourage the client to perform physical activities to the greatest extent possible.
CN: Psychosocial integrity; CNS: None; CL: Application

52. A client with somatoform disorder states that her frequent headaches result from a brain tumor. However, a tumor hasn't shown up on diagnostic tests. The nurse identifies the client's form of somatization as which disorder?

1. Conversion disorder
2. Pain disorder
3. Hypochondriasis
4. Body dysmorphic disorder

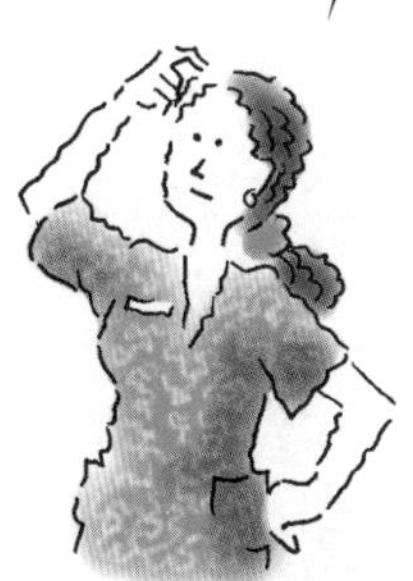

Have you sorted out the various forms of somatization? Don't try to rush. You can do it!

52. 3. In hypochondriasis, a physical symptom is interpreted as severe or life-threatening and causes exaggerated worry. In conversion disorder, the client loses a motor or sensory function but lacks appropriate concern about the loss. In pain disorder, pain is the dominant feature. In body dysmorphic disorder, the client is preoccupied with a perceived defect in appearance.
CN: Psychosocial integrity; CNS: None; CL: Application

53. A college student frequently visited the health center before course examinations. Physical causes for these visits have been eliminated. Based on the following progress note entry in the client's chart, the nurse suspects which disorder?

Progress notes

9/9/10 2130	19-year-old client states "I'm having abdominal discomfort. It happens on and off, especially the last week while I'm trying to study for mid-term exams. I know that there's something really wrong." Client denies that these symptoms are related to eating. Normal bowel sounds auscultated. Abdomen soft and nontender to palpation. Vital signs: Temp, 98.2°F; BP, 114/72 mm Hg; heart rate, 76 beats/minute; respiratory rate, 20 breaths/minute. Client denies nausea, vomiting, diarrhea or loss of appetite. ——— *Natalie Jones, RN*

1. Conversion disorder
2. Depersonalization
3. Hypochondriasis
4. Somatoform disorder

53. 3. Hypochondriasis in this case is shown by the client's belief that she has a serious illness, although pathologic causes have been eliminated. The disturbance usually lasts at least 6 months, and the GI system is commonly affected. Exacerbations are usually associated with identifiable life stressors that, in this case, can be related to the client's examinations. Conversion disorders are characterized by one or more neurologic symptoms. Depersonalization refers to persistent, recurrent, episodes of feeling detached from one's self or body. Somatoform disorders generally have a chronic course with few remissions.

CN: Psychosocial integrity; CNS: None; CL: Analysis

54. A 26-year-old client is diagnosed with somatoform disorder. When discussing the care plan with the client's wife, the nurse should give which instruction?

1. "Tell your husband that his symptoms are all in his head to force him to deal with reality."
2. "Tell your husband that his symptoms are an attempt to get attention and that you'll be more attentive."
3. "Accept the reality of the symptoms as your husband presents them, and don't dispute them."
4. "Realize that your husband is creating the symptoms on purpose."

54. 3. For a client with somatoform disorder, caregivers should accept the symptoms and avoid disputing them. The symptoms aren't contrived or all in the client's head. They're neither an attempt to get attention nor created "on purpose."

CN: Psychosocial integrity; CNS: None; CL: Application

55. A client with a diagnosis of somatoform disorder has been admitted to the psychiatric unit and has difficulty breathing, numbness, and loss of movement in his left arm. He seems unusually calm and unconcerned about his loss. The nurse recognizes these symptoms as which disorder?

1. Conversion disorder
2. Hypochondriasis
3. Body dysmorphic disorder
4. Pain disorder

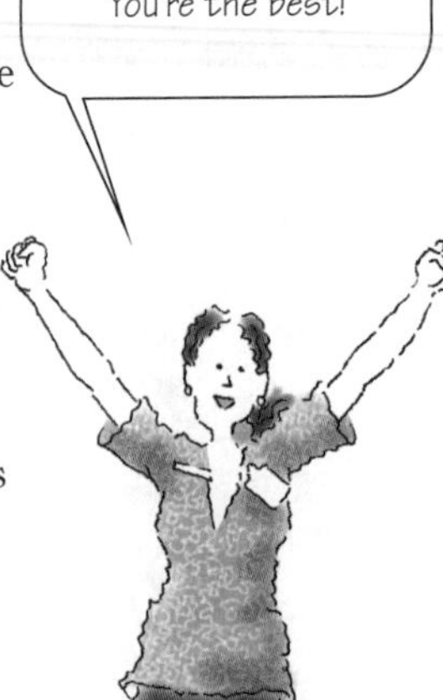
Hooray for you!
You're the best!

55. 1. Conversion disorder is characterized by loss of motor, sensory, or visceral functioning accompanied by the client's indifference to the loss. In hypochondriasis, the client interprets a physical symptom as severe or life-threatening and worries over it excessively. Body dysmorphic disorder is a preoccupation with a perceived defect in appearance. In pain disorder, pain is the dominant physical symptom.

CN: Psychosocial integrity; CNS: None; CL: Application

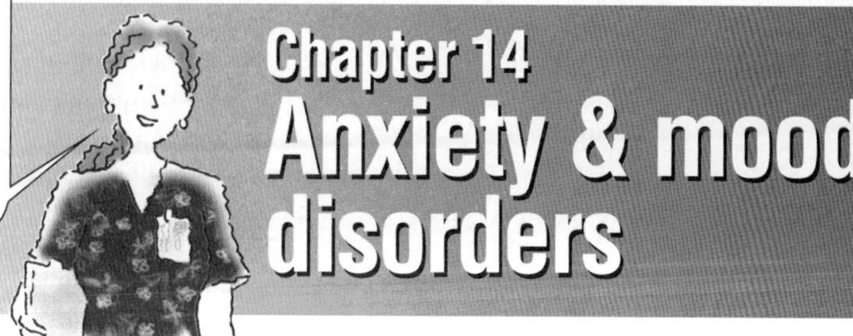

Want more information on anxiety and mood disorders to help you prepare for the NCLEX? Check out the Web site of the National Alliance for the Mentally Ill at **www.nami.org.**

Chapter 14
Anxiety & mood disorders

1. Which statement is typical of a client who experiences periodic panic attacks while sleeping?

1. "Yesterday, I sat up in bed and just felt so scared."
2. "I have difficulty sleeping because I'm so anxious."
3. "Sometimes I have the most wild and vivid dreams."
4. "When I drink beer, I fall asleep without any problems."

1. 1. A person who suffers a panic attack while sleeping experiences an abrupt awakening and feelings of fear. People with severe anxiety commonly have symptoms related to a sleep disorder; they wouldn't typically experience a sleep panic attack. A panic attack while sleeping often causes an inability to remember dreams. Intake of alcohol initially produces a drowsy feeling, but after a short period of time alcohol causes restless, fragmented sleep and strange dreams.

CN: Psychosocial integrity; CNS: None; CL: Analysis

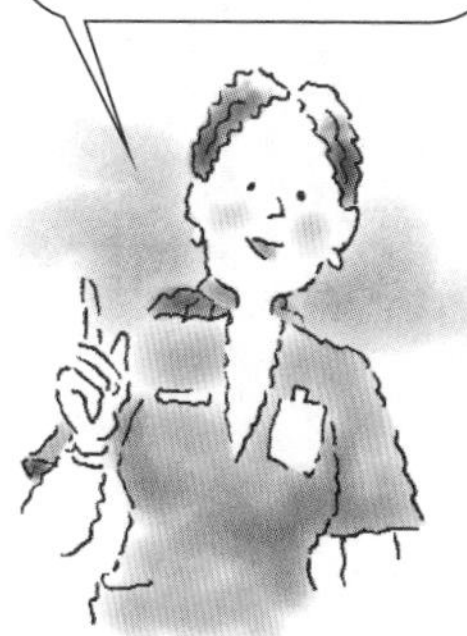

Question 1 is *typical* of what you'll be asked throughout the test.

2. A client with generalized anxiety disorder states, "I'm afraid I'm going to die from cancer. My mother had cancer." Which of the following responses by the nurse would be the most therapeutic?

1. "We all live in fear of dying from cancer."
2. "Did your father also have cancer?"
3. "I wouldn't worry about it just yet. You seem to be in good health."
4. "Has something happened that is causing you to worry?"

2. 4. By asking the client about what is making them worry, the nurse assists the client in determining the cause of the anxiety. The other responses deflect and minimize the client's concerns.

CN: Psychosocial integrity; CNS: None; CL: Analysis

3. A client with a history of panic attacks who says, "I felt so trapped," right after an attack most likely has which fear?

1. Loss of control
2. Loss of identity
3. Loss of memory
4. Loss of maturity

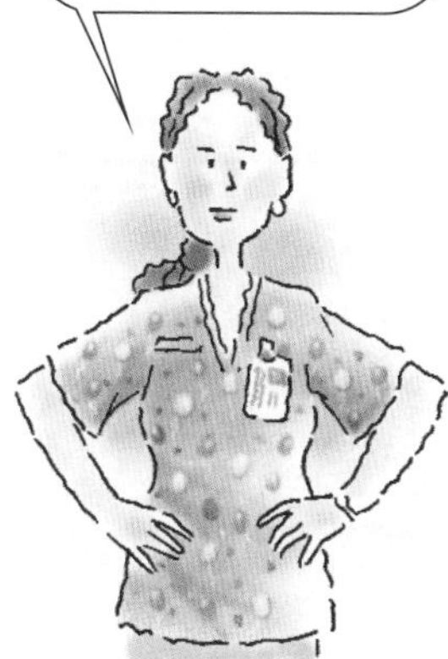

Remember: You're in control, so read the question carefully and choose the most likely response.

3. 1. People who fear loss of control during a panic attack commonly make statements about feeling trapped, getting hurt, or having little or no personal control over their situations. People who experience panic attacks don't tend to have loss of identity or memory impairment. People who have panic attacks also don't regress or become immature.

CN: Psychosocial integrity; CNS: None; CL: Application

CN: Client needs category CNS: Client needs subcategory CL: Cognitive level

4. A nurse is caring for a client with a panic disorder. On morning rounds, the physician orders alprazolam (Xanax). In reviewing the client's medical history, the nurse calls the physician regarding:

1. intermittent insomnia.
2. acute-angle glaucoma.
3. seizure disorder.
4. tartrazine hypersensitivity.

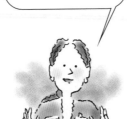

4. 2. Acute-angle glaucoma is a medical problem that contraindicates the use of alprazolam. Alprazolam causes drowsiness and sedation, so sleep shouldn't be interrupted. Seizure disorder isn't a contraindication for the use of alprazolam. Tartrazine hypersensitivity is associated with yellow dye used in some convenience foods and isn't a contraindication for the use of alprazolam.

CN: Physiological integrity; CNS: Pharmacological and parenteral therapies; CL: Application

Don't panic! Stay calm and remember to prioritize.

5. Which nursing intervention is given <u>priority</u> in a care plan for a client having an acute panic attack?

1. Tell the client to take deep breaths.
2. Have the client talk about the anxiety.
3. Encourage the client to verbalize feelings.
4. Ask the client about the cause of the attack.

5. 1. During a panic attack, the nurse should remain with the client and direct what's said toward changing the physiologic response, such as taking deep breaths. During an attack, the client is unable to talk about anxious situations and isn't able to address feelings, especially uncomfortable feelings and frustrations. While having a panic attack, the client is also unable to focus on anything other than the symptoms, so the client won't be able to discuss the cause of the attack.

CN: Safe, effective care environment; CNS: Management of care; CL: Analysis

6. Which instruction should a nurse include in a teaching session about panic disorder for clients and their families?

1. Identifying when anxiety is escalating
2. Determining how to stop a panic attack
3. Addressing strategies to reduce physical pain
4. Preventing the client from depending on others

6. 1. By identifying the presence of anxiety, it's possible to take steps to prevent its escalation. A panic attack can't be stopped. The nurse can take steps to assist the client safely through the attack. Later, the nurse can assist the client to alleviate the precipitating stressors. Clients who experience panic disorder don't tend to be in physical pain. The client experiencing a panic disorder may need to periodically depend on other people when having a panic attack.

CN: Psychosocial integrity; CNS: None; CL: Application

For the NCLEX, you should memorize the definitions of common fears such as agoraphobia.

7. Which question should a nurse ask to determine how <u>agoraphobia</u> affects the life of a client who has panic attacks?

1. How realistic are your goals?
2. Are you able to go shopping?
3. Do you struggle with impulse control?
4. Who else in your family has panic disorder?

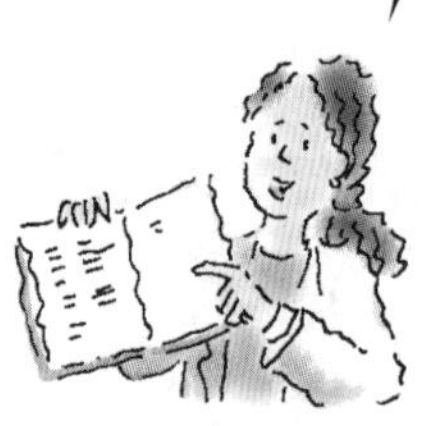

7. 2. The client with agoraphobia typically restricts himself to home and can't carry out normal socializing and life-sustaining activities. Clients with panic disorder are able to set realistic goals and tend to be cautious and reclusive rather than impulsive. Although there's a familial tendency toward panic disorder, information about client needs must be obtained to determine how agoraphobia affects the client's life.

CN: Psychosocial integrity; CNS: None; CL: Application

8. Which fact would be helpful to include when teaching a female client who's considering lifestyle changes as part of a behavior modification program to treat her panic attacks?
1. Cigarettes can trigger panic episodes.
2. Fermented foods can cause panic attacks.
3. Hormonal therapy can induce panic attacks.
4. Tryptophan can predispose a person to panic attacks.

8. 1. Cigarettes contain nicotine, which can be a stimulant, a depressant, or a tranquilizer, and can trigger panic attacks. None of the other options causes panic attacks.
CN: Psychosocial integrity; CNS: None; CL: Application

9. Which intervention should a nurse initially implement when caring for a client with panic disorder?
1. Make the client role-play the panic attack.
2. Assist the client to develop an exercise program.
3. Teach the client to identify cognitive distortions.
4. Teach the client to identify sources of anxiety.

9. 4. The client must be aware of the connection between sources of anxiety and the symptoms of a panic attack. Role-playing a panic attack isn't useful. Role-playing coping strategies would be useful for the client. Later in treatment, the client can develop an exercise program as part of the overall plan to handle stress. Learning to identify cognitive distortions is a useful strategy to teach the client after he's begun to work on identifying sources of anxiety.
CN: Psychosocial integrity; CNS: None; CL: Analysis

10. Which nursing intervention is appropriate to include when planning care for a client with panic disorder?
1. Identify childhood trauma.
2. Monitor nutritional intake.
3. Institute suicide precautions.
4. Monitor episodes of disorientation.

10. 3. Clients with panic disorder are at risk for suicide because they can be impulsive. Childhood trauma is associated with posttraumatic stress disorder, *not* panic disorder. Nutritional problems don't typically accompany panic disorder. Clients aren't typically disoriented; they may have a temporary altered sense of reality, but that lasts only for the duration of the attack.
CN: Psychosocial integrity; CNS: None; CL: Application

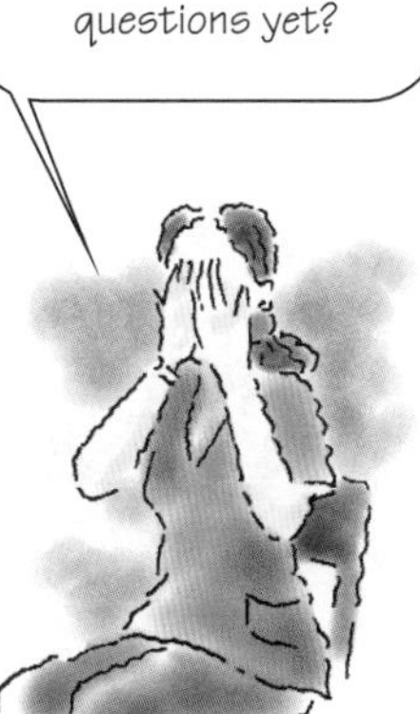

I'm too anxious to look. Have you finished 10 questions yet?

11. A client diagnosed with panic disorder with agoraphobia is talking with the nurse about the progress made in treatment. Which statement indicates a positive client response?
1. "I went to the mall with my friend last Saturday."
2. "I'm hyperventilating only when I have a panic attack."
3. "Today I decided that I can stop taking my medication."
4. "Last night I decided to eat more than a bowl of cereal."

11. 1. Clients with panic disorder tend to be socially withdrawn. Going to the mall is a sign of working on avoidance behaviors. Hyperventilation is a key symptom of panic disorder. Teaching breathing control is a major intervention for clients with panic disorder. The client taking medications for panic disorder, such as tricyclic antidepressants and benzodiazepines, must be weaned off these drugs. Most clients with panic disorder with agoraphobia don't have nutritional problems.
CN: Psychosocial integrity; CNS: None; CL: Analysis

12. Which group therapy intervention should be of primary importance to a client with panic disorder?

1. Explore how secondary gains are derived from the disorder.
2. Discuss new ways of thinking and feeling about panic attacks.
3. Work to eliminate manipulative behavior used for meeting needs.
4. Learn the risk factors and other demographics associated with panic disorder.

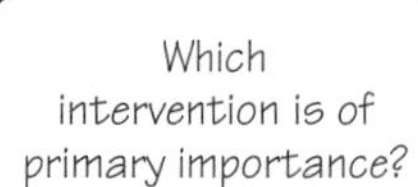
Which intervention is of primary importance?

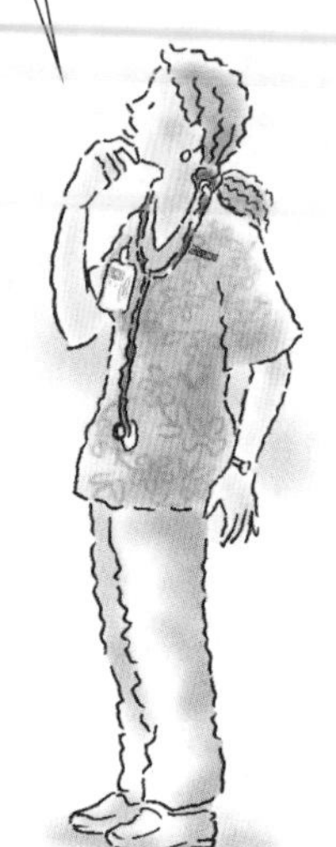

12. 2. Restructuring an anxiety-producing event allows the client to gain control over the situation. Discussing new ways of thinking and feeling about panic attacks can enable others to learn and benefit from a variety of intervention strategies. There are usually no secondary gains obtained from having a panic disorder. People with panic disorder aren't using the disorder as a way to manipulate others. Learning the risk factors could be accomplished in another format such as a psychoeducational program.

CN: Psychosocial integrity; CNS: None; CL: Analysis

13. A nurse is caring for a client with social phobia. A symptom that should be addressed in a team meeting is the client's tendency toward:

1. self-harm.
2. poor self-esteem.
3. compulsive behavior.
4. avoidance of social situations.

13. 4. Clients with social phobia avoid social situations for fear of being humiliated or embarrassed. They generally don't tend to be at risk for self-harm and usually don't demonstrate compulsive behavior. Not all individuals with social anxiety have low self-esteem.

CN: Psychosocial integrity; CNS: None; CL: Application

14. Which statement is typical of a client with social phobia?

1. "Without people around, I just feel so lost."
2. "There's nothing wrong with my behavior."
3. "I like to be the center of attention."
4. "I know I can't accept that award for my brother."

14. 4. People who have a social phobia usually undervalue themselves and their talents. They don't like to be in feared social situations or around many people. They tend to stay away from situations in which they may feel humiliated and embarrassed. They fear social gatherings and dislike being the center of attention. They're very critical of themselves and believe that others also will be critical.

CN: Psychosocial integrity; CNS: None; CL: Application

15. Clients with a social phobia would most likely fear which situation?

1. Dental procedures
2. Meeting strangers
3. Being bitten by a dog
4. Having a car collision

Don't be shy about answering this question.

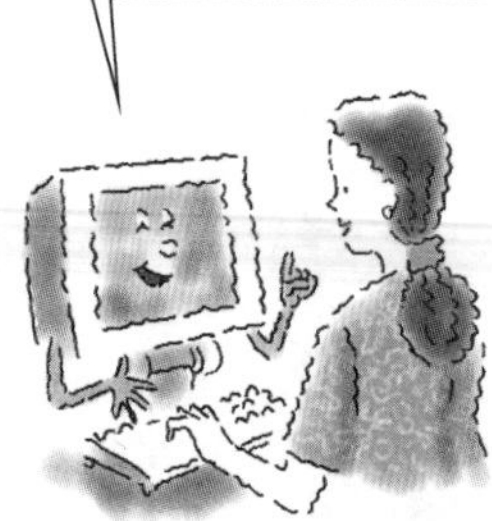

15. 2. Fear of meeting strangers is a common example of social phobia. Fears of having a dental procedure, being bitten by a dog, or having a collision are *not* social phobias.

CN: Psychosocial integrity; CNS: None; CL: Application

16. Which factor should the nurse find most helpful in assessing a client for a blood-injection-injury phobia?

1. Episodes of fainting
2. Gregarious personality
3. Difficulty managing anger
4. Dramatic, overreactive personality

16. 1. Many people with a history of blood-injection-injury phobia report frequently fainting when exposed to this type of situation. All personality styles can develop phobias, so personality type doesn't provide information for assessing phobias. Information about a client's difficulty managing anger isn't related to a specific phobic disorder. Individuals with blood-injection-injury phobias aren't being dramatic or overreactive.
CN: Psychosocial integrity; CNS: None; CL: Analysis

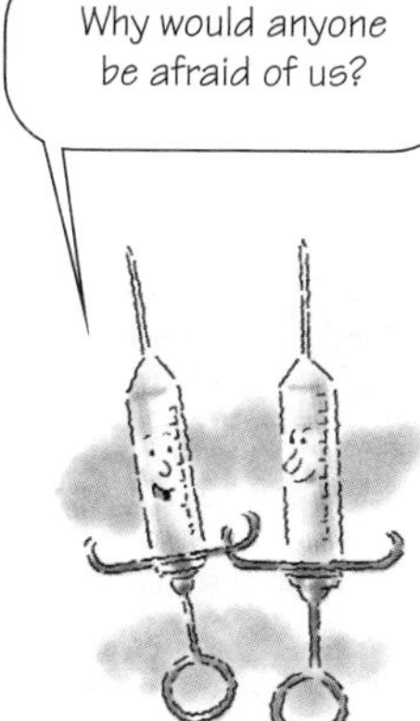

Why would anyone be afraid of us?

17. Which individual counseling approach should be used to assist a client with a phobic disorder?

1. Have the client keep a daily journal.
2. Help the client identify the source of the anxiety.
3. Teach the client effective ways to problem-solve.
4. Develop strategies to prevent the client from using substances.

17. 2. By understanding the source of the anxiety, the client will understand how this anxiety has been displaced as a phobic response. Keeping a journal is an effective method in many situations; however, its use is limited in the treatment of phobias. Problem solving is a more useful technique for clients with obsessive-compulsive disorder than for clients with phobias. People with phobias don't tend to self-medicate like clients with other psychiatric disorders.
CN: Psychosocial integrity; CNS: None; CL: Application

18. Which behavior modification technique is useful in the treatment of phobias?

1. Aversion therapy
2. Imitation or modeling
3. Positive reinforcement
4. Systematic desensitization

18. 4. Systematic desensitization is a common behavior modification technique successfully used to help treat phobias. Aversion therapy and positive reinforcement are *not* behavior modification techniques used with treatment of phobias. Imitation and modeling are social learning techniques, not behavior modification techniques.
CN: Psychosocial integrity; CNS: None; CL: Application

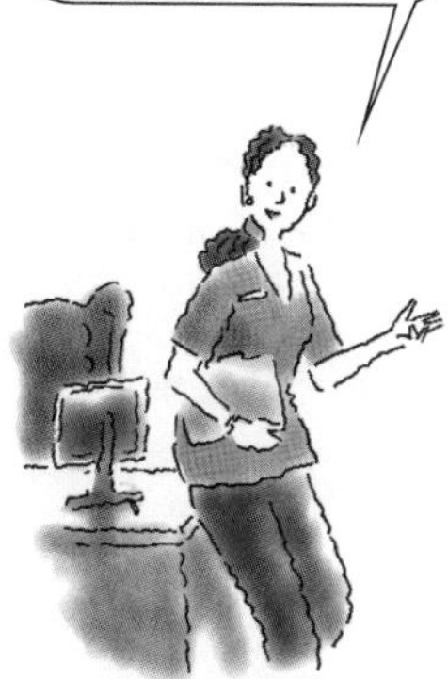

Along with assessment, you also need to familiarize yourself with common treatments.

19. Which statement would be useful when teaching the client and family about phobias and the need for a strong support system?

1. The use of a family support system is only temporary.
2. The need to be assertive can be reinforced by the family.
3. The family needs to set limits on inappropriate behaviors.
4. The family plays a role in promoting client independence.

19. 4. The family plays a vital role in supporting the client in treatment and preventing the client from using the phobia to obtain secondary gains. Family support must be ongoing, not temporary. The family can be more helpful by focusing on effective handling of anxiety, rather than focusing on developing assertiveness skills. People with phobias are already restrictive in their behavior; more restrictions aren't necessary.
CN: Psychosocial integrity; CNS: None; CL: Analysis

20. Which nursing intervention is of primary importance during the administration of paroxetine (Paxil) to a depressed client with a phobic disorder?

1. Monitor renal function.
2. Determine electrocardiogram (ECG) changes.
3. Assess for sleeping difficulties.
4. Observe for extrapyramidal symptoms.

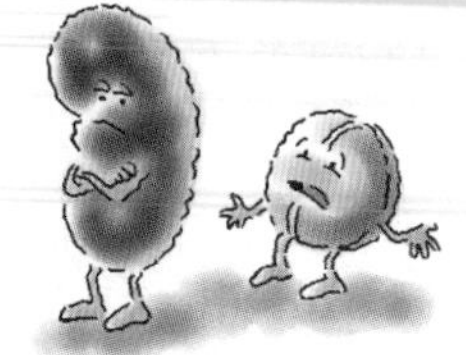

How do I know you aren't going to hurt me?

20. 1. Clients with impaired renal function shouldn't take paroxetine. ECG changes aren't adverse effects of paroxetine. Other than a transient period of drowsiness occurring when the client begins to take the drug, sleep difficulties don't tend to be a problem. Extrapyramidal symptoms aren't seen with paroxetine.
CN: Physiological integrity; CNS: Pharmacological and parenteral therapies; CL: Analysis

21. A client suspected of having posttraumatic stress disorder should be assessed for which problem?

1. Eating disorder
2. Schizophrenia
3. Suicide
4. "Sundown" syndrome

21. 3. Clients who experience posttraumatic stress disorder are at high risk for suicide and other forms of violent behaviors. Eating disorders are possible but aren't a common complication of posttraumatic stress disorder. Clients with posttraumatic stress disorder don't usually have their extreme anxiety manifest itself as schizophrenia. "Sundown" syndrome is an increase in agitation accompanied by confusion. It's commonly seen in clients with dementia, not clients with posttraumatic stress disorder.
CN: Psychosocial integrity; CNS: None; CL: Application

22. Which action explains why tricyclic antidepressant medication is given to a client who has severe posttraumatic stress disorder?

1. It prevents hyperactivity and purposeless movements.
2. It increases the client's ability to concentrate.
3. It helps prevent experiencing the trauma again.
4. It facilitates the grieving process.

22. 3. Tricyclic antidepressant medication will decrease the frequency of reenactment of the trauma for the client. It will help memory problems and sleeping difficulties and will decrease numbing. The medication won't prevent hyperactivity and purposeless movements nor increase the client's concentration. No medication will facilitate the grieving process.
CN: Physiological integrity; CNS: Pharmacological and parenteral therapies; CL: Application

23. Which nursing action should be included in a care plan for a client with posttraumatic stress disorder who states that the experience was "bad luck"?

1. Encourage the client to verbalize the experience.
2. Assist the client in defining the experience as a trauma.
3. Work with the client to take steps to move on with life.
4. Help the client accept positive and negative feelings.

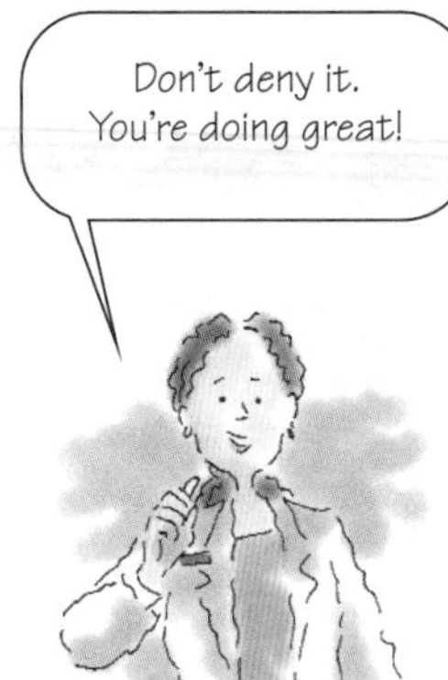

Don't deny it. You're doing great!

23. 2. The client must define the experience as traumatic to realize the situation wasn't under his personal control. Encouraging the client to verbalize the experience without first addressing the denial isn't a useful strategy. The client can move on with life only after acknowledging the trauma and processing the experience. Acknowledgment of the actual trauma and verbalization of the event should come *before* the acceptance of feelings.
CN: Psychosocial integrity; CNS: None; CL: Analysis

24. Which instruction should a nurse include about relationships for the client with posttraumatic stress disorder?

1. Encourage the client to resume former roles as soon as possible.
2. Assess the client's discomfort when talking about feelings to family members.
3. Explain that avoiding emotional attachment protects against anxiety.
4. Warn the client that he'll have a tendency to be overdependent in relationships.

24. 3. The client may tend to avoid interpersonal relationships to protect himself against unrelieved anxiety. Because relationships tend to be avoided, the client won't express feelings to family members at this time and won't resume roles and responsibilities for a while. Clients with posttraumatic stress disorder don't tend to become overdependent in relationships but do tend to withdraw from them.

CN: Psychosocial integrity; CNS: None; CL: Application

Caring for clients commonly means working with their families—a skill you can expect the exam to test.

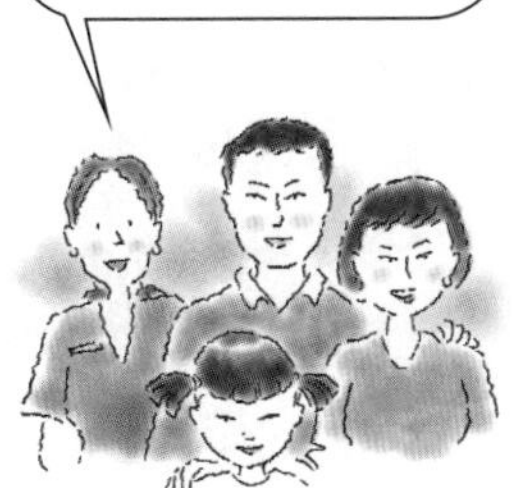

25. Which approach should a nurse use with the family when a posttraumatic stress disorder client states, "My family doesn't believe anything about posttraumatic stress disorder"?

1. Provide the family with information.
2. Teach the family about problem solving.
3. Discuss the family's view of the problem.
4. Assess for the presence of family violence.

25. 1. If the family can understand posttraumatic stress disorder, they can more readily participate in the client's care and be supportive. Learning problem-solving skills doesn't help clarify posttraumatic stress disorder. After being given information about posttraumatic stress disorder, the family can then ask questions and present its views. The family must first have information about posttraumatic stress disorder; then the discussion about violence to self or others can be addressed.

CN: Safe, effective care environment; CNS: Management of care; CL: Application

26. While caring for a client with posttraumatic stress disorder, the family notices that loud noises cause a serious anxiety response. Which explanation should help the family understand the client's response?

1. Environmental triggers can cause the client to become hyperaroused and have exaggerated startle reactions.
2. Clients commonly experience extreme fear about normal environmental stimuli.
3. After a trauma, the client can't respond to stimuli in an appropriate manner.
4. The response indicates that another emotional problem needs investigation.

26. 1. Repeated exposure to environmental triggers can cause the client to experience a hyperarousal state because there's a loss of physiologic control of incoming stimuli. After experiencing a trauma, the client may have strong reactions to stimuli similar to those that occurred during the traumatic event. However, not *all* stimuli will cause an anxiety response. The client's anxiety response is typically seen after a traumatic experience and doesn't indicate the presence of another problem.

CN: Psychosocial integrity; CNS: None; CL: Application

27. Which psychological symptom should a nurse expect to find in a hospitalized client who's the only survivor of a train collision?

1. Denial
2. Indifference
3. Perfectionism
4. Trust

27. 1. Denial can act as a protective response. The client tends to be overwhelmed and disorganized by the trauma, not indifferent to it. Perfectionism is more commonly seen in clients with eating disorders, not in clients with posttraumatic stress disorder. Clients who have had a severe trauma commonly experience an inability to trust others.

CN: Psychosocial integrity; CNS: None; CL: Analysis

28. If a client suffering from posttraumatic stress disorder says, "I've decided to just avoid everything and everyone," the nurse might suspect the client is at greatest risk for which behavior?
1. Becoming homeless
2. Exhausting finances
3. Terminating employment
4. Using substances

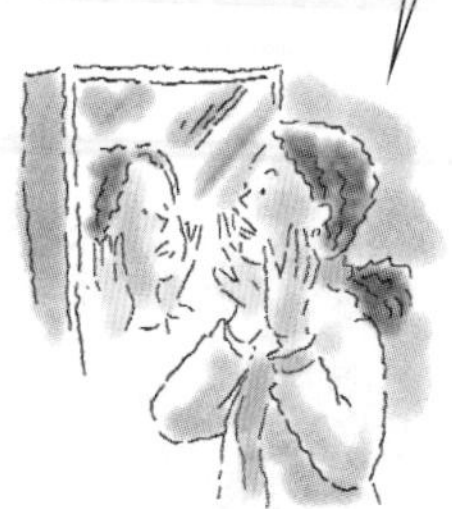

Mirror, mirror, on
the wall, what's the
greatest risk of all?

28. 4. The use of substances is a way for the client to deny problems and self-medicate distress. There are few homeless people with posttraumatic stress disorder as the cause of their homelessness. Most clients with posttraumatic stress disorder can manage money and maintain employment.
CN: Psychosocial integrity; CNS: None; CL: Application

29. Which action would be most appropriate when speaking with a client with posttraumatic stress disorder about the trauma?
1. Obtain validation of what the client says from another party.
2. Request that the client write down what's being said.
3. Ask questions to convey an interest in the details.
4. Listen attentively and remain with the client.

29. 4. An effective communication strategy for a nurse to use with a posttraumatic stress disorder client is listening attentively and staying with the client. There's no need to obtain validation about what the client says by asking for information from another party, asking the client to write what's being said, or distracting him by asking questions.
CN: Psychosocial integrity; CNS: None; CL: Application

30. Which client statement indicates an understanding of survivor guilt?
1. "I think I can see the purpose of my survival."
2. "I can't help but feel that everything is their fault."
3. "I now understand why I'm not able to forgive myself."
4. "I wish I could stop sabotaging my family relationships."

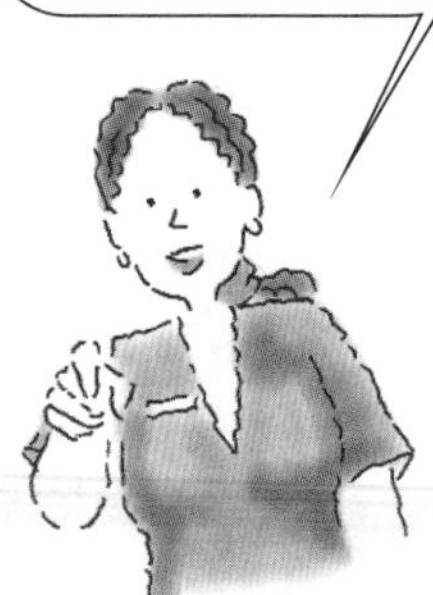

Thirty questions!
Your survival skills
are kicking in!

30. 3. Survivor guilt occurs when the person has almost constant thoughts about the other people who perished in the event. The survivor doesn't understand why he survived when a friend or loved one didn't. Blaming self, not others, is a component of survivor guilt. Survivor guilt and impaired interpersonal relationships are two different categories of responses to trauma.
CN: Psychosocial integrity; CNS: None; CL: Analysis

31. Which nursing intervention would best help a client with posttraumatic stress disorder and his family handle interpersonal conflict at home?
1. Have the family teach the client to identify defensive behaviors.
2. Have the family discuss how to change dysfunctional family patterns.
3. Have the family agree not to tell the client what to do about problems.
4. Have the family arrange for the client to participate in social activities.

31. 2. Discussion of dysfunctional family patterns allows the family to determine why and how these patterns are maintained. Having family members point out the defensive behaviors of the client may inadvertently produce more defensive behavior. Families can be a source of support and assistance; therefore, inflexible rules aren't useful to either the client or the family. The family shouldn't be encouraged to arrange social activities for the client. Social activities outside of the home don't help the family handle conflict within the home.
CN: Psychosocial integrity; CNS: None; CL: Application

32. The family members of a client diagnosed with posttraumatic stress disorder can't understand why the client has this disorder, especially because the client didn't directly experience a personal trauma. Which topic should the nurse discuss with the family?

1. Advise them to obtain a second psychiatric evaluation.
2. Ask them what they perceive the client's problem to be.
3. Explain the effect of learning about another's experience.
4. Identify the time period the client manifested symptoms.

32. 3. Posttraumatic stress disorder can occur if a person has experienced the traumatic event, witnessed the event happening to another person, or learned that trauma has happened to a family member or close friend. After educating the family about posttraumatic stress disorder, a second evaluation may not be necessary. Encouraging family members to discuss the situation and share their perceptions can be helpful, but it isn't their responsibility or within their abilities to diagnose the health problem. Symptoms of posttraumatic stress disorder usually appear 6 or more months after the event has occurred for at least a 1-month duration. This information isn't as important as an explanation of what constitutes a traumatic event.

CN: Psychosocial integrity; CNS: None; CL: Analysis

33. The effectiveness of monoamine oxidase (MAO) inhibitor drug therapy in a client with posttraumatic stress disorder can be demonstrated by which client self-report?

1. "I'm sleeping better and don't have nightmares."
2. "I'm not losing my temper as much."
3. "I've lost my craving for alcohol."
4. "I've lost my phobia for water."

33. 1. MAO inhibitors are used to treat sleep problems, nightmares, and intrusive daytime thoughts in individuals with posttraumatic stress disorder. MAO inhibitors aren't used to help control flashbacks or phobias or to decrease the craving for alcohol.

CN: Physiological integrity; CNS: Pharmacological and parenteral therapies; CL: Analysis

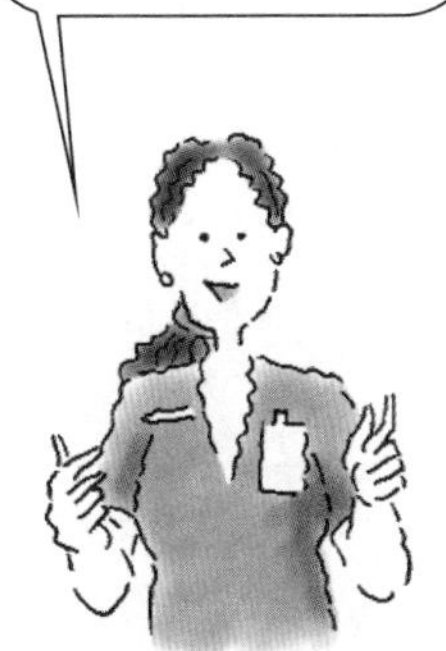

The term *major purpose* indicates that there may be more than one right answer. You need to choose the best answer.

34. Which result is the major purpose of group therapy for adolescents who witnessed the violent death of a peer?

1. To learn violence prevention strategies
2. To talk about appropriate expression of anger
3. To discuss the effect of the trauma on their lives
4. To develop trusting relationships among their peers

34. 3. By discussing the effect of the trauma on their lives, the adolescents can grieve and develop effective coping strategies. Learning violence prevention strategies isn't the most immediate concern after a trauma occurs nor is working on developing healthy relationships. It's appropriate to talk about how to express anger constructively after the trauma is addressed.

CN: Psychosocial integrity; CNS: None; CL: Application

35. Which symptom of posttraumatic stress disorder would indicate that hypnosis is an appropriate treatment modality?

1. Addiction
2. Confabulation
3. Dissociation
4. Hallucinations

35. 3. Hypnosis is one of the main therapies for clients who dissociate. Hypnosis isn't a treatment of choice for clients with addictive disorders or hallucinations. Confabulation isn't a symptom of posttraumatic stress disorder.

CN: Psychosocial integrity; CNS: None; CL: Application

36. Which nursing behavior would demonstrate caring to a client with a diagnosis of anxiety disorder?

1. Verbalize concern about the client.
2. Arrange group activities for the client.
3. Have the client sign the treatment plan.
4. Hold psychoeducational groups on medications.

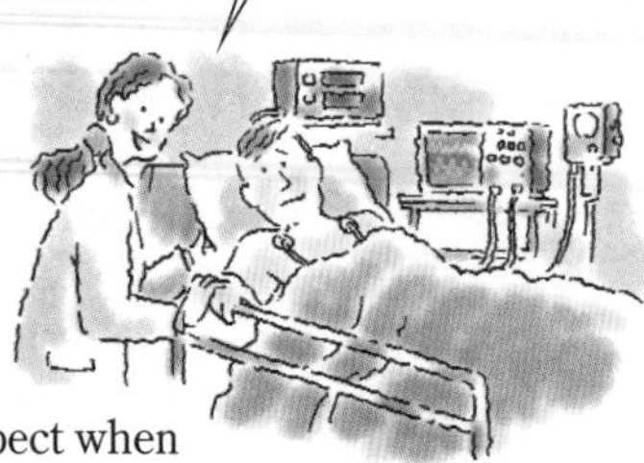

It's important for the client to know you care.

36. 1. The nurse who verbally expresses concern about a client's well-being is acting in a caring and supportive manner. Arranging for group activities may be an action where the nurse has no direct client contact and is therefore unable to have interpersonal contact with clients. Having a client sign the treatment plan may not be viewed as a sign of caring. Having a psychoeducational group on medications may be viewed by clients as a teaching experience and not interpersonal contact, because the nurse may have limited interactions with them.
CN: Psychosocial integrity; CNS: None; CL: Application

37. Which finding should a nurse expect when talking about school to a child diagnosed with a generalized anxiety disorder?

1. The child has been fighting with peers for the past month.
2. The child can't stop lying to parents and teachers.
3. The child has gained 15 (6.8 kg) pounds in the past month.
4. The child expresses concerns about grades.

37. 4. Children with generalized anxiety disorder will worry about how well they're performing in school. Children with generalized anxiety disorder don't tend to be involved in conflict. They're more oriented toward good behavior. Children with generalized anxiety disorder don't tend to lie to others. They would want to do their best and try to please others. A weight gain of 15 pounds isn't a typical characteristic of a child with anxiety disorder.
CN: Psychosocial integrity; CNS: None; CL: Analysis

38. A client with a generalized anxiety disorder also may have which concurrent diagnosis?

1. Bipolar disorder
2. Gender identity disorder
3. Panic disorder
4. Schizoaffective disorder

38. 3. Approximately 75% of clients with generalized anxiety disorder also may have a diagnosis of phobia, panic disorder, or substance abuse. Clients with generalized anxiety disorder don't tend to have a coexisting diagnosis of gender identity disorder, bipolar disorder, or schizoaffective disorder.
CN: Psychosocial integrity; CNS: None; CL: Application

39. Which statement indicates a positive response from a generalized anxiety disorder client to a nurse's teaching about nutrition?

1. "I've stopped drinking so much diet cola."
2. "I've reduced my intake of carbohydrates."
3. "I now eat less at dinner and before bedtime."
4. "I've cut back on my use of dairy products."

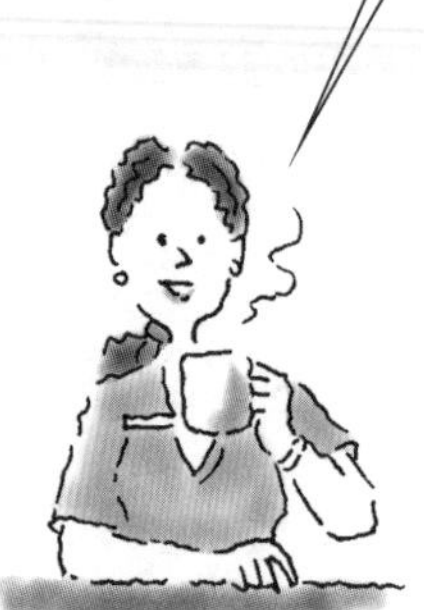

What do you know about the relationship between anxiety and caffeine?

39. 1. Clients with generalized anxiety disorder can decrease anxiety by eliminating caffeine from their diets. It isn't necessary for clients with generalized anxiety to decrease their carbohydrate intake, eat less at dinner or before bedtime (unless there are other compelling health reasons), or cut back on their use of dairy products.
CN: Physiological integrity; CNS: Basic care and comfort; CL: Application

40. A client with generalized anxiety disorder is prescribed a benzodiazepine, but the client doesn't want to take the medication. Which explanation by the client for this behavior would be most likely?

1. "I don't think the psychiatrist likes me."
2. "I want to solve my problems on my own."
3. "The voices tell me that I don't have to take the medication."
4. "I think my family gains by keeping me medicated."

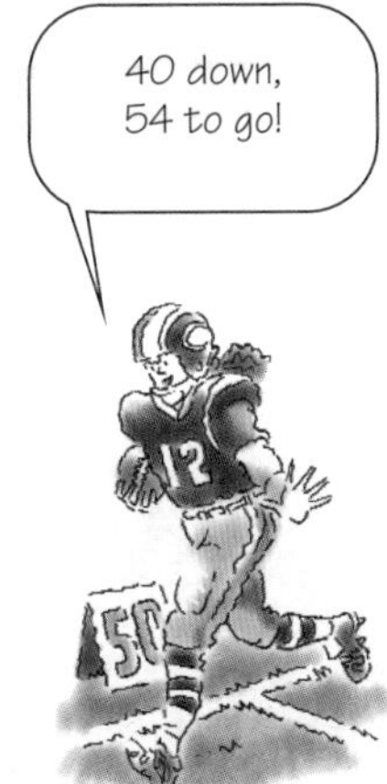

40 down,
54 to go!
12
50

40. 2. It's common for a client with generalized anxiety disorder to refuse to take medication because he believes that using a medication is a sign of personal weakness and that he can't solve problems by himself. Fear that the psychiatrist dislikes him reflects paranoid thinking that isn't usually seen in a client with generalized anxiety disorder. Auditory hallucinations and paranoia about the motives of friends and family members aren't characteristic of clients with generalized anxiety disorder.

CN: Psychosocial integrity; CNS: None; CL: Analysis

41. Which factor should a nurse consider when assisting a client with generalized anxiety disorder in verbalizing feelings?

1. The client may intellectualize the anxiety.
2. The client may regard the problem as genetic.
3. The client may decide that verbalizing feelings isn't beneficial.
4. The client may believe only medications are useful.

41. 1. Clients who experience generalized anxiety disorder commonly need assistance acknowledging anxiety instead of denying or intellectualizing it. Although scientists believe that there may be a tendency for anxiety to be familial, the problem isn't regarded as genetic. A client who's unwilling to express feelings may not view therapy as helpful. The most effective treatment of generalized anxiety disorder combines psychotherapy and pharmacotherapy.

CN: Psychosocial integrity; CNS: None; CL: Analysis

42. Which of the following statements would most likely be associated with an adult client who has a long-standing history of generalized anxiety disorder?

1. "I was, and still am, an impulsive person."
2. "I've always been hyperactive, but not in useful ways."
3. "When I was in college, I never thought I would finish."
4. "All my life I've had intrusive dreams and scary nightmares."

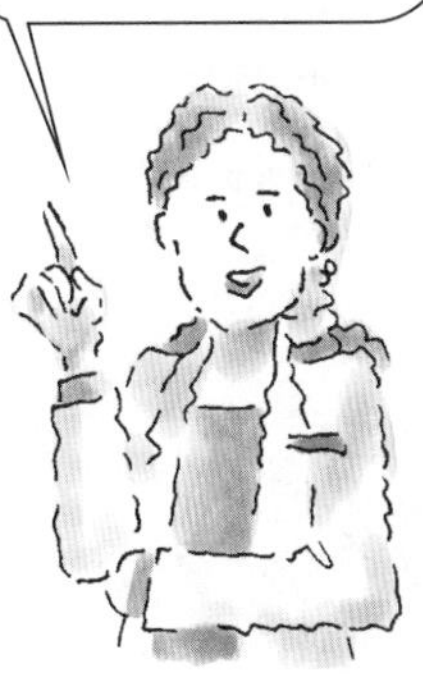

Certain psychological disorders tend to appear at particular ages—that's information to know for the NCLEX.

42. 3. For many people who have a generalized anxiety disorder, the age of onset is during young adulthood. The symptoms of impulsiveness and hyperactivity aren't commonly associated with a diagnosis of generalized anxiety disorder. Intrusive dreams and nightmares are associated with posttraumatic stress disorder rather than generalized anxiety disorder.

CN: Psychosocial integrity; CNS: None; CL: Analysis

43. Which symptom would a client with generalized anxiety disorder most likely display when assessed for muscle tension?

1. Difficulty sleeping
2. Restlessness
3. Strong startle response
4. Tachycardia

43. 2. Restlessness is a symptom associated with muscle tension. Difficulty sleeping and a strong startle response are considered symptoms of vigilance and scanning of the environment, not muscle tension. Tachycardia is classified as a symptom of autonomic hyperactivity, not muscle tension.

CN: Physiological integrity; CNS: Physiological adaptation; CL: Application

44. Which intervention should be given priority for a client with generalized anxiety disorder who's working to develop coping skills?

1. Determine whether the client has fears or obsessive thinking.
2. Monitor the client for overt and covert signs of anxiety.
3. Teach the client how to use effective communications skills.
4. Assist the client to identify coping mechanisms used in the past.

44. 4. To help a client develop effective coping skills, the nurse must know the client's baseline functioning. Determining whether the client has fears or obsessive thinking, monitoring for signs of anxiety, and teaching about effective communications skills are later priorities, not initial ones.

CN: Safe, effective care environment; CNS: Management of care; CL: Application

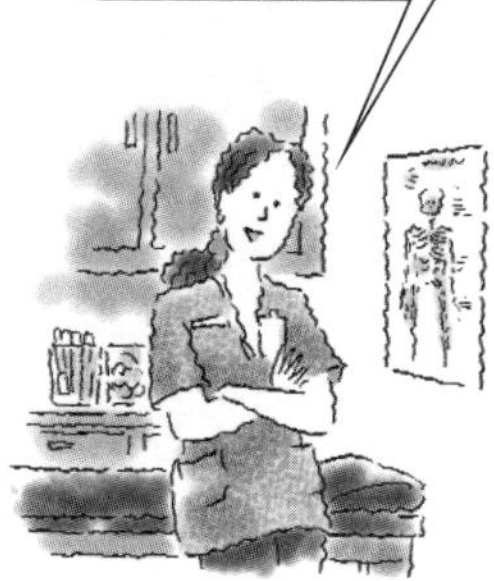

Thorough teaching plans typically include ways to contact support organizations.

45. Which instruction should help a nurse deal with escalating client anxiety?

1. Explore feelings about current life stressors.
2. Discuss the need to flee from painful situations.
3. Have the client develop a realistic view of self.
4. Provide appropriate phone numbers for hotlines and clinics.

45. 4. By having information on hotlines and clinics, the client can pursue help when the anxiety is escalating. Discussion about current life stressors isn't useful when focusing on how best to handle the client's escalating anxiety. Fleeing from painful situations and discussing views of oneself aren't the best strategies; neither allows for problem solving.

CN: Psychosocial integrity; CNS: None; CL: Application

46. Which of the following points would a nurse include in teaching for the family of an adult client with generalized anxiety disorder?

1. Explain how the family can handle the confusion related to memory loss.
2. Teach the family to assist the client with coping strategies as needed.
3. Teach the family how to cope with the client's sudden and unexpected travel behavior.
4. Have the family determine when and for what reasons the client should take medication.

46. 2. The family can be there for support, but they negate the client's ability to function if they take control of the situation and don't allow the client to use his own coping skills. A client who has confusion related to memory loss is commonly struggling with dissociative amnesia, not a generalized anxiety disorder. Sudden and unexpected travel behavior is a problem for families who have members with dissociative identity disorder, not generalized anxiety disorder. The client must handle and use medication as prescribed.

CN: Psychosocial integrity; CNS: None; CL: Application

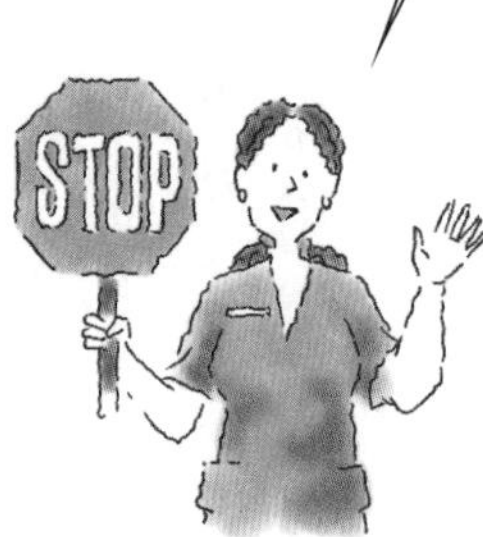

You should be familiar with the symptoms that discontinuing key medications may cause.
STOP

47. A client with a diagnosis of generalized anxiety disorder wants to stop taking his lorazepam (Ativan). Which important fact should the nurse discuss with the client about discontinuing the medication?

1. Stopping the drug may cause depression.
2. Stopping the drug increases cognitive abilities.
3. Stopping the drug decreases sleeping difficulties.
4. Stopping the drug can cause withdrawal symptoms.

47. 4. Stopping antianxiety drugs such as benzodiazepines can cause the client to have withdrawal symptoms. Stopping a benzodiazepine doesn't tend to cause depression, increase cognitive abilities, or decrease sleeping difficulties.

CN: Physiological integrity; CNS: Pharmacological and parenteral therapies; CL: Application

48. Five days after running out of medication, a client taking clonazepam (Klonopin) says to the nurse, "I know I shouldn't have just stopped the drug like that, but I'm OK." Which response would be best?

1. "Let's monitor you for problems, in case something else happens."
2. "You could go through withdrawal symptoms for up to 2 weeks."
3. "You have handled your anxiety, and you now know how to cope with stress."
4. "If you're fine now, chances are you won't experience withdrawal symptoms."

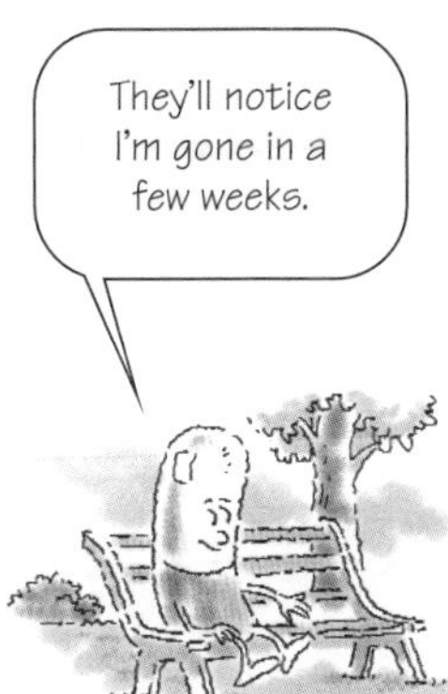

They'll notice I'm gone in a few weeks.

48. 2. Withdrawal syndrome symptoms can appear after 1 or 2 weeks because the benzodiazepine has a long half-life. Looking for another problem unrelated to withdrawal isn't the nurse's best strategy. The act of discontinuing an antianxiety medication doesn't indicate that a client has learned to cope with stress. Every client taking medication needs to be monitored for withdrawal symptoms when the medication is stopped abruptly.

CN: Physiological integrity; CNS: Pharmacological and parenteral therapies; CL: Analysis

49. A client taking alprazolam (Xanax) reports light-headedness and nausea every day while getting out of bed. Which action should the nurse take to objectively validate this client's problem?

1. Take the client's blood pressure.
2. Monitor body temperature.
3. Teach the Valsalva maneuver.
4. Obtain a blood chemical profile.

49. 1. The nurse should take a blood pressure reading to validate orthostatic hypotension. A body temperature reading or chemistry profile won't yield useful information about hypotension. The Valsalva maneuver is performed to lower the heart rate and isn't an appropriate intervention.

CN: Physiological integrity; CNS: Reduction of risk potential; CL: Application

50. A client with generalized anxiety disorder complains of a headache and upset stomach. In assessing this client, the nurse is aware that a client with generalized anxiety disorder may experience which of the following?

1. May have a variety of somatic symptoms.
2. Undergo an alteration in his self-care skills.
3. Is prone to unhealthy binge eating episodes.
4. Will experience secondary gains from mental illness.

50. 1. Clients with anxiety disorders commonly experience somatic symptoms. They don't usually experience problems with self-care. Eating problems aren't a typical part of the diagnostic criteria for anxiety disorders. Not all clients obtain secondary gains from mental illness.

CN: Psychosocial integrity; CNS: None; CL: Application

51. Which communication guideline should a nurse use when talking with a client experiencing mania?

1. Address the client in a light and joking manner.
2. Focus and redirect the conversation as necessary.
3. Allow the client to talk about several different topics.
4. Ask only open-ended questions to facilitate conversation.

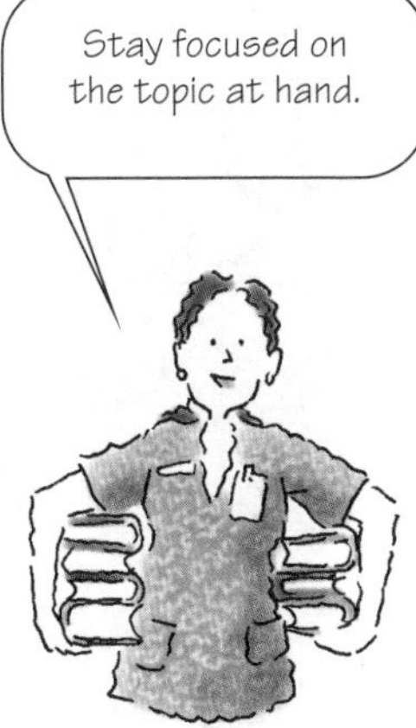

Stay focused on the topic at hand.

51. 2. To decrease stimulation, the nurse should attempt to redirect and focus the client's communication, not allow the client to talk about different topics. By addressing the client in a light and joking manner, the conversation may contribute to the client's feeling out of control. For a manic client, it's best to ask closed questions because open-ended questions may enable the client to talk endlessly, again possibly contributing to the client's feeling out of control.

CN: Psychosocial integrity; CNS: None; CL: Application

52. Which adverse effect should a nurse explain to a client with bipolar disorder and his family when providing preprocedure teaching for electroconvulsive therapy (ECT)?

1. Cholestatic jaundice
2. Hypertensive crisis
3. Mouth ulcers
4. Respiratory distress

52. 4. Respiratory distress or even arrest may occur as a complication of the anesthesia used with ECT. Cholestatic jaundice, hypertensive crisis, and mouth ulcers don't occur during or as a result of ECT.

CN: Physiological integrity; CNS: Physiological adaptation; CL: Application

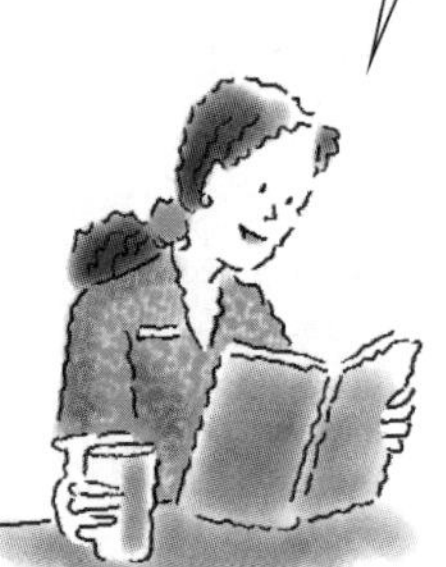
What harm could result from a glass of water?

53. A client who has just had electroconvulsive therapy (ECT) asks for a drink. Which assessment is a <u>priority</u> when meeting the client's request?

1. Take the client's blood pressure.
2. Monitor the gag reflex.
3. Obtain a body temperature.
4. Determine the level of consciousness.

53. 2. The nurse must check the client's gag reflex before allowing the client to have a drink after an ECT procedure. Blood pressure and body temperature don't influence whether the client may have a drink after the procedure. The client would obviously be conscious if he's requesting a glass of water.

CN: Physiological integrity; CNS: Physiological adaptation; CL: Analysis

54. A nurse is caring for a client with hypomania. In performing the assessment, which behavior should she expect?

1. A hypomanic client is on the verge of experiencing depression and crisis.
2. A hypomanic client is indecisive and vacillating, with a diminished ability to think.
3. A hypomanic client is irritable, with an elevated mood and symptoms of mania.
4. A hypomanic client is disorganized and tends to exhibit impaired judgment.

54. 3. When a client is hypomanic, there's evidence of an elevated and irritable mood, along with mild or beginning symptoms of mania. A hypomanic client is experiencing a period of mild elation, not a depression or crisis. Indecision and vacillation with a diminished ability to think are symptoms more likely seen in a major depressive episode than in a hypomanic episode. A client with hypomania tends to be creative and more productive than usual, rather than disorganized with impaired judgment.

CN: Psychosocial integrity; CNS: None; CL: Analysis

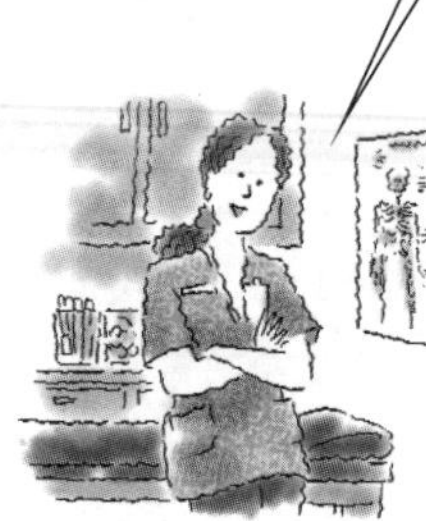
The words most likely can help you focus on the answer.

55. A client with bipolar disorder who complains of headache, agitation, and indigestion is <u>most likely</u> experiencing which of the following problems?

1. Depression
2. Cyclothymia
3. Hypomania
4. Mania

55. 4. Headache, agitation, and indigestion are symptoms suggestive of mania in a client with a history of bipolar disorder. These symptoms are *not* suggestive of depression, cyclothymia, or hypomania.

CN: Physiological integrity; CNS: Physiological adaptation; CL: Application

56. A client with bipolar disorder has abruptly stopped taking his prescribed medication. Which high-risk behavior would indicate the client has experienced a manic episode?

1. Binge eating
2. Relationship avoidance
3. Sudden relocation
4. Thoughtless spending

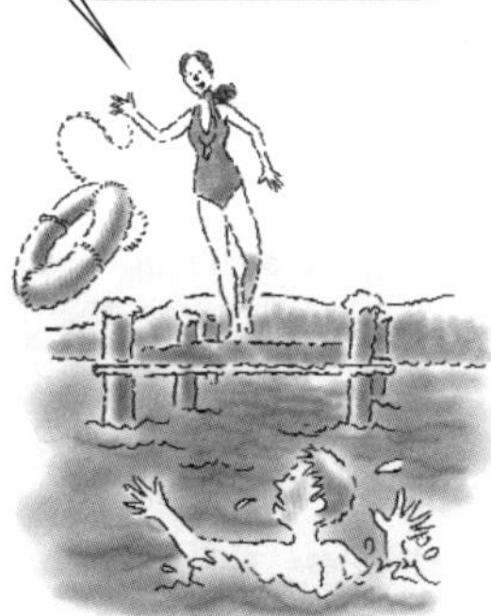

Know the high-risk behaviors associated with each disorder.

56. 4. Thoughtless or reckless spending is a common symptom of a manic episode. Binge eating isn't a behavior that's characteristic of a client during a manic episode. Relationship avoidance doesn't occur in a client experiencing a manic episode; during episodes of mania, a client may in fact interact with many people and participate in unsafe sexual behavior. Sudden relocation isn't a characteristic of impulsive behavior demonstrated by a client with bipolar disorder.

CN: Psychosocial integrity; CNS: None; CL: Application

57. Which intervention would assist a client with bipolar disorder to maintain adequate nutrition during a manic episode?

1. Determine the client's metabolic rate.
2. Make the client sit down for each meal and snack.
3. Give the client foods to be eaten while he's active.
4. Have the client interact with a dietitian twice a week.

57. 3. By giving the client high-caloric foods that can be eaten while he's active, the nurse facilitates the client's nutritional intake. Determining the client's metabolic rate isn't useful information when the client is experiencing mania. During a manic episode, the client can't be still or focused long enough to interact with a dietitian or sit still long enough to eat.

CN: Physiological integrity; CNS: Basic care and comfort; CL: Application

58. A nurse is providing discharge teaching to a client being discharged on lithium. The nurse would emphasize that the client should report which of the following?

1. Black tongue
2. Increased lacrimation
3. Periods of excitability
4. Persistent GI upset

58. 4. Persistent GI upset indicates a mild-to-moderate toxic reaction. Black tongue is an adverse reaction of mirtazapine (Remeron), not lithium. Increased lacrimation and periods of excitability aren't adverse effects of lithium.

CN: Physiological integrity; CNS: Pharmacological and parenteral therapies; CL: Application

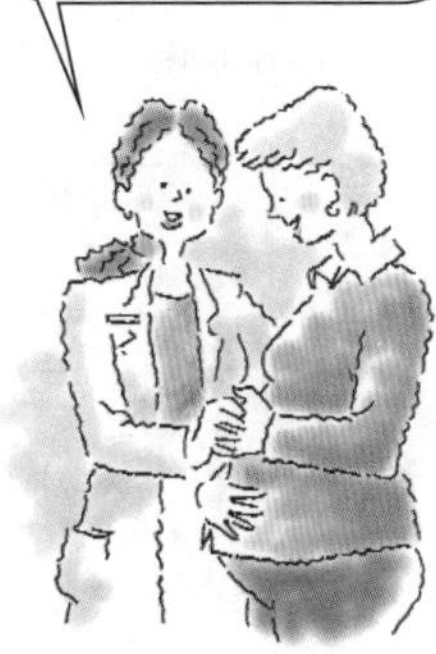

59. Which information is important to teach a client with bipolar disorder who's pregnant and taking lithium?

1. Use of lithium usually results in serious congenital problems.
2. Thyroid problems can occur in the first trimester of the pregnancy.
3. Lithium causes severe urine retention and increased risk of toxicity.
4. Women who take lithium are very likely to have a spontaneous abortion.

59. 1. Use of lithium during pregnancy results in congenital defects, especially cardiac defects. Thyroid problems don't occur in the first trimester of the pregnancy. In lithium toxicity, a condition called nontoxic goiter may occur. An adverse effect of lithium is polyuria, not urine retention. The rate of spontaneous abortion for women taking lithium is no greater than for non-users.

CN: Physiological integrity; CNS: Pharmacological and parenteral therapies; CL: Application

60. A nurse is teaching a client with bipolar disorder about the drug carbamazepine (Tegretol). The teaching has been effective when the client states which of the following?

1. "My hair will fall out if I take this drug."
2. "I will drink plenty of water so I don't develop kidney problems."
3. "I need to have my blood counts checked periodically."
4. "I can't take any other drugs with this one."

60. 3. The most dangerous adverse effect of carbamazepine is bone marrow depression. Other medications may be taken with carbamazepine. Hair loss doesn't occur in clients taking carbamazepine. Clients who take lithium, not carbamazepine, must be closely monitored for nephrogenic diabetes insipidus. The interactions of all drugs being taken must be monitored because some drugs can either increase or decrease the blood level of carbamazepine.

CN: Physiological integrity; CNS: Pharmacological and parenteral therapies; CL: Analysis

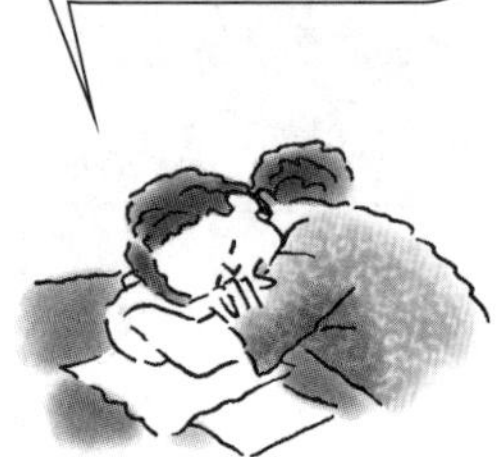

My immediate sleep goal is a 10-minute nap.

61. A nurse is leading a team conference. Suggestions are given for a client with bipolar disorder. Which one should the nurse enter on the care plan?

1. Obtain medication for sleep.
2. Work on solving a problem.
3. Exercise before bedtime.
4. Develop a sleep ritual.

61. 4. A sleep ritual or nighttime routine helps the client to relax and prepare for sleep. Obtaining sleep medication is a temporary solution. Working on problem solving may excite the client rather than tire him. Exercise before retiring is inappropriate.

CN: Physiological integrity; CNS: Reduction of risk potential; CL: Application

62. Which topic should the nurse discuss with the family of a client with bipolar disorder if the family is distressed about the client's episodes of manic behavior?

1. Ways to protect oneself from client's behavior
2. How to proceed with an involuntary commitment
3. How to confront the client about the reckless behavior
4. When to safely increase medication during manic periods

62. 1. Family members need to assess their needs and develop ways to protect themselves. Clients who have symptoms of impulsive or reckless behavior might not be candidates for hospitalization. Confronting the client during a manic episode may escalate the behavior. The family must never increase the dosage of prescribed medication without first consulting the primary health care provider.

CN: Safe, effective care environment; CNS: Safety and infection control; CL: Application

63. Which statement regarding lithium blood levels represents the most accurate client teaching for a bipolar client?

1. Lithium levels are obtained to determine liver and renal damage.
2. Lithium levels demonstrate whether the client is taking a therapeutic dose range of the drug.
3. Lithium levels indicate whether the drug has passed through the blood-brain barrier.
4. Lithium levels are unnecessary if the client takes the drug as ordered.

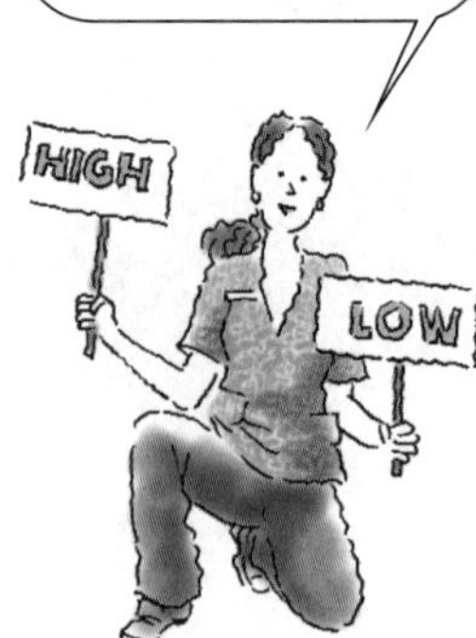

Monitoring blood levels helps ensure that adequate doses of lithium are being administered.
HIGH
LOW

63. 2. Lithium levels determine whether an effective dose of lithium is being given to maintain a therapeutic level of the drug. The drug is contraindicated for clients with renal, cardiac, or liver disease. Lithium levels aren't drawn for the purpose of determining whether the drug passes through the blood-brain barrier. Taking the drug as ordered doesn't eliminate the need for blood work.

CN: Physiological integrity; CNS: Pharmacological and parenteral therapies; CL: Application

64. What information is important to include in the nutritional counseling of a family with a member who has bipolar disorder?

1. If sufficient roughage isn't eaten while taking lithium, bowel problems will occur.
2. If the intake of carbohydrates increases, the lithium level will increase.
3. If the intake of calories is reduced, the lithium level will increase.
4. If the intake of sodium increases, the lithium level will decrease.

64. 4. Any time the level of sodium increases, such as with a change in dietary intake, the level of lithium will decrease. The intake of roughage and carbohydrates in the diet isn't related to the metabolism of lithium. Reducing the number of calories the client eats doesn't affect the lithium level in the body.

CN: Physiological integrity; CNS: Reduction of risk potential; CL: Analysis

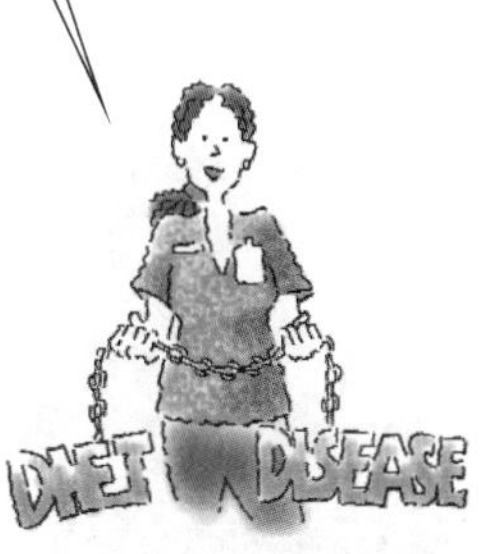

65. Which statement made by a client with bipolar disorder indicates that the nurse's teaching on coping strategies was effective?

1. "I can decide what to do to prevent family conflict."
2. "I can handle problems without asking for any help."
3. "I can stay away from my friends when I feel distressed."
4. "I can ignore things that go wrong instead of getting upset."

65. 1. The client should be focusing on his strengths and abilities to prevent family conflict. Not being able to ask for help is problematic and not a good coping strategy. Avoiding problems also isn't a good coping strategy. It's better to identify and handle problems as they arise. Ignoring situations that cause discomfort won't facilitate solutions or allow the client to demonstrate effective coping skills.

CN: Psychosocial integrity; CNS: None; CL: Analysis

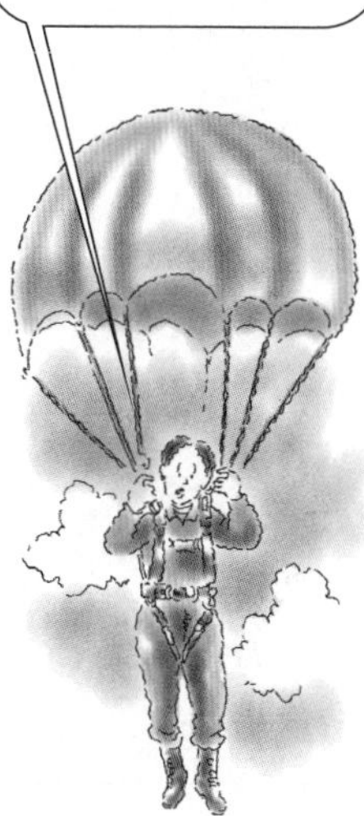

You shouldn't have to ask what short-term goal is most appropriate!

66. A client with depression is admitted to the inpatient unit because of attempted suicide. Which of the following nursing goals should be given the highest priority?

1. The client will seek out the nurse when feeling self-destructive.
2. The client will identify and discuss actual and perceived losses.
3. The client will learn strategies to promote relaxation and self-care.
4. The client will establish healthy and mutually caring relationships.

66. 1. By seeking out the nurse when feeling self-destructive, the client can feel safe and begin to see that there are coping skills to assist in dealing with self-destructive tendencies. Discussion of losses also is important when dealing with feelings of depression, but the priority intervention is still to promote immediate client safety. Although relationship building and learning strategies to promote relaxation and self-care are important goals, safety is the priority intervention.

CN: Safe, effective care environment; CNS: Management of care; CL: Analysis

67. A nurse is caring for a client who reports that he thinks about suicide every day. In conferring with the treatment team, which recommendation by the nurse would be the most appropriate for this client?

1. A no-suicide contract
2. Weekly outpatient therapy
3. A second psychiatric opinion
4. Intensive inpatient treatment

67. 4. For a client thinking about suicide on a daily basis, inpatient care would be the best intervention. Although a no-suicide contract is an important strategy, this client needs additional care. The client needs a more intensive level of care than weekly outpatient therapy. Immediate intervention is paramount, not a second psychiatric opinion.

CN: Safe, effective care environment; CNS: Management of care; CL: Application

68. Which short-term goal should a nurse focus on for a client who makes statements about not deserving things?
1. Identify distorted thoughts.
2. Describe self-care patterns.
3. Discuss family relationships.
4. Explore communication skills.

68. 1. It's important to identify distorted thinking because self-deprecating thoughts lead to depression. Self-care patterns don't necessarily reflect distorted thinking. Family relationships might not influence distorted thinking patterns. A form of communication called negative self-talk would be explored only after distorted thinking patterns were identified.
CN: Psychosocial integrity; CNS: None; CL: Application

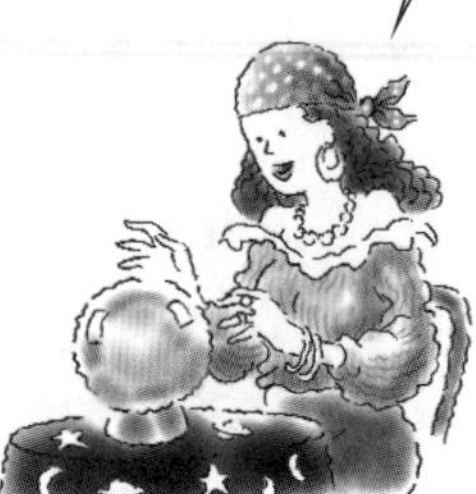

You're doing great in the short term, and your long-term goal is in sight.

69. Which intervention should be of primary importance to a nurse working with a client to modify the client's negative expectations?
1. Encourage the client to discuss spiritual matters.
2. Assist the client to learn how to problem-solve.
3. Help the client explore issues related to loss.
4. Have the client identify positive aspects of self.

69. 4. An important intervention used to counter negative expectations is to focus on the positive and have the client explore positive aspects of himself. Discussion of spiritual matters doesn't address the need to change negative expectations. Learning how to problem-solve won't modify the client's negative expectations. If the client dwells on the negative and focuses on loss, it will be natural to have negative expectations.
CN: Psychosocial integrity; CNS: None; CL: Application

70. Which intervention strategy is most appropriate to use with a client with depression who may be suicidal?
1. Speak to family members to ascertain whether the client is suicidal.
2. Talk to the client to determine whether the client is an attention seeker.
3. Arrange for the client to be placed on immediate suicidal precautions.
4. Ask a direct question such as, "Do you ever think about killing yourself?"

70. 4. The best approach to determining whether a client is suicidal is to ask about thoughts of suicide in a direct and caring manner. Assessing for attention-seeking behaviors doesn't deal directly with the problem. The client should be assessed directly, not through family members. Assessment must be performed before determining whether suicide precautions are necessary.
CN: Psychosocial integrity; CNS: None; CL: Application

71. Which instruction should a nurse include when teaching the family of a client with major depression?
1. Address how depression is a lifelong illness.
2. Explain that depression is an illness and can be treated.
3. Describe how depression masks a person's true feelings.
4. Teach how depression causes frequent disorganized thinking.

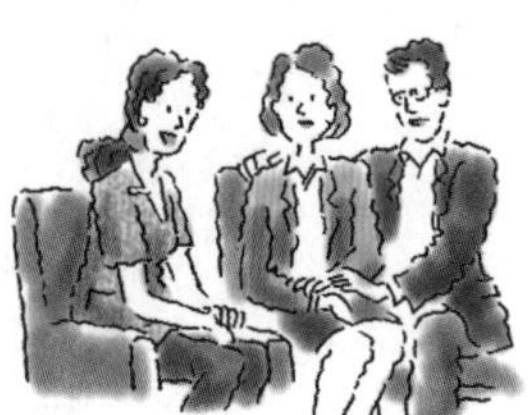

Depression affects the entire family.

71. 2. The nurse must help the family understand depression, its impact on the family, and recommended treatments. Depression doesn't need to be a lifelong illness. It's important to help families understand that depression can be successfully treated and that, in some situations, depression can reoccur during the life cycle. The feelings expressed by the client are genuine; they reflect cognitive distortions and disillusionment. Disorganized thinking is more commonly associated with schizophrenia rather than with depression.
CN: Psychosocial integrity; CNS: None; CL: Application

72. A client with major depression asks why he is taking mirtazapine (Remeron) instead of imipramine hydrochloride (Tofranil). Which explanation is most accurate?

1. The newer serotonin reuptake inhibitor drugs are better-tested drugs.
2. The serotonin reuptake inhibitors have few adverse effects.
3. The serotonin reuptake inhibitors require a low dose of antidepressant drug.
4. The serotonin reuptake inhibitors are as good as other antidepressant drugs.

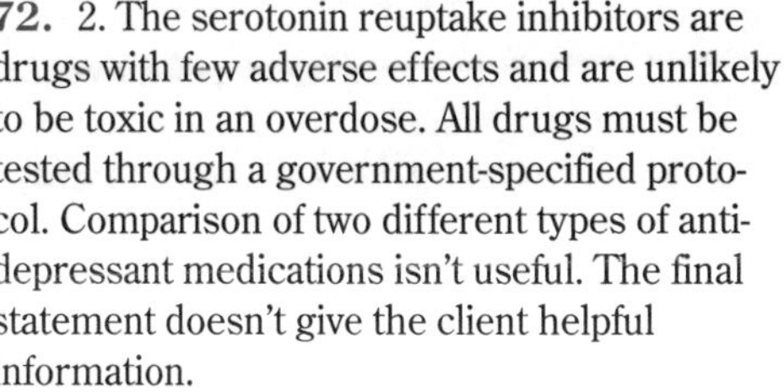

72. 2. The serotonin reuptake inhibitors are drugs with few adverse effects and are unlikely to be toxic in an overdose. All drugs must be tested through a government-specified protocol. Comparison of two different types of antidepressant medications isn't useful. The final statement doesn't give the client helpful information.

CN: Physiological integrity; CNS: Pharmacological and parenteral therapies; CL: Analysis

73. A nurse is caring for a client with depression. Which of the following interventions will best meet the client's goal of enhancing self-esteem?

1. Playing cards
2. Praying daily
3. Taking medication
4. Writing poetry

73. 4. Writing poetry or engaging in some other creative outlet will enhance self-esteem. Playing cards and praying don't necessarily promote self-esteem. Taking medication will decrease symptoms of depression after a blood level is established, but it won't, by itself, promote self-esteem.

CN: Psychosocial integrity; CNS: None; CL: Application

74. An adolescent who is depressed and is reported by his parents as having difficulty in school is brought to the community mental health center to be evaluated. Which other health problem should the nurse suspect?

1. Anxiety disorder
2. Behavioral difficulties
3. Cognitive impairment
4. Labile moods

74. 2. Adolescents tend to demonstrate severe irritability and behavioral problems rather than simply a depressed mood. Anxiety disorder is more commonly associated with small children rather than with adolescents. Cognitive impairment is typically associated with delirium or dementia. Labile mood is more characteristic of a client with cognitive impairment or bipolar disorder.

CN: Psychosocial integrity; CNS: None; CL: Analysis

75. Which nursing intervention is most effective in lowering a client's risk of suicide?

1. Using a caring approach
2. Developing a strong relationship with the client
3. Establishing a suicide contract to ensure his safety
4. Encouraging avoidance of overstimulating activities

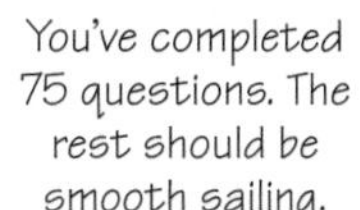

You've completed 75 questions. The rest should be smooth sailing.

75. 3. Establishing a suicide contract with the client demonstrates that the nurse's concern for his safety is a priority and that his life is of value. When a client agrees to a suicide contract, it decreases his risk of a successful attempt. Caring alone ignores the underlying mechanism of the client's wish to commit suicide. Merely developing a strong relationship with the client isn't addressing the potential the client has for harming himself. Encouraging the client to stay away from activities could cause isolation, which would be detrimental to the client's well-being.

CN: Psychosocial integrity; CNS: None; CL: Application

76. Which nursing diagnosis would the nurse expect to find on the care plan of a client with a phobia about elevators?
1. *Social isolation related to a lack of social skills*
2. *Disturbed sleep pattern related to a fear of elevators*
3. *Ineffective coping related to poor coping skills*
4. *Anxiety related to fear of elevators*

76. 3. Poor coping skills can cause ineffective coping. Such a client isn't relegated to social isolation, and lack of social skills has nothing to do with phobia. Fear of elevators is a manifestation, not the cause of altered thoughts and anxiety.
CN: Psychosocial integrity; CNS: None; CL: Analysis

No need to fear this question-focus on which technique would be useful.

77. Which behavior modification technique is useful in the treatment of phobias?
1. Aversion therapy
2. Imitation or modeling
3. Positive reinforcement
4. Systematic desensitization

77. 4. Systematic desensitization is a common behavior modification technique that has been successfully used to help treat phobia. Aversion therapy and positive reinforcement aren't behavior modification techniques used with the treatment of phobias. The techniques of imitation or modeling are social learning techniques, not behavior modification techniques.
CN: Psychosocial integrity; CNS: None; CL: Application

78. Which statement would be useful when teaching a client and her family about phobias and the need for a strong support system?
1. The use of a family support system is only temporary.
2. The need to be assertive can be reinforced by the family.
3. The family must set limit on inappropriate behaviors.
4. The family plays a role in promoting client independence.

78. 4. The family plays a vital role in supporting a client in treatment and in preventing the client from using the phobia to obtain secondary gains. Family support must be ongoing, not temporary. The family can be more helpful by focusing on effective handling of anxiety, rather than focusing energy on developing assertiveness skills. People with phobias are already restrictive in their behavior; more restrictions aren't necessary.
CN: Psychosocial integrity; CNS: None; CL: Analysis

79. A client with an anxiety disorder is taking alprazolam (Xanax). The nurse should instruct the client to avoid:
1. shellfish.
2. alcohol.
3. coffee.
4. cheese.

79. 2. Alcohol should be avoided because of additive depressive effects. Ingestion of shellfish, coffee, and cheese isn't problematic.
CN: Physiological integrity; CNS: Pharmacological and parenteral therapies; CL: Application

80. A female client describes her unpredictable episodes of acute anxiety as "just awful." She says that she feels like she's about to die and can hardly breathe. The nurse recognizes that the symptoms described by the client are associated with which condition?

1. Agoraphobia
2. Dissociative disorder
3. Posttraumatic stress disorder (PTSD)
4. Panic disorder

80. 4. This client is describing the characteristics of someone with panic disorder. Agoraphobia is characterized by fear of public places; dissociative disorder, by lost periods of time; and PTSD, by hypervigilance and sleep disturbance.
CN: Psychosocial integrity; CNS: None; CL: Application

Don't *panic* if the answer isn't immediately clear—read through the question carefully and eliminate the obvious incorrect options first.

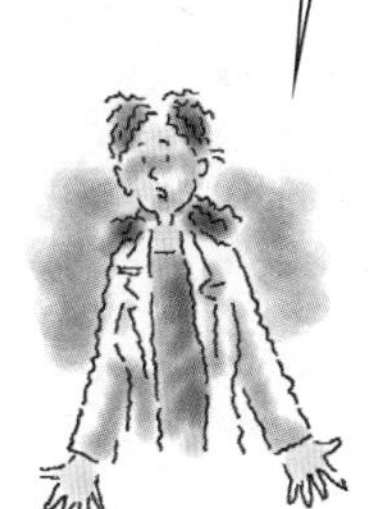

81. A client taking antidepressants for major depression for about 3 weeks is expressing that he's feeling better. Which complication should he now be assessed for?

1. Manic depression
2. Potential for violence
3. Substance abuse
4. Suicidal ideation

81. 4. After a client has been on antidepressants and is feeling better, he commonly then has the energy to harm himself. Manic depression isn't treated with antidepressants. Nothing in the client's history suggests a potential for violence. There are no signs or symptoms suggesting substance abuse.
CN: Safe, effective care environment; CNS: Safety and infection control; CL: Analysis

82. A 40-year-old female client has been brought to the hospital by her husband because she has refused to get out of bed for 2 days. She won't eat, she's been neglecting household responsibilities, and she's tired all the time. Her diagnosis on admission is major depression. Which question is most appropriate for the admitting nurse to ask at this point?

1. "What has been troubling you?"
2. "Why do you dislike yourself?"
3. "How do you feel about your life?"
4. "What can we do to help?"

82. 3. The nurse must develop nursing interventions based on the client's perceived problems and feelings. Asking the client to draw a conclusion may be difficult for her at this time. *Why* questions can place the client in a defensive position. Requiring the client to find possible solutions is beyond the scope of her present abilities.
CN: Psychosocial integrity; CNS: None; CL: Analysis

Timing is critical here. Read the question again if you have any doubts about what's being asked.

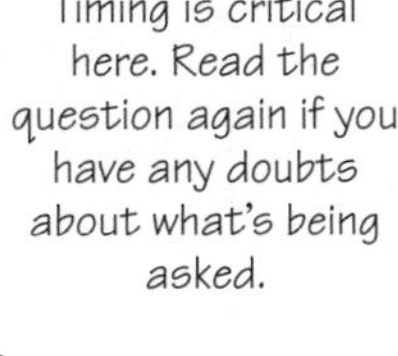

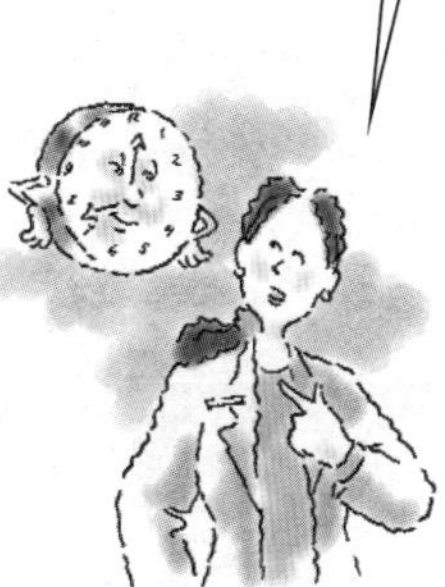

83. A client with bipolar disorder has been receiving lithium (Eskalith) for 2 weeks. He also has been taking chemotherapeutic drugs that cause him to feel nauseated and anorexic, making it difficult to distinguish early signs of lithium toxicity. Which sign would indicate lithium toxicity at serum drug levels below 1.5 mEq/L?

1. Hyperpyrexia
2. Marked analgesics and lethargy
3. Hypotonic reflexes with muscle weakness
4. Oliguria

83. 3. Lithium alters sodium transport in nerve and muscle cells, slowing the speed of impulse transmission, so look for hypotonic reflexes and muscle weakness. Lithium has no known effect on body temperature or on the transmission of pain impulses. The drug doesn't cause lethargy. Oliguria and other signs of renal failure occur late in severe lithium toxicity.
CN: Physiologic integrity; CNS: Pharmacological and parenteral therapies; CL: Application

84. A client came to the psychiatric unit 2 days ago. He has a history of bipolar disorder, is in the manic phase, and stopped taking lithium (Eskalith) 2 weeks ago. Which finding should the nurse be likely to see?

1. Flight of ideas
2. Echolalia
3. Clang associations
4. Neologism

84. 1. Flight of ideas is a speech pattern characterized by rapid transition from topic to topic, typically without finishing one idea. It's common in mania. Echolalia (repetition of words heard), clang associations (use of rhyming), and neologism (inverted words) aren't seen in mania states.

CN: Psychosocial integrity; CNS: None; CL: Application

85. An acutely manic client kisses a nurse on the lips and asks her to marry him. The nurse is taken by surprise. Which response would be best?

1. Seclude the client for his inappropriate behavior.
2. Ask the client what he's trying to prove by his behavior.
3. Ask the client to fold some laundry.
4. Tell the client his behavior is offensive.

85. 3. Having the client help with laundry rechannels his energy in a positive activity. The client needs direction and structure, not seclusion. Asking the client what he's trying to prove ignores his impaired judgment and poor impulse control. Telling the client that his behavior is offensive doesn't assist him in controlling his behavior.

CN: Psychosocial integrity; CNS: None; CL: Application

86. Which discharge instruction is most important for a client taking lithium (Eskalith)?

1. Limit fluids to 1,500 ml daily.
2. Maintain a high fluid intake.
3. Take advantage of the warm weather by exercising outside whenever possible.
4. When feeling a cold coming, it's OK to take over-the-counter (OTC) remedies.

86. 2. Clients taking lithium need to maintain a high fluid intake. Exercising outside may not be safe; photosensitivity occurs with lithium use, and activity in warm weather could increase sodium loss, predisposing the client to lithium toxicity. The client shouldn't take OTC drugs without the physician's approval.

CN: Physiological integrity; CNS: Pharmacological and parenteral therapies; CL: Application

87. A client in an outpatient psychiatric facility is diagnosed with dysthymic disorder. Which statement would the nurse include in the teaching for this client?

1. It involves a mood range from moderate depression to hypomania.
2. It involves a single manic episode.
3. It's a form of depression that occurs in the fall and winter.
4. It's a mood disorder similar to major depression but of mild to moderate severity.

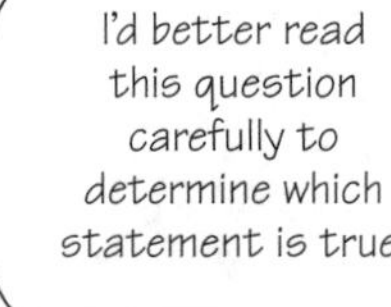

I'd better read this question carefully to determine which statement is true.

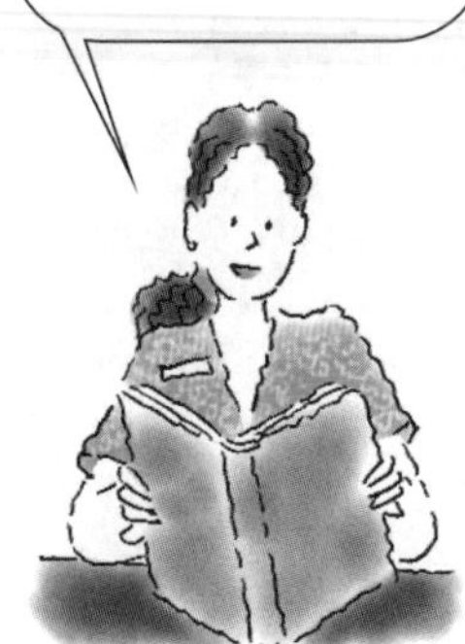

87. 4. Dysthymic disorder is a mood disorder similar to major depression, but it remains mild to moderate in severity. Cyclothymic disorder is a mood disorder characterized by a mood range from moderate depression to hypomania. Bipolar I disorder is characterized by a single manic episode with no past major depressive episodes. Seasonal affective disorder is a form of depression occurring in the fall and winter.

CN: Psychosocial integrity; CNS: None; CL: Application

88. A depressed client taking a prescribed tricyclic antidepressant tells a nurse he's sleepy all the time and doesn't feel like doing anything. Which nursing action is appropriate?

1. Tell the client to stop taking the drug until he sees his physician.
2. Advise the client to continue taking the drug to see whether these effects wear off.
3. Ask the physician whether the medication can be given in one dose at bedtime.
4. Advise the client to get another opinion.

88. 3. Many tricyclic antidepressants can be given safely in one dose; when an antidepressant is taken at bedtime, the adverse effect of drowsiness can help the client sleep. It's inappropriate for the nurse to tell the client to stop taking the drug, to continue taking it until the undesired effects wear off, or to seek a second opinion.

CN: Physiological integrity; CNS: Pharmacological and parenteral therapies; CL: Application

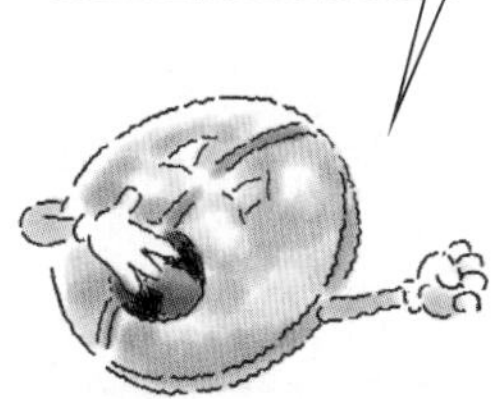
I just don't feel like doing anything.

89. A depressed client is taking trazodone (Desyrel), an atypical antidepressant. On discharge, the nurse will instruct the client to take the medication:

1. in the morning.
2. at bedtime.
3. at any time during the day.
4. when he has an urge for a cigarette.

89. 2. Trazodone has a strong sedative effect and is commonly prescribed as a sleep aid to be taken at bedtime. Wellbutrin is used for smoking cessation.

CN: Physiological integrity; CNS: Pharmacological and parenteral therapies; CL: Application

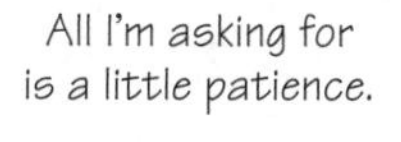
All I'm asking for is a little patience.

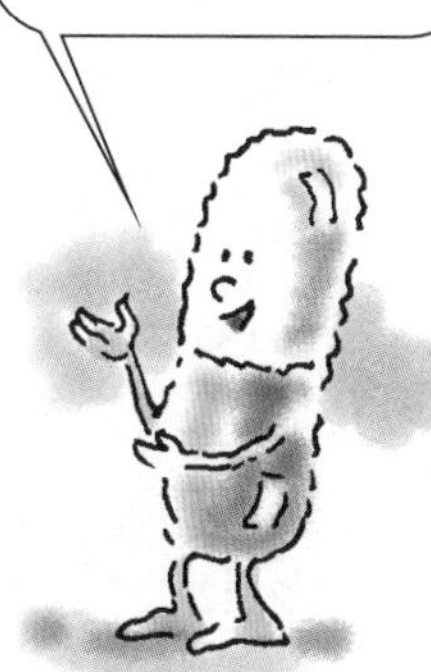

90. Which instruction should a nurse provide when teaching a client about tricyclic antidepressants?

1. "This drug causes photosensitivity."
2. "Avoid milk and dairy products."
3. "Notify your physician if your mood doesn't improve within 7 days."
4. "Mood improvement takes up to 28 days."

90. 4. The client's mood may not improve until the 3rd or 4th week of tricyclic antidepressant therapy. The client needs to be reassured that the drug works slowly. The drug doesn't cause photosensitivity or interact with milk and dairy products.

CN: Physiological integrity; CNS: Pharmacological and parenteral therapies; CL: Application

91. Which intervention by the nurse would be the most appropriate when caring for a client newly diagnosed with insulin-dependent diabetes mellitus who also has blood-injection-injury phobia?

1. Teach the client to avoid fainting by tensing the muscles of the legs and abdomen.
2. Quickly expose the client to feared situations.
3. Have the client avoid as much medical care as possible.
4. Focus on treating the symptoms with an antianxiety medication.

91. 1. The client may be able to avoid fainting and relieve hypotension by tensing the larger muscle groups. Desensitization by slowly, not quickly, exposing the client to blood injection is indicated to reduce fear. Clients with blood-injection-injury phobia may avoid all medical care, which is dangerous to their health. Antianxiety medications may help on a short-term basis only.

CN: Psychosocial integrity; CNS: None; CL: Application

92. A client with the nursing diagnosis of *Fear related to being embarrassed in the presence of others* exhibits symptoms of social phobia. What should the goals be for this client? Select all that apply:

1. Manage his fear in group situations.
2. Develop a plan to avoid situations that may cause stress.
3. Verbalize feelings that occur in stressful situations.
4. Develop a plan for responding to stressful situations.
5. Deny feelings that may contribute to irrational fears.
6. Use suppression to deal with underlying fears.

92. 1, 3, 4. Improving stress-management skills, verbalizing feelings, and anticipating and planning for stressful situations are adaptive responses to stress. Avoidance, denial, and suppression are maladaptive defense mechanisms.
CN: Psychosocial integrity; CNS: None; CL: Application

93. The nurse recognizes improvement in a client with the nursing diagnosis of *Ineffective role performance related to the need to perform rituals.* Which behavior indicates improvement? Select all that apply:

1. The client refrains from performing rituals during stress.
2. The client verbalizes that he uses "thought stopping" when obsessive thoughts occur.
3. The client verbalizes the relationship between stress and ritualistic behaviors.
4. The client avoids stressful situations.
5. The client rationalizes ritualistic behavior.
6. The client performs ritualistic behaviors in private.

93. 1, 2, 3. Refraining from rituals demonstrates that the client manages stress appropriately. Using "thought stopping" demonstrates the client's ability to employ appropriate interventions for obsessive thoughts. Verbalizing the relationship between stress and behaviors indicates that the client understands the disease process. Avoiding, rationalizing, and hiding behaviors demonstrate maladaptive methods for managing stress and anxiety.
CN: Psychosocial integrity; CNS: None; CL: Analysis

94. After interviewing a client diagnosed with recurrent depression, the nurse determines the client's potential to commit suicide. Which factors should the nurse consider as contributors to the client's potential for suicide? Select all that apply:

1. Psychomotor retardation
2. Impulsive behaviors
3. Overwhelming feelings of guilt
4. Chronic, debilitating illness
5. Decreased physical activity
6. Repression of anger

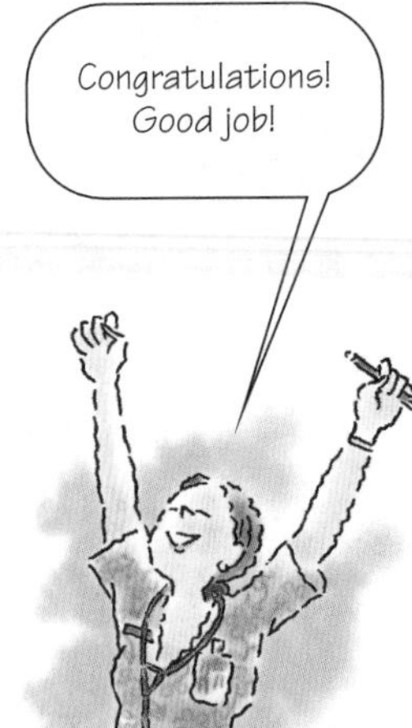
Congratulations!
Good job!

94. 2, 3, 4, 6. Impulsive behavior, overwhelming guilt, chronic illness, and anger repression are factors that contribute to suicide potential. Psychomotor retardation and decreased activity are symptoms of depression but don't typically lead to suicide because the client doesn't have the energy to harm himself.
CN: Psychosocial integrity; CNS: None; CL: Analysis

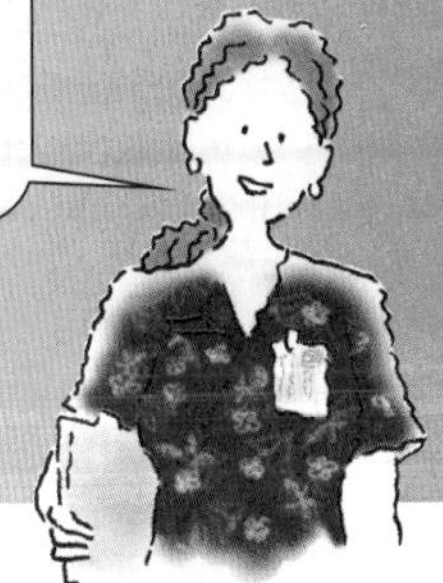

This chapter covers a host of cognitive disorders. Are your own cognitive powers ready? OK, let's go!

Chapter 15 Cognitive disorders

1. A nurse is assessing a client with dementia. Which disorder is the client most likely to have?

1. Alcohol withdrawal
2. Alzheimer's disease
3. Obsessive-compulsive disorder
4. Postpartum depression

1. 2. Dementia occurs in Alzheimer's disease and is generally progressive and deteriorating. The symptoms related to alcohol withdrawal result from alcohol intoxication. Effects of alcohol on the central nervous system include loss of memory, concentration, insight, and motor control. Obsessive-compulsive disorders are recurrent ideas, impulses, thoughts, or patterns of behavior that produce anxiety if resisted. Postpartum depression doesn't lead to dementia.

CN: Physiological integrity; CNS: Physiological adaptation; CL: Application

2. A physician diagnoses a client with dementia of the Alzheimer's type. Which statement about possible causes of this disorder is most accurate?

1. Alzheimer's disease is most commonly caused by cerebral abscess.
2. Chronic alcohol abuse plays a significant role in Alzheimer's disease.
3. Multiple small brain infarctions typically lead to Alzheimer's disease.
4. The cause of Alzheimer's disease is currently unknown.

2. 4. Several hypotheses suggest genetic factors, trauma, accumulation of aluminum, alterations in the immune system, or alterations in acetylcholine as contributing to the development of Alzheimer's disease, but the exact cause of Alzheimer's disease is unknown.

CN: Health promotion and maintenance; CNS: None; CL: Application

3. Of the following conditions that can cause symptoms similar to Alzheimer's disease, which is <u>reversible</u>?

1. Multiple sclerosis
2. Electrolyte imbalance
3. Multiple small brain infarctions
4. Human immunodeficiency virus infection

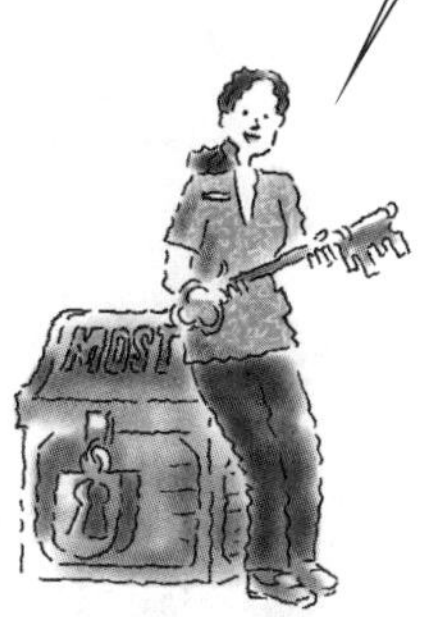

The key to the answer is the word *reversible*.

3. 2. Electrolyte imbalance is a correctable metabolic abnormality. The other conditions are irreversible.

CN: Physiological integrity; CNS: Physiological adaptation; CL: Application

CN: Client needs category CNS: Client needs subcategory CL: Cognitive level

4. In the early stages of Alzheimer's disease, which symptom is expected?
1. Dilated pupils
2. Rambling speech
3. Elevated blood pressure
4. Significant recent memory impairment

4. 4. Significant recent memory impairment, indicated by the inability to verbalize remembrances after several minutes to an hour, can be assessed in the early stages of Alzheimer's disease. Dilated pupils, rambling speech, and increased blood pressure are expected symptoms of delirium.

CN: Physiological integrity; CNS: Physiological adaptation; CL: Application

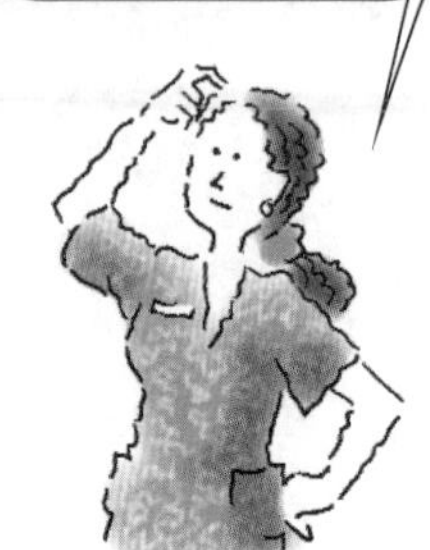

The answer is on the tip of my tongue, but I just can't remember.

5. A nurse is caring for a client with delirium. Which nursing intervention has the highest priority?
1. Providing a safe environment
2. Offering recreational activities
3. Providing a structured environment
4. Instituting measures to promote sleep

5. 1. The nurse's highest priority when caring for a client with delirium is to ensure client safety. Offering recreational activities, providing a structured environment, and promoting sleep are all appropriate interventions after safety measures are in place.

CN: Safe, effective care environment; CNS: Management of care; CL: Analysis

6. Which assessment finding shows impairment in abstract thinking and reasoning?
1. The client can't repeat a sentence.
2. The client has problems calculating simple problems.
3. The client doesn't know the name of the president of the United States.
4. The client can't find similarities and differences between related words or objects.

6. 4. Abstract thinking is assessed by noting similarities and differences between related words or objects. Not being able to repeat a sentence or do a simple calculation shows a client's inability to concentrate and focus on thoughts. Not knowing the president of the United States is a deficiency in general knowledge.

CN: Physiological integrity; CNS: Physiological adaptation; CL: Analysis

7. In addition to disturbances in cognition and orientation, a client with Alzheimer's disease may also show changes in which area?
1. Appetite
2. Energy levels
3. Hearing
4. Personality

7. 4. Personality change is common in dementia. There shouldn't be a remarkable change in appetite, energy level, or hearing.

CN: Physiological integrity; CNS: Physiological adaptation; CL: Application

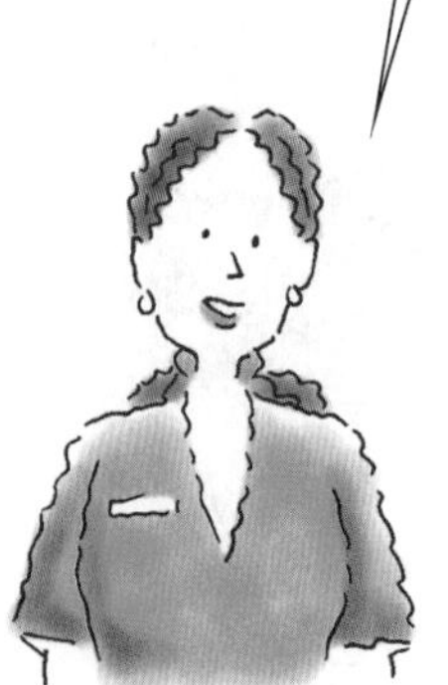

8. Which interventions should help a client diagnosed with Alzheimer's disease perform activities of daily living?
1. Have the client perform all basic care without help.
2. Tell the client morning care must be done by 9 a.m.
3. Give the client a written list of activities he's expected to do.
4. Encourage the client, and give ample time to complete basic tasks.

8. 4. Clients with Alzheimer's disease respond to the effect of those around them. A gentle, calm approach is comforting and nonthreatening, and a tense, hurried approach may agitate the client. The client has problems performing independently. The inherent expectations of deadlines and activity lists may lead to frustration.

CN: Physiological integrity; CNS: Basic care and comfort; CL: Application

9. Which of the following medications for Alzheimer's disease will improve cognition and functional autonomy?
1. Bupropion (Wellbutrin)
2. Haloperidol (Haldol)
3. Donepezil (Aricept)
4. Triazolam (Halcion)

9. 3. Donepezil is used to improve cognition and functional autonomy in mild to moderate dementia of the Alzheimer's type. Bupropion is used for depression. Haloperidol is used for agitation, aggression, hallucinations, thought disturbances, and wandering. Triazolam is used for sleep disturbances.

CN: Physiological integrity; CNS: Pharmacological and parenteral therapies; CL: Application

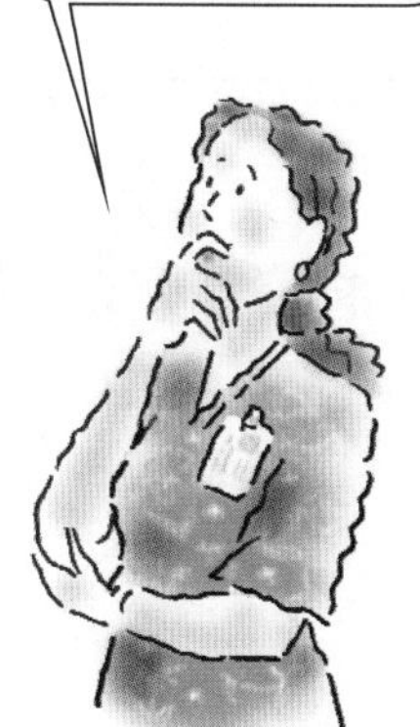

10. A nurse places an object in the hand of a client with Alzheimer's disease and asks the client to identify the object. Which term represents the client's inability to name the object?
1. Agnosia
2. Aphasia
3. Apraxia
4. Perseveration

10. 1. Agnosia is the inability to recognize familiar objects. Aphasia is characterized by an impaired ability to speak. Apraxia refers to the client's inability to use objects properly. All three impairments usually occur in stage 3 of Alzheimer's disease. Perseveration is continued repetition of a meaningless word or phrase that occurs in stage 2 of Alzheimer's disease.

CN: Health promotion and maintenance; CNS: None; CL: Application

11. Which nursing intervention will help a client with progressive memory deficit function in his environment?
1. Help the client do simple tasks by giving step-by-step directions.
2. Avoid frustrating the client by performing basic care routines for the client.
3. Stimulate the client's intellectual functioning by bringing new topics to the client's attention.
4. Promote the use of the client's sense of humor by telling jokes or riddles and discussing cartoons.

11. 1. Clients with cognitive impairment should do all the tasks they can. By receiving simple directions in a step-by-step fashion, the client can better process information and perform tasks. Stimulation of intellect can be accomplished by discussing familiar topics with them; changes in topics may add to their confusion. Clients with cognitive impairment may not be able to understand the joke or riddle, and cartoons may add to their confusion.

CN: Psychosocial integrity; CNS: None; CL: Application

12. Which intervention is an important part of providing care to a client diagnosed with Alzheimer's disease?
1. Avoid physical contact.
2. Confine the client to his room.
3. Provide a high level of sensory stimulation.
4. Monitor the client carefully.

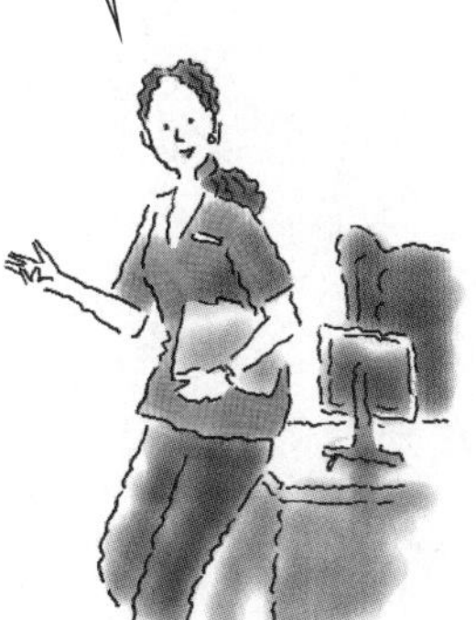

Look for the answer that makes the most safety sense.

12. 4. Whenever client safety is at risk, careful observation and supervision are of ultimate importance in avoiding injury. Physical contact is implemented during basic care. Confining the client may cause agitation and combativeness. A high level of sensory stimulation may be too stimulating and distracting.

CN: Safe, effective care environment; CNS: Management of care; CL: Application

13. Which nursing intervention is the most important in caring for a client diagnosed with Alzheimer's disease?

1. Make sure the environment is safe to prevent injury.
2. Make sure the client receives food she likes to prevent hunger.
3. Make sure the client meets other clients to prevent social isolation.
4. Make sure the client takes care of her daily physical care to prevent dependence.

13. 1. Providing client safety is the number one priority when caring for any client but particularly when a client is already compromised and at greater risk for injury. The other options may be part of caring for a client with Alzheimer's disease but they are not the priority.

CN: Safe, effective care environment; CNS: Safety and infection control; CL: Application

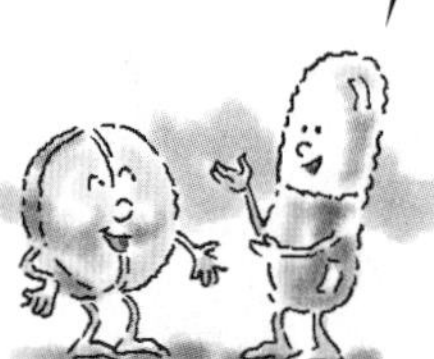

14. Which medication is used to decrease the agitation, violence, and bizarre thoughts associated with dementia?

1. Diazepam (Valium)
2. Ergoloid (Hydergine)
3. Haloperidol (Haldol)
4. Tacrine (Cognex)

14. 3. Haloperidol is an antipsychotic that decreases the symptoms of agitation, violence, and bizarre thoughts. Diazepam is used for anxiety and muscle relaxation. Ergoloid is an adrenergic blocker used to block vascular headaches. Tacrine is used for improvement of cognition.

CN: Physiological integrity; CNS: Reduction of risk potential; CL: Application

15. A client diagnosed with Alzheimer's disease tells the nurse that today she has a luncheon date with her daughter, *who is not visiting that day.* Which response by the nurse would be most appropriate for this situation?

1. "Where are you planning on having your lunch?"
2. "You're confused and don't know what you're saying."
3. "I think you need some more medication, and I'll bring it to you."
4. "Today is Monday, March 8, and we'll be eating lunch in the dining room."

15. 4. The best nursing response is to reorient the client to the date and environment. Humoring the client isn't therapeutic. Medication won't provide immediate relief for memory impairment. Confrontation can provoke an outburst.

CN: Psychosocial integrity; CNS: None; CL: Application

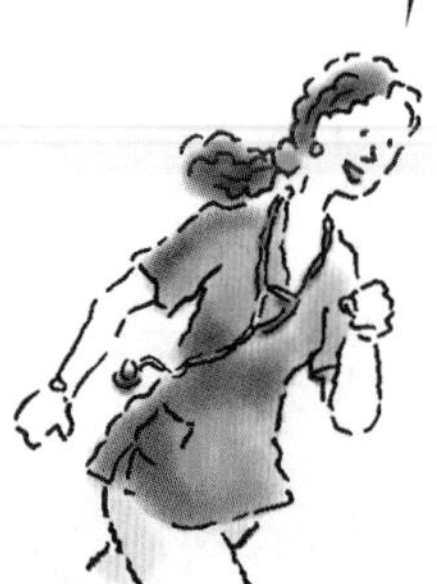

You're already at question 15 and doing great. Keep going!

16. Which feature is characteristic of cognitive disorders?

1. Catatonia
2. Depression
3. Feeling of dread
4. Deficit in memory

16. 4. Cognitive disorders represent a significant change in cognition or memory from a previous level of functioning. Catatonia is a type of schizophrenia characterized by periods of physical rigidity, negativism, excitement, and stupor. Depression is a feeling of sadness and apathy and is part of major depressive and other mood disorders. A feeling of dread is characteristic of an anxiety disorder.

CN: Physiological integrity; CNS: Physiological adaptation; CL: Application

17. A nurse is assessing an elderly client who is admitted with progressive deterioration in cognition. The client most likely has which degenerative disorder?
1. Delirium
2. Dementia
3. Neurosis
4. Psychosis

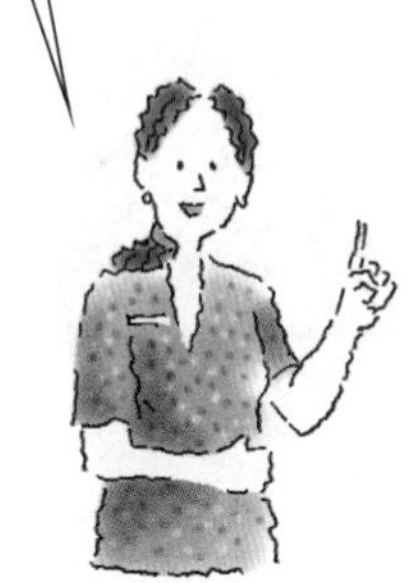

Only one of these disorders is degenerative.

17. 2. Dementia is progressive and often associated with aging or underlying metabolic or organic deterioration. Delirium is characterized by abrupt, spontaneous cognitive dysfunction with an underyling organic mental disorder. Neurosis and psychosis are psychological diagnoses.

CN: Physiological integrity; CNS: Physiological adaptation; CL: Application

18. A nurse is teaching the family of a client with dementia. Which of the following responses by the nurse would be the most accurate definition of dementia?
1. Personal neglect in self-care
2. Poor judgment, especially in social situations
3. Memory loss occurring as a natural consequence of aging
4. Loss of intellectual abilities sufficient to impair the ability to perform basic care

18. 4. The ability to perform self-care is an important measure of the progression of dementia. Memory loss reflects underlying physical, metabolic, and pathologic processes. Personal neglect and poor judgment typically occur in dementia but aren't considered defining characteristics.

CN: Physiological integrity; CNS: Physiological adaptation; CL: Application

19. Asking a client with a suspected dementia disorder to recall what she ate for breakfast would assess which area?
1. Food preferences
2. Recent memory
3. Remote memory
4. Speech

19. 2. Persons with dementia have difficulty in recent memory or learning, which may be a key to early detection. Assessing food preferences may be helpful in determining what the client likes to eat, but this assessment has no direct correlation in assessing dementia. Speech difficulties, such as rambling, irrelevance, and incoherence, may be related to delirium.

CN: Health promotion and maintenance; CNS: None; CL: Application

20. Which factor is the most important to determine when collecting data for a definitive diagnosis of a dementia disorder?
1. Prognosis
2. Genetic information
3. Degree of impairment
4. Implications for treatment

20. 4. The progression of biological impairment in the central nervous system is a function of the underlying pathologic states, so it's important to collect data and treat the underlying cause. Prognosis isn't the most important factor when making a diagnosis. Genetic information isn't relevant. The degree of impairment is necessary information for developing a care plan.

CN: Health promotion and maintenance; CNS: None; CL: Analysis

21. What is considered the primary causative factor for vascular dementia?
1. Head trauma
2. Genetic factors
3. Acetylcholine alteration
4. Interruption of blood flow to the brain

This question is asking specifically about vascular dementia.
STOP

21. 4. The cause of vascular dementia is directly related to an interruption of blood flow to the brain. Head trauma, genetic factors, and acetylcholine alteration are causative factors related to dementia of the Alzheimer's type.

CN: Physiological integrity; CNS: Physiological adaptation; CL: Application

22. The family of a client recently admitted with vascular dementia asks the nurse about the cause of the client's condition. Which of the following would be the most accurate response by the nurse?

1. "It is caused by high blood pressure."
2. "It is caused by low oxygen levels."
3. "It is caused by an infection."
4. "It is caused by toxins."

22. 1. Vascular dementia is a result of small strokes that can either destroy or damage cerebral tissue. Strokes may be caused by high blood pressure, high cholesterol levels, heart disease, or diabetes. Hypoxia, infection, and toxins aren't causes of dementia.

CN: Physiological integrity; CNS: Physiological adaptation; CL: Application

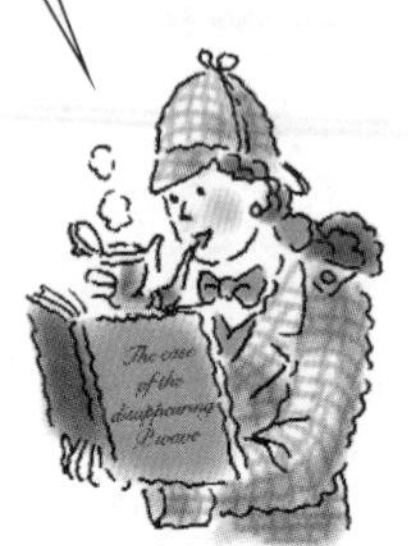

Let's see! What is the cause?

23. Which assessment finding is expected for a client with vascular dementia?

1. Hypersomnolence
2. Insomnia
3. Restlessness
4. Small-stepped gait

23. 4. Focal neurologic signs commonly seen with vascular dementia include weakness of the limbs, small-stepped gait, and difficulty with speech. Insomnia, hypersomnolence, and restlessness are symptoms related to delirium.

CN: Physiological integrity; CNS: Physiological adaptation; CL: Application

24. The spouse of a client diagnosed with vascular dementia asks the nurse how this disorder differs from Alzheimer's disease. Which response from the nurse is most appropriate?

1. "Vascular dementia has a more abrupt onset."
2. "Vascular dementia develops slowly."
3. "Personality change is common in vascular dementia."
4. "The inability to perform motor activities occurs in vascular dementia."

24. 1. Vascular dementia differs from Alzheimer's disease in that it has a more abrupt onset and runs a highly variable course. Personality change is common in Alzheimer's disease. The inability to carry out motor activities is common in Alzheimer's disease.

CN: Health promotion and maintenance; CNS: None; CL: Application

25. A progression of symptoms that occurs in steps rather than a gradual deterioration indicates which type of dementia?

1. Alzheimer's dementia
2. Parkinson's dementia
3. Substance-induced dementia
4. Vascular dementia

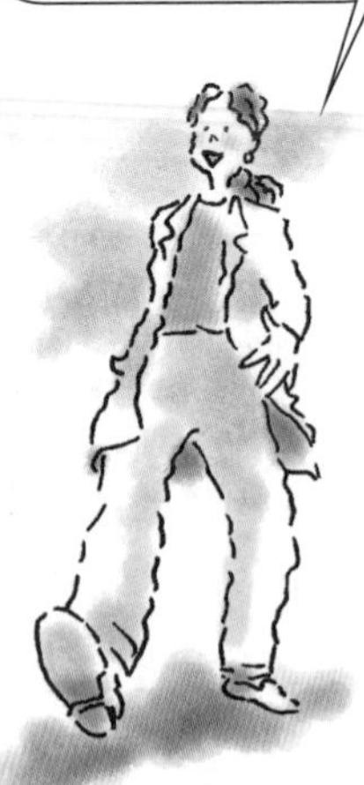

You've taken the first steps towards understanding the many types of dementia.

25. 4. Vascular dementia differs from Alzheimer's disease in that vascular dementia has a more abrupt onset and progresses in steps. At times the dementia seems to clear up, and the individual shows fairly lucid thinking. Dementia of the Alzheimer's type has a slow onset with a progressive and deteriorating course. Dementia of Parkinson's sometimes resembles the dementia of Alzheimer's disease. Substance-induced dementia is related to the persisting effects of use of a substance.

CN: Physiological integrity; CNS: Physiological adaptation; CL: Analysis

26. Which pathophysiological change in the brain causes the symptoms of Alzheimer's disease?

1. Glucose inadequacy
2. Atrophy of the frontal lobe
3. Degeneration of the cholinergic system
4. Intracranial bleeding in the limbic system

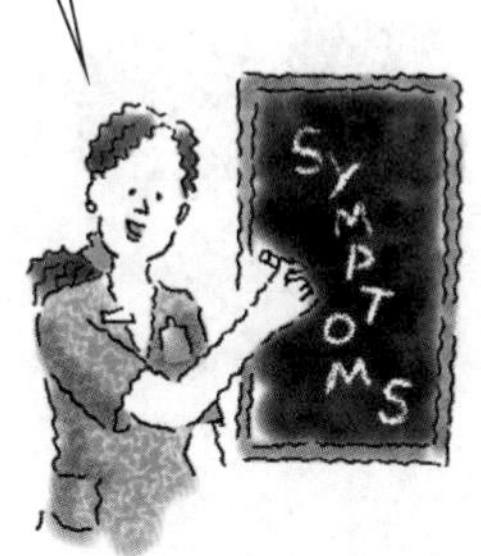

Which one of these changes is a cause of Alzheimer's symptoms?
SYMPTOMS

26. 3. Research related to Alzheimer's disease indicates that the enzyme needed to produce acetylcholine is dramatically reduced. The other pathophysiological changes don't cause the symptoms of Alzheimer's disease

CN: Physiological integrity; CNS: Physiological adaptation; CL: Analysis

27. An elderly client has experienced memory and attention deficits that developed over a 3-day period. These symptoms are characteristic of which disorder?

1. Alzheimer's disease
2. Amnesia syndrome
3. Delirium
4. Dementia

27. 3. Delirium is characterized by an abrupt onset of fluctuating levels of awareness, clouded consciousness, perceptual disturbances, and disturbed memory and orientation. Alzheimer's disease is a progressive dementia. Amnesia refers to recent short-term and long-term memory loss. Dementia is characterized by general impairment in intellectual functioning and occurs in a progressive, irreversible course.

CN: Physiological integrity; CNS: Physiological adaptation; CL: Application

28. Which age-group is at high risk for developing a state of delirium?

1. Adolescent
2. Elderly
3. Middle-aged
4. School-aged

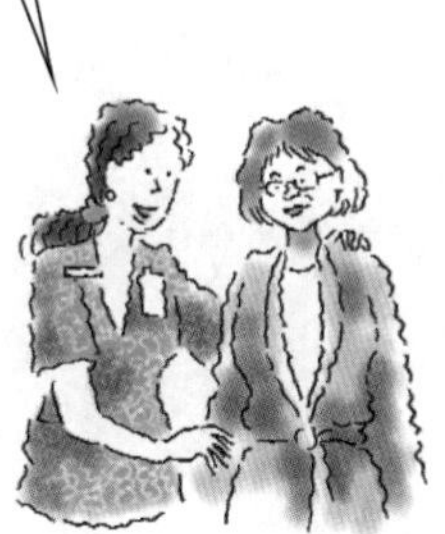

Age is an important factor when assessing a client.

28. 2. The elderly population, because of normal physiological changes, is highly susceptible to delirium. All the other options are incorrect.

CN: Health promotion and maintenance; CNS: None; CL: Application

29. Which nursing diagnosis is best for an elderly client experiencing visual and auditory hallucinations?

1. *Interrupted family processes*
2. *Ineffective role performance*
3. *Impaired verbal communication*
4. *Disturbed sensory perception (visual, auditory)*

29. 4. The client is experiencing visual and auditory hallucinations related to a sensory alteration. The other options don't address the hallucinations the client is experiencing.

CN: Health promotion and maintenance; CNS: None; CL: Application

30. Which intervention is the most appropriate for clients with cognitive disorders?
1. Promote socialization.
2. Maintain optimal physical health.
3. Provide frequent changes in personnel.
4. Provide an overstimulating environment.

30. 2. A client's cognitive impairment may hinder self-care abilities. More socialization, frequent changes in staff members, and an overstimulating environment would only increase anxiety and confusion.
CN: Health promotion and maintenance; CNS: None; CL: Application

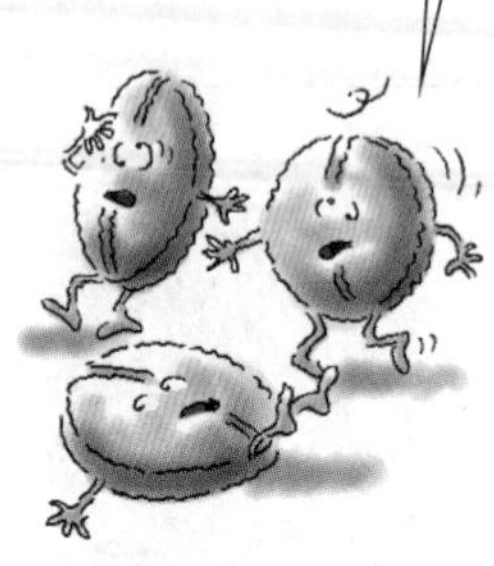

Sometimes we're not a good combination.

31. A newly admitted client diagnosed with delirium has a history of hypertension and anxiety. The client had been taking digoxin, furosemide (Lasix), and diazepam (Valium) for anxiety. This client's impairment may be related to which condition?
1. Infection
2. Metabolic acidosis
3. Drug intoxication
4. Hepatic encephalopathy

31. 3. This client was taking several medications that have a propensity for producing delirium; digoxin (a cardiac glycoside), furosemide (a thiazide diuretic), and diazepam (a benzodiazepine). Sufficient supporting data don't exist to suspect the other options as causes.
CN: Physiological integrity; CNS: Physiological adaptation; CL: Analysis

32. Which environment is the most appropriate for a client experiencing sensory-perceptual alterations?
1. A softly lit room around the clock
2. A brightly lit room around the clock
3. Sitting by the nurses' desk while out of bed
4. A quiet, well-lit room without glare during the day and a darkened room for sleeping

32. 4. A quiet, shadow-free environment produces the fewest sensory-perceptual distortions for a client with cognitive impairment associated with delirium.
CN: Psychosocial integrity; CNS: None; CL: Application

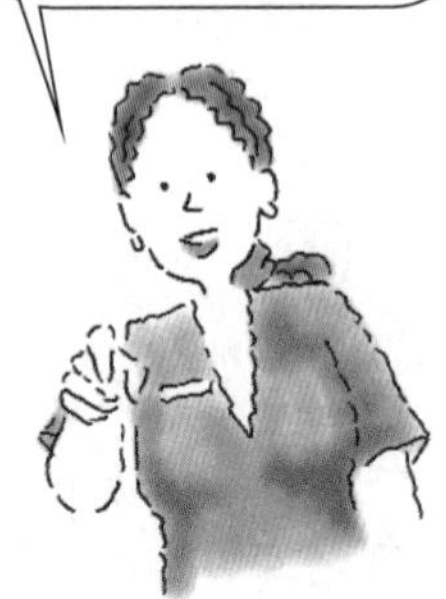

Your clients depend on you for meeting their environmental needs as well as their physical ones.

33. As a nurse enters a client's room, the client says, "They're crawling on my sheets! Get them off my bed!" Which assessment is the most accurate?
1. The client is experiencing aphasia.
2. The client is experiencing dysarthria.
3. The client is experiencing a flight of ideas.
4. The client is experiencing visual hallucinations.

33. 4. The presence of a sensory stimulus correlates with the definition of a hallucination, which is a false sensory perception. Aphasia refers to a communications problem. Dysarthria is difficulty in speech production. Flight of ideas is rapid shifting from one topic to another.
CN: Psychosocial integrity; CNS: None; CL: Application

34. A delirious client is shouting for someone to get the bugs off her. Which response is the most appropriate?

1. "Don't worry, I'll stay here and brush away the bugs for you."
2. "Try to relax. The crawling sensation will go away sooner if you can relax."
3. "There are no bugs on your legs. It's just your imagination playing tricks on you."
4. "I know you're frightened. I don't see bugs crawling on your legs, but I'll stay here with you."

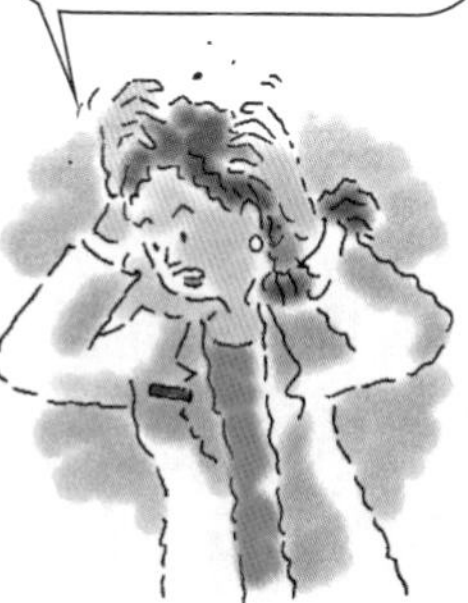

This question is really starting to bug me.

34. 4. Never argue about hallucinations with a client. Instead, promote an environment of trust and safety by acknowledging the client's perceptions.

CN: Physiological integrity; CNS: Basic care and comfort; CL: Application

35. Which description of a client's experience and behavior can be assessed as an illusion?

1. The client tries to hit the nurse when vital signs must be taken.
2. The client says, "I keep hearing a voice telling me to run away."
3. The client becomes anxious whenever the nurse leaves the bedside.
4. The client looks at the shadows on a wall and tells the nurse she sees frightening faces on the wall.

35. 4. An illusion is an inaccurate perception or false response to a sensory stimulus. Auditory hallucinations are associated with sound and are more common in schizophrenia. Anxiety and agitation can be secondary to illusions.

CN: Physiological integrity; CNS: Physiological adaptation; CL: Analysis

36. Which neurologic change is an <u>expected</u> characteristic of aging?

1. Widening of the sulci
2. Depletion of neurotransmitters
3. Neurofibrillary tangles and plaques
4. Degeneration of the frontal and temporal lobes

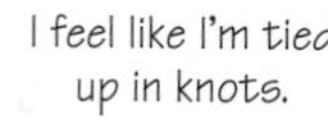

I feel like I'm tied up in knots.

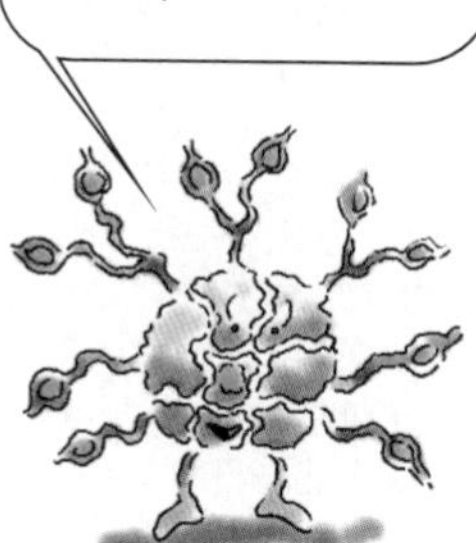

36. 3. Aging isn't necessarily associated with significant decline, but neurofibrillary tangles and plaques are expected changes. These normal occurrences are sometimes referred to as benign senescent forgetfulness of age-associated memory impairment.

CN: Physiological integrity; CNS: Physiological adaptation; CL: Analysis

37. A major consideration in assessing memory impairment in an elderly individual includes which factor?

1. Allergies
2. Past surgery
3. Age at onset of symptoms
4. Social and occupational lifestyle

37. 4. Minor memory problems are distinguished from dementia by their minor severity and their lack of significant interference with the client's social or occupational lifestyle. Other options would be included in the history data but don't directly correlate with the client's lifestyle.

CN: Psychosocial integrity; CNS: None; CL: Analysis

38. During morning care, a nursing assistant asks a client with dementia, "How was your night?" The client replies, "My husband and I went out to dinner and a movie and had a wonderful evening!" Which state best describes the client's actions?

1. Delirium
2. Perseveration
3. Confabulation
4. Showing a sense of humor

38. 3. Confabulation is the process in which an individual makes up stories to answer questions. It's considered a defense tactic to protect the individual's self-esteem and prevent others from noticing the memory loss. Delirium is a state of mental confusion and excitement characterized by disorientation to time and place, often with hallucinations, incoherent speech, and a continual state of aimless physical activity. Perseveration is persistent repetition of the same word or idea in response to different questions. The client's response isn't meant to be humorous.

CN: Psychosocial integrity; CNS: None; CL: Application

39. A nursing assistant tells a nurse, "The client with amnesia looks fine but responds to questions in a vague, distant manner. What should I be doing for her?" Which response is the most appropriate?

1. "Give her lots of space to test her independence."
2. "Keep her busy and make sure she doesn't take naps during the day."
3. "Whenever you think she needs direction, use short, simple sentences."
4. "Spend as much time with her as you can, and ask questions about her recent life."

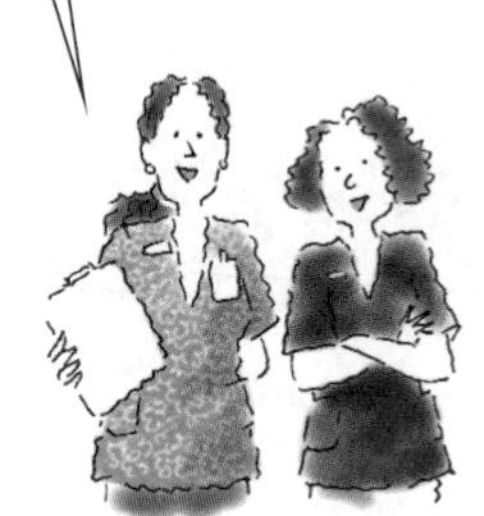

Teaching nursing assistants helps to improve the quality of care they provide.

39. 3. Disruptions in the ability to perform basic care, confusion, and anxiety are often apparent in clients with amnesia. Offering simple directions to promote daily functions and reduce confusion helps increase feelings of safety and security. Giving this client lots of space may make her feel insecure. Asking her many questions that she won't be able to answer just intensifies her anxiety level. There is no significant rationale for keeping her busy all day with no rest periods; the client may become more tired and less functional at other basic tasks.

CN: Safe, effective care environment; CNS: Management of care; CL: Application

40. With amnestic disorders, in which cognitive area is a change expected?

1. Speech
2. Concentration
3. Intellectual function
4. Recent short-term and long-term memory

40. 4. The primary area affected in amnesia is memory; all other areas of cognition are normal.

CN: Physiological integrity; CNS: Physiological adaptation; CL: Application

41. Which nursing action is the best way to help a client with mild Alzheimer's disease to remain functional?

1. Obtain a physician's order for a mild anxiolytic to control behavior.
2. Call attention to all mistakes so they can be quickly corrected.
3. Advise the client to move into a retirement center.
4. Maintain a stable, predictable environment and daily routine.

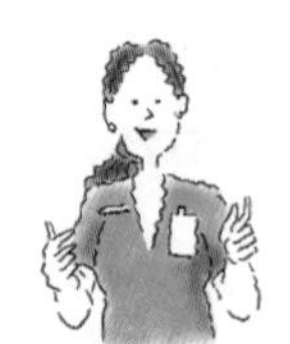

Question 41 is asking which action is best.

41. 4. Clients in the early stages of Alzheimer's disease remain fairly functional with familiar surroundings and a predictable routine. They become easily disoriented with surprises and social overstimulation. Anxiolytics can impair memory and worsen the problem. Calling attention to all the client's mistakes is nonproductive and serves to lower the client's self-esteem. Moving to an unfamiliar environment will heighten the client's agitation and confusion.

CN: Psychosocial integrity; CNS: None; CL: Application

CN: Client needs category CNS: Client needs subcategory CL: Cognitive level

42. The nurse is providing nursing care to a client with Alzheimer's-type dementia. Which nursing intervention takes top priority?

1. Establish a routine that supports former habits.
2. Maintain physical surroundings that are cheerful and pleasant.
3. Maintain an exact routine from day to day.
4. Control the environment by providing structure, boundaries, and safety.

42. 4. By controlling the environment and providing structure and boundaries, the nurse is helping to keep the client safe and secure, which is a top-priority nursing measure. Establishing a routine that supports former habits and maintaining cheerful, pleasant surroundings and an exact routine foster a supportive environment; however, keeping the client safe and secure takes priority.

CN: Safe, effective care environment; CNS: Management of care; CL: Application

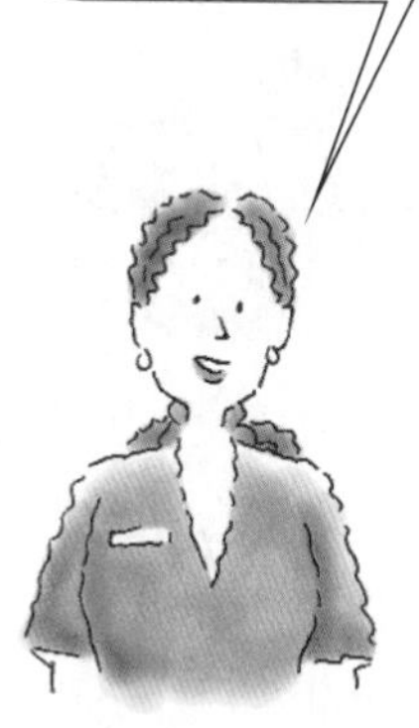

You need to determine which approach is best.

43. The nurse finds a 78-year-old client with Alzheimer's-type dementia wandering in the hall at 3 a.m. The client has removed his clothing and says to the nurse, "I'm just taking a stroll through the park." What's the best approach to this behavior?

1. Immediately help the client back to his room and into some clothing.
2. Tell the client that such behavior won't be tolerated.
3. Tell the client it's too early in the morning to be taking a stroll.
4. Ask the client if he would like to go back to his room.

43. 1. The nurse shouldn't allow the client to embarrass himself in front of others. Intervene as soon as the behavior is observed. Scolding the client isn't helpful because it isn't something the client can understand. Don't engage in social chatter. The interaction with this client should be concrete and specific. Don't ask the client to choose unnecessarily. The client may not be able to make appropriate choices.

CN: Psychosocial integrity; CNS: None; CL: Application

44. Which nursing diagnosis is appropriate for a client diagnosed with an amnestic disorder?

1. *Grieving*
2. *Ineffective denial*
3. *Ineffective coping*
4. *Risk for injury*

44. 4. Changes in cognitive ability place a client at high risk for injury. The client isn't aware of a loss and therefore doesn't grieve for it. The client isn't in denial but has an impaired ability to learn new information or to remember past information. The client isn't aware of a need to cope.

CN: Safe, effective care environment; CNS: Management of care; CL: Analysis

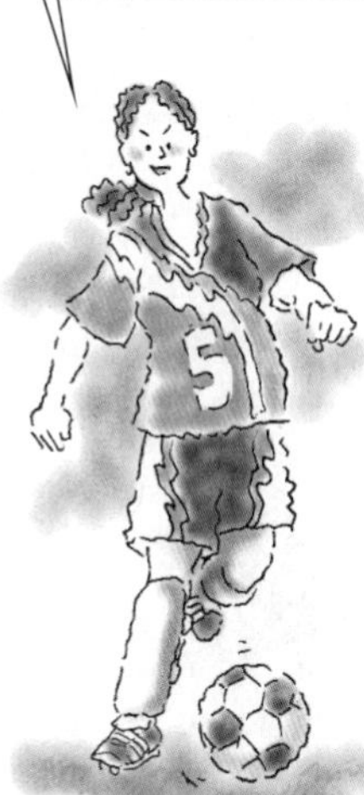

You've reached question 45. Now's the time to kick it into high gear!
5

45. The nurse is planning care for a client who was admitted with dementia due to Alzheimer's disease. The family reports that the client has to be watched closely for wandering behavior at night. Which nursing diagnosis is the nurse's top priority?

1. *Disturbed sleep pattern*
2. *Insomnia*
3. *Risk for injury*
4. *Activity intolerance*

45. 3. Providing a safe, effective care environment takes priority with this client. *Disturbed sleep pattern*, *Insomnia*, and *Activity intolerance* are important but not the priority.

CN: Safe, effective care environment; CNS: Management of care; CL: Application

46. Which medical condition may be associated with an amnestic disorder?

1. Drug overdose
2. Cerebral anoxia
3. Medications (anticonvulsants)
4. Lead, mercury, and carbon dioxide toxins

46. 2. A variety of medical conditions are related to amnestic disorders, such as head trauma, stroke, cerebral neoplastic disease, herpes simplex, encephalitis, poorly controlled insulin-dependent diabetes, and cerebral anoxia. The other three options are substance-induced.

CN: Physiological integrity; CNS: Physiological adaptation; CL: Application

47. Which laboratory evaluation is an expected part of the *initial* workup for an amnestic disorder?

1. Angiography
2. Cardiac catheterization
3. Electrocardiography
4. Metabolic and endocrine tests

47. 4. An amnesic disorder is caused by either physiological effects of a medical condition or effects of a substance, medication, or toxin, so metabolic and endocrine tests should be done. The other options are diagnostic tests related to the cardiovascular system.

CN: Health promotion and maintenance; CNS: None; CL: Application

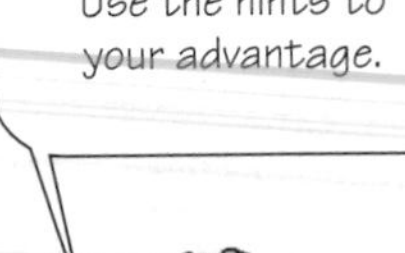

Use the hints to your advantage.

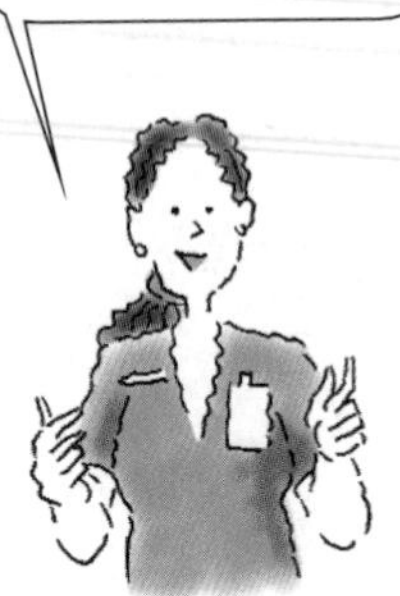

48. Which nursing intervention is appropriate for a client with memory impairment?

1. Speak to the client in a high-pitched tone.
2. Offer low-dose sedative-hypnotic drugs.
3. Ask a series of questions when obtaining information.
4. Identify yourself and look directly into the client's eyes.

48. 4. Clients with memory impairments need to reestablish the nurse's identification constantly. High-pitched tones may create more anxiety. A low-dose sedative-hypnotic medication may be used to promote rapid-eye-movement sleep. Asking a series of questions may create confusion; ask only one question at a time.

CN: Safe, effective care environment; CNS: Management of care; CL: Application

49. Transient global amnesia is generally associated with which disorder?

1. Adjustment disorders
2. Cardiac anomalies
3. Cerebrovascular disease
4. Sleep disorders

49. 3. Transient global amnesia is usually associated with cerebrovascular disease that involves transient impairment in blood flow through the vertebrobasilar arteries. No correlation exists with the other options.

CN: Physiological integrity; CNS: Physiological adaptation; CL: Analysis

50. During conversation with a client, the nurse observes that he shifts from one topic to the next on a regular basis. Which disorder is the client *most likely* to have?

1. Flight of ideas
2 Concrete thinking
3 Ideas of reference
4. Loose associations

50. 4. Loose associations are conversations that constantly shift in topic. Loose associations don't necessarily start in a disorganized way; the conversations can begin cogently, then become loose. Flight of ideas is characterized by conversation that's disorganized from the onset. Concrete thinking implies highly definitive thought processes. Ideas of reference is characterized by a delusional belief that things irrelevant to the client, such as newspaper headlines, are referring to the client directly.

CN: Psychosocial integrity; CNS: None; CL: Application

Hey! You've answered 50 questions. Awesome!

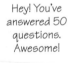

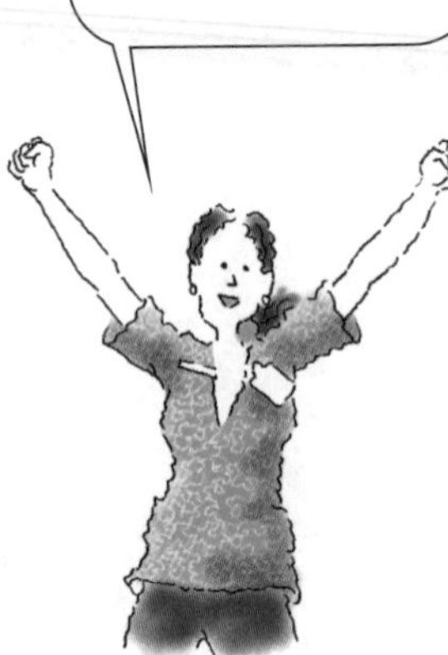

51. For a client with dementia, which assessment finding indicates worsening of dementia?
1. The client resists logical explanations.
2. The client stops redirecting negative energy.
3. The client stops maintaining a nondefensive position.
4. The client becomes increasingly agitated.

51. 4. A client with dementia who becomes increasingly agitated may be unable to perform expected tasks. Communication must be clear and concise; giving logical explanations is inappropriate. This client may revert to old ways of coping, and trying to change the client rarely proves successful; the nurse should try to decrease the source of negativity. The client with dementia is rarely defensive.

CN: Psychosocial integrity; CNS: None; CL: Analysis

52. For the family of a client with Alzheimer's disease, one goal is effective communication. Which outcome is successful for this goal?
1. Family members don't use humor with the client.
2. Family members speak to the client in a loud voice.
3. Family members give the client one-step commands.
4. Family members don't touch the client while speaking.

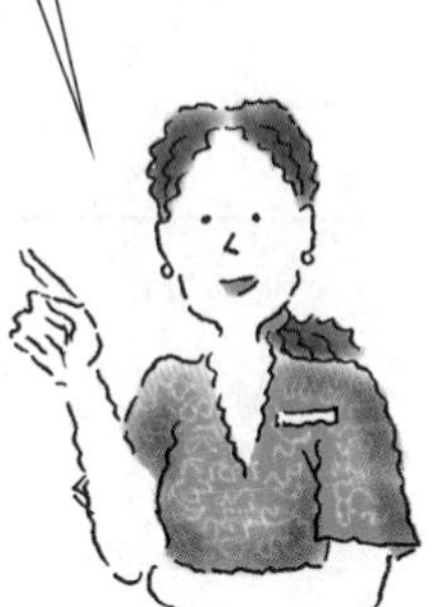

For effective communications, think clear and concise.

52. 3. Giving one-step commands keeps communication simple, clear, concise, and pleasant. Humor must be used judiciously so as not to confuse the client. Speaking in a loud voice may be interpreted as shouting and cause agitation. Depending on the situation, the use of touch may be appropriate, helping to reassure and soothe the client.

CN: Psychosocial integrity; CNS: None; CL: Application

53. Immediately after visiting hours, a nurse identifies wandering behavior in a client with Alzheimer's disease. The client is showing which behavior?
1. The client may need to walk after eating a complete meal.
2. The client may feel tense because of an uncomfortable situation.
3. The client may be demonstrating several eccentric behaviors.
4. The client may have difficulty following directions.

53. 2. Tension and stress may cause a client with Alzheimer's disease to want to get away from an uncomfortable situation. Exercise is an important health promotion activity, but it doesn't help explain wandering behavior. Eccentric behaviors are rarely related to wandering. Many clients with dementia have difficulty following directions; however, wandering typically results from disorientation.

CN: Psychosocial integrity; CNS: None; CL: Application

54. For a client with dementia who lives in a long-term care facility, which outcome takes the highest nursing care priority?
1. Maintaining the client's optimal level of functioning
2. Identifying coping methods the client can use to handle stress
3. Facilitating client conversation with five people each day
4. Having the client use physical activity to work off aggressive energy

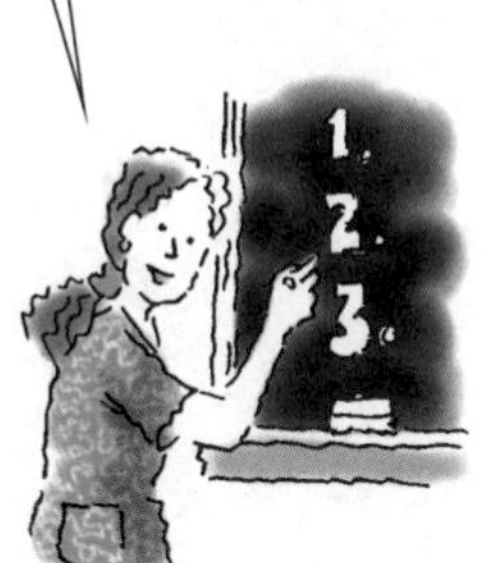

As a nurse, you will often need to prioritize!
1.
2.
3.

54. 1. The highest nursing care priority is to maintain the client's optimal level of functioning. Reducing the client's stress is the nurse's responsibility. Having a conversation with five people each day is unrealistic for this client. Expecting a client with dementia to use physical activity to decrease aggressive energy is also unrealistic.

CN: Safe, effective care environment; CNS: Management of care; CL: Application

55. A nurse is assessing a client for dementia. What history would the nurse expect to find in a client with dementia? Select all that apply:

1. There's a slow progression of symptoms.
2. The client admits to feelings of sadness.
3. The client acts apathetic and pessimistic.
4. The family can't determine when the symptoms first appeared.
5. There are changes in the client's basic personality.
6. The client has great difficulty paying attention to others.

55. 1, 4, 5, 6. Common characteristics of dementia are a slow onset of symptoms, which makes it difficult to determine when they first occurred. It progresses to noticeable changes in the client's personality and impaired ability to pay attention to other people. Feelings of sadness, apathy, and pessimism are symptoms of depression.

CN: Health promotion and maintenance; CNS: None; CL: Analysis

56. A delusional client approaches a nurse, states, "I am the Easter Bunny," and insists that the nurse refer to him as such. Which nursing interventions should the nurse implement when working with this client? Select all that apply:

1. Consistently use the client's name in interaction.
2. Smile at the humor of the situation.
3. Agree that the client is the Easter Bunny.
4. Logically point out why the client could not be the Easter Bunny.
5. Provide as-needed medication.
6. Provide the client with structured activities.

56. 1, 6. Continued reality-based orientation is necessary, so it is appropriate to use the client's name in any interaction. Structured activities can help the client refocus and resolve his delusion. The nurse shouldn't contribute to the delusion by going along with the situation. Logical arguments and as-needed medication aren't likely to change the client's beliefs.

CN: Psychosocial integrity; CNS: None; CL: Analysis

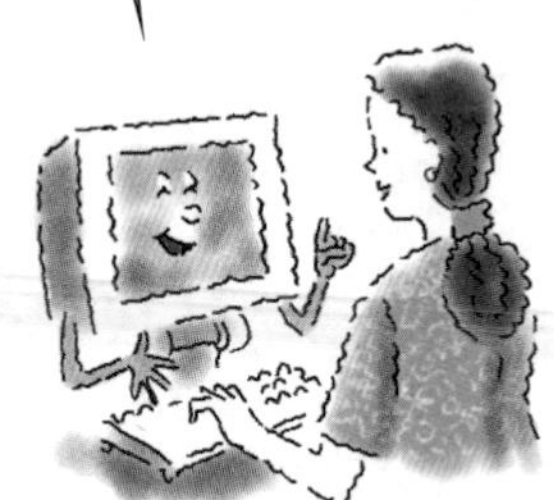

Wow! You completed this chapter in record time. There's nothing wrong with your cognitive skills!

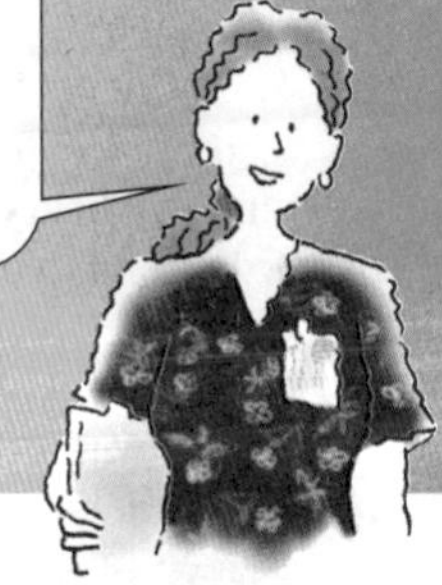

No, this chapter doesn't cover quirks of the rich and famous. It's all about mental disorders affecting the personality. Have a blast!

Chapter 16 Personality disorders

1. A client tells the nurse that her coworkers are sabotaging the computer. When the nurse asks questions, the client becomes argumentative. Which intervention would be most appropriate for the nurse to implement?

1. Encourage the client to vent his anger about his coworkers.
2. Tell the client that his coworkers haven't touched his computer.
3. Use clear and consistent speech when talking to the client.
4. Tell the client to go to his room and stay there until he calms down.

1. 3. Using clear and consistent speech when talking with the client helps him focus on reality and fosters a therapeutic relationship. Encouraging the client to vent his anger at his coworkers validates his suspicious thoughts and may make him more argumentative. Trying to convince him that his coworkers haven't touched his computer or telling him to go to his room may make him more defensive.

CN: Psychosocial integrity; CNS: None; CL: Analysis

2. A nurse observes that a client is mistrustful and shows hostile behavior. Which type of personality disorder is the client <u>most likely</u> to have?

1. Antisocial
2. Avoidant
3. Borderline
4. Paranoid

2. 4. Paranoid individuals have a need to constantly scan the environment for signs of betrayal, deception, and ridicule, appearing mistrustful and hostile. They expect to be tricked or deceived by others. The extreme suspiciousness is lacking in antisocial personalities, who tend to be more arrogant and self-assured despite their vigilance and mistrust. Individuals with avoidant personality disorders are guarded, fearing interpersonal rejection and humiliation. Clients with borderline personality disorders behave impulsively and tend to manipulate others.

CN: Psychosocial integrity; CNS: None; CL: Application

3. The nurse is caring for a client with paranoid personality disorder. Which behavior is a common characteristic of this disorder?

1. The client can't follow limits set on his behavior.
2. The client is afraid another person will inflict harm.
3. The client avoids responsibility for his health care.
4. The client depends on others to make important decisions.

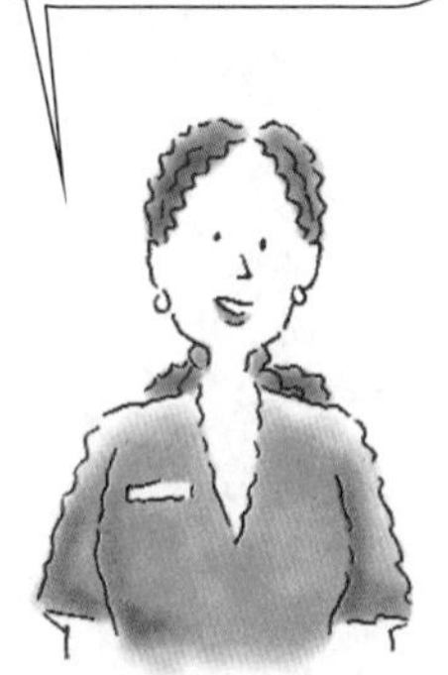

Understanding a client's traits will help you deal with him effectively.

3. 2. A client with paranoid personality disorder is afraid others will inflict harm. An individual with antisocial personality disorder won't be able to follow the limits set on behavior. An individual with an avoidant personality might avoid responsibility for health care because he tends to scan the environment for threatening things. A client with dependent personality disorder is likely to want others to make important decisions for him.

CN: Psychosocial integrity; CNS: None; CL: Analysis

CN: Client needs category CNS: Client needs subcategory CL: Cognitive level

4. Which statement is typical for a client diagnosed with paranoid personality disorder?
1. "I understand you're to blame."
2. "I must be seen first; it's not negotiable."
3. "I see nothing humorous in this situation."
4. "I wish someone would select the outfit for me."

4. 3. Clients with paranoid personality disorder tend to be extremely serious and lack a sense of humor. Clients with borderline personality disorder tend to blame others for their problems. Clients with narcissistic personality disorders have a sense of self-importance and entitlement. Clients with dependent personality disorder want others to make their decisions.
CN: Psychosocial integrity; CNS: None; CL: Analysis

5. Which characteristic is expected for a client with paranoid personality disorder who receives bad news?
1. The client is overly dramatic after hearing the facts.
2. The client focuses on self to not become overanxious.
3. The client responds from a rational, objective point of view.
4. The client doesn't spend time thinking about the information.

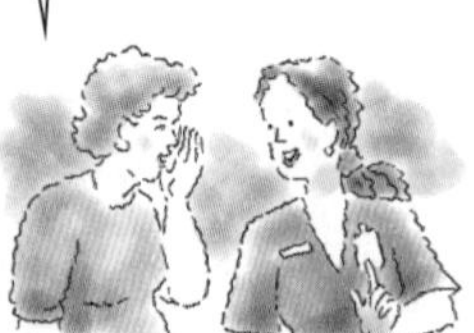

Pssst! Do you want to know the answer to this question?

5. 3. Clients with paranoid personality disorder are affectively restricted, appear unemotional, and appear rational and objective. Clients with histrionic personality disorder are overly dramatic in response to stress. Clients with narcissistic personality disorder focus on themselves and don't spend time thinking about bad news. Clients with an obsessive-compulsive personality disorder are preoccupied with the fear of becoming very anxious and losing control.
CN: Psychosocial integrity; CNS: None; CL: Analysis

6. A nurse is caring for a client with paranoid personality disorder. The nurse would expect to observe which of the following conditions?
1. Exhibitionism
2. Impulsiveness
3. Secretiveness
4. Self-destructiveness

6. 3. Clients with paranoid personality disorder tend to be secretive. Clients with histrionic personality disorder tend to be exhibitionists, and those with borderline personality disorder tend to be impulsive and self-destructive.
CN: Psychosocial integrity; CNS: None; CL: Application

7. Which type of behavior is expected from a client diagnosed with paranoid personality disorder?
1. Eccentric
2. Exploitative
3. Hypersensitive
4. Seductive

7. 3. People with paranoid personality disorders are hypersensitive to perceived threats. Schizotypal personalities appear eccentric and engage in activities others find perplexing. Clients with narcissistic personality disorder are interpersonally exploitative to enhance themselves or indulge their own desires. A client with histrionic personality disorder can be extremely seductive when in search of stimulation and approval.
CN: Psychosocial integrity; CNS: None; CL: Analysis

8. A client with paranoid personality disorder is discussing current problems with a nurse. Which nursing intervention has priority in the care plan?

1. Have the client look at sources of frustration.
2. Have the client focus on ways to interact with others.
3. Have the client discuss the use of defense mechanisms.
4. Have the client clarify thoughts and beliefs about an event.

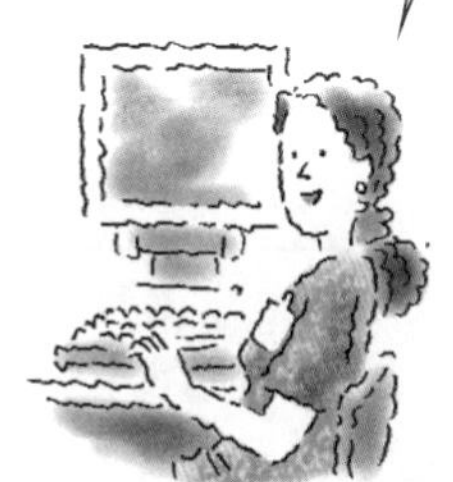

8. 4. Clarifying thoughts and beliefs helps the client avoid misinterpretations. Clients with a paranoid personality disorder tend to mistrust people and don't see interacting with others as a way to handle problems. They tend to be aggressive and argumentative rather than frustrated. The client's priority must be to interpret his thoughts and beliefs realistically, rather than discuss defensive mechanisms. A paranoid client will focus on defending self rather than acknowledging the use of defense mechanisms.
CN: Safe, effective care environment; CNS: Management of care; CL: Analysis

9. A client with a paranoid personality disorder makes an inappropriate and unreasonable report to a nurse. Which principle of good communication skills is important to use?

1. Use logic to address the client's concern.
2. Confront the client about the stated misperception.
3. Use nonverbal communication to address the issue.
4. Tell the client matter-of-factly that you don't share his interpretation.

9. 4. Telling the client you don't share his interpretation helps the client differentiate between realistic and emotional thoughts and conclusions. When the nurse uses logic to respond to a client's inappropriate statement, the nurse risks creating a power struggle with the client. The use of nonverbal communication will probably be misinterpreted and arouse the client's suspicion. It's unwise to confront a client with a paranoid personality disorder as the client will immediately become defensive.
CN: Psychosocial integrity; CNS: None; CL: Analysis

10. Which short-term goal is most appropriate for a client with paranoid personality disorder who has impaired social skills?

1. Obtain feedback from other people.
2. Discuss anxiety-provoking situations.
3. Address positive and negative feelings about self.
4. Identify personal feelings that hinder social interaction.

10. 4. The client must address the feelings that impede social interactions before developing ways to address impaired social skills. Feedback can only be obtained after action is taken to improve or change the situation. Discussion of anxiety-provoking situations is important but doesn't help the client with impaired social skills. Addressing the client's positive and negative feelings about self won't directly influence impaired social skills.
CN: Psychosocial integrity; CNS: None; CL: Application

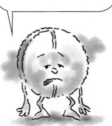

11. Which intervention is important for a client with paranoid personality disorder taking olanzapine (Zyprexa)?

1. Explain effects of serotonin syndrome.
2. Teach the client to watch for extrapyramidal adverse reactions.
3. Explain that the drug is less effective if the client smokes.
4. Discuss the need to report paradoxical effects such as euphoria.

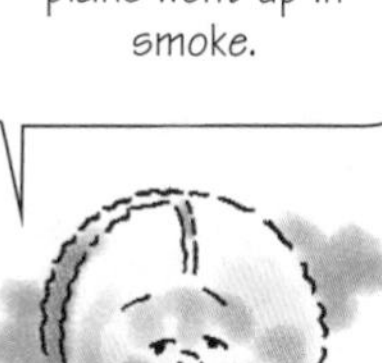

I tried to be effective but my plans went up in smoke.

11. 3. Olanzapine is less effective for clients who smoke cigarettes. Serotonin syndrome occurs with clients who take a combination of antidepressant medications. Olanzapine doesn't cause euphoria, and extrapyramidal adverse reactions aren't a problem. However, the client should be aware of adverse effects such as tardive dyskinesia.
CN: Physiological integrity; CNS: Pharmacological and parenteral therapies; CL: Application

12. Which approach should be used with a client with paranoid personality disorder who misinterprets many things the health care team says?

1. Limit interaction to activities of daily living.
2. Address only problems and causes of distress.
3. Explore anxious situations and offer reassurance.
4. Speak in simple messages without details.

12. 4. If the nurse speaks to the client with clear and simple messages, there's less chance information will be misinterpreted. Interaction can't be limited because it will interfere with working on identified treatment goals. Discussing complex topics creates a situation in which the client will have additional information to misinterpret. If the nurse addresses only problems and specific stressors, it will be difficult to establish a trust relationship.

CN: Psychosocial integrity; CNS: None; CL: Application

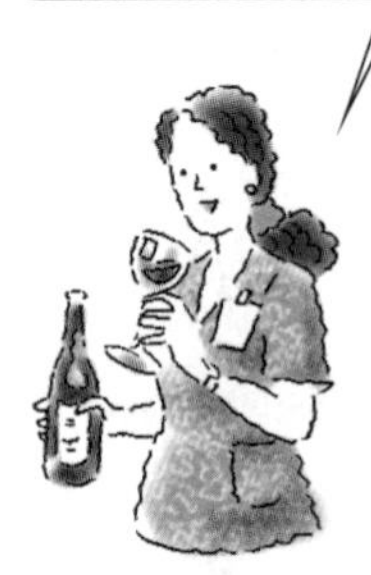
Cheers to you—
you're doing great!

13. A client with paranoid personality disorder responds aggressively during a psychoeducational group therapy to something another client said about him. Which explanation is the most likely?

1. The client doesn't want to participate in the group.
2. The client took the statement as a personal criticism.
3. The client is impulsive and was acting out of frustration.
4. The client was attempting to handle emotional distress.

13. 2. Clients with paranoid personality disorder tend to be hypersensitive and take what other people say as a personal attack on their character. The client is driven by the suspicion that others will inflict harm. Group participation would be minimal because the client is directing energy toward emotional self-protection. Clients with a paranoid personality disorder tend to be rigid and guarded rather than expressive and acting out. The client with a paranoid personality disorder is acting to defend himself, not handle emotional distress.

CN: Psychosocial integrity; CNS: None; CL: Analysis

14. A client with a paranoid personality disorder tells a nurse of his decision to stop talking to his wife. Which area should be assessed?

1. The client's doubts about the partner's loyalty
2. The client's need to be alone and have time for self
3. The client's decision to separate from the marital partner
4. The client's fears about becoming too much like the partner

14. 1. Clients with paranoid personality disorder are preoccupied with the loyalty or trustworthiness of people, especially family and friends. People commonly withdraw from a client with paranoid personality disorder due to the difficulty in maintaining a healthy relationship. The client's need to be alone and have time for self isn't related to the decision to stop talking to a partner. These clients focus on the belief that others will harm them, not that they may become like a marital partner.

CN: Psychosocial integrity; CNS: None; CL: Application

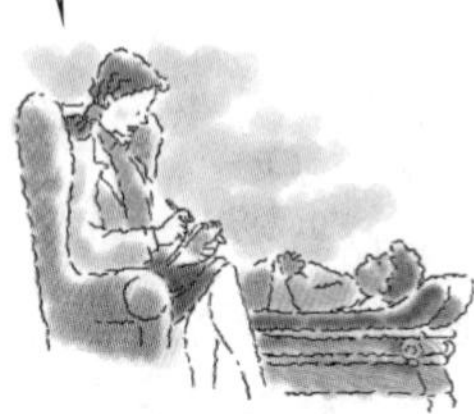
Try to establish a
therapeutic
relationship with the
client.

15. Which characteristic of a client with a paranoid personality disorder makes it difficult for a nurse to establish an interpersonal relationship?

1. Dysphoria
2. Hypervigilance
3. Indifference
4. Promiscuity

15. 2. Clients with paranoid personality disorder think others will harm, deceive, or exploit them in some way, and they're often guarded and ready to defend themselves from actual or perceived attacks. They don't tend to be dysphoric, indifferent, or promiscuous.

CN: Psychosocial integrity; CNS: None; CL: Application

CN: Client needs category CNS: Client needs subcategory CL: Cognitive level

16. The wife of a client diagnosed with paranoid personality disorder tells the client she wants a divorce. When discussing this situation with the couple, which factor should help the nurse form a care plan for this couple?
1. Denied grief
2. Intense jealousy
3. Exploitation of others
4. Self-destructive tendencies

16. 2. Clients with paranoid personality disorder are often extremely suspicious and jealous and make frequent accusations of partners and family members. Clients with paranoid personality disorder don't tend to struggle with the denial of grief. Clients with narcissistic personality disorder tend to exploit other people. Clients with borderline personality disorder have self-destructive tendencies.

CN: Psychosocial integrity; CNS: None; CL: Application

17. A client with a paranoid personality disorder tells a nurse that another nurse is out to get him. Which action by the nurse may cause this paranoid client distress?
1. Giving as-needed medication to another client
2. Taking the clients outside the unit for exercise
3. Checking vital signs of each person on the unit
4. Talking to another client in the corner of the lounge

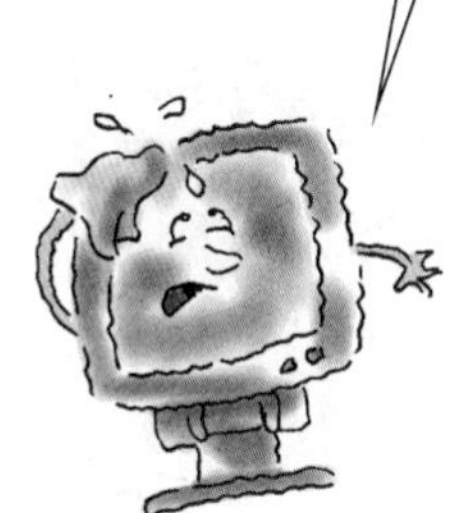

I wonder what they're saying about me?

17. 4. Clients with paranoid personality disorder tend to interpret any discussion that doesn't include them as evidence of a plot against them. Giving medication to another client wouldn't alarm the client. Checking vital signs on each client on the unit or taking the clients outside for exercise probably wouldn't be seen as a threat to the client's well-being.

CN: Psychosocial integrity; CNS: None; CL: Application

18. Which statement made by a client with paranoid personality disorder shows that teaching about social relationships is effective?
1. "As long as I live, I won't abide by social rules."
2. "Sometimes I can see what causes relationship problems."
3. "I'll find out what problems others have so I won't repeat them."
4. "I don't have problems in social relationships; I never really did."

18. 2. Progress is shown when the client addresses behaviors that negatively impact relationships. Clients with paranoid personality disorder tend to have impaired social relationships and are very uncomfortable in social settings. Clients with paranoid personality disorder struggle to understand and express their feelings about social rules. Knowing other people's problems isn't useful; the client must focus on his own issues. Not recognizing the problem indicates the client is in denial.

CN: Psychosocial integrity; CNS: None; CL: Application

19. Which <u>long-term</u> goal is appropriate for a client with paranoid personality disorder who is trying to improve peer relationships?
1. The client will verbalize a realistic view of self.
2. The client will take steps to address disorganized thinking.
3. The client will become appropriately interdependent on others.
4. The client will become involved in activities that foster social relationships.

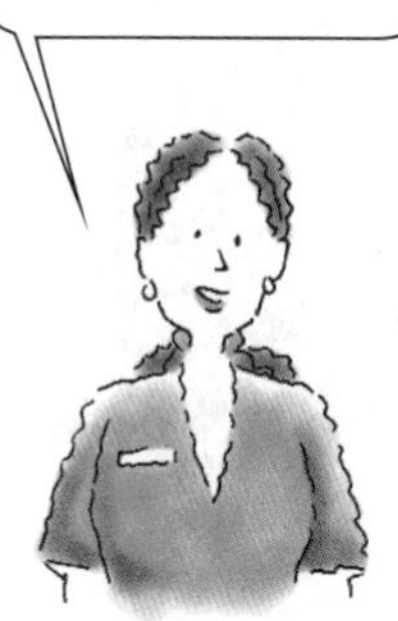

The word long-term is a clue to the correct choice.

19. 4. An appropriate long-term goal is for the client to increase interactions and social skills and make the commitment to become involved with others on a long-term basis. To verbalize a realistic view of self is a short-term goal. The client with a paranoid personality disorder doesn't tend to have disorganized thinking. A client with paranoid personality disorder won't allow himself to be interdependent on others.

CN: Psychosocial integrity; CNS: None; CL: Analysis

20. A family of a client with paranoid personality disorder is trying to understand the client's behavior. Which intervention should help the family?

1. Help the family find ways to handle stress.
2. Explore the possibility of finding respite care.
3. Help the family manage the client's eccentric action.
4. Encourage the family to focus on the client's strength.

20. 3. The family needs to know how to handle the client's symptoms and eccentric behaviors. All people need to learn strategies for handling stress, but the focus must be on helping the family learn how to handle symptoms. There's no need to find respite care for a client with a paranoid personality disorder. Focusing on the client's strengths is a positive action, but the family in this situation must learn how to manage the client's behavior.

CN: Psychosocial integrity; CNS: None; CL: Application

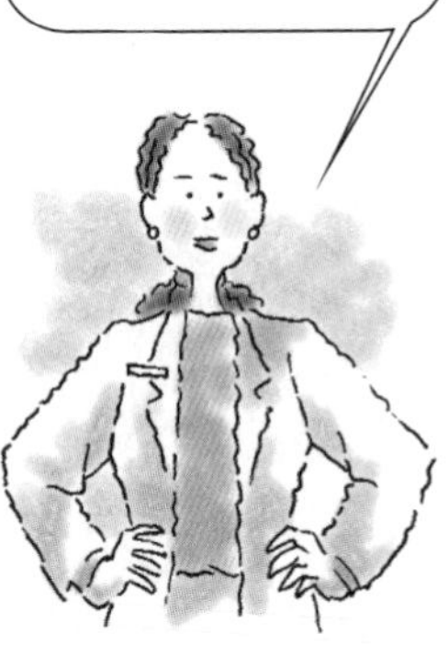

Therapeutic interventions must be appropriate for the client.

21. A client with antisocial personality disorder is trying to convince a nurse that he deserves special privileges and that an exception to the rules should be made for him. Which response is the most appropriate?

1. "I believe we need to sit down and talk about this."
2. "Don't you know better than to try to bend the rules?"
3. "What you're asking me to do for you is unacceptable."
4. "Why don't you bring this request to the community meeting?"

21. 3. These clients often try to manipulate the nurse to get special privileges or make exceptions to the rules on their behalf. By informing the client directly when actions are inappropriate, the nurse helps the client learn to control unacceptable behaviors by setting limits. By sitting down to talk about the request, the nurse is telling the client there's room for negotiation when there is none. The second option humiliates the client. The client's behavior is unacceptable and shouldn't be brought to a community meeting.

CN: Psychosocial integrity; CNS: None; CL: Application

22. A client with antisocial personality disorder tells a nurse, "Life has been full of problems since childhood." Which situation or condition should the nurse explore in the assessment?

1. Birth defects
2. Distracted easily
3. Hypoactive behavior
4. Substance abuse

22. 4. Clients with antisocial personality disorder often engage in substance abuse during childhood. They don't have a higher incidence of birth defects than other people. Clients with antisocial personality disorder are often manipulative and are no more distracted from issues than others. They tend to be hyperactive, not hypoactive.

CN: Psychosocial integrity; CNS: None; CL: Application

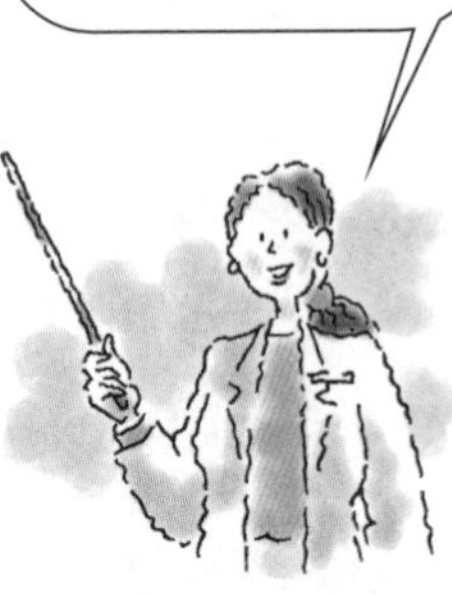

This is one of those further teaching questions. It asks you to identify a client behavior that signals the need for more teaching.

23. Which behavior by a client with antisocial personality disorder alerts the nurse to the need for teaching related to interaction skills?

1. Frequently crying
2. Having panic attacks
3. Avoiding social activities
4. Failing to follow social norms

23. 4. Failure to abide by social norms influences the client's ability to interact in a healthy manner with peers. Clients with antisocial personality disorders don't have frequent crying episodes or panic attacks. Avoiding social activities is more likely to be observed in avoidance personality style.

CN: Psychosocial integrity; CNS: None; CL: Analysis

24. When reviewing a client's chart, the nurse notes the progress note below. Which statement about the client's condition is most accurate?

Progress notes

9/15/10 1130	Client, age 28, admitted to unit with diagnosis of antisocial personality disorder and suicide attempt after cutting his right wrist. Right wrist dressing appears dry and intact. Client states, "I don't want to be here and I'm not following your treatment plan or any of your rules. I'm going to tell everyone here not to follow your rules." ——— Barbara Jones, RN

1. The client requires psychotropic drugs to treat his condition, which he refuses.
2. The client manipulates other clients but not his family.
3. The client may not be motivated to change his behavior or his lifestyle.
4. The client could quickly make behavior changes if motivated.

24. 3. Clients with antisocial personality disorder feel nothing is wrong with their behavior and have no desire to change. These clients don't benefit from psychotropic drug therapy. They attempt to manipulate all people with whom they come in contact. A quick behavior change isn't realistic expectation for clients with this disorder.

CN: Psychosocial integrity; CNS: None; CL: Application

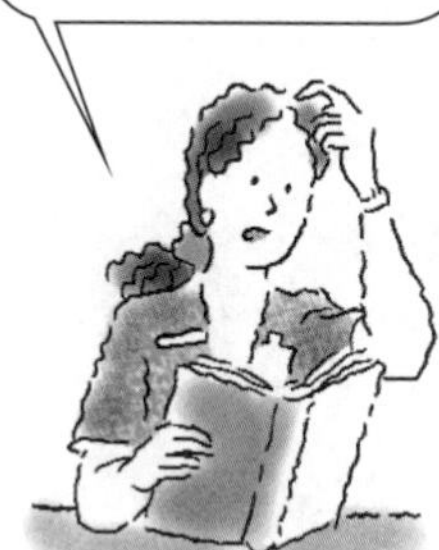
Which intervention should be done first?

25. Which intervention should be done first for a client who has an antisocial personality disorder and a history of polysubstance abuse?

1. Human immunodeficiency virus (HIV) testing
2. Electrolyte profile
3. Anxiety screening
4. Psychological testing

25. 1. A client who engages in high-risk behaviors such as polysubstance abuse should undergo HIV testing. This client would benefit from an entire chemistry profile as part of a complete medical examination, rather than a singular test for electrolytes. An anxiety screen isn't needed for a client with antisocial personality disorder. Information from psychological testing is valuable when developing a treatment but isn't an immediate concern.

CN: Safe, effective care environment; CNS: Management of care; CL: Application

26. Which short-term goal is appropriate for a client with an antisocial personality disorder who acts out when distressed?

1. Develop goals for personal improvement.
2. Identify situations that are out of the client's control.
3. Encourage the client to identify traumatic life events.
4. Learn to express feelings in a nondestructive manner.

26. 4. By working on appropriate expression of feelings, the client learns how to talk about what's stressful, rather than hurt himself or others. The most pressing need is to learn to cope and talk about problems rather than act out. Developing goals for personal improvement is a long-term goal, not a short-term one. Although it's important to differentiate what is and isn't under the client's control, the most important goal for handling distress is to talk about feelings appropriately. The identification of traumatic life events will occur only after the client begins to express feelings appropriately.

CN: Psychosocial integrity; CNS: None; CL: Application

27. A nurse notices other clients on the unit avoiding a client diagnosed with antisocial personality disorder. When discussing appropriate behavior in group therapy, which comment is expected about this client by his peers?
1. Lack of honesty
2. Belief in superstitions
3. Show of temper tantrums
4. Constant need for attention

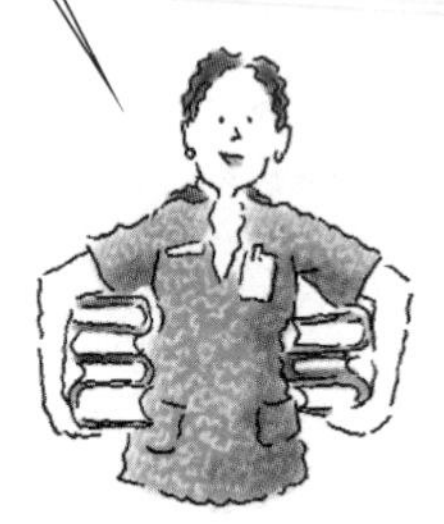

Read this question carefully. It seems to be asking you for a positive response, but it isn't.

27. 1. Clients with antisocial personality disorder tend to engage in acts of dishonesty, shown by lying. Clients with schizotypal personality disorder tend to be superstitious. Clients with histrionic personality disorders tend to overreact to frustrations and disappointments, have temper tantrums, and seek attention.
CN: Psychosocial integrity; CNS: None; CL: Application

28. During a family meeting for a client with antisocial personality disorder, which statement is expected from an exasperated family member?
1. "Today I'm the enemy, but tomorrow I'll be a saint to him."
2. "When he's wrong, he never apologizes or even acts sorry."
3. "Sometimes I can't believe how he exaggerates about everything."
4. "There are times when his compulsive behavior is too much to handle."

28. 2. The client with antisocial personality disorder has no remorse. The client with borderline personality disorder shows splitting. The client with antisocial personality disorder doesn't tend to exaggerate about life events or be compulsive.
CN: Psychosocial integrity; CNS: None; CL: Analysis

29. Which goal is most appropriate for a client with antisocial personality disorder with a high risk for violence directed at others?
1. The client will discuss the desire to hurt others rather than act.
2. The client will be given something to destroy to displace the anger.
3. The client will develop a list of resources to use when anger escalates.
4. The client will understand the difference between anger and physical symptoms.

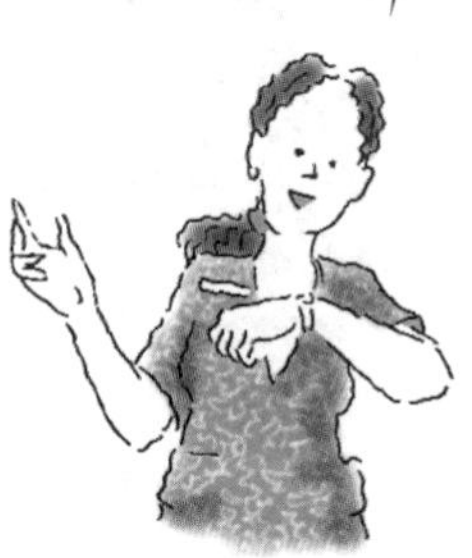

29. 1. By discussing the desire to be violent toward others, the nurse can help the client get in touch with the pain associated with the angry feelings. It isn't helpful to have the client destroy something. The client needs to talk about strong feelings in a nonviolent manner, not refer to a list of crisis references. Helping the client understand the relationship between feelings and physical symptoms can be done after discussing the desire to hurt others.
CN: Psychosocial integrity; CNS: None; CL: Analysis

30. A client with antisocial personality disorder says, "I always want to blow things off." Which response is the most appropriate?
1. "Try to focus on what needs to be done and just do it."
2. "Let's work on considering some options and strategies."
3. "Procrastinating is a part of your illness that we'll work on."
4. "The best thing to do is decide on some useful goals to accomplish."

30. 2. By considering options or strategies, the client gains skills to overcome ineffective behaviors. The client tends to be irresponsible and needs guidance on what specifically to focus on to change behavior. Clients with an antisocial personality disorder don't tend to struggle with procrastination; instead, they show reckless and irresponsible behaviors. It's premature to decide on goals when the client needs to address the mental mind-set and work to change the irresponsible behavior.
CN: Psychosocial integrity; CNS: None; CL: Analysis

31. Which goal for the family of a client with antisocial disorder should the nurse stress in her teaching?
1. The family must assist the client to decrease ritualistic behavior.
2. The family must learn to live with the client's impulsive behavior.
3. The family must stop reinforcing inappropriate negative behavior.
4. The family must start to use negative reinforcement of the client's behavior.

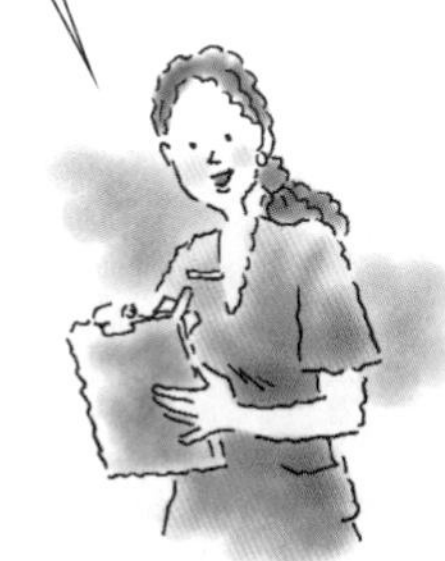
Teach the client skills to overcome ineffective behaviors.

31. 3. The family needs help learning how to stop reinforcing inappropriate client behavior. Negative reinforcement is an inappropriate strategy for the family to use to support the client. The family can set limits and reinforce consequences when the client shows shortsightedness and poor planning. Clients with antisocial personality disorder don't show ritualistic behaviors.
CN: Psychosocial integrity; CNS: None; CL: Analysis

32. Which nursing intervention has priority in the care plan for a client with antisocial personality disorder who shows defensive behaviors?
1. Help the client accept responsibility for his own decisions and behaviors.
2. Work with the client to feel better about himself by taking care of basic needs.
3. Teach the client to identify the defense mechanisms used to cope with distress.
4. Confront the client about the disregard of social rules and the feelings of others.

32. 1. Clients with antisocial personality disorder tend to blame other people for their behaviors and need to be taught how to take responsibility for their actions. Clients with antisocial personality disorder don't tend to have problems with self-care habits or meeting their basic needs. Clients with antisocial personality disorder will deny they're defensive or distressed. Most often, these clients feel justified with retaliatory behavior. To confront the client would only cause him to become even more defensive.
CN: Psychosocial integrity; CNS: None; CL: Analysis

33. A client with antisocial personality disorder is trying to manipulate the health care team. Which strategy is important for the staff to use?
1. Focus on how to teach the client more effective behaviors for meeting basic needs.
2. Help the client verbalize underlying feelings of hopelessness and learn coping skills.
3. Remain calm and don't emotionally respond to the client's manipulative actions.
4. Help the client eliminate the intense desire to have everything in life turn out perfectly.

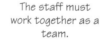

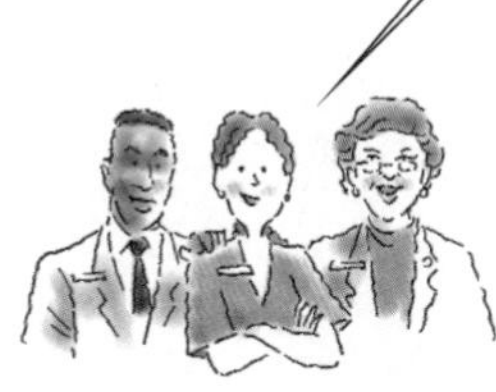
The staff must work together as a team.

33. 3. The best strategy to use with a client trying to manipulate staff is to stay calm and refrain from responding emotionally. Negative reinforcement of inappropriate behavior increases the chance it will be repeated. Later, it may be possible to address how to meet the client's basic needs. Clients with antisocial personality disorder don't tend to experience feelings of hopelessness or to desire life events to turn out perfectly. In most cases, these clients negate responsibility for their behavior.
CN: Psychosocial integrity; CNS: None; CL: Analysis

34. A client with dependent personality disorder is working to increase self-esteem. Which statement by the client shows teaching was <u>successful</u>?
1. "I'm not going to look just at the negative things about myself."
2. "I'm most concerned about my level of competence and progress."
3. "I'm not as envious of the things other people have as I used to be."
4. "I find I can't stop myself from taking over things others should be doing."

34. 1. As the client makes progress on improving self-esteem, self-blame and negative self-evaluations will decrease. Clients with dependent personality disorder tend to feel fragile and inadequate and would be extremely unlikely to discuss their level of competence and progress. These clients focus on self and aren't envious or jealous. Individuals with dependent personality disorders don't take over situations because they see themselves as inept and inadequate.
CN: Psychosocial integrity; CNS: None; CL: Application

35. A client is suspected of having antisocial personality disorder. Which finding most supports this diagnosis?

1. The client has delusional thinking.
2. The client has feelings of inferiority.
3. The client has disorganized thinking.
4. The client has multiple criminal charges.

35. 4. Clients with antisocial personality disorder are commonly sent for treatment by the court after multiple crimes or for the use of illegal substances. Clients with antisocial personality disorder don't tend to have delusional thinking, feelings of inferiority, or disorganized thinking.

CN: Psychosocial integrity; CNS: None; CL: Application

36. A client with antisocial personality disorder talks about personal life changes that need to occur. Which client statement shows group therapy is having a positive therapeutic effect?

1. "I'm not doing as bad as I thought I was."
2. "I wish I could believe I can change, but it's probably too late."
3. "I see all the problems, but I'm not sure there are good solutions."
4. "I'm finally learning how to live my life without living on the edge."

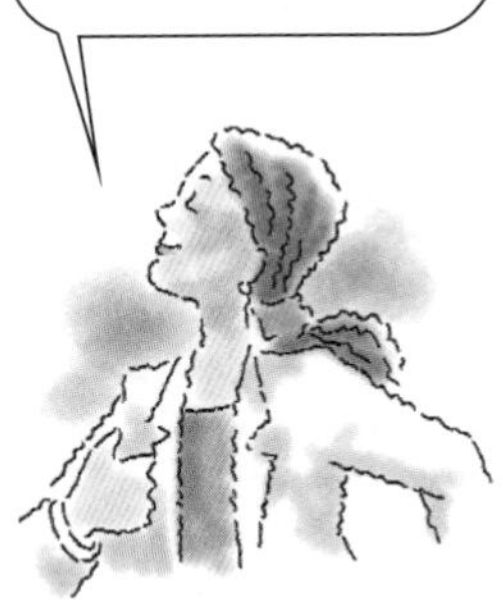
I think I've had a positive effect!

36. 4. The client is becoming aware of risky behaviors and how problematic these behaviors are. The first option indicates denial, and the client is somewhat defensive about making a change. The second option indicates defeat, and the client seems to feel stuck. The third option indicates problem identification but also uncertainty and ambivalence about the client's ability to change.

CN: Psychosocial integrity; CNS: None; CL: Analysis

37. A nurse tells a client with a personality disorder that he must clean his room before he can go to the dayroom. The client asks if he can play one game of pool first. What's the most appropriate response by the nurse?

1. "You can play one quick game. Then you have to clean your room."
2. "No, you may not."
3. "No, you may not play pool first. The rules were explained to you."
4. "Yes, you may play a quick game. But don't tell the other clients about this."

37. 3. This response is firm and reinforces the rules. Allowing the client to play one game before cleaning his room and telling him not to tell anyone else encourages manipulative behavior. Saying no to the client without an explanation doesn't outline or reinforce the rules.

CN: Psychosocial integrity; CNS: None; CL: Analysis

38. A nurse determines that a client with antisocial personality disorder is beginning to practice several socially acceptable behaviors in the group setting. Which behavior is the nurse most likely to observe in this client?

1. Fewer panic attacks
2. Acceptance of reality
3. Improved self-esteem
4. Decreased physical symptoms

38. 3. When clients with antisocial personality disorder begin to practice socially acceptable behaviors, they also frequently experience a more positive sense of self-esteem. Clients with antisocial personality disorder don't tend to have panic attacks, somatic manifestations of their illness, or withdrawal or alteration in their perception of reality.

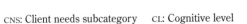

CN: Psychosocial integrity; CNS: None; CL: Application

39. A client with borderline personality disorder is admitted to the unit after slashing his wrist. Which goal is most important after promoting safety?

1. Establish a therapeutic relationship with the client.
2. Identify whether splitting is present in the client's thoughts.
3. Talk about the client's acting out and self-destructive tendencies.
4. Encourage the client to understand why he blames others.

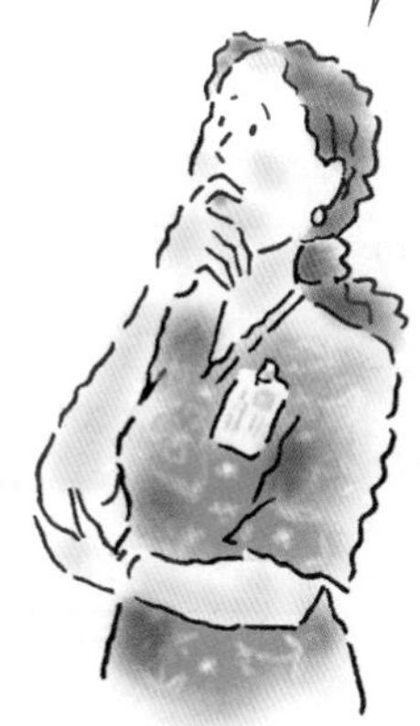

39. 1. After promoting client safety, the nurse establishes a rapport with the client to facilitate appropriate expression of feelings. A therapeutic relationship also must be established before working on the issue of splitting. At this time, the client isn't ready to address unhealthy behavior. A therapeutic relationship must be established before the nurse can effectively work with the client on self-destructive tendencies.

CN: Safe, effective care environment; CNS: Management of care; CL: Application

40. Which nursing intervention is most appropriate in helping a client with a borderline personality disorder identify appropriate behaviors?

1. Schedule a family meeting.
2. Place the client in seclusion.
3. Formulate a behavioral contract.
4. Perform a mental status assessment.

40. 3. The use of a behavioral contract establishes a framework for healthier functioning and places responsibility for actions back on the client. Seclusion will reinforce the fears of abandonment of clients with borderline personality. Performing a mental status assessment or scheduling a family meeting won't help the client identify appropriate behaviors.

CN: Psychosocial integrity; CNS: None; CL: Application

41. Which statement is typical of a client with borderline personality disorder who has recurrent suicidal thoughts?

1. "I can't believe how everyone has suddenly stopped believing in me."
2. "I don't care what other people say, I know how badly I looked to them."
3. "I might as well check out since my boyfriend doesn't want me anymore."
4. "I won't stop until I've gotten revenge on all those people who blamed me."

41. 3. This statement is typical for the borderline personality disorder client who is suicidal and reflects the tendency toward all-or-nothing thinking. The first option indicates the client has experienced a credibility problem, the second option indicates the client is extremely embarrassed, and the last option indicates the client has antisocial personality disorder. None of these is a characteristic of borderline personality disorder.

CN: Safe, effective care environment; CNS: Safety and infection control; CL: Application

42. The nurse is taking a health history on a client with borderline personality disorder. Which of the following findings would the nurse expect to observe?

1. A negative sense of self
2. A tendency to be compulsive
3. A problem with communication
4. An inclination to be philosophical

42. 1. Clients with a borderline personality disorder have low self-esteem and a negative sense of self. They have little or no problem expressing themselves and communicating with others, and although they have a tendency to be impulsive, they aren't usually compulsive or philosophical.

CN: Psychosocial integrity; CNS: None; CL: Application

43. Which characteristic or situation is indicated when a client with borderline personality disorder has a crisis?

1. Antisocial behavior
2. Suspicious behavior
3. Relationship problems
4. Auditory hallucinations

43. 3. Relationship problems can precipitate a crisis because they bring up issues of abandonment. Clients with borderline personality disorder aren't usually suspicious; they're more likely to be depressed or highly anxious. They don't have symptoms of antisocial behavior or auditory hallucinations.

CN: Psychosocial integrity; CNS: None; CL: Analysis

44. Which assessment finding is seen in a client diagnosed with borderline personality disorder?

1. Abrasions in various healing stages
2. Intermittent episodes of hypertension
3. Alternating tachycardia and bradycardia
4. Mild state of euphoria with disorientation

44. 1. Clients with borderline personality disorder tend to self-mutilate and have abrasions in various stages of healing. The other options don't tend to occur with this disorder.
CN: Psychosocial integrity; CNS: None; CL: Application

45. Which short-term goal is appropriate for a client with borderline personality disorder with low self-esteem?

1. Write in a journal daily.
2. Express fears and feelings.
3. Stop obsessive-compulsive behaviors.
4. Decrease dysfunctional family conflicts.

The word short-term is the key to the answer.

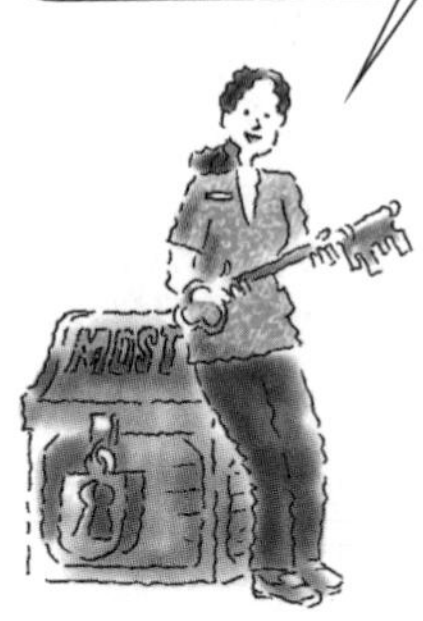

45. 2. Acknowledging fears and feelings can help the client identify parts of himself that are uncomfortable, and he can begin to work on developing a positive sense of self. Writing in a daily journal isn't a short-term goal to enhance self-esteem. A client with borderline personality disorder doesn't struggle with obsessive-compulsive behaviors. Decreasing dysfunctional family conflicts is a long-term goal.
CN: Psychosocial integrity; CNS: None; CL: Analysis

46. Which intervention is important to include in a teaching plan for a family with a member diagnosed with borderline personality disorder?

1. Teach the family methods for handling the client's anxiety.
2. Explore how the family reinforces the sick role with the client.
3. Encourage the family to have the client express intense emotions.
4. Help the family put pressure on the client to improve current behavior.

46. 1. The family needs to learn how to handle the client's intense stress and low tolerance for frustration. Family members don't want to reinforce the sick role; they're more concerned with preventing anxiety from escalating. Clients with borderline personality disorder already maintain intense emotions, and it isn't safe to encourage further expression of them. The family doesn't need to put pressure on the client to change behavior; this approach will only cause inappropriate behavior to escalate.
CN: Psychosocial integrity; CNS: None; CL: Application

47. In planning care for a client with borderline personality disorder, a nurse must be aware that this client is prone to develop which condition?

1. Binge eating
2. Memory loss
3. Cult membership
4. Delusional thinking

Clients with borderline personality disorder are likely to act out in self-destructive ways.

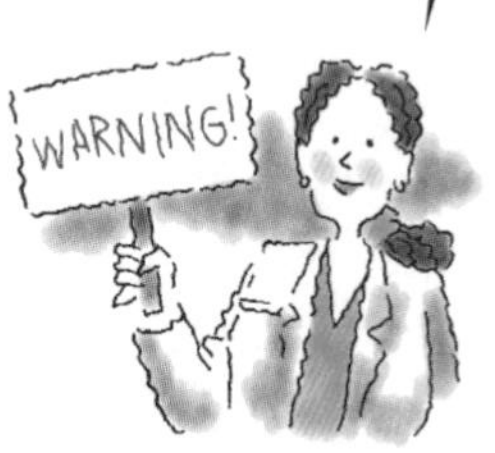

47. 1. Clients with borderline personality disorder are likely to develop dysfunctional coping and act out in self-destructive ways such as binge eating. They aren't prone to develop memory loss or delusional thinking. Becoming involved in cults may be seen in some clients with antisocial personality disorder.
CN: Psychosocial integrity; CNS: None; CL: Analysis

CN: Client needs category CNS: Client needs subcategory CL: Cognitive level

48. Which statement is expected from a client with borderline personality disorder with a history of dysfunctional relationships?

1. "I won't get involved in another relationship."
2. "I'm determined to look for the perfect partner."
3. "I've decided to learn better communication skills."
4. "I'm going to be an equal partner in a relationship."

48. 2. Clients with borderline personality disorder would decide to look for a perfect partner. This characteristic is a result of the dichotomous manner in which these clients view the world. They go from relationship to relationship without taking responsibility for their behavior. It's unlikely that an unsuccessful relationship will cause clients to make a change. They tend to be demanding and impulsive in relationships. There's no thought given to what one wants or needs from a relationship. Because they tend to blame others for problems, it's unlikely they would express a desire to learn communication skills.

CN: Psychosocial integrity; CNS: None; CL: Analysis

49. Which nursing intervention is <u>most appropriate</u> for a client with borderline personality disorder working on developing healthy relationships?

1. Have the client assess current behaviors.
2. Work with the client to develop outgoing behavior.
3. Limit the client's interactions to family members only.
4. Encourage the client to approach others for interactions.

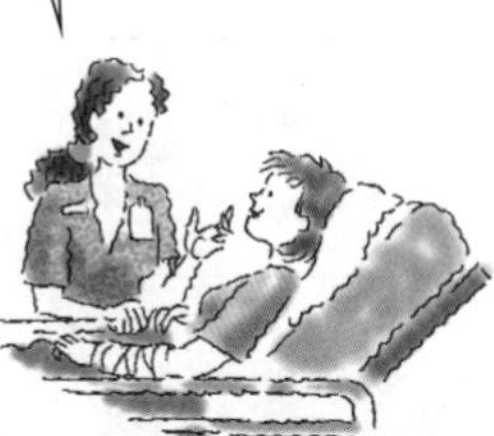
Appropriate care considers the client's best interests.

49. 1. Self-assessment of behavior enables the client to look at himself and identify social behaviors that need to be changed. It isn't useful to work on developing outgoing behavior. It's unrealistic to have clients with borderline personality disorder limit their interactions to family members only. Clients with borderline personality disorder don't tend to have difficulty approaching and interacting with other people; in fact, they tend to be demanding and the center of attention.

CN: Psychosocial integrity; CNS: None; CL: Analysis

50. Which defense mechanism is most likely to be seen in a client with borderline personality disorder?

1. Compensation
2. Displacement
3. Identification
4. Projection

50. 4. Clients with borderline personality disorder tend to blame and project their feelings and inadequacies onto others. They don't model themselves after other people or tend to use compensation to handle distress. Clients with borderline personality disorder are impulsive and tend to react immediately. It's unlikely they would displace their feelings onto others.

CN: Psychosocial integrity; CNS: None; CL: Analysis

51. What would be an important guideline for nurses working with clients with borderline personality disorder?

1. When behavioral problems emerge, calmly review the therapeutic goals and boundaries of treatment.
2. Try to prevent or reduce untoward effects of manipulation.
3. Remain neutral and avoid engaging in power struggles.
4. Respect a client's need for social isolation.

51. 1. Reminding the borderline client of the goals and boundaries of treatment helps the client to focus on therapy. Manipulation is an issue with antisocial personality clients. Power struggles are an issue for the narcissistic client and respecting the client's need for social isolation describes a client with schizotypal personality disorder.

CN: Safe, effective care environment; CNS: Safety & infection control; CL: Application

52. Which nursing intervention has <u>priority</u> for a client with borderline personality disorder?

1. Maintain consistent, realistic limits.
2. Give instructions for meeting basic self-care needs.
3. Engage in daytime activities to stimulate wakefulness.
4. Have the client attend group therapy on a daily basis.

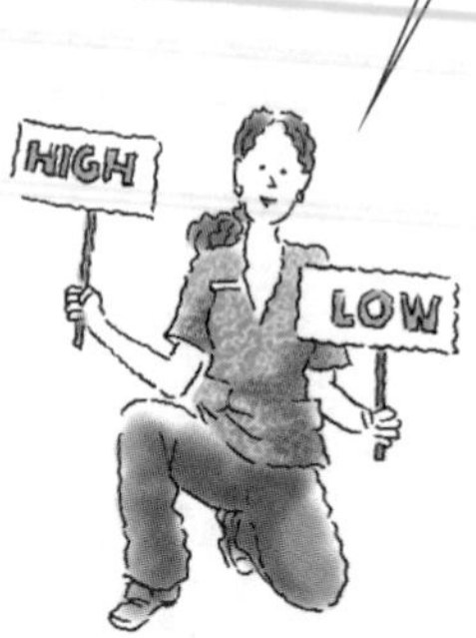

Prioritizing is a crucial part of nursing!
HIGH
LOW

52. 1. Clients with borderline personality disorder who are needy, dependent, and manipulative will benefit greatly from maintaining consistent, realistic limits. They don't tend to have difficulty meeting their self-care needs and don't tend to have sleeping difficulties. They enjoy attending group therapy because they typically attempt to use the opportunity to become the center of attention.

CN: Safe, effective care environment; CNS: Management of care; CL: Application

53. Which outcome indicates individual therapy has been effective for a client with borderline personality disorder?

1. The client accepts that medication isn't a treatment of choice.
2. The client agrees to undergo hypnosis for suppression of memories.
3. The client understands the organic basis for the problematic behavior.
4. The client verbalizes awareness of the consequences for unacceptable behaviors.

53. 4. An indication of effective individual therapy for this client is his expressed awareness of consequences for unacceptable behaviors. Medications can control symptoms. However, monitoring for reckless use or abuse of drugs must be done for the client with borderline personality disorder. Hypnosis isn't a treatment used with a client with borderline personality disorder. There's no organic basis for the development of this disorder.

CN: Psychosocial integrity; CNS: None; CL: Application

54. Which action by a client with borderline personality disorder indicates adequate learning about personal behavior?

1. The client talks about intense anger.
2. The client smiles while making demands.
3. The client decides never to engage in conflict.
4. The client stops the family from controlling finances.

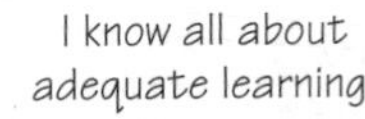

I know all about adequate learning.

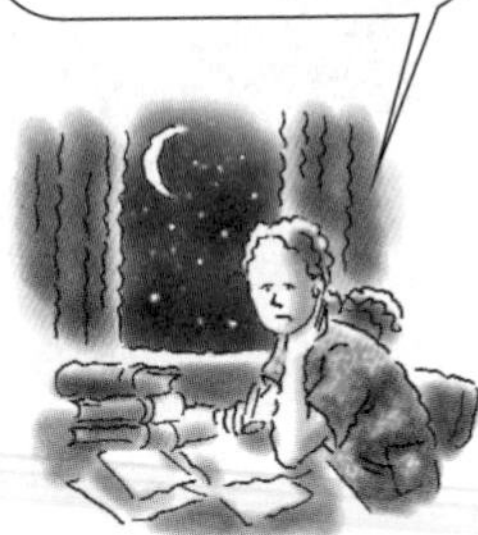

54. 1. Learning has occurred when anger is discussed rather than acted out in unhealthy ways. The behavior to change would be the demands placed on others. Smiling while making these demands shows manipulative behavior. Not engaging in conflict is unrealistic. It's important to help this client slowly develop financial responsibility rather than just stopping the family from monitoring the client's overspending.

CN: Psychosocial integrity; CNS: None; CL: Application

55. A nurse is planning care for a client with borderline personality disorder who has been agitated. Which instruction is included for the client and family?

1. Encourage the rebuilding of family relationships.
2. Help the client handle anxiety before it escalates.
3. Have the client participate in a weekly support group.
4. Discuss the client's bad habits that need to be changed.

55. 2. The client needs help handling anxiety because escalating anxiety can trigger self-destructive behaviors in clients with borderline personality disorder. When a client with borderline personality disorder is agitated, it's difficult to communicate, let alone rebuild family relationships. Participation in a weekly support group won't be enough to help the client handle agitation. When a client is agitated, it isn't appropriate to discuss bad habits that need to be changed. This action may further agitate the client.

CN: Psychosocial integrity; CNS: None; CL: Application

56. A client with a borderline personality disorder isn't making progress on the identified goals. Which client factor should be <u>reevaluated</u>?

1. Memory
2. Motivation
3. Orientation
4. Perception

56. 2. Clients with borderline personality disorders tend to be poorly motivated for treatment. They don't tend to have perception problems such as hallucinations or illusions, problems in orientation, or memory problems.

CN: Psychosocial integrity; CNS: None; CL: Analysis

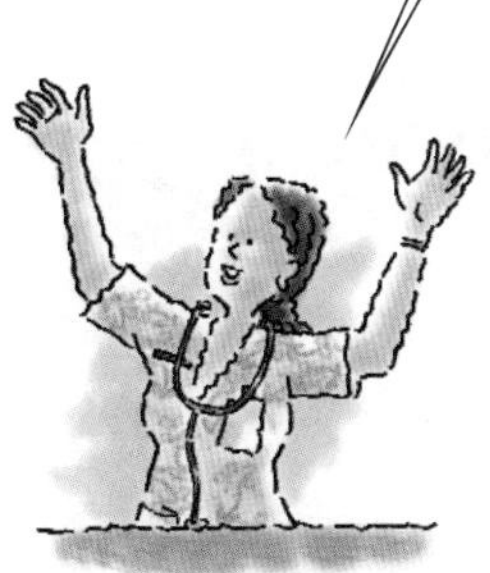

You've finished 56 questions. That should motivate you to keep going.

57. The nurse is performing an assessment on a client with dependent personality disorder. Which of the following characteristics would the nurse <u>most likely</u> assess in this client?

1. Abrasive to others
2. Indifferent to others
3. Manipulative of others
4. Overreliant on others

57. 4. Clients with dependent personality disorder are extremely overreliant on other people; they aren't abrasive, assertive, or indifferent. They're clinging and demanding of others; they don't manipulate. People with dependent personality disorder rely on others and want to be taken care of.

CN: Psychosocial integrity; CNS: None; CL: Application

58. A client with dependent personality disorder is working on goals for self-care. Which short-term goal is <u>most important</u> to the client's everyday activities of daily living?

1. Do all self-care activities independently.
2. Write a daily schedule for each day of the week.
3. Do self-care activities in a minimal amount of time.
4. Determine activities that can be performed without help.

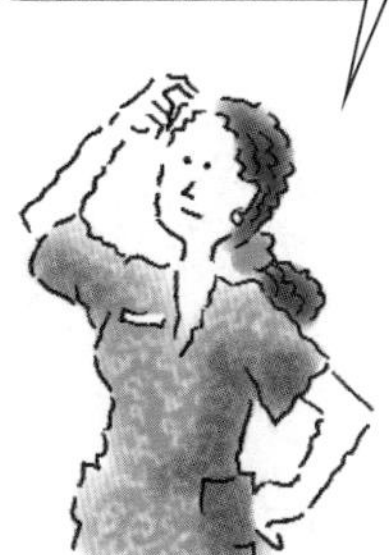

It's most important that I answer this question correctly.

58. 4. By determining activities that can be performed without assistance, the client can then begin to practice them independently. If the nurse only encourages a client to perform self-care activities independently, nothing may change. Writing a daily schedule doesn't help the client focus on what needs to be done to promote self-care. The amount of time needed to perform self-care activities isn't important. If time pressure is put on the client, there may be more reluctance to perform self-care activities.

CN: Psychosocial integrity; CNS: None; CL: Application

59. A nurse is teaching the family of a client diagnosed with dependent personality disorder. Which information would be most appropriate for the nurse to include?

1. Stress-reduction techniques
2. Panic attack prevention
3. Exercise program development
4. Aggressive outburst reduction

59. 1. The family needs information about coping skills to help the client learn to handle stress. Clients with dependent personality disorder don't tend to have panic attacks or aggressive outbursts; they tend to be passive and submit to others. Exercise is a health promotion activity for all clients. Clients with dependent personality disorder wouldn't need exercise promoted more than other people.

CN: Safe, effective care environment; CNS: Management of care; CL: Application

60. Which strategy is appropriate for a client with dependent personality disorder?
1. Orient the client to current surroundings.
2. Reassure the client about personal safety.
3. Ask questions to help the client recall problems.
4. Differentiate between positive and negative feedback.

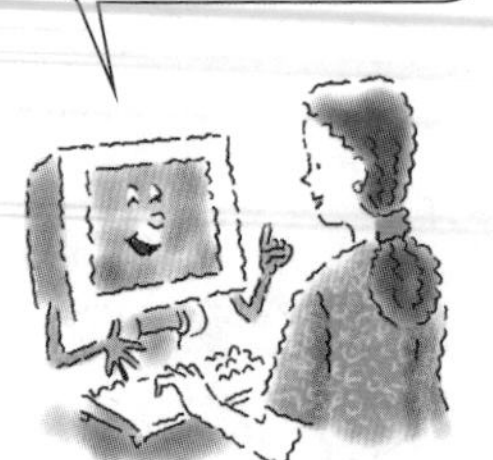

Think carefully.
You know the answer to this one.

60. 4. Clients with dependent personality disorder tend to view all feedback as criticism; they frequently misinterpret another's remarks. Clients with dependent personality disorder don't need orientation to their surroundings. Personal safety isn't an issue because a person with dependent personality disorder typically isn't self-destructive. Memory problems aren't associated with this disorder, so asking questions to stimulate the client's memory isn't necessary.

CN: Psychosocial integrity; CNS: None; CL: Application

61. A client with dependent personality disorder is crying after a family meeting. Which statement by a family member is most likely the cause of upset to this client?
1. "You take advantage of people, especially the people in our family."
2. "You act like you love me one minute but hate me the next minute."
3. "You feel like you deserve everything, whether you work for it or not."
4. "You always agree to everything, but deep down inside you feel differently."

61. 4. The client was confronted by a family member about behavior that doesn't represent the client's true feelings. Clients are afraid they won't be taken care of if they disagree. Clients with a dependent personality disorder don't have a sense of entitlement and don't take advantage of other people, but they subordinate their needs to others. They don't show the defense mechanism of splitting, where a person is valued and then devalued.

CN: Psychosocial integrity; CNS: None; CL: Analysis

62. A client with dependent personality disorder is having trouble performing activities of daily living. Which nursing intervention should help facilitate the client's daily activities?
1. Have the client eat three meals a day.
2. Work with the client to establish a budget.
3. Make a chart to document hygiene practices.
4. Discuss how the client can obtain a driver's license.

62. 2. Clients with dependent personality disorder tend to withdraw from adult responsibilities. Managing money through the use of a budget is a first step toward assuming adult responsibilities. These clients don't tend to have problems with nutritional intake. Hygiene issues usually aren't a problem for clients with dependent personality disorder. Clients with a dependent personality disorder don't have any special reasons for not obtaining a driver's license.

CN: Psychosocial integrity; CNS: None; CL: Application

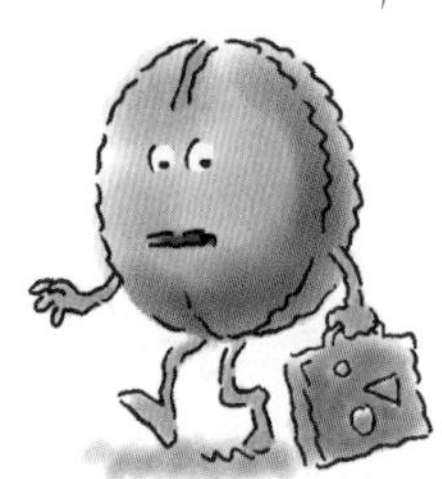

It takes me a while, but I'll get the job done.

63. A client with a dependent personality disorder is taking fluoxetine (Prozac) for depression. Which instruction is included in client teaching?
1. Drink only wine and beer when taking this drug.
2. Add as-needed doses if depression becomes worse.
3. Expect 3 to 4 weeks to go by before effects are seen.
4. Be aware that alterations in usual sleep patterns, especially nightmares, may occur.

63. 3. The client must take the drug for 3 to 4 weeks before therapeutic effects are seen. The nurse must caution the client against the use of alcohol, including wine and beer, when taking fluoxetine. The client is to take the drug as prescribed. Additional doses must not be self-administered. Fluoxetine treats disruptions in sleep and doesn't cause nightmares.

CN: Physiological integrity; CNS: Pharmacological and parenteral therapies; CL: Application

CN: Client needs category CNS: Client needs subcategory CL: Cognitive level

64. Which behavior by a client with dependent personality disorder shows the client has made progress toward the goal of increasing problem-solving skills?
1. The client is courteous.
2. The client asks questions.
3. The client stops acting out.
4. The client controls emotions.

64. 2. The client with dependent personality disorder is passive and tries to please others. By asking questions, the client is beginning to gather information, the first step of decision making. These clients don't tend to have emotional outbursts or to be impolite. They avoid expressing their feelings or acting out for fear of displeasing others.
CN: Psychosocial integrity; CNS: None; CL: Analysis

65. In planning care for a client with borderline personality disorder, the nurse must account for which behavioral trait?
1. An inability to make decisions independently
2. A propensity to act out when feeling afraid, alone, or devalued
3. A belief the client deserves special privileges not accorded to others
4. A display of inappropriately seductive appearance and behavior

65. 2. Clients with borderline personality disorder have an intense fear of abandonment. These clients are able to make decisions independently. Feeling deserving of special privileges is characteristic of a person with narcissistic personality disorder. Inappropriate seductive appearance and behavior is characteristic of someone with histrionic personality disorder.
CN: Psychosocial integrity; CNS: None; CL: Application

You're doing great!

66. Which short-term goal is appropriate for a client with dependent personality disorder experiencing excessive dependency needs?
1. Verbalize self-confidence in own abilities.
2. Decide relationships don't take energy to sustain.
3. Discuss feelings related to frequent mood swings.
4. Stop obsessive thinking that impedes daily social functioning.

66. 1. Individuals with dependent personalities believe they must depend on others to be competent for them. They need to gain more self-confidence in their own abilities. The client must realize that relationships take energy to develop and sustain. Clients with dependent personality disorder usually don't have obsessive thinking or mood swings to interfere with their socialization.
CN: Psychosocial integrity; CNS: None; CL: Application

67. A client with dependent personality disorder is thinking about getting a part-time job. Which nursing intervention will help this client when employment is obtained?
1. Help the client develop strategies to control impulses.
2. Explain that there are consequences for inappropriate behaviors.
3. Have the client work to sustain healthy interpersonal relationships.
4. Help the client decrease the use of regression as a defense mechanism.

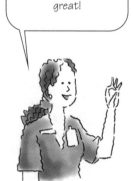

67. 3. Sustaining healthy relationships will help the client be comfortable with peers in the job setting. Clients with dependent personality disorder don't usually use regression as a defense mechanism. It's common to see denial and introjection used. They don't usually have trouble with impulse control or offensive behavior that would lead to negative consequences.
CN: Psychosocial integrity; CNS: None; CL: Analysis

68. A client with dependent personality disorder has difficulty expressing personal concerns. Which communication technique is <u>best</u> to teach the client?

1. Questioning
2. Reflection
3. Silence
4. Touch

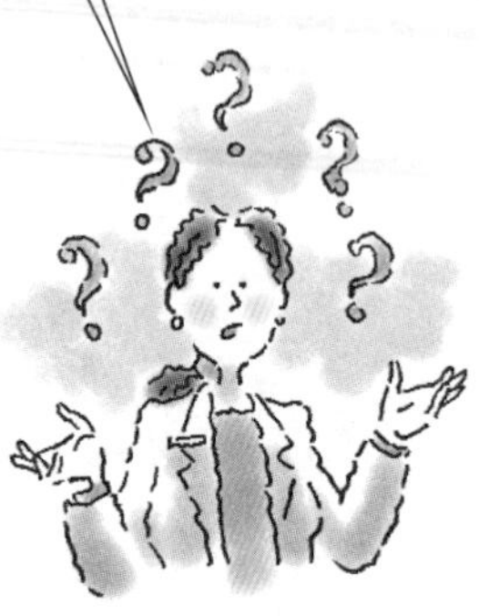

There are so many ways to communicate. How do I know which is the best?

68. 1. Questioning is a way to learn to identify feelings and express self. The use of reflection isn't a communication technique that will help the client express personal feelings and concerns. Using silence won't help the client identify and discuss personal concerns. The use of touch to express feelings and personal concerns must be used very judiciously.

CN: Psychosocial integrity; CNS: None; CL: Application

69. A nurse is evaluating the effectiveness of an assertiveness group that a client with dependent personality disorder attended. Which client statement indicates the group had therapeutic value?

1. "I can't seem to do the things other people do."
2. "I wish I could be more organized like other people."
3. "I want to talk about something that's bothering me."
4. "I just don't want people in my family to fight any more."

69. 3. By asking to talk about a bothersome situation, the client has taken the first step toward assertive behavior. To smooth over or minimize troubling events isn't an assertive position. The first option reflects a lack of self-confidence; it's not an assertive statement. Statements that express the client's wishes aren't assertive statements.

CN: Psychosocial integrity; CNS: None; CL: Analysis

70. After a family visit, a client with dependent personality disorder becomes anxious. Which situation is a possible cause of the anxiety?

1. Sensitivity to criticism
2. Discussion of family rules
3. Being asked personal questions
4. Identification of eccentric behavior

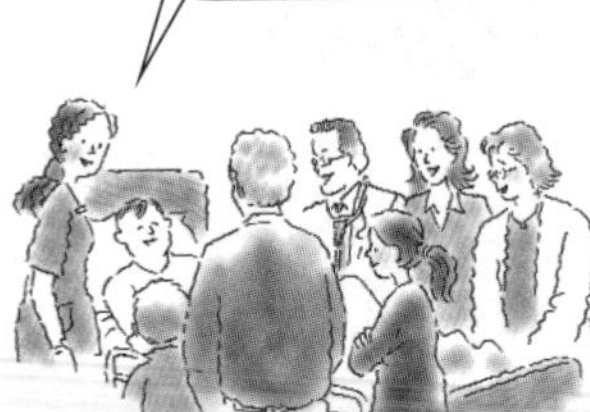

A family visit can be upsetting to the client.

70. 1. Clients with dependent personality disorder are extremely sensitive to criticism and can become very anxious when they feel interpersonal conflict or tension. When they have discussions about family rules, they try to become submissive and please others rather than become anxious. When they're asked personal questions, they don't necessarily become anxious. Clients with dependent personality disorder don't tend to show eccentric behavior that causes them anxiety.

CN: Psychosocial integrity; CNS: None; CL: Application

71. A client with dependent personality disorder has a history of minor GI problems. Which goal has <u>priority</u>?

1. Get a referral to a specialist.
2. Consult with a dietitian regularly.
3. Arrange for a family support meeting.
4. Examine the client's present level of coping skills.

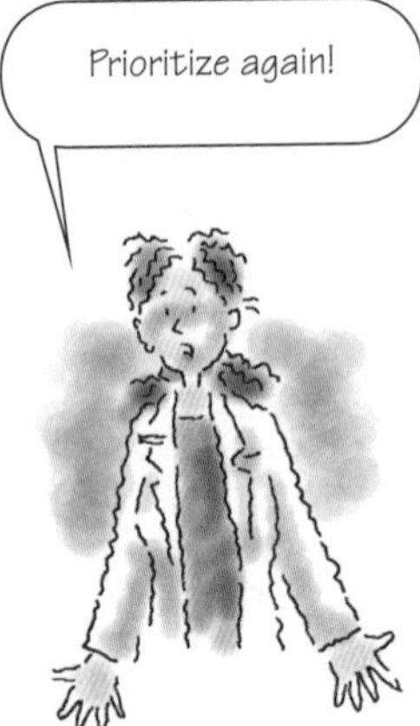

Prioritize again!

71. 4. Many clients with GI discomfort tend to be anxious and need help developing coping skills. Before a referral is obtained, other factors that could cause GI upset must be addressed. A client with dependent personality disorder usually is overdependent on family members and doesn't tend to need a nurse to advocate for client support. Consulting with a dietitian wouldn't be a priority goal. A consultation would be initiated only after other variables were assessed and a need was identified.

CN: Safe, effective care environment; CNS: Management of care; CL: Application

72. Which emotional health problem may potentially coexist in a client with dependent personality disorder?
1. Psychotic disorder
2. Anxiety disorder
3. Alcohol-related disorder
4. Posttraumatic stress disorder

72. 2. Because they've placed their own needs in the hands of others, clients with dependent personalities are extremely vulnerable to anxiety disorder. They don't tend to have coexisting problems of posttraumatic stress disorder, psychotic disorder, or alcohol-related disorder.
CN: Psychosocial integrity; CNS: None; CL: Analysis

73. A nurse notices that a client with dependent personality disorder is depressed. Which factor is assessed as contributing to depression?
1. Unmet needs
2. Sense of smothering
3. Messy, unkempt appearance
4. Difficulty delaying gratification

73. 1. Having many unmet needs is a precursor to depression. Clients with dependent personality disorder don't experience a sense of smothering, a problem seen in clients with panic disorder. Poor hygiene is often a *manifestation, not* a cause, of depression. Clients with problems delaying gratification tend to have anxiety problems, not problems with depression.
CN: Psychosocial integrity; CNS: None; CL: Analysis

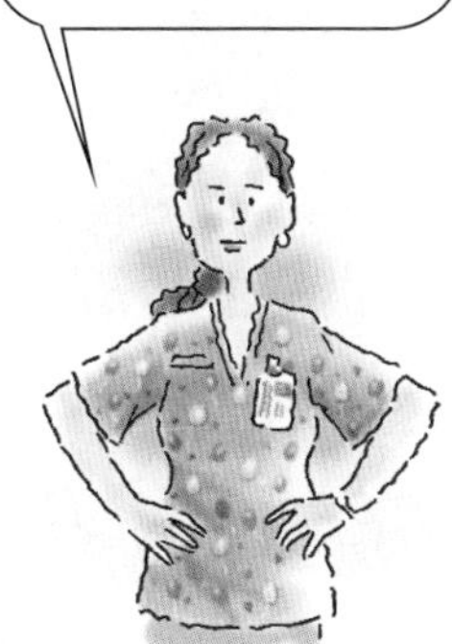

Keep in mind the type of personality this client has.

74. A client with dependent personality disorder makes the following statement, "I'll never be able to take care of myself." Which response is best?
1. "How can you say that? You can function."
2. "Let's talk about what's making you feel so fearful."
3. "I think we need to work on identifying your strengths."
4. "Can we talk about this tomorrow at the family meeting?"

74. 2. The client with dependent personality disorder is afraid of abandonment and being unable to care for himself. Talking about his fears is a useful strategy. The first option is inappropriate because the nurse doesn't recognize the client's feelings. When the client makes a desperate statement, the nurse must respond to the client's feelings, rather than insert her opinion. Working on identifying a client's strengths will add to his feelings of not being strong enough to care for himself. Waiting to talk about his concern until the family meeting minimizes its importance.
CN: Psychosocial integrity; CNS: None; CL: Analysis

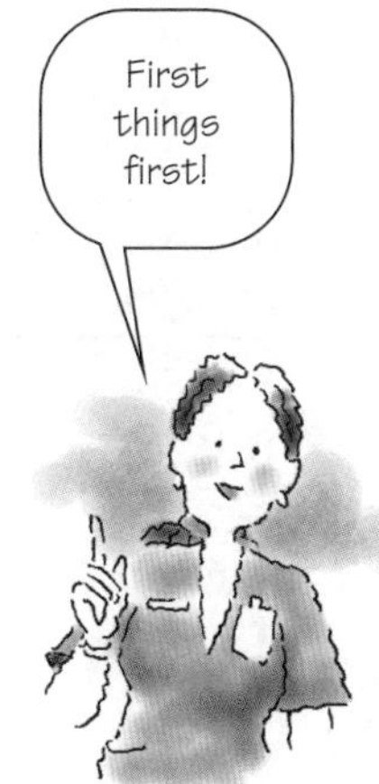

75. A client on your unit says the Mafia has a contract out on him. He refuses to leave his semiprivate room and insists on frisking his roommate before allowing him to enter. Which action should the nurse take first?
1. Transfer the client to a private room.
2. Acknowledge the client's fear when he refuses to leave his room or wants to frisk his roommate.
3. Transfer the roommate to another room.
4. Lock the client out of his room for a while each day so he can see he's safe.

75. 2. Acknowledging underlying feelings may help defuse the client's anxiety without promoting his delusional thinking. This, in turn, may help the client distinguish between his emotional state and external reality. Transferring either client to another room would validate the client's delusional thinking. Locking the client out of his room may further escalate the client's anxiety and stimulate aggressive acting-out behavior.
CN: Psychosocial integrity; CNS: None; CL: Application

76. A client with schizotypal personality disorder is sitting in a puddle of urine. He's playing in it, smiling, and softly singing a child's song. Which action would be best?

1. Admonish the client for not using the bathroom.
2. Firmly tell the client that her behavior is unacceptable.
3. Ask the client whether she's ready to get cleaned up now.
4. Help the client to the shower, and change the bedclothes.

76. 4. A client with a schizotypal personality disorder can experience high levels of anxiety and regress to childlike behaviors. This client may require help meeting self-care needs. The client may not respond to the other options or those options may generate more anxiety.
CN: Psychosocial integrity; CNS: None; CL: Application

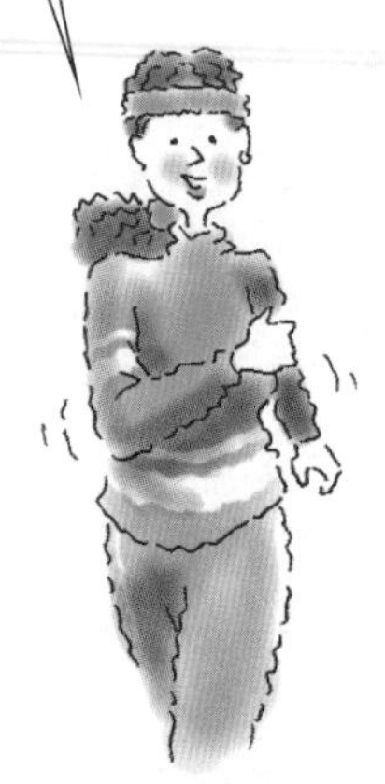

You've passed the 75 mark. Not too much more to go!

77. A client with avoidant personality disorder says occupational therapy (OT) is boring and he doesn't want to go. Which action would be best?

1. State firmly that you'll escort him to OT.
2. Arrange with OT for the client to do a project on the unit.
3. Ask the client to talk about why OT is boring.
4. Arrange for the client not to attend OT until he feels better.

77. 1. If given the chance, a client with avoidant personality disorder typically elects to remain immobilized. The nurse should insist that the client participate in OT. Arranging for the client to do a project on the unit validates and reinforces the client's desire to avoid going to OT. Addressing an invalid issue such as the client's perceived boredom avoids the real issue: the client's need for therapy. There's no indication that the client is incapable of participating in OT.
CN: Psychosocial integrity; CNS: None; CL: Application

78. A client with paranoid personality disorder works toward the goal of increasing social interaction. Which behavior indicates that the client is meeting this goal?

1. The client develops and follows a schedule of group activities.
2. The client verbalizes aggressive feelings to the nurse.
3. The client visits the consumer center to use the Internet.
4. The client explores somatic complaints with the staff.

78. 1. By developing and following a schedule of group activities, the client increases opportunities to use social skills and increase interactions with others. Verbalizing aggressive feelings doesn't give the client opportunities to increase social interaction. Using a computer at the consumer center is a solitary activity. Talking to the staff about somatic complaints doesn't provide opportunities for social interaction.
CN: Psychosocial integrity; CNS: None; CL: Application

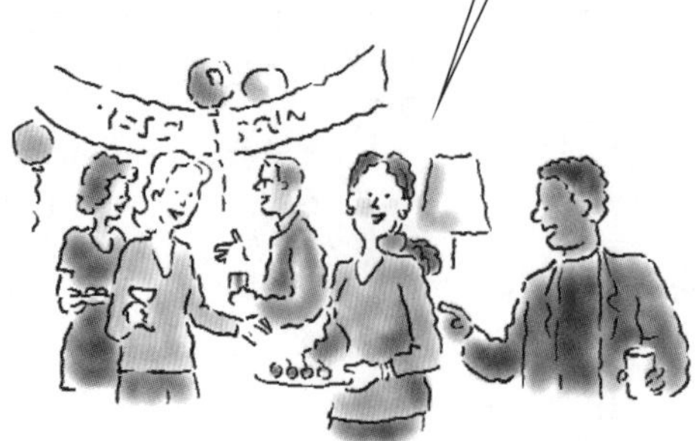

Which answer will help the client increase his social interaction?

79. A nurse works with the family of a client diagnosed with schizoid personality disorder, helping them to assist him in making decisions. Which outcome indicates the nurse's interventions have been successful?

1. The family prevents the client from experiencing disappointments.
2. The family encourages the client to talk about specific issues and concerns.
3. The family removes alcohol and unnecessary prescription drugs from the house.
4. The family doesn't let the client obtain secondary gains from illness.

80. A nurse discusses job possibilities with a client with schizoid personality disorder. Which suggestion by the nurse should be helpful?

1. "You could work in a family restaurant part-time on the weekends and holidays."
2. "Maybe your friend could get you that customer service job where you work only in the evenings."
3. "Your idea of applying for the position of filing and organizing records is worth pursuing."
4. "Being an introvert limits the employment opportunities you can pursue."

81. A client with borderline personality disorder is learning how to verbalize, rather than act on, the desire to hurt himself. Which intervention should the nurse use to help him recognize angry feelings?

1. Explain how pain triggers intense anger and causes the client to act out.
2. Determine how problems with the client's family cause her to act aggressively.
3. Teach the client that being volatile is a normal reaction to unfair events.
4. Have the client work on identifying speech and behavior that accompany anger.

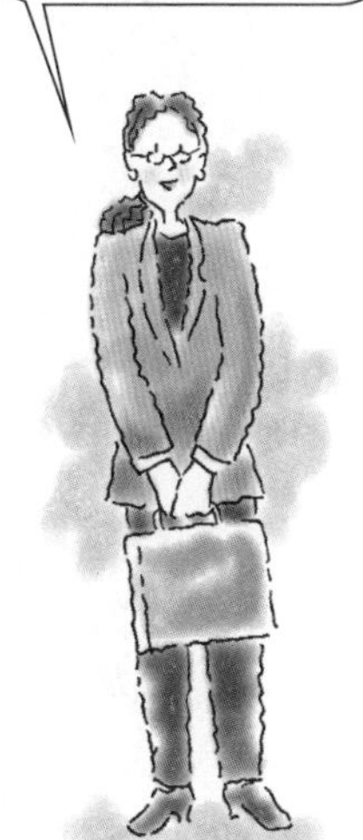

When trying to answer question 80, think about the type of activities this client prefers.

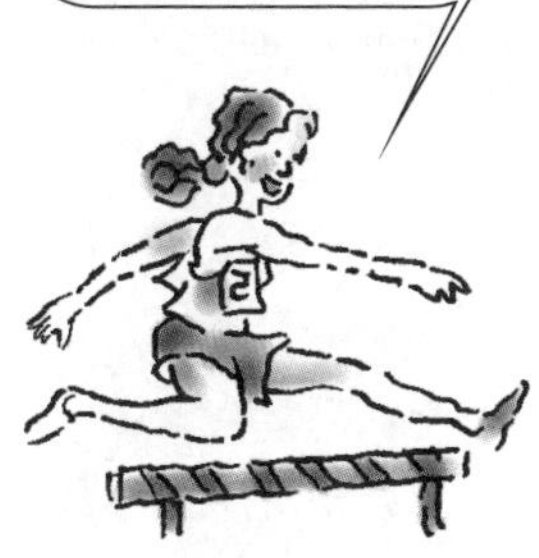

Three more hurdles...I mean questions...to go!

79. 2. A client with schizoid personality disorder typically is vague and has difficulty with self-expression; encouraging the client to talk about specific issues and concerns shows that the nurse's interventions were successful. It's neither realistic nor helpful for the family to protect the client from disappointments. Clients with schizoid personality disorder aren't at high risk for substance abuse and don't seek secondary gains from illness.

CN: Psychosocial integrity; CNS: None; CL: Application

80. 3. Clients with schizoid personality disorder prefer solitary activities, such as filing, to working with others. Working as a cashier or customer service representative would involve interacting with many people. Not all jobs require extensive interpersonal contact.

CN: Psychosocial integrity; CNS: None; CL: Analysis

81. 4. Aggressive speech and inappropriate behaviors indicate that the client is angry or upset; these feelings may trigger acting out. Pain rarely triggers intense anger or makes a client act out. Blaming one's family of origin for inappropriate handling of anger isn't helpful. Being volatile isn't a normal reaction to unfair life events. The client needs to express anger in safe and appropriate ways.

CN: Psychosocial integrity; CNS: None; CL: Analysis

82. A client with borderline personality disorder states that he doesn't know how to deal with his impulsive behavior. Which intervention should the nurse implement?

1. Teach the client that impulsive behavior is part of his illness.
2. Explore how depression influences impulsive situations.
3. Select an example of an impulsive situation and explore it.
4. Decrease interactions in which impulsive behavior occurs.

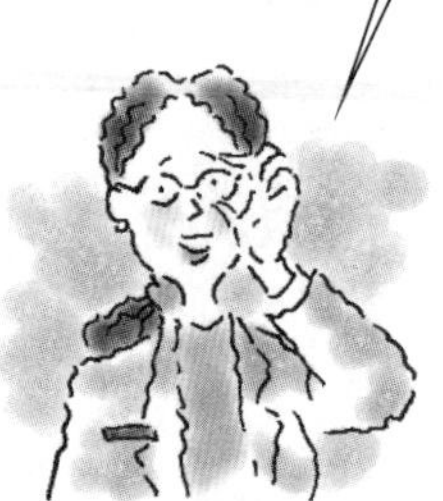

In question 82, focus on the client's impulsive behavior.

82. 3. By selecting an impulsive situation to explore with the client, the nurse can help him begin to understand the causes and consequences of his behavior and learn how to modify it. Although impulsive behavior is part of borderline personality disorder, the nurse's intervention needs to address ways to handle it. Anxiety, not depression, is strongly related to impulsive behavior. Decreasing social interactions is unrealistic; it's more useful to address the impulsive behavior.
CN: Psychosocial integrity; CNS: None; CL: Analysis

83. A nurse is monitoring a client who appears to be hallucinating. She notes paranoid content in the client's speech and that he appears agitated. The client is gesturing at a figure on the television. Which nursing interventions are appropriate? Select all that apply:

1. In a firm voice, instruct the client to stop the behavior.
2. Reinforce that the client is not in any danger.
3. Acknowledge the presence of the hallucinations.
4. Instruct other team members to ignore the client's behavior.
5. Immediately implement physical restraint procedures.
6. Use a calm voice and simple commands.

83. 2, 3, 6. Using a calm voice, the nurse should reassure the client that he's safe. She shouldn't challenge the client; rather, she should acknowledge his hallucinatory experience. It's not appropriate to request that the client stop the behavior. Implementing restraints isn't warranted at this time. Although the client is agitated, no evidence exists that he is at risk for harming himself or others.
CN: Psychosocial integrity; CNS: None; CL: Application

84. When assessing a client diagnosed with impulse control disorder, the nurse observes violent, aggressive, and assaultive behavior. Which assessment data is the nurse also likely to find? Select all that apply:

1. The client functions well in other areas of his life.
2. The degree of aggressiveness is out of proportion to the stressor.
3. The violent behavior is most often justified by the stressor.
4. The client has a history of parental alcoholism and chaotic, abusive family life.
5. The client has no remorse about the inability to control his behavior.

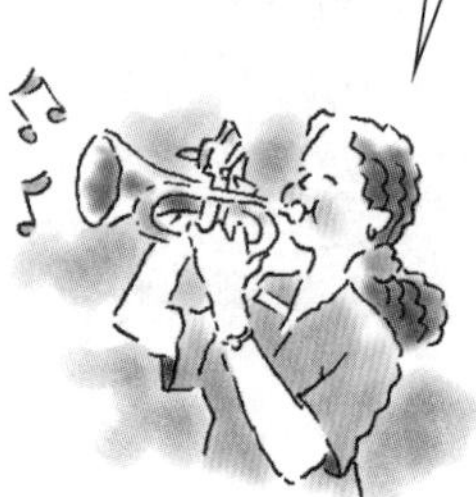

An incredible job! You've finished another big chapter! That's music to my ears!

84. 1, 2, 4. A client with an impulse control disorder who displays violent, aggressive, and assaultive behavior generally functions well in other areas of his life. The degree of aggressiveness is typically out of proportion with the stressor. Such a client commonly has a history of parental alcoholism and a chaotic family life, and often verbalizes sincere remorse and guilt for the aggressive behavior.
CN: Psychosocial integrity; CNS: None; CL: Application

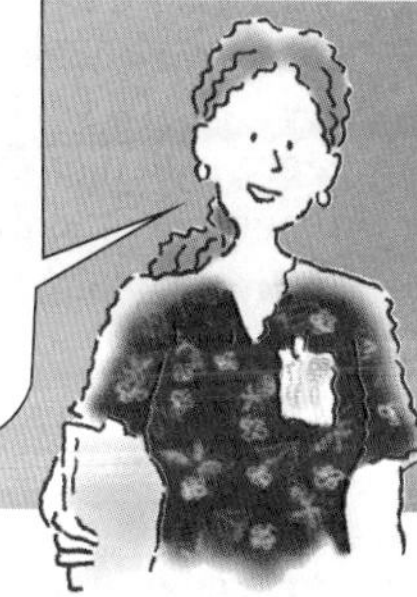

Chapter 17
Schizophrenic & delusional disorders

1. A schizophrenic client tells his primary nurse that he's scheduled to meet the King of Samoa at a special time, making it impossible for the client to leave his room for dinner. Which response by the nurse is most appropriate?

1. "It's meal time. Let's go so you can eat."
2. "The King of Samoa told me to take you to dinner."
3. "Your physician expects you to follow the unit's schedule."
4. "People who don't eat on this unit aren't being cooperative."

1. 1. A delusional client is so wrapped up in his false beliefs that he tends to disregard activities of daily living, such as nutrition and hydration. He needs clear, concise, firm directions from a caring nurse to meet his needs. The second option belittles and tricks the client, possibly evoking mistrust on the part of the client. The third option evades the issue of meeting his basic needs. The last option is demeaning and doesn't address the delusion.

CN: Health promotion and maintenance; CNS: None; CL: Application

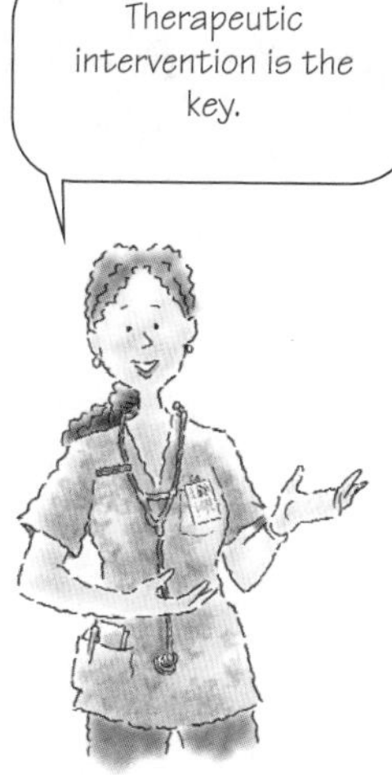

2. During breakfast, a client announces that he is still the President of the United States. What is the best response from the nurse?

1. "How are you, Mr. President?"
2. "The real president was on TV last night."
3. "How is your breakfast?"
4. "Is this the Oval Office then?"

2. 3. Asking about breakfast redirects the client and focuses him on a structured activity or reality-based task. The other responses focus attention on or support the client's delusion.

CN: Psychosocial integrity; CNS: None; CL: Application

3. A 40-year-old client with a diagnosis of chronic, undifferentiated schizophrenia lives in a rooming house that has a weekly nursing clinic. He scratches while he tells the nurse he feels creatures eating away at his skin. Which intervention should be done first?

1. Talk about his hallucinations and fears.
2. Refer him for anticholinergic adverse reactions.
3. Assess for possible physical problems such as rash.
4. Call his physician to get his medication increased to control his psychosis.

3. 3. Clients with schizophrenia generally have poor visceral recognition because they live so fully in their fantasy world. They need to have an in-depth assessment of physical complaints that may spill over into their delusional symptoms. Talking with the client won't provide an assessment of his itching, and itching isn't an adverse reaction of antipsychotic drugs. Calling the physician to get the client's medication increased doesn't address his physical complaints.

CN: Safe, effective care environment; CNS: Management of care; CL: Application

4. A 22-year-old schizophrenic client was admitted to the psychiatric unit during the night. The next morning, he began to misidentify the nurse and call her by his sister's name. Which intervention is best?

1. Assess the client for potential violence.
2. Take the client to his room, where he'll feel safer.
3. Assume the misidentification makes the client feel more comfortable.
4. Correct the misidentification, and orient the client to the unit and staff.

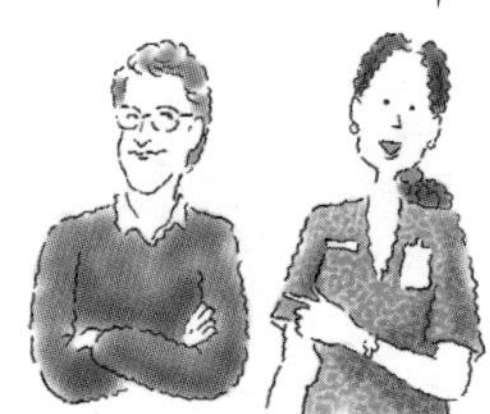

4. 4. Misidentification can contribute to anxiety, fear, aggression, and hostility. Orienting a new client to the hospital unit, staff, and other clients, along with establishing a nurse-client relationship, can decrease these feelings and help the client feel in control. Assessing for potential violence is an important nursing function for any psychiatric client, but a perceived supportive environment reduces the risk for violence. Withdrawing to his room, unless interpersonal relationships have become nontherapeutic for him, encourages the client to remain in his fantasy world.

CN: Psychosocial integrity; CNS: None; CL: Application

5. Which term describes an effect of isolation?

1. Delusions
2. Hallucinations
3. Lack of volition
4. Waxy flexibility

5. 2. Prolonged isolation can produce sensory deprivation, manifested by hallucinations. A delusion is a false, fixed belief that has no basis in reality. Lack of volition is a symptom associated with type I negative symptoms of schizophrenia. Waxy flexibility is a motor disturbance that's a predominant feature of catatonic schizophrenia.

CN: Psychosocial integrity; CNS: None; CL: Application

6. A client diagnosed with schizophrenia several years ago tells a nurse that he feels "very sad." The nurse observes that he's smiling when he says it. Which term best describes the nurse's observation?

1. Inappropriate affect
2. Extrapyramidal
3. Insight
4. Inappropriate mood

6. 1. Affect refers to behaviors such as facial expression that can be observed when a person is expressing and experiencing feelings. If the client's affect doesn't reflect the emotional content of the statement, the affect is considered inappropriate. Extrapyramidal symptoms are adverse effects of some categories of medication. Insight is a component of the mental status examination and is the ability to perceive oneself realistically and understand if a problem exists. Mood is an extensive and sustained feeling tone.

CN: Psychosocial integrity; CNS: None; CL: Application

7. A disorganized schizophrenic's symptoms include the distressing triad of extreme social withdrawal, odd mannerisms, and other regressive behaviors. The nurse's most therapeutic intervention is which of the following?

1. Require the client to attend one group activity each day.
2. Suggest that the client keeps up with his same gender peer group.
3. Interact with the client often and briefly, in a friendly manner.
4. Allow the client to come out when he is ready.

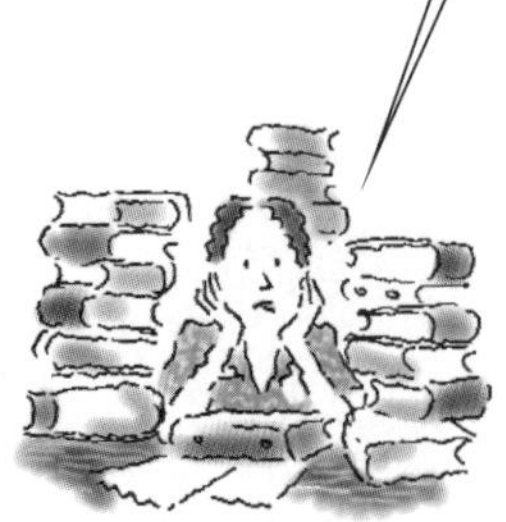

The word disorganized refers to a type of schizophrenia, and to me!

7. 3. Interacting with the client often and in a friendly manner suggests planned, short, frequent, and undemanding interactions. Clients with disorganized schizophrenia require one-on-one non-threatening activities and should not remain in social isolation.

CN: Psychosocial integrity; CNS: None; CL: Application

CN: Client needs category CNS: Client needs subcategory CL: Cognitive level

8. A client on the psychiatric unit is copying and imitating the movements of his primary nurse. During recovery, he says, "I thought the nurse was my mirror. I felt connected only when I saw my nurse." This behavior is known by which term?

1. Modeling
2. Echopraxia
3. Ego-syntonicity
4. Ritualism

8. 2. Echopraxia is the copying of another's behaviors and is the result of the loss of ego boundaries. Modeling is the conscious copying of someone's behaviors. Ego-syntonicity refers to behaviors that correspond with the individual's sense of self. Ritualistic behaviors are repetitive and compulsive.

CN: Psychosocial integrity; CNS: None; CL: Application

9. The teenage son of a father with schizophrenia is worried that he might have schizophrenia as well. Which behavior would be an indication that he should be evaluated for signs of the disorder?

1. Moodiness
2. Preoccupation with his body
3. Spending more time away from home
4. Changes in sleep patterns

9. 4. In conjunction with other signs, changes in sleep patterns are distinctive initial signs of schizophrenia. Other signs include changes in personal care habits and social isolation. Moodiness, preoccupation with the body, and spending more time away from home are normal adolescent behaviors.

CN: Health promotion and maintenance; CNS: None; CL: Application

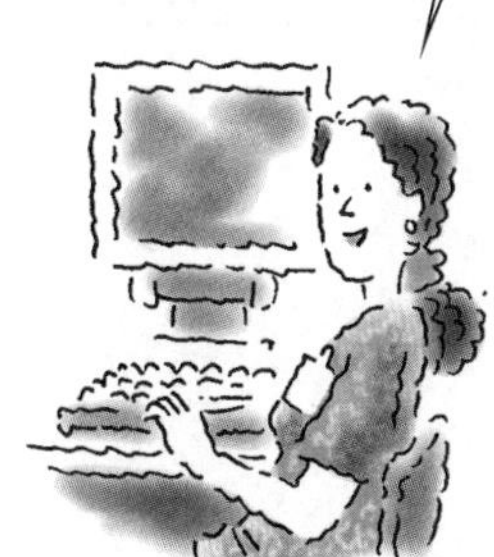
Pay attention to the key word in questions 10 and 11.

10. The nurse is teaching the family of a client with a psychiatric disorder about <u>traditional</u> antipsychotic drugs and their effect on symptoms. Which of the following symptoms would be most responsive to these types of drugs?

1. Apathy
2. Delusions
3. Social withdrawal
4. Attention impairment

10. 2. Positive symptoms, such as delusions, hallucinations, thought disorder, and disorganized speech, respond to traditional antipsychotic drugs. The other options are part of the category of negative symptoms, including affective flattening, restricted thought and speech, apathy, anhedonia, asociality, and attention impairment, and are more responsive to the new atypical antipsychotics, such as clozapine (Clozaril), risperidone (Risperdal), and olanzapine (Zyprexa).

CN: Physiological integrity CNS: Pharmacological and parenteral therapies; CL: Application

11. A client was hospitalized after his son filed a petition for involuntary hospitalization for safety reasons. The son seeks out the nurse because his father is angry and refuses to talk with him. He's frustrated and feeling very guilty about his decision. Which response to this client is the most <u>empathic</u>?

1. "Your father is here because he needs help."
2. "He'll feel differently about you as he gets better."
3. "It sounds like you're feeling guilty about leaving your father here."
4. "This is a stressful time for you, but you'll feel better as he gets well."

11. 3. This response focuses on the son and helps him discuss and deal with his feelings. Unresolved feelings of guilt, shame, isolation, and loss of hope impact on the family's ability to manage the crisis and be supportive to the client. The other options offer premature reassurance and cut off the opportunity for the son to discuss his feelings.

CN: Psychosocial integrity; CNS: None; CL: Application

12. A client followed her antipsychotic medication regimen for a number of years. Her physician treats her urinary tract infection with antibiotic therapy. Which action is a nursing responsibility?

1. Arrange for possible hospitalization.
2. Have a visiting nurse give the medication.
3. Give instructions on the medication, possible adverse effects, and a return demonstration for teaching effectiveness.
4. Develop a psychoeducational program to address the client's emotional and physical problems arising from physiologic problems.

12. 3. The client has been successful and reliable in carrying out her current medication regimen. The nurse should assume the competency includes self-administration of antibiotics if the instructions are understood. No evidence exists that the client is having a relapse as a result of the infection, so she wouldn't need a psychoeducational program or hospitalization. Having a community nurse give the medication encourages dependency as opposed to self-care.

CN: Safe, effective care environment; CNS: Management of care; CL: Application

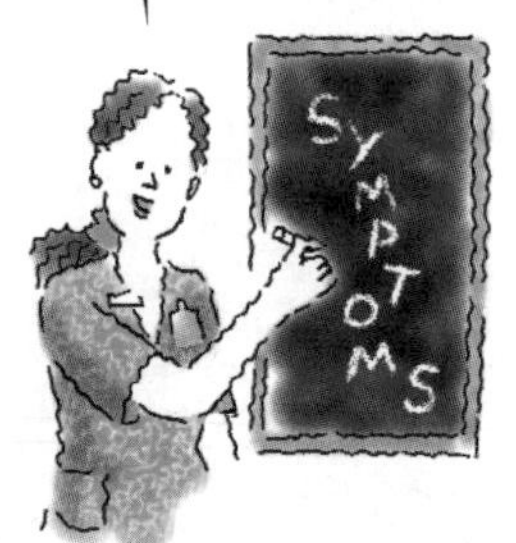

Signs and symptoms are big on NCLEX examinations. Better know them cold.
SYMPTOMS

13. Which sign indicates tardive dyskinesia?

1. Involuntary movements
2. Blurred vision
3. Restlessness
4. Sudden fever

13. 1. Symptoms of tardive dyskinesia include tongue protrusion, lip smacking, chewing, blinking, grimacing, choreiform movements of limbs and trunk, and foot tapping. Blurred vision is a common adverse reaction of antipsychotic drugs and usually disappears after a few weeks of therapy. Restlessness is associated with akathisia. Sudden fever is a symptom of a malignant neurologic disorder.

CN: Physiological integrity; CNS: Reduction of risk potential; CL: Application

14. A client approaches a nurse and tells her that he hears voices telling him that he's evil and deserves to die. Which response by the nurse is most appropriate?

1. "The voices aren't real, so ignore them."
2. "I don't see anyone in the room."
3. "I don't hear any voices, but I understand that you do."
4. "Tell the voices you won't listen to them."

14. 3. The nurse should let the client know that although she can't hear the voices, she understands that they are real to him. She should keep communication open and encourage him to talk. Telling the client that the voices aren't real may make him hold tighter to his belief and doesn't promote trust. Telling him to talk back to the voices validates their reality.

CN: Psychosocial integrity; CNS: None; CL: Application

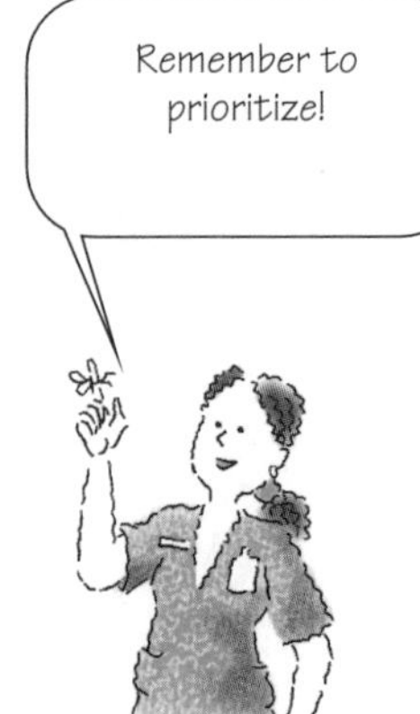

15. A 49-year-old client is admitted to the emergency department frightened and reporting that he's hearing voices telling him to do bad things. Which intervention should be the nurse's priority?

1. Tell the client he's safe and that the voices aren't real.
2. Tell the client he's safe now and promise the staff will protect him.
3. Assess the nature of the commands by asking the client what the voices are saying.
4. Administer a neuroleptic medication.

15. 3. Safety is the priority. The nurse should directly ask the client about the nature of the auditory commands to adequately assess the safety of the client and staff. The nurse should never make promises to the client that she may not be able to fulfill. The physician may order a neuroleptic, but the nurse's priority is to address safety.

CN: Safe, effective care environment; CNS: Management of care; CL: Application

16. Which pair of numbers of members in a therapy group is ideal?

1. 1 to 4
2. 4 to 7
3. 7 to 10
4. 10 to 15

16. 3. The ideal number of members in an inpatient group is 7 to 10. Having fewer than 7 members provides inadequate interaction and material for successful group process. Having more than 10 members doesn't allow for adequate time for individual participation.

CN: Psychosocial integrity; CNS: None; CL: Application

17. A client admitted to an inpatient unit approaches a nursing student saying he descended from a long line of people of a "superrace." Which action is correct?

1. Smile and walk into the nurse's station.
2. Challenge the client's false belief.
3. Listen for hidden messages in themes of delusion, indicating unmet needs.
4. Introduce yourself, shake hands, and sit down with the client in the day room.

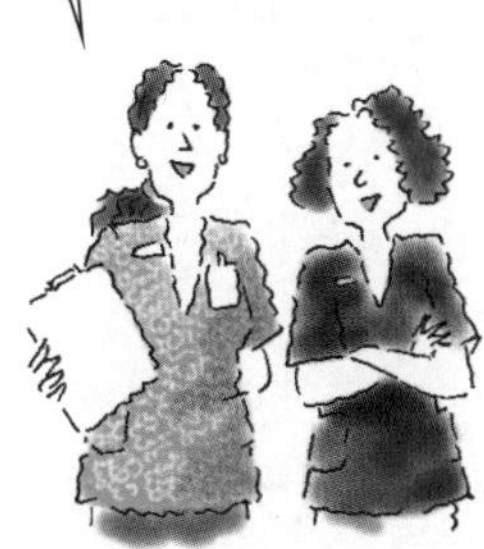

Teach nursing students the importance of genuine interest and concern for client's needs.

17. 4. The first goal is to establish a relationship with the client, which includes creating psychological space for the creation of trust. The student should sit and make herself available, reflecting concern and interest. Walking into the nurse's station would indicate disinterest and lack of concern about the client's feelings. After establishing a relationship and lessening the client's anxiety, the student can orient the client to reality, listen to his concerns and fears, and try to understand the feelings reflected in the delusions. Delusions are firmly maintained false beliefs, and attempts to dismiss them don't work.

CN: Safe, effective care environment; CNS: Management of care; CL: Application

18. Which nursing diagnosis is most appropriate for a client with acute schizophrenic reaction?

1. *Social isolation related to impaired ability to trust*
2. *Impaired physical mobility related to fear of hostile impulses*
3. *Disturbed sleep patterns related to impaired thinking ability*
4. *Risk for other-directed violence related to perceptual distortions*

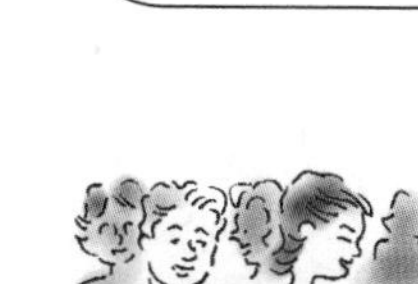
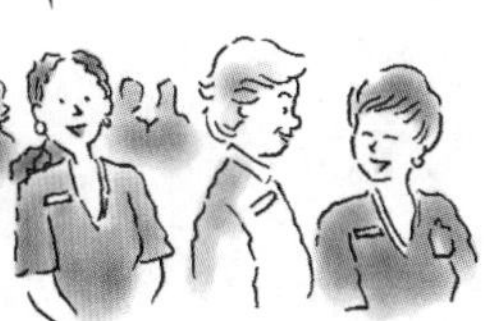

An accurate nursing diagnosis helps all nurses better understand the client.

18. 1. Clients with schizophrenia are mistrustful, which results in withdrawal and social isolation. Mobility isn't a common problem for persons with schizophrenia. Sleep disturbance may be present but isn't the most common symptom. Contrary to popular belief, persons with schizophrenia usually aren't violent.

CN: Safe, effective care environment; CNS: Management of care; CL: Analysis

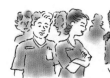

19. A nurse is assisting with morning care when a client suddenly throws off the covers and starts shouting, "My body is changing and disintegrating because I'm not of this world." Which term best describes this behavior?

1. Depersonalization
2. Ideas of reference
3. Looseness of association
4. Paranoid ideation

19. 1. Depersonalization is a state in which the client feels unreal or believes parts of the body are being distorted. Ideas of reference are beliefs unrelated to situations and hold special meaning for the individual. The term loose associations refers to sentences that have vague connections to each other. Paranoid ideations are beliefs that others intend to harm the client in some way.

CN: Psychosocial integrity; CNS: None; CL: Analysis

20. A 16-year-old client with a diagnosis of undifferentiated schizophrenia has become very clingy and begins sucking her thumb while interacting with the nurse. The nurse understands that these behaviors indicate which defense mechanism?

1. Repression
2. Regression
3. Rationalization
4. Projection

20. 2. Regression, a return to earlier behavior in order to reduce anxiety, is the basic defense mechanism in schizophrenia. Repression is the blocking of unacceptable thoughts or impulses from the consciousness. Rationalization is a defense mechanism used to justify one's behavior. Projection is a defense mechanism in which one blames others and attempts to justify actions.
CN: Psychosocial integrity; CNS: None; CL: Application

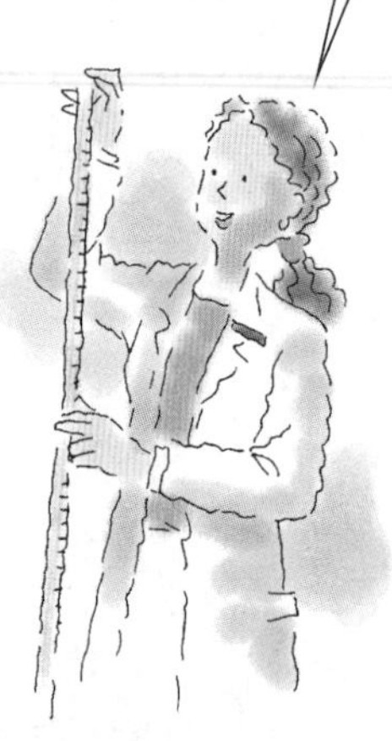

Any way you measure it, you're doing great.

21. Which assessment technique is best when interviewing a client with paranoia?

1. Using indirect questions
2. Using direct questions
3. Using lead-in remarks
4. Using open-ended sentences

21. 2. Direct questioning is the most appropriate technique to use when interviewing a client with paranoid schizophrenia. Specific questions, such as "Are you hearing voices right now?" provide the nurse useful information. The other forms of communication may be misunderstood by the client and his responses may be vague.
CN: Psychosocial integrity; CNS: None; CL: Application

22. A nurse on a psychiatric unit observes a client in the corner of the room moving his lips as if he were talking to himself. Which action is the most appropriate?

1. Ask him why he's talking to himself.
2. Leave him alone until he stops talking.
3. Tell him it isn't good for him to talk to himself.
4. Invite him to join in a card game with the nurse.

22. 4. Being with the nurse provides stimulation that competes with the hallucinations. The client doesn't think he's talking to himself, he's responding only to the voices he hears. Being alone keeps the client in his fantasy world. Telling the client that he shouldn't talk to himself fails to understand how real his fantasy world and hallucinations are.
CN: Psychosocial integrity; CNS: None; CL: Application

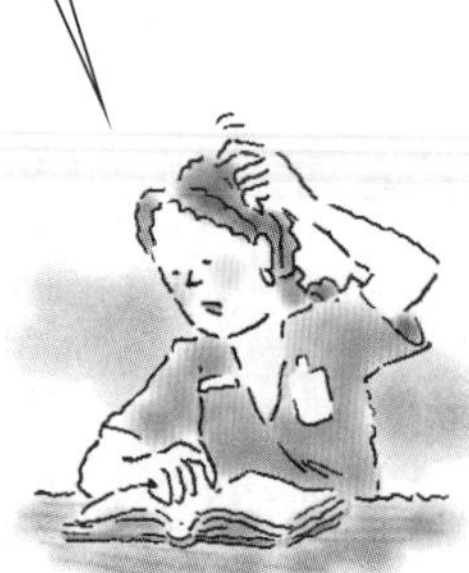

I'm trying to understand but sometimes it's difficult.

23. A client makes vague statements with no logical connections. He asks whether the nurse understands. Which response is best?

1. "Why don't we wait until later to talk about it?"
2. "You're not making sense, so I won't talk about this topic."
3. "Yes, I understand the overall sense of the logical connections from the idea."
4. "I want to understand what you're saying, but I'm having difficulty following you."

23. 4. The nurse needs to communicate that she wants to understand without blaming the client for the lack of understanding. Asking the client to wait because he's too confused cuts off an attempt to communicate and asks the client to do what he can't at present. Telling the client that he isn't making sense is judgmental and could impair the therapeutic relationship. Pretending to understand is a violation of trust and can damage the therapeutic relationship.
CN: Psychosocial integrity; CNS: None; CL: Application

24. A client asks a nurse if she hears the voice of the nonexistent man speaking to him. Which response is best?

1. "No one is in your room except you."
2. "Yes, I hear him, but I won't listen to him."
3. "What has he told you? Is it helpful advice?"
4. "No, I don't hear him, but I know you do. What is he saying?"

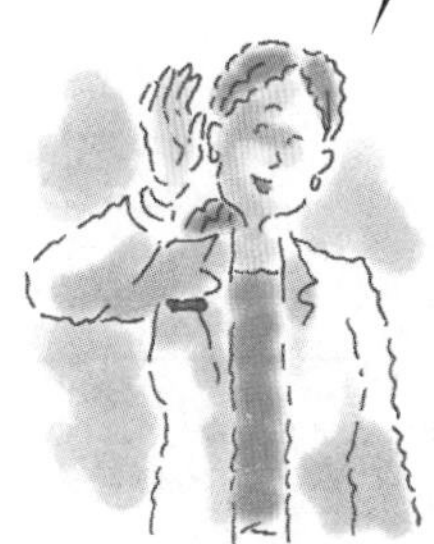

Do you hear what I hear?

24. 4. This response points out reality and shows concern and support. Attempting to argue the client out of the belief might entrench him more firmly in his belief, making him feel more out of control because of the negative and fearful nature of hallucinations. The other two options violate the trust of the therapeutic relationship.

CN: Safe, effective care environment; CNS: Management of care; CL: Application

25. Which instruction is correct for a client taking chlorpromazine?

1. Reduce the dosage if you feel better.
2. Occasional social drinking isn't harmful.
3. Stop taking the drug immediately if adverse reactions develop.
4. Schedule routine medication checks.

25. 4. Ongoing assessment by a primary health care provider is important to assess for adverse reactions and continued therapeutic effectiveness. The dosage should be changed only after checking with the primary care provider. Alcoholic beverages are contraindicated while taking an antipsychotic drug. Adverse reactions should be reported immediately to determine if the drug should be discontinued.

CN: Physiological integrity; CNS: Pharmacological and parenteral therapies; CL: Application

26. A 34-year-old male client is referred to a mental health clinic by the court. The client harassed a couple next-door to him with charges that the wife was in love with him. He wrote love notes and called her on the telephone throughout the night. The client is employed and has had no problems in his job. Which disorder is suspected?

1. Major depression
2. Paranoid schizophrenia
3. Delusional disorder
4. Bipolar affective disorder

26. 3. The client has a delusional disorder with erotomanic delusions as his primary symptom and believes he's loved intensely by a married person showing no interest in him. No symptoms of major depression exist. The client doesn't believe someone is trying to harm him, the hallmark characteristic of paranoia. Bipolar affective disorder is characterized by cycles of extreme emotional highs (mania) and lows (depression).

CN: Psychosocial integrity; CNS: None; CL: Application

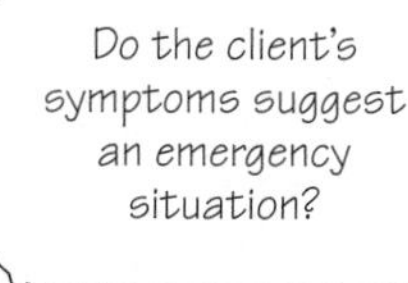

Do the client's symptoms suggest an emergency situation?

27. A homebound client taking clozapine (Clozaril) tells the nurse he has been feeling tired for 5 days. His temperature is 99.6° F; pulse, 110 beats/minute; and respirations, 20 breaths/minute. Which instruction is correct?

1. Take the medication with milk.
2. Stop the medication at once, and see the physician immediately.
3. Understand that the symptoms will disappear as soon as he gets more rest.
4. Stop the medication gradually, and see the physician next week.

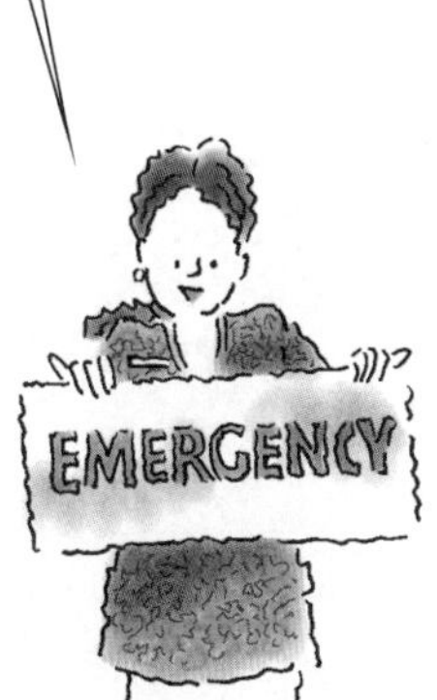

27. 2. He should stop the medication and see his physician immediately because fever can be a sign of agranulocytosis, which is a medical emergency. Taking antipsychotic medication with milk, nicotine, and caffeine will decrease the effectiveness. Rest will have no effect on this client's symptoms. Drowsiness and fatigue usually disappear with continued therapy.

CN: Physiological integrity; CNS: Pharmacological and parenteral therapies; CL: Application

28. A client who is delusional approaches the nurse and states, "You are my aunt and you live with my family." Which statement by the nurse would be the most therapeutic?

1. "I'm not your aunt."
2. "I don't live here."
3. "I'm honored."
4. "This is my name. What is your aunt's name?"

28. 4. By the nurse stating her name and asking the name of the client's aunt, the nurse acknowledges the client is speaking of family, while basing it in a realistic interaction. The other responses all focus on and respond directly to the client's fixed delusional system.
CN: Psychosocial integrity; CNS: None; CL: Application

29. A client tells the nurse that he can only drink bottled water since the water from his sink has been poisoned. The nurse understands that the client is exhibiting which behavior?

1. Paranoia
2. Auditory hallucinations
3. Delusions of grandeur
4. Perseveration

29. 1. This client is exhibiting extreme suspiciousness and distrust of others. Auditory hallucinations occur when a client hears voices that are often threatening or violent. Delusions of grandeur are an exaggerated sense of self-importance. A client with perseveration involuntarily repeats words.
CN: Psychosocial integrity; CNS: None; CL: Application

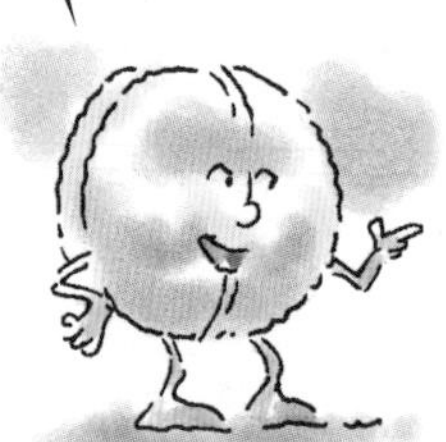
The words most likely can help you focus on the answer.

30. A client with a diagnosis of paranoid-type schizophrenia is receiving an antipsychotic medication. His physician has just prescribed benztropine (Cogentin). The nurse realizes that this medication was most likely prescribed in response to which possible adverse reaction?

1. Tardive dyskinesia
2. Hypertensive crisis
3. Acute dystonia
4. Orthostatic hypotension

30. 3. Benztropine is used as adjunctive therapy in parkinsonism and for all conditions and medications that produce extrapyramidal symptoms except tardive dyskinesia. Its anticholinergic effect reduces the extrapyramidal effects associated with antipsychotic drugs. Hypertensive crisis and orthostatic hypotension aren't associated with extrapyramidal symptoms.
CN: Psychosocial integrity; CNS: Pharmacological and parenteral therapies; CL: Analysis

31. Which action by a nurse is an appropriate therapeutic intervention for a client experiencing hallucinations?

1. Confine him in his room until he feels better.
2. Provide a competing stimulus that distracts from the hallucinations.
3. Discourage attempts to understand what precipitates his hallucinations.
4. Support perceptual distortions until he gives them up of his own accord.

31. 2. Providing competing stimuli acknowledges the presence of the hallucination and teaches ways to decrease the frequency of hallucinations. The other options support and maintain hallucinations or deny their existence.
CN: Psychosocial integrity; CNS: None; CL: Application

32. A client with schizophrenia reports that her hallucinations have decreased in frequency. Which intervention would be appropriate to begin addressing the client's problem with social isolation?

1. Have the client join in a group game.
2. Name the client as the leader of the client support group.
3. Have the client play solitaire.
4. Ask the client to participate in a group sing-along.

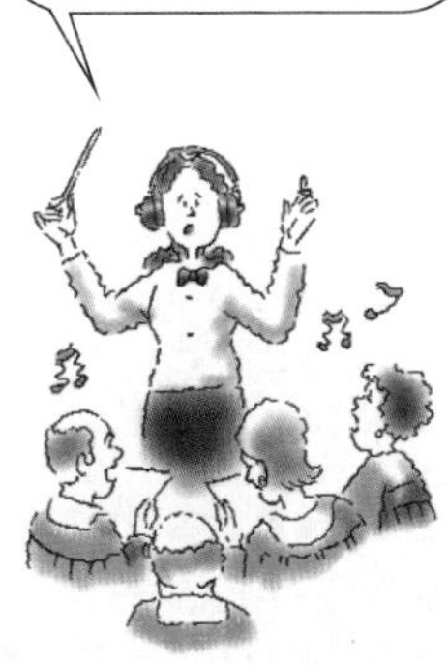
Music can be very therapeutic.

32. 4. Having the client participate in a noncompetitive group activity that doesn't require individual participation won't present a threat to the client. Games can become competitive and lead to anxiety or hostility. The client probably lacks sufficient social skills to lead a group at this time. Playing solitaire doesn't encourage socialization.

CN: Psychosocial integrity; CNS: None; CL: Application

33. A single 24-year-old client is admitted with acute schizophrenic reaction. Which method is appropriate therapy for this type of schizophrenia?

1. Counseling to produce insight into behavior
2. Biofeedback to reduce agitation associated with schizophrenia
3. Drug therapy to reduce symptoms associated with acute schizophrenia
4. Electroconvulsive therapy to treat the mood component of schizophrenia

33. 3. Drug therapy is usually successful in normalizing behavior and reducing or eliminating hallucinations, delusions, thought disorder, affect flattening, apathy, and asociality. Counseling isn't appropriate at this time. Electroconvulsive therapy might be considered for schizoaffective disorder, which has a mood component, and is a treatment of choice for clinical depression. Biofeedback reduces anxiety and modifies behavioral responses but isn't the major component in the treatment of schizophrenia.

CN: Psychosocial integrity; CNS: None; CL: Application

34. A client tells a nurse voices are telling him to do "terrible things." Which action is part of the initial therapy?

1. Find out what the voices are telling him.
2. Let him go to his room to decrease his anxiety.
3. Begin talking to the client about an unrelated topic.
4. Tell the client the voices aren't real.

34. 1. For safety purposes, the nurse must find out whether the voices are directing the client to harm himself or others. Further assessment can help identify appropriate therapeutic interventions. Isolating a person during this intense sensory confusion often reinforces the psychosis. Changing the topic indicates that the nurse isn't concerned about the client's fears. Dismissing the voices shuts down communication between the client and the nurse.

CN: Psychosocial integrity; CNS: None; CL: Application

35. A client is preoccupied with his belief that the CIA has been planning to take him away to save the agency from his influence. These delusions are a defense against which underlying feeling?

1. Aggression
2. Guilt
3. Inferiority
4. Persecution

35. 3. The delusional system contains grandiose ideation that allows the client to feel important rather than inferior. Feelings of aggression will appear as violent or hostile thoughts. Guilt results in beliefs that the person deserves to be punished. Persecution is the fear that others are trying to harm you.

CN: Psychosocial integrity; CNS: None; CL: Application

36. A client has started taking haloperidol (Haldol). Which instruction is most appropriate for a client taking haloperidol?

1. You should report feelings of restlessness or agitation at once.
2. Use a sunscreen outdoors on a year-round basis.
3. Be aware you'll feel increased energy taking this drug.
4. This drug will indirectly control essential hypertension.

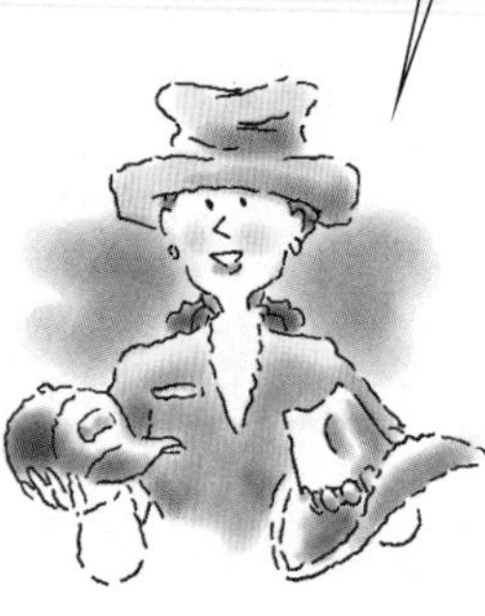

Which hat do you think is most appropriate?

36. 1. Agitation and restlessness are adverse effects of haloperidol and can be treated with anticholinergic drugs. Haloperidol isn't likely to cause photosensitivity or control essential hypertension. Although the client may experience increased concentration and activity, these effects are due to a decrease in symptoms, not the drug itself.
CN: Physiological integrity; CNS: Pharmacological and parenteral therapies; CL: Application

37. A 45-year-old client experiencing delusions has been admitted to the crisis center. When assessing the content of the delusions, the nurse should look for which aspect of the delusions?

1. Logic
2. Religious beliefs
3. Themes
4. True experiences

37. 3. Understanding the themes inherent in the client's psychotic symptoms may help the nurse learn what stresses trigger the symptoms. A delusion is a false, fixed belief that misrepresents perceptions or experiences and isn't open to rational argument. Assessing for logic, religious beliefs, or true experiences draws the nurse into the delusional thinking and therefore isn't therapeutic.
CN: Psychosocial integrity; CNS: None; CL: Analysis

38. The nurse is caring for a 58-year-old male client diagnosed with paranoid schizophrenia. When the client says, "The earth and the roof of the house rule the political structure with particles of rain," the nurse recognizes this as which type of expression?

1. Tangentiality
2. Perseveration
3. Loose association
4. Thought blocking

38. 3. Loose association refers to changing ideas from one unrelated theme to another, as exhibited by the client. Tangentiality is the wandering from topic to topic. Perseveration is involuntary repetition of the answer to a question in response to a new question. Thought blocking is having difficulty articulating a response or stopping midsentence.
CN: Psychosocial integrity; CNS: None; CL: Application

39. Which symptom indicates that schizophrenia is a thought disorder?

1. Faulty logic
2. Distorted but organized thinking
3. Organized but disruptive thoughts
4. Appropriate perception, but difficulty responding appropriately to people and events

39. 1. Thought disorders are characterized by problems in the form and organization of thinking. They appear as loose associations, word salad, tangentiality, illogicality, circumstantiality, pressure of speech, and poverty of speech that impairs communication. Thinking is disorganized and perceptions are often misinterpreted. The other options are inaccurate characteristics of schizophrenia.
CN: Psychosocial integrity; CNS: None; CL: Analysis

40. A client with schizophrenia tells the nurse that the President consults with him before making major decisions. Which is the best response by the nurse?

1. "How long have you known the President?"
2. "You're fortunate to know the President."
3. "How will you speak with the President from the hospital?"
4. "You must feel important. Now let's make your bed."

40. 4. Acknowledging that the client feels important addresses the underlying reason for the delusion. The other options reinforce the reality of the delusion.

CN: Psychosocial integrity; CNS: None; CL: Analysis

41. A client is admitted after being found on a highway, hitting at cars and yelling at motorists. When approached by the nurse, the client shouts, "You're the one who stole my husband from me!" Which term describes the client's condition?

1. Hallucinatory experience
2. Delusional experience
3. Disorientation to the environment
4. Phobic experience

41. 2. A delusion is a false, fixed belief manufactured without appropriate or sufficient evidence to support it. The client's statements don't represent hallucinations because they aren't perceptual disorders. No information in the question addresses orientation. The client's statements don't represent a phobia because they don't represent an irrational fear.

CN: Psychosocial integrity; CNS: None; CL: Application

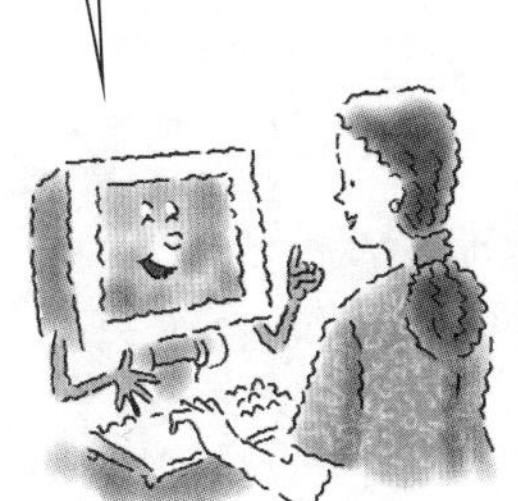

I'd be remiss if I didn't advise you to read this question carefully.

42. The nurse is teaching the family of a client with schizophrenia about symptoms of remission. Which of the following responses would be the most accurate?

1. The disease is in the prodromal phase.
2. The client no longer has prominent psychotic symptoms.
3. The client is free from all signs of illness and is no longer on medication.
4. The client is free from all signs of illness whether or not he's on medication.

42. 2. Schizophrenia is a chronic disorder with periods of remission and exacerbation. The prodromal phase is the precursor to an exacerbation. Clients aren't usually cured but are treated over time with case management, medication, symptom management skills, social skill training, network support, vocational training, and health-promoting practices.

CN: Psychosocial integrity; CNS: None; CL: Application

43. A client with schizophrenia is huddled on the floor and appears to be interacting with someone underneath the bed. The nurse notes that the client appears afraid. Which assessment by the nurse is most likely correct?

1. The client is having hallucinations.
2. The client is having suicidal ideations.
3. The client is having nightmares.
4. The client is having delusions.

43. 1. The client appears to be having auditory hallucinations and is hearing voices that he perceives to be coming from under the bed. There is no evidence that the client is having suicidal ideations, nightmares, or delusions.

CN: Psychosocial integrity; CNS: None; CL: Analysis

44. A nurse on an inpatient unit is having a discussion with a client with schizophrenia about his schedule for the day. The client comments that he was highly active at home and then explains the volunteer job he held. Which term describes the client's thinking?
1. Circumstantiality
2. Loose associations
3. Referential
4. Tangentiality

44. 4. Tangentiality describes thought patterns loosely connected but not directly related to the topic. In circumstantiality, the person digresses with unnecessary details. Loose associations are rapid shifts in the expression of ideas from one subject to another in an unrelated manner. Referential thinking is when an individual incorrectly interprets neutral incidents and external events as having a particular or special meaning for him.

CN: Psychosocial integrity; CNS: None; CL: Application

45. While talking to a client with schizophrenia, a nurse notes the client frequently uses unrecognizable words with no common meaning. Which term describes this?
1. Echolalia
2. Clang association
3. Neologisms
4. Word salad

45. 3. Neologisms are newly coined words with personal meanings to the client with schizophrenia. Echolalia is parrotlike echoing of spoken words or sounds. Clang association is the linking of words by sound rather than meaning. A word salad is stringing words in sequence that have no connection to one another.

CN: Psychosocial integrity; CNS: None; CL: Application

46. While caring for a hospitalized client diagnosed with schizophrenia, a nurse observes the client watching television. The client tells the nurse the television is speaking directly to him. Which term describes this belief?
1. Autistic thinking
2. Concrete thinking
3. Paranoid thinking
4. Referential thinking

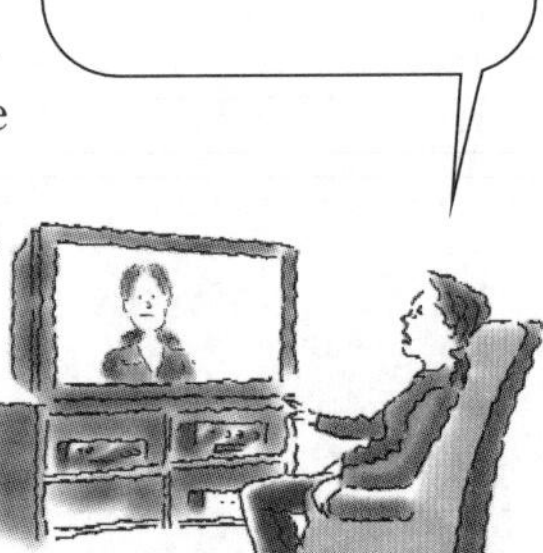

Are you talking to me?

46. 4. Referential, or primary process thinking, is a belief that incidents and events in the environment have special meaning for the client. Autistic thinking is a disturbance in thought due to the intrusion of a private fantasy world, internally stimulated, resulting in abnormal responses to people. Concrete thinking is the literal interpretation of words and symbols. Paranoid thinking is the belief that others are trying to harm you.

CN: Psychosocial integrity; CNS: None; CL: Application

47. A nurse is talking with a family of a client diagnosed with schizophrenia. The mother asks, "What causes this disorder?" Which explanation is the most widely accepted?
1. Prenatal or postpartum central nervous system damage
2. Bacterial infections in the mother during pregnancy or delivery
3. A biological predisposition exacerbated by environmental stressors
4. Lack of bonding and attachment during infancy, which leads to depression in later life

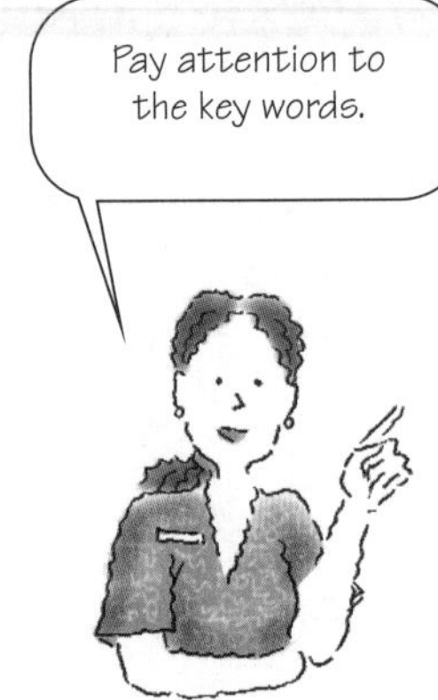

Pay attention to the key words.

47. 3. The holistic theory, currently the most widely accepted theory of its type, states that an interaction between biological predisposition and environmental stressors is the cause of schizophrenia. The biological explanation states that schizophrenia is caused by a brain disease, a bacterial infection in utero, or early brain damage. The psychoanalytic perspective involves the belief that the mother-infant bond is the source of the schizophrenia.

CN: Physiological integrity; CNS: Physiological adaptation; CL: Application

48. Which action should a nurse implement when caring for a client who is having a delusion?

1. Ask the client to describe his delusion.
2. Explain to the client that the delusion isn't real.
3. Act as if the delusion is real to reduce the client's anxiety.
4. Engage the client in an organized activity.

48. 4. Engaging the client in an organized activity reinforces reality. Asking the client to describe the delusion and acting as if the delusion is real reinforce the delusion's reality. Explaining that the delusion isn't real won't help and may make the client hold tighter to the delusion.

CN: Psychosocial integrity; CNS: Physiological adaptation; CL: Application

49. During the initial interview, a schizophrenic client states to the nurse, "I don't enjoy things anymore. I used to love to read mystery books, but even that isn't enjoyable now." The nurse correctly identifies the client is experiencing which of the following conditions?

1. Avolition
2. Anhedonia
3. Alogia
4. Flat affect

49. 2. Anhedonia is the loss of pleasure in things that are usually pleasurable. Avolition is the lack of motivation. Alogia, also called poverty of speech, is a decrease in the amount of richness of speech. A flat affect is the absence of emotional expression.

CN: Physiological integrity; CNS: None; CL: Application

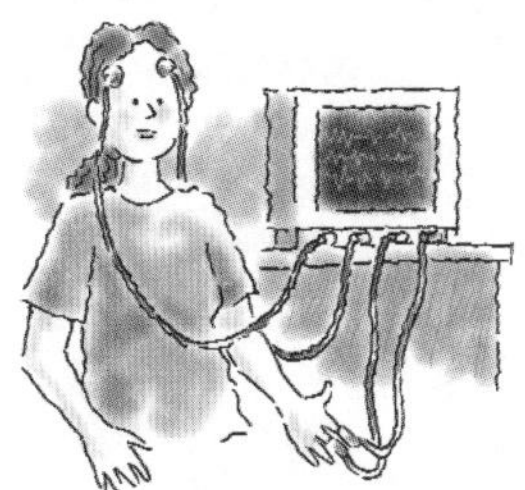

Feedback alerts you to a lack of understanding.

50. In preparation for discharge, a client diagnosed with schizophrenia was taught self-symptom management as part of a relapse prevention program. Which statement indicates the client understands symptom monitoring?

1. "When I hear voices, I become afraid I'll relapse."
2. "My parents aren't involved enough to be aware if I begin to relapse."
3. "My family is more protected from stress if I keep them out of my illness process."
4. "When I'm feeling stressed, I go to a quiet room by myself and do imagery."

50. 4. This statement indicates the client has learned a technique for coping with stress with the use of imagery technique. The other options don't show an understanding of self-symptom monitoring and may result in symptom intensification and possible relapse.

CN: Psychosocial integrity; CNS: None; CL: Application

51. A client diagnosed with schizophrenia has been taking haloperidol (Haldol) for 1 week when a nurse observes that the client's eyeball is fixated on the ceiling. Which specific condition is the client exhibiting?

1. Akathisia
2. Neuroleptic malignant syndrome
3. Oculogyric crisis
4. Tardive dyskinesia

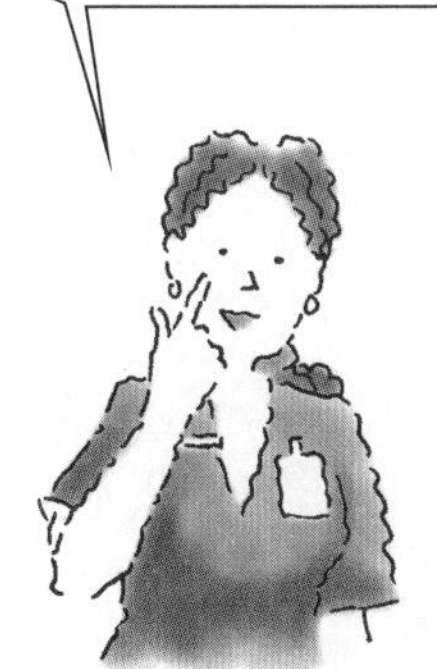

Keep your eye on question 51. It's asking for a specific condition.

51. 3. An oculogyric crisis involves a fixed positioning of the eyes, typically in an upward gaze. Neuroleptic malignant syndrome causes increased body temperature, muscle rigidity, and altered consciousness. Akathisia is a restlessness that can cause pacing and tapping of the fingers or feet. Stereotyped involuntary movements (tongue protrusion, lip smacking, chewing, blinking, and grimacing) characterize tardive dyskinesia.

CN: Physiological integrity; CNS: Pharmacological and parenteral therapies; CL: Application

52. A client taking antipsychotic medications shows dystonic reactions, including torticollis and oculogyric crisis. Which medication is given?
1. Benztropine (Cogentin)
2. Chlordiazepoxide (Librium)
3. Diazepam (Valium)
4. Fluoxetine (Prozac)

52. 1. Benztropine and trihexyphenidyl are anticholinergic drugs used to counteract the dystonic reactions and adverse reactions of antipsychotic drugs. The antihistamine diphenhydramine is also effective in treating extrapyramidal symptoms. Fluoxetine is an antidepressant, and diazepam and chlordiazepoxide are benzodiazepines.
CN: Physiological integrity; CNS: Pharmacological and parenteral therapies; CL: Application

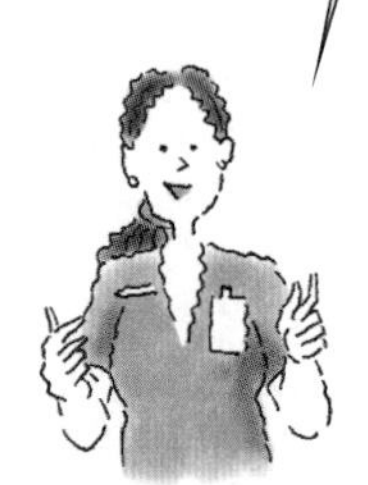

For question 53, you're looking for the most appropriate action.

53. A 50-year-old schizophrenic client becomes agitated and confronts the nurse with clenched fists. Which would be the most appropriate intervention by the nurse?
1. Take the client by the hand and lead him to the activity room for cards.
2. Step up to the client and tell him his behavior is inappropriate.
3. Call for security to take him to a seclusion room.
4. Speak to him in a quiet voice and offer him medication to help him calm down.

53. 4. Always use the least restrictive means to calm a client. Never touch an agitated client; touch can be misinterpreted as a threat and can further escalate the situation. Stepping up to an agitated client can be seen as an aggressive act. Seclusion is a last resort.
CN: Physiological integrity; CNS: Reduction of risk potential; CL: Application

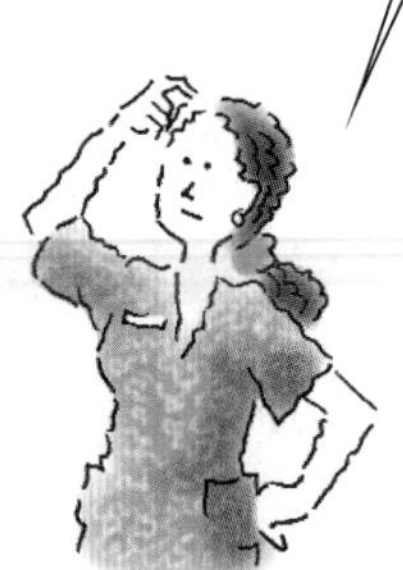

They're all important, but which one takes priority?

54. A 20-year-old client has been diagnosed with schizophrenia. He presently lives by himself, doesn't bathe, doesn't dress himself, and is erratic with eating, drinking, and taking prescribed medications. Which nursing diagnosis for this client has priority?
1. *Ineffective role performance related to isolation*
2. *Activity intolerance related to perceptual distortions*
3. *Ineffective coping*
4. *Imbalanced nutrition: Less than body requirements related to symptoms of schizophrenia*

54. 4. The deterioration of the client undergoing a schizophrenic crisis is manifested in multiple self-care deficits. Adequate nutrition in these instances is the primary concern of the nurse. The other problems can be addressed after the client has been stabilized.
CN: Safe, effective care environment; CNS: Management of care; CL: Application

55. As a nurse approaches the nursing station, a client with the diagnosis of delusional disorder raises his voice and says, "You're following me. What do you want?" To prevent escalating fear and anger, the nurse takes a nonthreatening posture and makes which response in a calm voice?
1. "Are you frightened?"
2. "You know I'm not following you."
3. "You'll have to go into seclusion if you continue to threaten me."
4. "I'm sorry if I frightened you. I was returning to the nursing station after going out for lunch."

55. 4. Being clear in communication, remaining calm, and showing concern increases the chance the client will cooperate, lessening potential for violence. The first option tries to identify the client's feelings but doesn't convey warmth and concern. The second option isn't empathic and shows no indication of trying to reach the client at a level beyond content of communication. The third option may increase the client's anxiety, fear, and mistrust when the nurse engages in a power struggle and triggers competitiveness within the client.
CN: Psychosocial integrity; CNS: None; CL: Application

56. Which action by a client with stable schizophrenia is most important for preventing relapse?
1. Attending group therapy sessions
2. Participating in family support meetings
3. Attending social skills training sessions
4. Consistently taking prescribed medications

The words *most important* in question 56 indicate the need to prioritize. As a matter of fact, there's lots of prioritizing on this page.

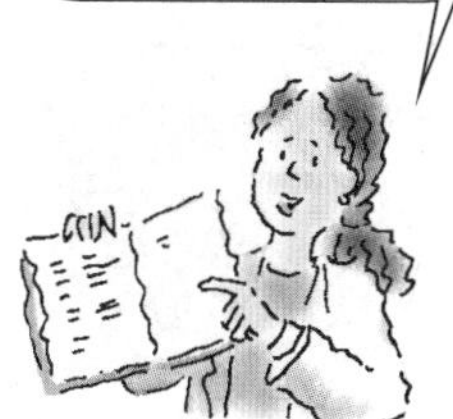

56. 4. Although all of the choices are important for preventing relapse, compliance with the medication regimen is central to the treatment of schizophrenia, a brain disease.
CN: Safe, effective care environment; CNS: Management of care; CL: Application

57. A client approaches the nurse and points at the sky, showing her where the men would be coming from to get him. Which response is most therapeutic?
1. "Why do you think the men are coming here?"
2. "You're safe here, we won't let them harm you."
3. "It seems like the world is pretty scary for you, but you're safe here."
4. "There are no bad men in the sky because no one lives that close to earth."

57. 3. This response acknowledges the client's fears, listens to his feelings, and offers a sense of security as the nurse tries to understand the concerns behind the symbolism. She reflects these concerns to the client, along with reassurance of safety. The first option validates the delusion, not the feelings and fears, and doesn't orient the client to reality. The second option gives false reassurance. Because the nurse isn't sure of the symbolism, she can't make this promise. The last option rejects the client's feelings and doesn't address the client's fears.
CN: Safe, effective care environment; CNS: Management of care; CL: Application

58. A client is brought to the crisis response center by his family. During evaluation, he reports being depressed for the last month and complains about voices constantly whispering to him. Which diagnosis is the most likely?
1. Catatonic schizophrenia
2. Disorganized schizophrenia
3. Paranoid schizophrenia
4. Schizoaffective disorder

58. 4. A client with major depressive episode who begins to hear voices and at times thinks someone is after him is most likely schizoaffective. The client who repeats phrases and shows waxy flexibility or stupor with prominent grimaces is most likely catatonic. The client with disorganized speech and behavior and a flat or inappropriate affect most likely has disorganized schizophrenia. The client who expresses thoughts of people spying on him, attributes ulterior motives to others, and has a flat affect is most likely paranoid schizophrenic.
CN: Psychosocial integrity; CNS: None; CL: Analysis

59. Which nursing intervention is most appropriate for use with a client with paranoid schizophrenia?
1. Defend yourself when the client is verbally hostile toward you.
2. Provide a warm approach by touching the client.
3. Explain everything you're doing before you do it.
4. Clarify the content of the client's delusions.

59. 3. Explaining everything you do will prevent misinterpretation of your actions. A nondefensive stance provides an atmosphere in which the client's angry feelings can be explored. Touching the paranoid client should be avoided because it can be interpreted as threatening. The content of delusions should not be the focus of your care because the content is illogical.
CN: Psychosocial integrity: CNS: None: CL: Analysis

60. The nurse is interviewing a client with a delusional disorder. Which of the following conditions would the nurse expect from this client?

1. Bizarre behavior
2. Agitation
3. Impaired short-term memory
4. Apparently normal functioning

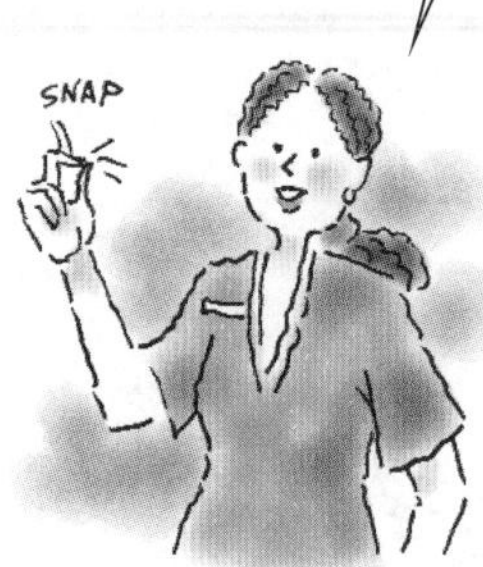

You've finished 60 questions. The rest of this test should be a snap.
SNAP

60. 4. The psychosocial functioning of the person with a delusional disorder may be relatively unimpaired. Another common characteristic of the client with a delusional disorder is the apparent normality of his behavior and appearance when his delusional ideas aren't being discussed or acted on. The client with delusional disorder doesn't have such symptoms as concrete thinking, bizarre or agitated behavior, and impaired memory, typical of a client with schizophrenia who functions at a lower level.
CN: Psychosocial integrity; CNS: None; CL: Application

61. A client is admitted to a psychiatric unit for a delusional disorder. He explains to a nurse that he made a contract with God to be the best minister on earth. Now that he has achieved the goal, most of his friends have stopped seeing him out of envy. On mental status examination, there is little impairment in psychosocial functioning. Which condition is expected?

1. Nonbizarre delusions
2. Fragmentary delusions
3. Regressive behavior
4. Regressive delusions

61. 1. The essential feature of delusional disorder is the presence of one or more nonbizarre delusions that persist for at least 1 month. The most common delusions by subtypes are erotomanic, grandiose, jealousy, persecutory, and somatic. Bizarre delusions are patently absurd beliefs with absolutely no foundation in reality. Fragmentary delusions are unconnected delusions not organized around a coherent theme. Regressive behaviors revert back to a less mature state and aren't associated with a mental disorder.
CN: Psychosocial integrity; CNS: None; CL: Application

62. Which statement made by a client taking fluphenazine tells the nurse that the client understands his discharge instructions?

1. "I need to stay out of the sun."
2. "I need to drink plenty of fluids."
3. "I can't eat cheese."
4. "I need to plan rest periods throughout the day."

62. 1. Fluphenazine is an antipsychotic drug that can cause photosensitivity and sunburn. Clients taking this drug don't need to increase fluid intake, avoid cheeses, or plan rest periods.
CN: Physiological integrity; CNS: Pharmacological and parenteral therapies; CL: Analysis

63. The nurse is teaching the family of a client who has been prescribed thiothixene (Navane). Which of the following adverse reactions concerning this medication would be the most accurate for the nurse to discuss?

1. Akinesia
2. Hypotension
3. Sedation
4. Weight gain

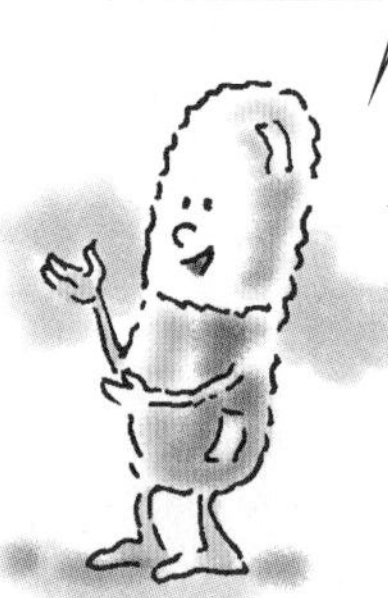

I didn't intend to cause any adverse reactions.

63. 1. Thiothixene is a high-potency agent with a high affinity for the dopamine-2 receptors, resulting in the increased likelihood of akinesia, a form of extrapyramidal symptoms. Although thiothixene targets other neurotransmitters responsible for hypotension, sedation, and weight gain, their affinity to these receptors is weak and more likely to occur with low-potency psychotropics.
CN: Physiological integrity; CNS: Pharmacological and parenteral therapies; CL: Application

64. Inability to carry out daily responsibilities typically occurs during the prodromal phase of schizophrenia. Which symptom may also occur during this phase?

1. Increased energy and motivation
2. Increased social interaction
3. Impaired role functioning and neglect of personal hygiene
4. Heightened work performance

64. 3. Prodromal (early) signs and symptoms of schizophrenia can occur 1 month to 1 year before the first psychotic break and represent a clear deterioration in functioning. They may include impaired role functioning and neglect of personal hygiene as well as social withdrawal and depression. Increases in energy and social interaction and heightened work performance don't occur during the prodromal phase.

CN: Psychosocial integrity; CNS: None; CL: Application

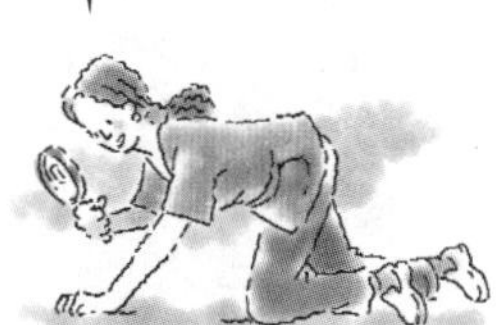

Families often search for the link to their loved one's disease.

65. The daughter of a client with schizophrenia states, "I'm afraid I may develop this disease, too." The nurse should teach the daughter that schizophrenia is linked to which factor?

1. Sexual abuse
2. A combination of genetic and other factors
3. Both parents having schizophrenia
4. Emotional trauma during childhood

65. 2. Experts believe schizophrenia results from a combination of genetic, environmental, and other factors—such as viruses, birth injuries, and nutritional factors. Schizophrenia incidence is higher among relatives of persons with the disease. It can occur even if both parents don't have schizophrenia. Emotional trauma during childhood hasn't been linked to schizophrenia.

CN: Psychosocial integrity; CNS: None; CL: Application

66. A nurse teaches a class of caregivers about the positive and negative behaviors of schizophrenia. Positive behaviors include:

1. limited spontaneous speech.
2. inability to initiate and persist in goal-directed activities.
3. misinterpretation of experiences and altered sensory input.
4. extremely brief replies to questions.

66. 3. Positive behaviors of schizophrenia include attention-getting behaviors, which can result from misinterpretation of experiences and altered sensing input (such as hallucinations, delusions, and bizarre behavior). Negative behaviors are those that render the client inert and unmotivated, such as lack of spontaneous speech, poverty of thought, apathy, and poor social functioning.

CN: Psychosocial integrity; CNS: None; CL: Application

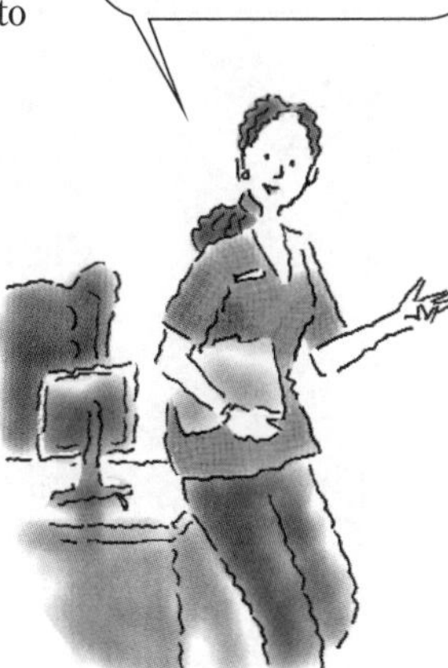

67. A nurse is facilitating a group of schizophrenic clients when one client says, "I like to drive my car, bar, tar, far." This pattern of speech is known as which disorder?

1. Clang association
2. Echolalia
3. Echopraxia
4. Neologisms

67. 1. Linking together words based on their sounds rather than their meanings is called clang association. Echolalia is the involuntary parrotlike repetition of words spoken by others. Echopraxia refers to meaningless imitation of others' motions. Neologisms are new words that a person invents.

CN: Psychosocial integrity; CNS: None; CL: Application

68. A schizophrenic client who's receiving antipsychotic medication paces, fidgets, and can't seem to stay still. The nurse recognizes these behaviors as which disorder?

1. Tardive dyskinesia
2. Dystonia
3. Akathisia
4. Akinesia

68. 3. Akathisia is an extrapyramidal adverse effect of some antipsychotic medications, manifested by restlessness and an inability to stay still. Tardive dyskinesia refers to involuntary abnormal movements of the mouth, tongue, face, and jaw. Dystonia refers to difficulty with movement. Akinesia is absence of movement.
CN: Physiological integrity; CNS: Pharmacological and parenteral therapies; CL: Analysis

69. Which nursing diagnosis is most appropriate for a client diagnosed with schizophrenia, disorganized type?

1. *Feeding self-care deficit*
2. *Disturbed sleep pattern*
3. *Impaired verbal communication*
4. *Social isolation*

69. 3. Schizophrenia, disorganized type, is characterized by disorganized speech, disorganized behavior, and inappropriate or flat affect. *Feeding self-care deficit*, *Disturbed sleep pattern*, and *Social isolation* aren't classic manifestations of this type of schizophrenia.
CN: Psychosocial integrity; CNS: None; CL: Analysis

70. A client with paranoid schizophrenia tells the nurse that two people talking in the hall are planning to kidnap and kill him. The client's thought pattern reflects which disorder?

1. Auditory hallucinations
2. Delusions of grandeur
3. Ideas of reference
4. Echolalia

70. 3. A client with ideas of reference mistakenly believes that other people's thoughts, speech, and behaviors refer to the client. Auditory hallucinations are sounds that aren't based in reality. Delusions of grandeur are false beliefs that arise without appropriate external stimuli. Echolalia refers to involuntary repetition of words spoken by others.
CN: Psychosocial integrity; CNS: None; CL: Application

71. A client with schizophrenia is taking the atypical antipsychotic medication clozapine (Clozaril). Which signs and symptoms indicate the presence of adverse effects associated with this medication? Select all that apply:

1. Sore throat
2. Pill-rolling movements
3. Polyuria
4. Fever
5. Polydipsia
6. Orthostatic hypotension

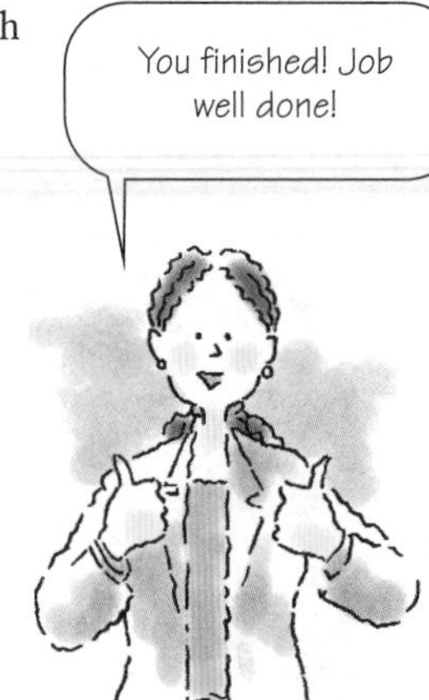
You finished! Job well done!

71. 1, 4. Sore throat, fever, and sudden onset of other flulike symptoms are signs of agranulocytosis. The condition is caused by a lack of sufficient granulocytes (a type of white blood cell), which causes the client to be susceptible to infection. The client's white blood cell count should be monitored at least weekly throughout the course of treatment. Pill-rolling movements can occur in those experiencing extrapyramidal adverse effects associated with antipsychotic medication that has been prescribed for a much longer time frame than clozapine. Polydipsia (excessive thirst) and polyuria (increased urine output) are common adverse effects of lithium. Orthostatic hypotension is an adverse effect of tricyclic antidepressants.
CN: Physiological integrity; CNS: Pharmacological and parenteral therapies; CL: Application

CN: Client needs category CNS: Client needs subcategory CL: Cognitive level

About the only substance of abuse this chapter *doesn't* cover is my personal weakness—chocolate mousse! Think of me as you work through this chapter. I'll be the one with chocolate smudges on her fingers. Tee-hee!

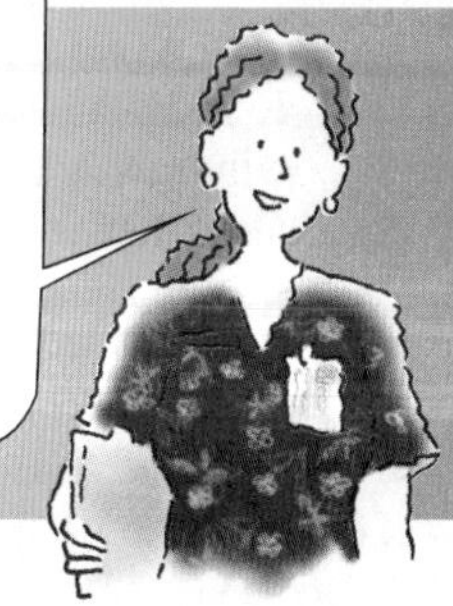

Chapter 18 Substance abuse disorders

1. Family members of a client who abuses alcohol asks a nurse to help them intervene. Which action is essential for a successful intervention?

1. All family members must tell the client they're powerless.
2. All family members must describe how the addiction affects them.
3. All family members must come up with their share of financial support.
4. All family members must become caregivers during the detoxification period.

1. 2. After the family is taught about addiction, they must write down examples of how the addiction has affected each of them and use this information during the intervention. It isn't necessary to tell the client the family is powerless. The family is empowered through this intervention experience. In many cases, a third-party payer will help with treatment costs. Doing an intervention doesn't make family members responsible for financial support or providing care and support during the detoxification period.

CN: Psychosocial integrity; CNS: None; CL: Analysis

2. A client who abuses alcohol tells a nurse, "I'm sure I can become a social drinker." Which response is <u>most appropriate</u>?

1. "When do you think you can become a social drinker?"
2. "What makes you think you'll learn to drink normally?"
3. "Does your alcohol use cause major problems in your life?"
4. "How many alcoholic beverages can a social drinker consume?"

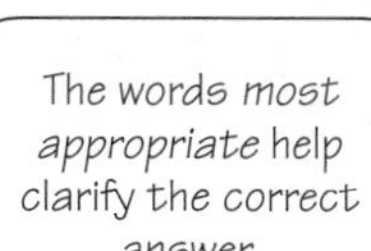

The words *most appropriate* help clarify the correct answer.

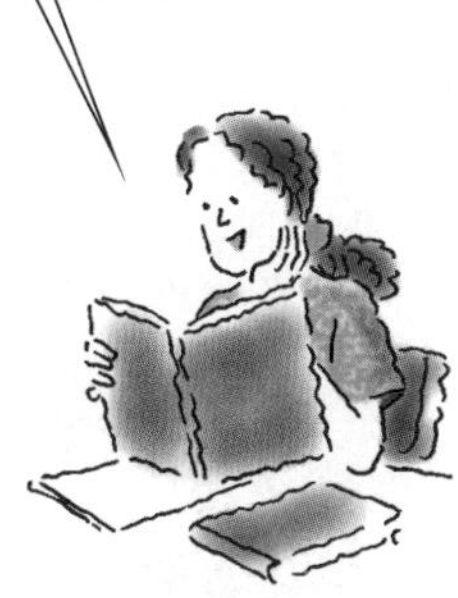

2. 3. This question may help the client recall the problematic results of using alcohol and the reasons the client began treatment. Asking when he believes he can become a social drinker will only encourage the addicted person to deny the problem and develop an unrealistic, self-defeating goal. Asking how many alcoholic beverages a social drinker can consume and why the client thinks he can drink normally will encourage the addicted person to defend himself and deny the problem.

CN: Psychosocial integrity; CNS: None; CL: Application

3. A client asks a nurse not to tell his parents about his alcohol problem. Which response is most appropriate?

1. "How can you not tell them? Is that being honest?"
2. "Don't you think you'll need to tell them someday?"
3. "Do alcohol problems run in either side of your family?"
4. "What do you think will happen if you tell your parents?"

3. 4. Clients who struggle with addiction problems often believe people will be judgmental, rejecting, and uncaring if they are told that the client is recovering from alcohol abuse. The first option challenges the client and will put him on the defensive. The second option will make the client defensive and construct rationalizations as to why his parents don't need to know. The third option is a good assessment question, but it isn't an appropriate question to ask a client who's afraid to tell others about his addiction.

CN: Psychosocial integrity; CNS: None; CL: Analysis

4. A nurse assesses a client with alcohol withdrawal. Which finding is of most concern to the nurse?

1. Hallucinations
2. Nervousness
3. Diaphoresis
4. Nausea

4. 1. Hallucinations are a sign of late alcohol withdrawal. The nurse should stay with the client, have someone notify the physician, and institute seizure precautions. Nervousness, diaphoresis, and nausea are signs of early withdrawal.

CN: Physiological integrity; CNS: Reduction of risk potential; CL: Analysis

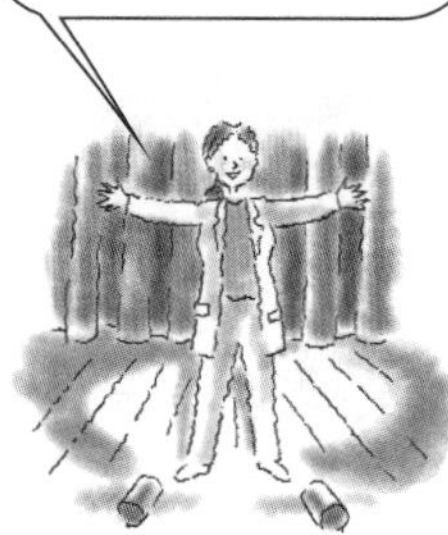

A disease can have many "stages," each with its own symptoms.

5. The nurse is assessing a client with prolonged, chronic alcohol intake. Which of the following findings would the nurse expect to find?

1. Enlarged liver
2. Nasal irritation
3. Muscle wasting
4. Limb paresthesia

5. 1. A major effect of alcohol on the body is liver impairment, and an enlarged liver is a common physical finding. Nasal irritation is commonly seen with clients who snort cocaine. Muscle wasting and limb paresthesia don't tend to occur with clients who abuse alcohol.

CN: Physiological integrity; CNS: Physiological adaptation; CL: Application

6. A client has an order for chlordiazepoxide (Librium) to be given as needed for signs and symptoms of alcohol withdrawal. Which symptoms indicate that the client needs this medication?

1. Mild tremors, hypertension, tachycardia
2. Bradycardia, hyperthermia, sedation
3. Hypotension, decreased reflexes, drowsiness
4. Hypothermia, mild tremors, slurred speech

6. 1. Chlordiazepoxide is given during alcohol withdrawal. Symptoms that indicate a need for this drug include tremors, hypertension, tachycardia, and elevated body temperature. Bradycardia, sedation, hypotension, decreased reflexes, hypothermia, and slurred speech aren't symptoms of alcohol withdrawal.

CN: Physiological integrity; CNS: Pharmacological and parenteral therapies; CL: Application

7. A client who abuses alcohol tells a nurse, "Alcohol helps me sleep." Which information about alcohol use and sleep is most accurate?

1. Alcohol doesn't help promote sleep.
2. Continued alcohol use causes insomnia.
3. One glass of alcohol at dinnertime can induce sleep.
4. Sometimes alcohol can make one drowsy enough to fall asleep.

7. 1. Alcohol use may initially promote sleep, but with continued use, it causes insomnia. Evidence shows that alcohol doesn't facilitate sleep. One glass of alcohol at dinnertime won't induce sleep. The last option doesn't give information about how alcohol affects sleep. It makes the client think alcohol use to induce sleep is an appropriate strategy to try.

CN: Physiological integrity; CNS: Physiological adaptation; CL: Analysis

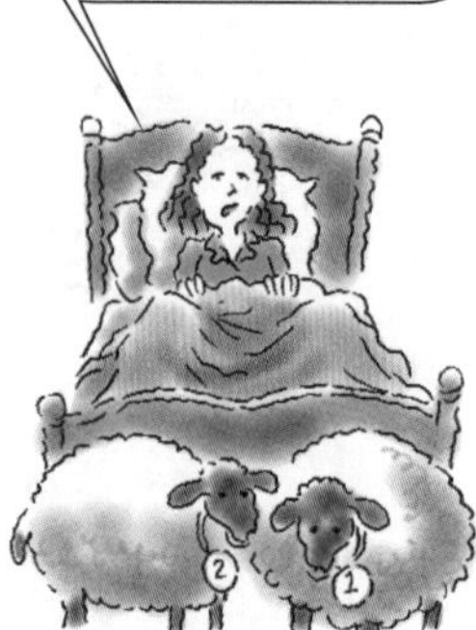

What I would give for a good night's sleep.
2
1

CN: Client needs category CNS: Client needs subcategory CL: Cognitive level

8. A client withdrawing from alcohol is given lorazepam (Ativan). The nurse teaches the client's family about the drug. Which response by a family member indicates that the nurse's teaching has been successful?

1. "Short-term use of lorazepam can lead to dependence."
2. "The lorazepam will reduce the symptoms of withdrawal."
3. "The lorazepam will make him forget about symptoms of withdrawal."
4. "The lorazepam will also help with his heart disease."

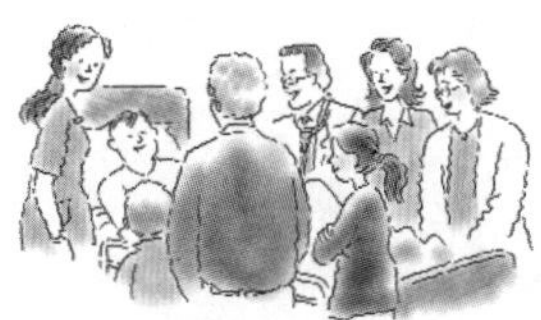
It's important to teach the family and the client.

8. 2. Lorazepam is a short-acting benzodiazepine usually given for 1 week to help the client in alcohol withdrawal. Long-term (not short-term) use of lorazepam can lead to dependence. The medication isn't given to help forget the experience; it lessens the symptoms of withdrawal. It isn't used to treat coexisting cardiovascular problems.
CN: Physiological integrity; CNS: Pharmacological and parenteral therapies; CL: Application

9. A client who abuses alcohol tells a nurse everyone in his family has an alcohol problem and nothing can be done about it. Which response is the most appropriate?

1. "You're right, it's much harder to become a recovering person."
2. "This is just an excuse for you so you don't have to work on becoming sober."
3. "Sometimes nothing can be done, but you may be the exception in this family."
4. "Alcohol problems can occur in families, but you can decide to take the steps to become and stay sober."

9. 4. This statement challenges the client to become proactive and take the steps necessary to maintain a sober lifestyle. The first option agrees with the client's denial and isn't a useful response. The second option confronts the client and may make him more adamant in defense of this position. The third option agrees with the client's denial and isn't a useful response.
CN: Psychosocial integrity; CNS: None; CL: Application

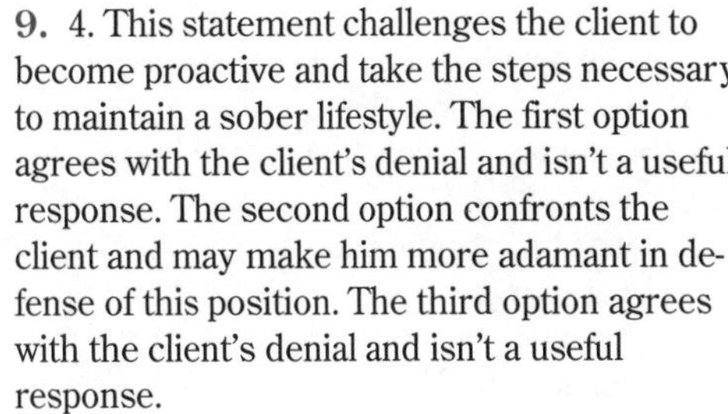

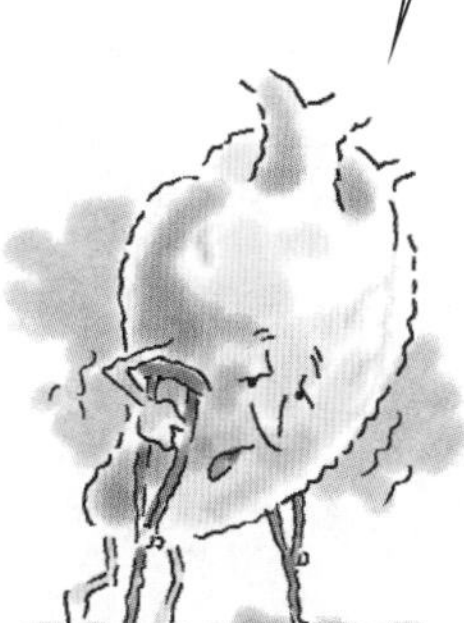
I feel like I'm failing fast.

10. A client with chronic alcoholism may be predisposed to develop which of the following conditions?

1. Arteriosclerosis
2. Heart failure
3. Heart valve damage
4. Pericarditis

10. 2. Heart failure is a severe cardiac consequence associated with long-term alcohol use. Arteriosclerosis, heart valve damage, and pericarditis aren't medical consequences of alcoholism.
CN: Physiological integrity; CNS: Reduction of risk potential; CL: Application

11. Which assessment finding is commonly associated with the abuse of alcohol in a young, depressed adult woman?

1. Defiant responses
2. Infertility
3. Memory loss
4. Sexual abuse

11. 4. Many women diagnosed with substance abuse problems also have a history of physical or sexual abuse. Alcohol abuse isn't a common finding in a young woman showing defiant behavior or experiencing infertility. Memory loss isn't a common finding in a young woman experiencing alcohol abuse.
CN: Psychosocial integrity; CNS: None; CL: Analysis

12. A nurse determines that a client who abused alcohol has nutritional problems. Which strategy is <u>best</u> for addressing the client's nutritional needs?

1. Encourage the client to eat a diet high in calories.
2. Help the client recognize and follow a balanced diet.
3. Have the client drink liquid protein supplements daily.
4. Have the client monitor the calories consumed each day.

12. 2. Clients who abuse alcohol are usually malnourished and need help to follow a balanced diet. Increasing calories may cause the client to just eat empty calories. The client must be involved in the decision to supplement the daily dietary intake. The nurse can't force the client to drink liquid protein supplements. Having the client monitor calorie intake could be done only after the client recognizes the need to maintain a balanced diet. Calorie counts usually aren't needed in most recovering clients who begin to eat from the basic food groups.

CN: Physiological integrity; CNS: Basic care and comfort; CL: Application

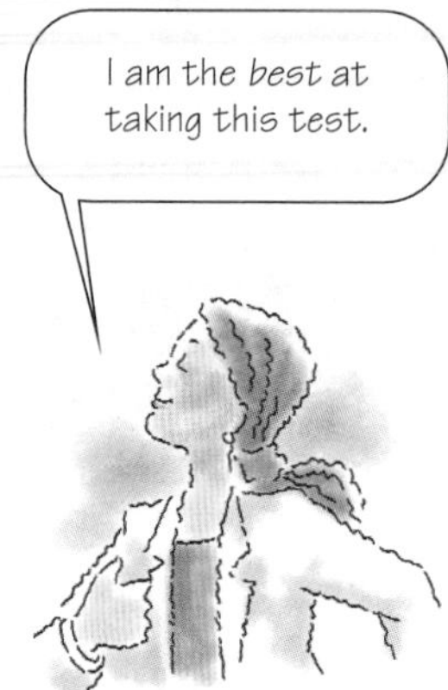

I am the *best* at taking this test.

13. A client with a history of alcohol abuse refuses to take vitamins. Which statement is most appropriate for explaining why vitamins are important?

1. "It's important to take vitamins to stop your craving."
2. "Prolonged use of alcohol can cause vitamin depletion."
3. "For every vitamin you take, you'll help your liver heal."
4. "By taking vitamins, you don't need to worry about your diet."

13. 2. Chronic alcoholism interferes with the metabolism of many vitamins. Vitamin supplements can prevent deficiencies from occurring. Taking vitamins won't stop a person from craving alcohol or help a damaged liver heal. A balanced diet is *essential* in addition to taking multivitamins.

CN: Health promotion and maintenance; CNS: None; CL: Application

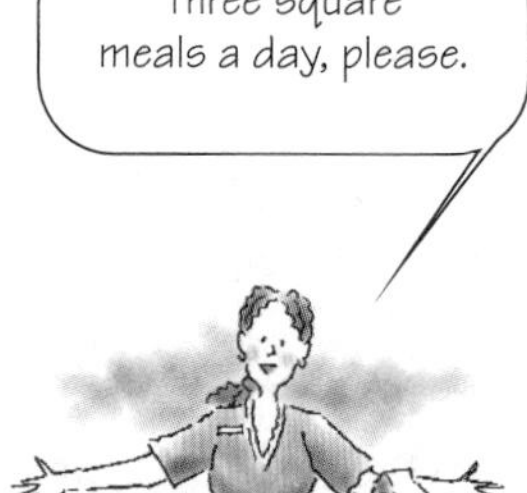

Three square meals a day, please.

14. Which statement by a client who abuses alcohol indicates a need for nutritional teaching?

1. "I should avoid foods high in fat."
2. "I should eat only one balanced meal per day."
3. "I should take vitamin and mineral supplements."
4. "I should eat large portions of food containing fiber."

14. 2. If the client eats only one adequate meal each day, there will be a deficit of essential nutrients. It's appropriate for the client to take vitamin and mineral supplements to prevent deficiency in these nutrients. Avoiding foods high in fat content and consuming large portions of foods containing fiber indicate the client has good knowledge about nutrition.

CN: Health promotion and maintenance; CNS: None; CL: Analysis

15. A client tells a nurse, "I've been drinking ever since they told me I had learning disabilities." Which rationale does this client's statement indicate?

1. The client is self-medicating.
2. The client has an excuse to drink.
3. The client isn't a productive person.
4. The client will be unable to stop drinking.

15. 1. A client with learning disabilities may experience frustration, depression, or overall feelings of low self-esteem and may self-medicate with alcohol. Many people with learning disabilities don't resort to alcohol but develop other coping skills to handle the disability. People with learning disabilities can be very productive. A person with a learning disability can successfully recover from alcohol addiction.

CN: Psychosocial integrity; CNS: None; CL: Application

16. A nurse is caring for a client undergoing treatment for acute alcohol dependence. The client tells the nurse, "I don't have a problem. My wife made me come here." Which defense mechanism is the client using?

1. Projection and suppression
2. Denial and rationalization
3. Rationalization and repression
4. Suppression and denial

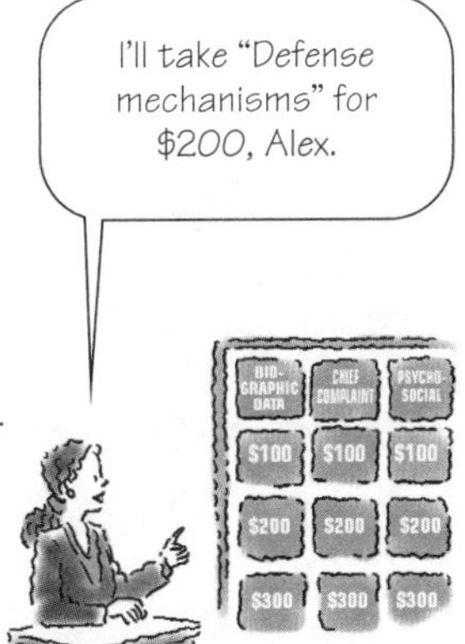

16. 2. The client is using denial and rationalization. Denial is the unconscious disclaimer of unacceptable thoughts, feelings, needs, or certain external factors. Rationalization is the unconscious effort to justify intolerable feelings, behaviors, and motives. The client isn't using projection, suppression, or repression.
CN: Psychosocial integrity; CNS: None; CL: Application

17. A nurse has a meeting with a family of a recovering client. The client tells a family member, "You made it easy for me to use alcohol. You always made excuses for my behavior." Which important issue should the family be encouraged to address?

1. Giving up enabling behaviors
2. Managing the client's self-care
3. Dealing with negative behaviors
4. Evaluating the home environment

17. 1. Enabling the behaviors of family members allows the client to continue the addiction by rationalizing, denying, or otherwise excusing the problem. Managing the client's self-care isn't an issue that needs to be addressed based on the client's statement. Dealing with negative behaviors and evaluating the home environment don't address the client's statement about the family's enabling behavior.
CN: Psychosocial integrity; CNS: None; CL: Application

18. Which short-term goal should be a priority for a client with a knowledge deficit about the effects of alcohol on the body?

1. Test blood chemistries daily.
2. Verbalize the results of substance use.
3. Talk to a pharmacist about the substance.
4. Attend a weekly aerobic exercise program.

18. 2. It's important for the client to talk about the health consequences of the continued use of alcohol. Testing blood chemistries daily gives the client minimal knowledge about the effects of alcohol on the body and isn't the most useful information in a teaching plan. A pharmacist isn't the appropriate health care professional to educate the client about the effects of alcohol use on the body. Although exercise is an important goal of self-care, it doesn't address the client's knowledge deficit about the effects of alcohol on the body.
CN: Safe, effective care environment; CNS: Management of care; CL: Application

19. A client recovering from alcohol abuse tells a nurse, "I feel so depressed about what I've done to my family that I feel like giving up." Assessment of which area is a priority?

1. Family support
2. A plan for self-harm
3. A sponsor for the client
4. Other ambivalent feelings

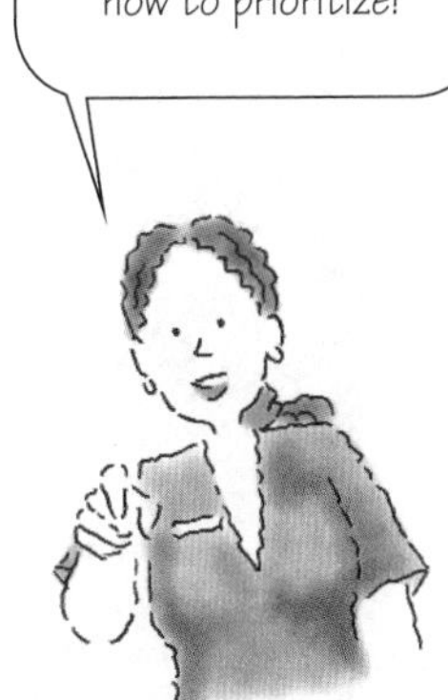

19. 2. When a client talks about giving up, the nurse must explore the potential for suicidal behavior. Although questioning the client about family support, the availability of a sponsor, or ambivalent feelings are important, the priority action is to assess for suicide.
CN: Psychosocial integrity; CNS: None; CL: Application

20. A client withdrawing from alcohol says he's worried about periodic hallucinations. Which intervention is best for this client's problem?

1. Point out that the sensation doesn't exist.
2. Allow the client to talk about the experience.
3. Encourage the client to wash the body areas well.
4. Determine if the client has a cognitive impairment.

20. 2. The client needs to talk about the periodic hallucinations to prevent them from becoming triggers to acting out behaviors and possible self-injury. The client's experience of sensory-perceptual alterations must be acknowledged; therefore, denying that the client's hallucinations exist isn't a helpful strategy. Determining if the client has a cognitive impairment and encouraging the client to wash the body areas well don't address the problem of periodic hallucinations.
CN: Psychosocial integrity; CNS: None; CL: Application

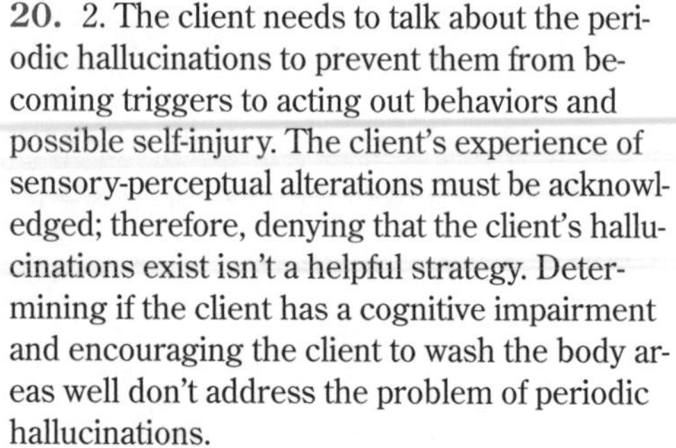

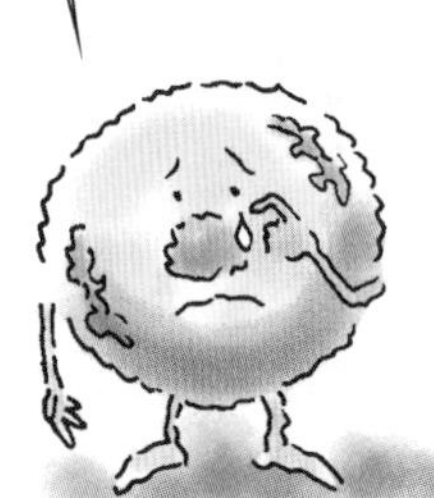

Alcohol can make me more susceptible to infections.

21. A client who has been drinking alcohol for 30 years asks a nurse if permanent damage has occurred to his immune system. Which response is the best?

1. "There is often less resistance to infections."
2. "Sometimes the body's metabolism will increase."
3. "Put your energies into maintaining sobriety for now."
4. "Drinking puts you at high risk for disease later in life."

21. 1. Chronic alcohol use depresses the immune system and causes increased susceptibility to infections. A nutritionally well-balanced diet that includes foods high in protein and B vitamins will help develop a strong immune system. The potential damage to the immune system doesn't increase the body's metabolism. The third option negates the client's concern and isn't an appropriate or caring response. Drinking alcohol may put the client at risk for immune system problems at any time in life.
CN: Psychosocial integrity; CNS: None; CL: Analysis

22. A client experiencing alcohol withdrawal is upset about going through detoxification. Which goal is a priority?

1. The client will commit to a drug-free lifestyle.
2. The client will work with the nurse to remain safe.
3. The client will drink plenty of fluids on a daily basis.
4. The client will make a personal inventory of strengths.

22. 2. The priority goal is for client safety. Although drinking enough fluids, identifying personal strengths, and committing to a drug-free lifestyle are important goals, the nurse's first priority must be to promote client safety.
CN: Safe, effective care environment; CNS: Management of care; CL: Application

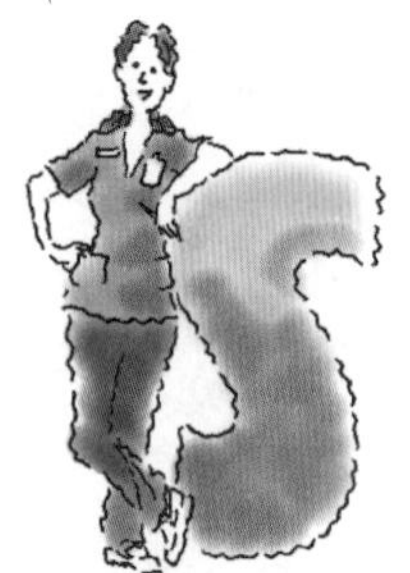

In this case, the "S" stands for "safety."

23. A client recovering from alcohol abuse needs to develop effective coping skills to handle daily stressors. Which intervention is most useful to the client?

1. Determine the client's level of verbal skills.
2. Help the client avoid areas that cause conflict.
3. Discuss examples of successful coping behavior.
4. Teach the client to accept uncomfortable situations.

23. 3. The client needs help to identify successful coping behavior and develop ways to incorporate that behavior into daily functioning. There are many skills for coping with stress, and determining the client's level of verbal skills may not be important. Encouraging the client to avoid conflict prevents him from learning skills to handle daily stressors.
CN: Psychosocial integrity; CNS: None; CL: Analysis

24. A client is struggling with alcohol dependence. Which communication strategy would be most effective?

1. Speak briefly and directly.
2. Avoid blaming or preaching to the client.
3. Confront feelings and examples of perfectionism.
4. Determine if nonverbal communication will be more effective.

24. 2. Blaming or preaching to the client causes negativity and prevents the client from hearing what the nurse has to say. Speaking briefly to the client may not allow time for adequate communication. Perfectionism doesn't tend to be an issue. Determining if nonverbal communication will be more effective is better suited for a client with cognitive impairment.

CN: Psychosocial integrity; CNS: None; CL: Analysis

25. A nurse is working with a client on recognizing the relationship between alcohol abuse and interpersonal problems. Which intervention has priority?

1. Help the client identify personal strengths.
2. Help the client decrease compulsive behaviors.
3. Examine the client's use of defense mechanisms.
4. Have the client work with peers who can serve as role models.

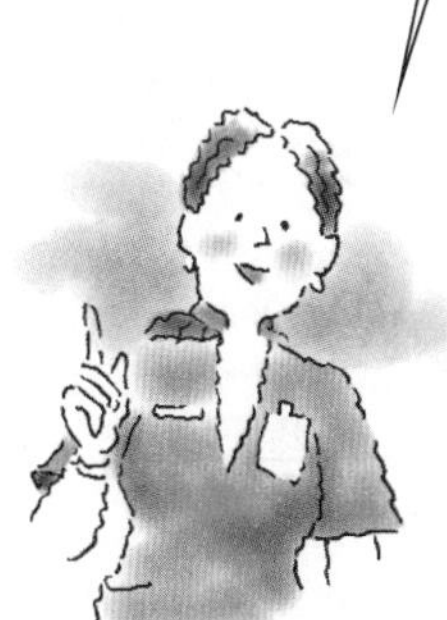
Remember to prioritize!

25. 3. Defense mechanisms can impede the development of healthy relationships and cause the client pain. After identifying barriers to relationship problems, it would be appropriate to identify or clarify personal strengths. Compulsive behavior doesn't tend to be a problem for alcoholic clients who struggle with interpersonal problems. Working with peers who are role models would be useful after the client recognizes and gains some insight into the problems. It isn't the priority intervention.

CN: Safe, effective care environment; CNS: Management of care; CL: Analysis

26. A client recovering from alcohol addiction has limited coping skills. Which characteristic would indicate relationship problems?

1. The client is prone to panic attacks.
2. The client doesn't pay attention to details.
3. The client has poor problem-solving skills.
4. The client ignores the need to relax and rest.

26. 3. To have satisfying relationships, a person must be able to communicate and problem solve. Relationship problems don't predispose people to panic attacks more than other psychosocial stressors. Paying attention to details isn't a major concern when addressing the client's relationship difficulties. Although ignoring the need for rest and relaxation is unhealthy, it shouldn't pose a major relationship problem.

CN: Psychosocial integrity; CNS: None; CL: Analysis

27. A nurse suggests to a client struggling with alcohol addiction that keeping a journal may be helpful. The journal helps the client:

1. identify stressors and responses to them.
2. understand the diagnosis.
3. help others by reading the journal to them.
4. develop an emergency plan for use in a crisis.

27. 1. Keeping a journal enables the client to identify problems and patterns of coping. From this information, the difficulties the client faces can be addressed. A journal isn't necessarily kept to promote better understanding of the client's illness, but it helps the client understand himself better. Journals aren't read to other people unless the client wants to share a particular part. Journals aren't typically used for identifying an emergency plan for use in a crisis.

CN: Psychosocial integrity; CNS: None; CL: Application

28. Which information is <u>most important</u> to use in a teaching plan for a client who abused alcohol?

1. Personal needs
2. Illness exacerbation
3. Cognitive distortions
4. Communication skills

28. 4. Addicted clients typically have difficulty communicating their needs in an appropriate way. Learning appropriate communication skills is a major goal of treatment. Next, behavior that focuses on the self and meeting personal needs will be addressed. The identification of cognitive distortions would be difficult if the client has poor communication skills. Teaching about illness exacerbation isn't a skill, but it is essential for relaying information about relapse.

CN: Psychosocial integrity; CNS: None; CL: Analysis

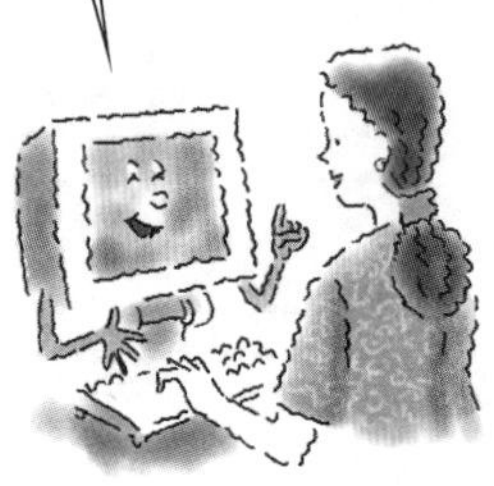

It is most important that you read this question carefully.

29. Which assessment must be done before starting a teaching session with a client who abuses alcohol?

1. Sleep patterns
2. Decision making
3. Note-taking skills
4. Readiness to learn

29. 4. It's important to know if the client's current situation helps or hinders the potential to learn. Decision making and sleep patterns aren't factors that must be assessed before teaching about addiction. Note-taking skills aren't a factor in determining whether the client will be receptive to teaching.

CN: Psychosocial integrity; CNS: None; CL: Application

30. A nurse is developing strategies to prevent relapse with a client who abuses alcohol. Which client intervention is important?

1. Avoid taking over-the-counter medications.
2. Limit monthly contact with the family of origin.
3. Refrain from becoming involved in group activities.
4. Avoid people, places, and activities from the former lifestyle.

30. 4. Changing the client's old habits is essential for sustaining a sober lifestyle. Certain over-the-counter medications that don't contain alcohol will probably need to be used by the client at certain times. It's unrealistic to have the client abstain from all such medications. Contact with the client's family of origin may not be a trigger to relapse, so limiting contact wouldn't be useful. Refraining from group activities isn't a good strategy to prevent relapse. Going to Alcoholics Anonymous and other support groups will help prevent relapse.

CN: Psychosocial integrity; CNS: None; CL: Analysis

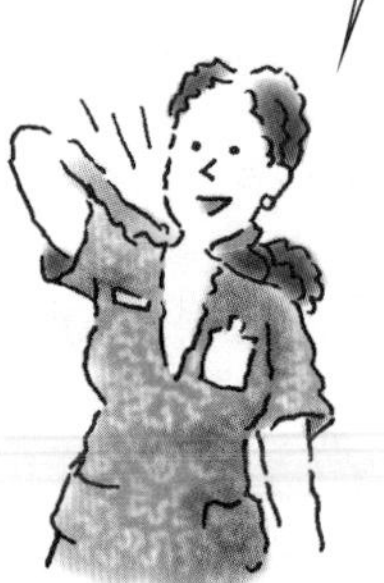

Congratulations! You've finished 30 questions!

31. A client recovering from alcohol abuse tells the nurse, "I get nothing out of Alcoholics Anonymous (AA) meetings." Which response is most appropriate?

1. "What were you told about going to AA meetings?"
2. "What do you want to get out of the AA meetings?"
3. "When do you think you'll stop going to the meetings?"
4. "Do you think you can control what happens in a meeting?"

31. 2. This response puts some of the responsibility for staying sober on the client and encourages the client to take a more active role. Asking what the client was told about AA meetings opens up a discussion that allows the client to continue to discuss disappointments rather than taking a proactive stand to support the value of AA meetings. The third option condones the client's desire to stop going to the meetings. The fourth option changes the issue from being responsible for staying sober to focusing on what the client can't control.

CN: Psychosocial integrity; CNS: None; CL: Analysis

32. A client asks a nurse, "Why does it matter if I talk to my peers in group therapy?" Which response is <u>most appropriate</u>?

1. "Group therapy lets you see what you're doing wrong in your life."
2. "Group therapy acts as a defense against your disorganized behavior."
3. "Group therapy provides a way to ask for support as well as to support others."
4. "In group therapy, you can vent your frustrations and others will listen."

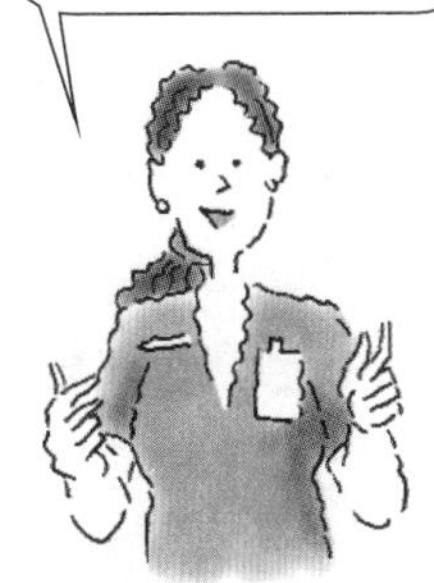

All answers may seem right, but choose the most appropriate one.

32. 3. The best response addresses how group therapy provides opportunities to communicate, learn, and give and get support. Group members will give a client feedback, not just point out what a client is doing wrong. Group therapy isn't a defense against disorganized behavior. People can express all kinds of feelings and discuss a variety of topics in group therapy. Interactions are goal oriented and not just vehicles to vent one's frustrations.

CN: Psychosocial integrity; CNS: None; CL: Application

33. A family meeting is held with a client who abuses alcohol. While listening to the family, which unhealthy communication pattern might be identified?

1. Use of descriptive jargon
2. Disapproval of behaviors
3. Avoidance of conflicting issues
4. Unlimited expression of nonverbal communication

33. 3. The interaction pattern of a family with a member who abuses alcohol often revolves around denying the problem, avoiding conflict, or rationalizing the addiction. Health care providers are more likely to use jargon. The family might have problems setting limits and expressing disapproval of the client's behavior. Nonverbal communication often gives the nurse insight into family dynamics.

CN: Psychosocial integrity; CNS: None; CL: Analysis

34. A client addicted to alcohol begins individual therapy with a nurse. Which intervention should be a <u>priority</u>?

1. Learn to express feelings.
2. Establish new roles in the family.
3. Determine strategies for socializing.
4. Decrease preoccupation with physical health.

34. 1. The client must address issues, learn ways to cope effectively with life stressors, and express his needs appropriately. After the client establishes sobriety, the possibility of taking on new roles can become a reality. Determining strategies for socializing isn't the priority intervention for an addicted client. Usually, these clients need to change former socializing habits. Clients addicted to alcohol don't tend to be preoccupied with physical health problems.

CN: Safe, effective care environment; CNS: Management of care; CL: Analysis

35. A client recovering from alcohol addiction asks a nurse how to talk to his children about the impact of his addiction on them. Which response is most appropriate?

1. "Try to limit references to the addiction, and focus on the present."
2. "Talk about all the hardships you've had in working to remain sober."
3. "Tell them you're sorry, and emphasize that you're doing so much better now."
4. "Talk to them by acknowledging the difficulties and pain your drinking caused."

35. 4. Part of the healing process for the family is to acknowledge the pain, embarrassment, and overall difficulties the client's drinking problem caused family members. The first option facilitates the client's ability to deny the problem. The second option prevents the client from acknowledging the difficulties the children endured. The third option leads the client to believe only a simple apology is needed. The addiction must be addressed and the children's pain acknowledged.

CN: Psychosocial integrity; CNS: None; CL: Application

36. A client with a diagnosis of alcohol dependency is being discharged from the hospital. Which goal will be a *priority* for successful outpatient therapy?

1. Find a way to drink socially.
2. Allow self to grieve recent losses.
3. Work to bring others into treatment.
4. Develop relapse-prevention strategies.

36. 4. The primary goal for a client in outpatient treatment is to focus on strategies that prevent relapse. Finding ways to drink socially and working to bring others into treatment aren't goals of outpatient therapy. Allowing self to grieve the losses the addiction caused is a part of the early work of inpatient therapy and may be continued in outpatient therapy.

CN: Safe, effective care environment; CNS: Management of care; CL: Analysis

37. A client addicted to alcohol tells a nurse, "Making friends used to be hard for me." Which statement by the client indicates that client teaching about relationships was successful?

1. "I've set limits on my behaviors toward others."
2. "I need to be judgmental of others."
3. "I won't become intimately involved with others."
4. "I can't bear to see myself hurt again in a relationship."

37. 1. When the client can set personal limits and maintain boundaries, the ability to have successful interpersonal relationships can occur. Being judgmental is contraindicated if a client wants to have successful relationships. Setting arbitrary limits on relationships indicates the client needs to learn more interpersonal relationship skills. The universal truth about relationships is that they bring both joy and pain. The last statement indicates a need to learn more about relationships.

CN: Psychosocial integrity; CNS: None; CL: Application

Your client teaching stems in part from an understanding of the severity of disease.

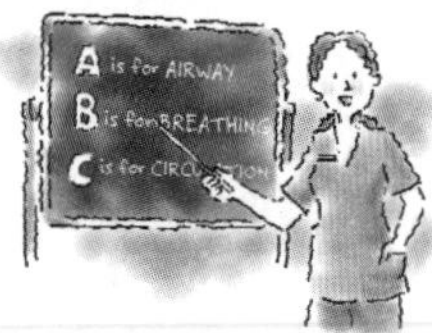

38. A client who abused alcohol for more than 20 years is diagnosed with cirrhosis of the liver. Which statement by the client shows that teaching has been effective?

1. "If I decide to stop drinking, I won't kill myself."
2. "If I watch my blood pressure, I should be okay."
3. "If I take vitamins, I can undo some liver damage."
4. "If I use nutritional supplements, I won't have problems."

38. 1. This statement reflects the client's perception of the severity of the condition and the life-threatening complications that can result from continued use of alcohol. Aggressive treatment is required, not merely watching one's blood pressure. At this point in the illness, there is little likelihood that liver damage from cirrhosis can be altered. The fourth option denies the severity of the problem and negates the life-threatening complications common with a diagnosis of cirrhosis.

CN: Psychosocial integrity; CNS: None; CL: Analysis

39. A client tells a nurse, "I'm not going to have problems from smoking marijuana." Which response is most appropriate?

1. "Evidence shows it can cause major health problems."
2. "Marijuana can cause reproductive problems later in life."
3. "Smoking marijuana isn't as dangerous as smoking cigarettes."
4. "Some people have minor or no reactions to smoking marijuana."

39. 2. Marijuana causes cardiac, respiratory, immune, and reproductive health problems. Most people who smoke marijuana don't have major health problems. All people who smoke marijuana have symptoms of intoxication. The residues from marijuana are more toxic than those from cigarettes.

CN: Psychosocial integrity; CNS: None; CL: Application

40. During an assessment of a client with a history of polysubstance abuse, which information is a priority to obtain after the names of the drugs?

1. Oral administration of any drug
2. Time of last use of each drug
3. How the drug was obtained
4. The place the drug was used

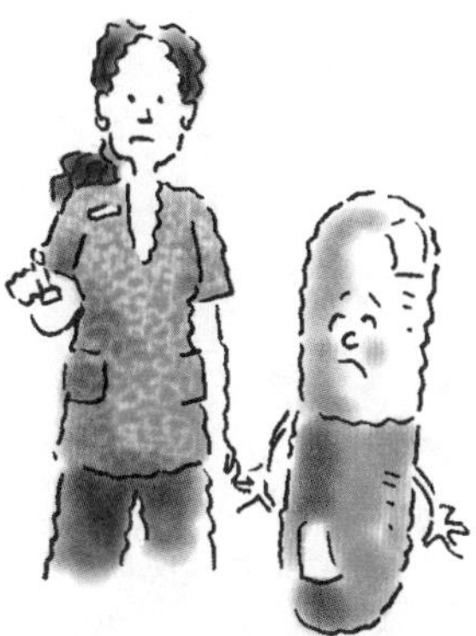

40. 2. The time of last use gives information about expected withdrawal symptoms of the drugs and what immediate treatment is necessary. How the drugs were obtained and the places the drugs were used aren't essential information for treatment, nor is oral administration.
CN: Psychosocial integrity; CNS: None; CL: Application

41. A client says, "I started using cocaine as a recreational drug, but now I can't seem to control the use." The nurse knows that the client's statement is *most* consistent with which drug behavior?

1. Toxic dose
2. Dual diagnosis
3. Cross-tolerance
4. Compulsive use

41. 4. Compulsive drug use involves taking a substance for a period of time significantly longer than intended. A toxic dose is the amount of a drug that causes a poisonous effect. Dual diagnosis is the coexistence of a drug problem and a mental health problem. Cross-tolerance occurs when the effects of a drug are decreased and the client takes larger amounts to achieve the desired drug effect.
CN: Psychosocial integrity; CNS: None; CL: Application

42. A client says he used amphetamines to be productive at work. Which symptom commonly occurs when the drug is abruptly discontinued?

1. Severe anxiety
2. Increased yawning
3. Altered perceptions
4. Amotivational syndrome

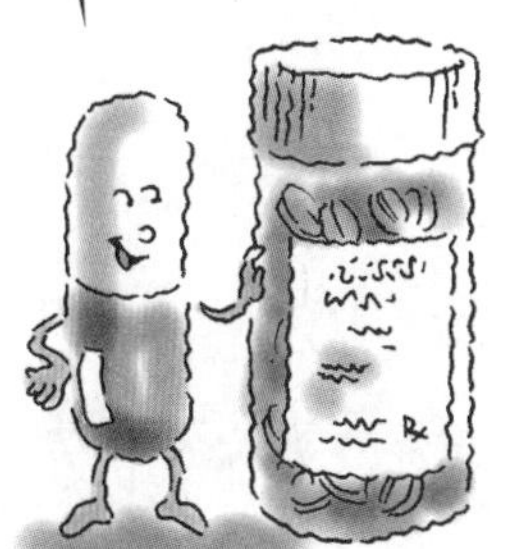

You should know which drugs cause which adverse effects!

42. 1. When amphetamines are abruptly discontinued, the client may experience severe anxiety or agitation. Increased yawning is a symptom of opioid withdrawal. Altered perceptions occur when a client is withdrawing from hallucinogens. Amotivational syndrome is seen with clients using marijuana.
CN: Psychosocial integrity; CNS: None; CL: Application

43. A 20-year-old client is admitted with bone marrow depression. He tells the nurse he's been abusing drugs since age 13. Which drug should the nurse expect to find in his history?

1. Amphetamines
2. Cocaine
3. Inhalants
4. Marijuana

43. 3. Inhalants cause severe bone marrow depression. Marijuana, cocaine, and amphetamines don't cause bone marrow depression.
CN: Physiological integrity; CNS: Pharmacological and parenteral therapies; CL: Application

44. Which reason best explains why it's important to monitor behavior in a client who has stopped using phencyclidine (PCP)?

1. Fatigue can cause feelings of being overwhelmed.
2. Agitation and mood swings can occur during withdrawal.
3. Bizarre behavior can be a precursor to a psychotic episode.
4. Memory loss and forgetfulness can cause unsafe conditions.

44. 3. Bizarre behavior and speech are associated with PCP withdrawal and can indicate psychosis. Fatigue isn't necessarily a problem when a client stops using PCP. Agitation, mood swings, memory loss, and forgetfulness don't tend to occur when a client has stopped using PCP.
CN: Psychosocial integrity; CNS: None; CL: Analysis

45. A client experiencing amphetamine withdrawal may commonly experience which of the following symptoms?

1. Disturbed sleep
2. Increased yawning
3. Psychomotor agitation
4. Inability to concentrate

45. 1. It's common for a person withdrawing from amphetamines to experience disturbed sleep and unpleasant dreams. Increased yawning is seen with clients withdrawing from opioids. Psychomotor agitation is seen in cocaine withdrawal, and the inability to concentrate is seen in caffeine withdrawal.
CN: Psychosocial integrity; CNS: None; CL: Application

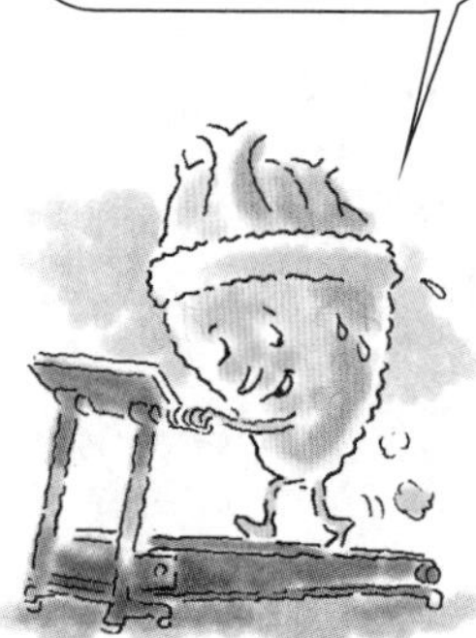

Somebody slow this thing down, please!

46. Which condition can occur in a client who has just used cocaine?

1. Tachycardia
2. Hyperthermia
3. Hypotension
4. Bradypnea

46. 1. Tachycardia is common because cocaine increases the heart's demand for oxygen. Cocaine doesn't cause hyperthermia (elevated temperature), hypotension (decreased blood pressure), or bradypnea (decreased respiratory rate).
CN: Psychosocial integrity; CNS: None; CL: Application

47. Which information is most important in teaching a client who abuses prescription drugs?

1. Herbal substitutes are safer to use.
2. Medication should be used only for the reason prescribed.
3. The client should consult a physician before using a drug.
4. Consider if family members influence the client to use drugs.

47. 2. People often take prescribed drugs for reasons other than those intended, primarily to self-medicate or experience a sense of euphoria. The safety and efficacy of most herbal remedies hasn't been established. Sometimes over-the-counter medications are necessary for minor problems. There may be a family history of substance abuse, but it isn't a priority when planning nursing care.
CN: Psychosocial integrity; CNS: None; CL: Application

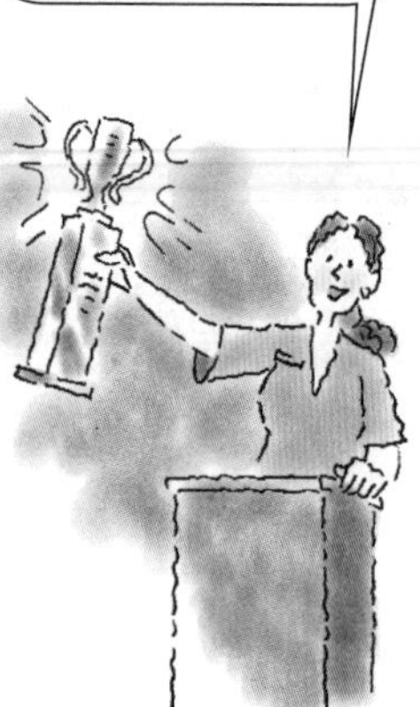

You're the best!

48. The family of an adolescent who smokes marijuana asks a nurse if the use of marijuana leads to abuse of other drugs. Which response is best?

1. "Use of marijuana is a stage your child will go through."
2. "Many people use marijuana and don't use other street drugs."
3. "Use of marijuana can lead to abuse of more potent substances."
4. "It's difficult to answer that question as I don't know your child."

48. 3. Marijuana is considered a "gateway drug" because it tends to lead to the abuse of more potent drugs. People who use marijuana tend to use or at least experiment with more potent substances. Marijuana isn't a part of a developmental stage that adolescents go through. It isn't important that the nurse knows the child.
CN: Psychosocial integrity; CNS: None; CL: Application

49. A pregnant client is thinking about stopping cocaine use. Which statement by the client indicates effective teaching about pregnancy and drug use?

1. "Right after birth, I'll give the baby up for adoption."
2. "I'll help the baby get through the withdrawal period."
3. "I don't want the baby to have withdrawal symptoms."
4. "It's scary to think the baby may have Down syndrome."

49. 3. Neonates born to mothers addicted to cocaine have withdrawal symptoms at birth. If the client says she'll give the baby up for adoption after birth or help the baby get through the withdrawal period, the teaching was ineffective because the mother doesn't see the impact of her drug use on the child. Use of cocaine during pregnancy doesn't contribute to the baby having Down syndrome.

CN: Psychosocial integrity; CNS: None; CL: Analysis

50. Which test might be ordered for a client with a history of cocaine abuse who exhibits behavior changes following a return from an inpatient treatment facility?

1. Antibody screen
2. Glucose screen
3. Hepatic screen
4. Urine screen

50. 4. A urine toxicology screen would show the presence of cocaine in the body. Glucose, hepatic, or antibody screening wouldn't show the presence of cocaine in the body.

CN: Psychosocial integrity; CNS: None; CL: Application

51. A nurse is assessing a client with a history of substance abuse who has pinpoint pupils, a heart rate of 56 beats/minute, a respiratory rate of 6 breaths/minute, and temperature of 96.4° F. Which substance should the nurse determine is the most likely cause of the client's symptoms?

1. Opioids
2. Amphetamines
3. Cannabis
4. Alcohol

51. 1. Opioids, such as morphine and heroin, can cause pinpont pupils and a reduced heart rate, respiratory rate, and body temperature with intoxication. Amphetamine intoxication can lead to tachycardia, euphoria, and irritability. Cannabis (marijuana) intoxication can cause slowed reflexes, lethargy, and tachycardia. Alcohol intoxication leads to slurred speech, unsteady gait, and uncoordination.

CN: Psychosocial integrity; CNS: None; CL: Application

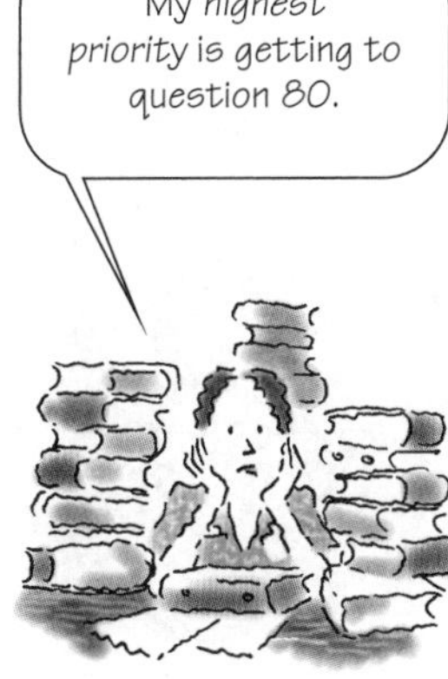
My highest priority is getting to question 80.

52. Which intervention is the <u>highest priority</u> in planning care for a client recovering from cocaine use?

1. Skin care
2. Suicide precautions
3. Frequent orientation
4. Nutrition consultation

52. 2. Clients recovering from cocaine use are prone to "postcoke depression" and have a likelihood of becoming suicidal if they can't take the drug. Frequent orientation and skin care are routine nursing interventions but aren't the most immediate considerations for this client. Nutrition consultation isn't the most pressing intervention for this client.

CN: Safe, effective care environment; CNS: Management of care; CL: Analysis

53. Which clinical condition is frequently seen with substance abuse clients who repeatedly use cocaine?

1. Panic attacks
2. Bipolar cycling
3. Attention deficits
4. Expressive aphasia

53. 2. Clients who frequently use cocaine will experience the rapid cycling effect of excitement and then severe depression. They don't tend to experience panic attacks, expressive aphasia, or attention deficits.

CN: Psychosocial integrity; CNS: None; CL: Analysis

54. A client who uses cocaine finally admits he also abused other drugs to equalize the effect of cocaine. Which substance might be included in the client's pattern of polysubstance abuse?

1. Alcohol
2. Amphetamines
3. Caffeine
4. Phencyclidine

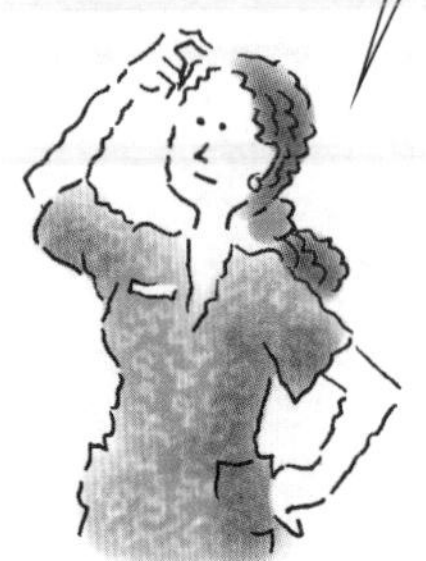

What would have
the opposite effect?

54. 1. A cocaine addict will commonly use alcohol to decrease or equalize the stimulating effects of cocaine. Caffeine, phencyclidine, and amphetamines aren't used to equalize the stimulating effects of cocaine.

CN: Psychosocial integrity; CNS: None; CL: Application

55. A group of teenagers tell the school nurse they used cocaine because they were bored. Which short-term goal is the most important for the nurse to immediately initiate?

1. Prepare a drug lecture.
2. Restrict school privileges.
3. Establish an activity schedule.
4. Report the incident to their parents.

55. 3. Having an activity schedule enables the adolescents to develop coping skills to make better choices about what to do with their free time. Preparing a drug lecture or restricting school privileges won't be seen as useful by the adolescents and may inadvertently contribute to their inappropriate behavior. As the nurse works with the adolescents, it would be more effective to have the children talk to their parents about their drug use.

CN: Psychosocial integrity; CNS: None; CL: Application

56. Which statement by a client indicates teaching about cocaine use has been effective?

1. "I wasn't using cocaine to feel better about myself."
2. "I started using cocaine more and more until I couldn't stop."
3. "I'm not addicted to cocaine because I don't use it every day."
4. "I'm not going to be a chronic user, I only use it on holidays."

56. 2. This statement reflects the trajectory or common pattern of cocaine use and indicates successful teaching. The first option reflects the client's denial. People gravitate to the drug and continue its use because it gives them a sense of well-being, competency, and power. Cocaine abusers tend to be binge users and can be drug-free for days or weeks between use, but they still have a drug problem. The fourth option indicates the client is in denial about the drug's potential to become a habit. Effective teaching didn't occur.

CN: Psychosocial integrity; CNS: None; CL: Analysis

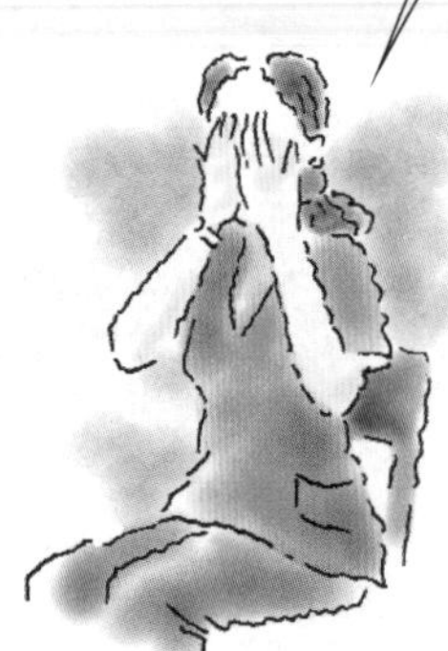

Don't panic now.
Just attack this
question with your
eyes wide open.

57. A client who formerly used lysergic acid diethylamide (LSD) is seeking counseling. Which characteristic or condition in the mental health history would be seen in this client?

1. Lack of trust
2. Panic attacks
3. Recurrent depression
4. Loss of ego boundaries

57. 2. Clients who used LSD typically have a history of panic attacks or psychotic behavior. This is often referred to as a "bad trip." Loss of ego boundaries, recurrent depression, and lack of trust don't tend to be problems for this type of client.

CN: Psychosocial integrity; CNS: None; CL: Analysis

58. A nurse is writing a nursing care plan for a client who has been using phencyclidine (PCP). Assessment for which emergency should be included?

1. Cardiac arrest
2. Seizure disorder
3. Violent behavior
4. Delirium reaction

58. 3. When a client is using phencyclidine, an acute psychotic reaction can occur. The client is capable of sudden, explosive, violent behavior. Phencyclidine doesn't tend to cause cardiac arrest or a seizure disorder. Delirium is associated with inhalant intoxication.

CN: Physiological integrity; CNS: Reduction of risk potential; CL: Application

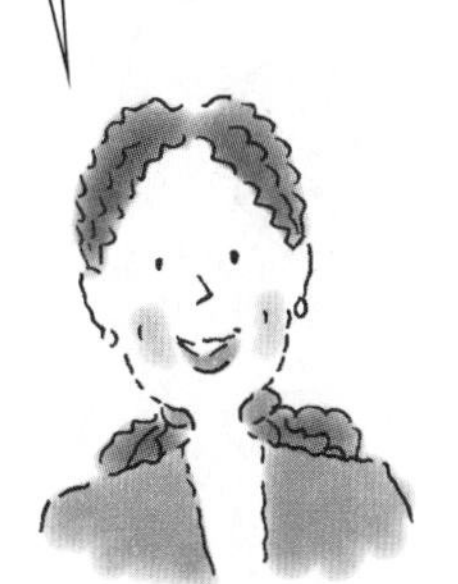

You're almost at question 60. That should motivate you to keep moving!

59. A client who smoked marijuana daily for 10 years tells a nurse, "I don't have any goals, and I just don't know what to do." Which communication technique is the most useful when talking to this client?

1. Focus the interaction.
2. Use nonverbal methods.
3. Use reflection techniques.
4. Ask open-ended questions.

59. 1. A client with amotivational syndrome from chronic use of marijuana tends to talk in tangents and needs the nurse to focus the conversation. Nonverbal communication or reflection techniques wouldn't be useful as this client must focus and learn to identify and accomplish goals. Using only open-ended questions won't allow the client to focus and establish specific goals.

CN: Psychosocial integrity; CNS: None; CL: Application

60. A nurse is assessing a client who uses heroin to determine if there are physical health problems. Which medical consequence of heroin use frequently occurs?

1. Hepatitis
2. Peptic ulcers
3. Hypertension
4. Chronic pharyngitis

60. 1. Hepatitis is the most common medical complication of heroin abuse. Peptic ulcers are more likely to be a complication of caffeine use, hypertension is a complication of amphetamine use, and chronic pharyngitis is a complication of marijuana use.

CN: Physiological integrity; CNS: Physiological adaptation; CL: Application

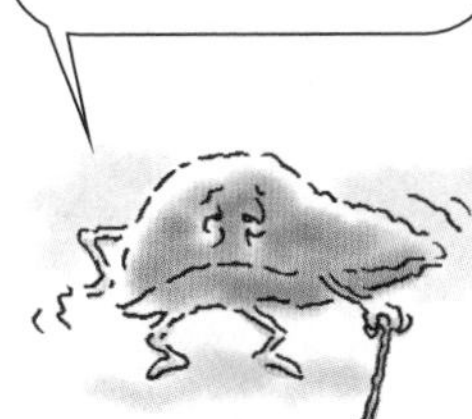

I feel so abused.

61. The family of a client in rehabilitation following heroin withdrawal asks a nurse why the client is receiving naltrexone (ReVia). Which response is correct?

1. To help reverse withdrawal symptoms
2. To keep the client sedated during withdrawal
3. To take the place of detoxification with methadone
4. To decrease the client's memory of the withdrawal experience

61. 1. Naltrexone is an opioid antagonist and helps the client stay drug-free. Keeping the client sedated during withdrawal isn't the reason for giving this drug. The drug doesn't decrease the client's memory of the withdrawal experience and isn't used in place of detoxification with methadone.

CN: Psychosocial integrity; CNS: None; CL: Application

62. Which nursing intervention has priority in a care plan for a client recovering from cocaine addiction?

1. Help the client find ways to be happy and competent.
2. Foster the creative use of self in community activities.
3. Teach the client to handle stresses in the work setting.
4. Help the client acknowledge the current level of dependency.

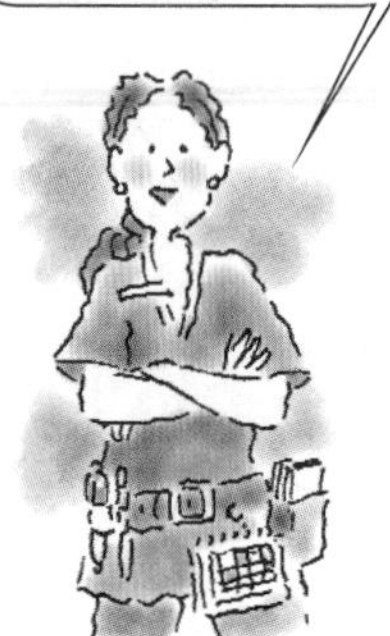

Maybe we should be called priority engineers instead of nurses.

62. 1. The major component of a treatment program for a client with cocaine addiction is to have the client feel happy and competent. Cocaine addiction is difficult to treat because the drug actions reinforce its use. There are often perceived positive effects. Clients often credit the drug with giving them creative energy instead of looking within themselves. Fostering the creative use of self may inadvertently reinforce the client's drug use. Teaching the client to handle stresses is appropriate but isn't the most immediate nursing action. Examining the client's level of dependency isn't the immediate choice, as the client needs to work on remaining drug free.

CN: Safe, effective care environment; CNS: Management of care; CL: Application

63. A client tells a nurse, "I've been clean from drugs for the past 5 years, but my life really hasn't changed." Which concept should be explored with this client?

1. Further education
2. Conflict resolution
3. Career development
4. Personal development

63. 4. True recovery involves changing the client's distorted thinking and working on personal and emotional development. Before the client pursues further education, career development, or conflict resolution skills, it's imperative the client devotes energy to emotional and personal development.

CN: Psychosocial integrity; CNS: None; CL: Analysis

64. A client discusses how drug addiction has made life unmanageable. Which information will help the client cope with the drug problem?

1. How peers have committed to sobriety
2. How to accomplish family of origin work
3. The addiction process and tools for recovery
4. How environmental stimuli serve as drug triggers

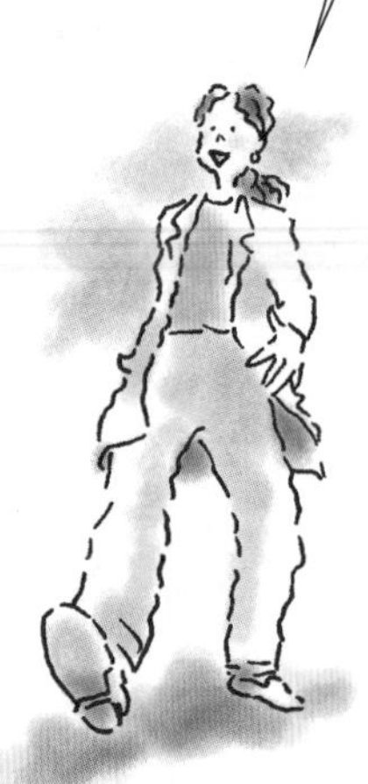

A journey of a thousand miles starts with one step.

64. 3. When the client admits life has become unmanageable, the best strategy is to teach about the addiction, how to obtain support, and how to develop new coping skills. Information about how peers committed to sobriety would be shared with the client as the treatment process begins. Identification of how environmental stimuli serve as drug triggers would be a later part of the treatment process and family of origin work. Initially, the client must commit to sobriety and learn skills for recovery.

CN: Psychosocial integrity; CNS: None; CL: Analysis

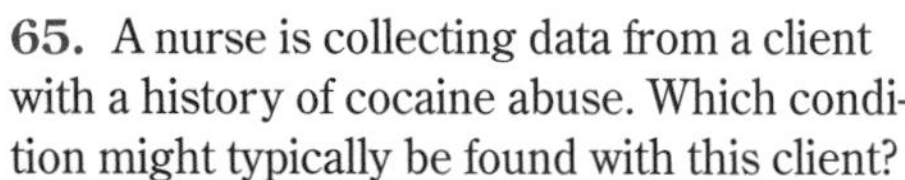

65. A nurse is collecting data from a client with a history of cocaine abuse. Which condition might typically be found with this client?

1. Glossitis
2. Pharyngitis
3. Bilateral ear infections
4. Perforated nasal septum

65. 4. When cocaine is snorted frequently, the client often develops a perforated nasal septum. Bilateral ear infections, pharyngitis, and glossitis aren't common physical findings for a client with a history of cocaine abuse.

CN: Psychosocial integrity; CNS: None; CL: Application

66. A client recovering from cocaine abuse is participating in group therapy. Which statement by the client indicates the client has benefited from the group?

1. "I think the laws about drug possession are too strict in this country."
2. "I'll be more careful about talking about my drug use to my children."
3. "I finally realize the short high from cocaine isn't worth the depression."
4. "I can't understand how I could get all these problems that we talked about in group."

66. 3. This is a realistic appraisal of a client's experience with cocaine and how harmful the experience is. The first option indicates the client was distracting self from personal issues and isn't working on goals in the group setting. Talking about drugs to children must be reinforced with nonverbal behavior, and not talking about drugs may give children the wrong message about drug use. The fourth option indicates the client is in denial about the consequences of cocaine use.

CN: Psychosocial integrity; CNS: None; CL: Analysis

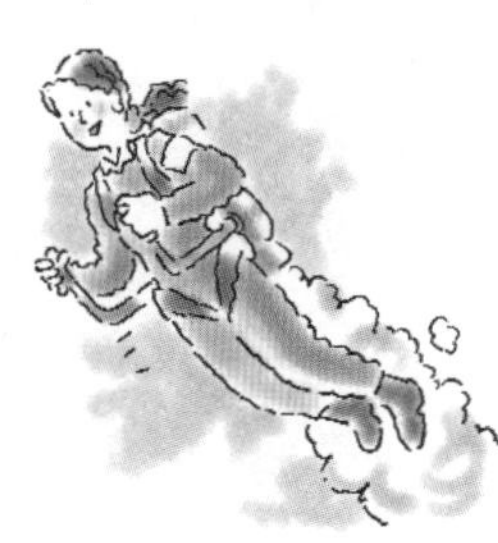
I'm flying high—
but not for long!

67. A family expresses concern that a member who stopped using amphetamines 3 months ago is acting paranoid. Which explanation is the best?

1. A person gets symptoms of paranoia with polysubstance abuse.
2. When a person uses amphetamines, paranoid tendencies may continue for months.
3. Sometimes family dynamics and a high suspicion of continued drug use make a person paranoid.
4. Amphetamine abusers may have severe anxiety and paranoid thinking.

67. 2. After a client uses amphetamines, there may be long-term effects that exist for months after use. Two common effects are paranoia and ideas of reference. Even with polysubstance abuse, the paranoia comes from the chronic use of amphetamines. The third option blames the family when the paranoia comes from the drug use. Severe anxiety isn't typically manifested in paranoid thinking.

CN: Psychosocial integrity; CNS: None; CL: Analysis

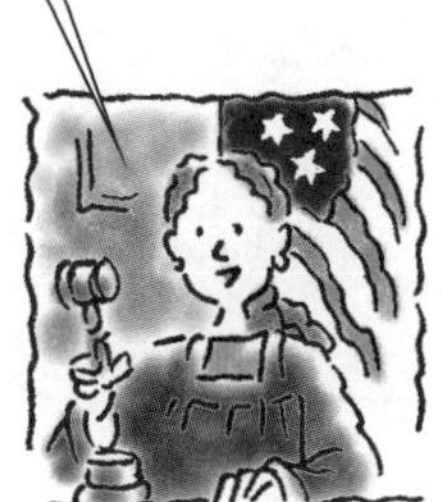
And the verdict is—the best answer.

68. A nurse is trying to determine if a client who abuses heroin has any drug-related legal problems. Which assessment question is the best to ask the client?

1. When did your spouse become aware of your use of heroin?
2. Do you have a probation officer that you report to periodically?
3. Have you experienced any legal violations while being intoxicated?
4. Do you have a history of frequent visits with the employee assistance program manager?

68. 3. This question focuses on obtaining direct information about drug-related legal problems. When a spouse becomes aware of a partner's substance abuse, the first action isn't necessarily to institute legal action. Even if the client reports to a probation officer, the offense isn't necessarily a drug-related problem. Asking if the client has a history of frequent visits with the employee assistance program manager isn't useful. It assumes any visit to the employee assistance program manager is related to drug issues.

CN: Psychosocial integrity; CNS: None; CL: Analysis

69. The severity of withdrawal symptoms for a client addicted to heroin may depend on which factor?

1. Ego strength
2. Liver function
3. Seizure history
4. Kidney function

69. 2. Liver function status is an important variable that can be used to indicate the severity of a client's drug withdrawal. Ego strength, seizure history, and kidney function aren't variables that can be used to predict the severity of withdrawal symptoms.

CN: Physiological integrity; CNS: Reduction of risk potential; CL: Analysis

70. A client who uses cocaine denies that drug use is a problem. Which intervention strategy would be best to confront the client's denial?

1. State ways to cope with stress.
2. Repeat the drug facts as needed.
3. Identify the client's ambivalence.
4. Use open-ended, factual questions.

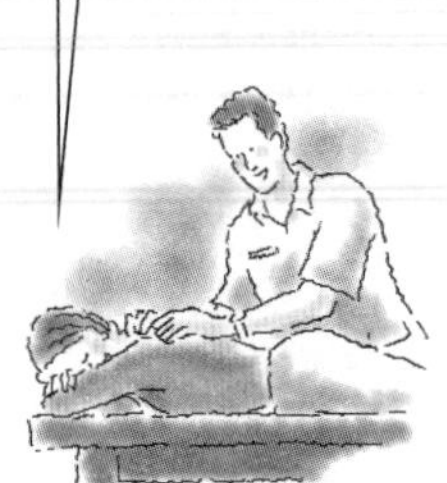
Think therapeutic.

70. 4. The use of open-ended, factual questions will help the client acknowledge that a drug problem is present. Stating ways to cope with stress and identifying the client's ambivalence won't be effective for breaking through a client's denial. Repeating drug facts won't be effective, as the client will perceive it as preaching or nagging.

CN: Psychosocial integrity; CNS: None; CL: Application

71. A nurse is working with parents of an adolescent client who abuses inhalants. Which information about consequences is best to include in a teaching plan?

1. Consequences must be enforceable.
2. Everything can become a consequence.
3. When setting consequences, be verbally forceful.
4. Consequences are seldom needed with adolescents.

71. 1. Consequences must be specific and enforceable. Sometimes parents are prone to make consequences that are too difficult to enforce or that actually become a punishment for the parents. Everything can't be made into a consequence. Being verbally forceful isn't appropriate because the consequence can occur in a civil tone of voice. A consequence can be used with every person regardless of developmental stage.

CN: Psychosocial integrity; CNS: None; CL: Analysis

72. A nurse is caring for a client undergoing treatment for cocaine abuse. The nurse should expect the client to make which statement if the client is pessimistic about treatment?

1. "I'll never get better. This is useless."
2. "I don't think I want to see my family anymore. They're not supportive."
3. "I'm fatigued all the time. My energy is low."
4. "I want to get better now. Can't we rush the treatment?"

72. 1. Clients withdrawing from drugs such as cocaine frequently experience depression. It's common for drug-addicted clients to experience fatigue without becoming pessimistic. Being impulsive or having feelings of estrangement aren't necessarily related to a client becoming pessimistic about treatment.

CN: Psychosocial integrity; CNS: None; CL: Analysis

73. A nurse is working with a client addicted to cocaine who is in denial. Which approach is most useful for dealing with the client's denial?

1. Ask whether the client sees the drug use as a problem.
2. Focus on the pain the client is having during withdrawal.
3. Reinforce the connection between drug use and harmful results.
4. Help the client recognize reality by pointing out withdrawal symptoms.

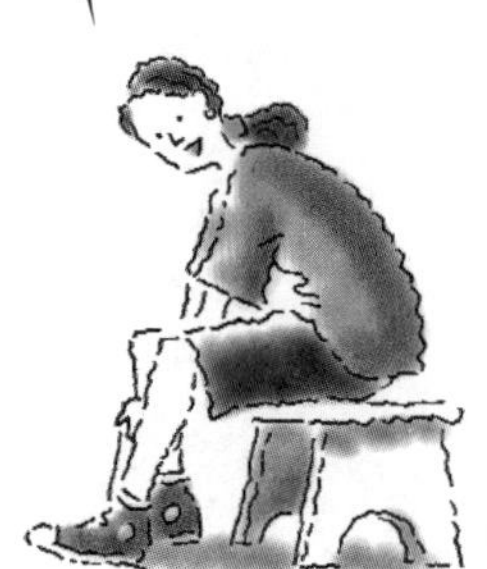
Only a handful of questions to go!

73. 3. To deal with the client's denial, the nurse must confront the drug use and point out the results of the behavior. Asking if the client sees the drug use as a problem will only reinforce the client's denial and provide a forum to intellectualize the problem or provide excuses for it. Pain isn't associated with withdrawal from cocaine. Pointing out withdrawal symptoms may not be the most effective strategy, as the client often downplays the significance of the problem.

CN: Psychosocial integrity; CNS: None; CL: Analysis

74. A client who uses cocaine is admitted to an intensive outpatient rehabilitation program. During cocaine withdrawal, which finding should the nurse expect when assessing the client?

1. GI distress
2. Blurred vision
3. Perceptual distortions
4. Increased appetite

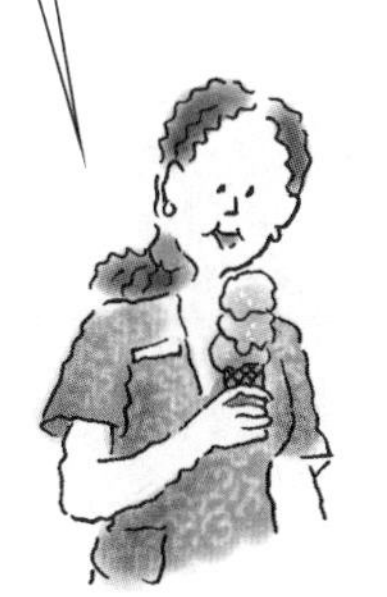

Which finding should you expect in question 74?

74. 4. Increased appetite is typical during cocaine or nicotine withdrawal. GI distress (especially nausea and vomiting) occurs during alcohol or opioid withdrawal. Blurred vision isn't typical in cocaine withdrawal. Perceptual distortions are common during withdrawal from phencyclidine (PCP, or "angel dust"), amphetamines, and hallucinogens.

CN: Physiological integrity; CNS: Physiological adaptation; CL: Application

75. A client who abuses alcohol is admitted to an outpatient drug and alcohol treatment facility. What's the most objective assessment method for determining if the client is still using alcohol?

1. Having the client walk a straight line
2. Smelling the client's breath
3. Giving the client a breath alcohol test
4. Asking the client if he has been drinking

75. 3. A breath alcohol test is the most objective way to determine if the client is still using alcohol. Having him walk a straight line and smelling his breath aren't objective tests. Asking him if he has been drinking may not elicit an honest answer (many clients who abuse alcohol deny alcohol use).

CN: Psychosocial integrity; CNS: None; CL: Application

76. During nicotine withdrawal, which client statement is typical?

1. "I sometimes feel like I'm seeing things."
2. "I feel lousy, and I'm grumpy with everybody."
3. "I can't believe I feel fine after just having stopped smoking."
4. "I'm always yawning now."

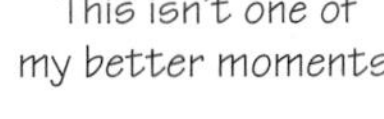

This isn't one of my better moments.

76. 2. During nicotine withdrawal, the client is typically irritable and nervous. Seeing things (hallucinations) isn't linked to nicotine withdrawal. A client going through nicotine withdrawal is unlikely to "feel fine." Yawning is associated with withdrawal from opioids, not nicotine.

CN: Physiological integrity; CNS: Physiological adaptation; CL: Application

77. A polyaddicted client is hospitalized for withdrawal complications. During his stay in a medical step-down unit, which immediate short-term goal takes <u>highest priority</u>?

1. The client will remain safe during the detoxification period.
2. The client will develop an accurate perception of his drug problem.
3. The client will abstain from mood-altering drugs.
4. The client will learn coping strategies to help him stop relying on drugs.

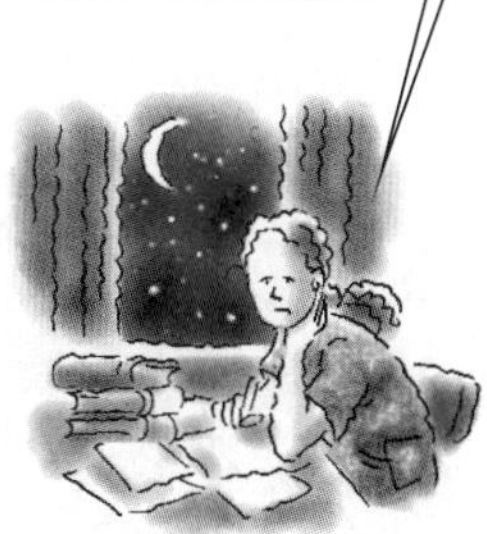

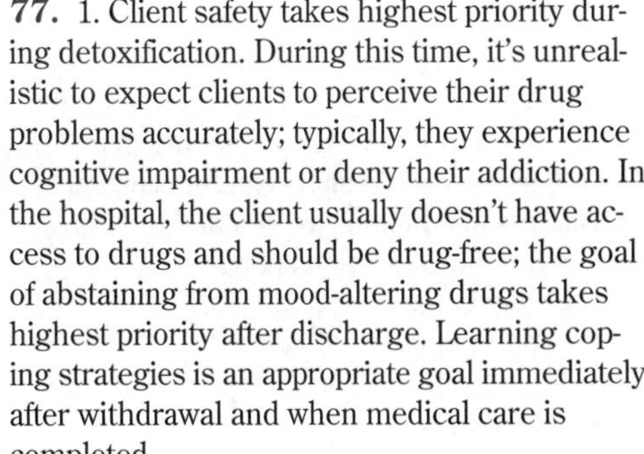

77. 1. Client safety takes highest priority during detoxification. During this time, it's unrealistic to expect clients to perceive their drug problems accurately; typically, they experience cognitive impairment or deny their addiction. In the hospital, the client usually doesn't have access to drugs and should be drug-free; the goal of abstaining from mood-altering drugs takes highest priority after discharge. Learning coping strategies is an appropriate goal immediately after withdrawal and when medical care is completed.

CN: Safe, effective care environment; CNS: Management of care; CL: Application

78. A client with an alcohol addiction requests a prescription for disulfiram (Antabuse). To determine the client's ability to take this drug appropriately, the nurse should focus on which factor?

1. Whether the client will take a prescription drug
2. Whether the client's family accepts the use of this treatment strategy
3. Whether the client is willing to follow the necessary dietary restrictions
4. Whether the client is motivated to stay sober

78. 4. A client with a strong craving for alcohol (and a lack of impulse control) isn't a good candidate for disulfiram therapy. Disulfiram is a prescription drug. Accepting the treatment strategy is a decision that the client and health care provider make; although family input may be welcome, family members don't make the final decision. Significant dietary restrictions aren't necessary during disulfiram therapy (except for alcohol and foods prepared or cooked in it).

CN: Psychosocial integrity; CNS: None; CL: Analysis

79. A nurse has developed a relationship with a client who has an addiction problem. Which information should indicate that the therapeutic interaction is in the working stage? Select all that apply:

1. The client addresses how the addiction has contributed to family distress.
2. The client reluctantly shares the family history of addiction.
3. The client verbalizes difficulty identifying personal strengths.
4. The client discusses financial problems related to the addiction.
5. The client expresses uncertainty about meeting with the nurse.
6. The client acknowledges the addiction's effects on the children.

79. 1, 3, 6. These statements are indicative of the nurse-client working phase, in which the client explores, evaluates, and determines solutions to identified problems. The remaining statements address what happens during the introductory phase of the nurse-client interaction.

CN: Psychosocial integrity; CNS: None; CL: Analysis

80. A client is receiving chlordiazepoxide (Librium) to control the symptoms of alcohol withdrawal. The chlordiazepoxide has been ordered as needed. Which symptoms may indicate the need for an additional dose of the medication? Select all that apply:

1. Tachycardia
2. Mood swings
3. Elevated blood pressure and temperature
4. Piloerection
5. Tremors
6. Increasing anxiety

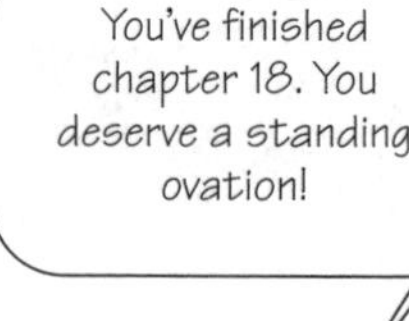

You've finished chapter 18. You deserve a standing ovation!

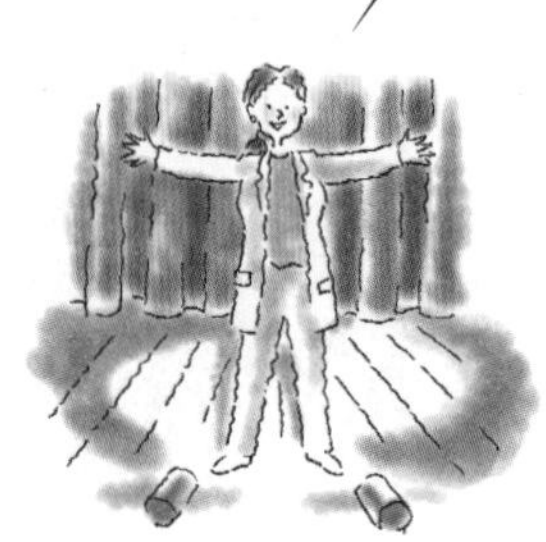

80. 1, 3, 5, 6. Benzodiazepines are usually administered based on elevations in heart rate, blood pressure, and temperature as well as on the presence of tremors and increasing anxiety. Mood swings are expected during the withdrawal period and are not an indication for further medication administration. Piloerection is not a symptom of alcohol withdrawal.

CN: Physiological integrity; CNS: Pharmacological and parenteral therapies; CL: Analysis

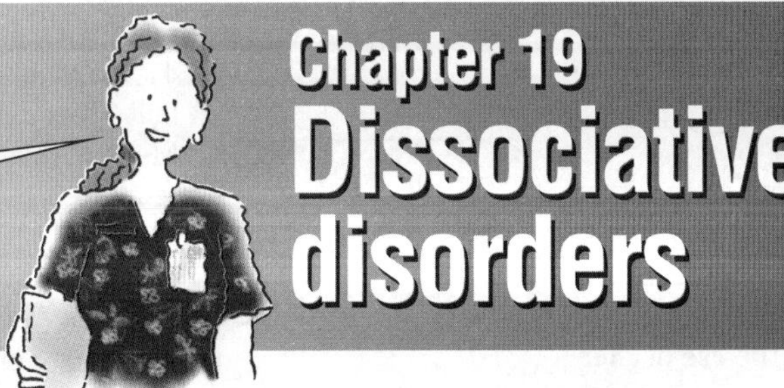
For more information
on dissociative
disorders, check this
independent
Web site:
www.mentalhealth.com.

Chapter 19
Dissociative disorders

1. When taking a history from a client with dissociative identity disorder (DID), the nurse should expect the client to make which statement?

1. "My father wasn't around much."
2. "I feel good about myself."
3. "I can recall many traumatic events from childhood."
4. "My father loved me one day and hit me the next day."

1. 4. Repeated exposure to a childhood environment that alternates between highly stressful and then loving and supportive can be a factor in the development of DID. Many children grow up in a household without a father but don't develop DID. Clients with DID commonly have low self-esteem. Because of dissociation from the trauma, a client with DID usually can't recall childhood traumatic events.
CN: Psychosocial integrity; CNS: None; CL: Application

2. A nursing care plan for a client with dissociative identity disorder (DID) should address which factor?

1. Ritualistic behavior
2. Out-of-body experiences
3. History of severe childhood abuse
4. Ability to give a thorough personal history

2. 3. DID is theorized to develop as a protective response to such traumatic experiences as severe child abuse. Ritualistic behavior is seen with obsessive-compulsive disorders. Out-of-body experiences are more commonly associated with depersonalization disorder. Because of the dissociative response to personal experiences, people with DID are usually unable to give a thorough personal history.
CN: Psychosocial integrity; CNS: None; CL: Application

3. Which nursing diagnosis is most appropriate for a client with dissociative identity disorder (DID)?

1. *Disturbed personal identity related to delusional ideations*
2. *Risk for self-directed violence related to suicidal ideations or gestures*
3. *Deficient diversional activity related to lack of environmental stimulation*
4. *Disturbed sensory perception: visual hallucinations related to altered sensory reception of visual stimulation*

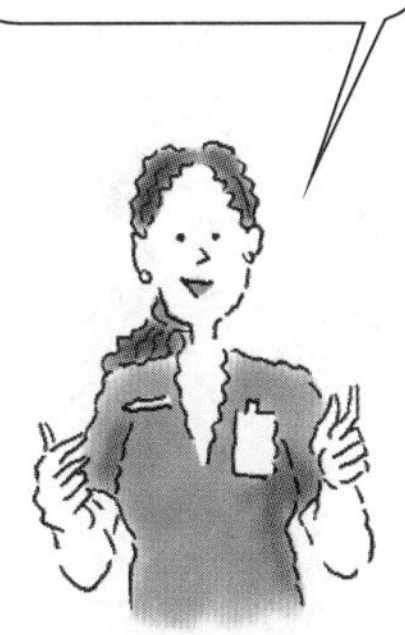
Nursing
diagnoses
standardize client
care.

3. 2. A common reason clients with DID are admitted to a psychiatric facility is because one of the alter personalities is trying to kill another personality. Hallucinations, delusions, and personal identity disturbances are commonly associated with schizophrenic disorders. Because of the assortment of alter personalities controlling the client with DID, diversional activity deficit is rarely a problem.
CN: Safe, effective care environment; CNS: Management of care; CL: Application

4. Which nursing intervention is important for a client with dissociative identity disorder (DID)?

1. Give antipsychotic medications as prescribed.
2. Maintain consistency when interacting with the client.
3. Confront the client about the use of alter personalities.
4. Prevent the client from interacting with others when one of the alter personalities is in control.

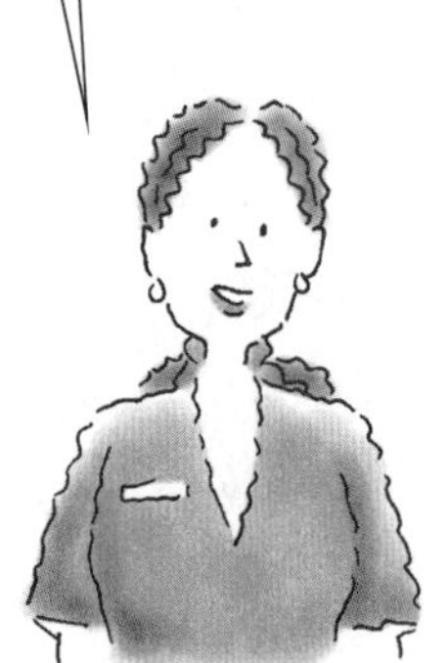

Understanding the client's problem allows you to provide more effective care.

4. 2. Establishing trust and support is important when interacting with a client with DID. Many of these clients have had few healthy relationships. Medication hasn't proven effective in the treatment of DID. Confronting the client about the alter personalities would be ineffective because the client has little, if any, knowledge of the presence of these other personalities. Isolating the client wouldn't be therapeutically beneficial.

CN: Safe, effective care environment; CNS: Management of care; CL: Analysis

5. A nurse notes a change in voice and mannerisms of a client with dissociative identity disorder (DID) after he learns that his wife has filed for a divorce. Which nursing intervention is most appropriate?

1. Avoid discussing the client's feelings.
2. Force the client to discuss his feelings.
3. Offer encouragement to the client that he'll be able to cope with the divorce.
4. Encourage the client to verbalize his feelings about the divorce.

5. 4. Encouraging a client with DID to verbalize his feelings will help him cope with his anxieties. Forcing the client to discuss his feelings can increase his level of anxiety. Avoiding discussion of feelings doesn't reduce anxiety and avoids the issue. Offering encouragement that the client will be able to cope with the divorce gives false reassurance and can erode the client's trust in the nurse.

CN: Psychosocial integrity; CNS: None; CL: Analysis

6. A nurse determines therapeutic interactions have been successful when a client with dissociative identity disorder (DID) shows which behavior or reaction?

1. Confronts the abuser
2. Attends the unit's milieu meetings
3. Prevents alter personalities from emerging
4. Reports no longer having feelings of anger about childhood traumas

6. 2. Attending milieu meetings decreases feelings of isolation and shows the client has begun to trust the nurse. Often the abuser was a part of the client's childhood, and confrontation in adulthood may not be possible or therapeutic. The client is often unaware of an alter personality and thus can't prevent these alter personalities from emerging. Clients with DID have dissociated from painful experiences, so the host personality often doesn't have negative feelings about such experiences.

CN: Psychosocial integrity; CNS: None; CL: Analysis

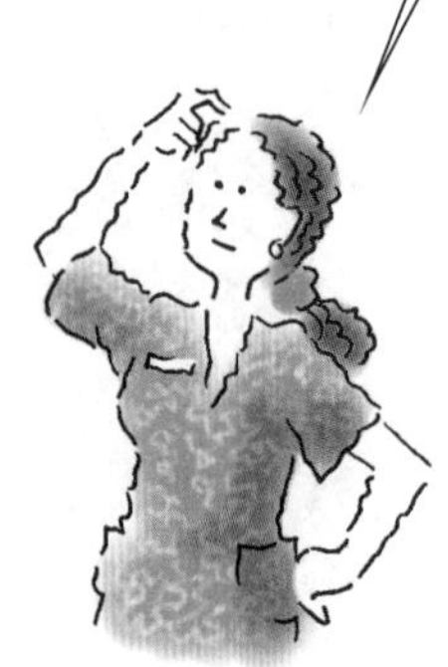

Sometimes I just can't remember anything.

7. Which of the following behaviors is indicative of a client with dissociative identity disorder (DID)?

1. Complaining of physical health problems with no organic basis
2. Being unable to account for certain times on a day-to-day basis
3. Participating in discussions about abusive incidents that occurred in the past
4. Being able to form a therapeutic relationship with the nurse after meeting twice

7. 2. When alter personalities are in control, periods of amnesia are common for clients with DID. Complaining of physical health problems with no organic basis describes clients with somatoform disorder. The client doesn't have memories of the abusive episodes, so he's unable to participate in discussions. These clients typically are slow in forming trusting relationships because many past relationships have been hurtful.

CN: Psychosocial integrity; CNS: None; CL: Application

8. A nurse is caring for a client with a dissociative disorder. Which intervention should the nurse include in the care plan?
1. Plan activities in which the client will be successful.
2. Offer praise whether or not the client has been successful.
3. Have the client engage in repetitive activities to reduce stress.
4. Encourage the client to keep a journal to recognize unsuccessful coping strategies.

8. 1. The care plan should include activities that will help the client be successful and feel a sense of accomplishment. Offering false praise can harm the nurse–client relationship and erode any sense of trust that develops. Repetitive activities and keeping a journal aren't appropriate therapeutic interventions for this client.
CN: Psychosocial integrity; CNS: None; CL: Application

9. A hospitalized client with dissociative identity disorder (DID) reports hearing voices. Which nursing intervention is most appropriate?
1. Tell the client to lie down and rest.
2. Give an as-needed dose of haloperidol (Haldol).
3. Encourage the client to continue with his daily activities.
4. Notify the physician that the client is having a psychotic episode.

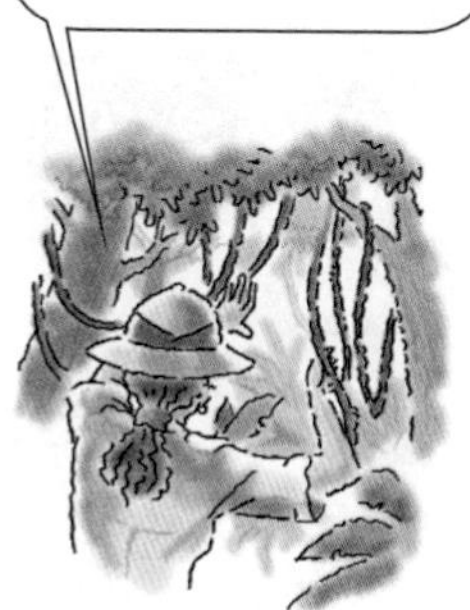
Which way is
most appropriate?

9. 3. Because many clients with DID hear voices, it's appropriate to have the client continue with daily activities. Having the client lie down and rest would have no therapeutic value. The voices the client hears are probably alter personalities communicating. This doesn't indicate a psychotic episode, so the physician wouldn't be notified to prescribe such antipsychotic medication as haloperidol.
CN: Safe, effective care environment; CNS: Management of care; CL: Application

10. Which goal would be the most important for a client with dissociative identity disorder (DID)?
1. Learning how to control periods of mania.
2. Learning how to integrate all the alternate personalities.
3. Developing coping strategies to deal with the traumatic childhood.
4. Determining what is causing them to feel they have periods of "lost time."

10. 4. The initial symptom many clients with DID experience, prompting them to seek health care, is the sensation of lost time. These are times the alter personalities are in control. Before therapeutic interventions, clients with DID may not even be aware of childhood trauma because of dissociation from the event. Initially, the client with DID isn't aware of the presence of alternate personalities. Depression, not mania, may be another early symptom of clients with DID.
CN: Psychosocial integrity; CNS: None; CL: Application

11. A client with dissociative identity disorder reports hearing voices and asks the nurse if that means he's "crazy." Which response would be the most appropriate?
1. "What do the voices tell you?"
2. "Why would you think you're crazy?"
3. "Clients with DID often report hearing voices."
4. "Hearing voices is often a symptom of schizophrenia."

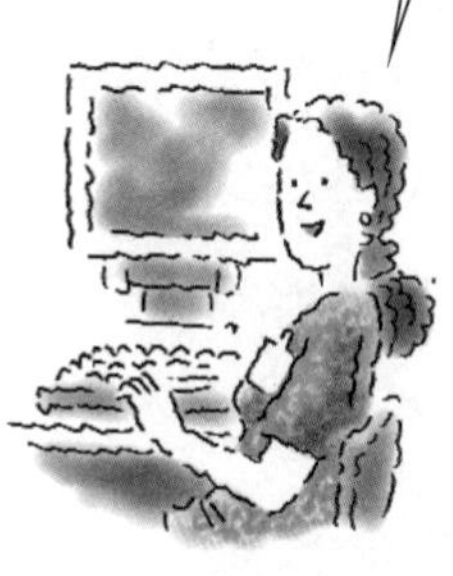
Think therapeutic
here.

11. 3. The most therapeutic answer is to give correct information. Asking what the voices tell the client would be changing the topic without answering the question. Asking "why" questions can put the client on the defensive. Schizophrenia isn't the only cause of hearing voices, and this response suggests the client may be schizophrenic.
CN: Psychosocial integrity; CNS: None; CL: Analysis

12. A nurse is preparing to admit a client with dissociative identity disorder (DID) to the inpatient psychiatric unit. Which intervention is most appropriate for this client?
1. Arrange to have staff check on the client every 15 to 30 minutes.
2. Prevent all family from visiting until the third day of hospitalization.
3. Make sure the staff understands the client will be on seizure precautions.
4. Place the client in a quiet room away from the noise of the nurse's station.

12. 1. A common reason for clients with DID to be hospitalized is for suicidal ideations or gestures. For the client's safety, frequent checks should be done. Family interactions might be therapeutic for the client, and the family may be able to provide a more thorough history because of the client's dissociation from traumatic events. Seizure activity isn't an expected symptom of DID. Because of the possibility of suicide, the client's room should be close to the nurse's station.
CN: Psychosocial integrity; CNS: None; CL: Application

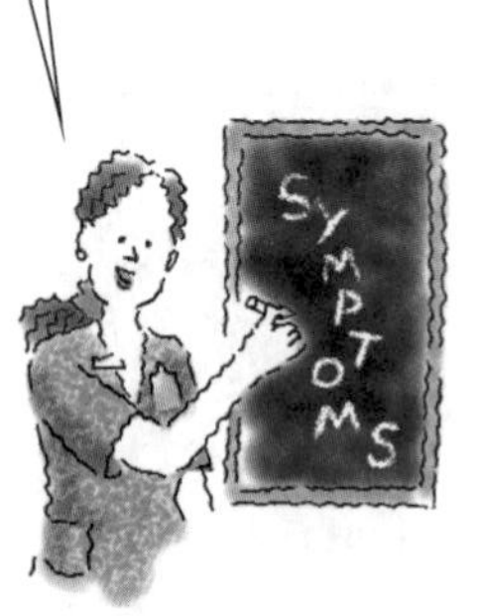

It helps to know what symptoms to watch for.
SYMPTOMS

13. A client is being treated at a community mental health clinic. A nurse has been instructed to observe for any behaviors indicating dissociative identity disorder (DID). Which behavior would be included?
1. Delusions of grandeur
2. Reports of often being very tired
3. Changes in dress, mannerisms, and voice
4. Refusal to make a follow-up appointment

13. 3. When alter personalities are in control, the person will have complete personality changes. Delusions of grandeur are more frequently associated with disorders such as manic states and schizophrenia. Complaints of fatigue aren't a main symptom of DID. The refusal to make a follow-up appointment could indicate many problems, including noncompliance.
CN: Psychosocial integrity; CNS: None; CL: Application

14. Which statement made by a client with dissociative identity disorder (DID) indicates an understanding of the nurse's teaching plan?
1. "I will never marry."
2. "I won't get better, even with treatment."
3. "I need to take my pills for anxiety."
4. "I need to attend my therapy sessions faithfully."

14. 4. Most clients with DID can be successfully treated with long-term therapy. For many of the conditions, pharmacologic therapy has little effect. Many clients with DID marry.
CN: Psychosocial integrity; CNS: None; CL: Application

15. When interacting with a client with a dissociative identity disorder, a nurse observes that one of the alter personalities is in control. Which intervention is the most appropriate?
1. Give recognition to the alter personality.
2. Notify the physician.
3. Immediately stop interacting with the client.
4. Ignore the alter personality, and ask to speak to the host personality.

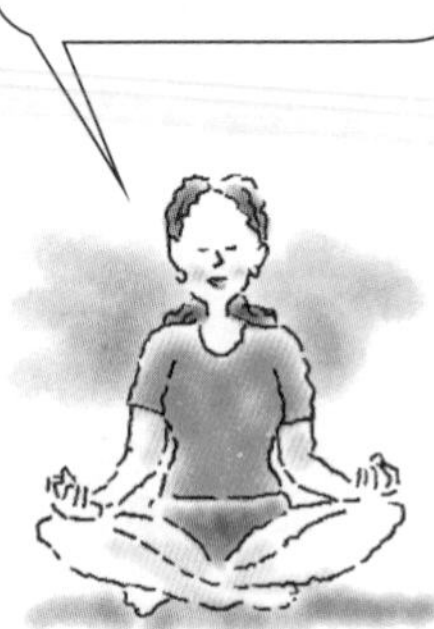

15. 1. By giving recognition to the alter personalities, the nurse conveys to the client that she believes the alter personalities exist. The physician doesn't need to be notified because this is an expected occurrence. Asking to speak to the host personality or immediately stopping interaction with the client won't stop the client from being controlled by alter personalities.
CN: Psychosocial integrity; CNS: None; CL: Application

CN: Client needs category CNS: Client needs subcategory CL: Cognitive level

16. A client with dissociative identity disorder (DID) indicates that he understands the need to continue therapy when he makes which statement?

1. "Therapy will help eliminate my family problems."
2. "I must continue going to outpatient treatment for the next 2 months."
3. "I understand that I need to integrate all my alter personalities into one."
4. "Once therapy is complete, I won't have the traits of my alter personalities."

16. 3. The main goal of therapy for clients with DID is to integrate, not eliminate, the alter personalities. Therapy is often long-term. Through therapy, the client can learn how to cope with family problems.
CN: Psychosocial integrity; CNS: None; CL: Application

17. A family member of a client with dissociative identity disorder (DID) asks a nurse if hypnotic therapy might help the client. Which response would be most appropriate?

1. "What would make you think that?"
2. "No, hypnosis is rarely used in the treatment of psychiatric conditions."
3. "Yes, but this treatment is used only after other types of therapy have failed."
4. "Yes, often the client doesn't have conscious awareness of alter personalities."

17. 4. Because of dissociation from painful events, hypnosis is often very effective in the treatment of clients with DID. It may be under hypnosis that alter personalities start to emerge. Hypnosis is used in a variety of psychiatric conditions. The first option could place the family member on the defensive. Hypnosis is often a first-line treatment for the client with DID.
CN: Psychosocial integrity; CNS: None; CL: Application

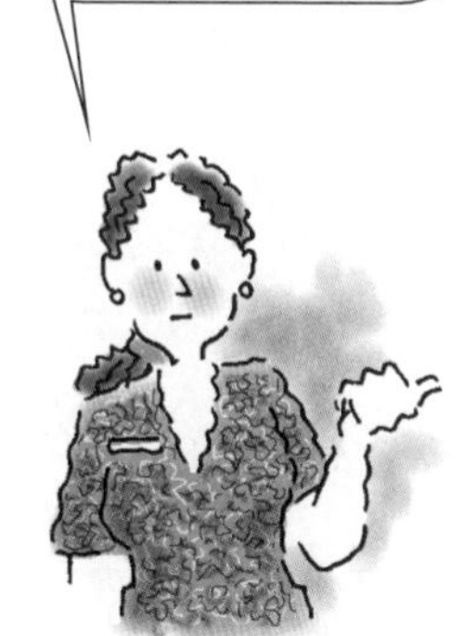

It's important to understand how the other person feels.

18. Which intervention is appropriate when caring for a client with dissociative identity disorder?

1. Remind the alter personalities they're part of the host personality.
2. Interact with the client only when the host personality is in control.
3. Establish an empathetic relationship with each emerging personality.
4. Provide positive reinforcement to the client when calm alter personalities are present instead of angry ones.

18. 3. Establishing an empathetic relationship with each emerging personality provides a therapeutic environment to care for the client. Interacting with the client only when the host personality is in control would be useless because the client has limited, if any, control or awareness when alter personalities are in control.
CN: Psychosocial integrity; CNS: None; CL: Application

19. While interacting with a client with dissociative identity disorder (DID), a nurse observes one of the alter personalities take over. The client goes from being very calm to angry and shouting. Which response would be most appropriate?

1. "Is one of you upset?"
2. "Why have you become angry?"
3. "Tell me what you're feeling right now."
4. "Let me speak to someone who isn't angry."

19. 3. This response encourages integration and discourages dissociation. When interacting with clients with DID, the nurse always wants to remind the client that the alter personalities are a component of one person. Responses reinforcing interaction with only one alter personality instead of trying to interact with the individual as a single person aren't appropriate. Asking "why" questions can put the client on the defensive and impede further communication.
CN: Psychosocial integrity; CNS: None; CL: Application

20. A client with dissociative identity disorder has been in therapy for 2 years and just learned her father passed away. Her father sexually abused her throughout her childhood. Which intervention would be most appropriate?

1. Have the client seek inpatient therapy.
2. Encourage the client's verbalization of feelings of anger and guilt.
3. Encourage the client's alter personalities to emerge during this stressful time.
4. Stress to the client that the death of the abuser should be very helpful in her healing process.

20. 2. The death of the abuser may cause the client to experience feelings of anger and guilt. Unless the client becomes suicidal or rapidly deteriorates, inpatient treatment won't be necessary. Encouraging the client's alter personalities to emerge could result in further dissociation. The death of the abuser can be a very stressful event and can leave the client with unresolved feelings.

CN: Health promotion and maintenance; CNS: None; CL: Analysis

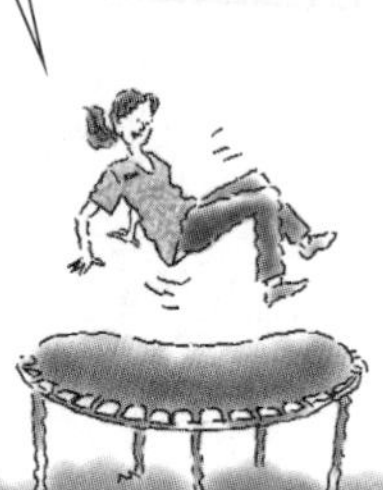

Keep it up, you're doing great!

21. Which activity is most appropriate for a client with dissociative identity disorder (DID)?

1. Group therapy with only clients who have DID
2. Inpatient therapy groups led by a psychologist
3. Support group with adult survivors of child abuse
4. Group therapy with clients who have a variety of diagnoses

21. 1. Homogenous group therapy has proven to be the most beneficial for clients with DID. In other groups, the members may find interacting on such an intimate level with a client with DID overwhelming and frightening. Not all victims of child abuse develop DID. Unless the client with DID is suicidal, hospitalization isn't required.

CN: Psychosocial integrity; CNS: None; CL: Application

22. A nurse observes that the alter personality of a client with a dissociative identity disorder is in control. The client is sitting in the dayroom, interacting with others. His voice becomes louder and more intense and he's tearful and confused. Which action would be most appropriate?

1. Allow the client to continue interacting with clients in the dayroom.
2. Ask to speak to one of the adult alter personalities of the host personality.
3. Remove the client from the dayroom, and allow the client to play with toys.
4. Remove the client from the dayroom, and reorient him that he's in a safe place.

22. 4. Removing the client at this time may protect him from future embarrassment. Asking to speak to an alter personality encourages dissociation. Allowing the client to play with toys also reinforces and encourages dissociation. Reorienting the client discourages dissociation and encourages integration.

CN: Safe, effective care environment; CNS: Safety and infection control; CL: Analysis

23. A nurse on the psychiatric unit is caring for a 51-year-old male client who's suicidal. Which nursing intervention takes priority?

1. Discouraging sleep except at bedtime
2. Making a verbal contract with the client to notify the staff of suicidal thoughts
3. Limiting time spent alone by encouraging the client to participate in group activities
4. Creating a safe physical and interpersonal environment

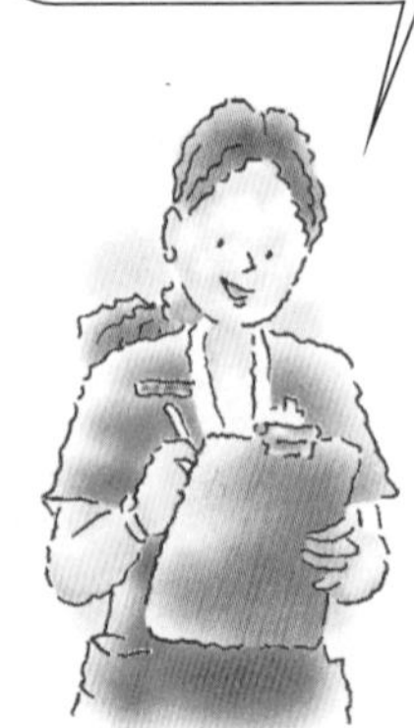

Take note: the question is asking which intervention has the priority.

23. 4. Creating a safe environment, including removing obvious hazards, recognizing non-obvious hazards, maintaining close observation, serving as a client advocate in interpersonal situations, and communicating concern to the client in verbal and non-verbal ways, is the nurse's highest priority. Other interventions, such as discouraging sleep except at bedtime, making a verbal contract, and encouraging participation in group activities, should be included in the client's plan, but these don't have top priority.

CN: Psychosocial integrity; CNS: None; CL: Application

CN: Client needs category CNS: Client needs subcategory CL: Cognitive level

24. A 14-year-old client is admitted to an inpatient adolescent unit. The treatment team believes he has dissociative identity disorder (DID). Based on this information, which intervention should the nurse anticipate using?

1. Request a social work consultation.
2. Institute elopement precautions.
3. Confront the parents about the staff's suspicion of child abuse.
4. Prevent the client from interacting with other clients on the unit.

24. 1. In many cases, clients with DID have been subjected to child abuse. The social worker is the appropriate person to investigate the child's home setting. The client isn't at any more risk for elopement than the other adolescent clients. Until there has been an investigation into the client's home setting, confrontation wouldn't be appropriate or therapeutic. Clients with DID are always encouraged to interact with other clients on the unit.

CN: Safe, effective care environment; CNS: Management of care; CL: Application

25. Which behavior reported by a family member of a client with dissociative identity disorder (DID) indicates that the client's therapy is effective?

1. The client is forgetful.
2. The client sleeps through the night.
3. The client has had several unsuccessful relationships.
4. The client hears voices.

25. 2. Because clients with DID often have sleep disorders, sleeping through the night is a sign of effective therapy. Forgetfulness, difficulty forming relationships, and hallucinations are signs of unsuccessful treatment.

CN: Psychosocial integrity; CNS: None; CL: Analysis

26. A client with dissociative identity disorder (DID) is admitted to an inpatient psychiatric unit. A nurse-manager asked all staff to attend a meeting. Which reason for the meeting is the <u>most likely</u>?

1. To review the restraint protocol with the staff
2. To inform the staff that no one should refuse to work with the client
3. To warn the staff that this client may be difficult and challenging to work with
4. To allow staff members to discuss concerns about working with a client with DID

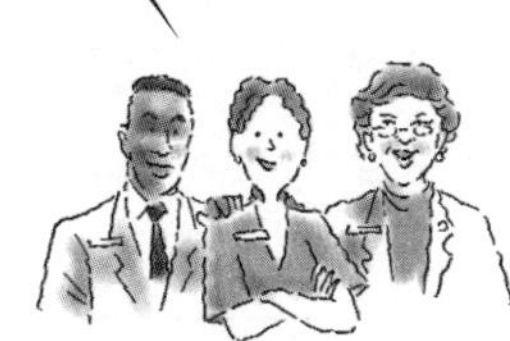

Know when to request a consultation from other medical professionals.

26. 4. Allowing all staff members to meet together may prevent the staff from splitting into groups of those who believe the validity of this diagnosis and those who don't. Unless this client shows behaviors harmful to himself or others, restraints aren't needed. Telling the staff no one should refuse to work with the client or this client will probably be very difficult and challenging sets a very negative tone as staff plan and provide care for the client.

CN: Safe, effective care environment; CNS: Management of care; CL: Application

27. A 26-year-old man is reported missing after being the victim of a violent crime. Two months later, a family member finds him working in a city 100 miles from his home. The man doesn't recognize the family member or recall being the victim of a crime. Which condition is the client <u>most likely</u> exhibiting?

1. Depersonalization disorder
2. Dissociative amnesia
3. Dissociative fugue
4. Dissociative identity disorder

27. 3. Dissociative fugue is sudden flight after a traumatic event. During the episode, the person may assume a new identity and not recognize people from his past. Depersonalization disorder is the sudden loss of the sense of one's own reality. Dissociative amnesia doesn't involve flight from work or home. Dissociative identity disorder is the coexistence of two or more personalities in one person.

CN: Psychosocial integrity; CNS: None; CL: Application

28. Which nursing intervention is most appropriate for a client who has just had an episode of dissociative fugue?

1. Let the client verbalize the fear and anxiety he feels.
2. Encourage the client to share his experiences during the episode.
3. Have the client sign a contract stating he won't leave the premises again.
4. Tell the client he won't resolve his problems by running away from them.

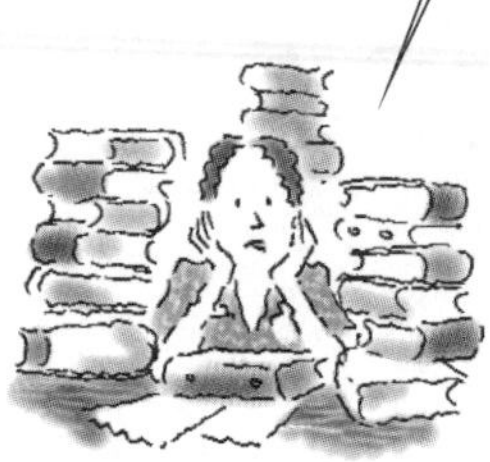

I'm feeling slightly overwhelmed—but it helps to tell someone.

28. 1. An episode of dissociative fugue can be a very frightening experience. The client rarely remembers the events during the episode. Signing a contract would have little effect because a dissociative fugue episode isn't something the client consciously wanted to do. Because the client isn't conscious of "running away," this response isn't helpful.
CN: Psychosocial integrity; CNS: None; CL: Analysis

29. Which statement about dissociative disorders by a family member of a client with a dissociative disorder indicates that the nurse's teaching has been successful?

1. "They occur as a result of incest."
2. "They occur as a result of substance abuse."
3. "They occur in more than 40% of all people."
4. "They occur as a result of the brain trying to protect the person from severe stress."

29. 4. Dissociative disorders are thought to be a form of coping with an extreme stressor or event that occurred in the client's life. Incest is only one of many reasons dissociative disorders occur. Typically, substance abuse isn't a cause (but may be an effect) of a dissociative disorder. Dissociative disorders are actually very rare.
CN: Psychosocial integrity; CNS: None; CL: Analysis

30. Which nursing intervention would be most appropriate when working with a client who had a recent episode of dissociative fugue?

1. Place the client on elopement precautions.
2. Help the client identify resources to deal with stressful situations.
3. Allow the client to share his experiences about the dissociative fugue episode.
4. Confront the client about his running away from problems instead of dealing with them.

30. 2. Dissociative fugue is precipitated by stressful situations. Helping the client identify resources could prevent recurrences. Once the dissociative fugue episode is over, the client returns to normal functioning; he wouldn't be an elopement risk. The client usually has amnesia about the events during the dissociative fugue episode, which limits his ability to share the experience. The client doesn't realize that he's running away from his problems.
CN: Psychosocial integrity; CNS: None; CL: Analysis

31. A 32-year-old client lost his home in a flood last month. When questioned about his feelings about the loss, he doesn't remember being in a flood or owning a home. Which of the following disorders is the client *most* likely exhibiting?

1. Depersonalization disorder
2. Dissociative amnesia
3. Dissociative fugue
4. Dissociative identity disorder

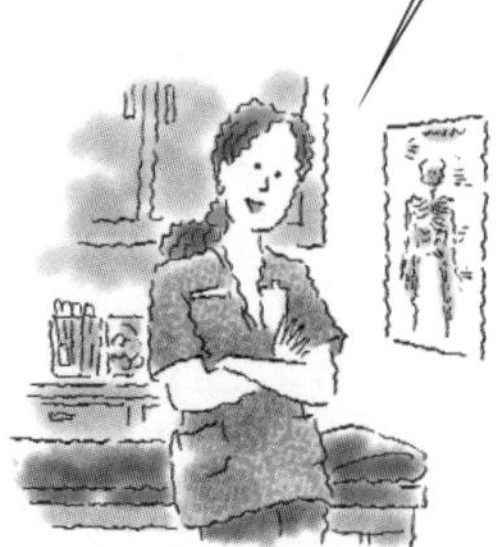

Helping the client help himself is an important aspect of teaching.

31. 2. Dissociative amnesia commonly occurs after a person has been in a traumatic event. Depersonalization disorder is characterized by recurrent sensations of loss of one's own reality. Dissociative fugue is the sudden departure from one's home or work. Dissociative identity disorder is the coexistence of two or more personalities within the same individual.
CN: Psychosocial integrity; CNS: None; CL: Analysis

32. The nurse is assessing a client with dissociative amnesia. Which of the following circumstances would most likely result in this condition?

1. Binge drinking
2. A hostage situation
3. A closed-head injury
4. A fight with a family member

32. 2. Dissociative amnesia typically occurs after the person has experienced a very stressful, traumatic situation. Binge drinking doesn't cause dissociative amnesia. A closed-head injury could result in physiologic but not dissociative amnesia. Having a fight with a family member typically wouldn't be stressful enough to cause dissociative amnesia.

CN: Psychosocial integrity; CNS: None; CL: Application

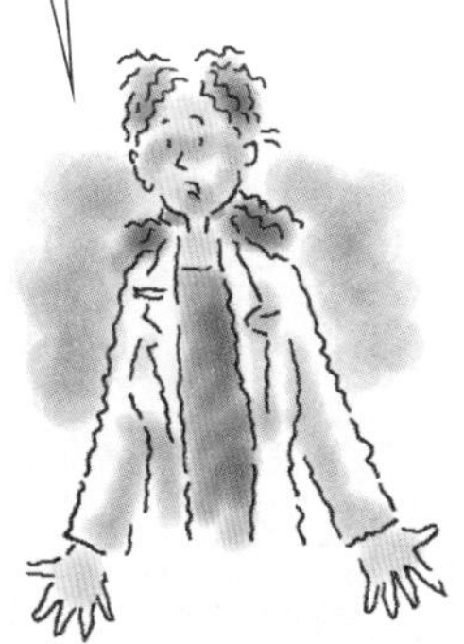

I feel like I'm a mess from all this stress!

33. A client was the driver in an automobile accident in which a 3-year-old boy was killed. The client now has dissociative amnesia. He verbalizes understanding of his treatment plan when he makes which statement?

1. "I won't drive a car again for at least a year."
2. "I'll take my Ativan anytime I feel upset about this situation."
3. "I'll visit the child's grave as soon as I'm released from the hospital."
4. "I'll attend my hypnotic therapy sessions prescribed by my psychiatrist."

33. 4. Hypnosis can be beneficial to this client because it allows repressed feelings and memories to surface. The client may be ready to drive again, and circumstances may dictate that he drives again before a year has passed. The client needs to learn other coping mechanisms besides taking a highly addictive drug such as lorazepam (Ativan). Visiting the child's grave on release from the hospital may be too traumatic and encourage continuation of the amnesia.

CN: Psychosocial integrity; CNS: None; CL: Application

34. A client with dissociative amnesia shows understanding of her condition when she makes which statement?

1. "I'll probably never be able to regain my memories of the fire."
2. "I have problems with my memory due to my abuse of tranquilizers."
3. "If I concentrate hard enough, I'll be able to bring up memories of the car accident."
4. "To protect my mental well-being, my brain has temporarily hidden my memories of the rape from me."

34. 4. One of the cardinal features of dissociative amnesia is that the person has loss of memory of a traumatic event. With therapy and time, the person will probably be able to recall the traumatic event. This type of amnesia isn't related to substance abuse. With this disorder, the loss of memory is a protective function performed by the brain and isn't within the person's conscious control.

CN: Psychosocial integrity; CNS: None; CL: Analysis

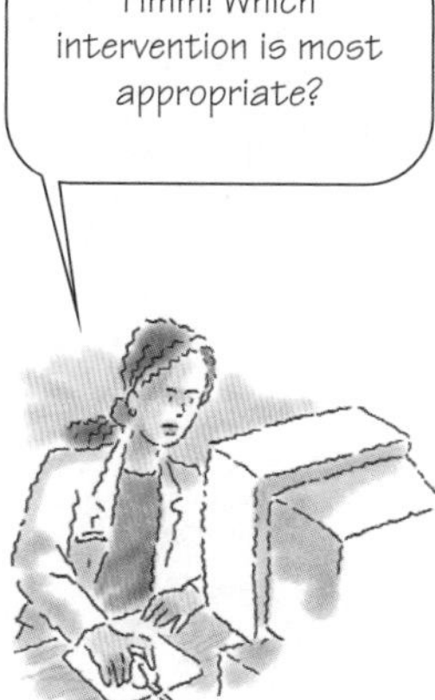

35. Which intervention is most appropriate in the treatment of a client admitted for a diagnostic workup for possible dissociative amnesia?

1. Restrain the client if he attempts to wander off the unit.
2. Question the client every hour about orientation to time, place, and person.
3. Provide teaching on computed tomography scans and other imaging tests.
4. Encourage the client not to dwell on the traumatic event that lead to his memory loss.

35. 3. Clients with a type of memory problem commonly have a diagnostic workup to rule out any physical cause. Clients with dissociative amnesia typically don't have a problem with wandering. Frequent attempts to assess the client's orientation level could easily make the client more distressed and agitated. In many cases, the client doesn't have memories of the traumatic events before amnesia.

CN: Health promotion and maintenance; CNS: None; CL: Application

36. A client with dissociative amnesia indicates understanding about the use of amobarbital (Amytal) in his treatment when he makes which statement?

1. "This medication helps me sleep."
2. "This medication helps me control my anxiety."
3. "I must take this drug once a day after discharge if the drug is to be therapeutically beneficial."
4. "I'm given this medication during therapy sessions to increase my ability to remember forgotten events."

36. 4. This drug is given to the client with dissociative amnesia to help her remember forgotten events. It isn't prescribed as a sleep aid or antianxiety agent. Because the drug is given during therapy to recall forgotten events, there would be no therapeutic benefit to taking this drug at home.

CN: Physiological integrity; CNS: Pharmacological and parenteral therapies; CL: Analysis

37. A client with dissociative amnesia says, "You must think I'm really stupid because I have no recollection of the accident." Which response would be most appropriate?

1. "Why would I think you're stupid?"
2. "Have I acted like I think you're stupid?"
3. "What kind of grades did you get in school?"
4. "As a protective measure, the brain sometimes doesn't let us remember traumatic events."

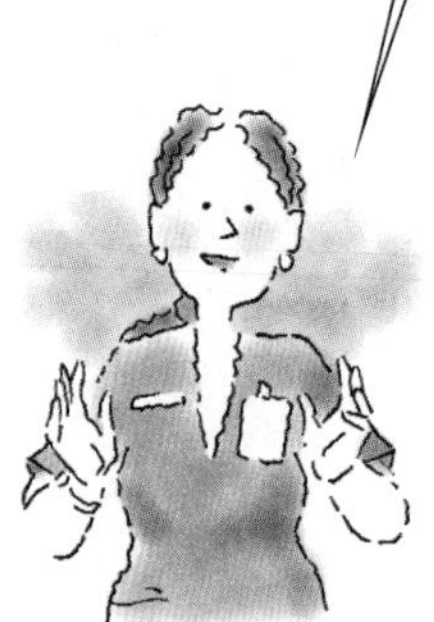
Sometimes a simple explanation is the best one.

37. 4. This provides a simple explanation for the client. The use of "why" can put someone on the defensive. The second option takes the focus off the client. The third option changes the topic.

CN: Psychosocial integrity; CNS: None; CL: Application

38. Which nursing intervention is important in caring for the client with a dissociative disorder?

1. Encourage the client to participate in unit activities and meetings.
2. Question the client about the events triggering the dissociative disorder.
3. Allow the client to remain in his room anytime he's experiencing feelings of dissociation.
4. Encourage the client to form friendships with other clients in his therapy groups to decrease his feelings of isolation.

38. 1. Attending unit activities and meetings helps decrease the client's sense of isolation. Often, the client can't recall the events that triggered the dissociative disorder, so questioning him would not be helpful. The client would need to be isolated from others only if he's unable to interact appropriately. A client with a dissociative disorder has typically had few healthy relationships. Forming friendships with others in therapy could be setting the client up to continue in unhealthy relationships.

CN: Safe, effective care environment; CNS: Management of care; CL: Application

39. The nurse is performing an assessment on a client with depersonalization disorder. Which of the following characteristics would the nurse most likely assess with this client?

1. Disorientation to time, place, and person
2. Sensation of detachment from body or mind
3. Unexpected and sudden travel to another location
4. A feeling that one's environment will never change

39. 2. In depersonalization disorder, the person feels detached from his body and mental processes. The person is usually oriented to time, place, and person. Unexpected and sudden travel to another location is one of the characteristics of dissociative fugue. Clients with depersonalization disorder often feel the outside world has changed.
CN: Psychosocial integrity; CNS: None; CL: Application

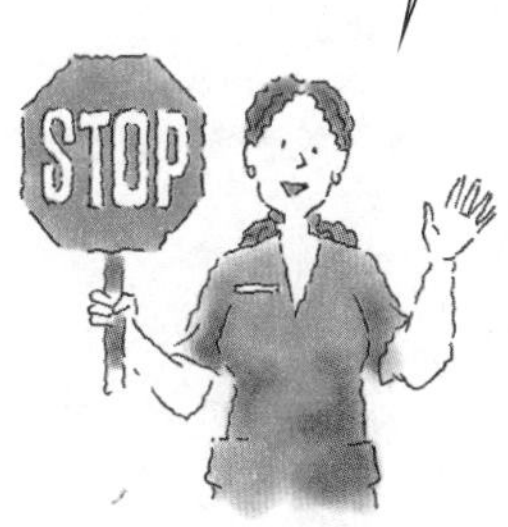

How can you tell when your client understands your instructions?
STOP

40. A client with depersonalization disorder verbalizes understanding of the ways to decrease his symptoms when he makes which statement?

1. "I'll avoid any stressful situation."
2. "Meditation will help control my symptoms."
3. "I'll need to practice relaxation exercises regularly."
4. "I may need to remain on antipsychotic medication for the rest of my life."

40. 3. Relaxation can lead to a decrease in maladaptive responses. Although stress can be a predisposing factor in depersonalization disorder, it's impossible to avoid all stressful situations. Meditation is the voluntary induction of the sensation of depersonalization. This isn't a psychotic disorder, so antipsychotic medication wouldn't be therapeutic or beneficial.
CN: Psychosocial integrity; CNS: None; CL: Analysis

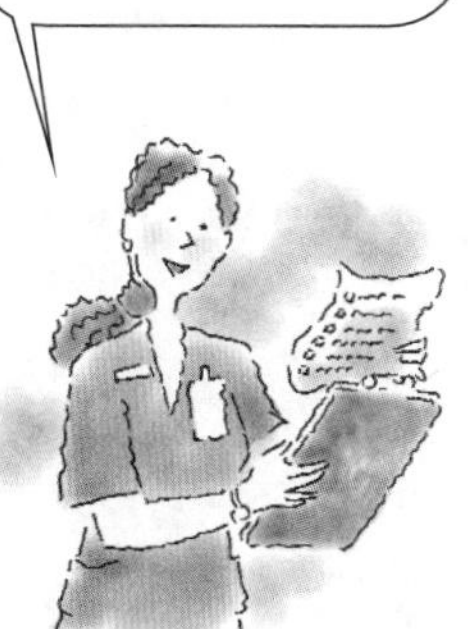

Making the right nursing diagnosis is critical for effective nursing care.

41. A client with depersonalization disorder spends much of his day in a dreamlike state during which he ignores personal care needs. Which nursing diagnosis is most appropriate for this client?

1. *Disturbed personal identity related to organic brain damage*
2. *Impaired memory related to frequently being in a dreamlike state*
3. *Dressing self-care deficit related to perceptual impairment*
4. *Deficient knowledge related to performance or personal care needs due to lack of information*

41. 3. Because of time spent in a dreamlike state, many clients with depersonalization disorder ignore self-care needs. There's no known organic brain damage with this disorder. Memory impairment is more of a problem with other dissociative disorders, such as dissociative identity disorder and dissociative amnesia. The dreamlike state can lead to problems meeting personal care needs, not a knowledge deficit.
CN: Safe, effective care environment; CNS: Safety and infection control; CL: Application

42. A client reports frequently feeling that he's floating above his body. During these times, he says he's aware of who he is and where he's located. Which of the following disorders is the client exhibiting?

1. Depersonalization disorder
2. Dissociative amnesia
3. Dissociative identity disorder
4. Dissociative fugue

42. 1. One of the cardinal symptoms of depersonalization disorder is feeling detached from one's body or mental processes. During the feelings of detachment, the person doesn't become disoriented. Dissociative amnesia is defined as one or more episodes of being unable to recall important information. Dissociative identity disorder is the existence of two or more personalities that take control of the person's behavior. In a dissociative fugue, the person has no memory of his life before the flight.
CN: Psychosocial integrity; CNS: None; CL: Analysis

43. The nurse is teaching the family of a client with depersonalization disorder. The family wants to know which setting has the most success in treating this disorder. Which of the following responses would be the most accurate?

1. Inpatient psychiatric hospital
2. Community mental health clinic
3. Family practice physician's office
4. Support group for clients with depersonalization disorder

43. 2. Most clients with depersonalization disorder can be treated successfully on an outpatient basis. These clients only need to be hospitalized if they become suicidal or have severe depression or anxiety. Because no organic basis for the disorder usually exists, these clients aren't treated in a family practice physician's office. Because the disorder is rare, few support groups are composed only of clients with this disorder.

CN: Psychosocial integrity; CNS: None; CL: Application

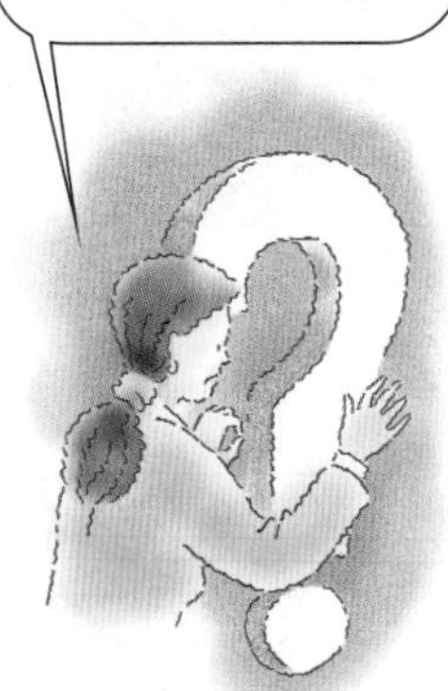

Which kinds of questions tend to encourage discussion?

44. A client with depersonalization disorder tells the nurse, "I feel like such a freak when I have an out-of-body experience." Which response would be most appropriate?

1. "How often do you have these feelings?"
2. "I don't understand what you mean by a freak."
3. "Tell me more about these out-of-body experiences."
4. "How does your husband feel about you having these experiences?"

44. 3. This open-ended response allows the client to focus and expand on this topic. Asking how often the experiences occur is a closed-ended question that doesn't encourage discussion of the experience. The second option could cause the client to focus too narrowly on only one aspect of the topic. Asking how the client's husband feels makes it appear that the nurse wants to change the topic.

CN: Psychosocial integrity; CNS: None; CL: Analysis

45. During an assessment on a client with dissociative disorder, which of the following characteristics would the nurse most likely assess?

1. A group of disorders with the common symptom of hallucinations
2. A group of disorders with a rapid disruption of the client's memory
3. A group of disorders with impairment of memory or identity due to the development of organic changes in the brain
4. A group of disorders with impairment of memory or identity due to an unconscious attempt to protect the person from emotional pain or traumatic experiences

45. 4. A group of disorders in which there's impairment of memory or identity due to an unconscious attempt to protect the client from emotional pain or traumatic experiences describes dissociative disorders. Hallucinations are associated with schizophrenic disorders. The onset of dissociative disorders may be gradual, sudden, or chronic. There's no known organic cause for dissociative disorders.

CN: Psychosocial integrity; CNS: None; CL: Application

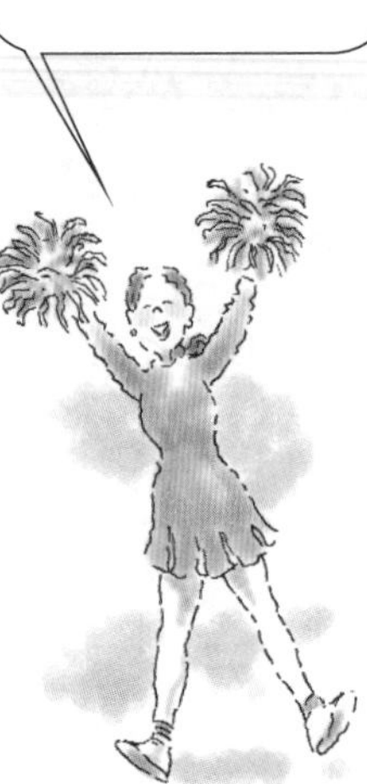

46. A client with depersonalization disorder tells the nurse, "I feel like my arm isn't attached to my body." Which response would be most appropriate?

1. "Do you know where you are?"
2. "What makes you feel that way?"
3. "Don't worry because I can see your arm is attached to your body."
4. "This disorder causes people to feel that body parts may be unattached to the rest of the body."

46. 4. Reinforcing that what the client feels is an expected result of the disease process would be most appropriate. Asking if the client knows where he is changes the topic. Asking why he feels that way could put the client on the defensive. Stating that his arm is attached to his body belittles the client's feelings.

CN: Psychosocial integrity; CNS: None; CL: Application

47. A client with a dissociative disorder suddenly wanders away from the facility. When the nurse finds him, he can't recall what happened. The nurse identifies this behavior as which dissociative disorder?

1. Repression
2. Depersonalization
3. Derealization
4. Dissociative fugue

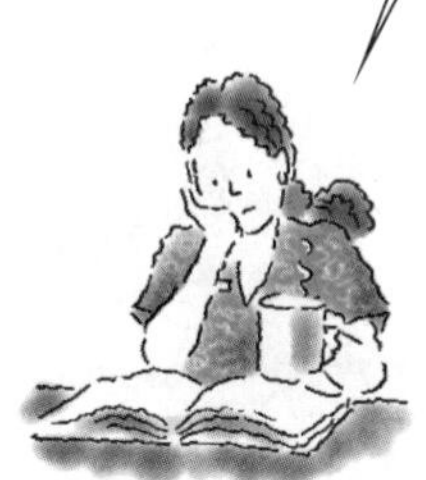
My mind keeps
wandering to
another place.

47. 4. Dissociative fugue is characterized by suddenly wandering away from one's usual place, accompanied by amnesia for all or part of the past. Repression is a defense mechanism in which thoughts and feelings are kept from consciousness. Depersonalization is a feeling of detachment or separation from one's self. Derealization is a feeling that the external world is unreal.
CN: Psychosocial integrity; CNS: None; CL: Application

48. A nurse conducts an admission assessment on a client diagnosed with dissociative identity disorder. Which sign or symptom supports this diagnosis?

1. A sense of being in a dream
2. Inability to remember a particular event
3. Having two or more personalities
4. Ritualistic behavior

48. 3. Dissociative identity disorder is characterized by having two or more distinct personalities, often in conflict with one another. A sense of being in a dream is common in depersonalization disorders. Selective amnesia refers to an inability to recall certain events that occurred during a specified period and is more common in traumatic stress disorders. Ritualistic behavior is seen in obsessive-compulsive disorders.
CN: Psychosocial integrity; CNS: None; CL: Application

49. Which set of circumstances indicates the highest risk of suicide?

1. Suicide plan, handy means of carrying out plan, and history of previous attempt
2. Preoccupation with morbid thoughts and limited support system
3. Suicidal ideation, active suicide planning, and family history of suicide
4. Threats of suicide, recent job loss, and intact support system

49. 1. A lethal plan with a handy means of carrying it out poses the highest risk and requires immediate intervention. Although all of the remaining risk factors can lead to suicide, they aren't considered as high a risk as a formulated, lethal plan and the means at hand. However, a client exhibiting any of these risk factors should be taken seriously and considered at risk for suicide.
CN: Psychosocial integrity; CNS: None; CL: Application

50. A nurse finds a suicidal client trying to hang himself in his room. To preserve the client's self-esteem and safety, what should the nurse do?

1. Place the client in seclusion with checks every 15 minutes.
2. Assign a nursing staff member to remain with the client at all times.
3. Make the client stay with the group at all times.
4. Refuse to let the client in his room.

50. 2. Implementing a one-on-one staff-to-client ratio is the nurse's highest priority. Doing so allows the client to maintain his self-esteem and keeps him safe. Seclusion would damage the client's self-esteem. Forcing the client to stay with the group and refusing to let him in his room don't guarantee his safety.
CN: Psychosocial integrity; CNS: None; CL: Application

51. A client with a dissociative identity disorder experiences amnesia. Which nursing diagnosis is <u>most</u> appropriate?
1. *Powerlessness*
2. *Ineffective coping*
3. *Disturbed sensory perception, visual*
4. *Risk for self-directed violence*

51. 2. Amnesia may result from an inability to cope with anxiety. *Powerlessness, Disturbed sensory perception*, and *Risk for self-directed violence* aren't appropriate in this situation.
CN: Psychosocial integrity; CNS: None; CL: Analysis

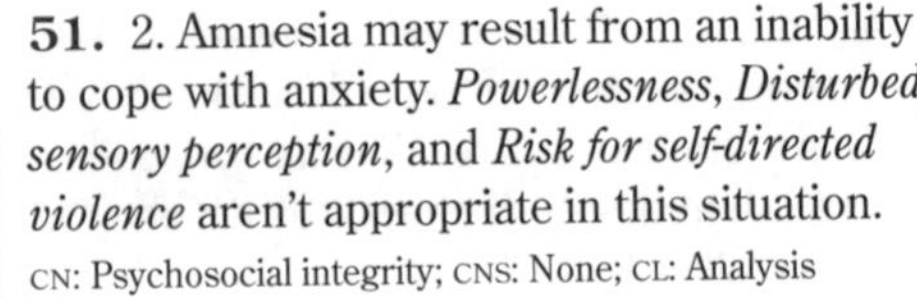

I know my highest priority at the moment.

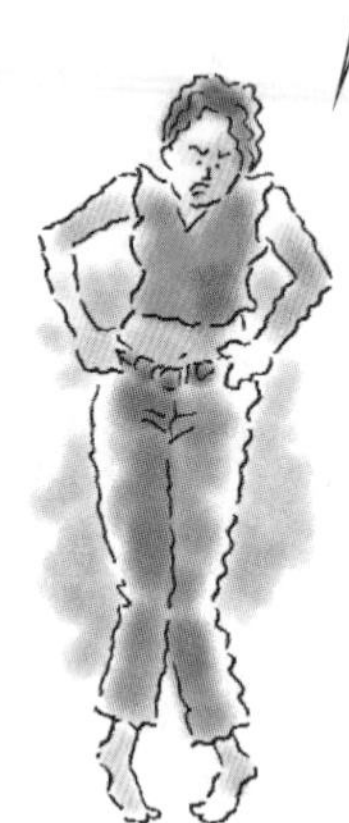

52. After taking a potentially lethal drug overdose, a client tells the nurse that his alter "did it." Which nursing diagnosis takes <u>highest priority</u>?
1. *Posttrauma syndrome*
2. *Anxiety*
3. *Risk for self-directed violence*
4. *Disturbed personal identity*

52. 3. Taking a potentially lethal drug overdose indicates that the client poses a danger to himself. Because the alter may act again, the risk for self-directed violence persists. The other nursing diagnoses either aren't relevant or take lower priority.
CN: Psychosocial integrity; CNS: None; CL: Analysis

53. A severely depressed client who has made multiple suicide attempts matter-of-factly tells the nurse that her family life was normal and uneventful. Which behaviors would lead the nurse to suspect a diagnosis of a dissociative identity disorder (DID) in this client? Select all that apply:
1. Inability to recall important personal information too severe to be explained by ordinary forgetfulness
2. Absence of any physiological effects of a substance, such as alcohol or drugs
3. Ability to selectively and consciously choose to avoid certain painful topics
4. A sense of grandiosity, that she's special and has a particular mission for mankind
5. Posttraumatic symptoms, such as flashbacks, nightmares, and an exaggerated startle response

53. 1, 2, 5. A dissociative disorder is a persistent state of being disconnected from the totality of one's personhood, particularly painful emotions. With dissociative disorder, the inability to recall personal information is far more extensive than ordinary forgetfulness; the symptoms occur apart from any chemical inducement, and the individual doesn't have the ability to consciously make a decision to separate from painful emotions or topics. A sense of grandiosity isn't characteristic of this disorder. Posttraumatic symptoms, such as flashbacks, nightmares, and an exaggerated startle response, are also signs and symptoms of DID.
CN: Psychosocial integrity; CNS: None; CL: Analysis

54. A client with dissociative identity disorder experiences frequent periods of memory loss. Which nursing intervention can help the client deal with the memory loss?
1. Orienting the client to time, place, person, and situation
2. Explaining to the client the circumstances surrounding the memory loss
3. Assessing for cues that the client is ready to discuss the memory loss
4. Telling the client not to worry because the memory loss has no physiologic base

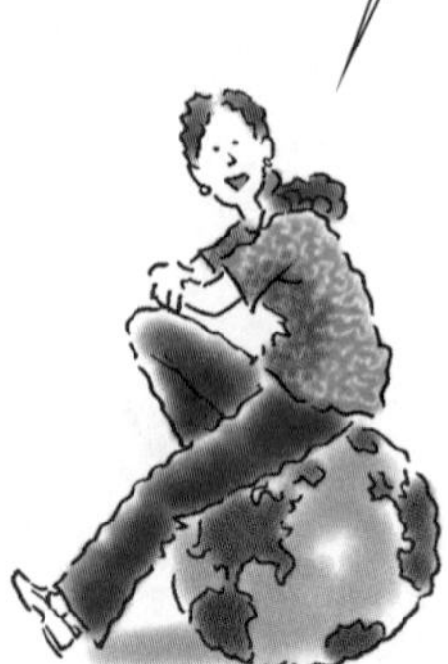

Congratulations! You should feel on top of the world!

54. 3. Memory loss serves as a protective mechanism for many clients with dissociative identity disorder; the nurse should wait until the client is ready to discuss the problem, as shown by certain cues. Orienting the client may force the client out of the protective mechanism of the memory loss (which the client may not be ready for and can result in further harm). Explaining the circumstances surrounding the memory loss and telling the client not to worry aren't therapeutic interventions.
CN: Psychosocial integrity; CNS: None; CL: Application

CN: Client needs category CNS: Client needs subcategory CL: Cognitive level

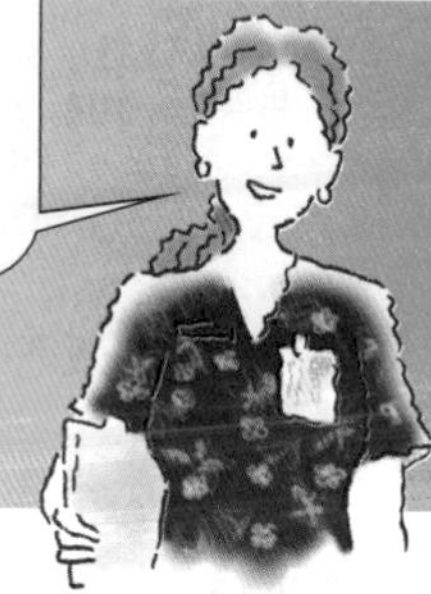

This chapter will test your knowledge of disorders of a highly sensitive nature. Remain professional at all times, and you'll do great. Good luck!

Chapter 20 Sexual & gender identity disorders

1. A client has undergone surgery for the repair of an abdominal aortic aneurysm. Which response is most appropriate to the client's wife when she asks if her husband will be impotent?

1. "Don't worry, he'll be all right."
2. "He has other problems to worry about."
3. "We'll cross that bridge when we come to it."
4. "There is a chance of impotence after repair of an abdominal aortic aneurysm."

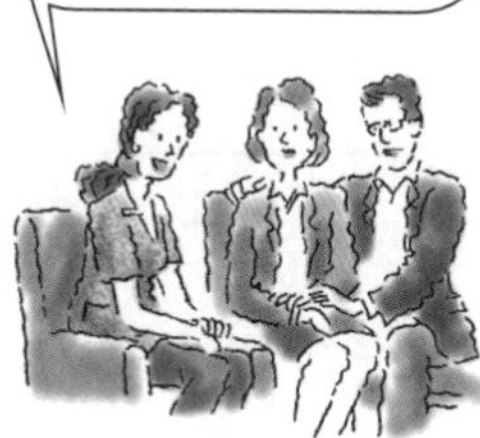

Therapeutic communication involves demonstrating sensitivity to your client's and his family's concerns.

1. 4. Impotence and retrograde ejaculation are sexual dysfunctions commonly experienced by male clients after abdominal aortic aneurysm. Telling a family member that the client will be all right is offering false assurance. Stating that he has other problems isn't therapeutic and doesn't address the wife's concern. Telling the client's wife to "cross that bridge when we come to it" ignores her concerns and isn't therapeutic.

CN: Psychosocial integrity; CNS: None; CL: Application

2. Which discharge instruction would be most accurate to provide to a female client who has suffered a spinal cord injury at the C4 level?

1. After a spinal cord injury, women usually remain fertile; therefore, you may consider contraception if you don't want to become pregnant.
2. After a spinal cord injury, women usually are unable to conceive a child.
3. Sexual intercourse shouldn't be different for you.
4. After a spinal cord injury, menstruation usually stops.

2. 1. After a spinal cord injury, women remain fertile and can conceive and deliver a child. If a woman doesn't want to become pregnant, she *must* use contraception. Menstruation isn't affected by a spinal cord injury, but sexual functioning may be different.

CN: Physiological integrity; CNS: Physiological adaptation; CL: Application

3. A nurse is caring for a 39-year-old male client who recently underwent surgery and is having difficulty accepting changes in his body image. Which nursing intervention is appropriate?

1. Actively listening to the client as he expresses positive and negative feelings about his body image
2. Restricting the client's opportunity to view the incision and dressing because it's upsetting
3. Assisting the client to focus on future plans for recovery
4. Assisting the client to repress anger while discussing the body image alteration

3. 1. The nurse must observe for any indication that the client is ready to address his body image change. The client should be allowed to look at the incision and dressing if he wants to do so. It's too soon to focus on the future with this client. The nurse should allow the client to express his feelings and not repress them, because repression prolongs recovery.

CN: Psychosocial integrity; CNS: None; CL: Application

CN: Client needs category CNS: Client needs subcategory CL: Cognitive level

4. A female client with chronic obstructive pulmonary disease (COPD) tells a nurse, "I no longer have enough energy to make love to my husband." Which nursing intervention would be <u>most appropriate</u>?

1. Refer the couple to a sex therapist.
2. Advise the woman to seek a gynecologic consult.
3. Suggest methods and measures that facilitate sexual activity.
4. Tell the client, "If you talk this over with your husband, he'll understand."

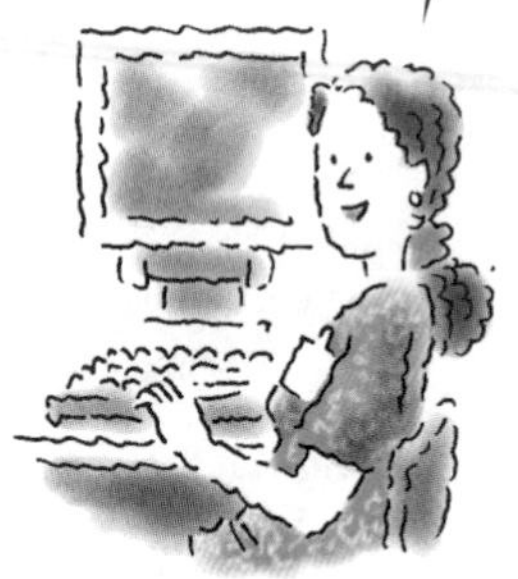

Several answers are possible. But which one is the most appropriate?

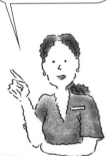

4. 3. Sexual dysfunction in COPD clients is the direct result of dyspnea and reduced energy levels. Measures to reduce physical exertion, enhance oxygenation, and accommodate decreased energy levels may aid sexual activity. If the problem persists, a consult with a sex therapist might be necessary. A gynecologic consult isn't necessary. Discussing this with her husband may not resolve the problem.

CN: Physiological integrity; CNS: Reduction of risk potential; CL: Application

5. A client with an ileostomy tells the nurse he can't have an erection. Which pertinent information should the nurse know?

1. The client will never regain functioning.
2. The client needs an abdominal X-ray.
3. The client has no problem with self-control.
4. Impotence is uncommon following an ileostomy.

5. 4. Sexual dysfunction is uncommon after an ileostomy. Psychological causes of impotence should be explored. An abdominal X-ray isn't indicated for sexual dysfunction. An ileostomy can change a person's self-control, making sexual functioning difficult.

CN: Physiological integrity; CNS: Physiological adaptation; CL: Analysis

6. A recently divorced 40-year-old client who has undergone radiation therapy for testicular cancer tells the nurse he is unable to achieve an erection. Which nursing diagnosis is <u>most appropriate</u>?

1. *Ineffective coping related to radiation therapy*
2. *Sexual dysfunction related to the effects of radiation therapy*
3. *Disturbed body image related to the effects of radiation therapy*
4. *Imbalanced nutrition: Less than body requirements related to radiation therapy*

6. 2. Radiation or chemotherapy may cause sexual dysfunction. Libido may only be temporarily affected, and the client should be provided with emotional support. The client may experience alopecia or skin changes as well as weight loss, but he isn't verbalizing concern in this area. The client hasn't verbalized fear or concern related to the cancer. Nutrition hasn't been mentioned.

CN: Psychosocial integrity; CNS: None; CL: Analysis

7. Which action should a nurse include in the teaching plan of a newly married female client with a cervical spinal cord injury who doesn't wish to become pregnant at this time?

1. Provide the client with brochures on sexual practice.
2. Provide the client's husband with material on vasectomy.
3. Instruct the client on the rhythm method of contraception.
4. Instruct the client's husband on inserting a diaphragm with contraceptive jelly.

7. 4. Because the client experienced a cervical spinal cord injury, she won't be able to insert any form of contraception protection by herself; therefore, it's vital to provide her husband with instruction on insertion of a diaphragm. Providing the couple with literature on sexual practice doesn't address the client's concerns. During this time of crisis, the couple doesn't wish to have children, but they may reconsider, so providing information on vasectomy isn't appropriate. The rhythm method isn't the most effective way to prevent pregnancy.

CN: Psychosocial integrity; CNS: None; CL: Application

8. A female client tells the nurse she is having her menstrual period every 2 weeks and it lasts for 1 week. Which term *best* defines this menstrual pattern?

1. Amenorrhea
2. Dyspareunia
3. Menorrhagia
4. Metrorrhagia

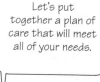

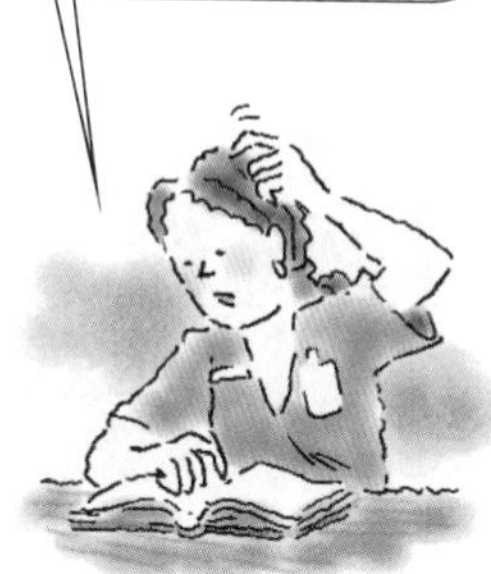

What's the difference between menorrhagia and metrorrhagia?

8. 3. Menorrhagia is an excessive menstrual period. Amenorrhea is lack of menstruation. Dyspareunia is painful intercourse. Metrorrhagia is uterine bleeding from another cause other than menstruation.

CN: Physiological integrity; CNS: Reduction of risk potential; CL: Application

9. Which aspect might be a major stressor for a couple being treated for infertility?

1. Examinations
2. Giving specimens
3. Scheduling intercourse
4. Finding out which partner is infertile

9. 3. The major cause of stress in infertile couples is planning sexual intercourse to correlate to fertility cycles. The inconvenience and discomfort of producing specimens and receiving examinations isn't a major stressor. Most couples undergoing fertility treatment understand that one partner is usually infertile.

CN: Health promotion and maintenance; CNS: None; CL: Application

10. A 38-year-old female client must undergo a hysterectomy for uterine cancer. The nurse planning her care should include which action to meet the client's body image changes?

1. Ask her if she is having pain.
2. Refer her to a psychotherapist.
3. Don't discuss the subject with her.
4. Encourage her to verbalize her feelings.

10. 4. Encourage the client to verbalize her feelings because loss of one's reproductive organs may bring on feelings of loss of sexuality. Pain is a concern after surgery, but it has no bearing on body image. Referring her to a psychotherapist may be premature; the client should be given time to work through her feelings. Avoidance of the subject isn't a therapeutic nursing intervention.

CN: Psychosocial integrity; CNS: None; CL: Application

11. A 50-year-old male client who had a myocardial infarction 8 weeks ago tells a nurse, "My wife wants to make love, but I don't think I can. I'm worried that it might kill me." Which response from the nurse would be most appropriate?

1. "Tell me about your feelings."
2. "Let's increase your rehabilitation schedule."
3. "Let me call the primary health care provider for you."
4. "Tell your wife when you're able you'll make love."

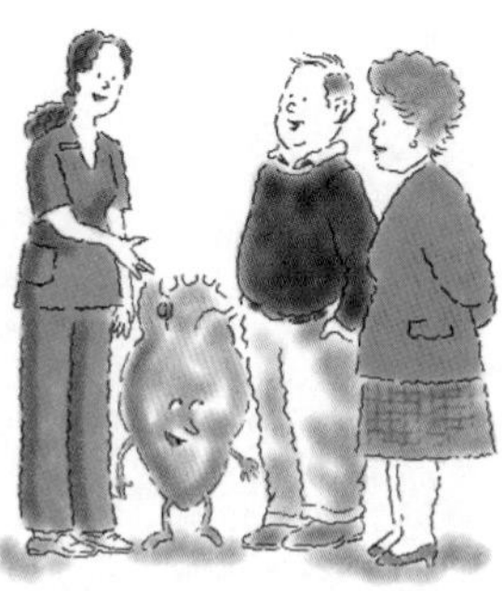

Let's put together a plan of care that will meet all of your needs.

11. 1. The nurse should address the client's concerns. Asking the client to verbalize his feelings will permit the nurse to gain insight into the problem. The rehabilitation schedule shouldn't be increased until the nurse assesses the situation and is sure no harm will come to the client. Calling the primary health care provider before a complete assessment is made is inappropriate. Telling the wife that eventually the client will make love may place strain on the marriage.

CN: Psychosocial integrity; CNS: None; CL: Application

12. A 55-year-old female client who's in cardiac rehabilitation tells a nurse that she's unable to make love to her husband because she often feels fatigued and has a sense of doom. Which nursing intervention is most appropriate?

1. Instruct her not to have intercourse until she is ready.
2. Instruct her to take a nitroglycerin tablet prior to intercourse.
3. Encourage her to learn additional methods to use for sexual intercourse.
4. Encourage her to verbalize her feelings while you perform a physical examination on her.

12. 4. Because the client has a complaint of fatigue, she should be examined and her feelings should be explored. Instructing her not to have intercourse doesn't address her concerns. She shouldn't take nitroglycerin before intercourse until her fatigue is evaluated. Before recommending alternative methods for intercourse, the client should be assessed physically and psychologically.
CN: Psychosocial integrity; CNS: None; CL: Application

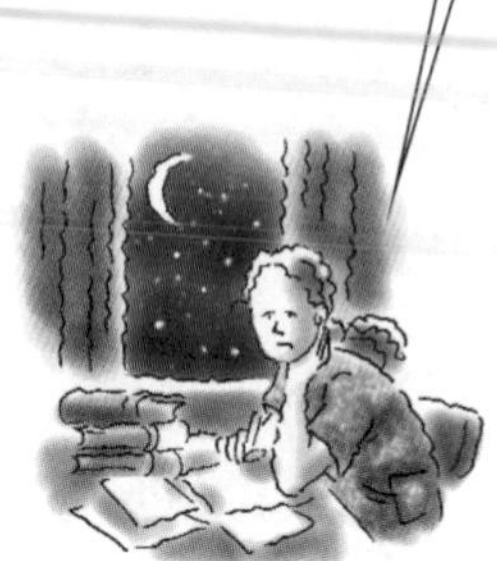

I know all about feeling fatigued.

13. A 33-year-old female client tells the nurse she has never had an orgasm and that her partner is upset that he's unable to meet her needs. Which nursing intervention is most appropriate?

1. Ask the client if she desires intercourse.
2. Assess the couple's perception of the problem.
3. Tell the client that most women don't reach orgasm.
4. Refer the client to a therapist because she has sexual aversion disorder.

13. 2. Assessing the couple's perception of the problem will define the problem and assist the couple and the nurse in understanding it. When assessing the client, the nurse should be professional and matter of fact and shouldn't make the client feel inadequate or defensive by asking if she desires intercourse. Most individuals can be taught to reach orgasm if there is no underlying medical condition. A nurse can't make a medical diagnosis such as sexual aversion disorder.
CN: Psychosocial integrity; CNS: None; CL: Application

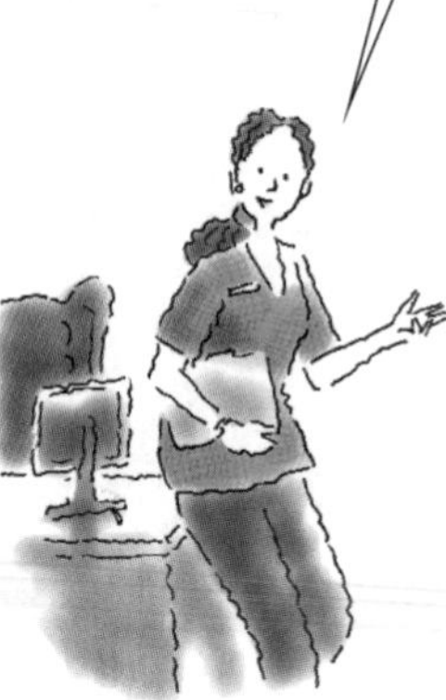

The NCLEX may include sexual identity questions for clients of different ages.

14. A 20-year-old female client is in the emergency department after being sexually assaulted by a stranger. Which nursing intervention has the highest priority?

1. Assisting the client in identifying which of her behaviors placed her at risk for the attack
2. Making an appointment for the client in 6 weeks at a local sexual assault crisis center
3. Encouraging discussion of the client's early childhood experiences
4. Assisting the client in identifying family or friends who could provide immediate support for her

14. 4. The client needs a lot of support to help her through this ordeal. Assisting the client in identifying behaviors that place her at risk for the attack places the blame on the client. Waiting 6 weeks to make an appointment is incorrect — the local crisis center must be called immediately. Some psychiatric disorders are related to early childhood experiences, but rape isn't.
CN: Psychosocial integrity; CNS: None; CL: Application

15. A 50-year-old client who is taking antihypertensive medication tells the office nurse who's monitoring his blood pressure that he can't have sexual intercourse with his wife anymore. Which problem is most likely the cause?

1. His advancing age
2. His blood pressure
3. His stressful lifestyle
4. His blood pressure medication

15. 4. Antihypertensive medication may cause impotence in men. Blood pressure itself doesn't cause impotence but its treatment does. Stress may cause erectile dysfunction, but there's no evidence that the client is under stress. Men are usually able to have an erection throughout their lives.
CN: Physiological integrity; CNS: Pharmacological and parenteral therapies; CL: Application

16. Adult victims of childhood sexual abuse need to be monitored for signs and symptoms of which disorder?

1. Depression and substance abuse disorders
2. Bipolar and somatization disorders
3. Narcissistic disorders and bulimia nervosa
4. Obsessive-compulsive and posttraumatic stress disorders

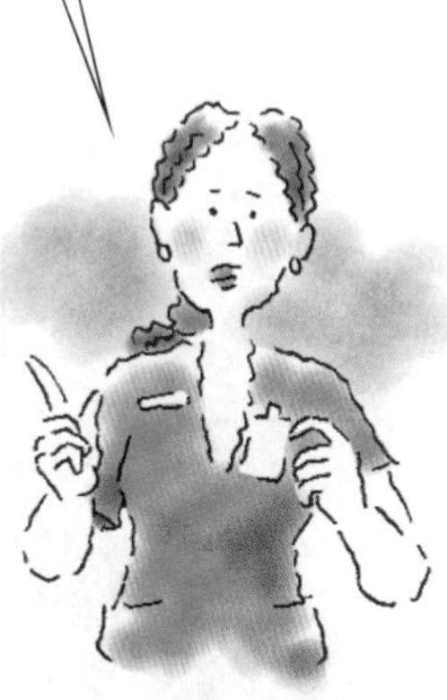

Don't despair over answering this question — focus on this disorder's symptoms.

16. 1. Childhood sexual abuse is closely linked to the development of depression and substance abuse disorders. It's also linked to the development of somatization and posttraumatic stress disorders and bulimia nervosa. Victims of childhood sexual abuse aren't predisposed to developing bipolar, narcissistic, or obsessive-compulsive disorders.

CN: Psychosocial integrity; CNS: None; CL: Analysis

17. Which intervention is important for a client who engages in sexual acts with animals (zoophilia)?

1. Place the client in the seclusion room.
2. Assess triggers that stimulate the behaviors.
3. Have the primary health care provider order antidepressant medication.
4. Counsel the client not to discuss his sexual behaviors with anyone.

17. 2. Assessing the triggers that stimulate inappropriate sexual behavior helps to prevent recurrence. The seclusion room should be used only to ensure the safety of the client and staff. Antidepressants aren't indicated for sexual disorders; hormonal therapy is the usual drug treatment. Clinical support and group therapy are used to teach sexually acceptable behavior.

CN: Psychosocial integrity; CNS: None; CL: Analysis

18. A 25-year-old client convicted of raping a female college student has completed his parole and has been attending a sex offenders group for 5 years. The client no longer wishes to participate in the group. Which action should the nurse take?

1. Insist that the client remain in therapy.
2. Perform a self-evaluation, and assess the discomfort level.
3. Call the parole board, and tell them of the client's decision.
4. Call the client's family, and tell them of his decision and progress.

18. 2. If the client has successfully completed therapy, then the nurse must evaluate her own value system. Insisting that the client remain in therapy may not prove to be successful, as he must be motivated to undergo therapy. Calling the parole board may be an inappropriate decision, especially if the client has met all of his requirements. A nurse can't release confidential information to the client's family without his permission and consent.

CN: Psychosocial integrity; CNS: None; CL: Analysis

19. A 32-year-old client who engages in voyeurism has come to the hospital for treatment so his family and friends don't find out. The nurse planning care for this client should include which intervention?

1. Encourage the client to inform his family and friends so that he isn't living a lie.
2. Suggest individual therapy to discuss socially unacceptable behavior.
3. Develop the care plan without input from the client.
4. Evaluate the client's defense mechanism.

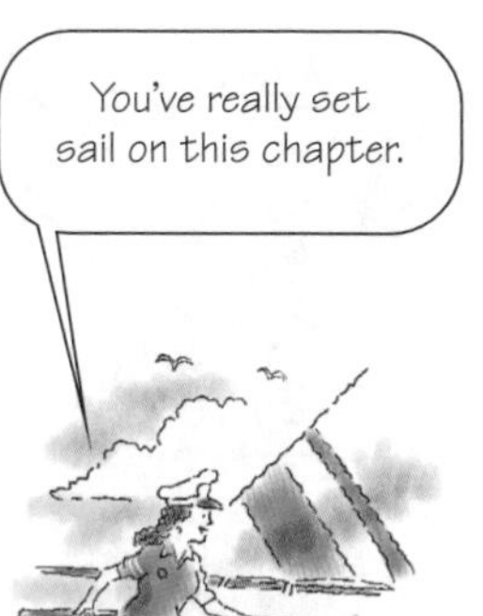

You've really set sail on this chapter.

19. 2. Discussing inappropriate sexual behavior with the client increases compliance with treatment and decreases the risk of relapse. Informing family and friends isn't an initial intervention; disclosure to family and friends is usually delayed until the client acknowledges his behavior. All care planning should involve the client. An initial evaluation should focus on the antecedents to the inappropriate behavior.

CN: Psychosocial integrity; CNS: None; CL: Application

20. A client is admitted to the psychiatric unit for paraphiliac coercive disorder: rape. Which assessment question will provide the nurse with insight toward this client's cognitive distortion?

1. "Tell me what you're feeling."
2. "Do you have any lifestyle problems?"
3. "What brings you to the hospital for treatment?"
4. "Do you believe you're here for a sexual disorder?"

20. 4. If a client had a cognitive disorder, then he would be using denial as a defense mechanism and would deny having a sexual disorder. Asking what a client is feeling is important, but it doesn't provide information on the use of defense mechanisms. Asking about lifestyle problems will provide the nurse with information related to problems with relationships. Asking why the client is at the hospital will tell the nurse if the client has insight into his illness.
CN: Psychosocial integrity; CNS: None; CL: Application

21. A 38-year-old female client was returning home from the store late one evening and was sexually assaulted. When she's brought to the emergency department, she's crying. Which concern for this client should be the nurse's first priority?

1. Filing a police report
2. Calling the client's family
3. Encouraging the client to enroll in a self-defense class
4. Remaining with the client and assisting her through the crisis

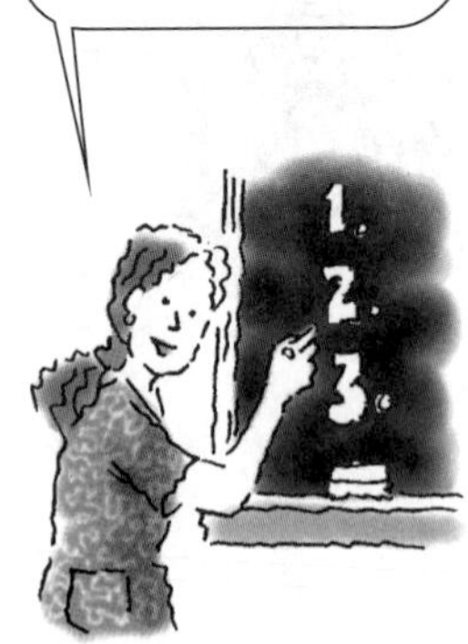

Prioritizing correctly is extremely important for question 21.

21. 4. Sexual assault is treated as a medical emergency, and the client requires constant attention and assistance during the crisis. Filing a police report wouldn't take precedence over a medical emergency. Comforting the client by contacting family should be carried out after the client's injuries are treated. Encouraging the client to enroll in a self-defense class isn't appropriate during crisis.
CN: Psychosocial integrity; CNS: None; CL: Application

22. A client is admitted to the psychiatric unit as part of his probation period for exhibitionism and fetishism. The client seems to be adjusting well, but several clients report that their undergarments are missing. Which action would be most appropriate?

1. Notify the primary health care provider.
2. Search the client's room.
3. Call a community meeting, and let the clients settle the matter.
4. Privately assess whether the client is engaging in sexual activities on the unit.

22. 4. Meeting with the client privately establishes trust. This client needs to be assessed for what triggers might be present to prompt this behavior. Notification of the primary health care provider shouldn't be done without assessment of the client. Searching the client's room without discussion is a violation of a trusting milieu. It isn't therapeutic to encourage the unit to confront one member of the community.
CN: Psychosocial integrity; CNS: None; CL: Application

23. A client is admitted to the hospital for scatophilia and tells the nurse that he doesn't want to talk to her about his sexual behaviors. Which response from the nurse is the most appropriate?

1. "I need to ask you the questions on the database."
2. "It's your right not to answer my questions."
3. "I know this must be difficult for you."
4. "OK, I'll just write 'no comment.'"

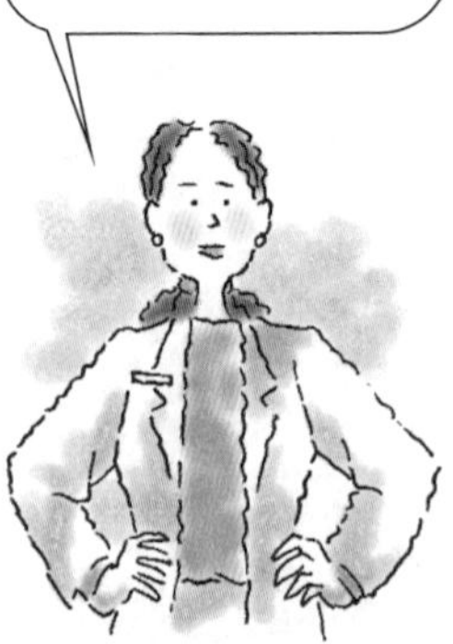

Clients with sexual disorders may be ashamed and unwilling to discuss the problem.

23. 3. Stating "I know this must be difficult for you" acknowledges the client's feelings and opens communications. Insisting that the form needs to be completed doesn't open up communications or acknowledge the client's feelings. Clients have rights, but data collection is necessary so that help with the problem can be offered. Writing "no comment" alone would be inappropriate.
CN: Psychosocial integrity; CNS: None; CL: Application

24. Which therapy may be used with a client who admits to frottage?

1. Electroconvulsive therapy
2. Relaxation therapy
3. Administration of psychotropic agents
4. Positive reinforcement and group therapy

24. 4. Frottage involves rubbing against someone in a public place. Positive reinforcement and group therapy are used to assist a client with frottage to develop new sexual response patterns. Electroconvulsive therapy and relaxation therapy aren't indicated for this condition. Psychotropic medications are used for dangerous and compulsive practices and aren't indicated for this condition.
CN: Psychosocial integrity; CNS: None; CL: Analysis

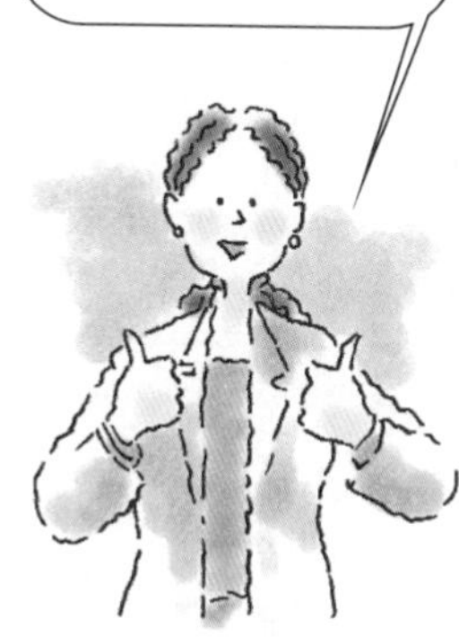
Keep going; you're doing great!

25. When treating a client admitted to the psychiatric unit for transvestic fetishism, the nurse should develop a care plan based on which diagnosis?

1. *Ineffective health maintenance*
2. *Ineffective sexuality patterns*
3. *Complicated grieving*
4. *Bathing self-care deficit*

25. 2. *Ineffective sexuality patterns* would be appropriate because transvestic fetishism refers to intense sexual arousal with cross-dressing. *Ineffective health maintenance* is an appropriate diagnosis for someone experiencing a health problem. *Complicated grieving* refers to the inability to recover from a loss. The client hasn't exhibited any problems with health, self-care, or loss. *Bathing self-care deficit* is a diagnosis for the inability to meet self-care needs.
CN: Psychosocial integrity; CNS: None; CL: Application

26. When working with a client with a paraphiliac disorder, which goal is appropriate for the client?

1. To attend all meetings on the unit
2. To use triggers to initiate sexual behaviors
3. To inform his employer of the reason for hospitalization
4. To verbalize appropriate methods to meet sexual needs upon discharge

26. 4. Upon discharge, the client should verbalize an alternative appropriate method to meet his sexual needs and effective strategies to prevent relapse. It isn't imperative that the client attend all meetings on the unit, but it's important that he attend the prescribed group sessions. A client with a paraphiliac disorder should recognize triggers that initiate inappropriate sexual behaviors and learn ways to direct his impulses. The client may wish to discuss the disorder with his spouse but not necessarily his employer.
CN: Psychosocial integrity; CNS: None; CL: Analysis

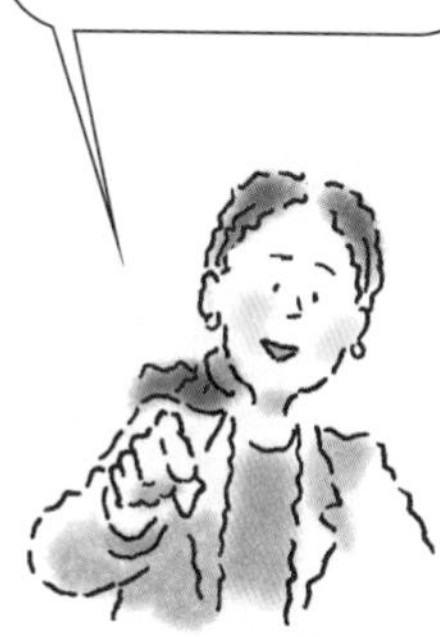
Effective care may involve managing interactions between clients.

27. A client admitted to the hospital with a diagnosis of pedophilia tells his roommate about his problems. His roommate runs down the hall yelling at the nurse, "I don't want to be in here with a child molester." Which response from the nurse is most appropriate?

1. "Stop acting out."
2. "Calm down, and go back to your room."
3. "Your roommate isn't a child molester."
4. "I can see you're upset. Sit down and we'll talk."

27. 4. Acknowledging that the client is upset and sitting down and talking with him will allow the client to verbalize his feelings. If a client were agitated or anxious over his roommate, it wouldn't be therapeutic or safe to keep those clients together without intervention. Telling the client to stop acting out or to calm down isn't a therapeutic response. Stating that the pedophile isn't a child molester doesn't acknowledge the client's feelings.
CN: Psychosocial integrity; CNS: None; CL: Application

28. When assigning rooms for clients, a nurse should not place which of the following clients with a client who has a diagnosis of sexual sadism?

1. A client with a diagnosis of sexual masochism
2. A client with a diagnosis of voyeurism
3. A client who's an exhibitionist
4. A client who's a homosexual

28. 1. A client who's admitted with a diagnosis of sexual masochism is aroused through suffering and, therefore, shouldn't be placed with a client who's diagnosed with sexual sadism, who's aroused by inflicted pain. A voyeur is aroused by secretly observing someone who's naked or engaged in sexual activity. An exhibitionist is aroused through the exposure of one's genitals to an unsuspecting person. A homosexual enjoys relationships with someone of the same sex.

CN: Safe, effective care environment; CNS: Management of care; CL: Application

29. A nurse is obtaining a health history from a client when he states he has been diagnosed with voyeurism. Which of the following actions would the nurse expect to assess in this client?

1. Observing others while they disrobe
2. Wearing clothing of the opposite sex
3. Rubbing against a nonconsenting person
4. Using rubber sheeting for sexual arousal

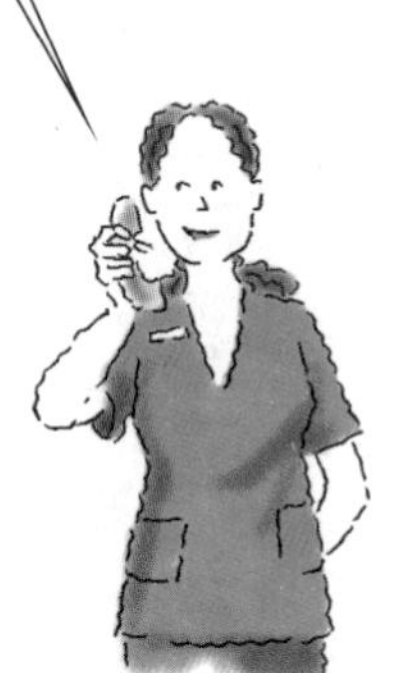

Hello, information? Do you know the answer to question 30?

29. 1. Voyeurism is sexual arousal from secretly observing someone who is disrobing. Transvestic fetishism describes someone who enjoys cross-dressing. Rubbing against someone who is nonconsenting is frottage. Using objects for sexual arousal is fetishism.

CN: Psychosocial integrity; CNS: None; CL: Application

30. The nurse is teaching the family of a client with scatophilia. Which response by the nurse is most accurate in teaching about the characteristics of this disorder?

1. The client uses the telephone for sexual arousal.
2. The client uses nonliving objects such as women's underwear for sexual gratification.
3. The client is aroused through contact with children.
4. The client is aroused by rubbing against a nonconsenting person.

30. 1. Telephone scatophilia is a paraphilia in which a person derives sexual arousal by engaging in lewd conversations on the telephone. Fetishism involves the use of nonliving objects whose presence are required or preferred for sexual excitement. Pedophiles engage in fondling or sexual activities with children under 13 years of age. Frottage is rubbing against a nonconsenting person for sexual arousal.

CN: Psychosocial integrity; CNS: None; CL: Application

31. A female being treated for infertility confides to the nurse that she hasn't told her partner she has been treated for a sexually transmitted disease in the past. What would be the most therapeutic response?

1. "Do you think withholding this information is the basis for a trusting relationship?"
2. "Don't you think your partner deserves to know?"
3. "What concerns do you have about sharing this information?"
4. "I can understand why you would want to keep this information from him."

31. 3. This response encourages the client to verbalize her concerns in a safe environment and begin to choose a course of action for how to deal with this issue now. Telling the client that she's withholding information that may cause distrust in her relationship or that her partner deserves to know conveys negative judgments. The fourth response doesn't encourage discussion or problem-solving.

CN: Psychosocial integrity; CNS: None; CL: Application

32. After learning that his gay roommate has tested positive for human immunodeficiency virus (HIV), a client asks the nurse about moving to another room on the psychiatric unit because the client doesn't feel "safe" now. What should the nurse do <u>first</u>?

1. Move the client to another room.
2. Ask the client to describe any fears.
3. Move the client's roommate to a private room.
4. Explain that such a move wouldn't be therapeutic for the client or his roommate.

32. 2. To intervene effectively, the nurse must first understand the client's fears. After exploring the client's fears, the nurse may move the client or his roommate or explain why such a move wouldn't be therapeutic.

CN: Psychosocial integrity; CNS: None; CL: Application

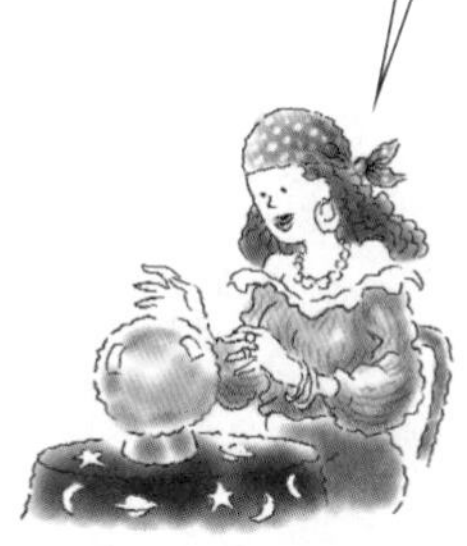

I predict you will be able to select which action should be performed first.

33. A nurse lecturing on paraphilias informs her audience that recidivism is high for clients with paraphilias. Which definition best describes recidivism?

1. Insight into treatment
2. Aggressive sexual assault
3. Behaviors associated with sexual deviation
4. Continued inappropriate behavior after treatment

33. 4. Recidivism is defined as continuing in an unacceptable behavior after completing treatment to correct that behavior. High level of insight isn't connected with any specific disorder. Aggressive sexual assault is a type of paraphilia. Sexually deviant behaviors are known as paraphilias.

CN: Psychosocial integrity; CNS: None; CL: Analysis

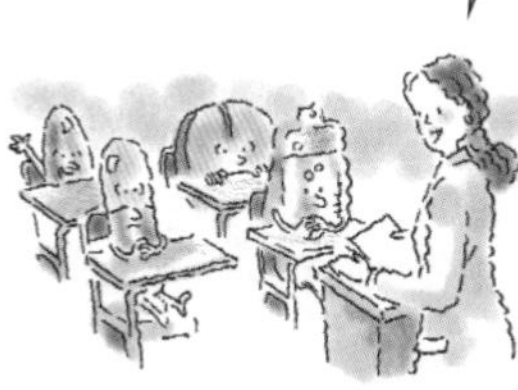

The NCLEX often tests your ability to educate accurately.

34. Which nursing diagnosis is most appropriate for a client with sexual masochism?

1. *Risk for self-mutilation*
2. *Ineffective role performance*
3. *Ineffective coping*
4. *Risk for other-directed violence*

34. 1. A person with sexual masochism is sexually aroused by being the receiver of pain and, therefore, may injure himself. A person diagnosed with transvestic fetishism may have ineffective role performance. There is no evidence that this client isn't coping. A sexual sadist would be a danger to others.

CN: Psychosocial integrity; CNS: None; CL: Analysis

35. Which statement made by a client with paraphilia indicates a potential for relapse?

1. "I am going to outpatient therapy."
2. "I am going to try to attend all therapy sessions."
3. "I don't need this, and I can't imagine why the judge sent me here."
4. "The physician wants me to take leuprolide acetate (Lupron). I think that will help."

35. 3. A lack of insight to the problem may indicate a potential for relapse. Attending all therapy sessions and outpatient therapy demonstrates compliance with the treatment plan. Leuprolide acetate is an anti-androgenic that lowers testosterone levels and decreases the libido.

CN: Psychosocial integrity; CNS: None; CL: Analysis

36. A female client taking antidepressant medication complains to the nurse that she has a decreased desire for sex, which is causing significant marital stress. Which response by the nurse would be the <u>most appropriate</u>?

1. "Don't stop taking the medication."
2. "What are your thoughts on how you should handle this?"
3. "Doesn't your husband understand the importance of your medication?"
4. "Have you discussed this with your physician?"

36. 2. Encouraging the client to verbalize her thoughts will help the client to problem solve and identify feelings related to different choices. The first response is too directive and doesn't encourage exploration on the part of the client. The third response conveys negative judgment. The fourth response might be appropriate, but it also may give the impression that the nurse doesn't want to discuss this issue with the client.

CN: Psychosocial integrity; CNS: None; CL: Application

More than one answer may seen correct, but choose the most appropriate.

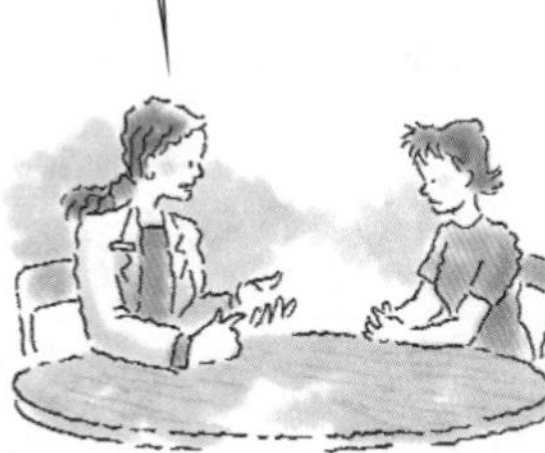

37. A mother brings her 14-year-old son to the psychiatric crisis room. The client's mother states, "He's always dressing in female clothing. There must be something wrong with him." Which response from the nurse would be most appropriate?

1. "Your son will be evaluated shortly."
2. "I'll tell your son that this isn't appropriate."
3. "I know you're upset. Would you like to talk?"
4. "I wouldn't want my son to dress in girl's clothing."

37. 3. Acknowledging the mother's feelings and offering her an opportunity to verbalize her concerns provides a forum for open communication. Telling the client's mother that he'll be evaluated shortly doesn't address her concerns. Telling the client that this behavior isn't appropriate doesn't assess his feelings nor does it analyze the behavior. The nurse shouldn't offer an opinion by stating she wouldn't want her son dressing in female clothing.
CN: Psychosocial integrity; CNS: None; CL: Application

38. A 17-year-old female who enjoys playing ball with boys and is most comfortable in jeans tells her mother she doesn't want to go to the prom if she has to wear a frilly dress. Her mother asks, "What should I do with my daughter?" Which response from the nurse would be most appropriate?

1. Tell the client's mother, "She'll grow out of it."
2. Offer to speak to the client about her dressing habits.
3. Ask the client's mother to talk about her fears for her daughter.
4. Tell the client's mother to make her go to the prom but not wear a dress.

38. 3. Asking the client's mother to verbalize her fears will permit the nurse to accurately assess the mother's distress. The client's mother may be upset over the behavior or the fact that her daughter doesn't wish to go to the prom. Telling the client's mother that her daughter will grow out of it may be offering the mother false reassurance. The nurse shouldn't speak to the client about her behavior as this implies a value judgment on the part of the nurse. Forcing her to go to the prom isn't therapeutic, and doesn't address the mother's fears.
CN: Psychosocial integrity; CNS: None; CL: Application

39. A 39-year-old male client wishes to undergo a sex-reassignment operation because he feels trapped in his male body. Which action is the next step the client should take if he wants to have the operation?

1. Tell his family and friends
2. Attend psychotherapy
3. Visit transsexual bars
4. See a surgeon

39. 2. Before having a sex-reassignment operation, the client should have several years of psychotherapy. The family, as well as friends, should be told of the client's plans. Visiting transsexual bars has no bearing on having a sex-reassignment operation. Seeing a surgeon isn't usually done on a regular basis until after the completion of psychotherapy.
CN: Psychosocial integrity; CNS: None; CL: Analysis

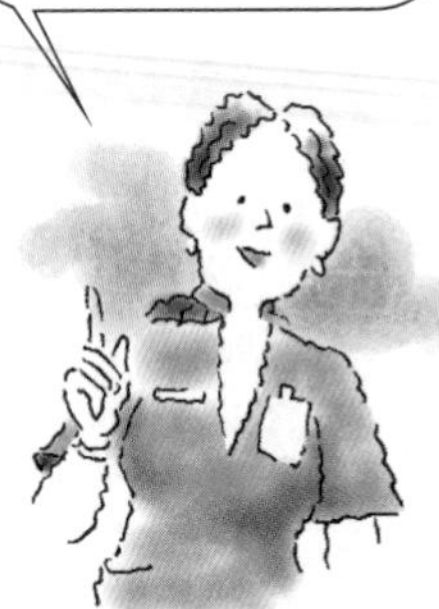

For question 40, you need to determine the best answer.

40. Which reason best explains the rationale for estrogen therapy for a male client who wishes to undergo sexual reassignment surgery?

1. To develop breasts
2. To cause menstruation
3. To assist with cross-dressing
4. To develop body hair and lack of menstruation

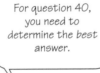

40. 1. A male who receives long-term estrogen therapy will develop female secondary sexual characteristics such as breasts. A male on estrogen won't menstruate because he doesn't have a uterus. Estrogen has no bearing on cross-dressing. Androgens would be taken by a female to develop body hair and stop menstruation.
CN: Psychosocial integrity; CNS: None; CL: Analysis

CN: Client needs category CNS: Client needs subcategory CL: Cognitive level

41. A nurse is caring for several clients with gender identity disorders. The nurse understands that which client is most at risk for anxiety related to transsexualism?

1. Elderly
2. Adolescent
3. Young adult
4. Prepubescent child

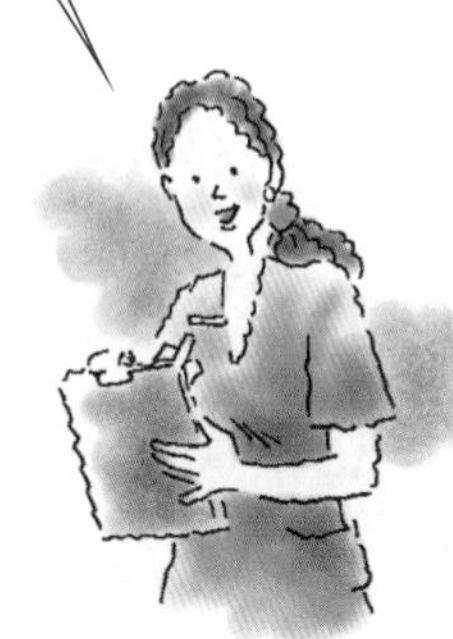

A client's age can affect his anxiety related to gender identity disorders.

41. 2. Adolescents who are transsexuals are usually very distraught over the changes occurring within their body. Elderly persons, young adults, and young children aren't experiencing rapidly developing secondary sexual characteristics in their bodies; therefore, they aren't at high risk for anxiety.
CN: Psychosocial integrity; CNS: None; CL: Analysis

42. What is the gender identity disorder that results in the person believing he or she is really the opposite sex?

1. Exhibitionism
2. Homosexuality
3. Transsexualism
4. Transvestitism

42. 3. Transsexuals believe they're really of the opposite sex. An exhibitionist is someone who's sexually aroused by displaying one's genitals in a public place. A homosexual enjoys sexual relations with a person of the same sexual orientation. A transvestite enjoys cross-dressing.
CN: Psychosocial integrity; CNS: None; CL: Application

43. A transsexual client wishes to have a sexual reassignment operation and tells the nurse he's ready to begin hormonal therapy. Which fact about the client must be true before estrogen therapy is administered?

1. He has cross-dressed and lived as the opposite sex for several years.
2. He has decided against undergoing the operation.
3. He has decided he needs more psychotherapy.
4. He has been functioning sexually as a female.

43. 1. Before a sexual reassignment operation, the client should live as the opposite sex after undergoing several years of psychotherapy. A client wishing to take hormonal therapy is in the final step before receiving the operation and therefore hasn't decided against the surgery. Psychotherapy is an ongoing modality for someone requesting a sexual reassignment operation. A male doesn't have female reproductive organs, so he couldn't have been functioning sexually as a female.
CN: Psychosocial integrity; CNS: None; CL: Analysis

44. According to Erikson, an adolescent who is suffering from gender identity disorder is unable to progress through which developmental task?

1. Initiative versus guilt
2. Intimacy versus isolation
3. Industry versus inferiority
4. Identity versus role confusion

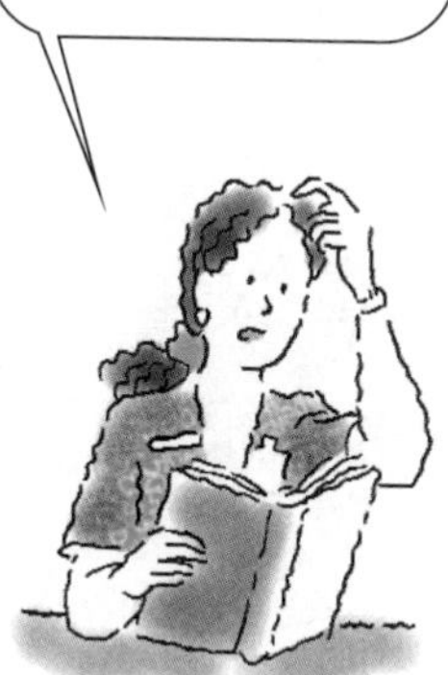

I remember reading about Erik Erikson. But now I'm confused.

44. 4. According to developmentalist Erik Erikson, adolescence is a time when role identity is found as a result of independence and sexual maturity; role confusion would result from the inability to integrate all experiences. Initiative versus guilt is when a child begins to conceptualize and interpersonalize relationships. Intimacy versus isolation is a stage in which the adult meets other adults and establishes relationships. Industry versus inferiority is when a child incorporates and acquires social skills.
CN: Health promotion and maintenance; CNS: None; CL: Analysis

45. A 35-year-old client who has been married for 10 years arrives at the psychiatric clinic stating, "I can't live this lie any more. I wish I were a woman. I don't want my wife. I need a man." Which initial action would be most appropriate from the nurse?

1. Call the primary health care provider.
2. Encourage the client to speak to his wife.
3. Have the client admitted.
4. Sit down with the client, and talk about his feelings.

45. 4. Sitting down with the client and exploring his feelings will allow the nurse to assess him. The primary health care provider shouldn't be notified until an assessment is made. The client shouldn't speak to his wife until he has processed his feelings. An assessment of the client should be made *before* admitting the client to the unit.

CN: Psychosocial integrity; CNS: None; CL: Application

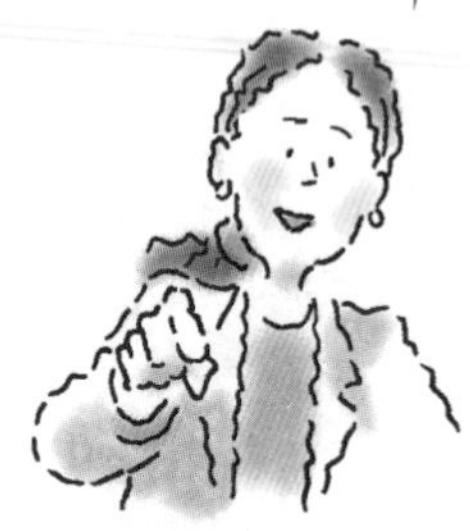

What should you do first?

46. A 14-year-old female client admits to having transsexual feelings and states, "I would rather die than live in this body." Which is the initial action most appropriate for the nurse to take?

1. Explain to her that she is too young to have these feelings.
2. Call her parents, and let them know about her feelings.
3. Encourage her to verbalize her feelings.
4. Ask her if she plans to kill herself.

46. 4. Whenever a client verbalizes feelings of preferring death to life, the nurse should always make sure that the client doesn't have a plan. Transsexual tendencies usually arise during the adolescent years, so it is appropriate for the client to have these feelings. Calling her parents wouldn't be a priority until after a psychological safety assessment is completed. Encouraging her to verbalize her feelings isn't an initial action for the nurse.

CN: Psychosocial integrity; CNS: None; CL: Application

47. A female client enjoys wearing men's clothing. Her sister tells the nurse that the client wishes for a sexual reassignment operation. The client tells the nurse she just wants to be left alone. Which initial nursing intervention is most appropriate?

1. Tell the client she is repressing her true feelings.
2. Encourage the client to verbalize her feelings.
3. Tell the client's sister to mind her own business.
4. Encourage the client to avoid her sister.

47. 2. The client needs to verbalize her feelings regarding wearing male attire as well as her desire to be left alone. Telling the client she is repressing her true feelings is judgmental. It's inappropriate for a nurse to tell a family member to mind her own business or to tell the client to avoid her sister.

CN: Psychosocial integrity; CNS: None; CL: Application

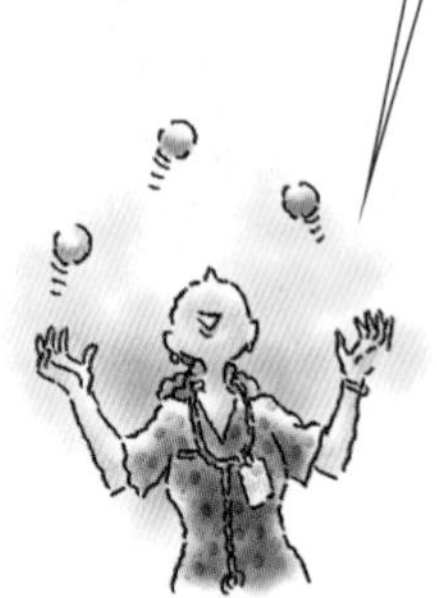

Keep going! Fewer than 10 questions to go!

48. A mother is concerned about her son and says he's 10 years old and has been playing with dolls since he was 2. Which initial strategy should be included in his care plan?

1. Providing counseling for his mother
2. Instructing the mother to throw away the dolls
3. Instructing the mother on play that's age-appropriate
4. Exploring with the child his feelings related to the dolls

48. 4. It's important to assess the child's feelings as well as to explore his preference for dolls rather than sports. The mother may need to be instructed on methods to cope with his behaviors but only after the child is permitted to verbalize. Until proper assessment is made, it's inappropriate to remove the dolls. There's no evidence of age-inappropriate play.

CN: Psychosocial integrity; CNS: None; CL: Application

49. A newly graduated nurse expresses concern to the nurse-manager about working with clients who want to discuss sexual problems. Which response by the nurse-manager is appropriate?

1. "It's part of the job. You'll get used to it."
2. "You can refer those types of questions to other health care professionals."
3. "If you've graduated from nursing school and passed the NCLEX, you qualify as a sex counselor."
4. "Tell me more about your concern."

49. 4. The nurse-manager would need to explore more what the nurse's specific concerns were before she could counsel her appropriately. Telling the nurse she'll get used to it doesn't allow the nurse to express her feeling or validate her concerns. Option 2 may be a possibility but the nurse-manager needs to understand the problem first. Passing the NCLEX doesn't qualify the nurse as a sex counselor. Sex therapists have additional training and education.

CN: Safe effective care environment; CNS: Management of care; CL: Analysis

50. A 57-year-old hypertensive male client expresses concern about his sexual functioning. Which question is <u>most</u> helpful in obtaining further assessment data?

1. Medication history
2. Sexual practices
3. Medical conditions
4. Family history

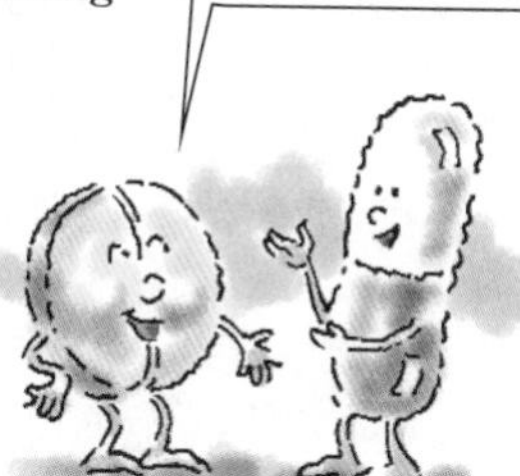

We have a history together.

50. 1. Many antihypertensive medications can affect sexual functioning; the nurse must assess if the client is taking other medications that may also alter sexual functioning. Sexual practices are part of the nursing assessment, as are other medical conditions and family history. However, obtaining a thorough medication history and reviewing effects on the client may help alleviate misconceptions and easily identify the source of the problem.

CN: Physiological integrity; CNS: Pharmacological and parenteral therapies; CL: Application

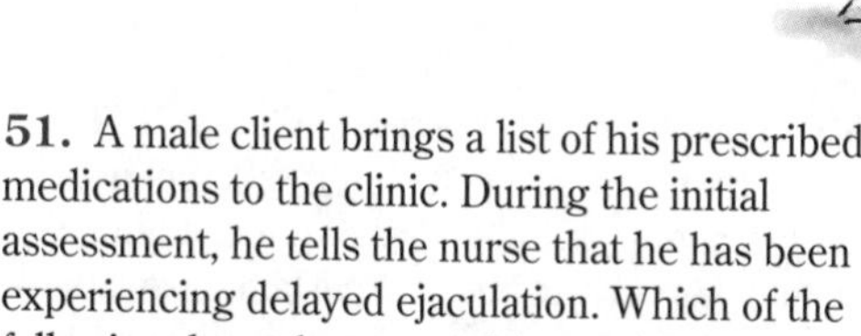

51. A male client brings a list of his prescribed medications to the clinic. During the initial assessment, he tells the nurse that he has been experiencing delayed ejaculation. Which of the following drug classes would <u>most likely</u> be associated with this condition?

1. Anticoagulants
2. Antibiotics
3. Antihypertensives
4. Steroids

51. 3. Antihypertensive agents can cause or contribute to sexual dysfunction. Anticoagulants, antibiotics, and steroids have no known effect on sexual function.

CN: Physiological integrity; CNS: Pharmacological and parenteral therapies; CL: Application

52. After a myocardial infarction (MI), a client tells the nurse he's afraid he'll have another heart attack if he attempts sexual intercourse. Which nursing diagnosis is <u>most</u> appropriate?

1. *Deficient knowledge related to sexual dysfunction*
2. *Disturbed body image related to lifestyle changes*
3. *Sexual dysfunction related to disturbances in self-esteem*
4. *Disturbed body image related to effects of treatment*

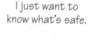

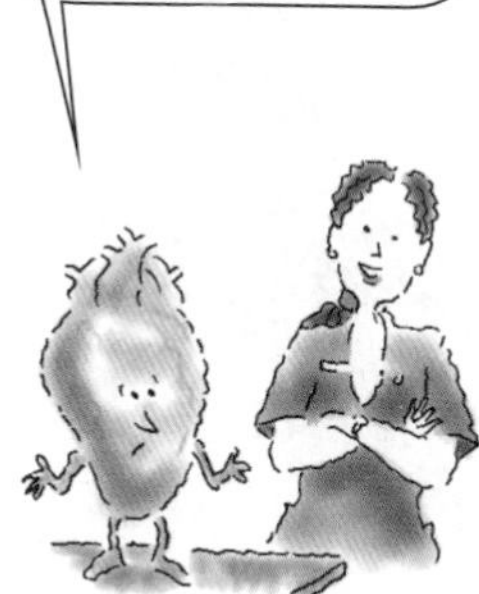

I just want to know what's safe.

52. 1. After an MI, many clients fear that engaging in sex will trigger another one. The nurse should teach the client about when he can safely resume sexual activity and which positions to use during intercourse to conserve energy. The client's fears result from lack of knowledge, not disturbances in self-esteem or body image.

CN: Psychosocial integrity; CNS: None; CL: Application

53. A 42-year-old female client complains of painful intercourse. Which nursing diagnosis is most useful in planning this client's care?

1. *Ineffective coping*
2. *Disturbed body image*
3. *Ineffective sexuality patterns*
4. *Sexual dysfunction*

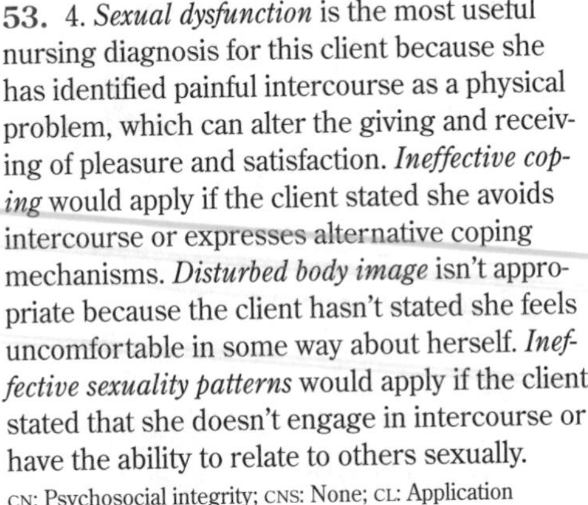

53. 4. *Sexual dysfunction* is the most useful nursing diagnosis for this client because she has identified painful intercourse as a physical problem, which can alter the giving and receiving of pleasure and satisfaction. *Ineffective coping* would apply if the client stated she avoids intercourse or expresses alternative coping mechanisms. *Disturbed body image* isn't appropriate because the client hasn't stated she feels uncomfortable in some way about herself. *Ineffective sexuality patterns* would apply if the client stated that she doesn't engage in intercourse or have the ability to relate to others sexually.

CN: Psychosocial integrity; CNS: None; CL: Application

54. A 46-year-old female client is diagnosed with a problem in sexual functioning. When planning her care, which nursing action takes highest priority?

1. Assessing the client's sexual functioning
2. Assessing the client's role in her sexual relationship
3. Determining the nurse's own beliefs and feelings about this issue
4. Interviewing the client's sexual partner

54. 3. The nurse must first identify her own beliefs and feelings about the issue and remain nonjudgmental. The other actions may be relevant but take lower priority.

CN: Safe, effective care environment; CNS: Management of care; CL: Application

55. A 35-year-old male client states he has little or no sexual desire. He also states that this is causing great distress in his marriage. What further information would be the most useful in assessing the situation? Select all that apply:

1. The client's age when he had his first girlfriend
2. When the problem first appeared and potential contributing factors
3. Medications and dosages
4. Report of recent bladder or prostate problems
5. Age of the client's wife

55. 2, 3. Option 2 is correct and provides opportunity to gather useful information in better understanding the client's current condition. Option 3 is correct because certain medications can have a profound effect on sexual desire. The client's age when he started dating has no bearing on the current problem. Reporting previous problems is useful but wouldn't provide a sufficient explanation for the lack of sexual desire. The age of the client's wife is irrelevant and doesn't provide assessment data.

CN: Psychosocial integrity; CNS: None; CL: Analysis

56. Pedophilia is diagnosed by the presence of specifically defined behaviors and characteristics. Which statements regarding pedophilia are true? Select all that apply:

1. A strong sexual attraction to prepubescent children exists.
2. Male children are more commonly the focus of attention than female children.
3. The pedophile is usually very attentive to a child's needs in order to gain the child's attention.
4. The disorder generally begins in early adulthood.
5. The pedophile must be age 16 or older or at least 5 years older than the child.

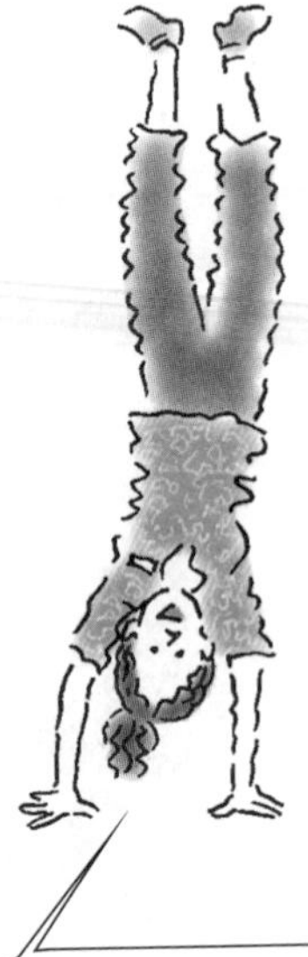
Time to celebrate! You finished chapter 20!

56. 1, 3, 5. Pedophilia is a disorder characterized by a strong sexual attraction to prepubescent children that generally begins to manifest itself in adolescence, not early adulthood. By definition, the pedophile must be age 16 or older or at least 5 years older than the child. The pedophile generally is attentive to the needs of children in order to gain their trust, loyalty, and attention. Female, not male, children are more commonly the focus of attention.

CN: Psychosocial integrity; CNS: None; CL: Application

CN: Client needs category CNS: Client needs subcategory CL: Cognitive level

New information about eating disorders is released almost continuously. For the latest about disorders of critical importance for young people, check the Web site of the National Eating Disorders Association at www.nationaleatingdisorders.org.

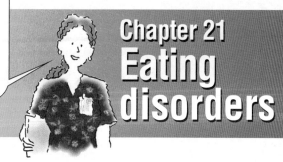

Chapter 21 Eating disorders

1. A parent with a daughter with bulimia nervosa asks a nurse, "How can my child have an eating disorder when she isn't underweight?" Which response is best?
   1. "A person with bulimia nervosa can maintain a normal weight."
   2. "It's hard to face this type of problem in a person you love."
   3. "At first there is no weight loss; it comes later in the disease."
   4. "This is a serious problem even though there is no weight loss."

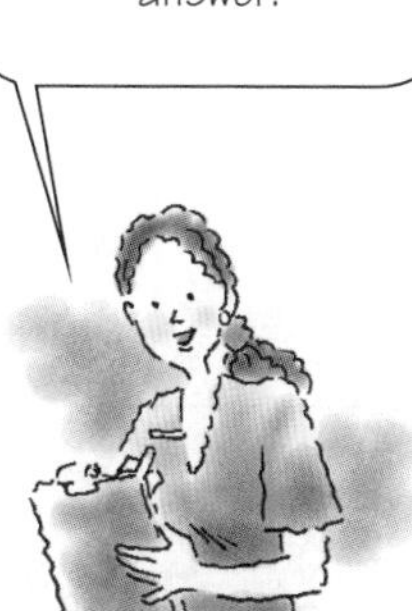

Choose the best answer!

1. 1. A client with bulimia nervosa may be of normal weight, overweight, or underweight. Weight loss isn't a clinical criterion for bulimia nervosa. The second option doesn't address the need for information about the relationship between weight change and bulimia nervosa. The third option is incorrect because there may be little or no weight loss. The fourth option doesn't address the issue of weight change in a client with bulimia nervosa.

CN: Psychosocial integrity; CNS: None; CL: Application

2. A 15-year-old female is brought to the clinic by her parents because of a significant amount of weight loss in the past 4 months. Which accompanying conditions would indicate that the client is suffering from anorexia nervosa?
   1. Hypertension
   2. Amenorrhea
   3. Hyperthermia
   4. Diarrhea

2. 2. Anorexia nervosa is characterized by profound weight loss caused by severe restriction of food intake by the client. If severe enough, it causes amenorrhea in females, along with decreased—not increased—body temperature. It usually doesn't produce diarrhea, but it may produce constipation because decreased oral intake leads to decreased GI motility.

CN: Physiological integrity; CNS: Reduction of risk potential; CL: Application

3. Which statement made by the client about the binge-purge cycle that occurs with bulimia nervosa indicates understanding of the disorder?
   1. "There are emotional triggers connected to bingeing."
   2. "Over time, people usually grow out of bingeing behaviors."
   3. "Bingeing isn't the problem; purging is the issue to address."
   4. "When a person gets too hungry, there's a tendency to binge."

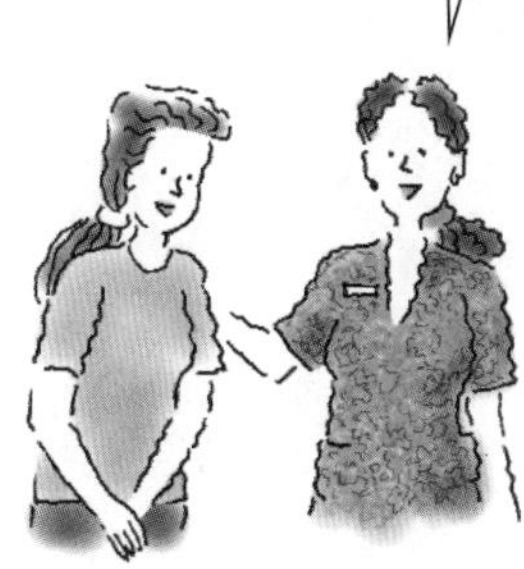

Help your client understand her behavior.

3. 1. It's important for the client to understand the emotional triggers to bingeing, such as disappointment, depression, and anxiety. People don't outgrow eating behaviors. This leads a person to believe binge eating is a normal part of growth and development when it definitely isn't. The third option negates the seriousness of bingeing and leads the client to believe only vomiting is a problem, not overeating. Physiologic hunger doesn't predispose a client to binge behaviors.

CN: Physiological integrity; CNS: Reduction of risk potential; CL: Application

4. A client with bulimia and a history of purging by vomiting is hospitalized for further observation because she's at risk for which of the following?

1. Diabetes mellitus
2. Electrolyte imbalance
3. GI obstruction
4. Septicemia

4. 2. Clients with bulimia who purge by vomiting are at greatest risk of electrolyte imbalances which can lead to cardiac arrhythmias. Purging by vomiting does not result in diabetes mellitus, GI obstruction, or septicemia.

CN: Physiological integrity; CNS: Physiological adaptation; CL: Application

5. A client with a diagnosis of bulimia nervosa is working on relationship issues. Which nursing intervention is the most important?

1. Have the client work on developing social skills.
2. Focus on how relationships cause bulimic behavior.
3. Help the client identify feelings about relationships.
4. Discuss how to prevent getting overinvolved in relationships.

5. 3. The client needs to address personal feelings, especially uncomfortable ones because they may trigger bingeing behavior. Social skills are important to a client's well-being, but they aren't typically a major problem for the client with bulimia nervosa. Relationships *don't cause* bulimic behaviors. It's the inability to handle stress or conflict that arises from interactions that causes the client to be distressed. The client isn't necessarily overinvolved in relationships; the issue may be the lack of satisfying relationships in the person's life.

CN: Psychosocial integrity; CNS: None; CL: Application

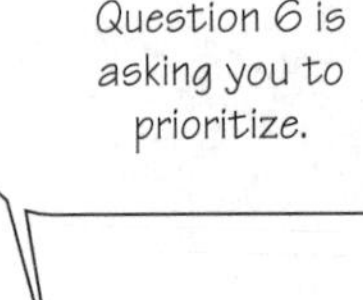
Question 6 is
asking you to
prioritize.

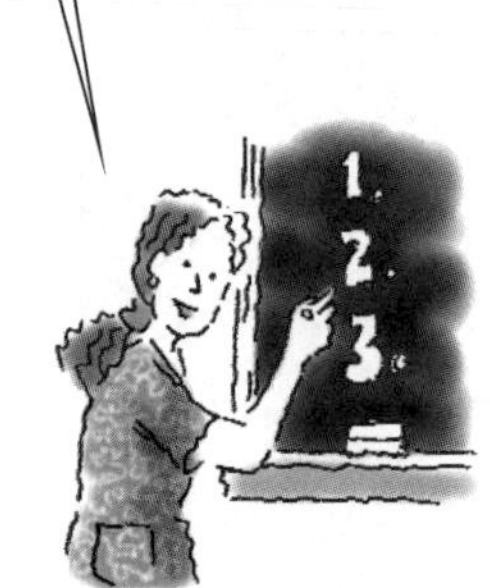
1.
2.
3.

6. A young female client with bulimia nervosa wants to lessen her feelings of powerlessness. Which short-term goal is most important initially?

1. Learn problem-solving skills.
2. Decrease symptoms of anxiety.
3. Perform self-care activities daily.
4. Verbalize how to set limits with others.

6. 1. If the client can learn effective problem-solving skills, she'll gain a sense of control and power over her life. Anxiety is commonly caused by feelings of powerlessness. Performing daily self-care activities won't reduce one's sense of powerlessness. Verbalizing how to set limits and protect self from the intrusive behavior of others is a necessary life skill, but problem-solving skills take priority.

CN: Psychosocial integrity; CNS: None; CL: Analysis

7. A female client with bulimia nervosa tells a nurse her parents don't know about her eating disorder. Which goal is appropriate for this client and her family?

1. Decrease the chaos in the family unit.
2. Learn effective communication skills.
3. Spend time together in social situations.
4. Discuss the client's need to be responsible.

7. 2. A major goal for the client and her family is to learn to communicate directly and honestly. To change the chaotic environment, the family must first learn to communicate effectively. Families with a member who has an eating disorder are often enmeshed and don't need to spend more time together. Before discussing the client's level of responsibility, the family needs to establish effective ways to communicate with each other.

CN: Psychosocial integrity; CNS: None; CL: Application

8. When discussing self-esteem with a client with bulimia nervosa, which area is the most important?

1. Personal fears
2. Family strengths
3. Negative thinking
4. Environmental stimuli

It is most important that you read question 8 carefully.

8. 3. Clients with bulimia nervosa need to work on identifying and changing their negative thinking and distortion of reality. Personal fears are related to negative thinking but isn't the most important. Exploring family strengths isn't a priority; it's more appropriate to explore the client's strengths. Environmental stimuli don't cause bulimic behaviors.

CN: Psychosocial integrity; CNS: None; CL: Application

9. Which complication of bulimia nervosa is life-threatening?

1. Serum calcium 10.1 mg/dl
2. Heart rate 56 beats/minute
3. Serum potassium 2.9 mEq/L
4. Respiratory rate 16 breaths/minute

9. 3. Electrolyte imbalance such as hypokalemia (normal serum potassium is 3.5 to 4.5 mEq/L) can be a life-threatening complication of bulimia nervosa due to purging behaviors. A serum calcium level of 10.1 mg/dl is within normal range. A heart rate of 56 beats/minute indicates bradycardia, but isn't life-threatening. A respiratory rate of 16 breaths/minute is within the normal range (16 to 20 breaths/minute) and not life-threatening.

CN: Physiological integrity; CNS: Reduction of risk potential; CL: Application

10. A nurse is talking to a client with bulimia nervosa about the complications of laxative abuse. Which statement by the client indicates that she's beginning to understand the risks associated with laxative abuse?

1. "I don't really have much taste for food, so there's no loss in getting it out of my system more quickly."
2. "Laxatives help me get rid of extra calories before they're added to my body. I know I just shouldn't eat the extra calories to begin with."
3. "Laxatives are over-the-counter medications that have no harmful effect."
4. "Using laxatives prevents my body from absorbing essential nutrients, such as protein, fat, and calcium."

10. 4. A serious complication of laxative abuse is malabsorption of nutrients, such as proteins, fats, and calcium. Laxative abuse doesn't tend to affect the client's sense of taste. Clients with bulimia nervosa need to change their negative thinking with respect to calories and the use of laxatives.

CN: Physiological integrity; CNS: Reduction of risk potential; CL: Application

11. A female client with bulimia nervosa tells a nurse she and her parents don't agree on anything. Which method is best to address this problem when the family comes for a family meeting?

1. Focus on conflict resolution skills.
2. Establish an internal locus of control.
3. Construct a three-generation genogram.
4. Discuss age-specific developmental problems.

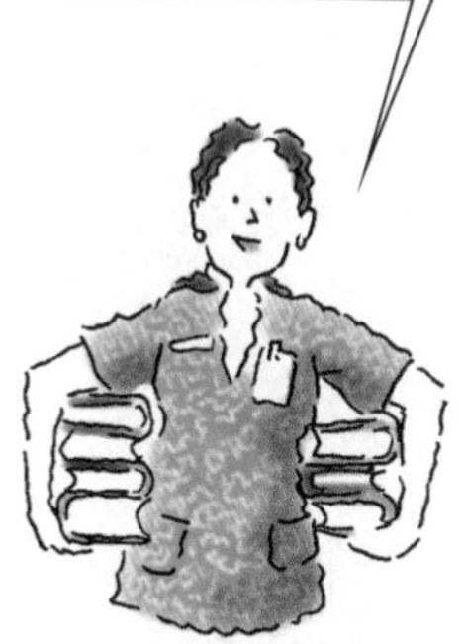

You're doing great! It looks like all your studying is paying off.

11. 1. To decrease conflict and promote family harmony, the nurse would teach the family conflict resolution skills. Establishing a plan to promote internal control or constructing a three-generation genogram won't help the family solve conflicts. Discussion of age-specific developmental problems won't promote conflict resolution or promote family harmony.

CN: Psychosocial integrity; CNS: None; CL: Application

12. A female client is talking to a nurse about her binge-purge cycle. Which question should the nurse ask about the cycle?

1. "Do you know how to stop the binge-purge cycle?"
2. "Does the binge-purge cycle help you lose weight?"
3. "Can the binge-purge cycle take away your anxiety?"
4. "How often do you go through the binge-purge cycle?"

12. 4. This is an important question because there's often a range of frequencies, such as from a once-a-week pattern to multiple times per day. The frequency of binge-purge cycles may also alert the nurse to the degree of risk from fluid and electrolyte imbalances. Asking the client if she knows how to stop the binge-purge cycle isn't appropriate as it will generate feelings of self-blame and shame. It's common for clients to experience daily fluctuations in weight (some report variations of up to 10 lb). Although the binge-purge behavior may decrease anxiety initially; it tends to generate overall negative feelings about self.

CN: Psychosocial integrity; CNS: None; CL: Application

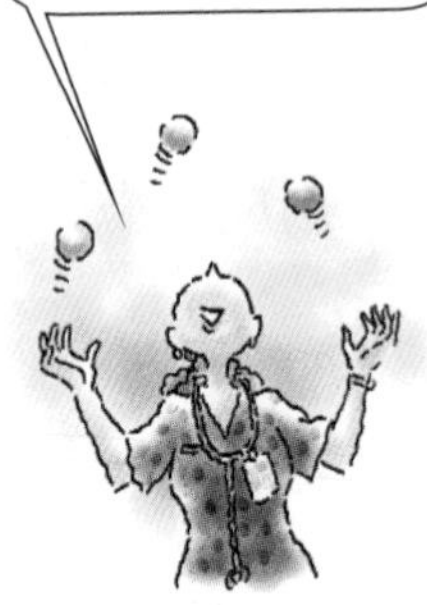

Consider all the answers. Then choose the best one.

13. A nurse is assessing a client with bulimia nervosa for possible substance abuse. Which question is best to obtain information about this possible problem?

1. "Have you ever used diet pills?"
2. "Where would you go to buy drugs?"
3. "At what age did you start drinking?"
4. "Do your peers ever offer you drugs?"

13. 1. Some clients with bulimia nervosa have a history of or actively use amphetamines to control weight. The use of alcohol and street drugs is also common. The second and fourth questions could be answered by the client without revealing drug use. The age the client started drinking may not show current substance use.

CN: Psychosocial integrity; CNS: None; CL: Application

14. A female client with bulimia nervosa is discussing her abnormal eating behaviors. Which statement by the client indicates she's beginning to understand this eating disorder?

1. "When my loneliness gets to me, I start to binge."
2. "I know that when my life gets better I'll eat right."
3. "I know I waste food and waste my money on food."
4. "After my parents divorce, I'll talk about bingeing and purging."

14. 1. Binge eating is a way to handle the uncomfortable feelings of frustration, loneliness, anger, and fear. The second option indicates the client is experiencing denial of the eating disorder. The third option addresses the client's guilt feelings; it doesn't reflect knowledge of her eating disorder. The fourth option shows the client isn't ready to discuss her eating disorder.

CN: Psychosocial integrity; CNS: None; CL: Analysis

15. A nurse is assessing a client with a history of recent binge eating. Which of the following symptoms would the nurse most likely observe in this client?

1. Ageusia
2. Headache
3. Pain
4. Sore throat

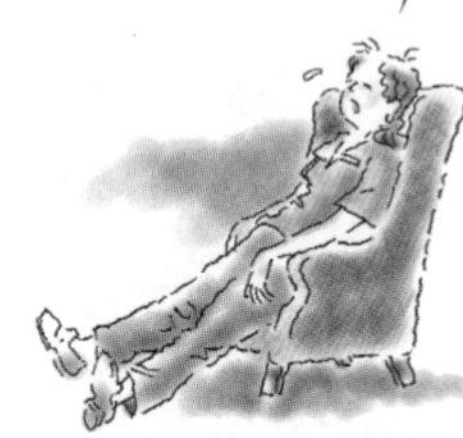

I think I ate too much!

15. 3. After a binge episode, the client commonly has abdominal distention and stomach pain. A sore throat is associated with vomiting. Ageusia (loss of taste) or headache aren't associated with binge eating.

CN: Physiological integrity; CNS: Physiological adaptation; CL: Application

CN: Client needs category CNS: Client needs subcategory CL: Cognitive level

16. A mother of a female client with bulimia nervosa asks a nurse if bulimia nervosa will stop her daughter from menstruating. Which response is best?

1. "All women with anorexia nervosa or bulimia nervosa will have amenorrhea."
2. "When your daughter is bingeing and purging, she won't have normal periods."
3. "The eating disorder must be ongoing for your daughter's menstrual cycle to change."
4. "Women with bulimia nervosa may have a normal or abnormal menstrual cycle, depending on the severity of the problem."

16. 4. Women with bulimia nervosa may have a normal or abnormal menstrual cycle, depending on the severity of the eating disorder. Not all women with eating disorders have amenorrhea. The eating disorder can disrupt the menstrual cycle at any point in the illness.

CN: Health promotion and maintenance; CNS: None; CL: Analysis

17. Which nursing diagnosis should have the highest priority in the plan of care for a client with an eating disorder?

1. *Interrupted family processes*
2. *Imbalanced nutrition: Less than body requirements*
3. *Disturbed body image*
4. *Ineffective coping*

17. 2. The most immediate priority is to meet the nutritional needs of the client to prevent complications. The other nursing diagnoses are all important long-term goals that can be addressed once the client's immediate physiologic needs have been met.

CN: Safe, effective care environment; CNS: Management of care; CL: Analysis

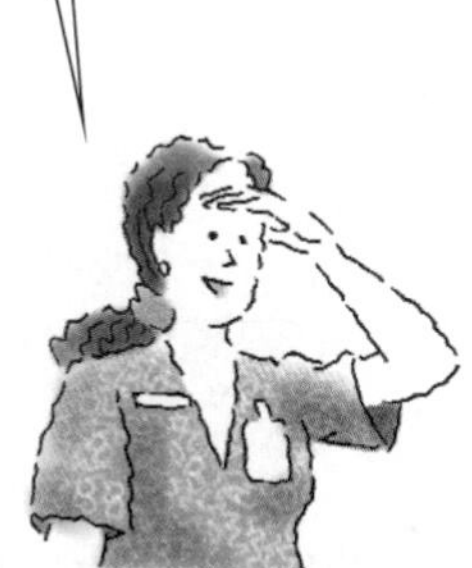

Help the client see the importance of reaching a short-term goal.

18. A female client with bulimia nervosa tells a nurse her major problem is eating too much food in a short period of time and then vomiting. Which short-term goal is the <u>most important</u>?

1. Help the client understand every person has a satiety level.
2. Encourage the client to verbalize fears and concerns about food.
3. Determine the amount of food the client will eat without purging.
4. Obtain a therapy appointment to look at the emotional causes of bulimia nervosa.

18. 3. The client must meet her nutritional needs to prevent further complications, so she must identify the amount of food she can eat without purging as her first short-term goal. Binge eaters can't recognize their satiety level or their feelings of fullness. Obtaining knowledge or verbalizing her fears and feelings about food are *not* priority goals for this client. After meeting immediate physiological needs, therapy is an important part of dealing with this disorder.

CN: Physiological integrity; CNS: Reduction of risk potential; CL: Application

19. Which statement indicates a female client with bulimia nervosa is making progress in interrupting the binge-purge cycle?

1. "I called my friend the last two times I got upset."
2. "I know I'll have this problem with eating forever."
3. "I started asking my mother or sister to watch me eat each meal."
4. "I can have my boyfriend bring me home from parties if I want to purge."

19. 1. A sign of progress is when the client begins to verbalize feelings and interact with people instead of going to food for comfort. The second option indicates the client needs more information on how to handle the disorder. Having another person watch the client eat isn't a helpful strategy as the client will depend on others to help control food intake. The last option indicates the client is in denial about the severity of the problem.

CN: Psychosocial integrity; CNS: None; CL: Analysis

20. A client with bulimia nervosa asks a nurse, "How can I ask for help from my family?" Which response is the most appropriate?

1. "When you ask for help, make sure you really need it."
2. "Have you ever asked for help before?"
3. "Ask family members to spend time with you at mealtime."
4. "Think about how you can handle this situation without help."

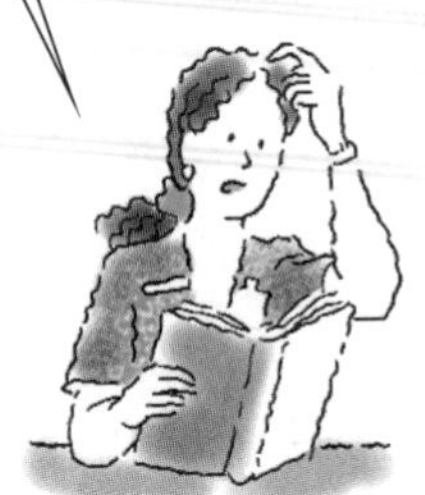

Is most appropriate the same as "prioritize?"

20. 2. Determine whether the client has ever been successful in asking for help. Previous experiences affect the client's ability to ask for help now. The client needs to ask for help anytime without analyzing the level of need. Having other people around at mealtime isn't the only way to ask for help. Developing a support system is imperative for this client.

CN: Psychosocial integrity; CNS: None; CL: Analysis

21. A female client with bulimia nervosa tells a nurse that she doesn't eat during the day, but after 5:00 p.m., she begins to binge and vomit. Which intervention should be the most useful to this client?

1. Help the client stop eating the foods on which she binges.
2. Discuss the effects of fasting on the client's pattern of eating.
3. Encourage the client to become involved in food preparation.
4. Teach the client to eat earlier in the day and decrease intake at night.

21. 2. If a person fasts for most of the day, it's common to become extremely hungry, overeat by bingeing, and then feel the need to purge. Restricting food intake can actually trigger the binge-purge cycle. In treatment, the client is taught to identify foods that trigger eating, discuss the feelings associated with these foods, and work to eat them in normal amounts. Involvement in food preparation won't promote changes in the client's behaviors. The last option doesn't address how fasting can trigger the binge-purge cycle.

CN: Psychosocial integrity; CNS: None; CL: Application

22. A female client with bulimia nervosa tells a nurse she was doing well until last week, when she had a fight with her father. Which nursing intervention should help most?

1. Examine the relationship between feelings and eating.
2. Discuss the importance of therapy for the entire family.
3. Encourage the client to avoid certain family members.
4. Identify daily stressors and learn stress management skills.

22. 1. The client needs to understand her feelings and develop healthy coping skills to handle unpleasant situations. Family therapy may be indicated but shouldn't be an immediate intervention. Avoidance isn't a useful coping strategy; eventually the underlying issues need to be explored. All clients can benefit from stress management skills, but for this client, care must focus on the relationship between feelings and eating behaviors.

CN: Psychosocial integrity; CNS: None; CL: Application

23. Which statement from a bulimic client shows that she understands the concept of relapse?

1. "If I can't maintain control over things, I'll have problems."
2. "If I have problems, then that says I haven't learned much."
3. "If this illness becomes chronic, I won't be able to handle it."
4. "If I have problems, I can start over again and not feel hopeless."

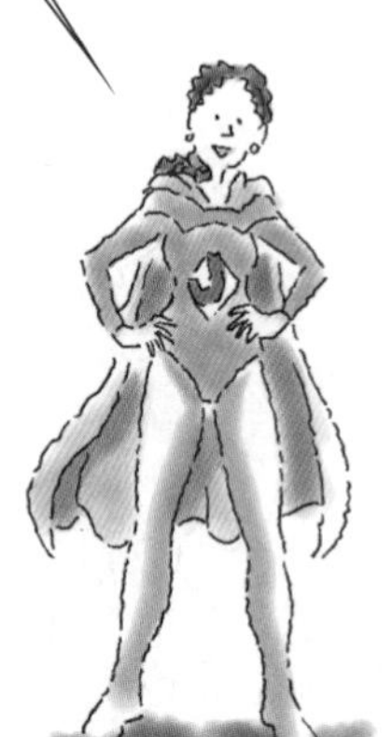

If at first you don't succeed. Try try again—to choose the correct answer.

23. 4. This statement indicates that the client knows a relapse is just a slip, and positive gains made from treatment haven't been lost. Negative self-statements can lead to relapse. Control issues relate to powerlessness, which contribute to relapse.

CN: Psychosocial integrity; CNS: None; CL: Application

24. What's the treatment team's <u>priority</u> in planning the care of a client with an eating disorder?

1. Preventing the client from performing any muscle-building exercises
2. Keeping the client on bedrest until she attains a specified weight
3. Meeting daily to discuss manipulation and countertransference
4. Monitoring the client's weight and vital signs daily

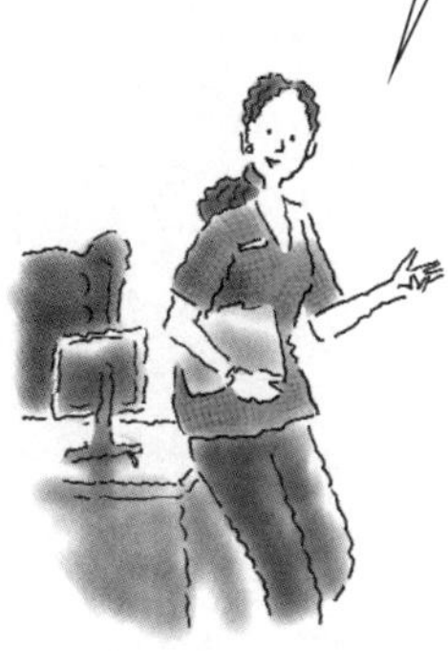

24. 3. Clients with eating disorders commonly use manipulative ploys and countertransference to resist weight gain (if they restrict food intake) or to maintain purging practices (if they're bulimic). Such clients commonly play staff members against one another. Muscle building is acceptable because it burns relatively few calories. Keeping the client on bedrest until a specified weight is reached may result in power struggles and prevent focusing on pertinent issues. Monitoring the client's weight and vital signs is important but not on a daily basis unless the client's condition warrants such scrutiny.

CN: Psychosocial integrity; CN: None; CL: Application

25. A nurse should be alert for which findings in a client with bulimia nervosa? Select all that apply:

1. Severe electrolyte imbalances
2. Damaged teeth due to the eroding effects of gastric acids on tooth enamel
3. Pneumonia from aspirated stomach contents
4. Cessation of menses
5. Esophageal tears and gastric rupture
6. Intestinal inflammation

25. 1, 2, 4, 5. Constant bingeing and purging behaviors can result in severe electrolyte imbalances, erosion of tooth enamel from constant exposure to gastric acids, menstrual irregularities, esophageal tears and, in severe cases, gastric rupture. Aspiration pneumonia is unlikely because the vomiting is controlled. Intestinal inflammation isn't typically associated with bulimia nervosa.

CN: Physiological integrity; CNS: Physiological adaptation; CL: Application

26. A client with anorexia nervosa attended psychoeducational sessions on principles of adequate nutrition. Which statement by the client indicates the teaching was effective?

1. "I eat while I'm doing things to distract myself."
2. "I eat all my food at night right before I go to bed."
3. "I eat small amounts of food slowly at every meal."
4. "I eat only when I'm with my family and trying to be social."

26. 3. Slowly eating small amounts of food facilitates adequate digestion and prevents distention. Healthy eating is best accomplished when a person isn't doing other things while eating. Eating right before bedtime isn't a healthy eating habit. If a client eats only when the family is present or when trying to be social, eating is tied to social or emotional cues rather than nutritional needs.

CN: Health promotion and maintenance; CNS: None; CL: Application

27. A client with anorexia nervosa tells a nurse, "I'll never have the slender body I want." Which intervention is <u>best</u> to handle this problem?

1. Call a family meeting to get help from the parents.
2. Help the client work on developing a realistic body image.
3. Make an appointment to see the dietitian on a weekly basis.
4. Develop an exercise program the client can do twice a week.

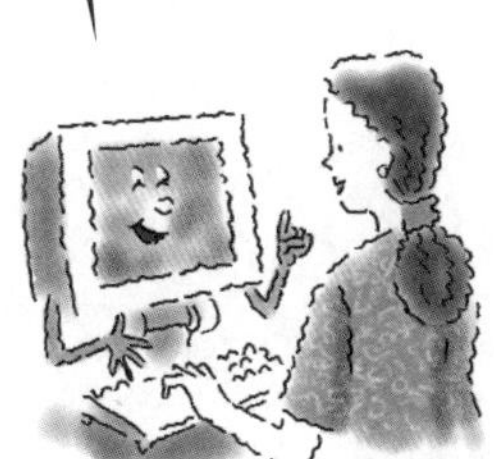

All options may
be good, but choose
the best one.

27. 2. With anorexia nervosa, the client pursues thinness and has a distorted view of self. A family meeting may not help the client develop a more realistic view of the body. Although meeting with a dietitian might be helpful, it isn't a priority. Clients with anorexia nervosa typically exercise excessively.

CN: Psychosocial integrity; CNS: None; CL: Application

28. A client with anorexia nervosa tells a nurse, "My parents never hug me or say I've done anything right." Which intervention is the best to use with this family?

1. Teach the family principles of assertive behavior.
2. Discuss the difficulties the family has in social situations.
3. Help the family convey a positive attitude toward the client.
4. Explore the family's ability to express affection appropriately.

28. 4. There's often a lack of affection and warmth in families who have a member with an eating disorder. Although assertiveness is an important skill, the family member needs to realize assertiveness isn't always rewarded. Difficulties in social situations are important to address, but the intervention must focus on how to express positive feelings and affection. A positive attitude helps a person become better able to handle the pressures of life, but it may not change the family's display of affection.
CN: Psychosocial integrity; CNS: None; CL: Application

29. Which communication strategy is best to use with a client with anorexia nervosa who is having problems with peer relationships?

1. Use concrete language and maintain a focus on reality.
2. Direct the client to talk about what is causing the anxiety.
3. Teach the client to communicate feelings and express self appropriately.
4. Confront the client about being depressed and self-absorbed.

29. 3. Clients with anorexia nervosa often communicate on a superficial level and avoid expressing feelings. Identifying feelings and learning to express them are initial steps in decreasing isolation. Clients with anorexia nervosa are usually able to discuss abstract and concrete issues. Discussions shouldn't be limited to the client's feelings of anxiety as the client may not be aware of the cause of the anxiety, which may result in misdirected self-reflection. Confrontation usually isn't an effective communication strategy as it may cause the client to withdraw and become more depressed.
CN: Psychosocial integrity; CNS: None; CL: Application

30. A nurse plans to include the parents of a client with anorexia nervosa in therapy sessions along with the client. What fact should the nurse remember about parents of clients with anorexia?

1. They tend to overprotect their children.
2. They usually have a history of substance abuse.
3. They maintain emotional distance from their children.
4. They alternate between loving and rejecting their children.

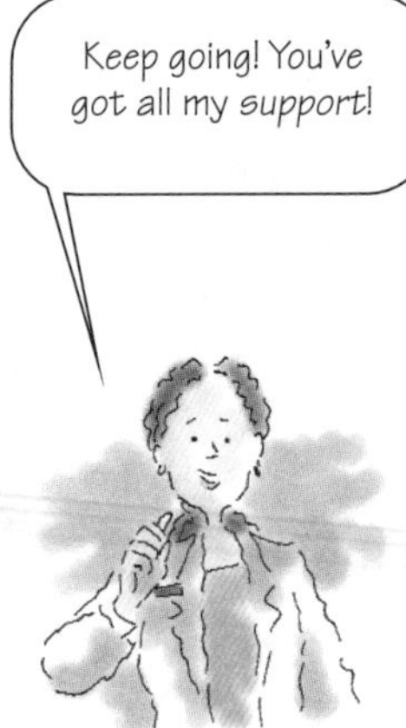

Keep going! You've got all my support!

30. 1. Clients with anorexia nervosa typically come from a family with parents who are controlling and overprotective. These clients use eating to gain control of an aspect of their lives. Having a history of substance abuse, maintaining an emotional distance, and alternating between love and rejection aren't typical characteristics of parents of children with anorexia nervosa.
CN: Psychological integrity; CNS: None; CL: Application

31. A nurse is talking to a family of a client with anorexia nervosa. Which family behavior is most likely to be seen during the family's interaction?

1. Sibling rivalry
2. Rage reactions
3. Parental disagreement
4. Excessive independence

31. 3. In many families with a member with anorexia nervosa, there is marital conflict and parental disagreement. Sibling rivalry is a common occurrence and not specific to a family with a member with anorexia nervosa. Emotions are overcontrolled and there's difficulty appropriately expressing negative feelings. In these families, the members tend to be enmeshed and dependent on each other.

CN: Psychosocial integrity; CNS: None; CL: Application

32. A nurse is working with a female client with anorexia nervosa who has acrocyanosis in her extremities. Which short-term goal is the most important for the client?

1. Do daily range-of-motion exercises.
2. Eat some fatty foods daily.
3. Check neurologic reflexes.
4. Promote adequate circulation.

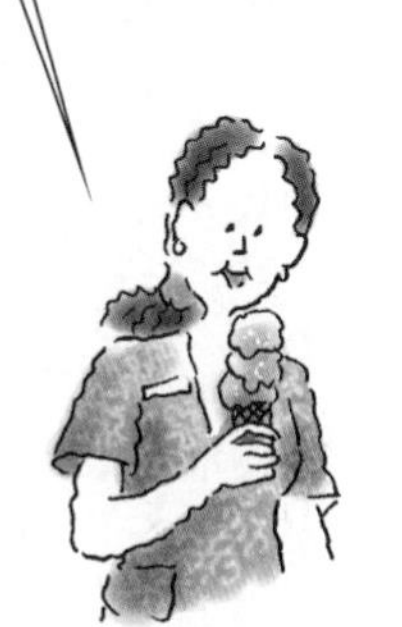

Fatty foods are almost never the right answer!

32. 4. Circulation changes will cause extremities to be cold, numb, and have dry and flaky skin. Exercise may help prevent contractures and muscle atrophy, but it may have only a limited secondary effect on promoting circulation. Intake of fatty foods won't have an impact on the client's skin problems. Checking neurologic reflexes won't necessarily assist with handling skin problems.

CN: Physiological integrity; CNS: Reduction of risk potential; CL: Application

33. A female client with anorexia nervosa is discharged from the hospital after gaining 12 lb. Which statement by the client best indicates that the nurse's reinforcement of discharge teachings has been effective?

1. "I plan to eat two small meals a day."
2. "I feel that this is scary, but I'm not going to write about it in my journal."
3. "I have to diet because I've gained 12 pounds."
4. "I'll need to attend therapy for support to stay healthy."

33. 4. The client is planning to attend therapy after discharge, which shows an understanding of the need for continued counseling. Eating only two small meals a day is an unrealistic plan for meeting nutritional needs. Feeling insecure when leaving a controlled environment is a common response to discharge. Gaining 12 pounds indicates that the client's nutritional needs are being met at the present caloric intake.

CN: Psychosocial integrity; CNS: None; CL: Analysis

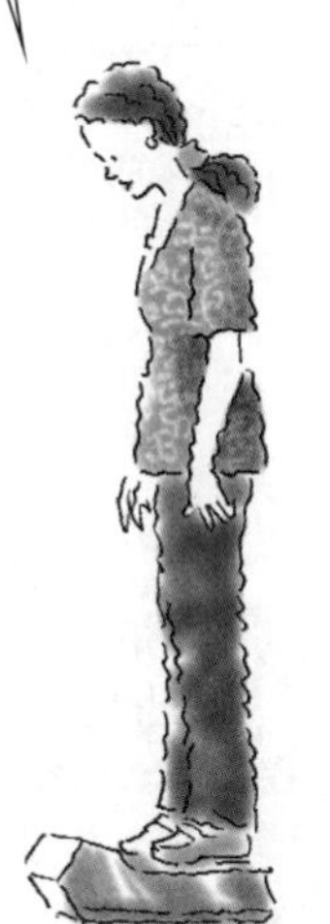

34. A female client with anorexia nervosa tells a nurse she always feels fat. Which intervention is the best for this client?

1. Talk about how important the client is.
2. Encourage her to look at herself in a mirror.
3. Address the dynamics of the disorder.
4. Talk about how she's different from her peers.

34. 3. The client can benefit from understanding the underlying dynamics of the eating disorder. The client with anorexia nervosa has low self-esteem and won't believe the positive statements. Although the client may look at herself in the mirror, in her mind she'll still see herself as fat. Pointing out differences will only diminish her already low self-esteem.

CN: Psychosocial integrity; CNS: None; CL: Application

35. The grandparents of a client with anorexia nervosa want to support the client, but aren't sure what they should do. Which intervention is best?

1. Promote positive expressions of affection.
2. Encourage behaviors that enhance socialization.
3. Discuss how eating disorders create powerlessness.
4. Discuss the meaning of hunger and body sensations.

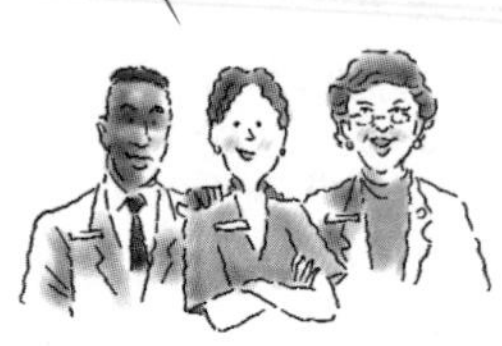

Care plans encourage staff to work toward the same goals.

35. 1. Clients with eating disorders need emotional support and expressions of affection from family members. It wouldn't be an appropriate strategy to have the grandparents promote socialization. Although clients with eating disorders feel powerless, it's better to have the grandparents focus on something positive. Talking about hunger and other sensations won't give the grandparents useful strategies.
CN: Psychosocial integrity; CNS: None; CL: Application

36. A nurse is analyzing the need for health teaching in a female client with anorexia nervosa who lives in a chaotic family situation. Which question is most important for the nurse to ask the client?

1. "How many months have your periods been irregular?"
2. "How often do you think about food in a 24-hour period?"
3. "What were the circumstances before your eating disorder?"
4. "How much and what kinds of exercise do you engage in every day?"

36. 3. This question lets the nurse get information about the family and background situations that influenced the client's needs and distorted eating. The other options deal with menstrual history, exercise patterns, and food obsessions. Although they're relevant, they don't provide information related to the family situation.
CN: Psychosocial integrity; CNS: None; CL: Analysis

37. An adolescent female client with anorexia nervosa tells a nurse about her outstanding academic achievements and her thoughts about suicide. Which factor must the nurse consider when making a care plan for this client?

1. Self-esteem
2. Physical illnesses
3. Paranoid delusions
4. Relationship avoidance

37. 1. The client lacks self-esteem, which contributes to her level of depression and feelings of personal ineffectiveness, which in turn may lead to suicidal thoughts. Physical illnesses are common with clients with anorexia nervosa, but they don't relate to this situation. Paranoid delusions refer to false ideas that others want to harm you. No evidence exists that this client is socially isolated.
CN: Psychosocial integrity; CNS: None; CL: Analysis

38. In making a care plan for a family with a member who has anorexia nervosa, which information should be included?

1. Coping mechanisms used in the past
2. Concerns about changes in lifestyle and daily activities
3. Rejection of feedback from family and significant others
4. Appropriate eating habits and social behaviors centering on eating

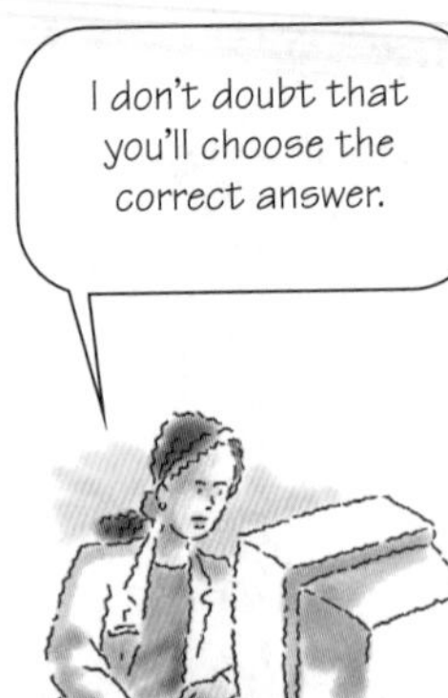

I don't doubt that you'll choose the correct answer.

38. 1. Examination of positive and negative coping mechanisms used by the family allows the nurse to build a care plan specific to the family's strengths and weaknesses. The way the family copes with concerns is more important than the concerns themselves. Feedback from the family and significant others is vital when building a care plan. Eating habits and behaviors are symptoms of the way people cope with problems.
CN: Psychosocial integrity; CNS: None; CL: Application

CN: Client needs category CNS: Client needs subcategory CL: Cognitive level

39. Which goal is best to help a client with anorexia nervosa recognize self-distortions?

1. Identify the client's misperceptions of self.
2. Acknowledge immature and childlike behaviors.
3. Determine the consequences of a faulty support system.
4. Recognize the age-appropriate tasks to be accomplished.

39. 1. Questioning the client's misperceptions and distortions will create doubt about how the client views himself. Acknowledging immature behaviors or determining the consequences of a faulty support system won't promote client recognition of self-distortions. Recognizing the age-appropriate tasks to be accomplished by the client won't help the client recognize distortions.
CN: Psychosocial integrity; CNS: None; CL: Analysis

40. Parents of a client with anorexia nervosa ask about the risk factors for this disorder. After the parents receive reinforcement of the teaching plan from the nurse, which statement by the parents best indicates that the teaching has been effective?

1. "Risk factors include the inability to be still and emotional lability."
2. "Risk factors include a high level of anxiety and disorganized behavior."
3. "Risk factors include low self-esteem and problems with family relationships."
4. "Risk factors include a lack of life experience and no opportunities to learn skills."

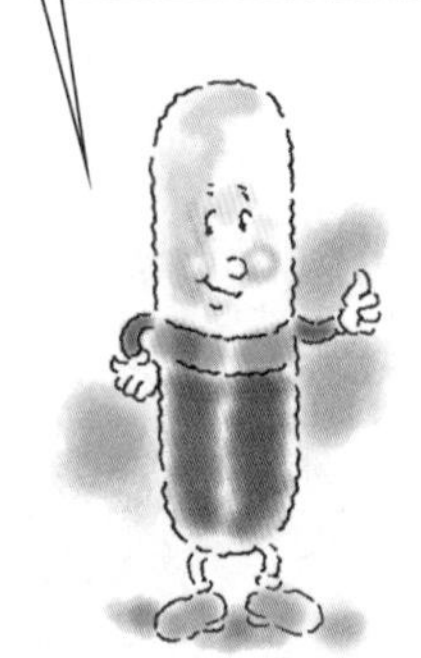

Knowing adverse reactions to key drugs is important.

40. 3. There are several risk factors for eating disorders, including low self-esteem, history of depression, substance abuse, and dysfunctional family relationships. Restlessness and emotional lability are symptoms of manic depressive illness. Anxiety and disorganized behavior could be signs of a psychotic disorder. A lack of life experiences and an absence of opportunities to learn life skills may be a result of anorexia nervosa.
CN: Psychosocial integrity; CNS: None; CL: Analysis

41. A client with anorexia nervosa has started taking fluoxetine hydrochloride (Prozac). The nurse should closely monitor the client for which adverse reaction?

1. Drowsiness
2. Dry mouth
3. Light-headedness
4. Nausea

41. 4. Nausea is an adverse reaction to the drug that compounds the eating disorder problem, and the client must be closely monitored. Although the adverse reactions of drowsiness, dry mouth, or light-headedness may occur, they aren't likely to interfere with treatment.
CN: Physiological integrity; CNS: Pharmacological and parenteral therapies; CL: Application

42. A client with anorexia nervosa is worried about rectal bleeding. Which question should be asked to obtain more information about this problem?

1. "How often do you use laxatives?"
2. "How many days ago did you stop vomiting?"
3. "Are you eating anything that causes irritation?"
4. "Do you have bleeding before or after exercise?"

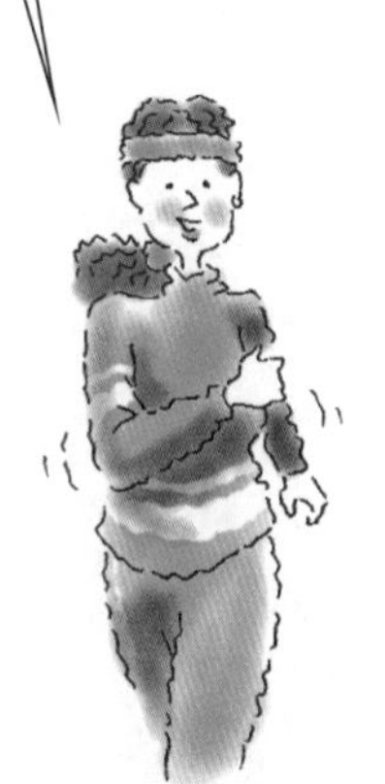

You're heading down the home stretch! Keep going!

42. 1. Excessive use of laxatives will cause GI irritation and rectal bleeding. If the client stopped vomiting but is still using laxatives, rectal bleeding can occur. Clients who are anorexic eat very little, and what they eat won't cause rectal bleeding. Exercise doesn't cause rectal bleeding.
CN: Health promotion and maintenance; CNS: None; CL: Application

43. A female client with anorexia nervosa tells a nurse that she has developed hair on most of her body. Which of the following disorders would the nurse most likely expect to be associated with anorexia nervosa?

1. Anemia
2. Osteoporosis
3. Dehydration
4. Electrolyte imbalance

43. 3. When a client with anorexia nervosa has fine hair all over her body (lanugo), the nurse would perform a more extensive assessment of the skin. Lanugo indicates dehydration due to starvation. Anemia is associated with hematologic complications. Osteoporosis is associated with the musculoskeletal system. Electrolyte imbalance is associated with body metabolism.
CN: Health promotion and maintenance; CNS: None; CL: Application

44. A female client with anorexia nervosa is talking to a nurse about her group therapy. Which statement shows the group experience has helped the client?

1. "I feel I'm different and I don't need a lot of friends."
2. "I'll tell my parents it's not just me who has problems."
3. "I can see how to do things better and become the best."
4. "I think I have some unrealistic expectations of myself."

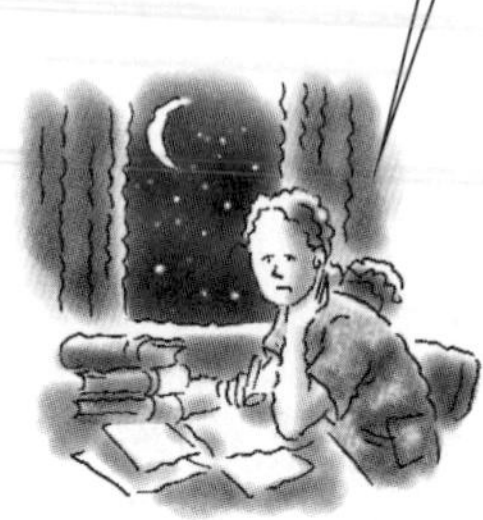

My plan to study
all night is starting
to seem unrealistic.

44. 4. A goal of group therapy is to provide methods to assess whether personal expectations are unrealistic. Other goals are to learn to handle problems; not to blame parents or others; decrease perfectionist tendencies; and decrease isolation and learn to have healthy peer relationships.

CN: Psychosocial integrity; CNS: None; CL: Application

45. A nurse and her female client who has anorexia nervosa are working on the goal of developing social relationships. Which action by the client is an indication the client is meeting her goal?

1. The client talks about the value of peer relationships.
2. The client decides to talk to her parents about her friends.
3. The client expresses the need to establish trust relationships.
4. The client attends an activity without prompting from others.

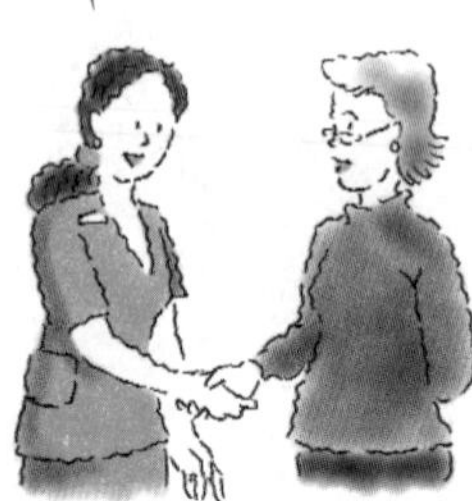

The client must
agree to the goal or
it won't work.

45. 4. When a client with anorexia nervosa attends an activity without prompting from others, it's a positive sign the client is working toward developing social relationships. Talking about the value of relationships is also beneficial but is only the first step in establishing them. Talking to parents about friends is a start but doesn't necessarily indicate that the client can establish relationships. Expressing the need to establish trust relationships is a first step, but an indication of success would be actually initiating such a relationship.

CN: Psychosocial integrity; CNS: None; CL: Application

46. What initial action should a nurse take when a young female client with anorexia nervosa says, "I'll try to eat something"?

1. Provide a small portion of a healthy food.
2. Weigh the client before and after eating.
3. Ask the client what she thinks she can eat.
4. Suggest the client drink something before eating.

46. 1. Small amounts of food won't overwhelm the client when given at frequent intervals. They also won't overtax the GI and cardiac systems. Weighing the client before and after meals is a useless, stress-provoking action. Asking the client questions may provoke anxiety. It's better to give the client food when she asks. Drinking something before eating isn't necessary; the fluid may prevent the client from being able to eat a sufficient amount of the food.

CN: Physiological integrity; CNS: Reduction of risk potential; CL: Application

47. A client with anorexia nervosa tells a nurse, "I feel so awful and inadequate." Which response is best?

1. "You're being too hard on yourself."
2. "Someday you'll feel better about things."
3. "Tell me something you like about yourself."
4. "Maybe relaxing by yourself will help you feel better."

47. 3. This statement redirects the client to talk about positive aspects of self. The other options minimize her feelings or don't address the client's concerns or encourage the client to change her self-image.

CN: Psychosocial integrity; CNS: None; CL: Application

48. Which of the following is the priority during assessment of a client with an eating disorder?
1. Cultural and gender needs
2. Substance abuse history
3. Academic achievement and performance
4. Level of danger to self or others

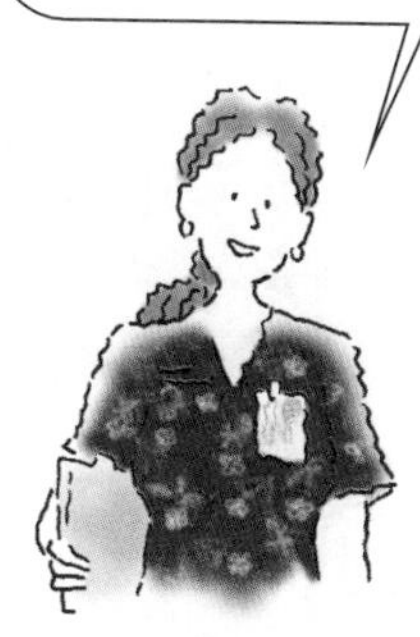

The term priority indicates that you should select the answer which would be of first concern during assessment.

48. 4. The priority in assessment should be to determine if the client is a danger to herself or to others. Cultural and gender needs, substance abuse history, and academic performance are an important part of assessment but not the priority.

CN: Safe, effective care environment; CNS: Management of care; CL: Analysis

49. An adolescent female client with anorexia nervosa starts outpatient treatment. Which client statement indicates that she has a basic understanding of her eating disorder?
1. "I'm not worried because no one ever dies from anorexia."
2. "I still feel fat even though I'm told that I'm not."
3. "My old school friends aren't important to me anymore."
4. "I don't feel right unless I do an intense workout every day."

49. 2. A client with anorexia nervosa shows a basic understanding of the disorder if she can talk about feeling fat even though she's actually underweight, or if she expresses an intense fear of gaining weight. Anorexia nervosa has a mortality of approximately 10% to 15%. People with eating disorders tend to isolate themselves from friends and family members because of their intense focus on food, weight, and exercise. A client with anorexia nervosa may exercise compulsively to prevent weight gain; this behavior indicates continuing presence of the eating disorder.

CN: Psychosocial integrity; CNS: None; CL: Analysis

50. Which question is most useful in assessing the self-esteem of a client with anorexia nervosa?
1. "How would you describe yourself to others?"
2. "What activities do you enjoy doing with your friends?"
3. "Do you play any sports at school or in your community?"
4. "How do you decide how to spend your free time?"

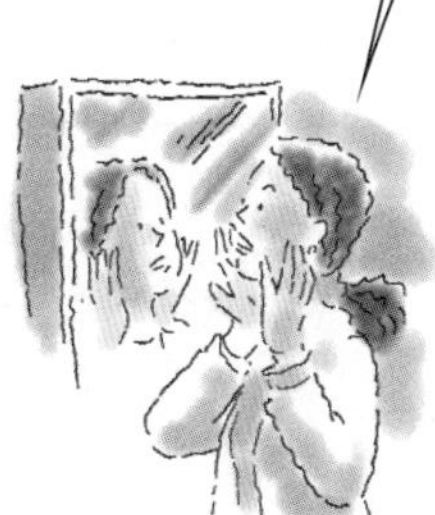

Do others see me as I see myself?

50. 1. Clients with anorexia nervosa tend to have low self-esteem even if they're high achievers in school, activities, and sports; asking for a self-description can uncover the client's distorted body image and low self-esteem. Questions about activities with friends, involvement in sports, or how the client decides to spend her free time don't necessarily elicit information about self-esteem.

CN: Psychosocial integrity; CNS: None; CL: Analysis

51. Which psychosocial finding should a nurse expect when assessing a client with anorexia nervosa?
1. Avoidant behavior
2. Antisocial behavior
3. Introverted behavior
4. Hypervigilant behavior

51. 3. Clients with anorexia nervosa typically demonstrate introverted behavior. Clients with bulimia, not anorexia nervosa, tend to show avoidant and dependent behaviors. Clients with eating disorders don't necessarily demonstrate antisocial behavior. Hypervigilant behavior is common in clients with posttraumatic stress disorder, not eating disorders.

CN: Psychosocial integrity; CNS: None; CL: Analysis

52. A nurse notes severe hypocalcemia in a client with anorexia nervosa. Which history finding supports a diagnosis of osteoporosis?

1. Eating a vegetarian diet
2. Drinking well water
3. Going scuba diving
4. Smoking cigarettes

52. 4. Hypocalcemia and cigarette smoking increase the risk for osteoporosis. Eating a vegetarian diet, drinking well water, and going scuba diving don't predispose the client to osteoporosis.
CN: Physiological integrity; CNS: Reduction of risk potential; CL: Analysis

53. A female client with anorexia nervosa is receiving care from her family after successfully completing the refeeding stage of treatment. Which nursing intervention takes priority at this time?

1. Providing a strong support system and opportunities to do reality testing
2. Teaching the family stress-reduction skills to help promote family harmony
3. Promoting anticipatory grieving over the loss each family member is experiencing
4. Assisting the family to work on the issues of autonomy and separation

53. 4. When a client with anorexia nervosa successfully completes the refeeding stage of treatment, the family must work on separation and individuation of the client and on decreasing family rigidity and overprotectiveness. Although the client needs a strong support system, developing a sense of self is more important at this time; also, reality testing isn't a typical problem in clients with eating disorders. All families can benefit from learning stress-reduction skills; however, at this time, these skills take lower priority than developing client independence. Anticipatory grieving isn't particularly relevant for family members of a client with an eating disorder.
CN: Psychosocial integrity; CNS: None; CL: Application

54. A client with bulimia nervosa has a history of severe GI problems caused by excessive purging. Based on this finding, the nurse must stay alert for which physiologic problem?

1. Renal calculi
2. Esophageal tears
3. Focal seizures
4. Muscle atrophy

54. 2. A bulimic client with severe GI problems from excessive purging is at increased risk for esophageal tears and irritation or esophagitis. Although clients with eating disorders may develop renal calculi, this client is at greater risk for developing esophageal tears. Focal seizures and muscle atrophy aren't related to severe GI problems.
CN: Physiological integrity; CNS: Reduction of risk potential; CL: Analysis

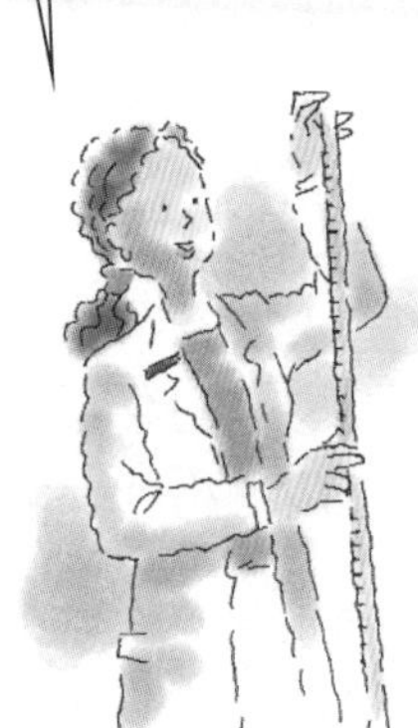

Good for you! It looks like you really measure up!

55. A nurse is caring for an anorexic client with a nursing diagnosis of *Imbalanced nutrition: Less than body requirements* related to dysfunctional eating patterns. Which interventions would be supportive for this client? Select all that apply:

1. Provide small, frequent meals.
2. Monitor weight gain.
3. Allow the client to skip meals until the anti-depressant levels are therapeutic.
4. Encourage the client to keep a journal.
5. Encourage the client to eat three substantial meals per day.

55. 1, 2, 4. Due to self-starvation, clients with anorexia can rarely tolerate large meals three times per day. Small, frequent meals may be tolerated better by the anorexic client and they provide a way to gradually increase daily caloric intake. The nurse should monitor the client's weight carefully because a client with anorexia may try to hide weight loss. The client may be emotionally restrained and afraid to express her feelings; therefore, keeping a journal can serve as an outlet for these feelings, which can assist recovery. An anorexic client is already underweight and shouldn't be permitted to skip meals.
CN: Health promotion and maintenance; CNS: None; CL: Analysis

Part IV Maternal-neonatal care

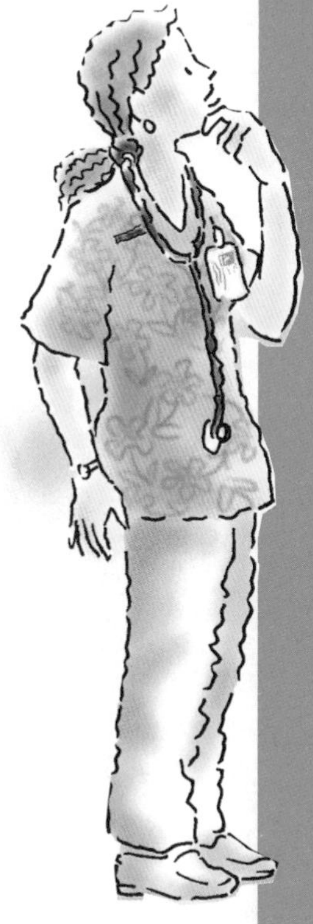

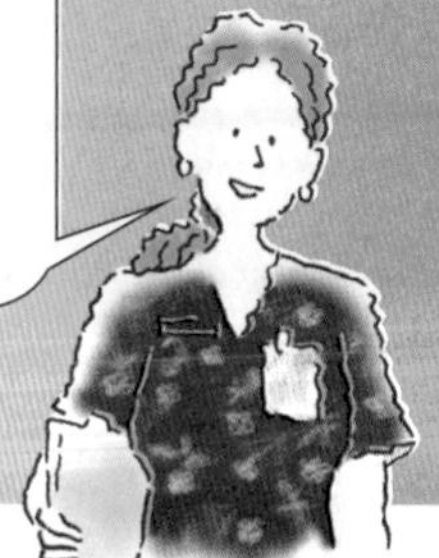

Chapter 22 Antepartum care

1. During an examination, a client who's 32 weeks pregnant becomes dizzy, lightheaded, and pale. While the client is lying supine, which nursing intervention should take priority?

1. Listen to fetal heart tones.
2. Take the client's blood pressure.
3. Ask the client to breathe deeply.
4. Turn the client on her left side.

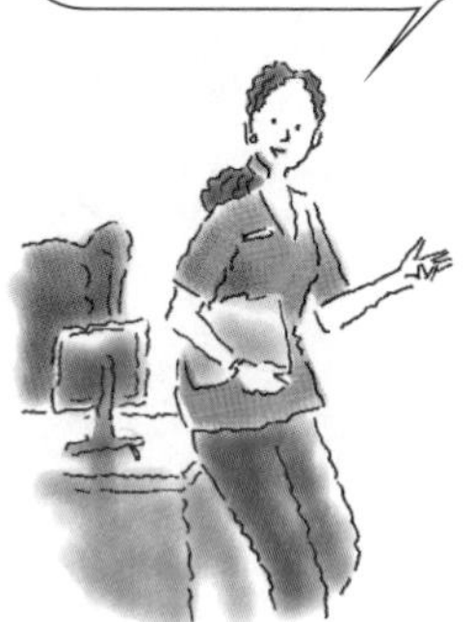

1. 4. As the enlarging uterus increases pressure on the inferior vena cava, it compromises venous return, which can cause dizziness, light-headedness, and pallor when the client is supine. The nurse can relieve these symptoms by turning the client on her left side, which relieves pressure on the vena cava and restores venous return. Although they're valuable assessments, fetal heart tone and maternal blood pressure measurements don't correct the problem. Because deep breathing has no effect on venous return, it can't relieve the client's symptoms.

CN: Safe, effective care environment; CNS: Management of care; CL: Analysis

2. A nurse is assessing a client at 33 weeks' gestation. Leopold's maneuvers indicate that the fetus is in a breech position. Which is the best location for the nurse to auscultate fetal heart tones?

1. Midway between the symphysis pubis and the umbilicus
2. Right lower quadrant of the abdomen
3. Right upper quadrant of the abdomen
4. Above the level of the umbilicus

2. 4. When the fetus is in the breech position, fetal heart tones are best heard at or above the level of the umbilicus.

CN: Health promotion and maintenance; CNS: None; CL: Application

3. In twin-to-twin transfusion syndrome, the arterial circulation of one twin is in communication with the venous circulation of the other twin. One fetus is considered the "donor" twin and one becomes the "recipient" twin. Assessment of the recipient twin would most likely show which condition?

1. Anemia
2. Oligohydramnios
3. Polycythemia
4. Small fetus

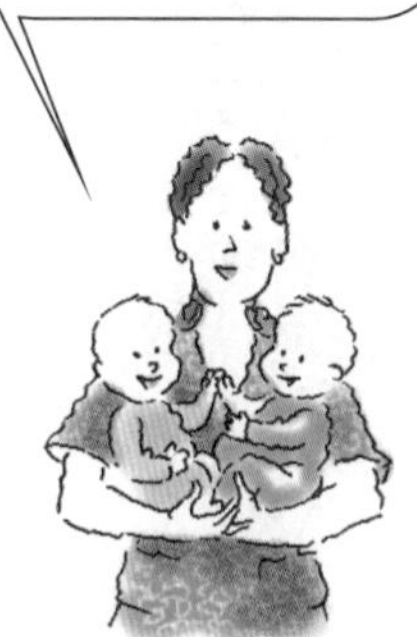

Careful. Question 3 asks about the *recipient* twin, not the donor.

3. 3. The recipient twin in twin-twin transfusion syndrome is transfused by the other twin. The recipient twin then becomes polycythemic and often has heart failure due to circulatory overload. The donor twin becomes anemic. The recipient twin has polyhydramnios, not oligohydramnios. The recipient twin is usually large, whereas the donor twin is often small.

CN: Physiological integrity; CNS: Physiological adaptation; CL: Analysis

4. A pregnant client who reports painless vaginal bleeding at 28 weeks' gestation is diagnosed with placenta previa. The placental edge reaches the internal os. The nurse would suspect the client has which type of placenta previa?

1. Low-lying placenta previa
2. Marginal placenta previa
3. Partial placenta previa
4. Total placenta previa

4. 2. A marginal placenta previa is characterized by implantation of the placenta in the margin of the cervical os, not covering the os. A low-lying placenta is implanted in the lower uterine segment but doesn't reach the cervical os. A partial placenta previa is the partial occlusion of the cervical os by the placenta. The internal cervical os is completely covered by the placenta in a total placenta previa.

CN: Physiological integrity; CNS: Physiological adaptation; CL: Analysis

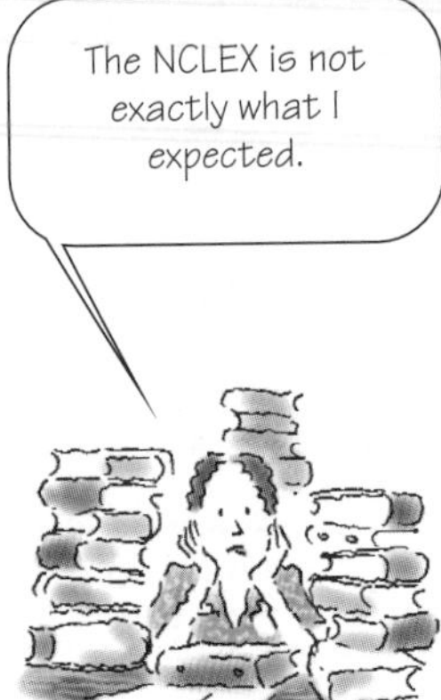

The NCLEX is not exactly what I expected.

5. Expectant management of the client with a placenta implanted in the lower uterine segment includes which procedure or treatment?

1. Stat culture and sensitivity
2. Antenatal steroids after 34 weeks' gestation
3. Ultrasound examination every 2 to 3 weeks
4. Scheduled delivery of the fetus before fetal maturity in a hemodynamically stable mother

5. 3. Placenta previa occurs when the placenta is implanted in the lower uterine segment. Fetal surveillance through ultrasound examination every 2 to 3 weeks is indicated to evaluate fetal growth, amniotic fluid, and placental location in clients with placenta previa being expectantly managed. A stat culture and sensitivity would be done for severe bleeding or maternal or fetal distress and isn't part of expectant management. Antenatal steroids may be given to clients between 26 and 32 weeks' gestation to enhance fetal lung maturity. In a hemodynamically stable mother, delivery of the fetus should be delayed until fetal lung maturity is attained.

CN: Physiological integrity; CNS: Reduction of risk potential; CL: Analysis

6. A client with painless vaginal bleeding at 28 weeks' gestation has just been diagnosed as having placenta previa. Which statement by the client indicates that she understands the nurse's teaching?

1. "I am still able to have sexual intercourse with my husband."
2. "I can continue to go to exercise class three times a week."
3. "I will still be able to fly to Florida for the holidays."
4. "I need to limit my activity and rest."

6. 4. The client with placenta previa needs to restrict her activities and may be placed on bed rest. She should avoid sexual intercourse, strenuous activity, and long-distance travel.

CN: Physiological integrity; CNS: Reduction of risk potential; CL: Analysis

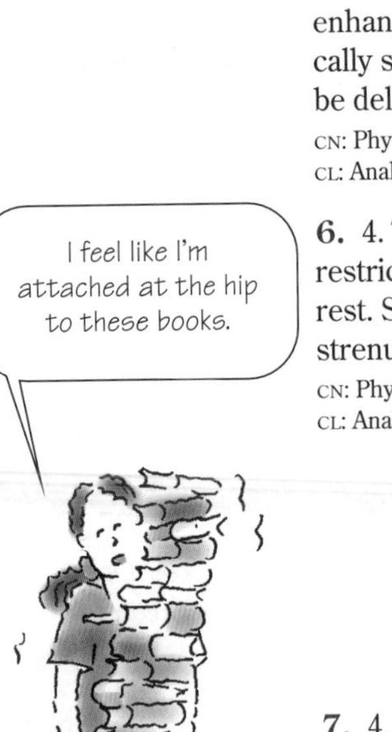

I feel like I'm attached at the hip to these books.

7. The nurse is teaching a client with placenta previa who has developed placenta accreta. Which statement concerning this condition would be the most correct?

1. The placenta invades the myometrium.
2. The placenta covers the cervical os.
3. The placenta penetrates the myometrium.
4. The placenta attaches to the myometrium.

7. 4. Placenta accreta is the abnormal attachment of the placenta to the myometrium of the uterus. When the placenta invades the myometrium, it's called placenta increta. When the placenta covers the cervical os, it's called placenta previa. Placenta percreta occurs when the villi of the placenta penetrate the myometrium to the serosa level.

CN: Physiological integrity; CNS: Physiological adaptation; CL: Application

8. The nurse is caring for a client suspected of having a hydatidiform mole. Which signs and symptoms would confirm this diagnosis?

1. Heavy, bright red bleeding every 21 days
2. Fetal cardiac motion after 6 weeks' gestation
3. Benign tumors found in the smooth muscle of the uterus
4. "Snowstorm" pattern on ultrasound with no fetus or gestational sac

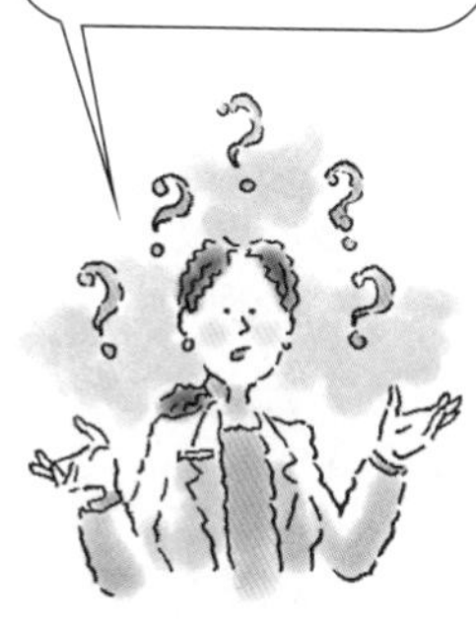

Sometimes it's hard to keep your symptoms straight, isn't it?

8. 4. Ultrasound is the technique of choice in diagnosing a hydatidiform mole. The chorionic villi of a molar pregnancy resemble a "snowstorm" pattern on ultrasound. Bleeding with a hydatidiform mole is often dark brown and may occur erratically for weeks or months. There's no cardiac activity because there's no fetus. Benign tumors found in the smooth muscle of the uterus are leiomyomas or fibroids.

CN: Physiological integrity; CNS: Reduction of risk potential; CL: Analysis

9. A 21-year-old client has just been diagnosed with having a hydatidiform mole. Which factor is considered a risk factor for developing a hydatidiform mole?

1. Age in 20s or 30s
2. High socioeconomic status
3. Primigravida
4. Prior molar gestation

9. 4. A previous molar gestation increases a woman's risk for developing a subsequent molar gestation by 4 to 5 times. Adolescents and women ages 40 years and older are at increased risk for molar pregnancies. Multigravidas, especially women with a prior pregnancy loss, and women with lower socioeconomic status are at an increased risk for this problem.

CN: Health promotion and maintenance; CNS: None; CL: Analysis

10. A 21-year-old female client arrives at the emergency department with complaints of cramping, abdominal pain, and mild vaginal bleeding. Pelvic examination shows a left adnexal mass that is tender when palpated. Culdocentesis shows blood in the cul-de-sac. This client probably has which condition?

1. Abruptio placentae
2. Ectopic pregnancy
3. Hydatidiform mole
4. Pelvic inflammatory disease (PID)

10. 2. Most ectopic pregnancies don't appear as obvious life-threatening medical emergencies. Ectopic pregnancies must be considered in any sexually active woman of childbearing age who complains of menstrual irregularity, cramping abdominal pain, and mild vaginal bleeding. The client with an ectopic pregnancy who is experiencing blood loss will have blood in the cul-de-sac. PID, abruptio placentae, and hydatidiform moles won't show blood in the cul-de-sac.

CN: Physiological integrity; CNS: Reduction of risk potential; CL: Analysis

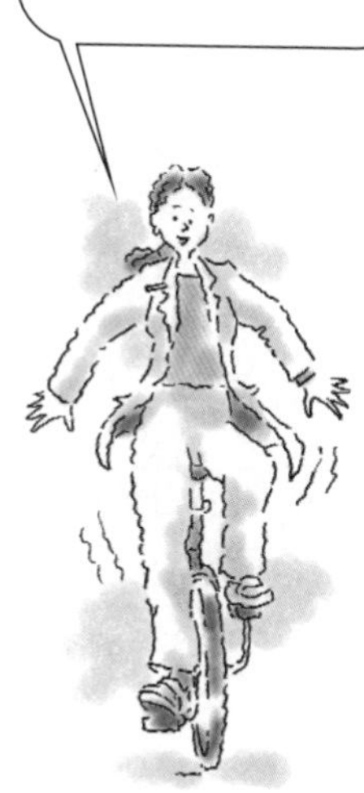

Now you're getting up to speed. Way to go!

11. A client at 34 weeks' gestation arrives at the emergency department with severe abdominal pain, uterine tenderness, and an increased uterine tone. The client denies vaginal bleeding. The external fetal monitor shows fetal distress with severe, variable decelerations. The client most likely has which condition?

1. Abruptio placentae
2. Ectopic pregnancy
3. Molar pregnancy
4. Placenta previa

11. 1. A client with severe abruptio placentae will often have severe abdominal pain. The uterus will have increased tone with little to no return to resting tone between contractions. The fetus will start to show signs of distress, with decelerations in the heart rate or even fetal death with a large placental separation. An ectopic pregnancy, which usually occurs in the fallopian tubes, would rupture well before 34 weeks. A molar pregnancy generally would be detected before 34 weeks' gestation and no fetal heart sounds would be present. Placenta previa usually involves painless vaginal bleeding without uterine contractions.

CN: Physiological integrity; CNS: Reduction of risk potential; CL: Analysis

12. During a routine visit to the clinic, a client tells the nurse that she thinks she may be pregnant. The physician orders a pregnancy test. Which result would most accurately confirm pregnancy?

1. Increase in human chorionic gonadotropin (HCG)
2. Decrease in HCG
3. Increase in luteinizing hormone (LH)
4. Decrease in LH

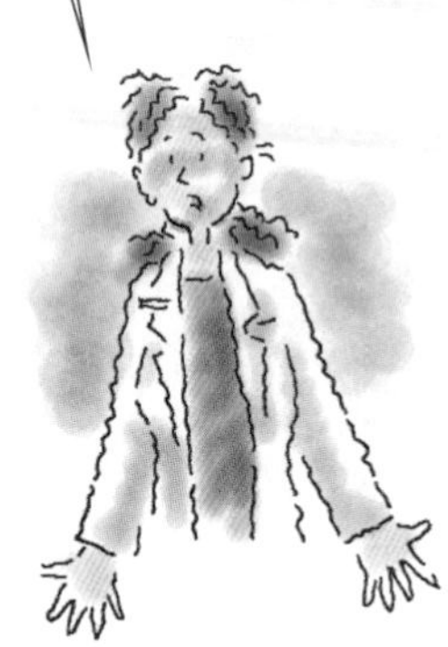

So many hormones to learn; so little time!

12. 1. HCG increases in a woman's blood and urine to fairly large concentrations until the 15th week of pregnancy. The other hormone values aren't indicative of pregnancy.
CN: Health promotion and maintenance; CNS: None; CL: Application

13. A nurse is assessing a pregnant client. Which symptom should the nurse expect to observe?

1. Increased tidal volume
2. Increased expiratory volume
3. Decreased inspiratory capacity
4. Decreased oxygen consumption

13. 1. A pregnant client breathes deeper, which increases the tidal volume of gas moved in and out of the respiratory tract with each breath. The expiratory volume and residual volume decrease as the pregnancy progresses. The inspiratory capacity increases during pregnancy. The increased oxygen consumption in the pregnant client is 15% to 20% greater than in the nonpregnant state.
CN: Health promotion and maintenance; CNS: None; CL: Application

14. Which intervention should the nurse implement in the client scheduled for amniocentesis?

1. Tell the client to drink 1L of water.
2. Have the client void.
3. Instruct the client to fast for 12 hours.
4. Place the client on her left side.

14. 2. Before amniocentesis, the client should void to empty the bladder, reducing the risk of bladder perforation. The client doesn't need to drink fluids before amniocentesis nor does she need to fast. The client should be placed in a supine position for the procedure.
CN: Health promotion and maintenance; CNS: None; CL: Application

15. A nurse is taking an initial history on a pregnant client, who asks about the chances of having dizygotic twins. Which statement by the nurse is correct?

1. "They occur most frequently in Asian women."
2. "There's a decreased risk with increased parity."
3. "There's an increased risk with increased maternal age."
4. "There's no increased risk with the use of fertility drugs."

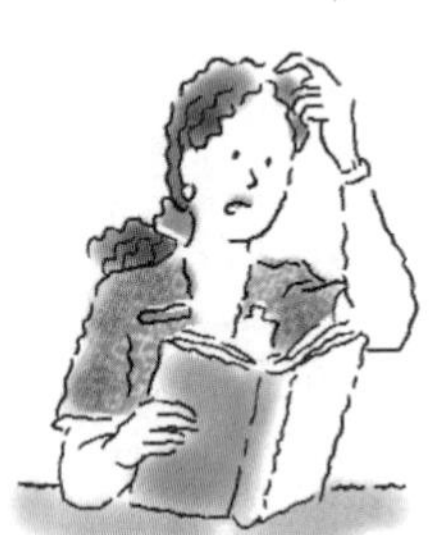

Which statement is true about dizygotic twins?

15. 3. Dizygotic twinning is influenced by race (most frequent in Black women and least frequent in Asian women), age (increased risk with increased maternal age), parity (increased risk with increased parity), and fertility drugs (increased risk with the use of fertility drugs, especially ovulation-inducing drugs). The incidence of monozygotic twins isn't affected by race, age, parity, heredity, or fertility medications.
CN: Health promotion and maintenance; CNS: None; CL: Application

16. A client in her fifth month of pregnancy is having a routine clinic visit. The nurse should assess the client for which common second trimester condition?

1. Mastitis
2. Metabolic alkalosis
3. Physiologic anemia
4. Respiratory acidosis

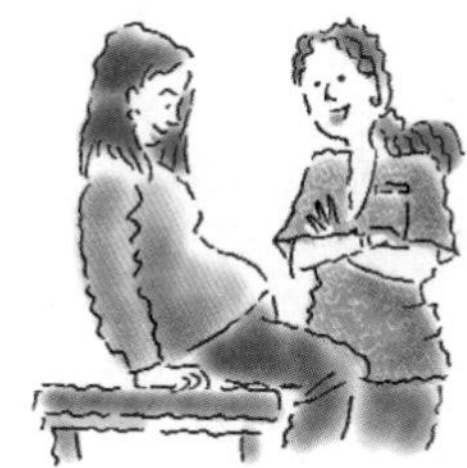

A pregnant client's needs may vary in each trimester.

16. 3. Hemoglobin and hematocrit values decrease during pregnancy as the increase in plasma volume exceeds the increase in red blood cell production. Mastitis is an infection in the breast characterized by a swollen tender breast and flulike symptoms. This condition is most frequently seen in breast-feeding clients. Alterations in acid-base balance during pregnancy result in a state of respiratory alkalosis, compensated by mild metabolic acidosis.

CN: Health promotion and maintenance; CNS: None; CL: Application

17. A 21-year-old client at 6 weeks' gestation is diagnosed with hyperemesis gravidarum. This excessive vomiting during pregnancy will often result in which condition?

1. Bowel perforation
2. Electrolyte imbalance
3. Miscarriage
4. Gestational hypertension

17. 2. Excessive vomiting in clients with hyperemesis gravidarum often causes weight loss and fluid, electrolyte, and acid-base imbalances. Clients with severe hyperemesis may have a low-birth-weight infant, but the disorder generally isn't life-threatening to the fetus. Gestational hypertension and bowel perforation aren't related to hyperemesis. The effects of hyperemesis on the fetus depend on the severity of the disorder.

CN: Physiological integrity; CNS: Reduction of risk potential; CL: Analysis

18. A 29-year-old client has gestational diabetes. The nurse is teaching her about managing her glucose levels. Which therapy would be most appropriate for this client?

1. Diet
2. Long-acting insulin
3. Oral hypoglycemic drugs
4. Glucagon

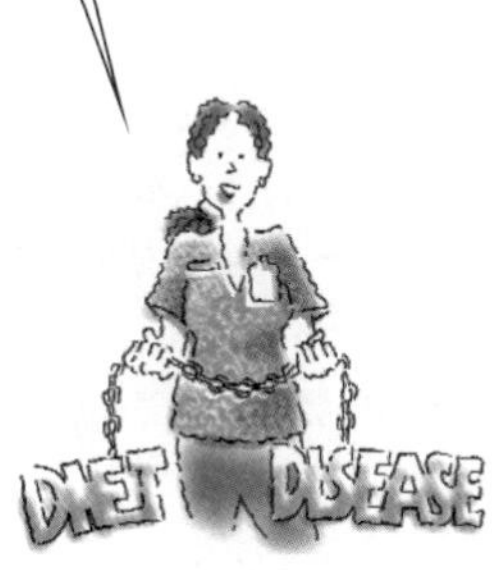

18. 1. Clients with gestational diabetes are usually managed by diet alone to control their glucose intolerance. Long-acting insulin usually isn't needed for blood glucose control in the client with gestational diabetes. Oral hypoglycemic drugs are contraindicated in pregnancy. Glucagon raises blood glucose and is used to treat hypoglycemic reactions.

CN: Health promotion and maintenance; CNS: None; CL: Application

19. Magnesium sulfate is given to pregnant clients with preeclampsia to prevent which condition?

1. Hemorrhage
2. Hypertension
3. Hypomagnesemia
4. Seizures

19. 4. The anticonvulsant mechanism of magnesium is believed to depress seizure foci in the brain and peripheral neuromuscular blockade. Magnesium doesn't help prevent hemorrhage in preeclamptic clients. Anti-hypertensive drugs other than magnesium are preferred for sustained hypertension. Hypomagnesemia isn't a complication of preeclampsia.

CN: Physiological integrity; CNS: Pharmacological and parenteral therapies; CL: Analysis

20. While assessing a client in her 24th week of pregnancy, the nurse learns that the client has been experiencing signs and symptoms of pregnancy-induced hypertension, or preeclampsia. Which sign or symptom helps differentiate preeclampsia from eclampsia?

1. Seizures
2. Headaches
3. Blurred vision
4. Weight gain

20. 1. The primary difference between preeclampsia and eclampsia is the occurrence of seizures, which occur when the client becomes eclamptic. Headaches, blurred vision, weight gain, increased blood pressure, and edema of the hands and feet are all indicative of preeclampsia.

CN: Physiological integrity; CNS: Physiological adaptation; CL: Application

21. A pregnant client has a negative contraction stress test (CST). Which statement most accurately describes these test results?

1. Persistent late decelerations in fetal heartbeat occurred, with at least three contractions in a 10-minute window.
2. Accelerations of fetal heartbeat occurred, with at least 15 beats/minute, lasting 15 to 30 seconds in a 20-minute period.
3. Accelerations of fetal heartbeat were absent or didn't increase by 15 beats/minute for 15 to 30 seconds in a 20-minute period.
4. There was good fetal heart rate (FHR) variability and no decelerations from contraction in a 10-minute period in which there were three contractions.

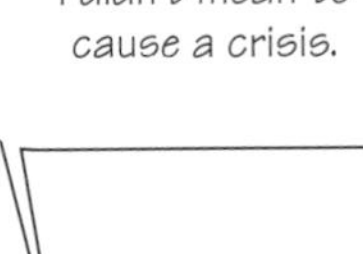
I didn't mean to cause a crisis.

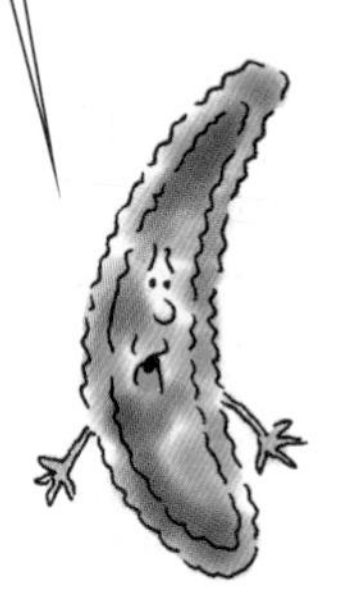

21. 4. A CST measures the fetal response to uterine contractions. A client must have three contractions in a 10-minute period. A negative CST shows good FHR variability with no decelerations from uterine contractions. Persistent late decelerations with contractions is a positive CST. Reactive NSTs have accelerations in the fetal heartbeat of at least 15 beats/minute lasting 15 to 30 seconds in a 20-minute period. No accelerations in the heartbeat of at least 15 beats/minute for 15 to 30 seconds in a 20 minute period indicate a nonreactive nonstress test (NST).

CN: Physiological integrity; CNS: Reduction of risk potential; CL: Analysis

22. A pregnant client with sickle cell anemia is at an increased risk for having a sickle cell crisis during pregnancy. Aggressive management of a sickle cell crisis includes which measure?

1. Antihypertensive agents
2. Diuretic agents
3. I.V. fluids
4. Acetaminophen (Tylenol) for pain

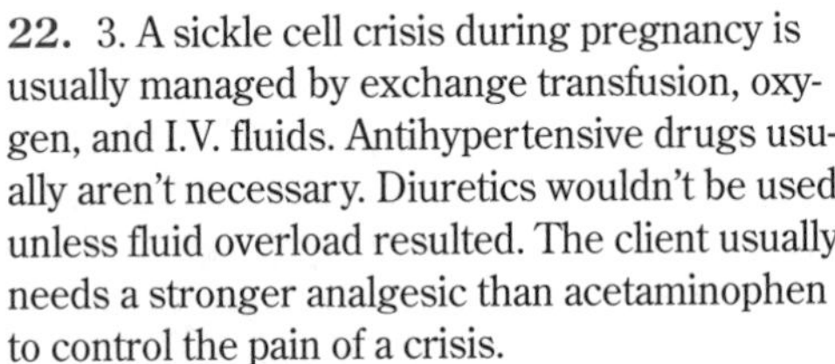

22. 3. A sickle cell crisis during pregnancy is usually managed by exchange transfusion, oxygen, and I.V. fluids. Antihypertensive drugs usually aren't necessary. Diuretics wouldn't be used unless fluid overload resulted. The client usually needs a stronger analgesic than acetaminophen to control the pain of a crisis.

CN: Physiological integrity; CNS: Reduction of risk potential; CL: Analysis

23. A nurse is assessing a pregnant client. Which cardiac condition should the nurse realistically expect in a normal pregnancy?

1. Cardiac tamponade
2. Heart failure
3. Endocarditis
4. Systolic murmur

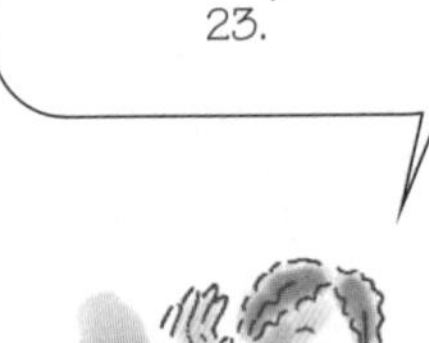
I think I hear the answer to question 23.

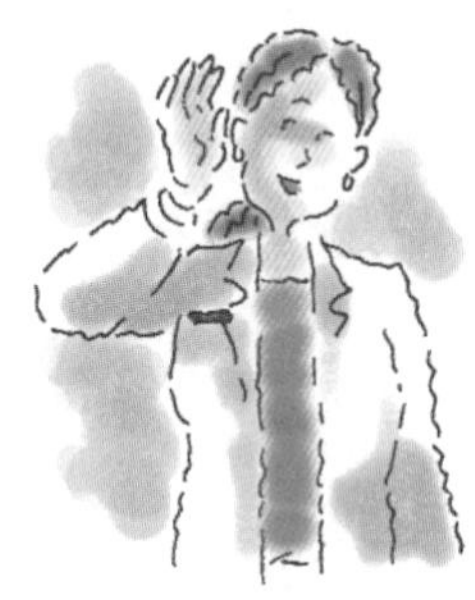

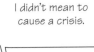

23. 4. Systolic murmurs are heard in up to 90% of pregnant clients, and the murmur disappears soon after the delivery. Cardiac tamponade, which causes effusion of fluid into the pericardial sac, isn't normal during pregnancy. Despite the increases in intravascular volume and workload of the heart associated with pregnancy, heart failure isn't normal in pregnancy. Endocarditis is most often associated with I.V. drug use and isn't a normal finding in pregnancy.

CN: Health promotion and maintenance; CNS: None; CL: Application

24. A 42-year-old pregnant client presents for her first prenatal visit at 16 weeks gestation. She has severe morning sickness and no fetal heart tones. Her B/P is 150/100. Fundal height is 24 cm. These signs are most likely indicative of which condition?
1. Abruptio placenta
2. Placenta previa
3. Normal pregnancy
4. Hydatidiform mole

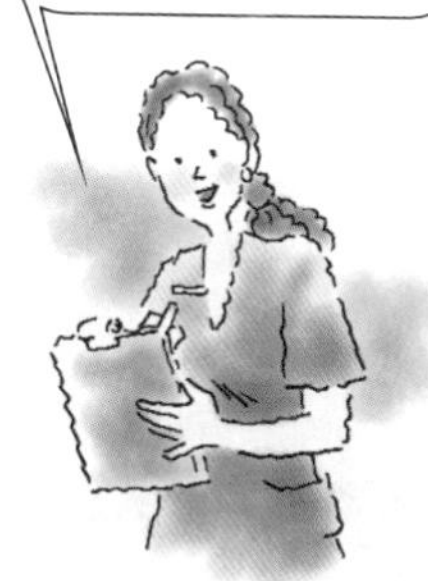

The words most likely can help you focus on the correct answer.

24. 4. The incidence of hydatidiform mole, also known as gestational trophoblastic disease, is higher in women who are older than 35 years of age, have low protein intake, or of Asian heritage. Molar pregnancy should be suspected in clients who have bleeding during the first half of pregnancy, hyperemesis, pregnancy-induced hypertension, absent fetal heart tones, and enlarged uterus for the time of pregnancy. The signs and symptoms do not pertain to the other conditions.

CN: Health promotion and maintenance; CNS: None; CL: Application

25. A client with gestational hypertension is receiving magnesium sulfate to prevent seizure activity. Which magnesium level is therapeutic for clients with preeclampsia?
1. 4 to 7 mEq/L
2. 8 to 10 mEq/L
3. 10 to 12 mEq/L
4. Greater than 15 mEq/L

25. 1. The therapeutic level of magnesium for clients with gestational hypertension is 4 to 7 mEq/L. A serum level of 8 to 10 mEq/L may cause the absence of reflexes in the client. Serum levels of 10 to 12 mEq/L may cause respiratory depression, and a serum level of magnesium greater than 15 mEq/L may result in respiratory paralysis.

CN: Physiological integrity; CNS: Pharmacological and parenteral therapies; CL: Application

26. A client is receiving I.V. magnesium sulfate for severe preeclampsia. Which adverse effect is associated with magnesium sulfate?
1. Anemia
2. Decreased urine output
3. Hyperreflexia
4. Increased respiratory rate

26. 2. Decreased urine output may occur in clients receiving I.V. magnesium and should be monitored closely to keep urine output at greater than 30 ml/hour because magnesium is excreted through the kidneys and can easily accumulate to toxic levels. Anemia isn't associated with magnesium therapy. Magnesium infusions may cause depression of deep tendon reflexes or hyporeflexia. The client should be monitored for respiratory depression and paralysis when serum magnesium levels reach approximately 15 mEq/L.

CN: Physiological integrity; CNS: Pharmacological and parenteral therapies; CL: Analysis

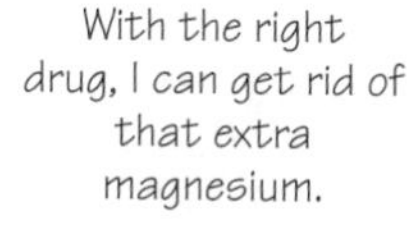

With the right drug, I can get rid of that extra magnesium.

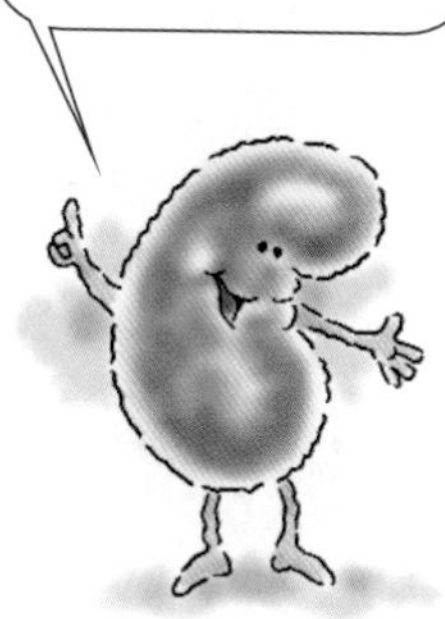

27. The antagonist for magnesium sulfate should be readily available to any client receiving I.V. magnesium. Which drug is the antidote for magnesium toxicity?
1. Calcium gluconate (Kalcinate)
2. Hydralazine
3. Naloxone
4. Rh_0(D) immune globulin (RhoGAM)

27. 1. Calcium gluconate is the antidote for magnesium toxicity. Ten milliliters of 10% calcium gluconate is given I.V. push over 3 to 5 minutes. Hydralazine is given for sustained elevated blood pressures in preeclamptic clients. Naloxone is used to correct narcotic toxicity. Rh_0(D) immune globulin is given to women with Rh-negative blood to prevent antibody formation from Rh-positive conceptions.

CN: Physiological integrity; CNS: Pharmacological and parenteral therapies; CL: Analysis

28. A pregnant client is screened for tuberculosis during her first prenatal visit. An intradermal injection of purified protein derivative (PPD) of the tuberculin bacilli is given. The client is considered to have a positive test for which result?

1. An indurated wheal under 10 mm in diameter appears in 6 to 12 hours.
2. An indurated wheal over 10 mm in diameter appears in 48 to 72 hours.
3. A flat circumcised area under 10 mm in diameter appears in 6 to 12 hours.
4. A flat circumcised area over 10 mm in diameter appears in 48 to 72 hours.

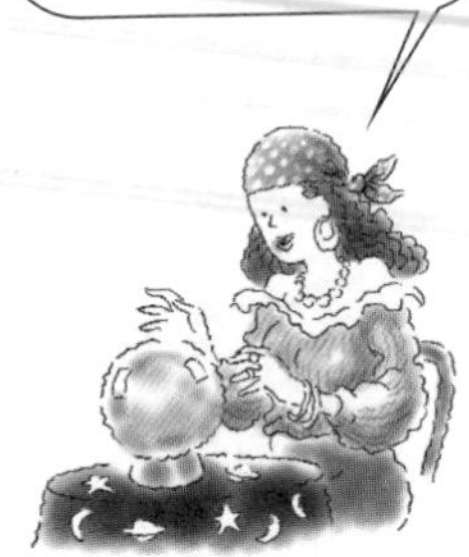

A mysterious wheal will appear within the next few days.

28. 2. A positive PPD result would be an indurated wheal over 10 mm in diameter that appears in 48 to 72 hours. The area must be a raised wheal, not a flat circumcised area, to be considered positive.

CN: Physiological integrity; CNS: Reduction of risk potential; CL: Application

29. A 23-year-old client who is at 27 weeks' gestation arrives at her physician's office with complaints of fever, nausea, vomiting, malaise, unilateral flank pain, and costovertebral angle tenderness. Which diagnosis is most likely?

1. Asymptomatic bacteriuria
2. Bacterial vaginosis
3. Pyelonephritis
4. Urinary tract infection (UTI)

29. 3. The symptoms indicate acute pyelonephritis, a serious condition in a pregnant client. Asymptomatic bacteriuria doesn't cause symptoms. Bacterial vaginosis causes milky white vaginal discharge but no systemic symptoms. UTI symptoms include dysuria, urgency, frequency, and suprapubic tenderness.

CN: Physiological integrity; CNS: Reduction of risk potential; CL: Analysis

30. Clients with which condition would be appropriate for a trial of labor after a prior cesarean delivery?

1. Complete placenta previa
2. Invasive cervical cancer
3. Premature rupture of membranes
4. Prior classical cesarean delivery

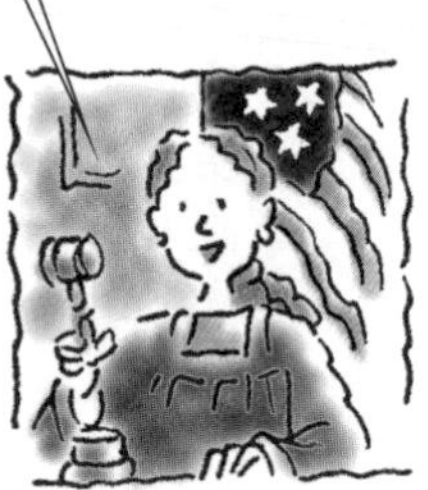

This isn't my kind of trial.

30. 3. Clients with premature rupture of membranes are permitted a trial of labor after a previous cesarean delivery. Clients with placenta previa or a prior classical cesarean delivery shouldn't be given a trial of labor due to the risk of uterine rupture or severe bleeding. A client with invasive cervical cancer should be scheduled for a cesarean delivery.

CN: Physiological integrity; CNS: Physiological adaptation; CL: Analysis

31. A nurse is teaching a client who receives a dose of RhoGAM (human Rh_0[D] immune globulin) at 28 weeks gestation to prevent Rh isoimmunization. Which statement is most accurate about the development of this condition?

1. Rh-positive maternal blood crosses into fetal blood, stimulating fetal antibodies.
2. Rh-positive fetal blood crosses into maternal blood, stimulating maternal antibodies.
3. Rh-negative fetal blood crosses into maternal blood, stimulating maternal antibodies.
4. Rh-negative maternal blood crosses into fetal blood, stimulating fetal antibodies.

31. 2. Rh isoimmunization occurs when Rh-positive fetal blood cells cross into the maternal circulation and stimulate maternal antibody production. In subsequent pregnancies with Rh-positive fetuses, maternal antibodies may cross back into the fetal circulation and destroy the fetal blood cells.

CN: Physiological integrity; CNS: Reduction of risk potential; CL: Application

32. Which dose of Rh_0(D) immune globulin (RhoGAM) is appropriate for a pregnant client at 28 weeks' gestation?

1. 50 mcg in a sensitized client
2. 50 mcg in an unsensitized client
3. 300 mcg in a sensitized client
4. 300 mcg in an unsensitized client

32. 4. An Rh-negative unsensitized woman should be given 300 mcg of RhoGAM at 28 weeks' gestation after an indirect Coombs, test is done to verify that sensitization hasn't occurred. For a first-trimester abortion or ectopic pregnancy, 50 mcg of RhoGAM is given. The administration of RhoGAM to a sensitized client isn't effective.

CN: Physiological integrity; CNS: Pharmacological and parenteral therapies; CL: Analysis

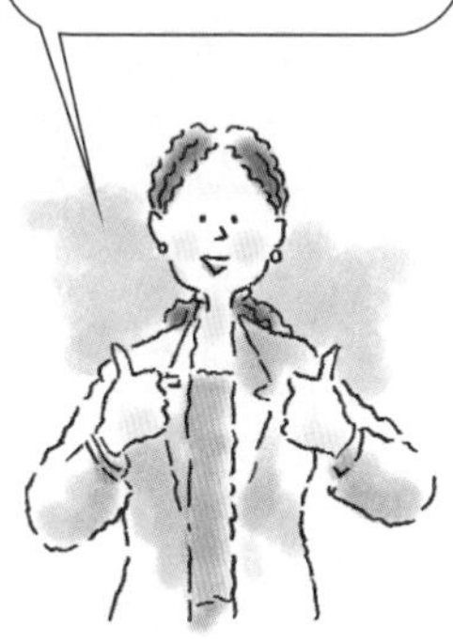

It may be premature. But I think you're doing great!

33. A client hospitalized for preterm labor tells the nurse she's having occasional contractions. Which nursing intervention would be the most appropriate?

1. Teach the client the possible complications of preterm birth.
2. Tell the client to walk to see if she can get rid of the contractions.
3. Encourage her to empty her bladder and drink plenty of fluids, and give I.V. fluids.
4. Notify anesthesia for immediate epidural placement to relieve the pain associated with contractions.

33. 3. An empty bladder and adequate hydration may help decrease or stop labor contractions. Teaching the potential complications is likely to increase the client's anxiety rather than help her relax. Walking may encourage contractions to become stronger. It would be inappropriate to call anesthesia and have an epidural placed because further assessment of contractions is necessary.

CN: Physiological integrity; CNS: Reduction of risk potential; CL: Application

34. A client's prenatal history shows her to be a 23-year-old gravida 4, para 2. The nurse has correctly interpreted this information when she makes which statement?

1. "The client has been pregnant four times and has had two miscarriages."
2. "The client has been pregnant four times and has had two children born after 20 weeks' gestation."
3. "The client has been pregnant four times and has had two cesarean deliveries."
4. "The client has been pregnant four times and has had two spontaneous abortions."

34. 2. *Gravida* refers to the number of times a client has been pregnant; *para* refers to the number of viable children born after 20 weeks' gestation. Therefore, the client who is *gravida 4, para 2* has been pregnant four times and had two live-born children.

CN: Health promotion and maintenance; CNS: None; CL: Analysis

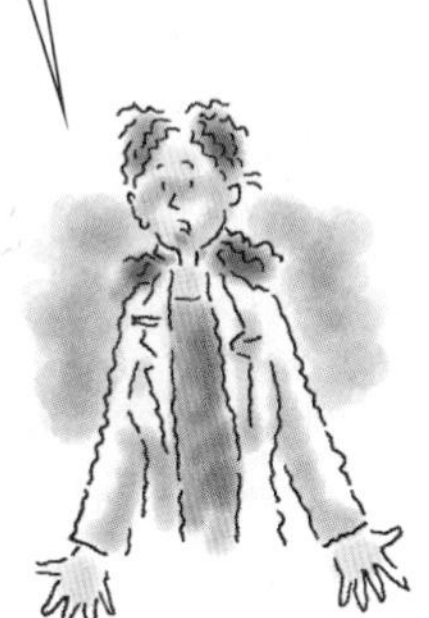

Nobody told me that I'd have to know Latin!

35. A nurse is planning the care of a pregnant client. Which condition would require more frequent visits?

1. Blood type O positive
2. First pregnancy at age 33 years
3. History of allergy to honey bee pollen
4. History of insulin-dependent diabetes mellitus

35. 4. A woman with a history of diabetes has an increased risk for perinatal complications, including hypertension, preeclampsia, and neonatal hypoglycemia and, therefore, needs to be more closely monitored. The age of 33 years without other risk factors doesn't increase risk, nor does type O positive blood or environmental allergens.

CN: Safe, effective care environment; CNS: Management of care; CL: Application

36. To detect life-threatening complications as early as possible in a client receiving a tocolytic agent; the nurse should be alert for which finding?

1. Serum blood glucose level of 140 mg/dl
2. Maternal heart rate of 54 beats/minute
3. Bilateral crackles on lung auscultation
4. Weakened carotid pulse

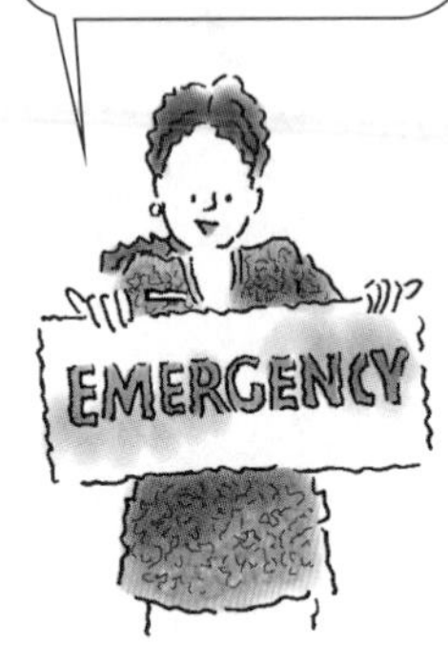

36. 3. Tocolytics are used to stop labor contractions. The most common adverse effect associated with the use of these drugs is pulmonary edema. Therefore, bilateral crackles on lung auscultation, a sign of pulmonary edema, require prompt action. A serum glucose level of 140 mg/dl is elevated and should be reported, however, it isn't life-threatening. Tocolytics may cause tachycardia and increased cardiac output with bounding arterial pulsations.

CN: Physiological integrity; CNS: Pharmacological and parenteral therapies; CL: Analysis

37. What would be the most appropriate medication to administer for a client who has been in early labor (contractions every 10–12 minutes) for 12 hours without progression to help stimulate uterine contractions?

1. Estrogen
2. Fetal cortisol
3. Oxytocin
4. Progesterone

37. 3. Oxytocin is the hormone responsible for stimulating uterine contractions. Pitocin, the synthetic form, may be given to clients to induce or augment uterine contractions. Although estrogen has a role in uterine contractions, it isn't given in a synthetic form to help uterine contractility. Fetal cortisol is believed to slow the production of progesterone by the placenta. Progesterone has a relaxing effect on the uterus.

CN: Physiological integrity; CNS: Pharmacological and parenteral therapies; CL: Application

38. A pregnant client asks the nurse about the pregnancy stage in which maternal and fetal blood are exchanged. Which response by the nurse would be most accurate?

1. Conception
2. 9 weeks' gestation, when the fetal heart is well developed
3. 32 to 34 weeks' gestation (third trimester)
4. Maternal and fetal blood are never exchanged

38. 4. Only nutrients and waste products are transferred across the placenta. Blood exchange never occurs. Complications and some medical procedures can cause an exchange to occur accidentally.

CN: Physiological integrity; CNS: Physiological adaptation; CL: Application

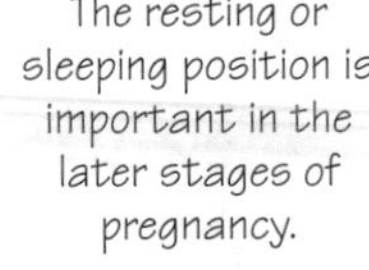

The resting or sleeping position is important in the later stages of pregnancy.

39. Which rationale best explains why a pregnant client should lie on her left side when resting or sleeping in the later stages of pregnancy?

1. To facilitate digestion
2. To facilitate bladder emptying
3. To prevent compression of the vena cava
4. To avoid the development of fetal anomalies

39. 3. The weight of the pregnant uterus is sufficiently heavy to compress the vena cava, which could impair blood flow to the uterus, possibly decreasing oxygen to the fetus. The side-lying position hasn't been shown to prevent fetal anomalies, nor does it facilitate bladder emptying or digestion.

CN: Physiological integrity; CNS: Reduction of risk potential; CL: Analysis

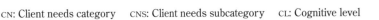

40. A pregnant client is concerned about lack of fetal movement. What instructions should the nurse give that might offer reassurance?

1. Start taking two prenatal vitamins.
2. Take a warm bath to facilitate fetal movement.
3. Eat foods that contain a high sugar content to enhance fetal movement.
4. Lie down once a day and count the number of fetal movements for 15 to 30 minutes.

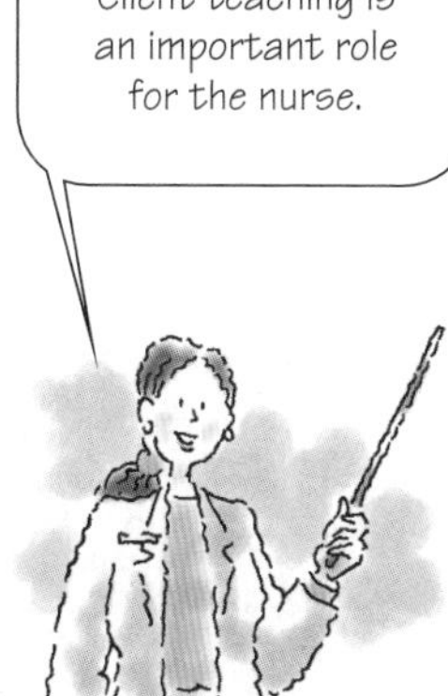

Client teaching is an important role for the nurse.

40. 4. Having the client lie down once during the day will allow her to concentrate on detecting fetal movement, which can be reassuring. Additionally, when the mother is up and actively walking around, it tends to be soothing to the fetus, resulting in sleep promotion. Lying down will make it easier for the client to detect movement. Instructing her to take additional prenatal vitamins isn't recommended as vitamins can be toxic when taken in excess. Taking a warm bath is also likely to be soothing to the fetus. There's also a risk for hyperthermia if the water is too warm or the client is immersed too long. Eating additional sugary foods isn't recommended as some pregnant clients are more susceptible to cavities.

CN: Health promotion and maintenance; CNS: None; CL: Application

41. What would be the most appropriate recommendation to a pregnant client who complains of swelling in her feet and ankles?

1. Limit fluid intake.
2. Buy walking shoes.
3. Sit and elevate the feet.
4. Start taking a diuretic as needed daily.

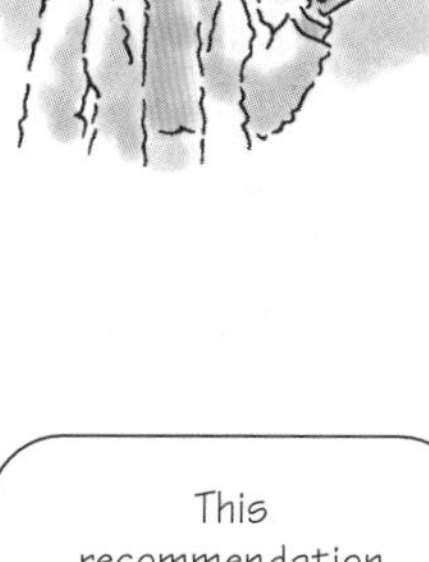

This recommendation works for me!

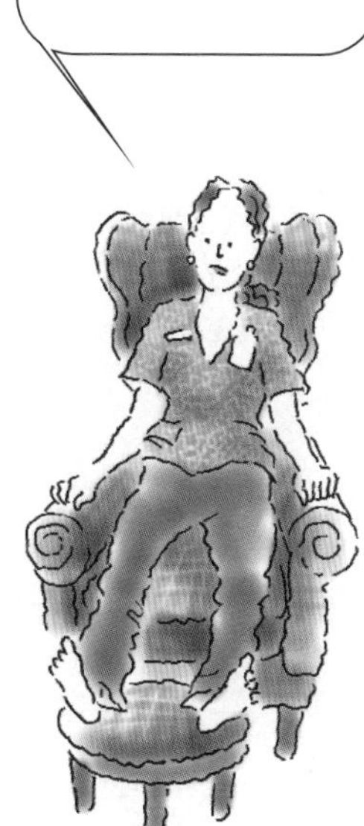

41. 3. Sitting down and putting up her feet will promote venous return and therefore decrease edema. Limiting fluid intake isn't recommended unless there are additional medical complications such as heart failure. Buying walking shoes won't necessarily decrease edema. Diuretics aren't recommended during pregnancy because it's important to maintain an adequate circulatory volume.

CN: Physiological integrity; CNS: Basic care and comfort; CL: Application

42. Which intervention should a nurse recommend to a client having severe heartburn during her pregnancy?

1. Eat several small meals daily.
2. Eat crackers on waking every a.m.
3. Drink a preparation of salt and vinegar.
4. Drink orange juice frequently during the day.

42. 1. Eating small frequent meals will place less pressure on the esophageal sphincter, reducing the likelihood of the regurgitation of stomach contents into the lower esophagus. None of the other suggestions have been shown to decrease heartburn.

CN: Physiological integrity; CNS: Basic care and comfort; CL: Application

43. Which maternal complication is associated with obesity in pregnancy?

1. Mastitis
2. Placenta previa
3. Preeclampsia
4. Rh isoimmunization

43. 3. The incidence of preeclampsia in obese clients is about seven times more than that in nonobese pregnant clients. Mastitis, placenta previa, and Rh isoimmunization aren't associated with increased incidence in obese pregnant clients.

CN: Physiological integrity; CNS: Reduction of risk potential; CL: Analysis

44. Because uteroplacental circulation is compromised in clients with preeclampsia, a nonstress test (NST) is performed to assess which condition?

1. Anemia
2. Fetal well-being
3. Intrauterine growth retardation (IUGR)
4. Oligohydramnios

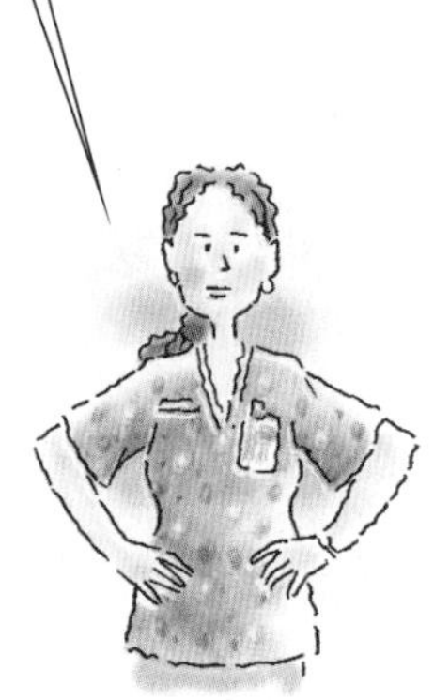

44. 2. An NST is based on the theory that a healthy fetus will have transient fetal heart rate accelerations with fetal movement. A fetus with compromised uteroplacental circulation usually won't have these accelerations, which indicate a nonreactive NST. An NST can't detect anemia in a fetus. Serial ultrasounds will detect IUGR and oligohydramnios in a fetus.

CN: Health promotion and maintenance; CNS: None; CL: Analysis

45. A client is at 33 weeks' gestation and has had diabetes since she was 21. When checking her fasting blood sugar level, which value would indicate the client's disease was controlled?

1. 45 mg/dl
2. 85 mg/dl
3. 120 mg/dl
4. 136 mg/dl

45. 2. Recommended fasting blood sugar levels in pregnant clients with diabetes are 60 to 90 mg/dl. A fasting blood sugar level of 45 mg/dl is low and may result in symptoms of hypoglycemia. A blood sugar level below 120 mg/dl is recommended for 1-hour postprandial values. A blood sugar level above 136 mg/dl in a pregnant client indicates hyperglycemia.

CN: Health promotion and maintenance; CNS: None; CL: Analysis

46. A client with diabetes, who is in the late third trimester, has a nonstress test twice weekly. The 20-minute test showed three fetal heart rate accelerations that exceeded the baseline by 15 beats/minute and that lasted longer than 15 seconds. The nurse knows these results are consistent with which interpretation of a nonstress test?

1. Reactive test
2. Nonreactive test
3. Positive test
4. Negative test

46. 1. The nonstress test is the preferred antepartum heart-rate screening test for pregnant clients with diabetes. A reactive nonstress test is two or more fetal heart rate accelerations that exceed the baseline by at least 15 beats/minute and that last longer than 15 seconds within a 20-minute period. A nonreactive nonstress test lacks accelerations in the fetal heart rate with fetal movement. The terms positive and negative aren't used to describe the interpretation of nonstress tests.

CN: Physiological integrity; CNS: Reduction of risk potential; CL: Analysis

47. A client is diagnosed with preterm labor at 28 weeks' gestation. Later, she comes to the emergency department saying, "I think I'm in labor." The nurse should expect her physical examination to show which condition?

1. Painful contractions with no cervical dilation
2. Regular uterine contractions with cervical dilation
3. Irregular uterine contraction with no cervical dilation
4. Irregular uterine contractions with cervical effacement

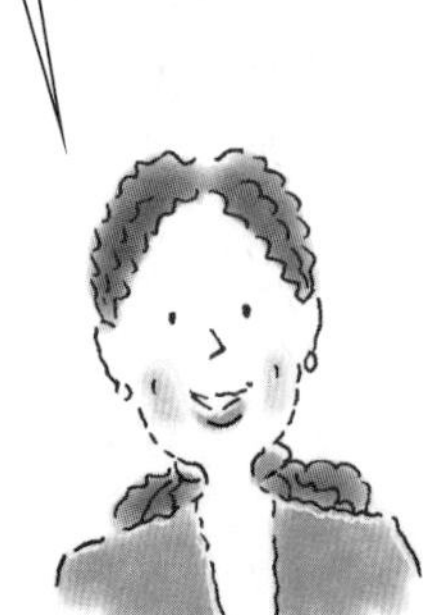

You're almost at question 50 and you're doing great.

47. 2. Regular uterine contractions (every 10 minutes or more) along with cervical dilation change before 36 weeks is considered preterm labor. No cervical change with uterine contractions isn't considered preterm labor.

CN: Health promotion and maintenance; CNS: None; CL: Application

48. A client at 18 weeks' gestation reports fluttering sensations in her abdomen. Which statement made by the client indicates that the nurse's teaching was successful?

1. "This is my baby moving."
2. "I will seek prompt medical attention if this happens again."
3. "This is an early sign of labor."
4. "I will avoid spicy foods."

48. 1. Fluttering in the abdomen, also called *quickening,* begins between 16 and 22 weeks' gestation and is caused by fetal movement. It doesn't require medical attention, nor is it a sign of early labor. Eating spicy foods has no effect on quickening.

CN: Health promotion and maintenance; CNS: None; CL: Analysis

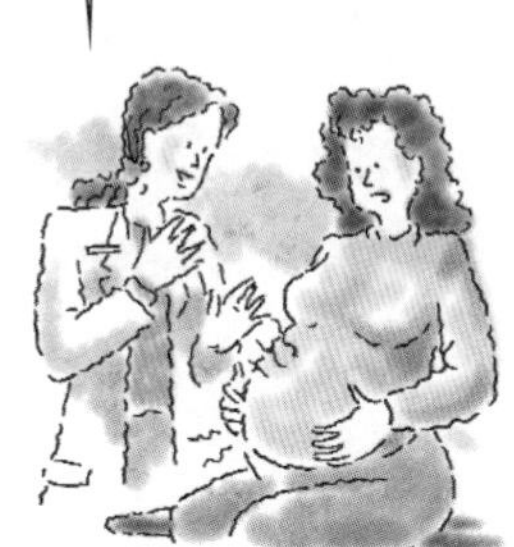
Oh my! I think your baby just moved.

49. A pregnant client is visiting the clinic and complains about the tiny, blanched, slightly raised end arterioles on her face, neck, arms, and chest. The nurse should explain that these are normal during pregnancy and referred to as which finding?

1. Epulis
2. Linea nigra
3. Striae gravidarum
4. Telangiectasias

49. 4. The dilated arterioles that occur during pregnancy are due to the elevated level of circulating estrogen and are called telangiectasias. An epulis is a red raised nodule on the gums that may develop at the end of the first trimester and continue to grow as the pregnancy progresses. The linea nigra is a pigmented line extending from the symphysis pubis to the top of the fundus during pregnancy. Striae gravidarum, or stretch marks, are slightly depressed streaks that commonly occur over the abdomen, breast, and thighs during the second half of pregnancy.

CN: Health promotion and maintenance; CNS: None; CL: Application

50. Which nursing intervention for a pregnant adolescent client has the highest priority during the first trimester?

1. Schedule the client for a screening glucose tolerance test.
2. Refer the client to a dietitian for nutritional counseling.
3. Tell the client that she will most likely need a cesarean delivery due to the head size of the fetus.
4. Assess the client for signs and symptoms of placenta previa.

50. 2. Adolescent clients are at risk for delivering low-birth-weight neonates, not macrosomic neonates. Nutritional counseling should be included as part of prenatal care for adolescent clients. The final head size of the fetus is unknown at this time. Adolescents aren't at increased risk for developing gestational diabetes or placenta previa.

CN: Health promotion and maintenance; CNS: None; CL: Analysis

51. A nurse is discussing nutrition with a primagravida client. The client states that she knows that calcium is important during pregnancy; however, she and her family don't consume many milk or dairy products. What advice should the nurse give?

1. "The prenatal vitamins that are recommended will satisfy all dietary requirements."
2. "You could supplement your diet with 1800 mg of over-the-counter calcium tablets."
3. "You should consume other non-dairy foods that are high in calcium."
4. "After the first trimester, calcium intake isn't significant because all fetal organ structures are formed."

51. 3. Food is considered the ideal source of nutrients. However, milk and dairy aren't the only sources of calcium. While prenatal vitamins are generally recommended, they don't satisfy all requirements. The calcium requirement for pregnancy is 1300 mg/day and over-the-counter supplements aren't always safe and should be specifically recommended by the healthcare practitioner. While it's true that all fetal organs are formed by the end of the first trimester, development continues throughout pregnancy.

CN: Health promotion and maintenance; CNS: None; CL: Application

52. Which drug should a nurse choose to utilize as an antagonist for magnesium sulfate?
1. Oxytocin (Pitocin)
2. Terbutaline
3. Calcium gluconate
4. Naloxone

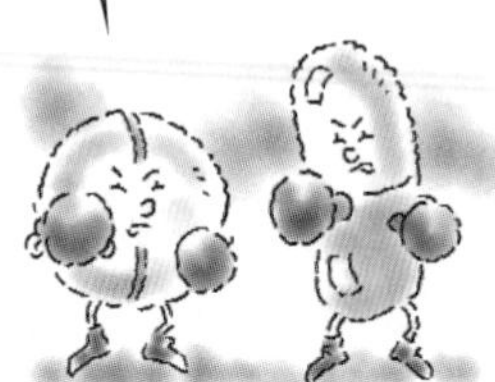
Who are you calling an antagonist?

52. 3. Calcium gluconate should be kept at the bedside while a client is receiving a magnesium infusion. If magnesium toxicity occurs, calcium gluconate is administered as an antidote. Oxytocin is the synthetic form of the naturally occurring pituitary hormone used to initiate or augment uterine contractions. Terbutaline is a beta$_2$-adrenergic agonist that may be used to relax the smooth muscle of the uterus, especially for preterm labor and uterine hyperstimulation. Naloxone is an opiate antagonist administered to reverse the respiratory depression that may follow administration of opiates.

CN: Physiological integrity; CNS: Pharmacological and parenteral therapies; CL: Analysis

53. A nurse receives an order to start an infusion for a client who's hemorrhaging due to a placenta previa. What supplies will be needed?
1. Y tubing, normal saline solution, and a 20G catheter
2. Y tubing, lactated Ringer's solution, and an 18G catheter
3. Y tubing, normal saline solution, and an 18G catheter
4. Y tubing, lactated Ringer's solution, and a 20G catheter

53. 3. Blood transfusions require Y tubing, normal saline solution to mix with the blood product, and an 18G catheter to avoid lysing (breaking) the red blood cells. A 20G catheter lumen isn't large enough for a blood transfusion. Lactated Ringer's solution isn't the I.V. solution of choice with a blood transfusion.

CN: Physiological integrity; CNS: Pharmacological and parenteral therapies; CL: Application

54. Which change should a nurse expect to assess in a client experiencing a normal pregnancy?
1. A 10 beat/minute drop in heart rate
2. A 2 breath/minute increase in respiratory rate
3. A 15 mm Hg increase in systolic blood pressure
4. A 2,000/µl drop in leukocyte count

54. 2. During pregnancy there is a slight increase (2 breaths/minute) in respiratory rate. Heart rate may increase up to 15 beats/minute by the end of pregnancy. Systolic and diastolic pressures may decrease by 5 to 10 mm Hg. The leukocyte count rises in pregnancy and may range from 10,000 to 12,000/µl.

CN: Physiological integrity; CNS: Reduction of risk potential; CL: Application

55. The nurse is teaching a student nurse about the GTPAL system, which documents a client's previous pregnancies. Which statement most accurately describes this system?

1. Total neonates, Preterm neonates, Anacephalic neonates, and Live births
2. Total neonates, Problem pregnancies, Abortions, and Live births
3. Term neonates, Preterm neonates, Anacephalic neonates, and Live births
4. Term neonates, Preterm neonates, Abortions, and Living children

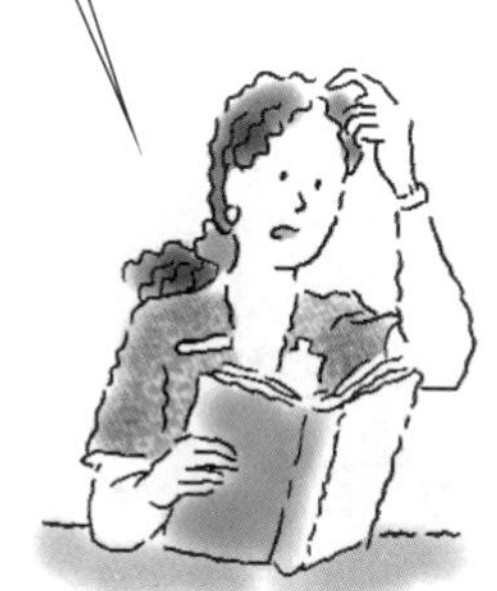

55. 4. In GTPAL, G stands for gravida; T denotes the number of term neonates born after 37 weeks' gestation; P, the number of preterm neonates born before 37 weeks' gestation; A, the number of pregnancies ending with spontaneous or therapeutic abortion; and L, the number of children currently living.

CN: Health promotion and maintenance; CNS: None; CL: Application

56. Which glucose tolerance test results in a client at 26 weeks' gestation requires further action?

1. A glucose level of 120 mg/dl during a 1-hour glucose tolerance test
2. A 1-hour glucose level of 160 mg/dl during a 3-hour glucose tolerance test
3. A 2-hour glucose level of 180 mg/dl during a 3-hour glucose tolerance test
4. A 3-hour glucose level of 130 mg/dl during a 3-hour glucose tolerance test

56. 2. Gestational diabetes is diagnosed when a 2-hour glucose level is 165 mg/dl or greater during a 3-hour glucose tolerance test. Other abnormal results include a 1-hour glucose tolerance test with a glucose level greater than 140 mg/dl, a 3-hour glucose tolerance test with a 1-hour glucose level of 140 mg/dl or greater, a 3-hour glucose tolerance test with a 2-hour glucose level of 165 mg/dl or greater, or a 3-hour glucose tolerance test with a 3-hour glucose level of 145 mg/dl or greater.

CN: Physiological integrity; CNS: Reduction of risk potential; CL: Application

57. A 32-year-old woman is at 15 weeks' gestation when admitted to the labor unit. According to the GTPAL system, she is a G5 P1212. Which description does this indicate?

1. Total of 5 pregnancies, 1 full-term pregnancy, 2 problem pregnancies, 1 spontaneous abortion, and 2 live births
2. Total of 5 children, 1 full-term pregnancy, 2 preterm pregnancies, 1 abortion, 2 live births
3. Total of 5 pregnancies, 1 full-term pregnancy, 2 preterm pregnancies, 1 abortion, 2 living children
4. Total of 5 pregnancies, 1 full-term pregnancy, 2 problem pregnancies, 1 abortion, 2 living children

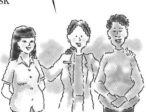

57. 3. T indicates the number of term neonates born at 37 weeks' gestation or after; P, the number of preterm neonates born before 37 weeks' gestation; A, the number of pregnancies ending with spontaneous or therapeutic abortion; and L, the number of children currently living. In this case, the client has been pregnant five times (including the current pregnancy); has had one pregnancy of at least 37 weeks' gestation, two preterm pregnancies, and one abortion; and has two living children.

CN: Health promotion and maintenance; CNS: None; CL: Application

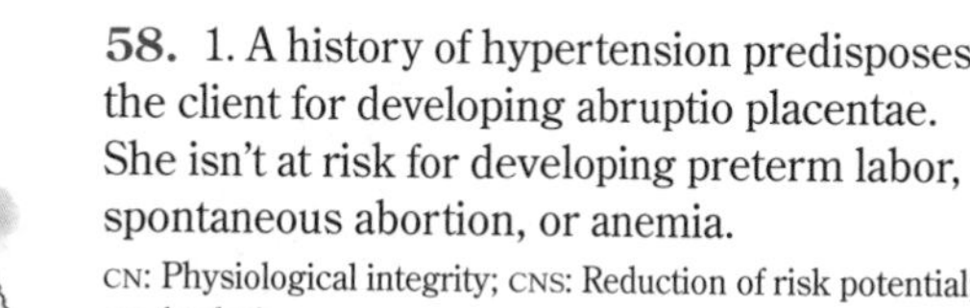

It's important to know the medical history of a pregnant client.

58. Which condition poses the greatest risk to a 32-year-old woman who is 15 weeks' pregnant and has a history of hypertension?

1. Abruptio placentae
2. Preterm labor
3. Spontaneous abortion
4. Anemia

58. 1. A history of hypertension predisposes the client for developing abruptio placentae. She isn't at risk for developing preterm labor, spontaneous abortion, or anemia.

CN: Physiological integrity; CNS: Reduction of risk potential; CL: Analysis

59. A 32-year-old female client has her first prenatal visit at 15 weeks' gestation. Which finding during this visit is abnormal?

1. Fundal height of 18 cm
2. Blood pressure of 124/72 mm Hg
3. Urine negative for protein
4. Weight of 144 lb (65.3 kg)

59. 1. Fundal height (in centimeters) should equal the number of weeks' gestation between 18 and 34 weeks; however, it shouldn't be used alone to determine weeks of gestation. This client should have a fundal height of 15 to 16 cm. The blood pressure, urine, and weight findings are within normal limits for the information given.

CN: Physiological integrity; CNS: Reduction of risk potential; CL: Analysis

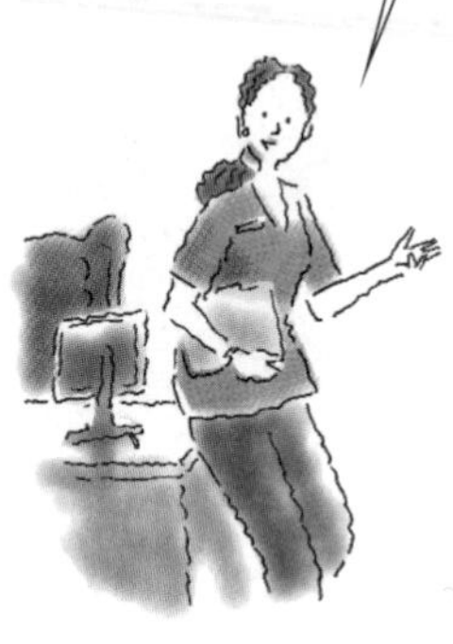

Question 59 is
asking for an
abnormal finding.

60. A 25-year-old primiparous client arrives for her first prenatal visit at 10 weeks' gestation. She seems nervous and has many questions. Which action should the nurse take first?

1. Assess the client's concerns while taking a comprehensive history.
2. Ask the client to undress to prepare for the physical examination.
3. Reassure the client that all her questions will be answered during the visit.
4. Tell the client there's nothing to worry about; the physician will take care of her.

60. 3. Providing initial reassurance helps set the client's mind at ease. Assessing the client's concerns while taking a history would be appropriate only if the client wrote down her questions in advance. Asking her to disrobe immediately may make the client even more nervous. She should be treated as a partner in her care rather than be told that the physician will take care of everything.

CN: Safe, effective care environment; CNS: Management of care; CL: Application

61. Accompanied by her father, a primiparous 15-year-old client arrives for her first prenatal visit at 30 weeks' gestation. Her father refuses to leave the room, stating that the girl is shy and he will answer the questions for her. Which aspect of this situation should be of most concern to the nurse?

1. The possibility of preterm labor with an adolescent pregnancy
2. Lack of prenatal care until this visit
3. Possible child abuse or domestic violence
4. Difficulties of an overprotective parent in dealing with his daughter

61. 3. Generally, a father would be somewhat uncomfortable staying in a room while his pregnant daughter is examined. If he insists on staying during the history and physical examination, the nurse should gently but firmly ask him to wait in another room. If the nurse suspects possible child abuse or domestic violence, the father may not want the girl to be alone with the nurse, fearing that she might reveal the abuse or violence. (Typically, a victim of domestic violence says nothing if the perpetrator is in the room with her.) The possibility of preterm labor and lack of prenatal care should be considered—but they aren't the primary concerns in this situation. An overprotective parent can be supported and taught how to let go of a child as time goes by; a social work referral may be warranted.

CN: Psychosocial integrity; CNS: None; CL: Analysis

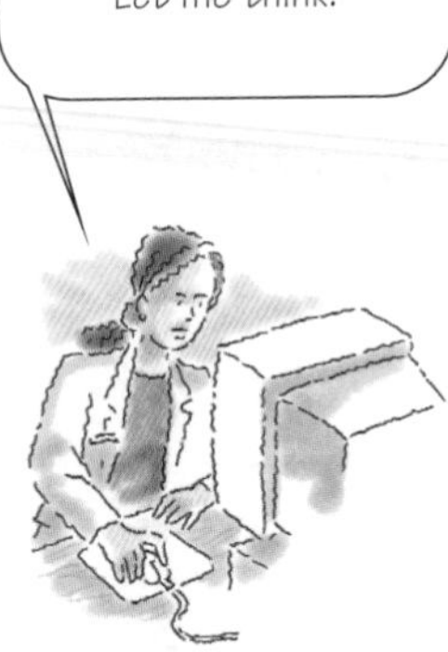

62. Which statement describes the best way for a nurse to determine if a pregnant client is the victim of domestic abuse or violence?

1. Interview the client with her partner in the room.
2. Interview the client with the physician present.
3. Interview the client alone in a nonjudgmental way.
4. Interview the client in a nonjudgmental way, with the partner present.

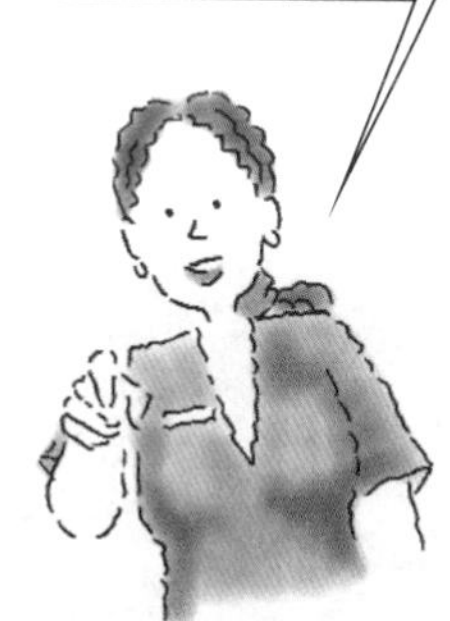

It's up to you to do your best.

62. 3. To help the client feel protected and develop enough trust in the nurse to share her "secret," the nurse should interview her alone in a nonjudgmental way. If the partner is present, the client is likely to clam up for fear of retaliation the next time they're alone together.

CN: Psychosocial integrity; CNS: None; CL: Application

63. A client with gestational hypertension is experiencing abdominal pain and vaginal bleeding. Which assessment should the nurse perform first?

1. Assess fetal heart tones
2. Assess strength of contractions
3. Assess urinary output
4. Assess serum electrolytes

63. 1. Since the findings suggest that the client is experiencing abruptio placentae, fetal heart tones should immediately be assessed to determine fetal well-being. The other interventions should also be implemented, but after the fetus is assessed.

CN: Physiological integrity; CNS: Reduction of risk potential; CL: Analysis

64. During the second and third trimesters, common pregnancy discomforts may increase in number and severity. Which discomforts would the nurse normally expect to see?

1. Ankle edema, hemorrhoids, nausea and vomiting, and shortness of breath
2. Ankle edema, shortness of breath, leg cramps, and increased vaginal discharge
3. Leg cramps, Braxton Hicks contractions, and nausea and vomiting
4. Leg cramps, ankle edema, and shortness of breath

64. 4. Leg cramps, ankle edema, and shortness of breath are normal during the second and third trimesters. The nurse should teach the client how to relieve minor discomforts and what to report if the discomfort becomes unbearable. Nausea and vomiting should subside by the end of the first trimester; if they don't, the nurse should suspect an undiagnosed problem, such as hyperemesis gravidarum or emotional factors that may be exacerbating the nausea and vomiting. Increased vaginal discharge generally occurs during the first trimester and decreases at the end of this period. A yellow, curdlike, or malodorous discharge suggests an abnormal vaginal infection, which should be reported to the physician.

CN: Health promotion and maintenance; CNS: None; CL: Application

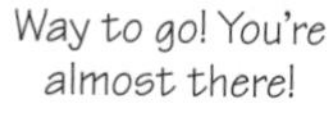

Way to go! You're almost there!

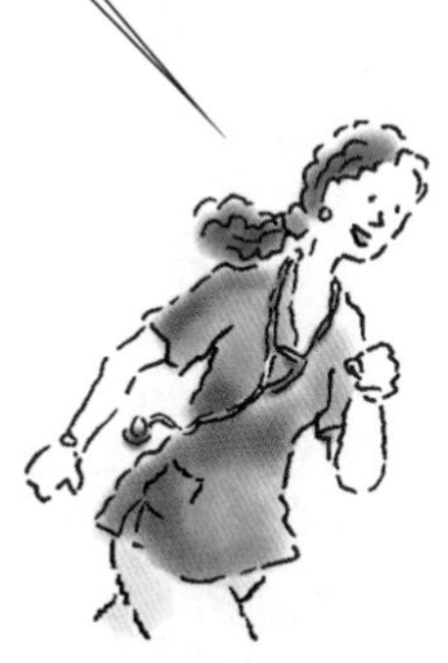

65. Which statement by a client with mild preeclampsia indicates an understanding of discharge instructions?

1. "I will be on my left side."
2. "I should increase my sodium intake."
3. "I will take acetaminophen for a headache."
4. "I will monitor my weight each week."

65. 1. The client should lie on her left side to improve uterine and renal blood flow and enhance venous return. Sodium intake should be limited in the client with preeclampsia. A headache should be reported to the health care provider since it can signal a worsening of the eclampsia. Weight should be monitored daily to assess for fluid retention.

CN: Physiological integrity; CNS: Reduction of risk potential; CL: Analysis

66. When teaching an antepartum client about the passage of the fetus through the birth canal during labor, the nurse describes the cardinal mechanisms of labor. Place these events in the proper sequence in which they occur.

1. Flexion
2. External rotation
3. Descent
4. Expulsion
5. Internal rotation
6. Extension

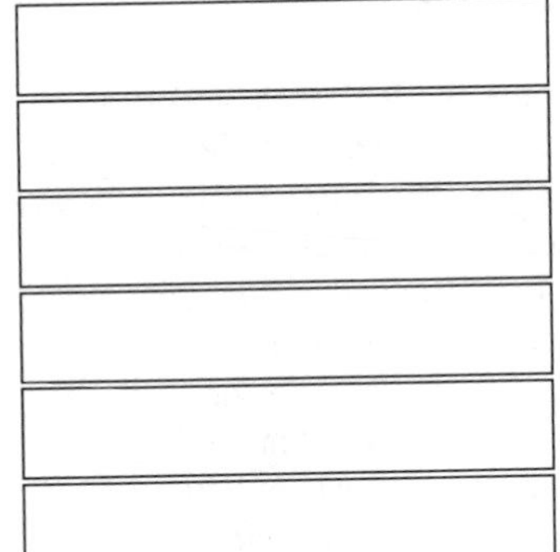

66.

3. Descent
1. Flexion
5. Internal rotation
6. Extension
2. External rotation
4. Expulsion

As the fetus moves through the birth canal, it goes through position changes to ensure that the smallest diameter of fetal head presents to the smallest diameter of the birth canal. Termed the cardinal mechanisms of labor, these position changes occur in the following sequence: descent, flexion, internal rotation, extension, external rotation, and expulsion.

CN: Health promotion and maintenance; CNS: None; CL: Application

67. A nurse is palpating the uterus of a client who is at 20 weeks' gestation to measure fundal height. Identify the area of the abdomen where the nurse should expect to feel the uterine fundus.

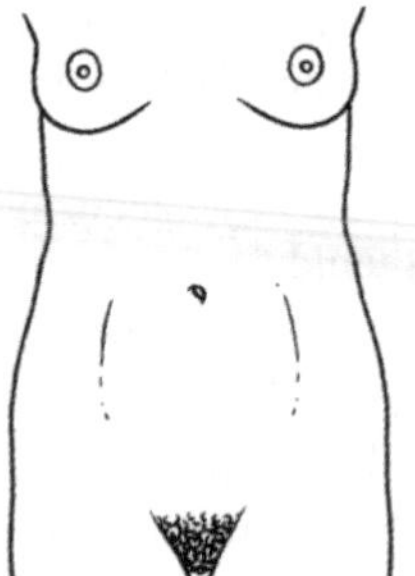

67. At 20 weeks' gestation, fundal height should be at about the umbilicus. Fundal height should be measured from the symphysis pubis to the top of the uterus. Serial measurements assess fetal growth over the course of the pregnancy. Between weeks 18 and 34, the centimeters measured correlate roughly with the week of gestation.

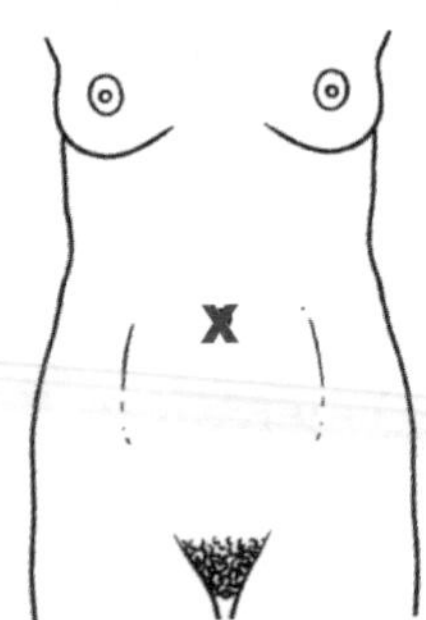

CN: Health promotion and maintenance; CNS: None; CL: Application

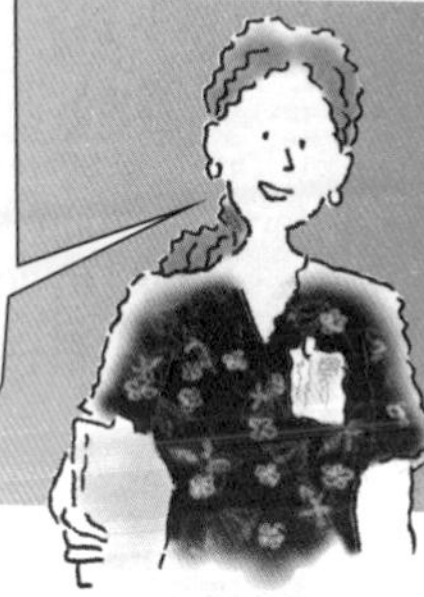

The prepartum and postpartum periods are important to know about. However, the intrapartum period—that's where the action is! This chapter covers the intrapartum period, perhaps the most critical of the three.

Chapter 23 Intrapartum care

1. A client with a term, uncomplicated pregnancy comes into the labor-and-delivery unit in early labor saying that she thinks her water has broken. Which action by a nurse would be most appropriate?

1. Prepare the woman for delivery.
2. Note the color, amount, and odor of the fluid.
3. Immediately contact the physician.
4. Collect a sample of the fluid for microbial analysis.

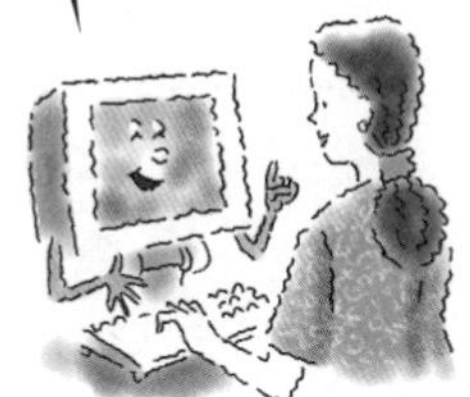

Pay attention to the words most appropriate. They're the key to the answer.

1. 2. Noting the color, amount, and odor of the fluid, as well as the time of the rupture, will help guide the nurse in her next action. There's no need to call the client's physician immediately or prepare the client for delivery if the fluid is clear and delivery isn't imminent. Rupture of membranes isn't unusual in the early stages of labor. Fluid collection for microbial analysis isn't routine if there's no concern for infection (maternal fever).

CN: Physiological integrity; CNS: Reduction of risk potential; CL: Application

2. A client who's at 36 weeks' gestation comes into the labor-and-delivery unit with mild contractions. Which complication should a nurse watch for when the client informs her that she has placenta previa?

1. Sudden rupture of membranes
2. Vaginal bleeding
3. Emesis
4. Fever

2. 2. Contractions may disrupt the microvascular network in the placenta of a client with placenta previa and result in bleeding. If the separation of the placenta occurs at the margin of the placenta, the blood will escape vaginally. Sudden rupture of the membranes isn't related to placenta previa. Fever would indicate an infectious process, and emesis isn't related to placenta previa.

CN: Physiological integrity; CNS: Reduction of risk potential; CL: Application

3. A client's labor doesn't progress. After ruling out cephalopelvic disproportion, the physician orders I.V. administration of 1,000 ml normal saline solution with oxytocin (Pitocin) 10 units to run at 2 milliunits/minute. Two milliunits/minute is equivalent to how many ml/minute?

1. 0.002
2. 0.02
3. 0.2
4. 2

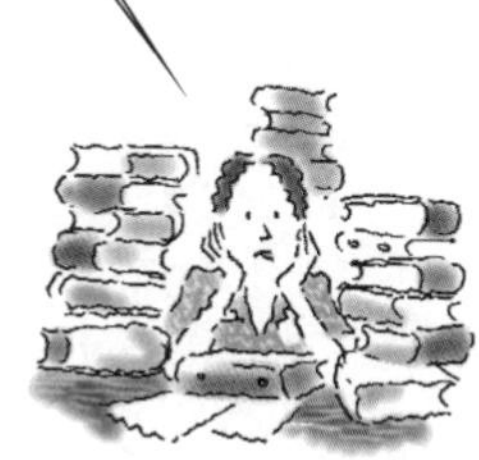

3. 3. The answer is found by setting up a ratio and following through with the calculations, shown below. Each unit of oxytocin contains 1,000 milliunits. Therefore, 1,000 ml of I.V. fluid contains 10,000 milliunits (10 units) of Pitocin. All other options are incorrect.

$$\frac{10{,}000}{1{,}000} = \frac{2}{X}$$

$$10{,}000X = 2{,}000$$

$$X = \frac{2{,}000}{10{,}000}$$

$$X = 0.2 \text{ ml}$$

CN: Physiological integrity; CNS: Pharmacological and parenteral therapies; CL: Analysis

CN: Client needs category CNS: Client needs subcategory CL: Cognitive level

4. A client in labor has been receiving oxytocin (Pitocin) to aid her progress. The nurse caring for her notes that contractions are lasting 100 seconds. Which action should the nurse take <u>first</u>?
1. Stop the oxytocin infusion.
2. Notify the physician.
3. Monitor fetal heart tones as usual.
4. Turn the client on her left side.

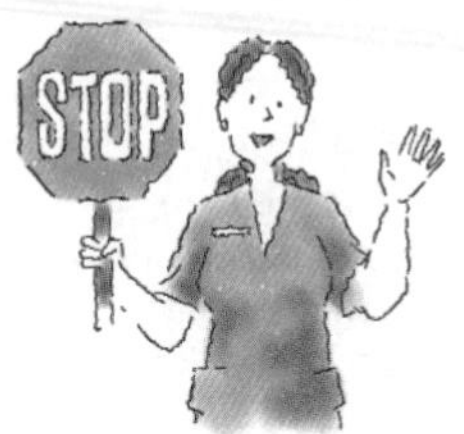

Don't underestimate the importance of the word first.
STOP

4. 1. Oxytocin stimulates contractions and should be stopped. A contraction that continues for more than 90 seconds signals tetany and could lead to decreased placental perfusion and, possibly, uterine rupture. The nurse should monitor the fetal heart tones and notify the physician, but only after stopping the oxytocin. The client should be turned on her left side to increase blood flow to the fetus, which can be decreased with tetany. This decreased blood flow can potentially compromise the fetus.
CN: Physiological integrity; CNS: Reduction of risk potential; CL: Application

5. A client at term arrives in the labor unit experiencing contractions every 4 minutes. After a brief assessment, she's admitted and an electriconic fetal monitor is applied. Which observation should alert the nurse to an increased potential for fetal distress?
1. Total weight gain of 30 lb (13.6 kg)
2. Maternal age of 32 years
3. Blood pressure of 146/90 mm Hg
4. Treatment for syphilis at 15 weeks' gestation

5. 3. A blood pressure of 146/90 mm Hg may indicate gestational hypertension. Over time, gestational hypertension reduces blood flow to the placenta and can cause intrauterine growth restriction and other problems that make the fetus less able to tolerate the stress of labor. A weight gain of 30 lb is within expected parameters for a healthy pregnancy. A woman over age 30 doesn't have a greater risk of complications if her general condition is healthy before pregnancy. Syphilis that has been treated doesn't pose an additional risk.
CN: Physiological integrity; CNS: Reduction of risk potential; CL: Application

6. To detect fetal distress during labor, a nurse should be alert for which finding?
1. Fetal scalp pH of 7.14
2. Fetal heart rate of 144 beats/minute
3. Acceleration of fetal heart rate with contractions
4. Presence of long-term variability

6. 1. A scalp pH below 7.25 indicates acidosis and fetal hypoxia. A fetal heart rate of 144 beats/minute, acceleration of the fetal heart rate with contractions, and long-term variability are normal responses of a healthy fetus to labor.
CN: Physiological integrity; CNS: Reduction of risk potential; CL: Application

7. During the labor of a client with a breech presentation, the amniotic membranes rupture. Meconium is present in the amniotic fluid. Which statement by a nurse is most appropriate?
1. "This often happens during a prolonged delivery."
2. "This indicates a blood incompatibility between the fetus and mother."
3. "This is a sign of fetal distress."
4. "This is normal in a breech delivery."

7. 4. Meconium in a breech presentation may be caused by compression of the fetus's intestinal tract during descent. Meconium in the amniotic fluid is a sign of fetal distress in a cephalic presentation and isn't a normal finding, even during a prolonged delivery. Yellow-stained amniotic fluid is a sign of a possible blood incompatibility between fetus and mother and is due to bilirubin from the breakdown of red blood cells.
CN: Physiological integrity; CNS: Reduction of risk potential; CL: Analysis

8. A client at 42 weeks' gestation is 3 cm dilated, 30% effaced, with membranes intact and the fetus at +2 station. Fetal heart rate (FHR) is 140 beats/minute. After 2 hours, the nurse notes on the external fetal monitor that, for the past 10 minutes, the FHR ranged from 160 to 190 beats/minute. The client states that her baby has been extremely active. Uterine contractions are strong, occurring every 3 to 4 minutes and lasting 40 to 60 seconds. Which finding would indicate fetal hypoxia?

1. Abnormally long uterine contractions
2. Abnormally strong uterine intensity
3. Excessively frequent contractions, with rapid fetal movement
4. Excessive fetal activity and fetal tachycardia

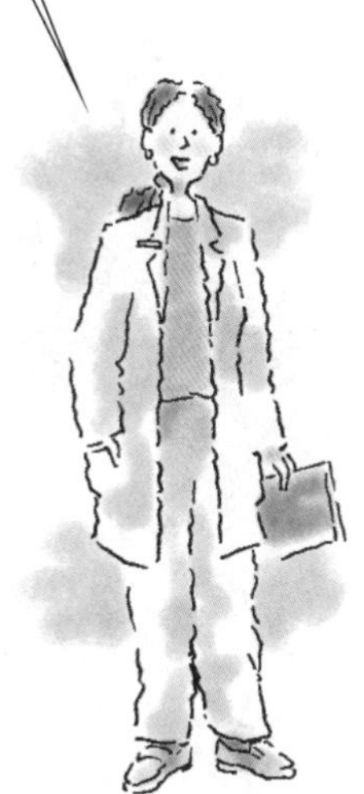

Remember that every piece of information provided may not be necessary to answer the question.

8. 4. Fetal tachycardia and excessive fetal activity are the first signs of fetal hypoxia. The duration of uterine contractions is within normal limits. Uterine intensity can be mild to strong and still be within normal limits. The frequency of contractions is within the normal limits for the active phase of labor.

CN: Physiological integrity; CNS: Reduction of risk potential; CL: Analysis

9. A client at 33 weeks' gestation and leaking amniotic fluid is placed on an external fetal monitor. The monitor indicates uterine irritability, and contractions are occurring every 4 to 6 minutes. The physician orders terbutaline. Which teaching statement is appropriate for this client?

1. "This medicine will make you breathe better."
2. "You may feel a fluttering or tight sensation in your chest."
3. "This will dry your mouth and make you feel thirsty."
4. "You'll need to replace the potassium lost by this drug."

9. 2. A fluttering or tight sensation in the chest is a common adverse reaction to terbutaline. Terbutaline relieves bronchospasm, but the client is receiving it to reduce uterine motility. Mouth dryness and thirst occur with the inhaled form of terbutaline but are unlikely with the subcutaneous form. Hypokalemia is a potential adverse reaction following large doses of terbutaline but not at doses of 0.25 mg.

CN: Health promotion and maintenance; CNS: None; CL: Application

10. A 17-year-old primigravida with severe hypertension of pregnancy has been receiving magnesium sulfate I.V. for 3 hours. The latest assessment reveals deep tendon reflexes (DTR) of +1, blood pressure of 150/100 mm Hg, a pulse of 92 beats/minute, a respiratory rate of 10 breaths/minute, and urine output of 20 ml/hour. Which action would be most appropriate?

1. Continue monitoring per standards of care.
2. Stop the magnesium sulfate infusion.
3. Increase the infusion rate by 5 gtt/minute.
4. Decrease the infusion rate by 5 gtt/minute.

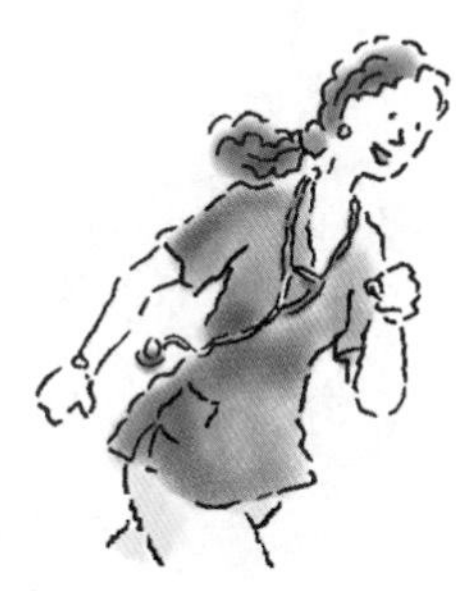

Sometimes you have to think fast on your feet.

10. 2. Magnesium sulfate should be withheld if the client's respiratory rate or urine output falls or if reflexes are diminished or absent, all of which are true for this client. The client also shows other signs of impending toxicity, such as flushing and feeling warm. Inaction won't resolve the client's suppressed DTRs and low respiratory rate and urine output. The client is already showing central nervous system depression because of excessive magnesium sulfate, so increasing the infusion rate is inappropriate. Impending toxicity indicates that the infusion should be stopped rather than just slowed down.

CN: Physiological integrity; CNS: Pharmacological and parenteral therapies; CL: Application

11. During a vaginal examination of a client in labor, the nurse palpates the fetus's larger, diamond-shaped fontanelle toward the anterior portion of the client's pelvis. Which statement best describes this situation?

1. The client can expect a brief and intense labor with potential for lacerations.
2. The client is at risk for uterine rupture and needs constant monitoring.
3. The client may need interventions to ease back pain and change the fetal position.
4. The fetus will be delivered using forceps or a vacuum extractor.

11. 3. The fetal position is occiput posterior, a position that commonly produces intense back pain during labor. Most of the time, the fetus rotates during labor to occiput anterior position. Positioning the client on her side can facilitate this rotation. An occiput posterior position would most likely result in prolonged labor. Occiput posterior alone doesn't create a risk of uterine rupture. The fetus would be delivered with forceps or vacuum extractor only if its presenting part doesn't rotate and descend spontaneously.

CN: Health promotion and maintenance; CNS: None; CL: Analysis

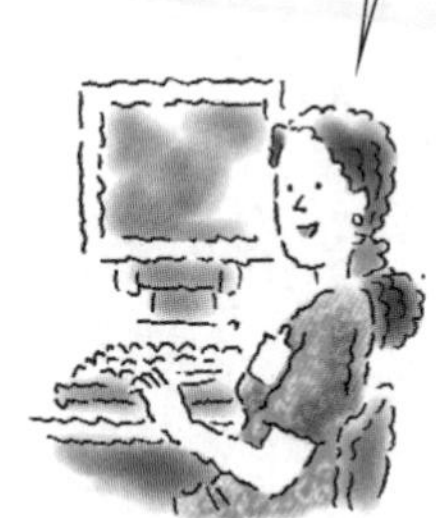

Be careful of the words will be in option 4. They indicate an absolute, a near rarity in health care.

12. The cervix of a 26-year-old primigravida in labor is 5 cm dilated and 75% effaced, and the fetus is at 0 station. The physician prescribes an epidural regional block. Into which position should the nurse place the client when the epidural is administered?

1. Lithotomy
2. Supine
3. Prone
4. Lateral

12. 4. The client should be placed on her left side or sitting upright, with her shoulders parallel and legs slightly flexed. Her back shouldn't be flexed because this position increases the possibility that the dura may be punctured and the anesthetic will accidentally be given as spinal, not epidural, anesthesia. None of the other positions allows proper access to the epidural space.

CN: Physiological integrity; CNS: Reduction of risk potential; CL: Application

13. A nurse administers oxytocin (Pitocin) to a client to induce labor. Which finding should cause the nurse to stop the infusion and notify the physician?

1. Contractions longer than 70 seconds, occurring every 2 minutes or less
2. Dry mucous membranes and decreased skin turgor
3. Fetal heart rate of 160 beats/minute
4. Maternal heart rate of 56 beats/minute

13. 1. Oxytocin, given to induce labor, may cause uterine tetany, which increases the risk of uterine rupture. Therefore, the infusion should be stopped and the physician notified if contractions last greater than 70 seconds and occur every 2 minutes or less. Oxytocin has an antidiuretic effect and can cause fluid overload, not dehydration indicated by dry mucous membranes and decreased skin turgor. A normal fetal heart rate is 120 to 160 beats/minute. Oxytocin may cause maternal tachycardia, not bradycardia.

CN: Physiological integrity; CNS: Pharmacologic parenteral therapies; CL: Application

14. Which fetal position is <u>most favorable</u> for birth?
1. Vertex presentation
2. Transverse lie
3. Frank breech presentation
4. Posterior position of the fetal head

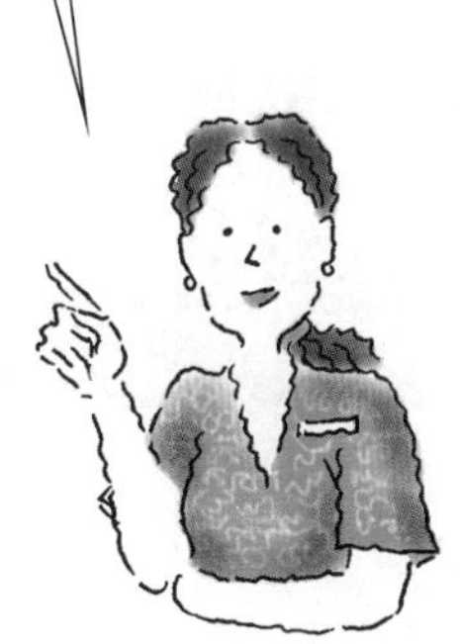

Question 14 is asking for the optimal birthing position.

14. 1. Vertex presentation (flexion of the fetal head) is the optimal presentation for passage through the birth canal. Transverse lie is an unacceptable fetal position for vaginal birth and requires a cesarean birth delivery. Frank breech presentation, in which the buttocks present first, is a high-risk situation and cesarean birth is recommended. Posterior positioning of the fetal head can make it difficult for the fetal head to pass under the maternal symphysis pubis bone.

CN: Physiological integrity; CNS: Reduction of risk potential; CL: Analysis

15. A nurse is preparing a client in the labor-and-delivery unit and is teaching her about the stages of labor. The client demonstrates an understanding of these stages when she states that birth occurs during which stage?
1. First stage of labor
2. Second stage of labor
3. Third stage of labor
4. Fourth stage of labor

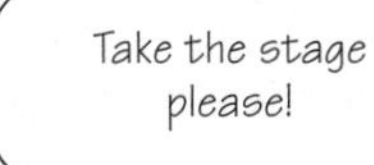

Take the stage please!

15. 2. The second stage of labor begins with complete dilation (10 cm) and ends with the expulsion of the fetus. The first stage of labor is the stage of dilation, which is divided into three distinct phases: latent, active, and transition. The third stage of labor begins with the birth of the infant and ends with the expulsion of the placenta. The fourth stage of labor is the first 4 hours after placental expulsion, in which the client's body begins the recovery process.

CN: Health promotion and maintenance; CNS: None; CL: Application

16. Which laboratory value would be critical for a client admitted to the labor-and-delivery unit?
1. Blood type
2. Calcium
3. Iron
4. Oxygen saturation

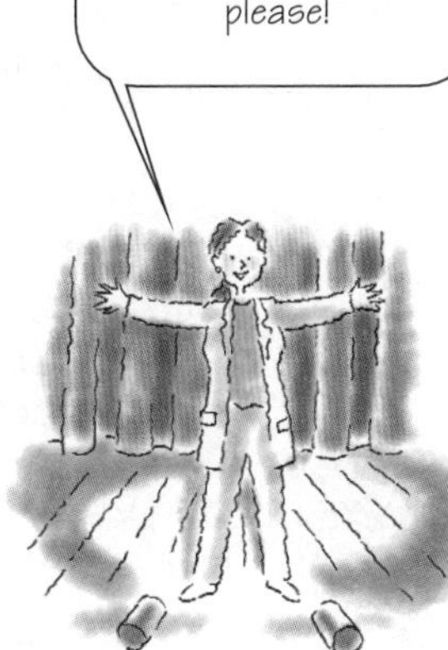

16. 1. Blood type is a critical value to have because the risk of blood loss is always a potential complication during the labor-and-delivery process. Approximately 40% of a woman's cardiac output is delivered to the uterus, therefore, blood loss can occur quite rapidly in the event of uncontrolled bleeding. Calcium and iron aren't critical values and oxygen saturation isn't a laboratory value.

CN: Physiological integrity; CNS: Reduction of risk potential; CL: Analysis

17. Which fetal heart rate would be expected in the fetus of a laboring woman who is full-term?
1. 80 to 100 beats/minute
2. 100 to 120 beats/minute
3. 120 to 160 beats/minute
4. 160 to 180 beats/minute

17. 3. A rate of 120 to 160 beats/minute in the fetal heart is appropriate for filling the heart with blood and pumping it out to the system. Faster or slower rates don't accomplish perfusion adequately and could indicate fetal compromise.

CN: Health promotion and maintenance; CNS: None; CL: Knowledge

18. A nurse has connected a laboring client to an external electronic fetal monitor. What data can the nurse expect to obtain from the monitor?

1. Gender of the fetus
2. Fetal position
3. Labor progress
4. Oxygenation

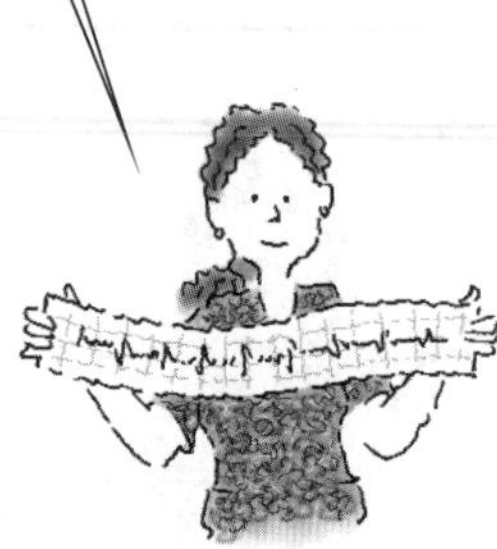

18. 4. Oxygenation of the fetus may be indirectly assessed through fetal monitoring by closely examining the fetal heart rate strip. Accelerations in the fetal heart rate strip indicate good oxygenation, while decelerations in the fetal heart rate sometimes indicate poor fetal oxygenation. The fetal heart rate strip can't determine the gender of the fetus or assess fetal position. Labor progress can be directly assessed only through cervical examination.

CN: Physiological integrity; CNS: Reduction of risk potential; CL: Application

19. Which nursing action is required before a client in labor receives an epidural?

1. Give a fluid bolus of 500 ml.
2. Check for maternal pupil dilation.
3. Assess maternal reflexes.
4. Assess maternal gait.

19. 1. One of the major adverse effects of epidural administration is hypotension. Therefore, a 500-ml fluid bolus is usually administered to help prevent hypotension in the client who wishes to receive an epidural for pain relief. Assessments of maternal reflexes, pupil response, and gait aren't necessary.

CN: Physiological integrity; CNS: Reduction of risk potential; CL: Analysis

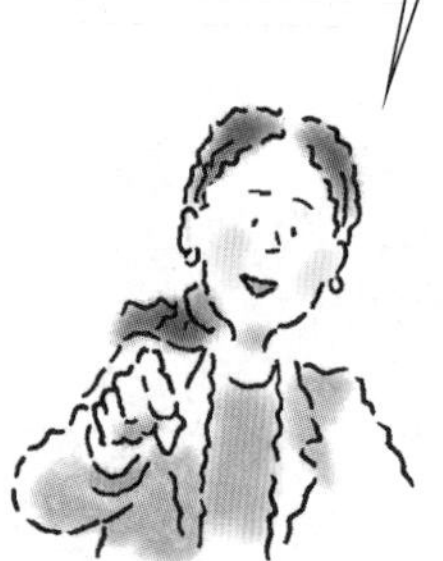

It's important to know the adverse effects of a procedure, and how to offset them.

20. Which complication is possible with an episiotomy?

1. Blood loss
2. Uterine disfigurement
3. Prolonged dyspareunia
4. Hormonal fluctuation postpartum

20. 3. Prolonged dyspareunia (painful intercourse) may result when complications such as infection interfere with wound healing. Minimal blood loss occurs when an episiotomy is performed. The uterus isn't affected by episiotomy because it's the perineum that is cut to accommodate the fetus. Hormonal fluctuations that occur during the postpartum period aren't the result of an episiotomy.

CN: Physiological integrity; CNS: Reduction of risk potential; CL: Analysis

21. A client in early labor states that she has a thick, yellow discharge from both of her breasts. Which action by the nurse would be most appropriate?

1. Tell her that her milk is starting to come in because she's in labor.
2. Complete a thorough breast examination, and document the results in the chart.
3. Perform a culture on the discharge, and inform the client that she might have mastitis.
4. Inform the client that the discharge is colostrum, normally present after the 4th month of pregnancy.

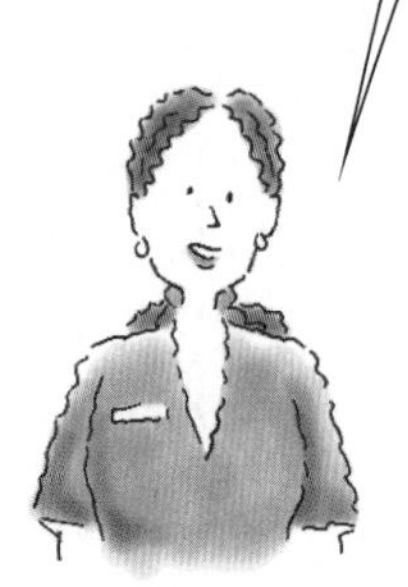

Teaching is an important part of a nurse's role.

21. 4. After the 4th month, colostrum may be expressed. The breasts normally produce colostrum for the first few days after delivery. Milk production begins 1 to 3 days postpartum. A clinical breast examination isn't usually indicated in the intrapartum setting. Although a culture may be indicated, it requires advanced assessment as well as a medical order.

CN: Health promotion and maintenance; CNS: None; CL: Application

22. While performing an admission nursing assessment of a client in early labor, the nurse observes a brown, raised lesion resembling a mole, 2″ (5 cm) below the left breast. Which observation by the nurse would be most appropriate?

1. "That looks like a mole and is clinically insignificant."
2. "That looks like seborrhea keratosis and is a precancerous lesion."
3. "That's a supernumerary nipple, a common finding."
4. "That's a skin tag and is clinically insignificant."

22. 3. Supernumerary nipples are common in men and women and are usually located 2″ to 2½″ (5 to 6 cm) below the breast near the midline. A supernumerary nipple resembles a mole, although closer inspection will reveal a small nipple and areola and is clinically insignificant. A mole (nevus) may be macular or papular, tan to brown in color, and usually has smooth borders. Keratosis lesions are raised, thickened areas of pigmentation that look scaly and warty. They don't become cancerous. Skin tags (acrochordons) are overgrowths of normal skin that form a stalk and are polyplike.

CN: Health promotion and maintenance; CNS: None; CL: Analysis

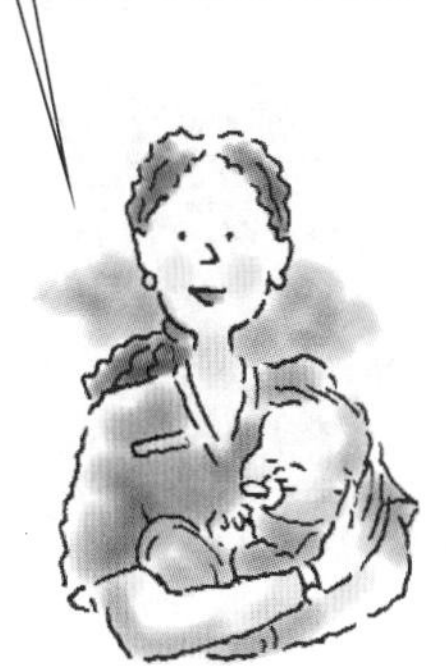

Stretch marks are yet another reminder of the joy of giving birth!

23. A client in early labor is concerned about the pinkish "stretch marks" on her abdomen. Which statement by the client indicates that the nurse's teaching has been effective?

1. "My stretch marks will completely fade away within 6 weeks."
2. "My stretch marks will fade but not disappear after delivery."
3. "An emollient cream will help fade my stretch marks."
4. "A regular exercise program will help my stretch marks go away."

23. 2. Striae are wavy, depressed streaks that may occur over the abdomen, breasts, or thighs as pregnancy progresses. They fade with time to a silvery color but won't disappear. Creams may soften the skin but won't remove the striae. Regular exercise won't affect the stretch marks.

CN: Health promotion and maintenance; CNS: None; CL: Application

24. Which position increases cardiac output and stroke volume of a client in labor?

1. Supine
2. Sitting
3. Side-lying
4. Semi-Fowler's

24. 3. In the side-lying position, cardiac output increases, stroke volume increases, and the pulse rate decreases. In the supine position, the blood pressure can drop severely, due to the pressure of the fetus and enlarged uterus on the vena cava, resulting in supine hypotensive or vena caval syndrome. Neither the sitting nor semi-Fowler's position increases cardiac output or stroke volume.

CN: Health promotion and maintenance; CNS: None; CL: Application

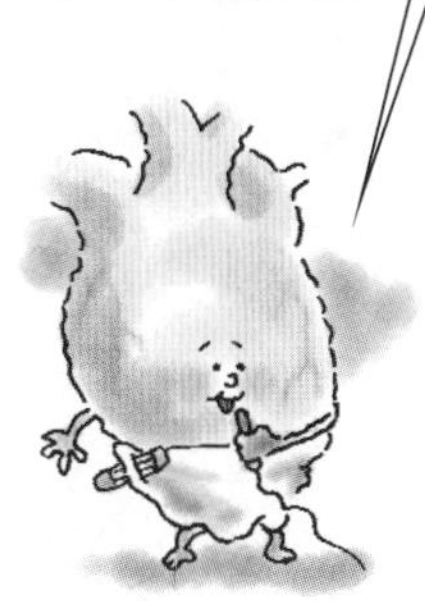

Things are sure getting slow around here.

25. A nurse is caring for a full-term pregnant client in active labor. The electronic fetal monitor reveals a fetal heart rate of less than 70 beats/minute. This finding is considered:

1. Severe fetal bradycardia
2. Normal fetal heart rate
3. Fetal tachycardia
4. Moderate fetal bradycardia

25. 1. A fetal heart rate (FHR) below 70 beats/minute is considered severe fetal bradycardia and is associated with rapidly occurring fetal acidosis. FHR from 70 to 100 beats/minute is considered moderate fetal bradycardia. Normal FHR for a full-term fetus is 120 to 160 beats/minute. Fetal tachycardia is an FHR above 160 beats/minute.

CN: Health promotion and maintenance; CNS: None; CL: Application

26. A nurse is performing Leopold's maneuvers on a client in the early stages of labor. Which finding should alert the nurse to a potential problem?

1. Palpation of the upper fundus reveals a firm, round shape.
2. Palpation of the upper fundus reveals a soft, less-defined shape.
3. Palpation of the side of the fundus reveals a smooth, firm shape.
4. Palpation of the lower fundus reveals a firm, round shape.

26. 1. Palpation of the upper fundus reveals a firm, round head in a breech presentation and a soft less-defined shape in a cephalic delivery. The firm, smooth back of the fetus is palpated on the side of the fundus and may be palpated with cephalic and breech presentations. In a cephalic presentation, palpation of the lower fundus reveals a firm, round head.

CN: Health promotion and maintenance; CNS: None; CL: Application

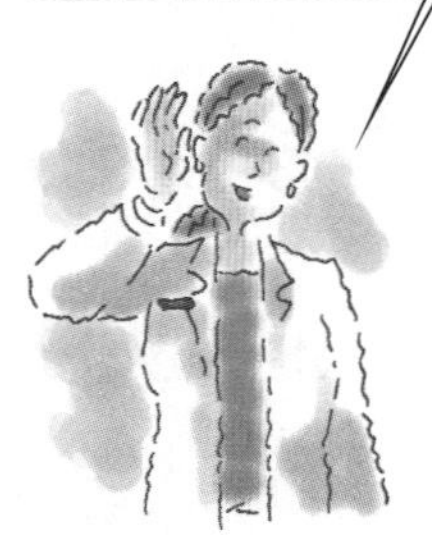

Ah, the sweet sound of most appropriate.

27. A client who's at 35 weeks' gestation arrives at a labor-and-delivery unit leaking clear fluid from her vagina. Which intervention would be most appropriate?

1. Perform a cervical examination.
2. Obtain a catheterized urine specimen.
3. Encourage the client to ambulate.
4. Obtain a sterile speculum sample of the fluid.

27. 4. A sterile speculum examination is performed to identify ruptured membranes. Confirmation is done with nitrazine paper and a positive ferning test. With premature rupture of membranes in a client under 37 weeks' gestation, cervical examinations are contraindicated to reduce the incidence of infection. Clean catch urine specimens, not catheterized specimens, would be appropriate to rule out infection. The client should ambulate only after a thorough nursing assessment and examination to determine the safety of walking for the client and fetus.

CN: Physiological integrity; CNS: Reduction of risk potential; CL: Application

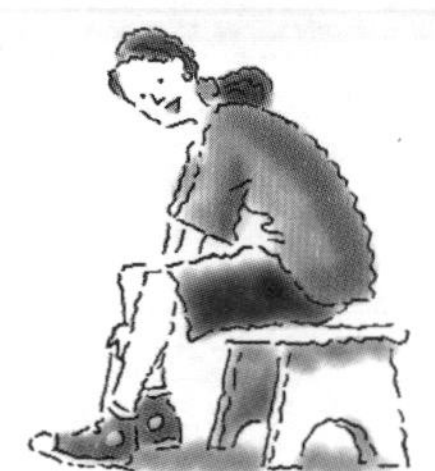

Walking is a great way to relieve stress, and other things!

28. A client at 28 weeks' gestation tells the nurse she's having abdominal contractions that started occurring irregularly and have remained irregular. Which statement should the nurse tell the client?

1. "These contractions will disappear when you walk."
2. "These contractions will increase in frequency and intensity."
3. "These contractions will become regular."
4. "These contractions will move to the lower back."

28. 1. Braxton Hicks contractions begin and remain irregular. They're felt in the abdomen and remain confined to the abdomen and groin. They commonly disappear with ambulation. True contractions begin irregularly but become regular and predictable increasing in frequency and intensity, causing cervical effacement and dilation. True contractions are felt initially in the lower back and radiate to the abdomen in a wavelike motion.

CN: Physiological integrity; CNS: Physiological adaptation; CL: Analysis

29. While in the first stages of labor, a client with active genital herpes is admitted to the labor-and-delivery area. Which type of birth should the nurse anticipate for this client?

1. Mid-forceps
2. Low forceps
3. Induction
4. Cesarean

29. 4. For a client with active genital herpes, cesarean delivery helps avoid infection transmission to the neonate, which could occur during a vaginal birth. Mid-forceps and low forceps are types of vaginal births that could transmit the herpes infection to the neonate. Induction is used only during vaginal birth; therefore, it's inappropriate for this client.

CN: Physiological integrity; CNS: Reduction of risk potential; CL: Application

CN: Client needs category CNS: Client needs subcategory CL: Cognitive level

30. A nurse is monitoring a client in labor and notes on the external fetal monitor that the fetal heart rate (FHR) drops with each contraction. Which action should the nurse take?

1. Turn the client to the left side.
2. Continue to observe FHR.
3. Administer oxygen by face mask.
4. Place the client in Trendelenburg position.

30. 2. Decelerations in FHR, called *early decelerations,* occur with the onset of uterine contractions. They're caused by head compression during the contraction and aren't a sign of fetal distress. Therefore, no action is necessary and the nurse should continue to monitor the FHR.
CN: Physiological integrity; CNS: Reduction of risk potential; CL: Application

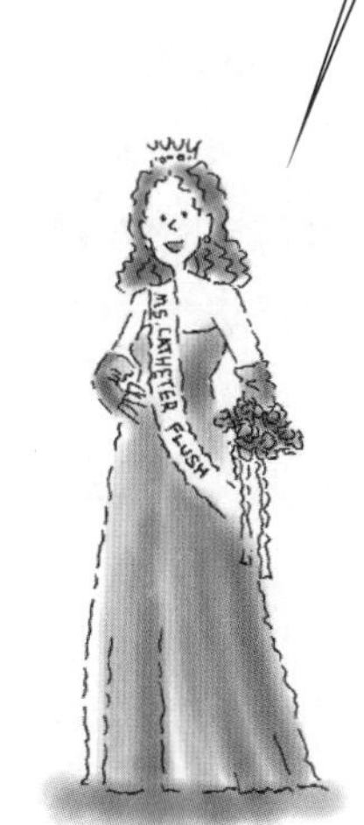

Would you like to know when my crowning took place?

31. The nurse is teaching the stages of labor to a 26-year-old pregnant client. The client would demonstrate that teaching has been effective when she states that crowning occurs during which stage of labor?

1. First
2. Second
3. Third
4. Fourth

31. 2. The second stage of labor begins at full cervical dilation (10 cm) and ends when the infant is born. Crowning is present during this stage as the fetal head, pushed against the perineum, causes the vaginal introitus to open, allowing the fetal scalp to be visible. The first stage begins with true labor contractions and ends with complete cervical dilation. The third stage is from the time the infant is born until the delivery of the placenta. The fourth stage is the first 1 to 4 hours following delivery of the placenta.
CN: Health promotion and maintenance; CNS: None; CL: Application

32. A nurse suspects that the laboring client may have been physically abused by her male partner. Which intervention by the nurse would be most appropriate?

1. Confront the male partner.
2. Question the woman in front of her partner.
3. Contact hospital security.
4. Collaborate with the physician to make a referral to social services.

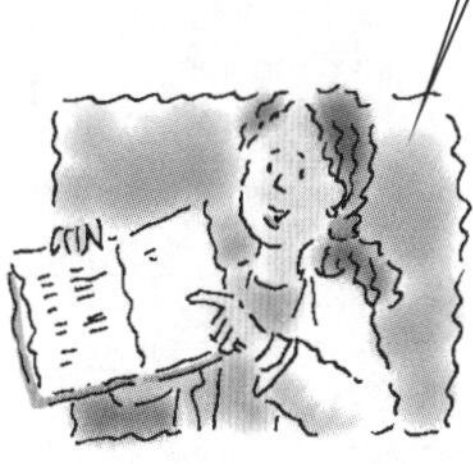

Did you notice the words most appropriate in question 32? Another hint!

32. 4. Collaborating with the physician to make a referral to social services will aid the client by creating a plan and providing support. Additionally, by law, the nurse or nursing supervisor must report the suspected abuse to the police and follow up with a written report. Although confrontation can be used therapeutically, this action will most likely provoke anger in the suspected abuser. Questioning the woman in front of her partner doesn't allow her the privacy required to address this issue and may place her in greater danger. If the woman isn't in imminent danger, there's no need to call hospital security.
CN: Physiological integrity; CNS: Reduction of risk potential; CL: Analysis

33. During a vaginal examination of a client in labor, it is determined that the biparietal diameter of the fetal head has reached the level of the ischial spines. The most accurate documentation of this fetal station would be:

1. −1.
2. 0.
3. +1.
4. +2.

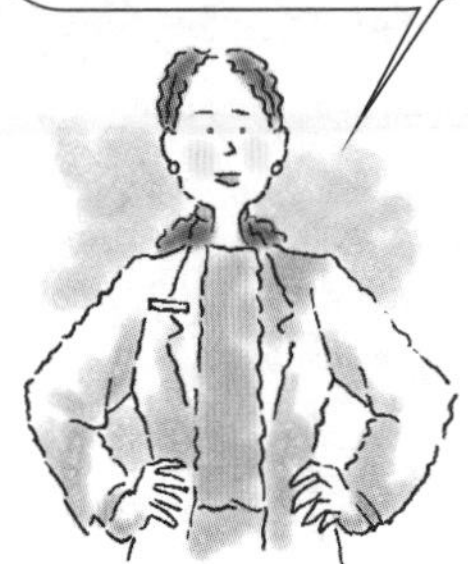

The words most accurate help clarify the correct answer.

33. 2. When the largest diameter of the presenting part (typically the biparietal diameter of the fetal head) is level with the ischial spines, the fetus is at station 0. A station of −1 indicates that the fetal head is 1 cm above the ischial spines. At +1, it's 1 cm below the ischial spines. At +2, it's 2 cm below the ischial spines.

CN: Health promotion and maintenance; CNS: None; CL: Application

34. A nurse has just admitted a client in the labor-and-delivery unit who has been diagnosed by her physician as having diabetes mellitus. Which measure would be most appropriate for this situation?

1. Ask the client about her most recent blood glucose levels.
2. Prepare oral hypoglycemic medications for administration during labor.
3. Notify the neonatal intensive care unit that you've admitted a client with diabetes.
4. Prepare the client for cesarean delivery.

34. 1. As part of the history, asking about the client's most recent blood glucose levels will indicate how well her diabetes has been controlled. Oral hypoglycemic drugs are never used during pregnancy because they cross the placental barrier, stimulate fetal insulin production, and are potentially teratogenic. Plans to admit the infant to the neonatal intensive care unit are premature. Cesarean delivery is no longer the preferred delivery for clients with diabetes. Vaginal birth is preferred and presents a lower risk to the mother and fetus.

CN: Physiological integrity; CNS: Reduction of risk potential; CL: Application

35. A client is admitted to the labor-and-delivery unit with a known anencephalic fetus. Which measure would be appropriate for the nurse to perform?

1. Assess fetal heart tones.
2. Reassure the client that she'll get pregnant again soon.
3. Avoid talking about the baby.
4. Provide privacy.

35. 4. Providing privacy is an appropriate therapeutic intervention for the client and family to grieve their loss. Fetal heart tones are rarely assessed in a client with an anencephalic fetus; most fetuses won't survive due to lack of cerebral function. Reassuring the client that she will get pregnant again dismisses how she is feeling about her current loss and also provides false reassurance. The nurse should take the lead from the client and family as some people want to talk about their loss and others don't.

CN: Psychosocial integrity; CNS: None; CL: Application

36. A 30-year-old multiparous client admitted to the labor-and-delivery unit hasn't received prenatal care for this pregnancy. Which data is most relevant to the nursing assessment?

1. Date of last menstrual period (LMP)
2. Family history of sexually transmitted diseases (STDs)
3. Name of insurance provider
4. Number of siblings

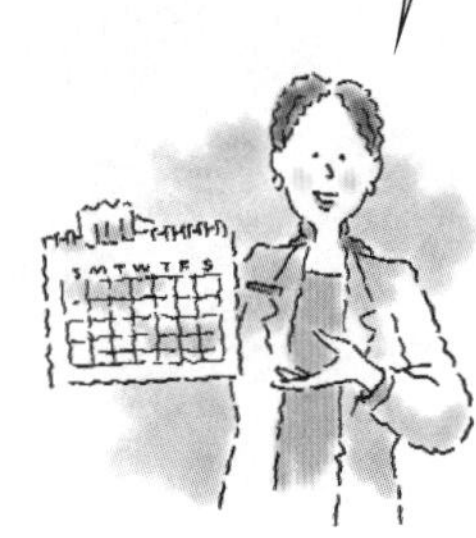

The estimated date of delivery can be determined with the proper information.
SMTWTFS

36. 1. The date of the LMP is essential to estimate the date of delivery. The nursing history would also include subjective information, such as personal (but not necessarily family) history of STDs, gravidity, and parity. Although beneficial to the hospital for financial reimbursement, the insurance provider has no bearing on the nursing history. Likewise, the number of siblings isn't pertinent to the assessment.

CN: Health promotion and maintenance; CNS: None; CL: Analysis

CN: Client needs category CNS: Client needs subcategory CL: Cognitive level

37. Which symptom, when observed in laboring clients with hypertension of pregnancy, would most likely indicate a worsening condition?

1. Decreasing blood pressure
2. Increasing oliguria
3. Decreasing edema
4. Trace levels of protein in the urine

37. 2. Renal plasma flow and glomerular filtration are decreased in gestational hypertension, so increasing oliguria indicates a worsening condition. Blood pressure increases (not decreases) as a result of increased peripheral resistance. Increasing (not decreasing) edema would suggest a worsening condition. Trace levels to +1 proteinuria are acceptable levels. Higher levels would indicate a worsening condition.

CN: Health promotion and maintenance; CNS: None; CL: Application

38. While performing a cervical examination, a nurse's fingertips feel pulsating tissue. What would be the most appropriate nursing intervention?

1. Leave the client and call the physician.
2. Put the client in a semi-Fowler's position.
3. Ask the client to push with the next contraction.
4. Leave the fingers in place and press the nurse call light.

38. 4. When the umbilical cord precedes the fetal presenting part, it's known as a prolapsed cord. Leaving the fingers in place and calling for assistance is the safest intervention for the fetus, as you'll need to keep the fetus off the cord to reduce cord compression. The nursing staff will contact the physician, and the client will probably need a cesarean delivery because of the risk of fetal demise with the fetus pressing against the cord during delivery. Placing the client in the semi-Fowler's position would increase the pressure of the fetus on the umbilical cord. Asking the client to push with the next contraction would be contraindicated, as it would also force the presenting part against the cord, causing severe bradycardia and possible fetal demise.

CN: Physiological integrity; CNS: Reduction of risk potential; CL: Application

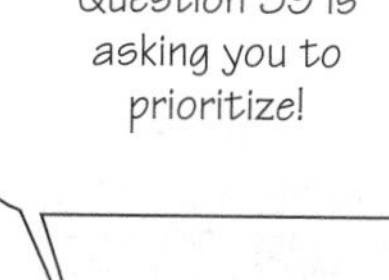
Question 39 is
asking you to
prioritize!

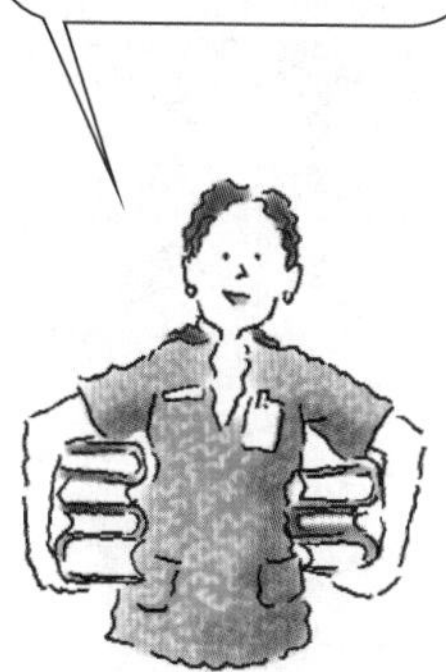

39. A client is admitted to the labor-and-delivery unit in labor, with blood flowing down her legs. Which nursing intervention would be most appropriate?

1. Place an indwelling catheter.
2. Monitor fetal heart tones.
3. Perform a cervical examination.
4. Prepare the client for cesarean delivery.

39. 2. Monitoring fetal heart tones would be the first step because it's necessary to establish fetal well-being due to a possible placenta previa or abruptio placentae. Although an indwelling catheter may be placed, it isn't an early intervention. Performing a cervical examination would be contraindicated because any agitation of the cervix with a previa can result in hemorrhage and death for the mother or fetus. Preparing the client for a cesarean delivery may not be indicated. A sonogram will need to be performed to determine the cause of bleeding. If the diagnosis is a partial placenta previa, the client may still be able to deliver vaginally.

CN: Physiological integrity; CNS: Reduction of risk potential; CL: Application

40. A client in labor is receiving magnesium sulfate to treat hypertension of pregnancy. How should this drug be administered?

1. As a loading dose of 4 g in normal saline solution, followed by a continuous infusion of 1 to 2 g/hour
2. As a loading dose of 2 g in normal saline solution, followed by a continuous infusion of 2 g/hour
3. As a loading dose of 4 g in dextrose 5% in water (D_5W), followed by a continuous infusion of 1 to 2 g/hour
4. As a loading dose of 4 grams in D_5W, followed by a continuous infusion of 4 g/hour

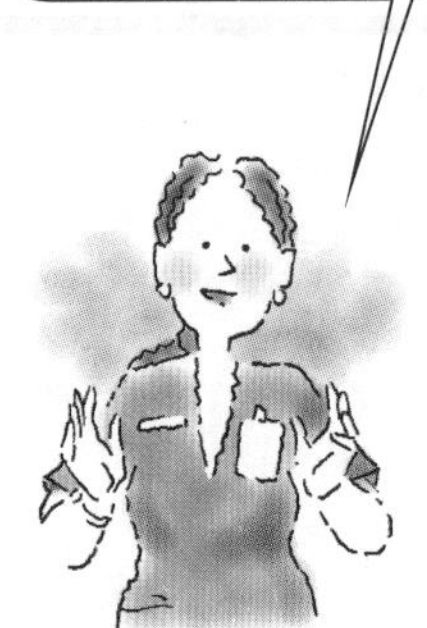

You're really "delivering" the right answers. Keep going!

40. 3. A loading dose of magnesium sulfate should be given as a 4-g bolus, followed by a continuous infusion of 1 to 2 g/hour in D_5W for maintenance. Magnesium sulfate shouldn't be administered in normal saline solution.

CN: Physiological integrity; CNS: Pharmacological and parenteral therapies; CL: Application

41. A multiparous client who has been in labor for 2 hours states that she feels the urge to move her bowels. How should the nurse respond?

1. Let the client get up to use the toilet.
2. Allow the client to use a bedpan.
3. Perform a pelvic examination.
4. Check the fetal heart rate (FHR).

41. 3. A complaint of rectal pressure usually indicates a low presenting fetal part, signaling imminent delivery. The nurse should perform a pelvic examination to assess the dilation of the cervix and station of the presenting fetal part. Don't let the client use the toilet or a bedpan before she's examined because she could deliver on the toilet or in the bedpan. Checking the FHR is important but comes after the nurse evaluates the client's complaint.

CN: Health promotion and maintenance; CNS: None; CL: Application

42. The physician has ordered an I.V. of 5% dextrose in lactated Ringer's solution at 125 ml/hr. The I.V. tubing delivers 10 drops per ml. How many drops per minute should fall into the drip chamber?

1. 10 to 11
2. 12 to 13
3. 20 to 21
4. 22 to 24

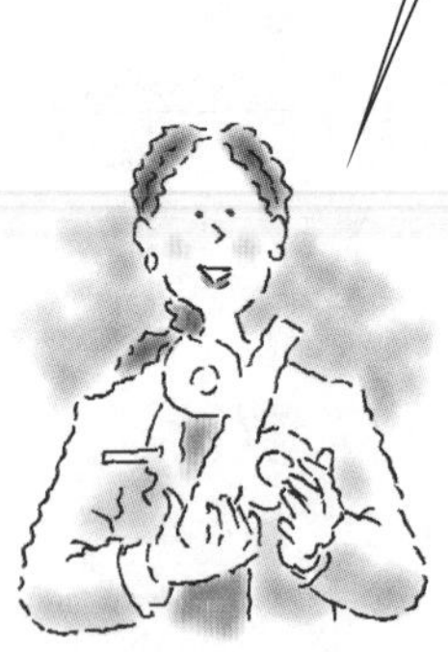

Your math skills are being tested on this one!
You can do it!

42. 3. Multiply the number of milliliters to be infused (125) by the drop factor (10); $125 \times 10 = 1{,}250$. Then divide the answer by the number of minutes to run the infusion (60); $1{,}250 \div 60 = 20.83$, or 20 to 21 gtt/minute.

CN: Physiological integrity; CNS: Pharmacological and parenteral therapies; CL: Application

43. An amniotomy is performed on a client in labor. Following this procedure what is the priority nursing intervention?

1. Encourage the client to use breathing exercises as contractions increase.
2. Assess fetal heart tones.
3. Assist the client to ambulate to promote labor.
4. Position the client on her left side.

43. 2. The nurse's priority is to assess fetal heart tones. When the amniotic membrane is ruptured, the umbilical cord may enter the birth canal with the gush of fluid and the presenting part may cause cord compression. After amniotomy, contractions may intensify; however, helping the client with her breathing should be done after fetal well-being is assessed. Ambulation may also promote labor, but should only be done after fetal well-being is established. While the left lateral position enhances blood flow, it isn't a priority until fetal heart tones are assessed.

CN: Physiological integrity; CNS: Reduction of risk potential; CL: Application

44. The effectiveness of drug therapy for a client at 34 weeks' gestation with hypertension of pregnancy can be determined by which finding?

1. Absence of seizures
2. Weight gain of 4 lb (1.8 kg)/week
3. Blood pressure of 154/90 mm Hg
4. Urinary output of 25 ml/hour

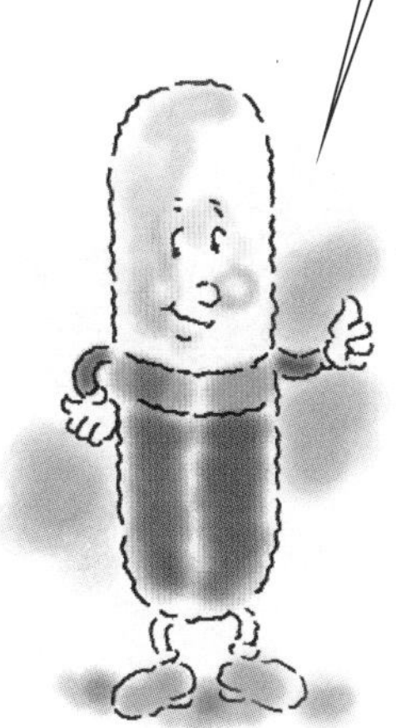

It's important to know how to measure a drug's effectiveness.

44. 1. Therapeutic effects of drugs used to treat hypertension of pregnancy in a client at 34 weeks' gestation, such as magnesium sulfate, include an absence of seizures, a weight gain of 2 lb (0.9 kg)/week, a normal blood pressure, and a urinary output greater than 30 ml/hour.

CN: Physiological integrity; CNS: Pharmacological and parenteral therapies; CL: Analysis

45. A laboring client in the latent stage of labor begins complaining of pain in the epigastric area, blurred vision, and a headache. The nurse knows that which medication should be prepared for administration?

1. Terbutaline
2. Oxytocin (Pitocin)
3. Magnesium sulfate
4. Calcium gluconate

45. 3. Magnesium sulfate is the drug of choice to treat hypertension of pregnancy because it reduces edema by causing a shift from the extracellular spaces into the intestines. It also depresses the central nervous system, which decreases the incidence of seizures. Terbutaline is a smooth-muscle relaxant used to relax the uterus. Oxytocin is the synthetic form of the pituitary hormone used to stimulate uterine contractions. Calcium gluconate is the antagonist for magnesium toxicity.

CN: Physiological integrity; CNS: Pharmacological and parenteral therapies; CL: Analysis

46. A nurse is assisting in monitoring a client in labor. Which monitoring data are indicative of fetal well-being?

1. Fetal heart rate of 145 to 155 beats/minute with 15-second accelerations to 160.
2. Fetal heart rate of 130 to 140 beats/minute with late decelerations to 110.
3. Fetal heart rate of 110 to 120 beats/minute with variable deceleration to 90.
4. Fetal heart rate of 165 to 175 beats/minute with late decelerations to 140.

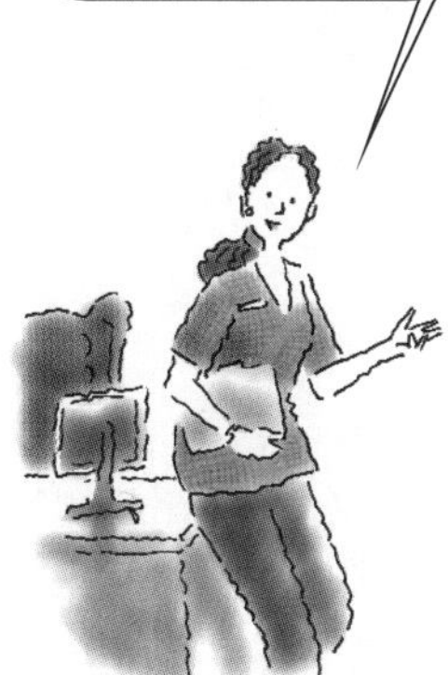

Remembering when different decelerations occur is important!

46. 1. Accelerations of up to 15 beats/minute above baseline for a duration of 15 seconds are signs of fetal well-being. Decelerations initiated 30 to 40 seconds after the onset of the contraction are termed late decelerations and are due to uteroplacental insufficiency from decreased blood flow during uterine contractions. Variable decelerations are an indication of cord compression. Variable decelerations can occur with or without contractions.

CN: Physiological integrity; CNS: Physiological adaptation; CL: Analysis

47. A nurse is examining a client in active labor who has had spontaneous rupture of the amniotic membrane and notes a protruding umbilical cord. What is the priority nursing action the nurse should take?

1. Push the umbilical cord into the uterus.
2. Place the client in Trendelenburg position.
3. Instruct the client to begin to push.
4. Wrap the cord in a dry sterile dressing.

47. 2. A Trendelenburg or knee-chest position takes the weight of the fetus off the umbilical cord, allowing blood to flow. The cord should never be pushed back into the uterus, as this could damage the cord, obsruct the flow of blood through the cord to the fetus, or introduce infection into the uterus. The client shouldn't be instructed to push as she is only in active labor and emergency surgery may be necessary. The cord should be wrapped in a sterile saline soaked gauze.

CN: Physiological integrity; CNS: Reduction of risk potential; CL: Application

48. The first day of a client's last menstrual period (LMP) was October 10. Using Nägele's rule, what is the estimated date of delivery?
1. July 10
2. July 17
3. August 10
4. August 17

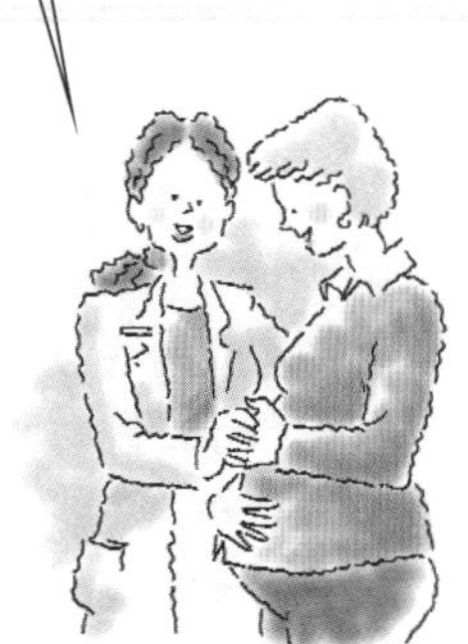

Can you figure out this little one's estimated time of arrival?

48. 2. After determining the first day of the LMP, the nurse would subtract 3 months and add 7 days. If the client's LMP was October 10, subtracting 3 months is July 10, and adding 7 days brings the date to July 17.
CN: Health promotion and maintenance; CNS: None; CL: Analysis

49. At 1 minute of life, a neonate is crying vigorously, has a heart rate of 98, is active with normal reflexes, and has a pink body and blue extremities. Which Apgar score would be correct for this neonate?
1. 6
2. 7
3. 8
4. 9

49. 3. Heart rate, respiratory effort, muscle tone, reflex irritability, and color are used to assess the Apgar score. Each of the signs is assigned a score of 0, 1, or 2. The highest possible score is 10. This neonate lost 1 point for a heart rate less than 100 beats/minute and 1 point for its acrocyanosis, a common finding in which the trunk is pink but the extremities are bluish.
CN: Health promotion and maintenance; CNS: None; CL: Analysis

50. A client in labor suddenly sits upright, clutches her chest, and gasps for breath. Which laboratory finding indicates that the client's condition is worsening?
1. Increased fibrinogen level
2. Increased platelet count
3. Prolonged prothrombin time
4. Reduced partial thromboplastin time

50. 3. The client most likely has an amniotic fluid embolism. Disseminated intravascular coagulation is a life-threatening complication of this condition and is marked by a decreased platelet count and fibrinogen level, and a prolonged prothrombin time and partial thromboplastin time.
CN: Physiological integrity; CNS: Reduction of risk potential; CL: Analysis

51. Immediately after delivery, a nurse assesses the neonate's respiratory effort as slow. The neonate is actively moving but grimaces in response to stimulation. His fingers and toes are bluish, and his heart rate is 130 beats/minute. Which step should the nurse take next?
1. Tell the physician that the neonate appears abnormal.
2. Assign an Apgar score of 8.
3. Assign an Apgar score of 10.
4. Provide oxygen and stimulate the baby to cry.

51. 4. The nurse should stimulate the baby to cry, provide oxygen, and call the physician to evaluate reflex irritability. It would be inappropriate to tell the physician that the neonate appears abnormal. The neonate's Apgar score is 7. Of a maximum possible score of 10, the nurse deducts 1 point for acrocyanosis, 1 point for slow respiratory effort, and 1 point for the grimace (indicating reflex irritability).
CN: Safe, effective care environment; CNS: Management of care; CL: Application

52. A pregnant client has a total hemoglobin level of 9 g/dl. Which risk is greatest during the intrapartum period?

1. Small-for-gestational-age neonate
2. Fetal distress
3. Excessive postpartum bleeding
4. Shortness of breath

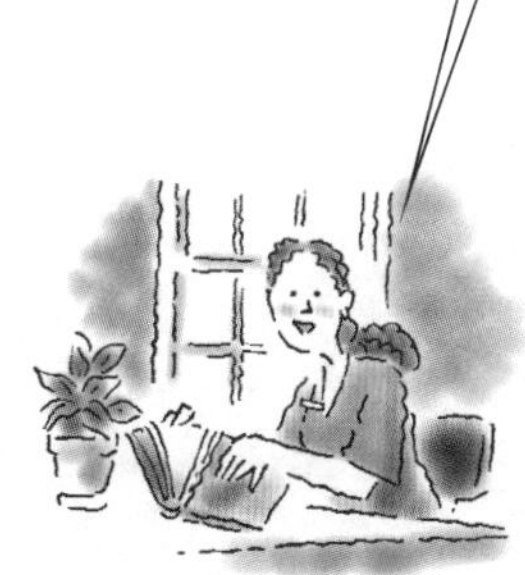

What do you think is the greatest risk?

52. 2. Fetal distress is more common in women with anemia than in the general non-anemic population. A small-for-gestational-age neonate and excessive postpartum bleeding are diagnosed after the intrapartum period. Shortness of breath occurs more commonly antepartally; the risk for developing shortness of breath doesn't increase during the intrapartum period.

CN: Physiological integrity; CNS: Reduction of risk potential; CL: Application

53. Which is the most common and popular method for assessing fetal status throughout labor?

1. Fetal heart rate (FHR) auscultation using a stethoscope
2. FHR auscultation and recording using electronic fetal monitoring
3. Asking the client how she feels and whether the fetus is moving
4. Doing pelvic examinations to check the location of the fetal presenting part

53. 2. The most common and popular method for fetal assessment throughout labor is electronic monitoring, which records the FHR and maternal contractions and shows how the fetus reacts to the stress of contractions. Although FHR auscultation can be done with a stethoscope, it's less common because it requires advanced skills. Asking the client how she feels and whether the fetus is moving are important but don't provide specifics about fetal well-being. A pelvic examination reveals cervical dilation and fetal station but doesn't reveal fetal well-being.

CN: Health promotion and maintenance; CNS: None; CL: Analysis

54. Which finding in a client who is at 36 weeks' gestation indicates that premature rupture of the membranes has occurred?

1. Fernlike pattern when vaginal fluid dries on a glass slide
2. Nitrogen paper indicates acidic pH of fluid
3. Cervical dilation of 8 cm
4. Contractions occurring every 3 minutes

54. 1. A fernlike pattern that forms when vaginal fluid is dried on a glass slide is a sign of ruptured membranes. Amniotic fluid is alkaline when tested with nitrogen paper. Cervical dilation and length of contractions don't indicate the condition of the membranes.

CN: Physiological integrity; CNS: Reduction of risk potential; CL: Application

55. The nurse is teaching an intrapartum client about fetal presentation. Which statement would be the most accurate?

1. Fetal body part that enters the maternal pelvis first
2. Relationship of the presenting part to the maternal pelvis
3. Relationship of the long axis of the fetus to the long axis of the mother
4. A classification according to the fetal part

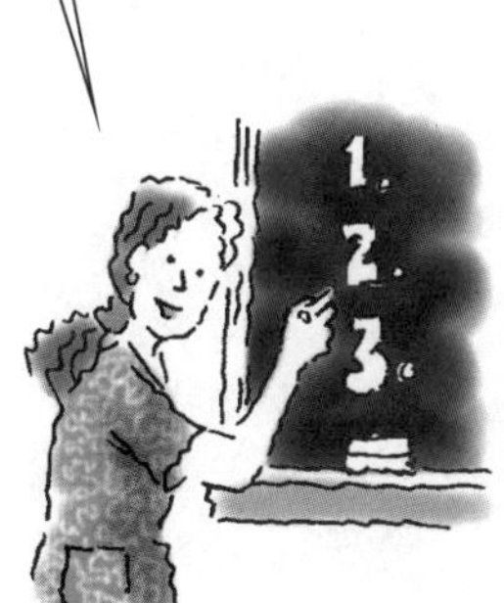

55. 1. Presentation is the fetal body part that enters the pelvis first; it's classified by the presenting part; the three main presentations are cephalic, breech, and shoulder. The relationship of the presenting fetal part to the maternal pelvis refers to fetal position. The relationship of the long axis of the fetus to the long axis of the mother refers to fetal lie; the three possible lies are longitudinal, transverse, and oblique.

CN: Physiological integrity; CNS: Physiological adaptation; CL: Application

56. A client with gestational diabetes has just delivered a 10-lb, 2-oz neonate at 39 weeks' gestation. Which priority nursing intervention should be included in the care plan?

1. Teach the mother about the nutritional needs of the neonate.
2. Obtain a serum neonatal glucose level.
3. Obtain a serum neonatal bilirubin level.
4. Prepare to administer insulin to the neonate.

56. 2. The priority nursing intervention is to monitor the neonate's serum glucose level due to the increased risk of hypoglycemia. During pregnancy the fetus secretes high levels of insulin to counteract the high maternal glucose levels. This elevated insulin secretion in the neonate can lead to severe hypoglycemia after birth. While it is important to discuss the neonate's nutritional needs with the mother, it isn't an immediate priority. The newborn of a mother with diabetes may develop hyperbilirubinemia, but not as quickly as hypoglycemia may develop. Since the neonate is at risk for hypoglycemia, insulin wouldn't be appropriate.
CN: Safe, effective care environment; CNS: Management of care; CL: Application

57. The nurse is caring for a client in labor. Which components of labor contractions would be the most accurate for the nurse to assess with this client?

1. Pelvic type, duration, and frequency
2. Contraction type and frequency, and pelvic type
3. Contraction duration, frequency, and intensity
4. Contraction type, duration, and intensity

57. 3. The three components of a contraction that the nurse must evaluate are the duration, frequency, and intensity of each contraction. Pelvic type has no bearing on contractions.
CN: Health promotion and maintenance; CNS: None; CL: Application

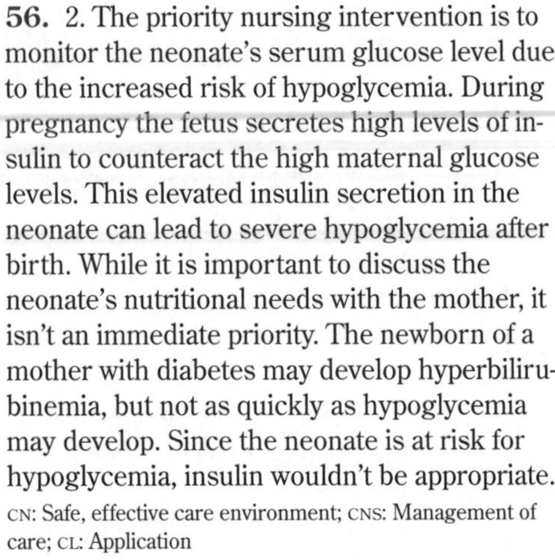

The Lamaze method of prepared childbirth uses breathing techniques to ease delivery.

58. A client in labor is using the Lamaze method of prepared childbirth. Her cervix is dilated 5 cm, with contractions occurring 2 to 3 minutes apart. The nurse should instruct the client to breathe at which level?

1. Level 1
2. Level 2
3. Level 3
4. Level 4

58. 2. Level 2 breathing techniques are useful when cervical dilation is between 4 and 6 cm. Level 1 breathing techniques are useful for early contractions; level 3 and level 4 breathing techniques are used in the transition stage of labor.
CN: Health promotion and maintenance; CNS: None; CL: Application

59. A client has received dinoprostone (Prostin E2) for cervical ripening. The nurse should assess her for which adverse drug effect?

1. Vomiting
2. Euphoria
3. Uterine inversion
4. Constipation

59. 1. Headache, nausea and vomiting, chills, fever, and hypertension are adverse effects of dinoprostone. Euphoria and uterine inversion are rare adverse effects of this drug. Diarrhea, not constipation, is a possible adverse effect.
CN: Physiological integrity; CNS: Pharmacological and parenteral therapies; CL: Analysis

60. A nurse is caring for a client with short, mild contractions and cervical dilation of 4 cm. Using an external fetal monitor, the nurse observes variable decelerations. Which action should the nurse take first?

1. Prepare for imminent delivery.
2. Place the client on her left side.
3. Administer oxygen by face mask.
4. Prepare the client for a still birth.

60. 2. Variable decelerations in fetal heart rate are caused by compression of the umbilical cord. Typically, variable decelerations are corrected by placing the client in a left lateral position to alleviate cord pressure. Since variable decelerations are usually transient and correctable, the nurse wouldn't prepare for an imminent or still birth. If other measures have been ineffective in correcting the variable deceleration, oxygen may be administered.

CN: Physiological integrity; CNS: Reduction of risk potential; CL: Analysis

61. At 39 weeks' gestation, a primiparous client arrives at the labor-and-delivery unit complaining of lower back pain that started 6 hours ago. A pelvic examination reveals that her cervix is dilated 3 cm and 75% effaced. Which action would be appropriate for the nurse to take?

1. Instruct the client to push.
2. Determine the Apgar score.
3. Monitor the fetal heart rate.
4. Assess the lochia.

61. 3. This client is in the latent phase of the first stage of labor. The nurse should monitor the fetal heart in this stage and all stages of labor. Pushing is appropriate during the second stage of labor when the cervix is fully dilated. The nurse determines the Apgar score on the neonate immediately after delivery. During the fourth stage the nurse assesses the amount, color, and consistency of lochia.

CN: Health promotion and maintenance; CNS: None; CL: Application

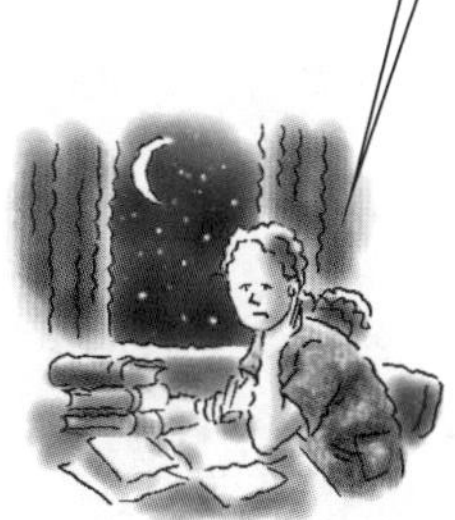

Don't give up now. Only three questions left!

62. A nurse is assisting in monitoring a client who's receiving oxytocin (Pitocin) to induce labor. The nurse should be alert to which maternal adverse reactions? Select all that apply:

1. Hypertension
2. Jaundice
3. Dehydration
4. Fluid overload
5. Uterine tetany
6. Bradycardia

62. 1, 4, 5. Adverse effects of oxytocin in the mother include hypertension, fluid overload, and uterine tetany. Oxytocin's antidiuretic effect increases renal reabsorption of water, leading to fluid overload, not dehydration. Jaundice and bradycardia are adverse effects that may occur in the neonate. Tachycardia, not bradycardia, is a maternal adverse effect.

CN: Physiological integrity; CNS: Pharmacology and parenteral therapies; CL: Application

63. A client is admitted to the labor-and-delivery unit at 36 weeks' gestation. She has a history of cesarean delivery and complains of severe abdominal pain that started less than 1 hour earlier. When the nurse palpates tetanic contractions, the client again complains of severe pain. After the client vomits, she states that the pain is better and then passes out. Which nursing intervention takes the highest priority?

1. Assess the client's level of pain.
2. Place the client in a left lateral position.
3. Administer I.V. antibiotics.
4. Prepare the client for immediate surgery.

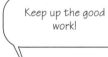

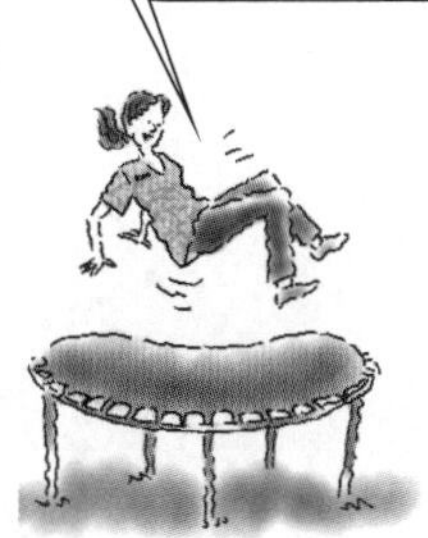

63. 4. Uterine rupture is a medical emergency that may occur before or during labor. Signs and symptoms typically include abdominal pain that may ease after uterine rupture, vomiting, vaginal bleeding, hypovolemic shock, and fetal distress. The client should be prepared for immediate surgery to save her life and that of the fetus. While assessing and relieving pain are important interventions, they aren't priorities in this life-threatening situation. Placing the client in a left lateral position won't affect her condition. Antibiotics may be administered but aren't the highest priority in this situation.

CN: Safe, effective care environment; CNS: Management of care; CL: Application

64. Which illustration represents a right occiput posterior (ROP) fetal position?

1. 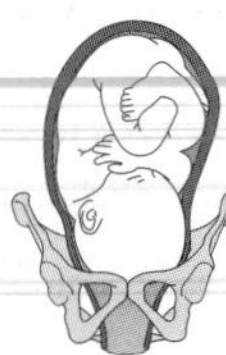
2. 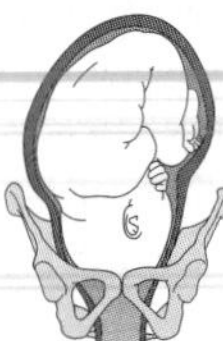
3. 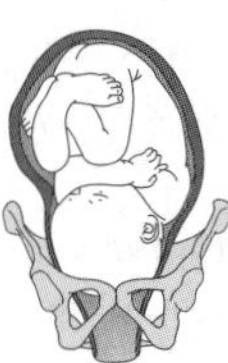
4. 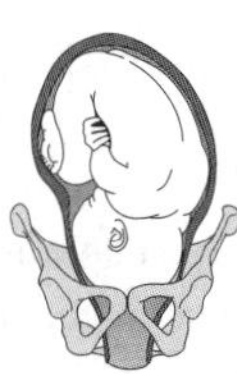

64. 1. Fetal positioning is determined by how the fetus presents in relation to the mother's pelvis, which is divided into four quadrants: right anterior, left anterior, right posterior, and left posterior. In a ROP position, the fetus' occiput points to the maternal right posterior quadrant. Option 2 shows a right occiput anterior (ROA) position, option 3 shows a left occiput posterior (LOP), and option 4 shows a left occiput anterior (LOA).

CN: Health promotion and maintenance; CNS: None; CL: Application

65. The nurse is evaluating an external fetal monitoring strip of a client in labor. What condition is the nurse concerned about?

1. Cephalopelvic disproportion
2. Oligohydramines
3. Uteroplacental insufficiency
4. Hydramnios

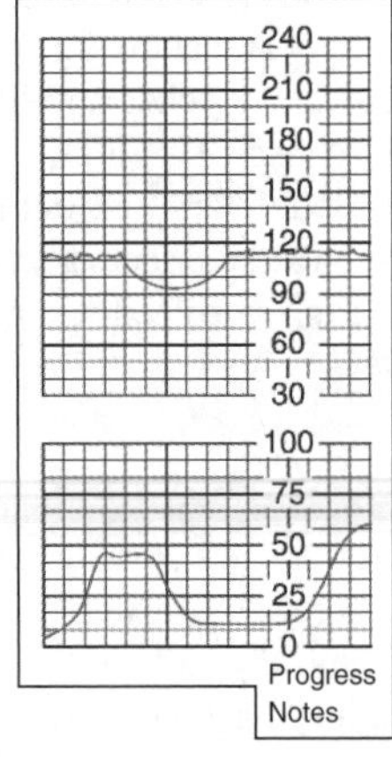

65. 3. This fetal monitoring strip illustrates a late deceleration. The decrease in fetal heart rate begins after the peak of the contraction and doesn't return to baseline until the contraction is over. Late decelerations are associated with uteroplacental insufficiency, shock, or fetal metabolic acidosis. Cephalopelvic disproportion may cause early not late decelerations early in labor. Oligohydramines (less than the normal amount of amniotic fluid) may be associated with variable decelerations. Hydramnios (excessive amniotic fluid) may be associated with uterine rupture.

CN: Physiological integrity; CNS: Reduction of risk potential; CL: Analysis

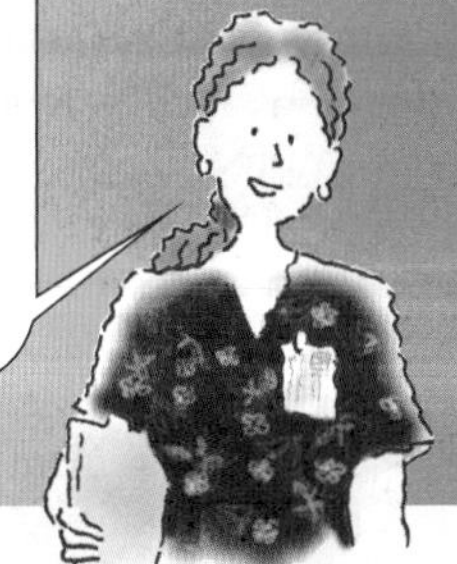

Before taking off through this chapter, why not spend a few minutes browsing the birthing stories at **www.birthstories.com.** It'll get you in just the right mood to tackle care of the postpartum client. Enjoy!

Chapter 24 Postpartum care

1. When completing the morning postpartum assessment, a nurse notices a client's perineal pad is completely saturated with lochia rubra. Which action should be the nurse's <u>first</u> response?

1. Vigorously massage the fundus.
2. Immediately call the physician.
3. Have the charge nurse review the assessment.
4. Ask the client when she last changed her perineal pad.

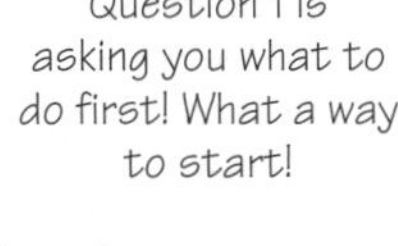

Question 1 is asking you what to do first! What a way to start!

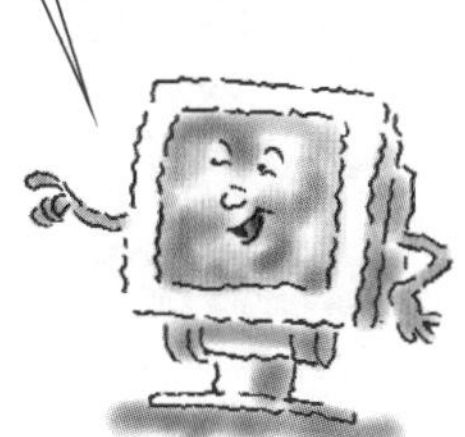

1. 4. If the morning assessment is done relatively early, it's possible that the client hasn't yet been to the bathroom, in which case her perineal pad may have been in place all night. Secondly, her lochia may have pooled during the night, resulting in a heavy flow in the morning. Vigorous massage of the fundus isn't recommended for heavy bleeding or hemorrhage. The nurse wouldn't want to call the physician unnecessarily. If the nurse were uncertain, it would be appropriate to have another qualified individual check the client but only after a complete assessment of the client's status.

CN: Safe, effective care environment; CNS: Management of care; CL: Analysis

2. Which factor might result in a decreased supply of breast milk in a postpartum mother?

1. Supplemental feedings with formula
2. Maternal diet high in vitamin C
3. An alcoholic drink
4. Frequent feedings

2. 1. Routine formula supplementation may interfere with establishing an adequate milk volume because suckling by the baby at the breast stimulates prolactin production, the hormone responsible for milk production. Vitamin C levels haven't been shown to influence milk volume. One drink containing alcohol generally tends to relax the mother, facilitating letdown. Excessive consumption of alcohol may block letdown of milk to the infant, though supply isn't necessarily affected. Frequent feedings are likely to increase milk production.

CN: Health promotion and maintenance; CNS: None; CL: Application

3. Which intervention should be helpful to a breast-feeding mother with engorged breasts?

1. Applying ice
2. Applying a breast binder
3. Teaching how to express her breasts in a warm shower
4. Administering bromocriptine (Parlodel)

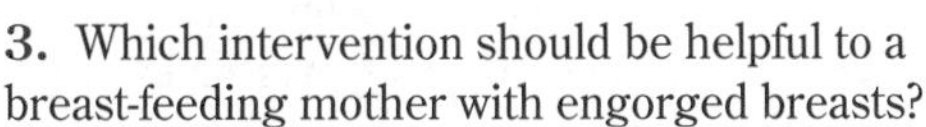

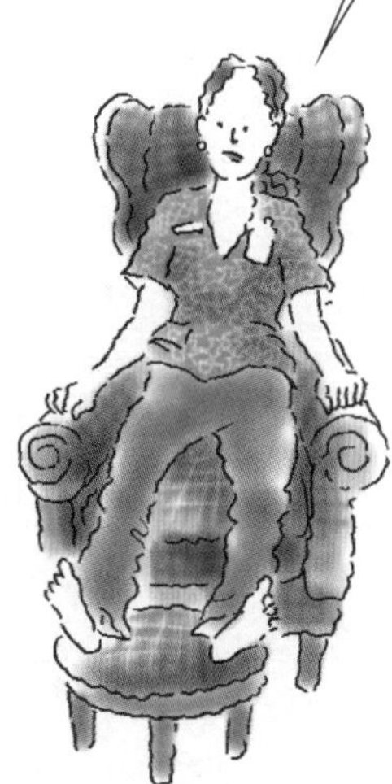

Which of these options would promote comfort best?

3. 3. Teaching the client how to express her breasts in a warm shower aids with letdown and will give temporary relief. Ice can promote comfort by decreasing blood flow (vasoconstriction), numbing, and discouraging further letdown of milk; however, this is followed by a rebound reaction of more letting down once the ice is removed. Breast binders aren't effective in relieving the discomforts of engorgement. Bromocriptine is no longer indicated for lactation suppression.

CN: Physiological integrity; CNS: Basic care and comfort; CL: Application

CN: Client needs category CNS: Client needs subcategory CL: Cognitive level

4. Which assessment should be performed routinely in the postpartum client?
1. Antibody screen
2. Babinski's reflex
3. Homans' sign
4. Patellar reflex

4. 3. Homans' sign, or pain on dorsiflexion of the foot, may indicate deep vein thrombosis (DVT). Postpartum women are at increased risk of DVT because of changes in clotting mechanisms to control bleeding at delivery. An antibody screen wouldn't be classified as an assessment technique. Both Babinski's reflex and the patellar reflex need not be routinely assessed in the postpartum woman.
CN: Health promotion and maintenance; CNS: None; CL: Analysis

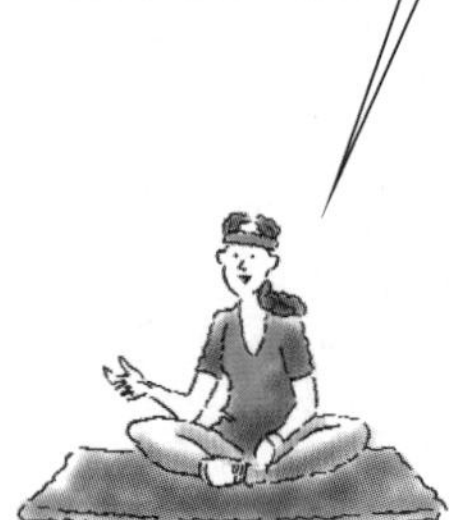

If you know what Kegel exercises are, you should get question 5 correct easily.

5. Which reason explains why Kegel exercises are advantageous to women after they deliver a child?
1. They assist with lochia removal.
2. They promote the return of normal bowel function.
3. They promote blood flow, allowing for healing and strengthening the musculature.
4. They assist the woman in burning calories for rapid postpartum weight loss.

5. 3. Exercising the pubococcygeal muscle increases blood flow to the area. The increased blood flow brings oxygen and other nutrients to the perineal area to aid in healing. Additionally, these exercises help to strengthen the musculature, thereby decreasing the risk of future complications, such as incontinence and uterine prolapse. Performing Kegel exercises may assist with lochia removal but that isn't their main purpose. Bowel function isn't influenced by Kegel exercises. Kegel exercises don't expend sufficient energy to burn many calories.
CN: Health promotion and maintenance; CNS: None; CL: Analysis

6. To detect pulmonary embolus in a client in the immediate postpartum period, a nurse should be alert to which symptoms?
1. Sudden dyspnea and chest pain
2. Chills and fever
3. Bradycardia and hypertension
4. Confusion and bradypnea

6. 1. Signs of pulmonary embolus include sudden dyspnea and chest pain. Chills and fever signal an infection. The client with a pulmonary embolus would have tachycardia, hypotension, confusion, and tachypnea.
CN: Physiological integrity; CNS: Reduction of risk potential; CL: Analysis

7. Which practice should a nurse recommend to a client who has had a cesarean delivery?
1. Frequent douching after she's discharged
2. Coughing and deep-breathing exercises
3. Sit-ups at 2 weeks postoperatively
4. Side-rolling exercises

7. 2. As for any postoperative client, coughing and deep-breathing exercises should be taught to keep the alveoli open and prevent infection. Frequent douching isn't recommended for women and is contraindicated in women who have just given birth. Sit-ups at 2 weeks postpartum could potentially damage the healing of the incision. Side-rolling exercises aren't an accepted medical practice.
CN: Physiological integrity; CNS: Reduction of risk potential; CL: Application

8. Which reason explains why a client might express disappointment after having a cesarean delivery instead of a vaginal delivery?

1. Cesarean deliveries cost more.
2. Depression is more common after a cesarean delivery.
3. The client is usually more fatigued after cesarean delivery.
4. The client may feel a loss for not having experienced a "normal" birth.

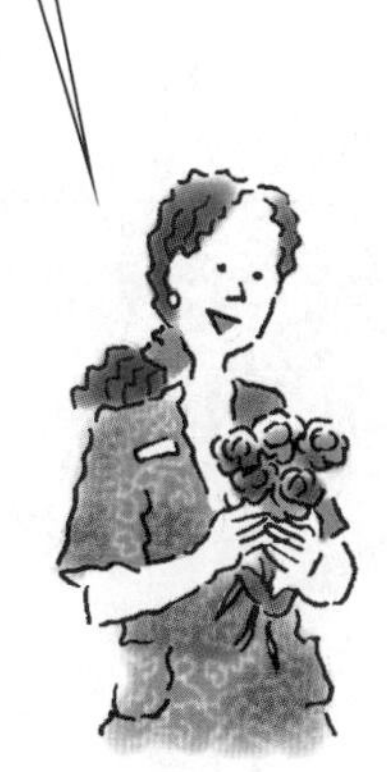

Remember to be sensitive to your postpartum client's needs.

8. 4. Clients occasionally feel a loss after a cesarean delivery especially if it was unplanned. They may feel they're inadequate because they couldn't deliver their infant vaginally. The cost of cesarean delivery doesn't generally apply because the woman isn't directly responsible for payment. No conclusive studies support the theory that depression is more common after cesarean delivery when compared to vaginal delivery. Although clients are usually more fatigued after a cesarean delivery, fatigue hasn't been shown to cause feelings of disappointment over the method of delivery.

CN: Psychosocial integrity; CNS: None; CL: Analysis

9. Which finding is normal for a postpartum client who has experienced a vaginal birth?

1. Redness or swelling in the calves
2. A palpable uterine fundus beyond 10 days postpartum
3. Vaginal dryness after the lochial flow has ended
4. Dark red lochia for approximately 6 weeks after the birth

9. 3. Vaginal dryness is a normal finding during the postpartum period due to hormonal changes. Redness or swelling in the calves may indicate thrombophlebitis. The fundus shouldn't be palpable beyond 10 days. Dark red lochia (indicating fresh bleeding) should only last 2 to 3 days postpartum.

CN: Health promotion and maintenance; CNS: None; CL: Application

10. On completing a fundal assessment, the nurse notes the fundus is situated on the client's left abdomen. Which action is appropriate?

1. Ask the client to empty her bladder.
2. Straight catheterize the client immediately.
3. Call the client's primary health care provider for direction.
4. Straight catheterize the client for half of her urine volume.

10. 1. A full bladder may displace the uterine fundus to the left or right side of the abdomen. A straight catheterization is unnecessarily invasive if the woman can urinate on her own. Nursing interventions should be completed before notifying the primary health care provider in a nonemergency situation.

CN: Physiological integrity; CNS: Reduction of risk potential; CL: Application

11. A client who is positive for human immunodeficiency virus (HIV) tells a nurse she would like to breast-feed. Which is the best response by the nurse?

1. "Breast-feeding will help reduce the risk of hemorrhage."
2. "Breast milk is better than formula for the baby."
3. "Breast-feeding will help with bonding."
4. "Breast milk can transmit HIV to the baby."

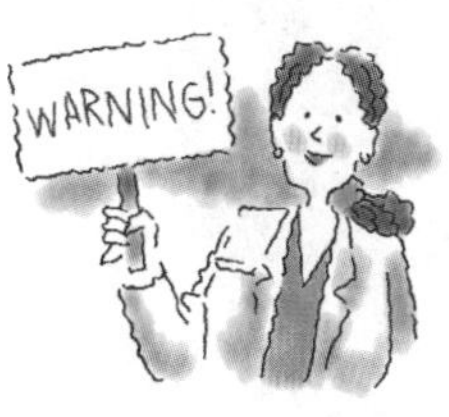

Make sure a client with HIV is aware of the risks of breast-feeding.
WARNING!

11. 4. Since HIV can be transmitted to the baby through breast milk, the client shouldn't breast-feed. Breast-feeding does stimulate uterine contractions, but in this case, breast-feeding should be discouraged. It wouldn't be appropriate to tell a client who shouldn't breast-feed that breast milk is best for the baby. In this case, formula is best. The client should be shown other ways to bond with her baby, such as holding, playing, and talking to the baby.

CN: Physiologic integrity; CNS: Reduction of risk potential; CL: Analysis

12. A client had a spontaneous vaginal delivery after 18 hours of labor. Her excessive vaginal bleeding has now become a postpartum hemorrhage. Immediate nursing care of this client should include which intervention?

1. Avoiding massaging the uterus
2. Monitoring vital signs every hour
3. Placing the client in Trendelenburg's position
4. Elevating the head of the bed to increase blood flow

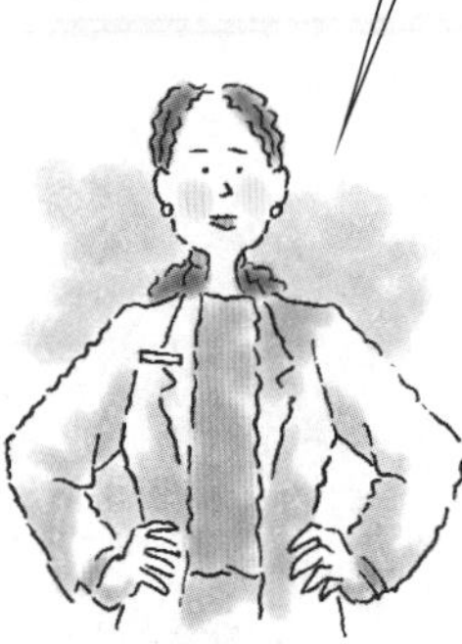

This question requires your immediate attention.

12. 3. The client should be placed in Trendelenburg's position to prevent or control hypovolemic shock. The uterus should be palpated to determine if it's contracting and should be massaged if it's boggy or not contracting. Vital signs should be monitored continuously, or at least every 10 to 15 minutes, until the client's condition stabilizes. The head of the bed shouldn't be elevated because this will further lower the blood pressure.

CN: Safe, effective care environment; CNS: Management of care; CL: Analysis

13. Which complication should a nurse assess for in a client with type 1 diabetes mellitus whose delivery was complicated by polyhydramnios and macrosomia?

1. Postpartum mastitis
2. Increased insulin needs
3. Postpartum hemorrhage
4. Gestational hypertension

13. 3. The client is at risk for a postpartum hemorrhage from the overdistention of the uterus because of the extra amniotic fluid and the large baby. The uterus may not be able to contract as well as it would normally. The diabetic mother usually has decreased insulin needs for the first few days postpartum. Neither polyhydramnios nor macrosomia would increase the client's risk of mastitis or gestational hypertension.

CN: Physiological integrity; CNS: Reduction of risk potential; CL: Application

14. The nurse is caring for a diabetic, postpartum client who has developed an infection. The nurse is aware that infections in diabetic clients tend to be more severe and can quickly lead to complications. For which complication should the nurse assess this client?

1. Anemia
2. Ketoacidosis
3. Respiratory acidosis
4. Respiratory alkalosis

14. 2. Diabetic clients who become pregnant tend to become sicker and develop illnesses quicker than pregnant women without diabetes. Severe infections in diabetes can lead to diabetic ketoacidosis. Anemia, respiratory acidosis, and respiratory alkalosis aren't generally associated with infections in diabetic clients.

CN: Physiological integrity; CNS: Reduction of risk potential; CL: Analysis

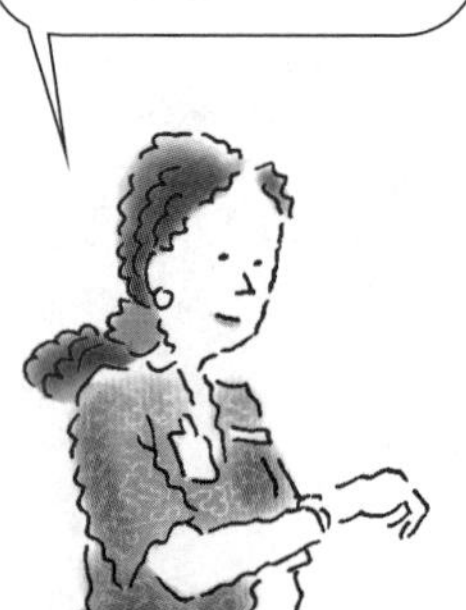

Uh oh. It's time to feed the baby again.

15. Which client action should alert a nurse to a potential problem in a client with mastitis?

1. Breast-feeding every 6 hours
2. Breast-feeding on the affected breast first
3. Increasing daily fluid intake
4. Emptying the affected breast completely with each feeding

15. 1. Mastitis is an infection of the breast characterized by flulike symptoms, along with redness and tenderness in the breast. Since mastitis may be due to milk stasis, the breast-feeding client should breast-feed every 2 to 3 hours. Other measures that the client with mastitis should follow include breast-feeding on the affected side first, drinking plenty of fluids, and completely emptying the affected breast with each feeding expressing milk by hand or using a pump, if necessary.

CN: Physiological integrity; CNS: Physiological adaptation; CL: Analysis

16. A nurse is assessing a client on the sixth postpartum day. Which condition requires prompt nursing action?

1. Blood loss in excess of 300 ml, occurring 24 hours to 6 weeks after delivery
2. Blood loss in excess of 500 ml, occurring 24 hours to 6 weeks after delivery
3. Blood loss in excess of 800 ml, occurring 24 hours to 6 weeks after delivery
4. Blood loss in excess of 1,000 ml, occurring 24 hours to 6 weeks after delivery

16. 2. Postpartum hemorrhage involves blood loss in excess of 500 ml. Most delayed postpartum hemorrhages occur between the fourth and ninth days postpartum. The most frequent causes of a delayed postpartum hemorrhage include retained placental fragments, intrauterine infection, and fibroids.

CN: Physiological integrity; CNS: Reduction of risk potential; CL: Application

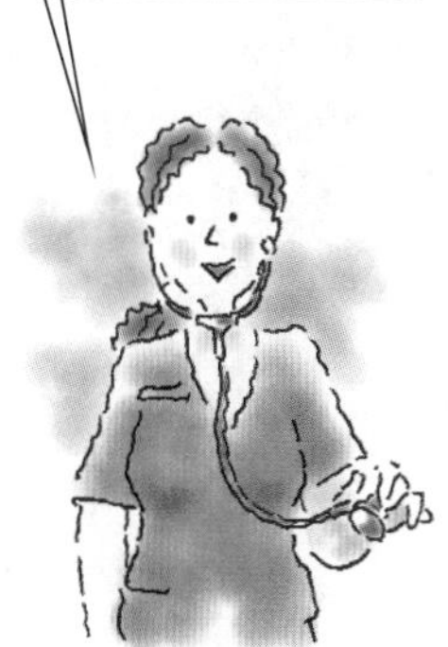

Question 17 requires your *immediate* attention.

17. Which assessment of the mother should be made in the <u>immediate</u> postpartum period (first 2 hours)?

1. Blood glucose level
2. Electrocardiogram (ECG)
3. Height of fundus
4. Stool test for occult blood

17. 3. A focused physical assessment should be performed every 15 minutes for the first 1 to 2 hours postpartum, including assessment of the fundus, lochia, perineum, blood pressure, pulse, and bladder function. A blood glucose level needs to be obtained only if the woman has risk factors for an unstable blood glucose level or if she has symptoms of an altered blood glucose level. An ECG would be necessary only if the woman is at risk for cardiac difficulty. A stool test for occult blood generally wouldn't be valid during the immediate postpartum period; it's difficult to sort out lochial bleeding from rectal bleeding.

CN: Health promotion and maintenance; CNS: None; CL: Application

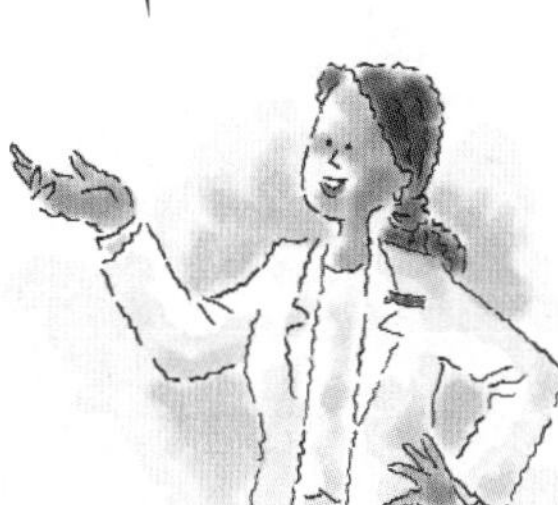

First things first! The word *initially* is a clue in this one.

18. In performing an assessment of a postpartum client 2 hours after delivery, a nurse notices heavy bleeding with large clots. Which response is most appropriate <u>initially</u>?

1. Massaging the fundus firmly
2. Performing bimanual compressions
3. Administering ergonovine (Ergotrate)
4. Notifying the physician

18. 1. Initial management of excessive postpartum bleeding is firm massage of the fundus along with a rapid infusion of oxytocin or lactated Ringer's solution. Bimanual compression is performed by a physician. Ergotrate should be used only if the bleeding doesn't respond to massage and oxytocin. The physician should be notified if the client doesn't respond to fundal massage, but other measures can be taken in the meantime.

CN: Safe, effective care environment; CNS: Management of care; CL: Analysis

19. A nurse is about to give a client with type 2 diabetes mellitus her insulin before breakfast on her first day postpartum. Which statement by the client indicates an understanding of insulin requirements immediately postpartum?

1. "I will need less insulin now than during my pregnancy."
2. "I will need more insulin now than during my pregnancy."
3. "I will need less insulin now than before I was pregnant."
4. "I will need more insulin now than before I was pregnant."

19. 3. Postpartum insulin requirements are usually significantly lower than prepregnancy requirements. Occasionally, clients may require little to no insulin during the first 24 to 48 hours postpartum.

CN: Physiological integrity; CNS: Reduction of risk potential; CL: Analysis

20. Which assessment finding in a postpartum client requires further nursing assessment?

1. Fundus at the umbilicus 1 hour postpartum
2. Fundus 3 cm below the umbilicus on postpartum day 3
3. Fundus not palpable in the abdomen at 2 weeks postpartum
4. Fundus slightly to right; 2 cm above umbilicus on postpartum day 2

20. 4. A uterus that isn't midline or is above the umbilicus on postpartum day 2 might be caused by a full, distended bladder or a uterine infection, requiring further assessment by the nurse. Within the first 12 hours postpartum, the fundus usually is at or below the umbilicus. The fundus should descend approximately 1 cm/day, thereafter. The fundus shouldn't be palpated in the abdomen after day 10.

CN: Health promotion and maintenance; CNS: None; CL: Analysis

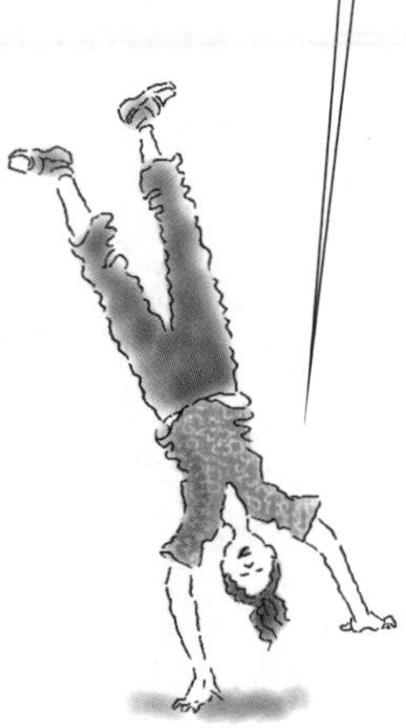

You're doing great! Keep up the good work!

21. Which condition should the nurse look for in a client's history that may explain an increase in the severity of afterpains?

1. Bottle-feeding
2. Diabetes
3. Multiple gestation
4. Primiparity

21. 3. Multiple gestation, breast-feeding, multiparity, and conditions that cause overdistention of the uterus will increase the intensity of afterpains. Bottle-feeding and diabetes aren't directly associated with increasing severity of afterpains, unless the client has delivered a macrosomic infant.

CN: Health promotion and maintenance; CNS: None; CL: Analysis

22. When giving a postpartum client self-care instructions, a nurse instructs her to report heavy or excessive bleeding. Which statement by the client indicates, she understands the nurse's instructions?

1. "I will call the doctor if I saturate a pad in 1 hour or less."
2. "I will call the doctor if I partially saturate a pad in 1 hour."
3. "I will call the doctor if I saturate a pad in 4 to 6 hours."
4. "I will call the doctor if I saturate a pad in 8 hours."

22. 1. Bleeding is considered heavy when a woman saturates a sanitary pad in 1 hour. Excessive bleeding occurs when a postpartum client saturates a pad in 15 minutes. Moderate bleeding occurs when the bleeding saturates less than 6″ (15 cm) of a pad in 1 hour.

CN: Health promotion and maintenance; CNS: None; CL: Application

23. The nurse is assessing a postpartum client who has *lochia serosa* (old blood, serum, leukocytes, and tissue debris). When the client asks the nurse how long to expect this type of bleeding, the nurse's response should be?

1. Days 3 and 4 postpartum
2. Days 3 to 10 postpartum
3. Days 10 to 14 postpartum
4. Days 14 to 42 postpartum

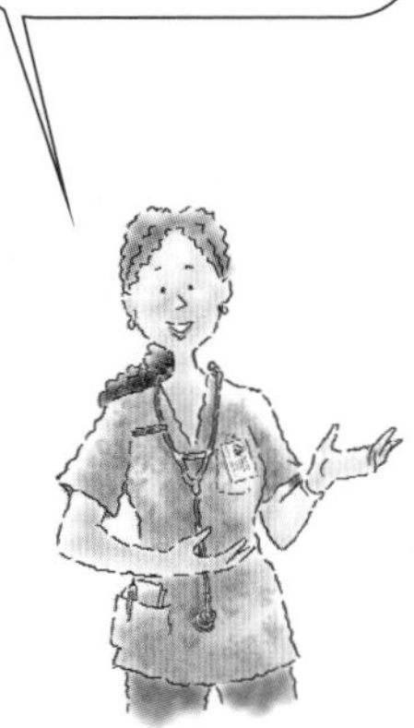

Remember: There are 3 types of lochia. Which type is this question referring to?

23. 2. On the third and fourth postpartum days, the lochia becomes a pale pink or brown and contains old blood, serum, leukocytes, and tissue debris. This type of lochia usually lasts until postpartum day 10. Lochia rubra usually last for the first 3 to 4 days postpartum and consists of blood, decidua, and trophoblastic debris. Lochia alba, which contains leukocytes, decidua, epithelial cells, mucus, and bacteria, may continue for 2 to 6 weeks postpartum.

CN: Health promotion and maintenance; CNS: None; CL: Application

24. A client and her neonate have a blood incompatibility, and the neonate has had a positive direct Coombs' test. Which nursing intervention is appropriate?

1. Because the woman has been sensitized, give $Rh_0(D)$ immune globulin (RhoGAM).
2. Because the woman hasn't been sensitized, give RhoGAM.
3. Because the woman has been sensitized, don't give RhoGAM.
4. Because the woman hasn't been sensitized, don't give RhoGAM.

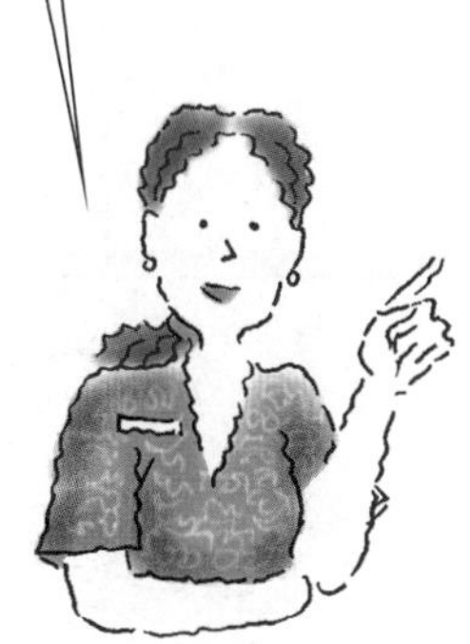
Blood incompatibility between a client and her neonate is serious business.

24. 3. A positive Coombs' test means that the Rh-negative woman is now producing antibodies to the Rh-positive blood of the neonate. RhoGAM shouldn't be given to a sensitized client because it won't be able to prevent antibody formation.

CN: Physiological integrity; CNS: Reduction of risk potential; CL: Analysis

25. The nurse is teaching a client with newly-diagnosed mastitis about her condition. The nurse would inform the client that she most likely contracted the disorder from which organism?

1. *Escherichia coli (E. coli)*
2. Group beta-hemolytic streptococci (GBS)
3. *Staphylococcus aureus (S. aureus)*
4. *Staphylococcus pyogenes (S. pyogenes)*

25. 3. The most common cause of mastitis is *S. aureus*, transmitted from the neonate's mouth. Mastitis isn't harmful to the neonate. *E. coli*, GBS, and *S. pyogenes* aren't associated with mastitis. GBS infection is associated with neonatal sepsis and death.

CN: Health promotion and maintenance; CNS: None; CL: Analysis

26. A nurse should expect to observe which behavior in a client on the 4th postpartum day?

1. The client asks many questions about the baby's care.
2. The client wants to relate her birth experience.
3. The client asks the nurse to select her meals for her.
4. The client asks the nurse to help her bathe herself.

26. 1. The taking-hold phase usually lasts from days 3 to 10 postpartum. During this stage, the mother strives for independence and autonomy; she also becomes curious and interested in the care of the baby and is most ready to learn. During the taking-in phase, which usually lasts 2 to 3 days, the mother is passive and dependent and expresses her own needs rather than the neonate's needs. During this taking-in phase, the client may ask the nurse to help her with self-care, wants to talk about the birth experience, and lets others make decisions for her.

CN: Psychosocial integrity; CNS: None; CL: Application

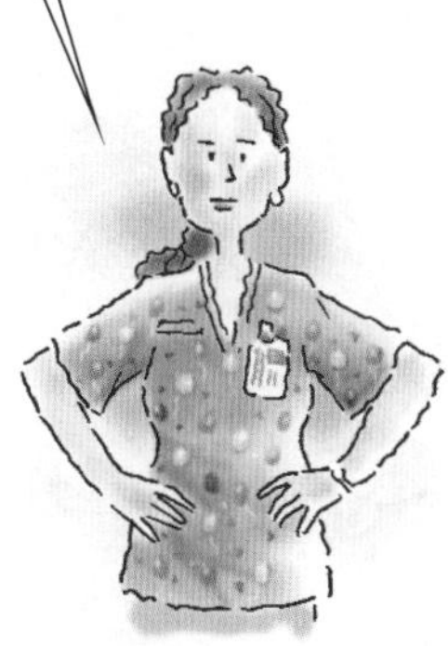
It's important to listen to the feelings and concerns of a postpartum client.

27. Which verbalization should be cause for concern to a nurse treating a postpartum client within a few days of delivery?

1. The client is nervous about taking the baby home.
2. The client feels empty since she delivered the baby.
3. The client would like to watch the nurse give the baby her first bath.
4. The client would like the nurse to take her baby to the nursery so she can sleep.

27. 2. A mother experiencing postpartum blues may say she feels empty now that the infant is no longer in her uterus. She may also verbalize that she feels unprotected now. Many first-time mothers are nervous about caring for their neonates by themselves after discharge. New mothers may want a demonstration before doing a task themselves. A client may want to get some uninterrupted sleep so she may ask that the baby be taken to the nursery.

CN: Psychosocial integrity; CNS: None; CL: Analysis

28. Which complication may be indicated by continuous seepage of blood from the vagina of a postpartum client, when palpation of the uterus reveals a firm uterus 1 cm below the umbilicus?

1. Retained placental fragments
2. Urinary tract infection (UTI)
3. Cervical laceration
4. Uterine atony

28. 3. Continuous seepage of blood may be due to cervical or vaginal lacerations if the uterus is firm and contracting. Retained placental fragments and uterine atony may cause subinvolution of the uterus, making it soft, boggy, and larger than expected. UTI won't cause vaginal bleeding, although hematuria may be present.

CN: Physiological integrity; CNS: Reduction of risk potential; CL: Application

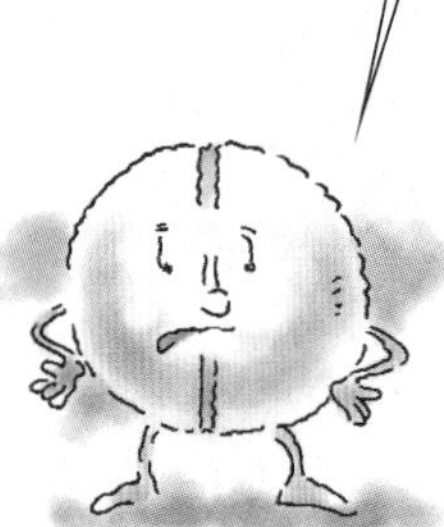

Why is everyone avoiding me?

29. Which statement indicates to a nurse that a client needs further instruction on the use of anticoagulant therapy for deep vein thrombosis?

1. "I will continue to take my iron replacement therapy."
2. "I will take aspirin for headaches."
3. "I will avoid restrictive clothing."
4. "I will report shortness of breath immediately."

29. 2. Discharge teaching should include informing the client to avoid salicylates, which may potentiate the effects of anticoagulant therapy. Iron won't affect anticoagulation therapy. Restrictive clothing should be avoided to prevent the recurrence of thrombophlebitis. Shortness of breath should be reported immediately because it may be a symptom of pulmonary embolism.

CN: Physiological integrity; CNS: Reduction of risk potential; CL: Analysis

30. A pregnant client is very upset when she hears that her TORCH panel has returned positive. She is distraught and says, "This means the baby has HIV!" The nurse replies that the *H* in TORCH represents which of the following disorders?

1. Hemophilia
2. Hepatitis B virus
3. Herpes simplex virus
4. Human immunodeficiency virus

30. 3. TORCH represents the following maternal infections: **T**oxoplasmosis; **O**thers, such as gonorrhea, syphilis, varicella, hepatitis, and human immunodeficiency virus; **R**ubella; **C**ytomegalovirus; and **H**erpes simplex virus. Hemophilia is a clotting disorder in which factors VII and X are deficient.

CN: Physiological integrity; CNS: Reduction of risk potential; CL: Application

31. Which sign of grieving is dysfunctional in a client 3 days after a perinatal loss?

1. Lack of appetite
2. Denial of the death
3. Blaming herself
4. Frequent crying spells

31. 2. Denial of the perinatal loss is dysfunctional grieving in the client. Lack of appetite, blaming oneself, and frequent crying spells are part of a normal grieving process.

CN: Psychosocial integrity; CNS: None; CL: Application

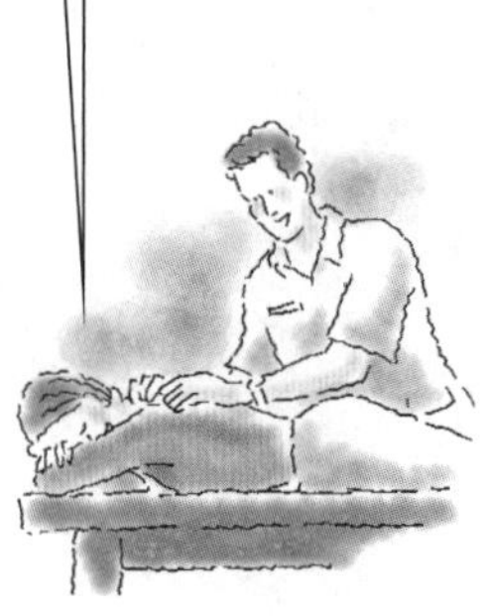

A good massage is just what the doctor, or in this case the nurse, ordered.

32. A nurse is assessing the fundus of a postpartum client and finds that the fundus is boggy. Which action should the nurse take first?

1. Prepare the client for surgery.
2. Administer blood replacement products.
3. Massage the fundus.
4. Administer methylergonovine, as ordered.

32. 3. The nurse should first massage the boggy uterus to stimulate it to contract. The client may need surgery, but only if other measures fail to cause the uterus to contract and control bleeding. Blood replacement products may be given if the client has a significant blood loss. Methylergonovine may be ordered if massage fails to firm the uterus.

CN: Physiological integrity; CNS: Reduction of risk potential; CL: Analysis

33. An RH-positive client delivers a 6 lb, 10 oz neonate vaginally after 17 hours of labor. Which condition puts this client at risk for infection?

1. Length of labor
2. Maternal Rh status
3. Method of delivery
4. Size of the baby

33. 1. A prolonged length of labor places the mother at increased risk for developing an infection. The average size of the baby, vaginal delivery, and Rh status of the client don't place the mother at increased risk.

CN: Physiological integrity; CNS: Physiological adaptation; CL: Analysis

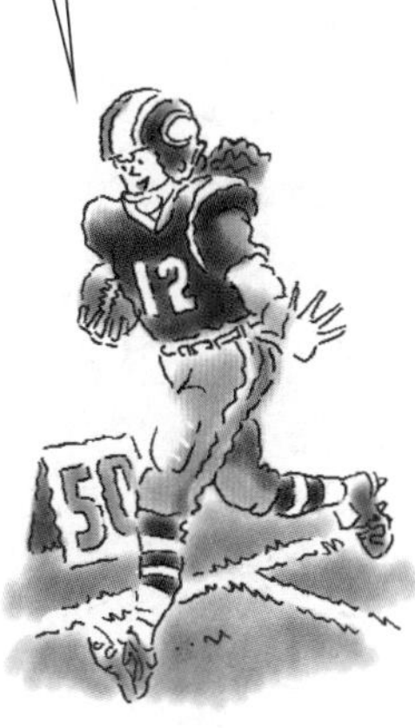

So that's what the coach meant by "holding."
12
50

34. When caring for a breast-feeding client who delivers by cesarean section, the nurse should teach the client to:

1. delay breast-feeding until 24 hours after delivery.
2. breast-feed frequently during the day and every 4 to 6 hours at night.
3. use the cradle hold position to avoid incisional discomfort.
4. use the football hold position to avoid incisional discomfort.

34. 4. When breast-feeding after a cesarean delivery, the client should be encouraged to use the football hold to avoid incisional discomfort. Breast-feeding should be initiated as soon after birth as possible. The mother should be encouraged to breast-feed her infant every 2 to 3 hours throughout the night as well as during the day to increase the milk supply.

CN: Health promotion and maintenance; CNS: None; CL: Analysis

35. Which client behavior indicates an understanding of the nurse's teaching plan for breast-feeding?

1. The client washes her nipples with soap and water.
2. The client lets her nipples air-dry.
3. The client lets the baby attach to the nipple only.
4. The client pulls the baby off the nipple when feeding is done.

35. 2. The nipples should be allowed to air dry after breast-feeding to keep them dry and prevent irritation. Only water should be used to wash the nipples since soap removes natural oils and dries out the nipples. When breast-feeding, the baby should grasp both the nipple and areola. When the baby is done with a breast, the baby's grasp on the nipple should be released before removing the baby from the breast.

CN: Health promotion and maintenance; CNS: None; CL: Application

36. Which recommendation should be given to a client with mastitis who is concerned about breast-feeding her neonate?

1. She should stop breast-feeding until completing the antibiotic.
2. She should supplement feeding with formula until the infection resolves.
3. She shouldn't use analgesics because they aren't compatible with breast-feeding.
4. She should continue to breast-feed; mastitis won't infect the infant.

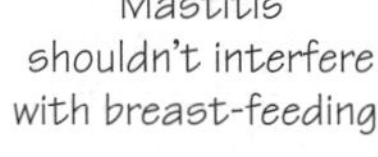

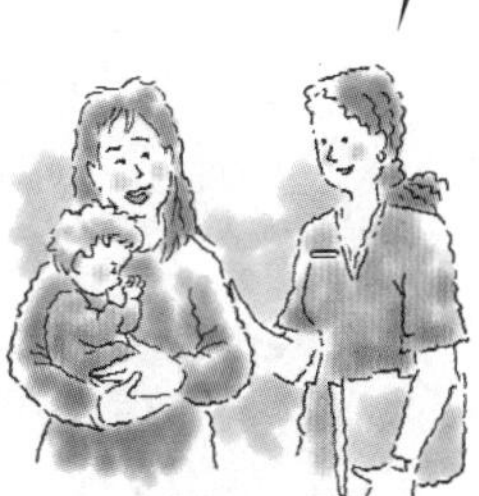

36. 4. The client with mastitis should be encouraged to continue breast-feeding while taking antibiotics for the infection. No supplemental feedings are necessary because breast-feeding doesn't need to be altered and actually encourages resolution of the infection. Analgesics are safe and should be administered as needed.

CN: Health promotion and maintenance; CNS: None; CL: Analysis

37. The nurse is assessing a 6-week-postpartum client in the obstetrician's office. In the exam room, the nurse asks the client how she's feeling. The client bursts into tears and reports she can barely get out of bed to dress, is crying most of the time, and feels like a failure. The nurse suspects the client is experiencing which of the following conditions?

1. Postpartum blues
2. Postpartum depression
3. Postpartum neurosis
4. Postpartum psychosis

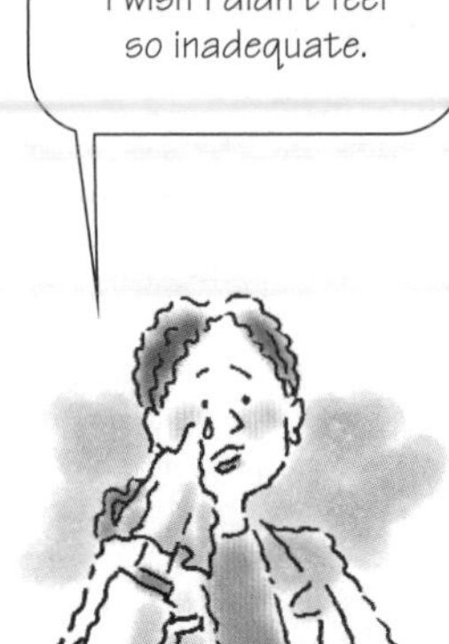

I wish I didn't feel so inadequate.

37. 2. Postpartum depression occurs in approximately 10% to 15% of all postpartum women. This depression is characterized by disabling feelings of inadequacy and an inability to cope that can last up to 3 years. The client is often tearful and despondent. The client with postpartum blues experiences crying and sadness, generally between 3 to 5 days postpartum, but this condition resolves itself quickly. Postpartum neurosis includes neurotic behavior during the initial 6 weeks after birth. Postpartum psychosis includes hallucinations, delusions, and phobias.

CN: Psychosocial integrity; CNS: None; CL: Application

38. A client who is breast-feeding reports pain, redness, and swelling in her right breast. Which instruction should the nurse give the client?

1. Wear a tight-fitting brassiere while breast-feeding.
2. Breast-feeding should be stopped permanently.
3. Continue antibiotic until pain, redness, and swelling subside.
4. Apply moist heat compresses to the right breast.

38. 4. Moist heat compresses reduce inflammation and swelling of the affected area and relieves pain. The client shouldn't wear a tight or constrictive brassiere while breast-feeding to allow the milk to flow freely and empty the breast. There's no need to stop breast-feeding permanently. Antibiotics should be taken for the prescribed cause of therapy and shouldn't be stopped when symptoms subside.

CN: Health promotion and maintenance; CNS: None; CL: Application

39. A 6-week-postpartum client is being assessed by the nurse at the obstetrician's office. The nurse notes that the uterus is enlarged and soft and that the client is experiencing vaginal bleeding. The nurse suspects the client has which of the following conditions?

1. Cervical laceration
2. Clotting deficiency
3. Perineal laceration
4. Uterine subinvolution

39. 4. Late postpartum bleeding is typically the result of subinvolution of the uterus. Retained products of conception or infection often cause subinvolution. Cervical or perineal lacerations can cause an immediate postpartum hemorrhage. A client with a clotting deficiency may also have an immediate postpartum hemorrhage, if the deficiency isn't corrected at the time of delivery.

CN: Physiological integrity; CNS: Physiological adaptation; CL: Application

40. A client needs to void 3 hours after a vaginal delivery. Which risk factor necessitates assisting her out of bed?

1. Chest pain
2. Breast engorgement
3. Orthostatic hypotension
4. Separation of episiotomy incision

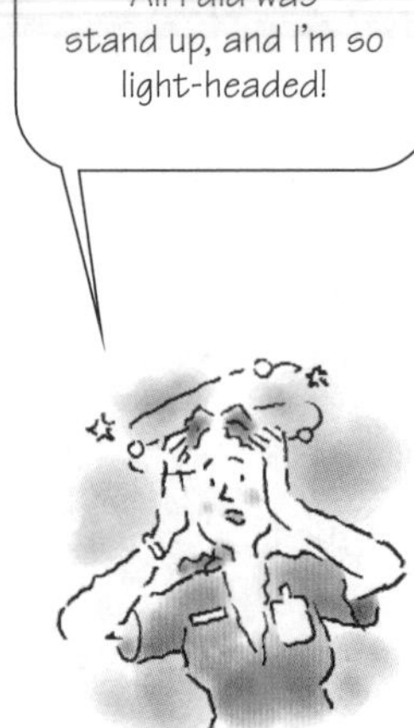

All I did was stand up, and I'm so light-headed!

40. 3. The rapid decrease in intra-abdominal pressure occurring after birth causes splanchnic engorgement. The client is at risk for orthostatic hypotension when standing due to the blood pooling in this area. Breast engorgement is caused by vascular congestion in the breast before true lactation. The client shouldn't experience separation of the episiotomy incision or chest pain when standing.

CN: Health promotion and maintenance; CNS: None; CL: Analysis

41. Before giving a postpartum client the rubella vaccine, which fact should the nurse include in client teaching?

1. The vaccine is safe in clients with egg allergies.
2. Breast-feeding isn't compatible with the vaccine.
3. Transient arthralgia and rash are uncommon adverse effects.
4. The client should avoid getting pregnant for 3 months after the vaccination because the vaccine has teratogenic effects.

41. 4. The client must understand that she must not become pregnant for 2 to 3 months after the vaccination because of its potential teratogenic effects. The rubella vaccine is made from duck eggs so an allergic reaction may occur in clients with egg allergies. The virus isn't transmitted into the breast milk, so clients may continue to breast-feed after vaccination. Transient arthralgia and rash are common adverse effects of the vaccine.

CN: Health promotion and maintenance; CNS: None; CL: Application

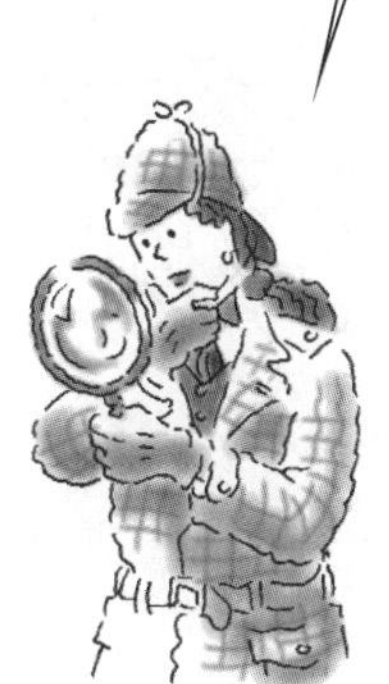
Don't lose your focus.

42. The nurse is caring for a postpartum client who develops preeclampsia. Which medication should the nurse expect to administer?

1. Diazepam (Valium)
2. Hydralazine
3. Magnesium sulfate
4. Nifedipine (Procardia)

42. 3. Magnesium sulfate is commonly used in the treatment of preeclampsia to prevent seizures. It also produces a smooth muscle depression effect, which can lower blood pressure. Diazepam may also be given for seizure activity. Nifedipine and hydralazine are used for severely hypertensive preeclamptic women.

CN: Physiological integrity; CNS: Pharmacological and parenteral therapies; CL: Application

43. Which complication is associated with magnesium sulfate therapy?

1. Hypotension
2. Postpartum depression
3. Postpartum hemorrhage
4. Uterine infection

43. 3. Because magnesium sulfate relaxes smooth muscle, the uterus should be assessed for uterine atony, which would increase the risk of postpartum hemorrhage. Postpartum depression and uterine infection aren't associated with magnesium sulfate therapy. Magnesium sulfate is considered more of an anticonvulsant than an antihypertensive.

CN: Physiological integrity; CNS: Pharmacological and parenteral therapies; CL: Comprehension

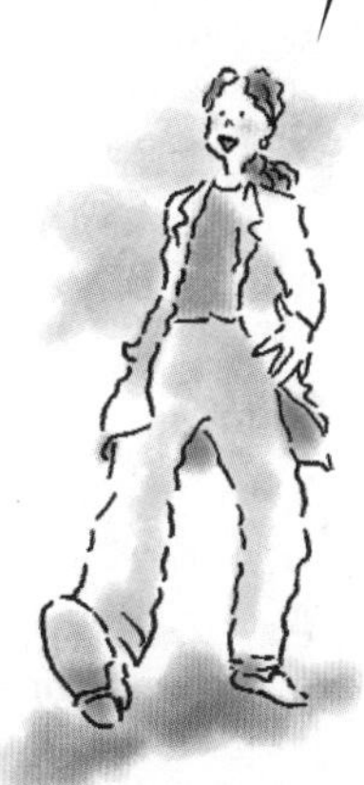
You're making great strides. Keep going!

44. Which intervention should be included in the plan of care for a client with an episiotomy on the third postpartum day?

1. Apply ice to the perineum.
2. Encourage the use of sitz baths.
3. Avoid tightening the pelvic muscles.
4. Massage the perineal area.

44. 2. A sitz bath reduces inflammation and relaxes the perineum, promoting healing and reducing discomfort. Ice should only be used for the first 24 hours following delivery. Kegel exercises, which involve tightening and relaxing the pelvic muscles, improve circulation and reduce edema. Massaging the perineum may disrupt the suture line and cause more pain.

CN: Physiological integrity; CNS: Physiological adaptation; CL: Analysis

45. Which response is most appropriate for a mother with diabetes who wants to breast-feed but is concerned about the effects of breast-feeding on her health?

1. Mothers with diabetes who breast-feed have a hard time controlling their insulin needs.
2. Mothers with diabetes shouldn't breast-feed because of potential complications.
3. Mothers with diabetes shouldn't breast-feed; insulin requirements are doubled.
4. Mothers with diabetes may breast-feed; insulin requirements may decrease from breast-feeding.

45. 4. Breast-feeding has an antidiabetogenic effect. Insulin needs are decreased because carbohydrates are used in milk production. Breast-feeding mothers are at a higher risk of hypoglycemia in the first postpartum days after birth because the glucose levels are lower. Mothers with diabetes should be encouraged to breast-feed.

CN: Physiological integrity; CNS: Pharmacological and parenteral therapies; CL: Application

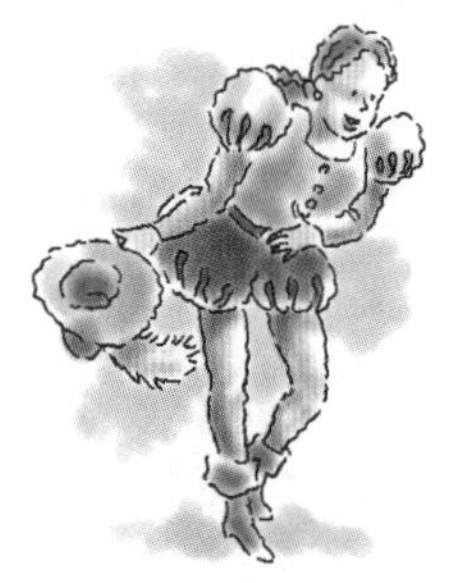

To breast-feed or not to breast-feed, that is the question.

46. Which activity by a client indicates that a nurse's teaching about perineal care has been effective?

1. The client uses a spray bottle to cleanse the perineum after urination and bowel movements.
2. The client wipes the perineum from back to front after urinating or a bowel movement.
3. The client douches after urination or a bowel movement.
4. The client changes perineal pads three times a day.

46. 1. The client should cleanse the perineal area after urinating or a bowel movement using a spray or peri-bottle. The client should wipe from front to back after urination or a bowel movement to avoid contaminating the perineal area. Perineal pads should be changed when they are soiled to keep the perineum clean.

CN: Health promotion and maintenance; CNS: None; CL: Application

47. Which factor puts a multiparous client on her first postpartum day at risk for developing hemorrhage?

1. Hemoglobin level of 12 g/dl
2. Uterine atony
3. Thrombophlebitis
4. Moderate amount of lochia rubra

47. 2. Multiparous women often experience a loss of uterine tone due to frequent distentions of the uterus from past pregnancies. As a result, this client is also at higher risk for hemorrhage. Thrombophlebitis doesn't increase the risk of hemorrhage during the postpartum period. The hemoglobin level and lochia flow are within acceptable limits.

CN: Health promotion and maintenance; CNS: None; CL: Analysis

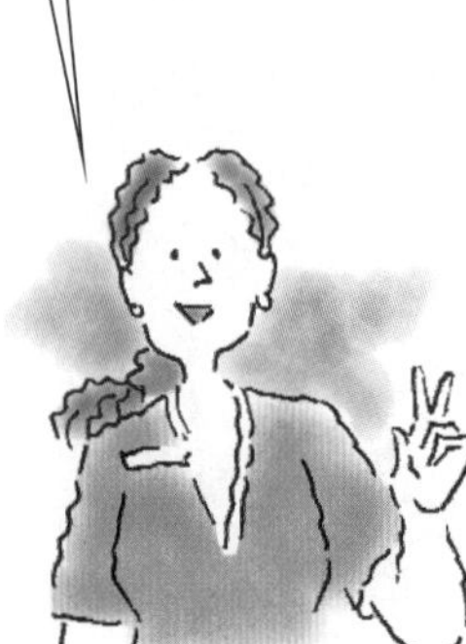

Remember, when you're dealing with a postpartum client, you've got two clients to think about.

48. On the first postpartum night, a client requests that her baby be sent back to the nursery so she can get some sleep. The client is most likely in which phase?

1. Depression phase
2. Letting-go phase
3. Taking-hold phase
4. Taking-in phase

48. 4. The taking-in phase occurs in the first 24 hours after birth. The mother is concerned with her own needs and requires support from staff and relatives. The depression phase isn't an appropriate answer. The letting-go phase begins several weeks later, when the mother incorporates the new infant into the family unit. The taking-hold phase occurs when the mother is ready to take responsibility for her care as well as her infant's care.

CN: Health promotion and maintenance; CNS: None; CL: Analysis

49. Four clients each gave birth 12 hours ago. Which one would most likely suffer complications after birth?

1. Gravida 2 Para 2002, cesarean birth, incisional site intact, hemoglobin level 9.8 g/dl
2. Gravida 2 Para 1011, cesarean birth, incisional site intact, pulse 84 beats/minute
3. Gravida 1 Para 1001, vaginal delivery, midline episiotomy, temperature 99.8° F (37.7° C)
4. Gravida 1 Para 1001, vaginal delivery, ruptured membranes 10 hours before delivery

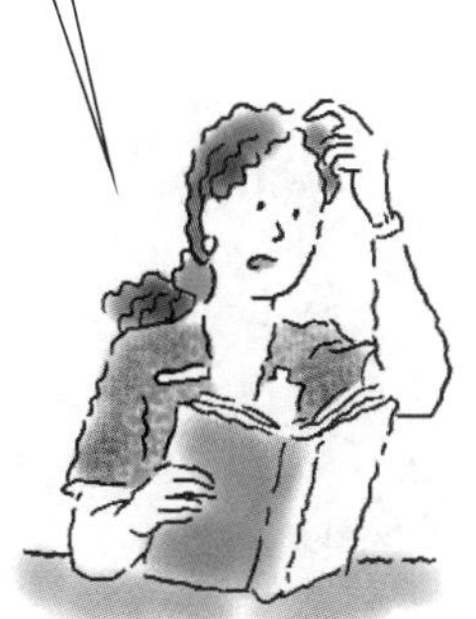

Which client is at the greatest risk for complications?

49. 1. Women who are anemic in pregnancy (defined as a hemoglobin < 10 g/dl) may experience more complications, such as poor wound healing and inability to tolerate activity. The vital signs in answers 2 and 3 are within normal limits. Dehydration can cause a slightly elevated temperature. Women whose membranes are ruptured more than 24 hours before birth are more prone to developing chorioamnionitis.

CN: Health promotion and maintenance; CNS: None; CL: Analysis

50. Which statement by a client shows she understands how to prevent breast engorgement while breast-feeding?

1. "I will apply moist heat to my breasts three times a day."
2. "I will breast-feed every 1 to 3 hours."
3. "I will use a breast pump to obtain milk for feedings."
4. "I will wear a tight bra continually."

50. 2. Frequent breast-feeding empties the breast, decreasing the risk of engorgement. Moist heat can stimulate the let-down reflex, leading to engorgement. A breast pump isn't necessary if a baby is able to breast-feed regularly. A tight brassiere may prevent the breasts from emptying completely when breast-feeding, increasing the risk of engorgement.

CN: Health promotion and maintenance; CNS: None; CL: Application

51. A client has delivered twins. Which intervention would be most important for a nurse to perform?

1. Assess fundal tone and lochia flow.
2. Apply a cold pack to the perineal area.
3. Administer analgesics, as ordered.
4. Encourage voiding by offering the bedpan.

51. 1. Women who deliver twins are at a higher risk for postpartum hemorrhage due to overdistention of the uterus, which causes uterine atony. Assessing fundal tone and lochia flow helps to determine risks for hemorrhage. Applying cold packs to the perineum, administering analgesics as ordered, and offering the bedpan are all significant nursing interventions but not as important as preventing postpartum hemorrhage.

CN: Health promotion and maintenance; CNS: None; CL: Analysis

52. Which physiological response is considered <u>normal</u> in the early postpartum period?

1. Urinary urgency and dysuria
2. Rapid diuresis
3. Decrease in blood pressure
4. Increased motility of the GI system

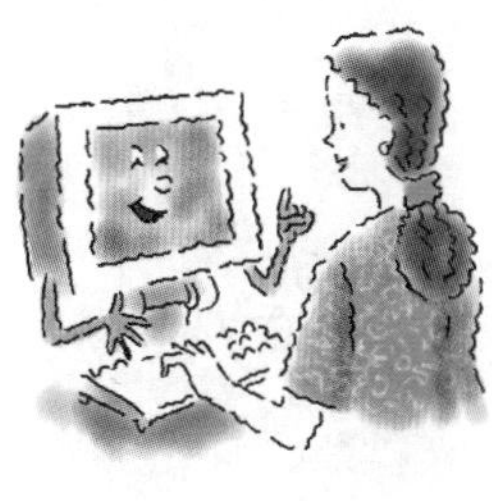

Question 52 is looking for a normal response.

52. 2. In the early postpartum period, there's an increase in the glomerular filtration rate and a drop in progesterone levels, which result in rapid diuresis. There should be no urinary urgency, though a woman may feel anxious about voiding. There's minimal change in blood pressure following childbirth, and a residual decrease in GI motility.

CN: Physiological integrity; CNS: Physiological adaptation; CL: Application

53. During the third postpartum day, which observation about a client should the nurse be most likely to make?

1. The client appears interested in learning more about neonatal care.
2. The client talks a lot about her birth experience.
3. The client sleeps whenever the neonate isn't present.
4. The client requests help in choosing a name for the neonate.

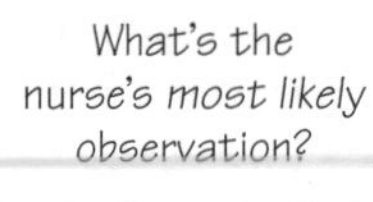

What's the nurse's most likely observation?

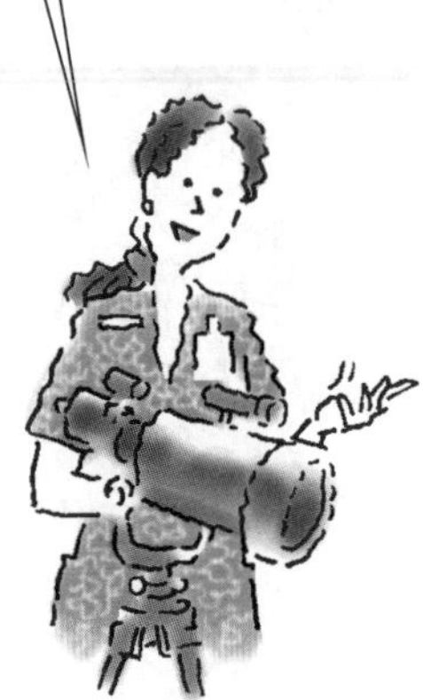

53. 1. By the third postpartum day, the client should be in the taking-hold phase, in which the new mother strives for independence and is eager for her neonate. The other options describe the phase in which the mother relives her birth experience.

CN: Health promotion and maintenance; CNS: None; CL: Analysis

54. Which circumstance is most likely to cause uterine atony and lead to postpartum hemorrhage?

1. Hypertension
2. Cervical and vaginal tears
3. Urine retention
4. Endometritis

54. 3. Urine retention causes a distended bladder to displace the uterus above the umbilicus and to the side, which prevents the uterus from contracting. The uterus needs to remain contracted if bleeding is to stay within normal limits. Cervical and vaginal tears can cause postpartum hemorrhage but are less common occurrences in the postpartum period. Maternal hypertension and endometritis don't cause postpartum hemorrhage.

CN: Health promotion and maintenance; CNS: None; CL: Application

55. Which assessment requires immediate action by a nurse in a client 22-hours following a cesarean delivery?

1. Heart rate of 132 beats/minute and blood pressure of 84/60 mm Hg
2. Oral temperature of 100.2° F
3. A gush of blood from the vagina when the client stands up
4. Complaints of abdominal pain and cramping

55. 1. Tachycardia (heart rate of 132 beats/minute) and hypotension (blood pressure of 84/60 mm Hg) may be a sign of hemorrhage. An oral temperature of 100.2° F may be due to dehydration, when it occurs on the first postpartum day. A gush of blood from the vagina when a client stands is a normal finding on the first postpartum day. Complaints of abdominal pain and cramping are expected following cesarean delivery.

CN: Physiological integrity; CNS: Reduction of risk potential; CL: Application

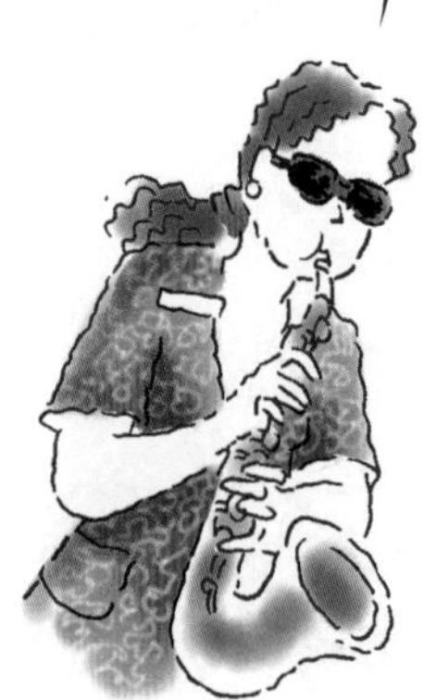

Have you ever heard the postpartum blues?

56. Which percentage of postpartum clients experiences "postpartum blues"?

1. 20% to 25%
2. 50% to 80%
3. 30% to 45%
4. 100%

56. 2. "Postpartum blues"—a transient mood alteration that arises during the first 3 weeks postpartum and is typically self-limiting—affects 50% to 80% of postpartum clients. A more severe mood alteration, seen in approximately 20% of clients, involves changes that occur within a few days after delivery and may last for a few days to more than 1 year.

CN: Psychosocial integrity; CNS: None; CL: Application

57. When performing a comprehensive fundal check during a postpartum assessment, a nurse evaluates which fundal state?

1. Fundal consistency, location, and height
2. Fundal consistency and height
3. Fundal location and potential fundal distention
4. Fundal location and height

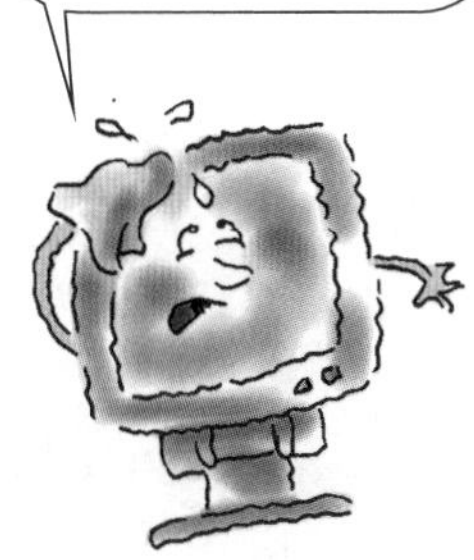

57. 1. A comprehensive fundal check includes evaluation of fundal consistency, height, and location. Normal results are a firm fundus that's at the correct height for the postpartum day and located in the center of the pelvis. Options 2, 3, and 4 don't reflect a comprehensive fundal check because they're missing valuable components.

CN: Physiological integrity; CNS: Physiological adaptation; CL: Analysis

58. A nurse is performing an assessment on a postpartum client. The assessment reveals that the fundus is firm. This data indicates which condition?

1. A firm tumor at the top of the uterus
2. Contraction of the uterus
3. Continuing labor contractions
4. Bladder distention

58. 2. A firm postpartum fundus means that the uterus has contracted and is constricting blood vessels, thereby decreasing lochial flow. A uterine tumor doesn't necessarily cause a firm fundus. The client wouldn't experience labor contractions during the postpartum period. Bladder distention restricts the uterus from contracting downward, resulting in a soft, boggy uterus and increased vaginal bleeding.

CN: Physiological integrity; CNS: Physiological adaptation; CL: Analysis

59. A primipara who is Rho(D)-negative has just given birth to an Rh-positive baby. Which priority nursing intervention should be included in the plan of care?

1. Administer Rh_0(D) immune globulin to the neonate within 3 days.
2. Administer Rh_0(D) immune globulin to the client within 3 days.
3. Administer Rh_0(D) immune globulin to the client at her first postpartum visit in 6 weeks.
4. Administer Rh_0(D) immune globulin to the neonate at the first well-baby visit.

59. 2. Administering Rh_0(D) immune globulin to the client within 72 hours of delivery prevents antibodies from forming that can destroy fetal blood cells in the next pregnancy. Rh_0(D) immune globulin isn't given to the baby. The client shouldn't wait 6 weeks to receive Rh_0(D) immune globulin as antibodies will already have formed.

CN: Safe, effective care environment; CNS: Management of care; CL: Application

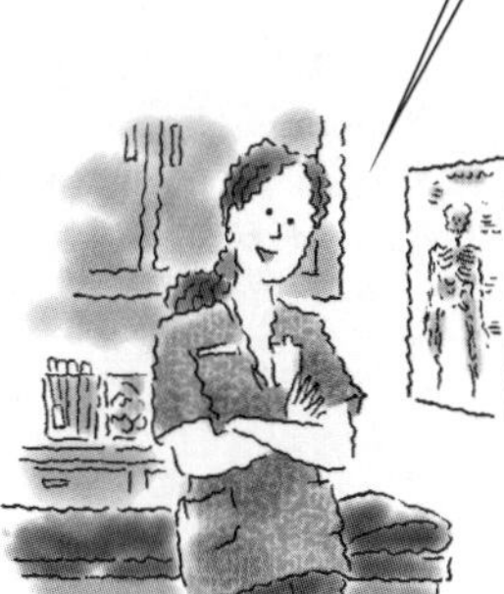

Discharge teaching is important. Which instruction should you include for your clients with DVT?

60. A postpartum client is receiving anticoagulant therapy for deep vein thrombophlebitis. Discharge teaching should include which instruction?

1. Avoid iron replacement therapy.
2. Wear a girdle and knee-high stockings whenever possible.
3. Avoid over-the-counter salicylates.
4. Be aware that shortness of breath is a common adverse effect of anticoagulants.

60. 3. Discharge teaching should include an instruction to avoid salicylates, which may magnify the effects of anticoagulant therapy. Iron doesn't affect anticoagulant therapy. The client should avoid restrictive clothing to prevent recurrence of thrombophlebitis. She should report shortness of breath immediately because it may indicate pulmonary embolus.

CN: Health promotion and maintenance; CNS: Reduction of risk potential; CL: Application

61. For a breast-feeding client on the fourth postpartum day, which breast examination findings are normal?

1. Soft, nontender breasts
2. Engorged breasts with inflamed, radiating areas that are sore to the touch
3. Slightly tender, cracked nipples; slightly firm, nontender breasts; transitional milk
4. Tender, intact nipples; firm, tender breasts; transitional milk

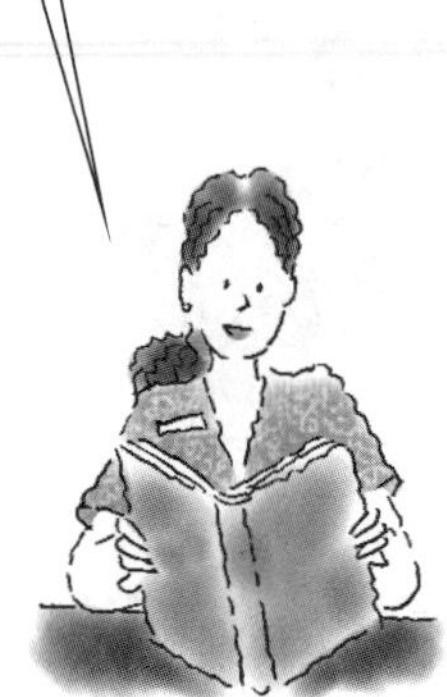

I need to determine which findings are normal for this client.

61. 4. Tender, intact nipples; firm, tender breasts; and transitional milk are normal in a breast-feeding client on the fourth postpartum day. Engorged, inflamed breasts signal mastitis. Tender, cracked nipples aren't a normal finding; they require intervention and client teaching to help the nipples heal and help the client avoid the problem in the future.

CN: Physiological integrity; CNS: Physiological adaptation; CL: Application

62. Which client statement should alert the nurse to a potential problem in a breast-feeding primiparous client?

1. "I will consume an additional 500 calories/day."
2. "I will increase my intake of protein."
3. "I will limit my fluid intake."
4. "I will eat foods high in vitamins and minerals."

62. 3. A breast-feeding client who states that fluid intake should be limited should alert the nurse that more education is needed. Increased fluids are needed for milk production. The breast-feeding client should consume an additional 500 calories/day, increase protein intake, and eat foods high in vitamins and minerals.

CN: Health promotion and maintenance; CNS: None; CL: Application

63. A nurse is teaching a breast-feeding primiparous client how to prevent sore nipples. Which client statement indicates the need for further instruction?

1. "I should breast-feed for only 3 to 4 minutes at a time until my milk flow is established."
2. "I should position the baby properly during feedings."
3. "I should pull the baby gently away from my nipple after the feeding."
4. "I should prevent the baby from feeding after my breast has been emptied."

63. 1. In some cases, it takes 7 minutes for the letdown reflex to cause milk to fill the breast. The other answers indicate that the client understands the nurse's instructions.

CN: Physiological integrity; CNS: Reduction of risk potential; CL: Application

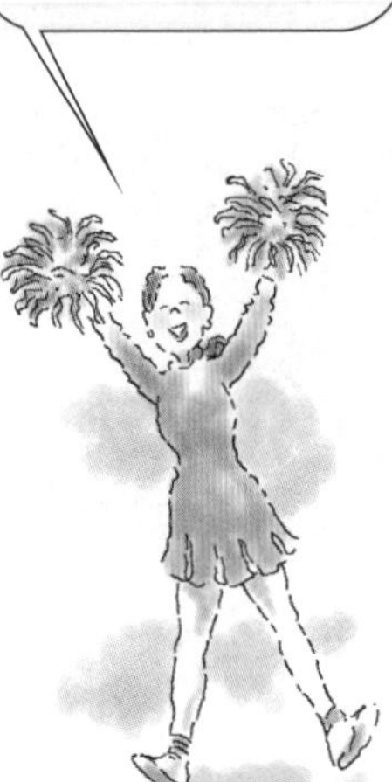

Only 7 more questions to go!

64. A client is 2 days postpartum and is talking with her nurse about the bleeding she's having, asking, "Will it always be so heavy?" Which statement by the nurse would be the <u>most accurate</u>?

1. "This is lochia alba and will last 4 weeks."
2. "This is lochia serosa and will last 2 days."
3. "This is lochia rubra and will last 3–4 days."
4. "This is your menstrual cycle and it will last 6 weeks."

64. 3. Lochia rubra, which is made up of blood, mucus, and tissue debris, lasts 3–4 days. Lochia serosa, which consists of blood, mucus, and leukocytes, lasts from day 3 to day 10 postpartum. Lochia alba, which consists largely of mucus, lasts from day 10 to day 14 postpartum. Lochia alba may last up to 6 weeks postpartum. Postpartum bleeding is not the menstrual cycle.

CN: Physiological integrity; CNS: Physiological adaptation; CL: Application

65. On examining a client who gave birth 3 hours ago, the nurse finds that the client has completely saturated a perineal pad within 15 minutes. Which actions should the nurse take? Select all that apply:

1. Begin an IV infusion of lactated Ringer's solution.
2. Assess the client's vital signs.
3. Palpate the client's fundus.
4. Place the client in high Fowler's position.
5. Administer a pain medication.

65. 2, 3. Assessing vital signs provides information about the client's circulatory status and identifies significant changes to report to the physician. By palpating the client's fundus, the nurse also gains valuable assessment data. A boggy uterus may lead to excessive bleeding. Starting an IV infusion requires a physician's order. Placing the client in high Fowler's position may lower blood pressure and be harmful to the client. Administration of a pain medication doesn't address the current problem.

CN: Physiological integrity; CNS: Reduction of risk potential; CL: Application

66. Which characteristic of lochia should a nurse expect in a client two weeks postpartum?

1. It's creamy white to brown and may have a stale odor.
2. It's creamy white to brown, contains decidual cells, and may have a stale odor.
3. It's brown to red, contains tissue fragments, and may have an odor.
4. It's brown to red and contains decidual cells and leukocytes.

66. 2. Lochia alba occurs from one to three weeks postpartum. Lochia alba is creamy white to brown, contains decidual cells, and may have a stale odor. It also contains leukocytes. Lochia alba shouldn't contain tissue fragments or have a foul odor.

CN: Physiological integrity; CNS: Physiological adaptation; CL: Application

67. In a client one week postpartum with retained placental fragments, which finding should alert a nurse of a common complication?

1. Puerperal infection
2. Postpartum depression
3. Postpartum hemorrhage
4. Uterine subinvolution

67. 3. Retained placental fragments, which prevent the uterus from contracting properly, increase postpartum blood loss. This loss may be dramatic and lead to postpartum hemorrhage of 500 ml of blood or more. Although retained placental fragments may also lead to uterine subinvolution or infection, these are less common complications. Postpartum depression is a psychiatric disorder not related to retained placental fragments.

CN: Health promotion and maintenance; CNS: None; CL: Application

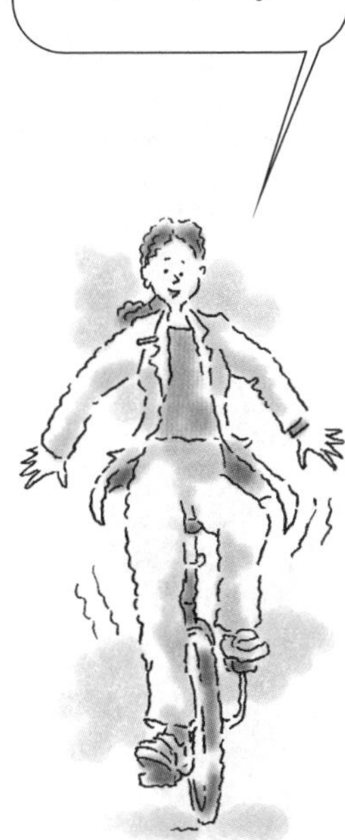

Stay with it! Just a few more to go!

68. The nurse is assisting in developing a care plan for a client who had an episiotomy. Which interventions would be included for the nursing diagnosis *Acute pain related to perineal sutures*? Select all that apply:

1. Apply an ice pack intermittently to the perineal area for 3 days.
2. Avoid the use of topical pain gels.
3. Administer sitz baths three to four times per day.
4. Encourage the client to do Kegel exercises.
5. Limit the number of times the perineal pad is changed.

68. 3, 4. Sitz baths help decrease inflammation and tension in the perineal area. Kegel exercises improve circulation to the area and help reduce edema. Ice packs should be applied to the perineum for the first 24 hours only; after that time, heat should be used. Topical pain gels should be applied to the suture area to reduce discomfort, as ordered. The perineal pad should be changed frequently to prevent irritation caused by the discharge.

CN: Physiological integrity; CNS: Basic care and comfort; CL: Application

69. A nurse is palpating the uterine fundus of a client who delivered a baby 8 hours ago. At what level in the abdomen would the nurse expect to feel the fundus?

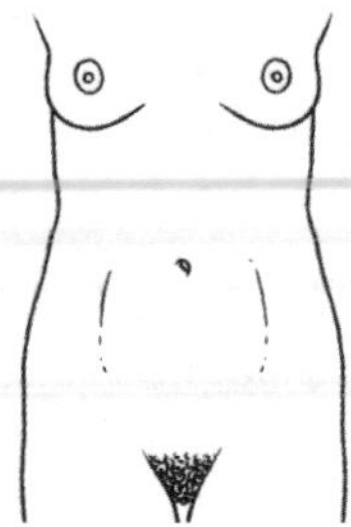

70. A mother with a past history of varicose veins has just delivered her first baby. A nurse suspects that the mother has developed pulmonary embolus. Which of the data below would lead to this nursing judgment? Select all that apply:

1. Sudden dyspnea
2. Chills, fever
3. Diaphoresis
4. Bradycardia
5. Confusion

71. A nurse observes several interactions between a mother and her neonate son. Which maternal behaviors should the nurse identify as evidence of mother-infant attachment? Select all that apply:

1. Talks and coos to her son.
2. Cuddles her son close to her.
3. Doesn't make eye contact with her son.
4. Requests that the nurse take the baby to the nursery for feedings.
5. Encourages the father to hold the baby.
6. Takes a nap when the baby is sleeping.

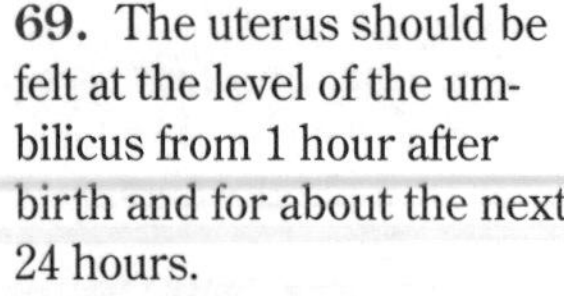

69. The uterus should be felt at the level of the umbilicus from 1 hour after birth and for about the next 24 hours.

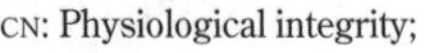

CN: Physiological integrity;
CNS: Reduction of risk potential;
CL: Application

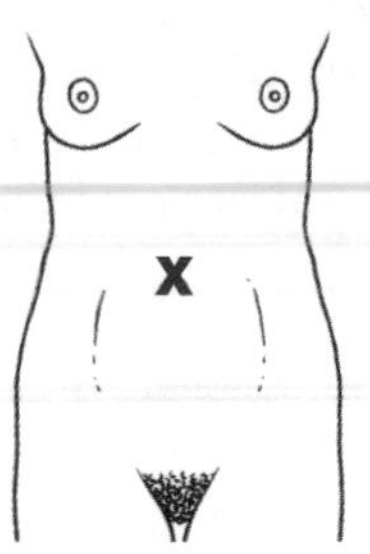

70. 1, 3, 5. Sudden dyspnea along with diaphoresis and confusion are classic symptoms that develop when a thrombus (stationary blood clot) from a varicose vein becomes an embolus (moving clot) that lodges in the pulmonary circulation. Chills and fever would indicate infection. A client with an embolus usually develops tachycardia.

CN: Physiological integrity; CNS: Physiological adaptation; CL: Analysis

71. 1, 2. Talking, cooing, and cuddling with her son are positive signs of mother-infant attachment. Avoiding eye contact is a nonbonding behavior. Eye contact, touching, and speaking help establish attachment with a neonate. Feeding a neonate is an important role of a new mother and facilitates attachment. Encouraging the father to hold the neonate will facilitate attachment. Resting while the neonate is sleeping will conserve needed energy and allow the mother to be alert.

CN: Psychosocial integrity; CNS: None; CL: Analysis

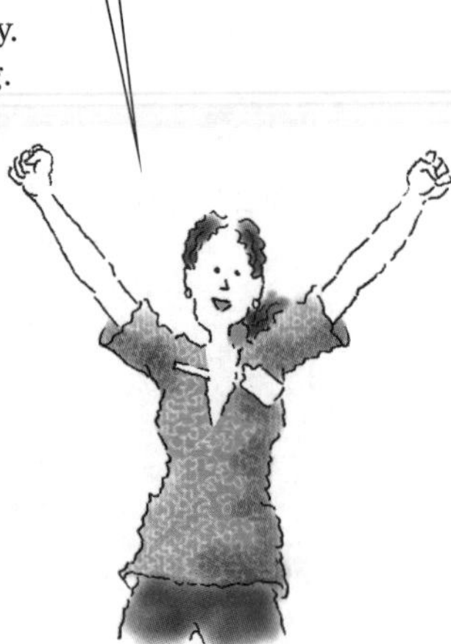

You did it! A star is born (no pun intended)!

CN: Client needs category CNS: Client needs subcategory CL: Cognitive level

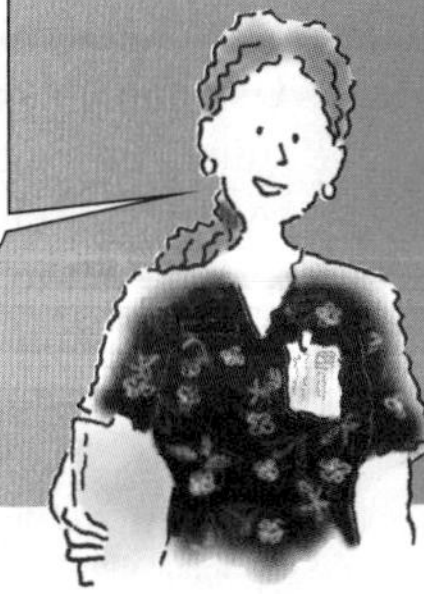

Neonates depend on you for everything. Let's show 'em you've got what it takes for neonatal care!

Chapter 25 Neonatal care

1. A client has given birth to a preterm male neonate. The client tells the nurse that she still wants to breast-feed her neonate. The nurse should explain to the mother that:

1. breast milk contains antibodies that help protect her neonate.
2. commercial formula will provide better nutrition for the neonate.
3. breast-feeding can be started when the neonate is ready for discharge.
4. the neonate will be less likely to develop an infection on commercial formula.

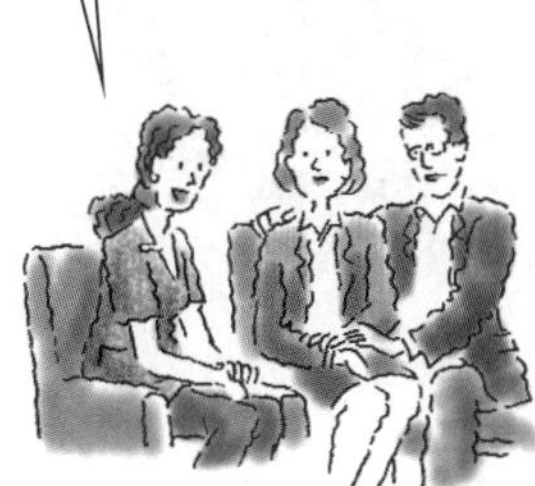

You need to keep the parents informed of the whats and whys of their baby's care.

1. 1. Studies have proven that breast milk provides preterm neonates with better protection from infection, such as necrotizing enterocolitis, because of the antibodies contained in breast milk. Commercial formula doesn't provide any better nutrition than breast milk. Breast milk feedings can be started as soon as the neonate is stable. The neonate is more likely to develop infections when fed formula rather than breast milk.

CN: Health promotion and maintenance; CNS: None; CL: Application

2. The parents of a neonate admitted to the NICU ask why the physician has ordered surfactant therapy. Which statement would be most accurate for parent education?

1. Surfactant will help regulate the baby's breathing pattern.
2. Surfactant helps clear mucus and fluid from the respiratory system to make breathing easier.
3. Surfactant helps mature the upper airways to make breathing easier.
4. Surfactant helps in keeping the lungs expanded after the baby starts breathing on its own.

2. 4. Surfactant works by reducing surface tension in the lung. It allows the lung to remain slightly expanded, decreasing the amount of work required for inspiration. Surfactant hasn't been shown to influence upper airway maturation, regulate the neonate's breathing pattern or clear the respiratory tract.

CN: Physiological integrity; CNS: Pharmacological and parental therapies; CL: Application

3. While assessing a 2-hour-old neonate, a nurse observes the neonate to have acrocyanosis. Which nursing action should be performed <u>initially</u>?

1. Activate the code blue or emergency system.
2. Do nothing because acrocyanosis is normal in the neonate.
3. Immediately take the neonate's temperature according to facility policy.
4. Notify the physician of the need for a cardiac consult.

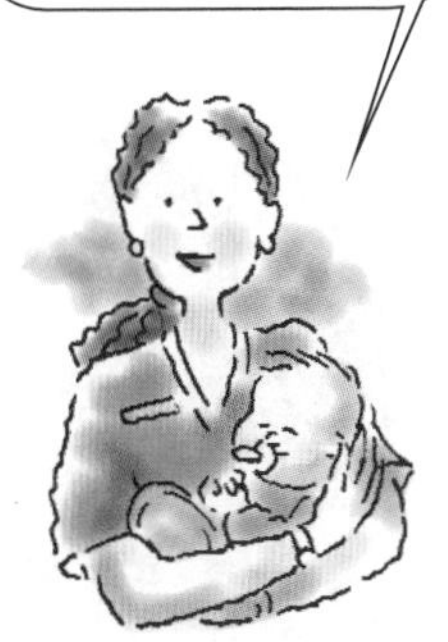

What do you need to do first?

3. 2. Acrocyanosis, or bluish discoloration of the hands and feet in the neonate (also called *peripheral cyanosis*), is a normal finding and shouldn't last more than 24 hours after birth. The other choices are inappropriate.

CN: Physiological integrity; CNS: Physiological adaptation; CL: Application

4. When teaching parents of a neonate the proper position for the neonate's sleep, a nurse stresses the importance of placing the neonate on his back to reduce the risk of which of the following?

1. Aspiration
2. Sudden infant death syndrome (SIDS)
3. Suffocation
4. Gastroesophageal reflux (GER)

4. 2. Supine positioning is recommended to reduce the risk of SIDS in infancy. The risk of aspiration is slightly increased with the supine position. Suffocation would be less likely with an infant supine than prone, and the position for GER requires the head of the bed to be elevated.

CN: Health promotion and maintenance; CNS: None; CL: Application

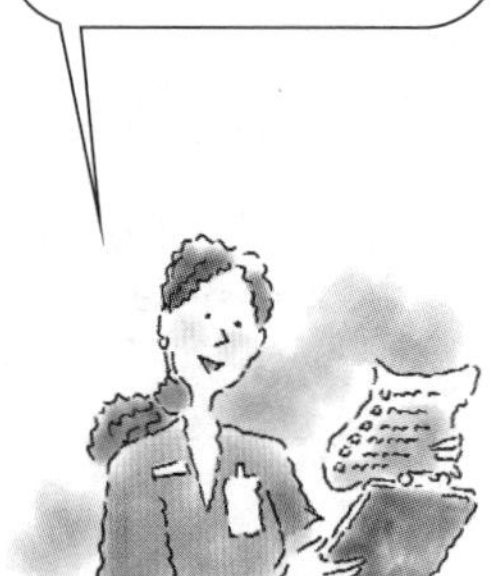

Knowing the risk factors can help guide your assessment.

5. A nurse is caring for a client with gestational diabetes. Which complication is the neonate most at risk of developing?

1. Anemia
2. Hypoglycemia
3. Nitrogen loss
4. Thrombosis

5. 2. Neonates of mothers with diabetes are at risk for hypoglycemia due to increased insulin levels. During gestation, an increased amount of glucose is transferred to the fetus through the placenta. The neonate's liver can't initially adjust to the changing glucose levels after birth. This may result in an overabundance of insulin in the neonate, resulting in hypoglycemia. Neonates of mothers with diabetes aren't at increased risk for anemia, nitrogen loss, or thrombosis.

CN: Physiological integrity; CNS: Physiological adaptation; CL: Analysis

6. Which complication is common in neonates who receive prolonged mechanical ventilation at birth?

1. Bronchopulmonary dysplasia
2. Esophageal atresia
3. Hydrocephalus
4. Renal failure

6. 1. Bronchopulmonary dysplasia commonly results from the high pressures that must sometimes be used to maintain adequate oxygenation. Esophageal atresia, a structural defect in which the esophagus and trachea communicate with each other, doesn't relate to mechanical ventilation. Hydrocephalus and renal failure don't typically occur in these clients.

CN: Physiological integrity; CNS: Physiological adaptation; CL: Analysis

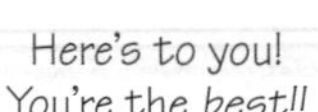

Here's to you!
You're the best!!

7. When performing neonatal assessment, which is the best indication of adequate hydration?

1. Soft, smooth skin
2. A sunken fontanel
3. Bradycardia
4. No urine output in the first 24 hours of life

7. 1. Soft, smooth skin is a sign of adequate hydration. A sunken fontanel and no urine output in the first 24 hours of life are signs of poor hydration. In the case of no urine output, kidney dysfunction would also be a concern. Tachycardia, not bradycardia, may occur with dehydration.

CN: Physiological integrity; CNS: Physiological adaptation; CL: Analysis

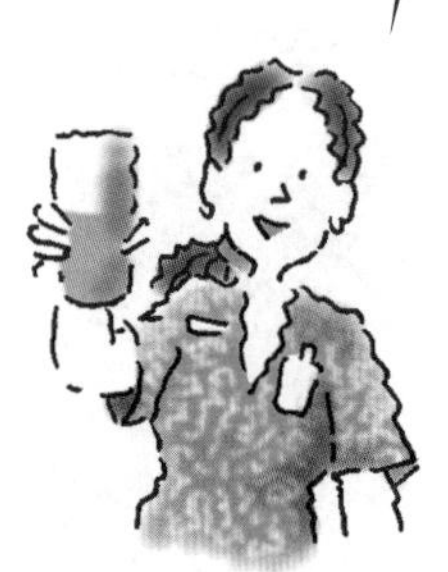

8. When performing a neurologic assessment, which sign is considered a normal finding in a neonate?

1. Doll eyes
2. "Sunset" eyes
3. Positive Babinski's sign
4. Pupils that don't react to light

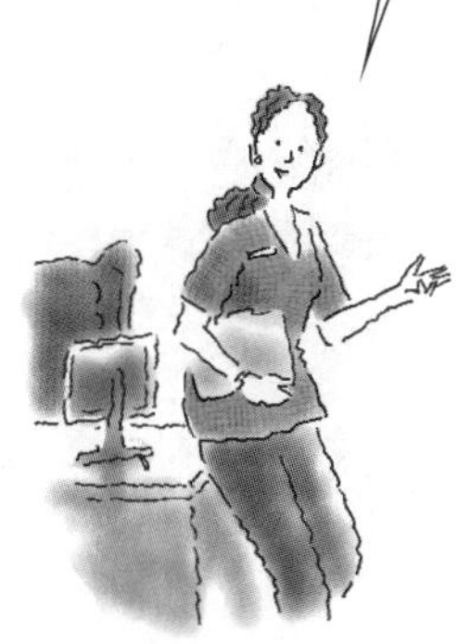

Question 8 asks what's normal versus what's abnormal. Be careful!

8. 3. A positive Babinski's sign is present in infants until approximately age 1. A positive Babinski's reflex is normal in neonates but abnormal in adults. Doll eyes is a neurologic response, but it's noted in adults. The appearance of "sunset" eyes, in which the sclera is visible above the iris, results from cranial nerve palsies and may indicate increased intracranial pressure. A neonate's pupils normally react to light as in an adult.

CN: Health promotion and maintenance; CNS: None; CL: Analysis

9. A nurse is caring for four clients on an antepartum unit. Which client would be carrying a viable conceptus at the earliest stage?

1. A client at 9 weeks' gestation
2. A client at 14 weeks' gestation
3. A client at 24 weeks' gestation
4. A client at 30 weeks' gestation

9. 3. At approximately 23 to 24 weeks' gestation, the lungs are developed enough to sometimes maintain extrauterine life. The lungs are the most immature system during the gestational period. Medical care for premature labor begins much earlier (aggressively at 21 weeks' gestation).

CN: Health promotion and maintenance; CNS: None; CL: Analysis

10. A client's mother asks the nurse why her newborn grandson is getting an injection of vitamin K. Which best explains why this drug is given to neonates?

1. Vitamin K assists with coagulation.
2. Vitamin K assists the gut to mature.
3. Vitamin K initiates the immunization process.
4. Vitamin K protects the brain from excess fluid production.

10. 1. Vitamin K, deficient in the neonate, is needed to activate clotting factors II, VII, IX, and X. In the event of trauma, the neonate would be at risk for excessive bleeding. Vitamin K doesn't assist the gut to mature, but the gut produces vitamin K after maturity is achieved. Vitamin K doesn't influence fluid production in the brain or the immunization process.

CN: Physiological integrity; CNS: Pharmacological and parenteral therapies; CL: Application

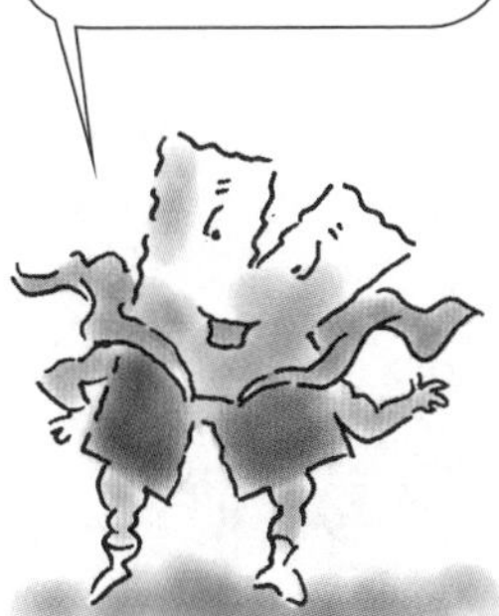

I'm very important to the well-being of a neonate. Do you know why?

11. A neonate is born to a woman infected with hepatitis B. Which treatment should be administered to this neonate?

1. Hepatitis B vaccine at birth and 1 month
2. Hepatitis B immune globulin at birth; no hepatitis B vaccine
3. Hepatitis B immune globulin within 48 hours of birth and hepatitis B vaccine at 1 month
4. Hepatitis B immune globulin within 12 hours of birth and hepatitis B vaccine at birth, 1 month, and 6 months

11. 4. Hepatitis B immune globulin should be given as soon as possible after birth but within 12 hours. Neonates should also receive hepatitis B vaccine at regularly scheduled intervals. This sequence of care has been determined as superior to the others provided.

CN: Health promotion and maintenance; CNS: None; CL: Analysis

12. When a neonate is delivered with meconium staining in the amniotic fluid, which sequence of events will most effectively decrease the risk of meconium aspiration?
1. Deliver the thorax; then suction the nose.
2. Clamp the umbilical cord; then suction the neonate's mouth.
3. Deliver the head; then suction the mouth and then the nose.
4. Deliver the thorax; then suction the nose and then the mouth.

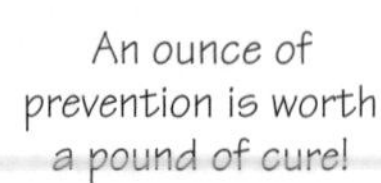

An ounce of prevention is worth a pound of cure!

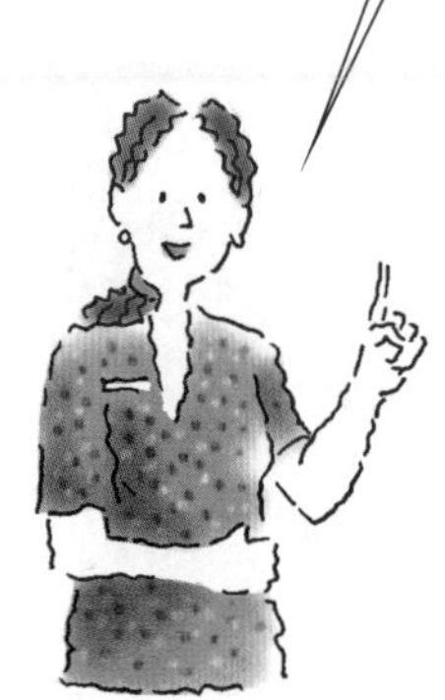

12. 3. To minimize the risk of aspiration of meconium after delivery, the neonate's mouth, then nose, should be suctioned after delivery of the head. This suctioning shouldn't be delayed until after delivery of the thorax because the neonate will take its first breath with meconium in its mouth.
CN: Physiological integrity; CN: Reduction of risk potential; CL: Analysis

13. Erythromycin ointment is administered to a neonate's eyes shortly after birth. The neonate's mother asks the nurse why this is done. The nurse tells the mother it is ordered to prevent which condition?
1. Cataracts
2. Diabetic retinopathy
3. Ophthalmia neonatorum
4. Strabismus

13. 3. Eye prophylaxis is administered to the neonate immediately or soon after birth to prevent ophthalmia neonatorum. Cataracts are opacity of the lens of the eye associated with children with congenital rubella, galactosemia, and cortisone therapy. Diabetic retinopathy occurs in clients with diabetes when the retina bleeds into the vitreous, causing scarring, after which neovascularization occurs. Strabismus is neuromuscular incoordination of the eye alignment.
CN: Physiological integrity; CNS: Pharmacological and parenteral therapies; CL: Application

14. A client with group AB blood whose husband has group O blood has just given birth. Which signs would indicate ABO blood incompatibility in the neonate?
1. Negative Coombs' test
2. Bleeding from the nose or ear
3. Jaundice after the first 24 hours of life
4. Jaundice within the first 24 hours of life

14. 4. The neonate with an ABO blood incompatibility with its mother will have jaundice within the first 24 hours of life. The neonate would have a positive Coombs' test result. Bleeding from the nose and ear should be investigated for possible causes but probably isn't related to ABO incompatibility. Jaundice after the first 24 hours of life is physiologic jaundice.
CN: Physiological integrity; CNS: Reduction of risk potential; CL: Analysis

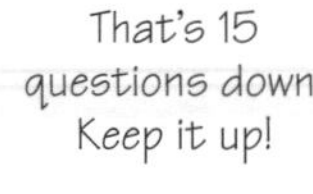

That's 15 questions down. Keep it up!

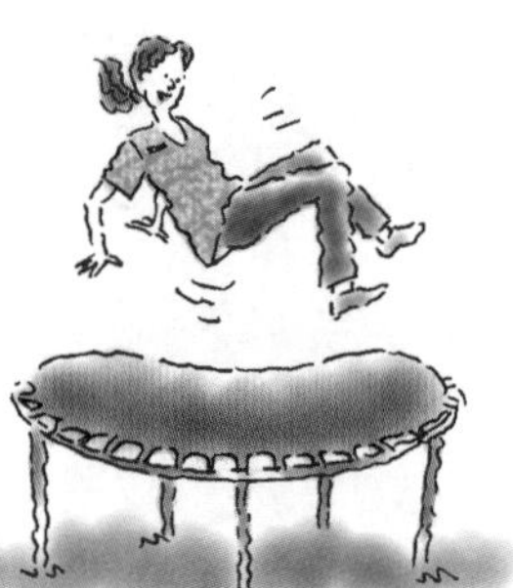

15. Which circumstance of delivery would predispose a neonate to respiratory distress syndrome (RDS)?
1. Preterm birth
2. Vaginal delivery
3. First born of twins
4. Postdate pregnancy

15. 1. Preterm birth is the single most important risk factor for developing RDS. The second born of twins and neonates born by cesarean delivery are also at increased risk for RDS. Surfactant deficiency, which commonly results in RDS, isn't a problem for postdate neonates.
CN: Physiological integrity; CNS: Physiological adaptation; CL: Analysis

16. Two days after circumcision, a nurse notes a yellow-white exudate around the head of the neonate's penis. What would be the <u>most</u> appropriate nursing intervention?

1. Leave the area alone.
2. Report the findings to the physician.
3. Take the neonate's temperature.
4. Remove the exudate with a warm washcloth.

17. A client has just given birth at 42 weeks' gestation. When assessing the neonate, which physical finding is expected?

1. A sleepy, lethargic baby
2. Lanugo covering the body
3. Desquamation of the epidermis
4. Vernix caseosa covering the body

18. A client delivers a small-for-gestation neonate. Which complication is this neonate most at risk for developing?

1. Anemia probably due to chronic fetal hypoxia
2. Hyperthermia due to decreased glycogen stores
3. Hyperglycemia due to decreased glycogen stores
4. Polycythemia probably due to chronic fetal hypoxia

19. Which finding might be seen in a neonate suspected of having an infection?

1. Flushed cheeks
2. Increased temperature
3. Decreased temperature
4. Increased activity level

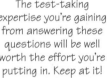

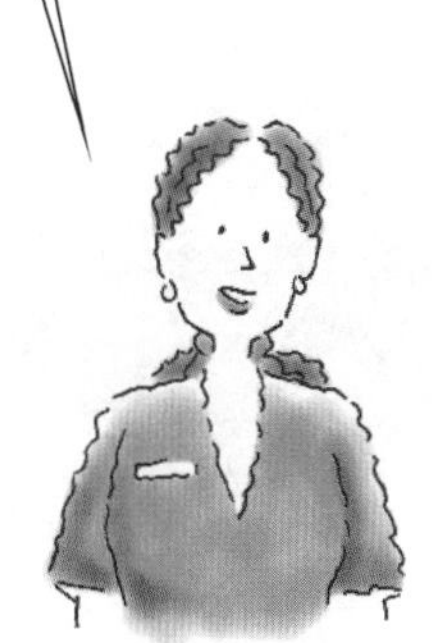

The color of an exudate helps determine its cause.

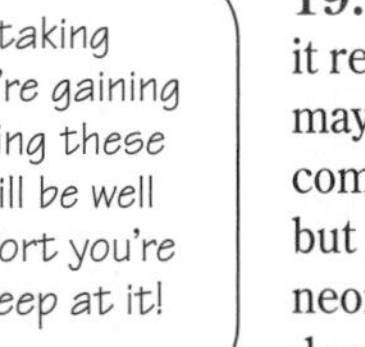

The test-taking expertise you're gaining from answering these questions will be well worth the effort you're putting in. Keep at it!

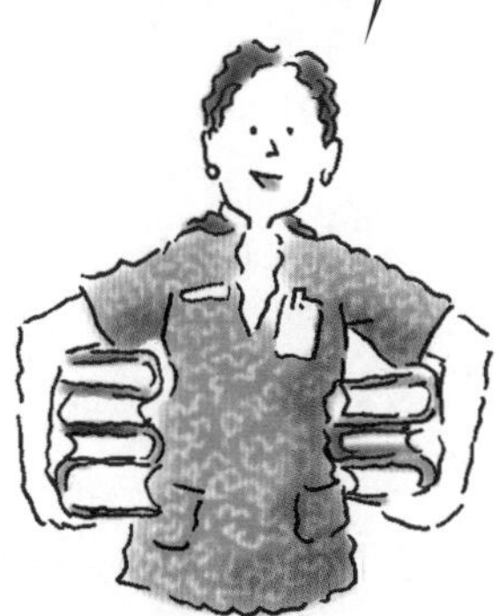

16. 1. The yellow-white exudate is part of the granulation process and a normal finding for a healing penis after circumcision. Therefore, notifying the physician isn't necessary. There's no indication of an infection that would necessitate taking the neonate's temperature. The exudate shouldn't be removed.

CN: Health promotion and maintenance; CNS: None; CL: Analysis

17. 3. Postdate fetuses lose the vernix caseosa, and the epidermis may become desquamated. These neonates are usually very alert. Lanugo is missing in the postdate neonate.

CN: Health promotion and maintenance; CNS: None; CL: Application

18. 4. The small-for-gestation neonate is at risk for developing polycythemia (not anemia) because of a state of anoxia during intrauterine life. The neonates are also at increased risk for developing hypoglycemia and hypothermia due to decreased glycogen stores.

CN: Health promotion and maintenance; CNS: None; CL: Analysis

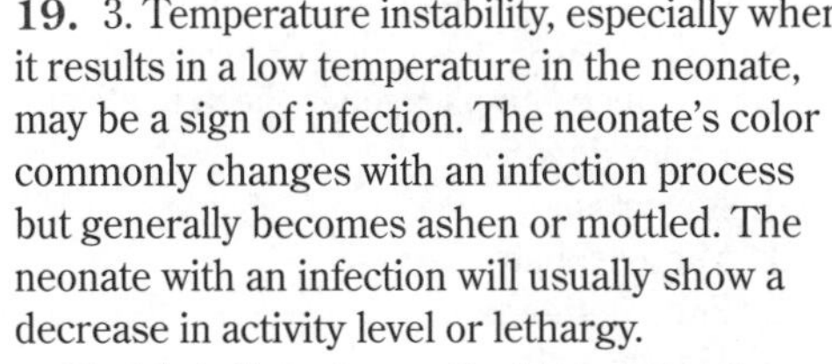

19. 3. Temperature instability, especially when it results in a low temperature in the neonate, may be a sign of infection. The neonate's color commonly changes with an infection process but generally becomes ashen or mottled. The neonate with an infection will usually show a decrease in activity level or lethargy.

CN: Physiological integrity; CNS: Physiological adaptation; CL: Analysis

20. A neonate has just been delivered without incident. Which symptom would indicate successful adaptation to extrauterine life?

1. Nasal flaring
2. Light audible grunting
3. Respiratory rate 40 to 60 breaths/minute
4. Apgar score of 5

20. 3. A respiratory rate 40 to 60 breaths/minute is normal for a neonate during the transitional period. Nasal flaring and audible grunting are signs of respiratory distress. An Apgar score of 5 or less indicates a need for resuscitative efforts.

CN: Health maintenance and promotion; CNS: None; CL: Analysis

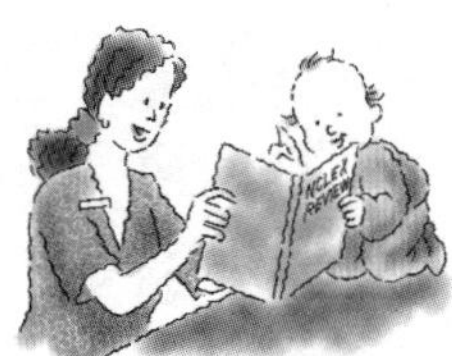

It's time to adapt to the "outside of the womb" world.

21. After reviewing the client's maternal history of magnesium sulfate during labor, which condition should the nurse anticipate as a potential problem in the neonate?

1. Hypoglycemia
2. Jitteriness
3. Respiratory depression
4. Tachycardia

21. 3. Magnesium sulfate crosses the placenta, and adverse neonatal effects are respiratory depression, hypotonia, and bradycardia. The serum blood sugar isn't affected by magnesium sulfate. The neonate would be floppy, not jittery.

CN: Physiological integrity; CNS: Pharmacological and parenteral therapies; CL: Analysis

22. Which intervention is helpful for the neonate experiencing drug withdrawal?

1. Place the isolette in a quiet area of the nursery.
2. Withhold all medication to improve the liver's metabolization of drugs.
3. Dress the neonate in loose clothing so he won't feel restricted.
4. Place the isolette near the nurses' station for frequent contact with health care workers.

22. 1. Neonates experiencing drug withdrawal commonly have sleep disturbance. The neonate should be moved to a quiet area of the nursery to minimize environmental stimuli. Medications, such as phenobarbital and paregoric, should be given as needed. The neonate should be swaddled to prevent him from flailing and stimulating himself.

CN: Psychosocial integrity; CNS: None; CL: Analysis

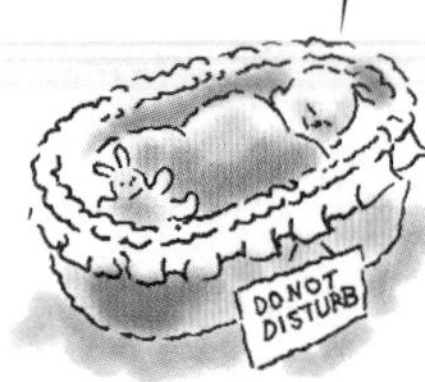

I need special interventions... whatever that means.

23. A client with gestational diabetes delivers a neonate. Because of the client's gestational diabetes, which complication is the neonate at risk for following birth?

1. Atelectasis
2. Microcephaly
3. Pneumothorax
4. Macrosomia

23. 4. Neonates of mothers with diabetes are at increased risk for macrosomia (excessive fetal growth) as a result of the combination of the increased supply of maternal glucose and an increase in fetal insulin. Along with macrosomia, neonates of diabetic mothers are at risk for respiratory distress syndrome, hypoglycemia, hypocalcemia, hyperbilirubinemia, and congenital anomalies. They aren't at greater risk for atelectasis or pneumothorax. Microcephaly is usually the result of cytomegalovirus or rubella virus infection.

CN: Health promotion and maintenance; CNS: None; CL: Analysis

24. A neonate is diagnosed with hemorrhagic disease. Which medication should have been given to the neonate as a preventive measure?

1. Vitamin K
2. Heparin
3. Iron
4. Warfarin

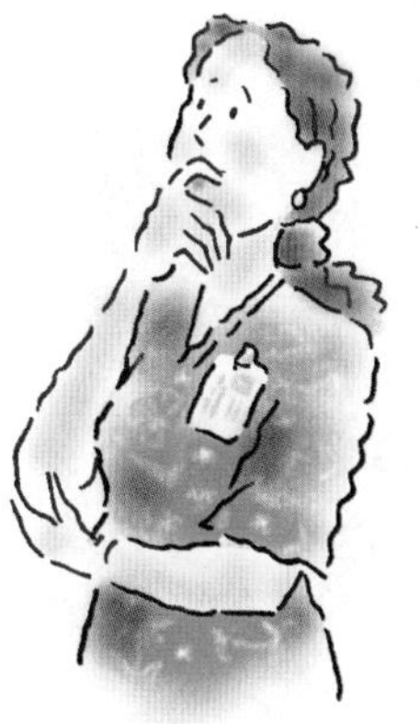

Which measure is preventive, rather than curative or restorative?

24. 1. Neonates have coagulation deficiencies because of a lack of organisms that help produce vitamin K in the intestines, which helps the liver synthesize clotting factors II, VII, IX, and X. Heparin and warfarin are given as anticoagulant therapy, not to prevent hemorrhagic disease in the neonate. Iron is stored in the fetal liver; hemoglobin binds to iron and carries oxygen.

CN: Health promotion and maintenance; CNS: None; CL: Application

25. Which places a neonate at an increased risk for losing heat during the transition period?

1. Placing a cap on the neonate's head immediately after delivery
2. Preheating the radiant warmer prior to delivery
3. Placing the thermometer on the shelf of the radiant warmer
4. Wrapping the neonate in the same blankets used for drying

25. 4. Wrapping the infant in the previously used wet blankets causes continued heat loss by evaporation. Placing a cap on the neonate's head immediately after delivery, preheating the radiant warmer, and placing objects outside of the crib helps prevent heat loss.

CN: Health promotion and maintenance; CNS: None; CL: Application

26. A nursery nurse wraps a neonate in a blanket and keeps the nursery temperature warm. Which type of heat loss is she trying to prevent in the neonate?

1. Conduction
2. Convection
3. Evaporation
4. Radiation

26. 2. Convection heat loss is the flow of heat from the body surface to cooler air. Conduction is the loss of heat from the body surface to cooler surfaces in direct contact. Evaporation is the loss of heat that occurs when a liquid is converted to a vapor. Radiation is the loss of heat from the body surface to cooler solid surfaces not in direct contact but in relative proximity.

CN: Health promotion and maintenance; CNS: None; CL: Application

27. A nurse is explaining physiologic hyperbilirubinemia to the parents of a neonate. Which statement made by one of the parents would demonstrate a correct understanding of the concept?

1. "The neonate usually also has a medical problem."
2. "In term neonates, it usually appears after 24 hours."
3. "It's caused by elevated conjugated bilirubin levels."
4. "It's usually progressive from the neonate's feet to his head."

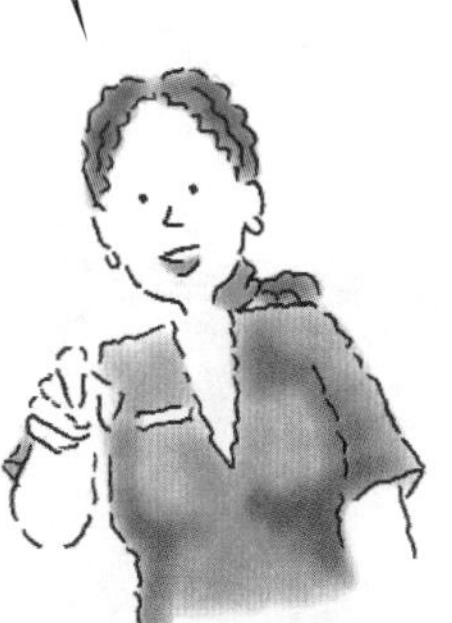

Be careful with this prefix. Hyper is almost identical to hypo, but its meaning, of course, is vastly different.

27. 2. Physiologic jaundice in term neonates first appears after 24 hours. Neonates are otherwise healthy and have no medical problems. Hyperbilirubinemia is caused almost exclusively from unconjugated bilirubin. Jaundice usually appears in a cephalocaudal progression from head to feet.

CN: Physiological integrity; CNS: Reduction of risk potential; CL: Analysis

28. A neonate has been diagnosed with caput succedaneum. Which information should the nurse include while teaching the mother about caput succedaneum?

1. It usually resolves in 3 to 6 weeks.
2. It doesn't cross the cranial suture line.
3. It's a collection of blood between the skull and periosteum.
4. It involves swelling of the tissue over the presenting part of the fetal head.

28. 4. Caput succedaneum is the swelling of tissue over the presenting part of the fetal scalp due to sustained pressure. This boggy edematous swelling is present at birth, crosses the suture line, and most commonly occurs in the occipital area. A cephalhematoma is a collection of blood between the skull and periosteum that doesn't cross cranial suture lines and resolves in 3 to 6 weeks. Caput succedaneum resolves within 3 to 4 days.

CN: Physiological integrity; CNS: Physiological adaptation; CL: Application

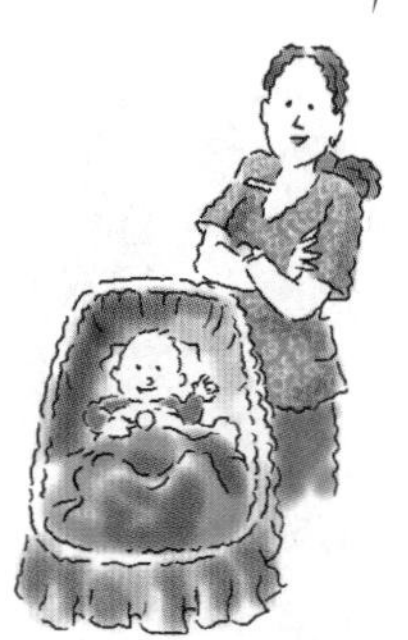

When you're teaching a new mom, it helps to know what to expect at each stage in a neonate's development!

29. A postpartum client expresses concern about the look of her baby's first stool, which she describes as "dark and slimy." Which is the best statement for the nurse to make for patient education?

1. "These types of stools occur when the baby is dehydrated in utero."
2. "The physician will be notified about this abnormal occurrence when he examines the infant."
3. "This bowel movement is called meconium and is considered normal."
4. "The type of first stool for your baby is determined by your diet during pregnancy."

29. 3. Meconium collects in the GI tract during gestation and is initially sterile. Meconium is greenish black because of occult blood and is viscous. Dehydration in utero does not occur. Physician notification is not necessary, as this is a normal occurrence for the first bowel movement. The stool of a neonate is not affected by the mother's antenatal diet.

CN: Health promotion and maintenance; CNS: None; CL: Analysis

30. A 3-day-old neonate needs phototherapy for hyperbilirubinemia. Nursery care of a neonate receiving phototherapy should include which nursing intervention?

1. Tube feedings
2. Feeding the neonate under phototherapy lights
3. Mask over the eyes to prevent retinal damage
4. Temperature monitored every 6 hours during phototherapy

30. 3. The neonate's eyes and genitalia must be covered with eye patches to prevent damage. The neonate can be removed from the lights and held for feeding. The neonate's temperature should be monitored at least every 2 to 4 hours because of the risk of hyperthermia with phototherapy.

CN: Physiological integrity; CNS: Physiological adaptation; CL: Analysis

31. A nurse is caring for four neonates. Which neonate is most likely to develop hyperbilirubinemia?

1. Neonate of an African-American mother
2. Neonate of an Rh-positive mother
3. Neonate with ABO incompatibility
4. Neonate with Apgar scores 9 and 10 at 1 and 5 minutes

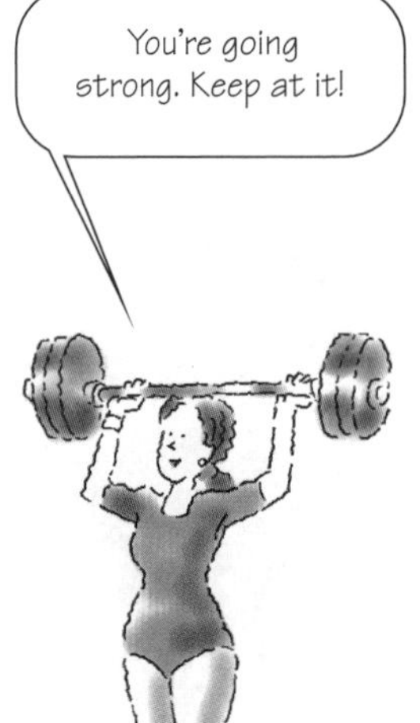

You're going strong. Keep at it!

31. 3. The mother's blood type, which is different from the neonate's, has an impact on the neonate's bilirubin level because of the antigen-antibody reaction. African-American neonates tend to have lower mean levels of bilirubin. Chinese, Japanese, Korean, and Greek neonates tend to have higher incidences of hyperbilirubinemia. Neonates of Rh-negative, not Rh-positive, mothers tend to have hyperbilirubinemia. Low Apgar scores may indicate a risk of hyperbilirubinemia.

CN: Physiological integrity; CNS: Physiological adaptation; CL: Analysis

32. A neonate has developed a major infection. Which gram-positive bacteria most likely contributed to this problem?
1. *Escherichia coli*
2. Group B streptococci
3. *Klebsiella* species
4. *Pseudomonas aeruginosa*

32. 2. Group B streptococci are gram-positive cocci that the neonate is exposed to if these bacteria are colonized in the vaginal tract. *E. coli, Klebsiella,* and *P. aeruginosa* species are gram-negative rods that produce 78% to 85% of the bacterial infection in neonates.

CN: Physiological integrity; CNS: Physiological adaptation; CL: Analysis

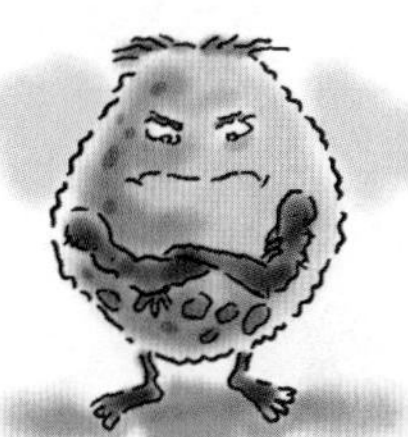

I'm responsible and proud of it!

33. A neonate develops sepsis 18 hours after birth. Which organism most likely contributed to this problem?
1. *Candida albicans*
2. *Chlamydia trachomatis*
3. *Escherichia coli*
4. Group B beta-hemolytic streptococci

33. 4. Transmission of group B beta-hemolytic streptococci to the fetus results in respiratory distress that can rapidly lead to septic shock. *E. coli* is the second most common cause. Candidiasis may be acquired from the birth canal and causes infection later than 24 hours. *C. trachomatis* infection causes neonatal conjunctivitis and pneumonia.

CN: Physiological integrity; CNS: Physiological adaptation; CL: Analysis

34. A nurse administers erythromycin ointment to a neonate's eyes to:
1. eliminate the incidence of viral infections.
2. prevent chlamydia infections.
3. prevent syphilis infection of the eyes.
4. reduce the incidence of group B streptococcal conjunctivitis.

34. 2. Both chlamydia and gonorrhea are common causes of neonatal conjunctival infections, and eryhromycin effectively treats these infections. Viral infections aren't treated with antibiotics, and syphilis and group B streptococcal infections are treated with other antibiotics.

CN: Physiological integrity; CNS: Pharmacological and parenteral therapies; CL: Analysis

35. When attempting to interact with a neonate experiencing drug withdrawal, which behavior would indicate that the neonate is willing to interact?
1. Gaze aversion
2. Hiccups
3. Quiet, alert state
4. Yawning

35. 3. When caring for a neonate experiencing drug withdrawal, the nurse needs to be alert for distress signals from the neonate. Stimuli should be introduced one at a time when the neonate is in a quiet alert state. Gaze aversion, yawning, sneezing, hiccups, and body arching are distress signals that the neonate can't handle stimuli at that time.

CN: Psychosocial integrity; CNS: None; CL: Analysis

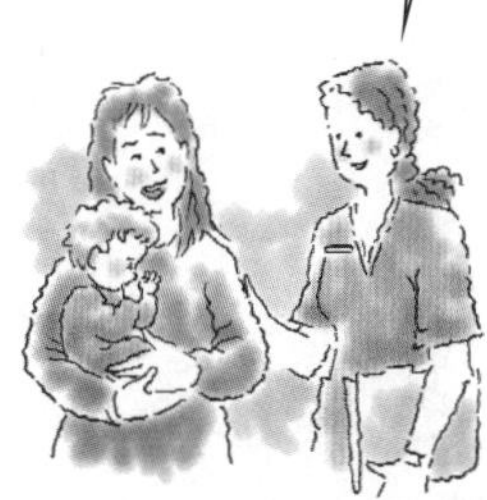

The stump of the umbilical cord will fall off later.

36. When teaching umbilical cord care to a new mother, a nurse would include which information?
1. Apply peroxide to the cord with each diaper change.
2. Cover the cord with petroleum jelly after bathing.
3. Use alcohol on the cord; keep it dry and open to air.
4. Wash the cord with soap and water each day during a tub bath.

36. 3. Using alcohol on the cord and keeping it dry and open to air helps reduce infection and hastens drying. Peroxide could be painful and isn't recommended. Petroleum jelly prevents the cord from drying and encourages infection. Infants aren't given tub baths but are sponged off until the cord falls off.

CN: Health promotion and maintenance; CNS: None
CL: Application

37. When caring for an infant of a mother with diabetes, which physiological finding is most indicative of a hypoglycemic episode?

1. Hyperalert state
2. Jitteriness
3. Excessive crying
4. Serum glucose level of 60 mg/dl

37. 2. Hypoglycemia in a neonate is expressed as jitteriness, lethargy, diaphoresis, and a serum glucose level below 40 mg/dl. A hyperalert state in a neonate is more suggestive of neurologic irritability and has no correlation to blood glucose levels. Excessive crying isn't found in hypoglycemia. A serum glucose level of 60 mg/dl is a normal level.

CN: Physiological integrity; CNS: Physiological adaptation; CL: Analysis

38. A mother of a term neonate asks what the thick, white, cheesy coating is on his skin. Which statement correctly describes the function of this coating for the neonate?

1. It helps keep the neonate warm after birth.
2. It prevents neonatal dehydration after birth.
3. It serves as a protective coating in utero.
4. It decreases the development of birth marks.

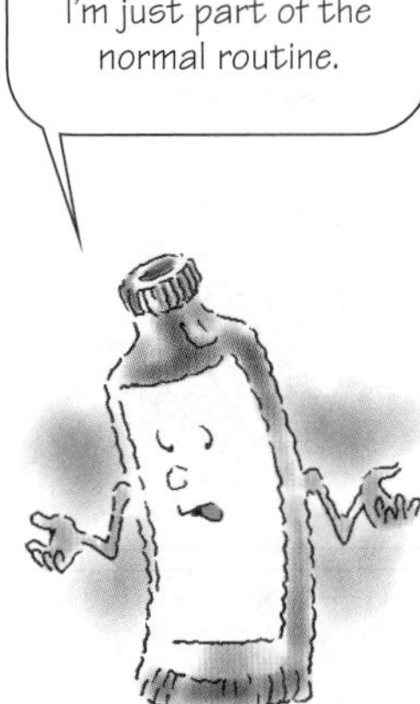

What can I say?
I'm just part of the
normal routine.

38. 3. Vernix caseosa is a white, cheesy material present on the neonate's skin at birth. The purpose of the vernix caseosa is to protect the fetus in utero. It does not prevent dehydration or keep the neonate warm after birth. There is no association between vernix caseosa and birthmarks.

CN: Health promotion and maintenance; CNS: None; CL: Analysis

39. Which drug is routinely given to the neonate within 1 hour of birth?

1. Erythromycin ophthalmic ointment
2. Gentamicin
3. Nystatin
4. Vitamin A

39. 1. Erythromycin ophthalmic ointment is given for prophylactic treatment of ophthalmic neonatorum. Gentamicin is an antibiotic used in the treatment of an infection of the neonate. Nystatin is used for treatment of neonate thrush. Vitamin K, not vitamin A, is given.

CN: Physiological integrity; CNS: Pharmacological and parenteral therapies; CL: Analysis

40. Which condition or treatment best ensures lung maturity in a neonate?

1. Meconium in the amniotic fluid
2. Glucocorticoid treatment just before delivery
3. Lecithin to sphingomyelin ratio more than 2:1
4. Absence of phosphatidylglycerol in amniotic fluid

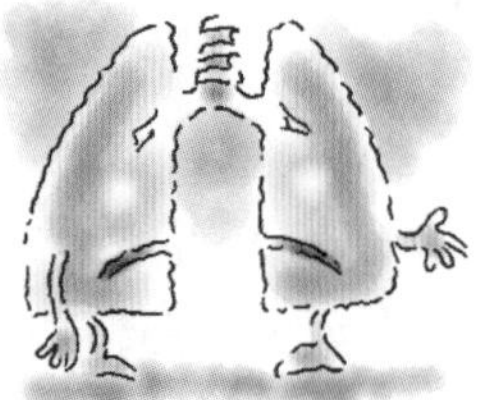

Why do they think
I'm immature?

40. 3. Lecithin and sphingomyelin are phospholipids that help compose surfactant in the lungs; lecithin peaks at 36 weeks, and sphingomyelin concentrations remain stable. Meconium is released because of fetal stress before delivery, but it's chronic fetal stress that matures lungs. Glucocorticoids must be given at least 48 hours before delivery. The presence of phosphatidylglycerol indicates lung maturity.

CN: Physiological integrity; CNS: Physiological adaptation; CL: Analysis

41. Which assessment finding would place the neonate at the least risk for developing respiratory distress syndrome (RDS)?

1. Second born of twins
2. Neonate born at 34 weeks
3. Neonate of a diabetic mother
4. Chronic maternal hypertension

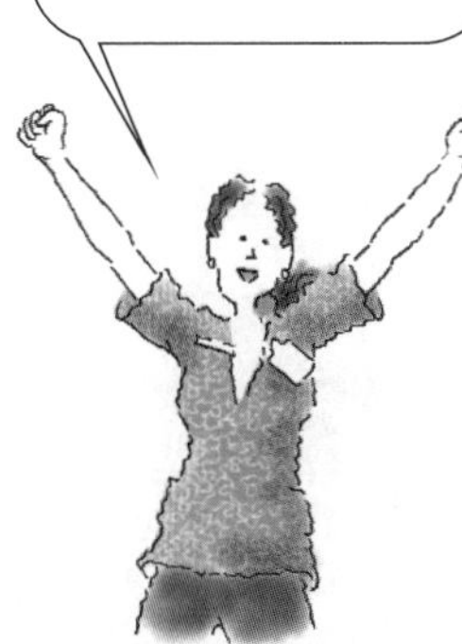

Congratulations! You're halfway through this chapter.

41. 4. Chronic maternal hypertension is an unlikely factor because chronic fetal stress tends to increase lung maturity. The second born of twins may be prone to greater risk of asphyxia leading to RDS. Premature neonates younger than 36 weeks are associated with RDS. Even with a mature lecithin to sphingomyelin ratio, neonates of mothers with diabetes may still develop respiratory distress.

CN: Physiological integrity; CNS: Physiological adaptation; CL: Analysis

42. A nurse is performing an assessment on a neonate. Which finding is considered common in the healthy neonate?

1. Simian crease
2. Conjunctival hemorrhages
3. Cystic hygroma
4. Bulging fontanelle

42. 2. Conjunctival hemorrhages are commonly seen in neonates secondary to the cranial pressure applied during the birth process. Simian creases are present in 40% of the neonates with trisomy 21. Cystic hygroma is a neck mass that can affect the airway. Bulging fontanelles are a sign of intracranial pressure.

CN: Health promotion and maintenance; CNS: None; CL: Analysis

43. When performing nursing care for a neonate after a birth, which intervention has the <u>highest</u> nursing <u>priority</u>?

1. Obtain a Dextrostix.
2. Give the initial bath.
3. Give the vitamin K injection.
4. Cover the neonate's wet head with a cap.

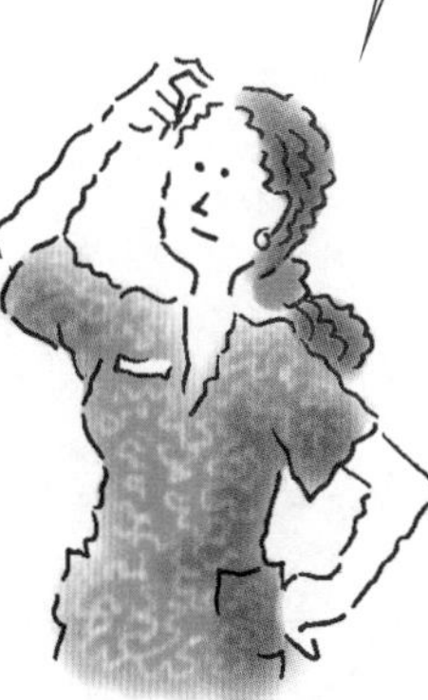

Which one of these actions is a priority right after birth?

43. 3. The American Academy of Pediatrics recommends that vitamin K be given in the delivery room within 1 hour of birth. Dextrostix, appropriate for neonates with risk factors, are obtained at 30 minutes to 1 hour of age. Initial baths aren't given until the neonate's temperature is stable. The head shouldn't be covered until the hair is dried under a radiant warmer.

CN: Safe, effective care environment; CNS: Management of care; CL: Analysis

44. When assessing a neonate's skin, the nurse observes small, white papules surrounded by erythematous dermatitis. Which most accurately describes this condition?

1. Cutis marmorata
2. Epstein's pearls
3. Erythema toxicum
4. Mongolian spots

44. 3. Erythema toxicum has lesions that come and go on the face, trunk, and limbs. They're small, white or yellow papules or vesicles with erythematous dermatitis and resemble flea bites. Cutis marmorata is bluish mottling of the skin. Epstein's pearls, found in the mouth, are similar to facial milia. Mongolian spots are large macules or patches that are gray or blue green.

CN: Health promotion and maintenance; CNS: None; CL: Application

45. Which nursing consideration is most important when giving a neonate his initial bath?

1. Give a tub bath.
2. Use water and mild soap.
3. Give it right after delivery.
4. Use hexachlorophene soap.

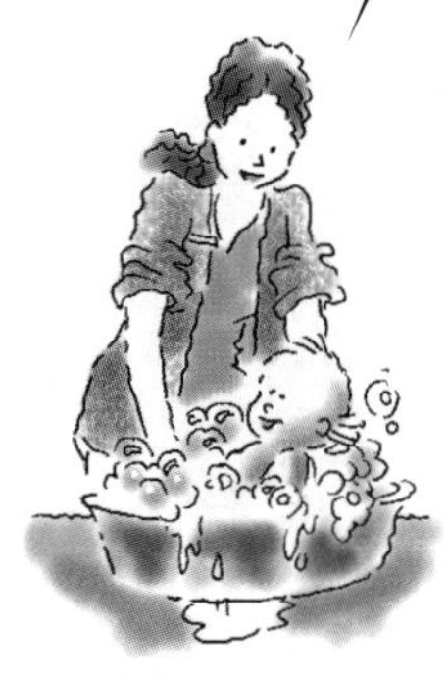

What's most important for baby's first bath?

45. 2. Use only water and mild soap on a neonate to prevent drying out the skin. The initial bath is given when the neonate's temperature is stable. Tub baths are delayed until the umbilical cord falls off. Hexachlorophene soaps should be avoided; they're neurotoxic and may be absorbed through a neonate's skin.
CN: Health promotion and maintenance; CNS: None; CL: Application

46. The nurse is teaching the parents of a neonate about the Centers for Disease Control and Prevention (CDC) recommendations for hepatitis B vaccine. Which statement would be the most accurate concerning these recommendations?

1. "It should be given to all neonates."
2. "It should be given to neonates exposed to hepatitis B only."
3. "It should be given to neonates showing symptoms of hepatitis B."
4. "It should be given to neonates whose mothers have human immunodeficiency virus."

46. 1. The CDC recommends hepatitis B vaccine be given to all neonates, including those born to hepatitis B surface antigen–negative mothers, before hospital discharge.
CN: Health promotion and maintenance; CNS: None; CL: Application

47. A male neonate has just been circumcised. Which nursing intervention is part of the initial care of a circumcised neonate?

1. Apply alcohol to the site.
2. Change the diaper as needed.
3. Keep the neonate in the supine position.
4. Apply petroleum gauze to the site for 24 hours.

47. 4. Petroleum gauze is applied to the site for the first 24 hours to prevent the skin edges from sticking to the diaper. Alcohol is contraindicated for circumcision care. Diapers are changed more frequently to inspect the site. Neonates are initially kept in the prone position.
CN: Health promotion and maintenance; CNS: None; CL: Application

48. When performing an assessment on a neonate, which assessment finding is most suggestive of hypothermia?

1. Bradycardia
2. Hyperglycemia
3. Metabolic alkalosis
4. Shivering

48. 1. Hypothermic neonates become bradycardic proportional to the degree of core temperature. Hypoglycemia is seen in hypothermic neonates. Metabolic acidosis, not alkalosis, is seen as a result of slowed respirations. Neonates use nonshivering thermogenesis.
CN: Health promotion and maintenance; CNS: None; CL: Analysis

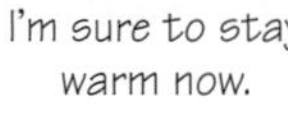

I'm sure to stay warm now.

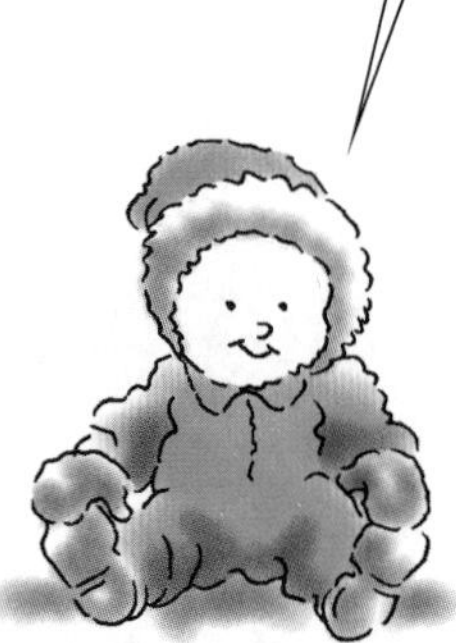

49. Which nursing intervention helps prevent evaporative heat loss in the neonate immediately after birth?

1. Administering warm oxygen
2. Controlling the drafts in the room
3. Immediately drying the neonate
4. Placing the neonate on a warm, dry towel

49. 3. Immediately drying the neonate decreases evaporative heat loss from his moist body from birth. Controlling the drafts in the room and administering warmed oxygen help reduce convective loss. Placing the neonate on a warm, dry towel decreases conductive losses.
CN: Health promotion and maintenance; CNS: None; CL: Analysis

CN: Client needs category CNS: Client needs subcategory CL: Cognitive level

50. A nurse is performing an assessment on a neonate. Which assessment finding would indicate a metabolic response to cold stress?

1. Arrhythmias
2. Hypoglycemia
3. Increase in liver function
4. Increase in blood pressure

50. 2. Hypoglycemia occurs as the consumption of glucose increases with the increase in metabolic rate. Arrhythmias and increases in blood pressure occur because of cardiorespiratory manifestations. Liver function declines in cold stress.

CN: Health promotion and maintenance; CNS: None; CL: Analysis

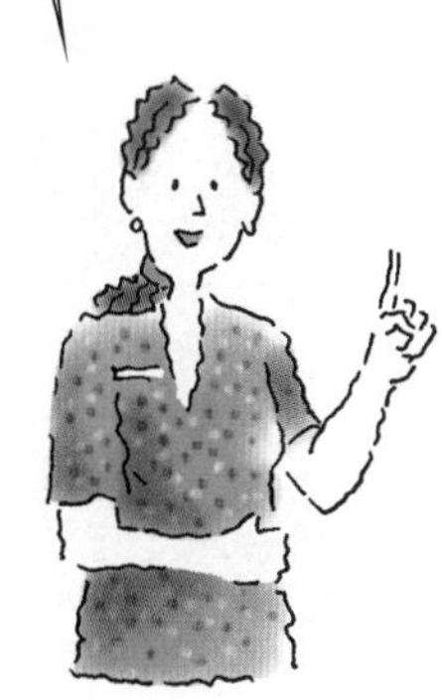

The word highest is a clue to the answer!

51. Which would be the highest priority in regulating the temperature of a neonate?

1. Supply extra heat sources to the neonate.
2. Keep the ambient room temperature less than 100° F (37.8°C).
3. Minimize the energy needed for the neonate to produce heat.
4. Block radiant, convective, conductive, and evaporative losses.

51. 4. Prevention of heat loss is always the first goal in thermoregulation to avoid hypothermia. The second goal is to minimize the energy necessary for neonates to produce heat. Adding extra heat sources is a means of correcting hypothermia. The ambient room temperature should be kept at approximately 100°F.

CN: Safe, effective care environment; CNS: Management of care; CL: Application

52. Which neonate would be most at risk for a problem with thermoregulation?

1. A term neonate born to a diabetic mother.
2. A preterm neonate born at 36 weeks' gestation.
3. A preterm neonate born at 39 weeks' gestation.
4. A term neonate with signs of jaundice at 36 hours of age.

52. 2. Preterm neonates are not able to thermoregulate due to the lack of brown fat. The more premature the infant, the more immature the thermoregulation system. Infants born to diabetic mothers and those with jaundice are not more at risk for problems with thermoregulation than a premature infant.

CN: Physiological integrity; CNS: Reduction of risk potential; CL: Analysis

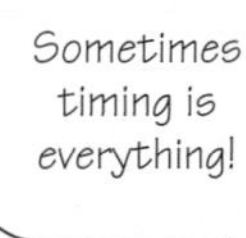

53. Which clinical finding is most suggestive of physiologic hyperbilirubinemia in a neonate?

1. Clinical jaundice before 36 hours of age
2. Clinical jaundice lasting beyond 14 days
3. Bilirubin levels of 12 mg/dl by 3 days of life
4. Serum bilirubin level increasing by more than 5 mg/dl/day

53. 3. Increased bilirubin levels in the liver usually cause bilirubin levels of 12 mg/dl by the 3rd day of life. This is from the impaired conjugation and excretion of bilirubin and difficulty clearing bilirubin from plasma. The other answers suggest pathologic jaundice.

CN: Physiological integrity; CNS: Reduction of risk potential; CL: Analysis

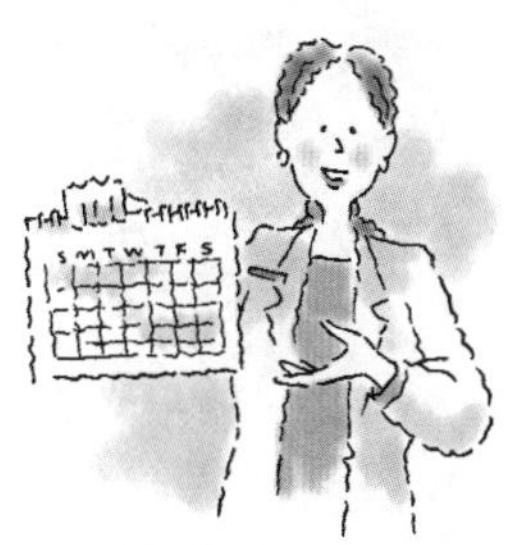

54. A nurse is caring for a full-term neonate who's receiving phototherapy for hyperbilirubinemia. She should notify the physician immediately if which finding is noted?

1. Maculopapular rash
2. Absent Moro reflex
3. Greenish stools
4. Bronze-colored skin

54. 2. An absent Moro reflex, lethargy, and seizures are symptoms of bilirubin encephalopathy which can be life-threatening. A maculopapular rash, greenish stools, and bronze-colored skin are minor side effects of phototherapy that should be monitored but don't require immediate intervention.

CN: Physiological integrity; CNS: Physiological adaptation; CL: Analysis

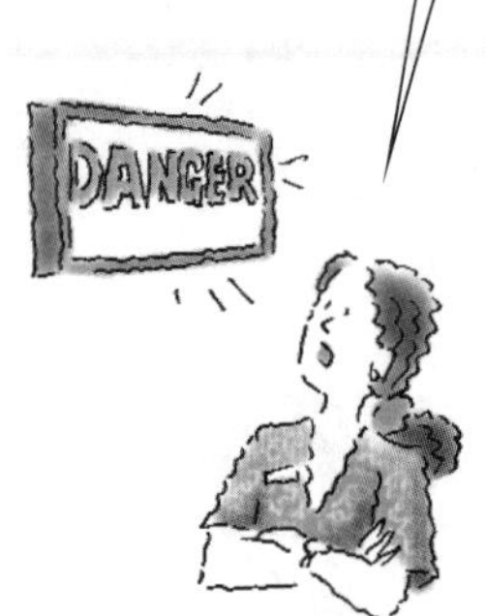

The signs are pointing to a dangerous situation.
DANGER

55. A neonate undergoing phototherapy treatment needs to be monitored for which adverse effect?

1. Hyperglycemia
2. Increased insensible water loss
3. Severe decrease in platelet count
4. Increased GI transit time

55. 2. Increased insensible water loss is due to absorbed photon energy from the lights. Hyperglycemia isn't a characteristic effect of phototherapy treatment. There may be a mild decrease in platelet count. GI transit time may decrease with use of phototherapy.

CN: Health promotion and maintenance; CNS: None; CL: Analysis

56. Which assessment finding might be seen in a neonate suspected of having early breast-milk jaundice?

1. History of being a poor feeder
2. Decreased bilirubin level around day 3 of life
3. Clinical jaundice evident after 24 hours
4. Interruption of breast-feeding resulting in decreased bilirubin levels between 24 and 72 hours

56. 4. The exact cause of early breast-milk jaundice is unknown. If bilirubin levels don't decrease after 3 days, human milk is eliminated as a cause. These babies are typically good eaters with good weight gain. Bilirubin levels increase, rather than decrease, at day 3. Jaundice in the first 24 hours of life is characteristic of hemolytic disease.

CN: Health promotion and maintenance; CNS: None; CL: Analysis

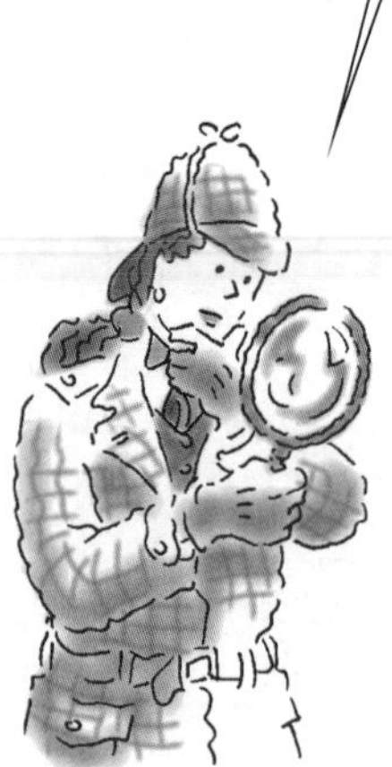

It's important to recognize the earliest clue.

57. Which sign is the earliest indication of respiratory distress syndrome (RDS) in a neonate?

1. Bilateral crackles
2. Pale gray color
3. Tachypnea more than 60 breaths/minute
4. Poor capillary filling time (3 to 4 seconds)

57. 3. Tachypnea and expiratory grunting occur early in RDS to help improve oxygenation. Crackles occur as the respiratory distress progressively worsens. A pale gray skin color obscures earlier cyanosis as respiratory distress symptoms persist and worsen. Poor capillary filling time, a later manifestation, occurs if signs and symptoms aren't treated.

CN: Health promotion and maintenance; CNS: None; CL: Analysis

58. A nurse is caring for a neonate with respiratory problems. Which condition is most likely to be caused by fluid remaining in the lungs of the neonate after delivery?

1. Choanal atresia
2. Meconium aspiration
3. Pulmonary hemorrhage
4. Transient tachypnea of a newborn

58. 4. Transient tachypnea of a newborn is caused by a delay in removing excessive amounts of lung fluid. Choanal atresia is caused by a protrusion of bone or membrane into nasal passages, causing blockage or narrowing. Meconium aspiration is meconium aspirated into the lungs during birth. Pulmonary hemorrhage is bleeding into the alveoli.

CN: Physiological integrity; CNS: Physiological adaptation; CL: Analysis

59. A neonate is admitted to the neonatal intensive care unit with persistent pulmonary hypertension. Which pulmonary vasodilator is the drug of choice for this disorder?

1. Dobutamine
2. Isoproterenol (Isuprel)
3. Prostaglandin E_2
4. Inhaled nitric oxide

59. 4. Inhaled nitric oxide is a potent selective pulmonary vasodilator. Dobutamine is a vasopressor, not a vasodilator. Isoproterenol dilates pulmonary arteries but doesn't decrease pulmonary vascular resistance. Prostaglandin E_2 is an oxytocic substance used to induce abortion and doesn't affect pulmonary vasodilation.

CN: Physiological integrity; CNS: Pharmacological and parenteral therapies; CL: Analysis

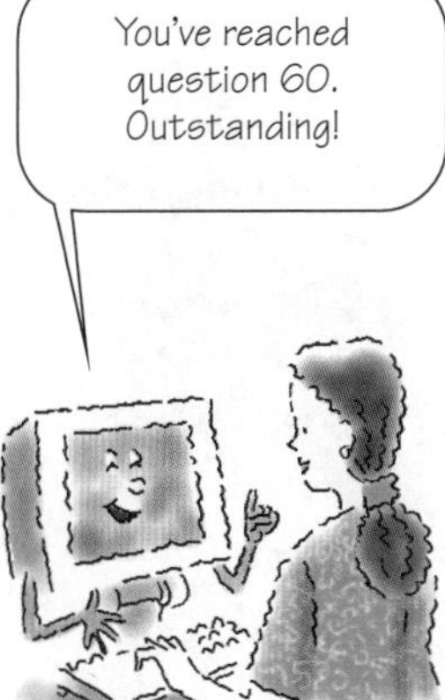
You've reached question 60. Outstanding!

60. Which neonatal respiratory disorder is usually mild and runs a self-limited course?

1. Pneumonia
2. Meconium aspiration syndrome
3. Transient tachypnea of newborn
4. Persistent pulmonary hypertension

60. 3. Transient tachypnea has an invariably favorable outcome after several hours to several days. The outcome of pneumonia depends on the causative agent involved and may have complications. Meconium aspiration, depending on severity, may have long-term adverse effects. In persistent pulmonary hypertension, the mortality rate is more than 50%.

CN: Physiological integrity; CNS: Physiological adaptation; CL: Analysis

61. Which procedure should be avoided in a neonate born with diaphragmatic hernia?

1. Chest X-ray
2. Mask ventilation
3. Placement of orogastric tube
4. Immediate endotracheal intubation

61. 2. Mask ventilation should be avoided to prevent air from being introduced into the GI tract by this technique. An emergency chest X-ray will help in diagnosing this defect. An orogastric tube is needed to decompress the bowel and stomach within the chest. Intubation is needed to ventilate the neonate because of the defect.

CN: Physiological integrity; CNS: Physiological adaptation; CL: Application

62. A nurse is preparing to administer Survanta (Beractant) to a preterm infant. The order is for 4 ml/kg. The neonate weighs 2000 grams. How many total ml will be used for one dose? Record your answer as a whole number:

______________________________ml

62. 8. The answer is 8 ml.

First, convert the weight from grams to kilograms using the conversion:

1000 gm = 1 kg
1000 gm/1 kg = 2000 gm/x kg
X = 2 kg

Then, determine how many ml are needed by using the following formula:

$4 \text{ ml} \times 2 \text{ kg} = 8 \text{ ml}$ total dose.

CN: Physiological integrity; CNS: Pharmacological and parenteral therapies; CL: Application

63. A nurse is caring for a neonate with fetal alcohol syndrome (FAS). Which craniofacial change is most indicative of FAS?

1. Macrocephaly
2. Microophthalmia
3. Wide palpebral fissures
4. Well-developed philtrum

63. 2. Distinctive facial dysmorphology of children with FAS most commonly involves the eyes (microophthalmia). Microcephaly is generally seen, as are short palpebral fissures and a poorly developed philtrum.

CN: Physiological integrity; CNS: Physiological adaptation; CL: Analysis

64. A 36-week neonate born weighing 1,800 g has microcephaly and microophthalmia. Based on these findings, which risk factor might be expected in the maternal history?
1. Use of alcohol
2. Use of marijuana
3. Gestational diabetes
4. Positive group B streptococci

64. 1. The most common sign of the effects of alcohol on fetal development is retarded growth in weight, length, and head circumference. Intrauterine growth retardation isn't characteristic of marijuana use. Gestational diabetes usually produces large-for-gestational-age neonates. Positive group B streptococcus isn't a relevant risk factor.
CN: Health promotion and maintenance; CNS: None; CL: Analysis

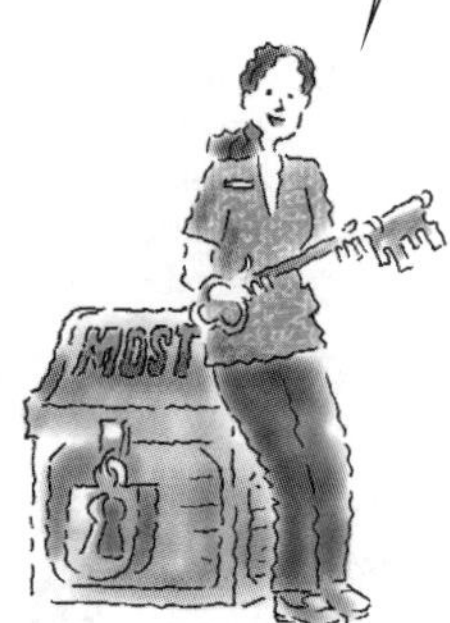

The mother's history may be the key to the neonate's current condition.
MOST

65. Which condition requires intervention when displayed by a neonate born to a mother with a history of chronic alcohol abuse?
1. Hypoactivity
2. High birth weight
3. Poor wake and sleep patterns
4. High threshold of stimulation

65. 3. Altered sleep patterns are caused by disturbances in the central nervous system from alcohol exposure in utero. Hyperactivity is a characteristic deficit generally associated with fetal alcohol syndrome (FAS). Low birth weight is a physical defect seen in neonates with FAS. Neonates with FAS generally have a low threshold for stimulation.
CN: Physiological integrity; CNS: Physiological adaptation; CL: Application

66. A neonate is admitted to rule out a diagnosis of cystic fibrosis. Which GI disorder most likely indicates this diagnosis?
1. Duodenal obstruction
2. Jejunal atresia
3. Malrotation
4. Meconium ileus

66. 4. Meconium ileus is a luminal obstruction of the distal small intestine by abnormal meconium seen in neonates with cystic fibrosis. Duodenal obstruction, jejunal atresia, and malrotation aren't characteristic findings in neonates with cystic fibrosis.
CN: Physiological integrity; CNS: Physiological adaptation; CL: Analysis

67. During discharge instructions, which statement by the nurse would be the most correct for the safety of the neonate? Select all that apply:
1. "Heavy blankets or stuffed animals can be placed in the crib."
2. "The car seat used should be a front-facing model."
3. "Never leave your infant alone in the tub."
4. "Verify that you babysitter knows CPR."
5. "The car seat used should be a rear-facing model."

67. 3, 4, 5. Infants should never be left alone in the tub, as they can easily drown. All caretakers should be trained in CPR. Car seats should be rear-facing models, not front-facing models, until the infant weights 20 pounds and/or is one-year-old. Heavy blankets or stuffed animals in the crib increase the risk of sudden infant death syndrome (SIDS).
CN: Health promotion and maintenance; CNS: None; CL: Application

Keep reading each question carefully and you'll do well.

68. A neonate has an imperforate anus, tracheoesophageal fistula, and a single umbilical artery. A nurse suspects that the neonate might have which congenital disorder?
1. Beckwith-Wiedemann syndrome
2. Trisomy 13
3. Turner's syndrome
4. VATER association

68. 4. VATER association clinically presents with three or more defects, including the three mentioned. These defects aren't associated with Beckwith-Wiedemann syndrome. Trisomy 13 and Turner's syndrome are chromosomal aberrations that aren't typically seen with the other defects.
CN: Physiological integrity; CNS: Physiological adaptation; CL: Analysis

CN: Client needs category CNS: Client needs subcategory CL: Cognitive level

69. An initial assessment of a female neonate shows pink-streaked vaginal discharge. This data indicates which condition?
1. Cystitis
2. Birth trauma
3. Neonatal candidiasis
4. Withdrawal of maternal hormones

69. 4. Withdrawal of maternal estrogen can produce pseudomenstruation. Cystitis or a urinary tract infection in a neonate would show generalized signs of sepsis. Birth trauma may cause surface abrasions but not vaginal discharge. Neonates with candidal infections usually have oral lesions (thrush) or monilial diaper rash.
CN: Health promotion and maintenance; CNS: None; CL: Application

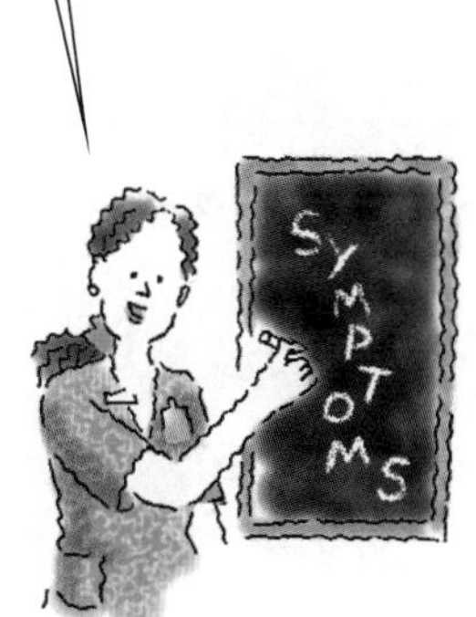

70. When assessing for congenital anomalies in a neonate, which symptom is seen first with tracheoesophageal atresia?
1. Torticollis
2. Nasal stuffiness
3. Oligohydramnios
4. Excessive oral secretions

70. 4. Accumulated secretions are copious in neonates with this disorder because the neonate can't swallow. Torticollis would be present only if there was a defect of muscle or bone. Nasal stuffiness is very common in neonates and doesn't indicate esophageal abnormalities. Atresia will produce polyhydramnios because the fetus can't swallow the amniotic fluid.
CN: Physiological integrity; CNS: Physiological adaptation; CL: Analysis

71. A new mother states to the nurse, "My baby spits up after every feeding." Which intervention would be appropriate to teach the mother initially for this problem?
1. Feed the baby every hour.
2. Change the infant to a soy formula.
3. Lay the infant on its stomach after every feeding.
4. Burp the infant more frequently during each feeding.

71. 4. Frequent burping decreases the amount of air the infant has in it stomach. Laying an infant on its back or side after feeding is preferred. Formula may have to be changed if it is determined that the spitting is related to milk intolerance, but this is not the initial reaction. Infants should be fed every 2–4 hours.
CN: Health promotion and maintenance; CNS: None; CL: Analysis

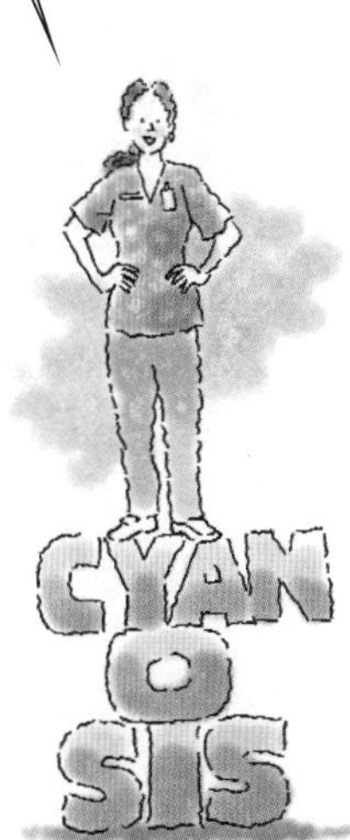

You need to stay on top of central cyanosis in a neonate.
CYAN
O
SIS

72. Maintaining thermoregulation in the neonate is an important nursing intervention because cold stress in the neonate can lead to which condition?
1. Anemia
2. Hyperglycemia
3. Metabolic alkalosis
4. Increased oxygen consumption

72. 4. The neonate's metabolic rate increases as a result of cold stress, which leads to an increased oxygen requirement. Cold stress doesn't increase erythrocyte destruction. Cold stress leads to anaerobic glycolysis, which results in metabolic acidosis. The increased metabolic rate leads to the use of glycogen stores and produces hypoglycemia.
CN: Physiological integrity; CNS: Reduction of risk potential; CL: Analysis

73. Which initial nursing intervention best addresses the needs of a term neonate with adequate respiratory and heart rates but who has central cyanosis?
1. Provide tactile stimulation.
2. Give supplemental free-flow oxygen.
3. Assist ventilation with a bag and mask.
4. Intubate and suction the lower airway.

73. 2. Room air is currently insufficient, seen by the central cyanosis. Tactile stimulation is needed only if the neonate is apneic or gasping. Bag and mask ventilation is indicated only if the heart rate is less than 100 beats/minute. Intubation is indicated only in special circumstances, such as prematurity or a diaphragmatic hernia.
CN: Health promotion and maintenance; CNS: None; CL: Application

74. A woman delivers a 3,250-g neonate at 42 weeks' gestation. Which physical finding is expected during an examination of this neonate?

1. Abundant lanugo
2. Absence of sole creases
3. Breast bud of 1 to 2 mm in diameter
4. Leathery, cracked, and wrinkled skin

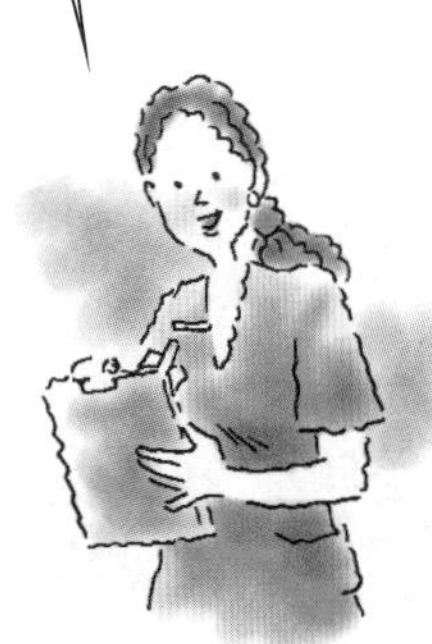

Question 74 asks about an *expected* finding, not necessarily an abnormal one.

74. 4. Neonatal skin thickens with maturity and is typically peeling by postterm. Lanugo disappears as pregnancy progresses, with very little remaining on the postterm neonate. Because sole creases increase in number and depth with gestational age, a postterm neonate would have deep sole creases. A postterm neonate would have a well-developed breast bud of 5 to 10 mm in diameter.

CN: Health promotion and maintenance; CNS: None; CL: Analysis

75. While performing an initial assessment on a term neonate with an Asian mother, a bluish marking is observed across the neonate's lower back. What does this finding signify?

1. It's probably a sign of birth trauma.
2. It's probably a telangiectatic hemangioma.
3. It's probably a typical marking in dark-skinned races.
4. It probably indicates that hyperbilirubinemia may follow.

75. 3. This is a Mongolian spot, commonly found over the lumbosacral area in neonates of Black, Asian, Latin American, or Native American origin. The coloration is due to the deposition of melanocytes, not erythrocytes, and, without other findings, isn't a bruise resulting from a birth trauma. A telangiectatic hemangioma is a salmon pink coloration found at the nape of the neck, eyelids, and forehead. A Mongolian spot is a deep dermal infiltration of melanocytes, so there would be no breakdown of erythrocytes to cause hyperbilirubinemia.

CN: Health promotion and maintenance; CNS: None; CL: Analysis

76. A nurse in the neonate nursery is serving as preceptor for a student nurse. The student asks the nurse why a neonate's head is cone-shaped. Which response is accurate?

1. "It results from caput succedaneum. The difficult labor caused bruising and swelling of the neonate's head."
2. "It results from molding. Overriding of the cranial sutures allows the neonate's head to pass though the birth canal."
3. "It results from cephalohematoma. Some blood has collected between the skull bone and periosteum."
4. "It results from hydrocephalus. Either too much cerebrospinal fluid (CSF) is being formed, or too little is being absorbed."

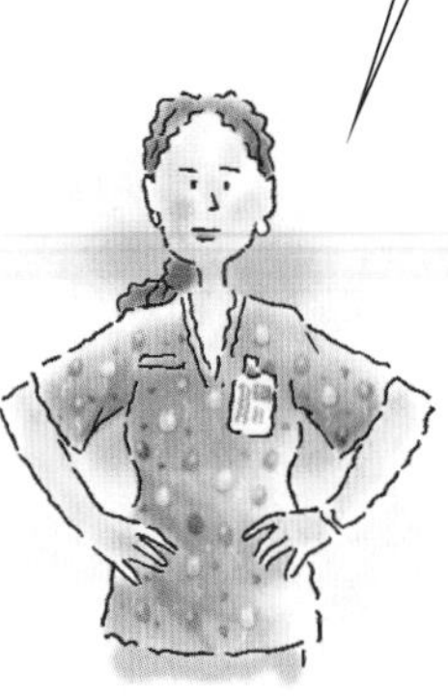

Your role as a preceptor is to help "mold" future nurses.

76. 2. Molding refers to overlapping of the cranial sutures, which causes the neonate's head to appear cone-shaped. Caput succedaneum, cephalohematoma, and hydrocephalus don't result in a cone-shaped head. Caput succedaneum is an area of localized swelling and bruising over a presenting part. Cephalohematoma is a collection of blood between the skull bone and periosteum. Hydrocephalus is an increase in the size of the entire head as a result of increased CSF volume.

CN: Health promotion and maintenance; CNS: None; CL: Analysis

77. A neonate receiving formula feedings is discharged from the neonate nursery. Twenty-four hours later, the mother calls the hospital, stating that the neonate is vomiting most of his feedings. Which statement by the mother indicates that she needs further discharge instructions?

1. "Every time I feed him, he spits up about a teaspoonful of formula onto his bib."
2. "I'm using prepared formula, and he takes ½ oz to 1 oz every 3 to 4 hours."
3. "I feed him every time he cries. Sometimes he eats 4 oz at a time every couple of hours."
4. "I burp him after each ½ oz of formula."

77. 3. Feeding the neonate every time he cries results in overfeeding. A neonate's crying doesn't always signal hunger; sometimes it means his diaper is wet, he needs to suck, or he wants to be held. A neonate who's spitting up should be burped after every ounce of formula or less. For the first few days, the neonate's normal stomach capacity is 15 ml, so he should be fed every 3 to 4 hours. All neonates spit up a small amount because of an immature cardiac sphincter.

CN: Physiological integrity; CNS: Basic care and comfort; CL: Application

78. A healthy term neonate born by cesarean delivery was admitted to the transitional nursery 30 minutes ago and placed under a radiant warmer. The neonate has an axillary temperature of 99.5° F (37.5° C), a respiratory rate of 80 breaths/minute, and a heelstick glucose value of 60 mg/dl. Which action should the nurse take?

1. Wrap the neonate warmly and place him in an open crib.
2. Administer an oral glucose feeding of dextrose 10% in water.
3. Increase the temperature setting on the radiant warmer.
4. Obtain an order for I.V. fluid administration.

78. 4. Assessment findings indicate that the neonate is in respiratory distress—most likely from transient tachypnea, which is common after cesarean delivery. The normal respiratory rate is 30 to 60 breaths/minute; a neonate with a rate of 80 breaths/minute shouldn't be fed but should receive I.V. fluids until the respiratory rate returns to normal. To allow close observation for worsening respiratory distress, the neonate should be kept unclothed in the radiant warmer. Temperature is in the normal range; raising the warmer's temperature setting would cause overheating and worsen the neonate's respiratory distress.

CN: Physiological integrity; CNS: Basic care and comfort; CL: Application

79. A home health nurse assesses a neonate who is 48 hours old and was discharged from the hospital 24 hours ago. Which assessment finding indicates a potential problem?

1. The neonate cries but no tears appear.
2. Small papules appear all over the neonate's skin.
3. The neonate doesn't turn his head in the direction that his cheek is stroked.
4. The neonate produces a greenish brown stool.

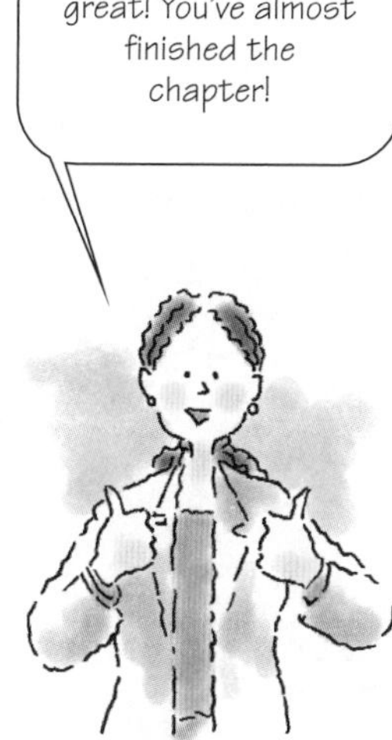

You're doing great! You've almost finished the chapter!

79. 3. A normal, healthy neonate turns in the direction that the cheek is stroked. Failure to do so may indicate a neurologic problem, which the nurse should report to the physician. A neonate's lacrimal glands are immature, resulting in tearless crying for up to 2 months. Erythema toxicum neonatorum causes a transient maculopapular rash—a normal finding in all neonates. Greenish brown stools at 48 hours are normal and indicate that the neonate is eliminating formula or breast milk instead of meconium.

CN: Health promotion and maintenance; CNS: None; CL: Application

80. A nurse is administering vitamin K (AquaMEPHYTON) to a preterm neonate following delivery. The medication comes in a concentration of 2 mg/ml, and the ordered dose is 0.5 mg to be given subcutaneously. How many milliliters should the nurse administer? Record your answer using two decimal points.

_______________ milliliters

81. A nurse is eliciting reflexes in a neonate during a physical examination. Identify the area the nurse would touch to elicit a plantar grasp reflex.

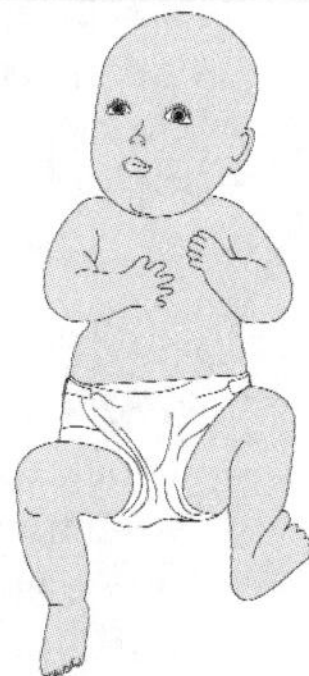

82. What information should a nurse include when teaching postcircumcision care to parents of a neonate prior to discharge from the hospital? Select all that apply:

1. The infant must void before being discharged.
2. Petroleum jelly should be applied to the glans of the penis with each diaper change.
3. The infant can take tub baths while the circumcision heals.
4. Any blood noted on the front of the diaper should be reported.
5. The circumcision will require care for 2 to 4 days after discharge.

80. 0.25. Use the following formula to calculate drug dosages: Dose on hand/Quantity on hand = Dose desired/X. Plug in the values and the equation is as follows: 2 mg/ml = 0.5 mg/X. X = 0.25 ml.

CN: Physiological integrity; CNS: Pharmacological and parenteral therapies; CL: Application

81. To elicit a plantar grasp reflex, the nurse should touch the sole of the foot near the base of the digits, causing flexion or grasping. This reflex disappears around age 9 months.

CN: Health promotion and maintenance; CNS: None; CL: Application

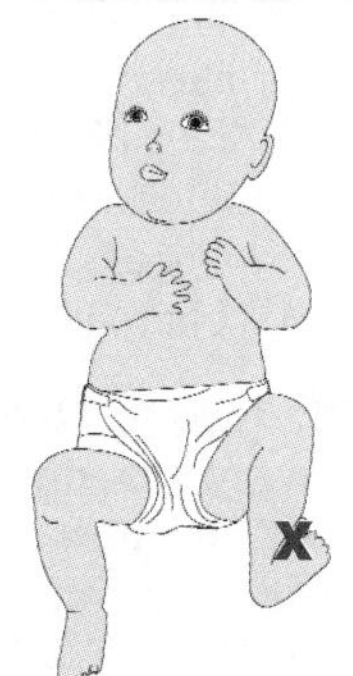

82. 1, 2, 5. It's necessary for the infant to void prior to discharge to ensure that the urethra isn't obstructed. A lubricating ointment is appropriate and is applied with each diaper change. Typically, the penis heals within 2 to 4 days, and circumcision care is required for that period only. To prevent infection, avoid giving the infant tub baths until the circumcision is healed; sponge baths are appropriate. A small amount of bleeding is expected following a circumcision; parents should report only a large amount of bleeding.

CN: Health promotion and maintenance; CNS: None; CL: Application

Part V Care of the child

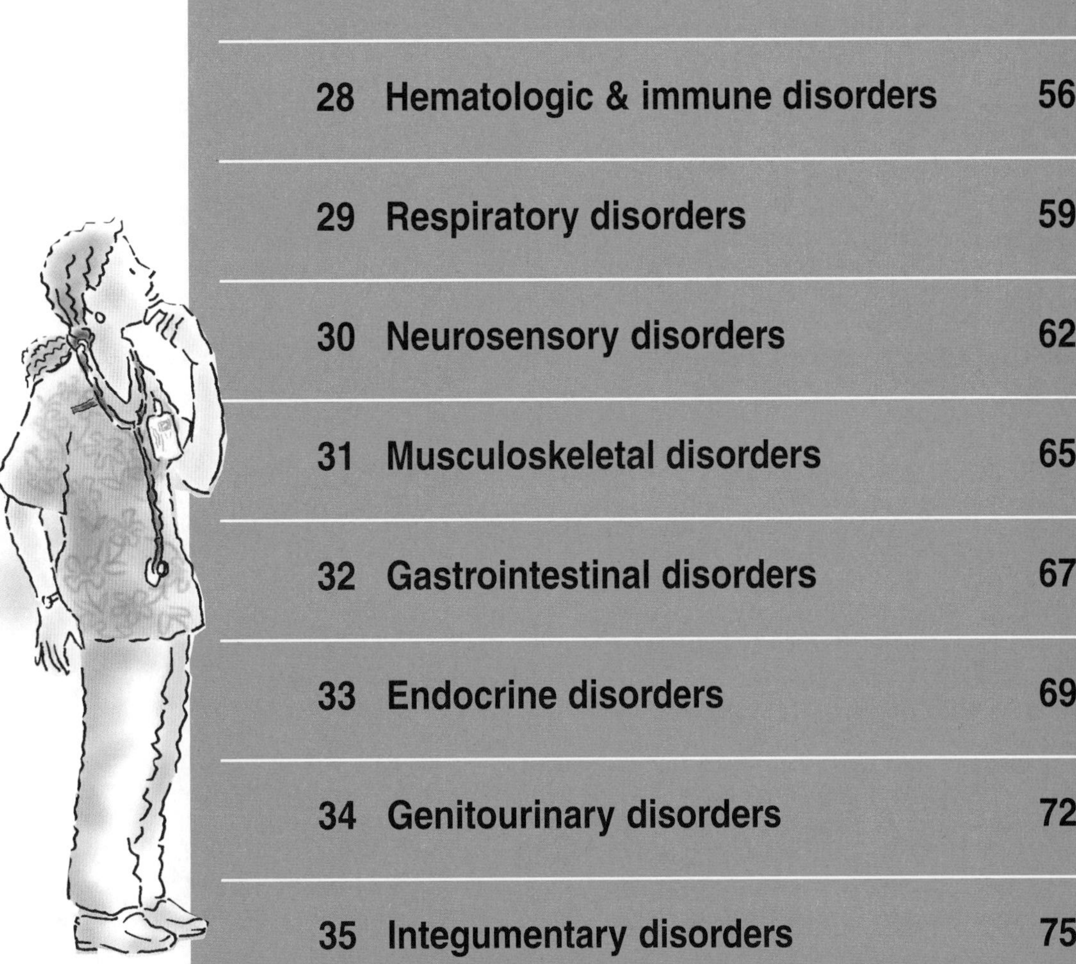

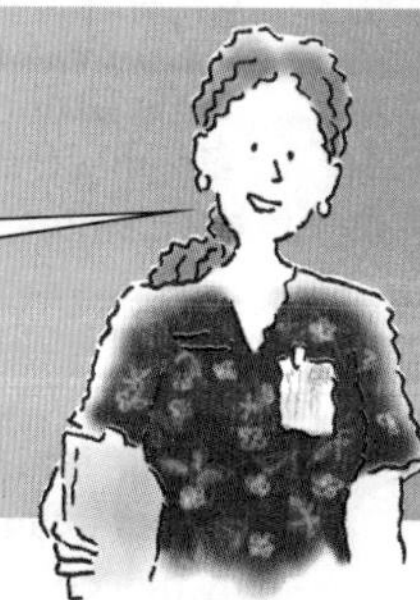

Here's a short but important chapter that covers growth and development of children. Enjoy!

Chapter 26
Growth & development

1. A mother tells a nurse that her 22-month-old child says "no" to everything. When scolded, the toddler becomes angry and starts crying loudly but then immediately wants to be held. What is the best interpretation of this behavior?

1. The toddler isn't effectively coping with the stress.
2. The toddler's need for affection isn't being met.
3. This is normal behavior for a 2-year-old child.
4. This behavior suggests the need for counseling.

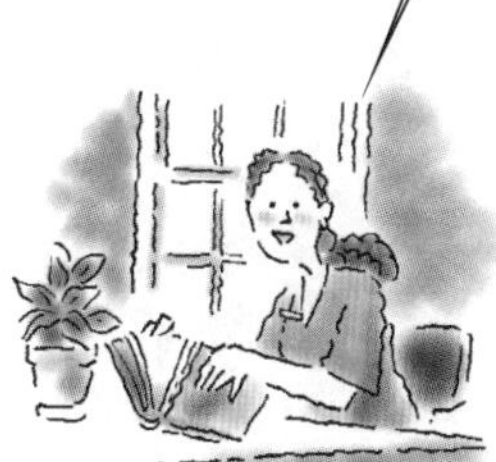

Question 1 wants you to read the rest, but go with the best.

1. 3. Toddlers are confronted with the conflict of achieving autonomy yet relinquishing the much-enjoyed dependence on—and affection of—others. As a result, their negativism is a necessary part of their growth and development. Nothing about this behavior indicates that the child is under stress, isn't receiving sufficient affection, or requires counseling.
CN: Health promotion and maintenance; CNS: None; CL: Analysis

2. The mother of a 12-month-old infant expresses concern about the effect of frequent thumb sucking on her child's teeth. After the nurse teaches her about this matter, which response by the mother indicates that the teaching has been effective?

1. "Thumb sucking should be discouraged at 12 months."
2. "I'll give the baby a pacifier instead."
3. "Sucking is important to the baby."
4. "I'll wrap the thumb in a bandage."

2. 3. Sucking is the infant's chief pleasure. However, thumb sucking can cause malocclusion if it persists after age 4. Many fetuses begin sucking their fingers in utero and, as infants, refuse a pacifier as a substitute. A young child is likely to chew on a bandage, which could lead to airway obstruction.
CN: Health promotion and maintenance; CNS: None; CL: Analysis

3. An adolescent client has just had surgery and has a dressing on the abdomen. Which question should the nurse expect the client to ask initially?

1. "Did the surgery go OK?"
2. "Will I have a large scar?"
3. "What complications can I expect?"
4. "When can I return to school?"

3. 2. Adolescents are deeply concerned about their body image and how they appear to others. An adolescent wouldn't ask how the surgery went or what complications to expect, although an adult probably would. Although an adolescent may be curious as to when he can return to school, it probably wouldn't be his primary concern.
CN: Health promotion and maintenance; CNS: None; CL: Application

CN: Client needs category CNS: Client needs subcategory CL: Cognitive level

4. For an 8-month-old infant, the nurse should plan to provide which toy to promote the child's cognitive development?

1. Blocks to stack
2. Jack-in-the-box
3. Small rubber ball
4. Play gym strung across the crib

4. 2. According to Piaget's theory of cognitive development, an 8-month-old child will look for an object after it disappears from sight to develop the cognitive skill of object permanence. Stacking blocks and small balls are inappropriate because infants frequently put their fingers or objects into their mouth. Anything strung across an infant's crib is a safety hazard, especially to a child who may use it to pull to a standing position.

CN: Health promotion and maintenance; CNS: None; CL: Application

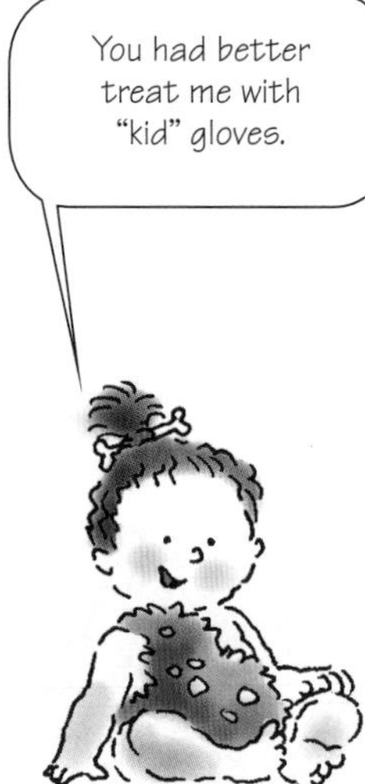
You had better
treat me with
"kid" gloves.

5. A 14-month-old is admitted to the pediatric unit with a diagnosis of croup. Which characteristics would the nurse expect the toddler to demonstrate if he's developing normally? Select all that apply:

1. Strong hand grasp
2. Tendency to hold one object while looking for another
3. Recognition of familiar voices (smiles in recognition)
4. Presence of Moro reflex
5. Weight that's triple his birth weight
6. Closed anterior fontanel

5. 1, 2, 3, 5. A strong hand grasp is demonstrated within the first month of life. Holding one object while looking for another is accomplished by the 20th week. Within the first year of life, the toddler masters smiling at familiar faces and voices, the toddler's birth weight triples, and the Moro reflex disappears. The anterior fontanel closes at approximately age 18 months.

CN: Health promotion and maintenance; CNS: None; CL: Application

6. Which comment by a 7-year-old boy to his friend best typifies his developmental stage?

1. "Girls are so yucky."
2. "My mommy and I are always together."
3. "I can't decide if I like Amy or Heather better."
4. "I can turn into Batman when I come out of my closet."

6. 1. During the school-age years, the most important social interactions typically are those with peers. Peer-to-peer interactions lead to the formation of intimate friendships between same-sex children. Friendships with opposite-sex children are uncommon. At this age, children socialize more frequently with friends than with parents. Interest in peers of the opposite sex generally doesn't begin until ages 10 to 12. Magical thinking and fantasy play are more characteristic during the preschool years.

CN: Health promotion and maintenance; CNS: None; CL: Application

7. A nurse should expect a 3-year-old child to be able to perform which action?

1. Ride a tricycle
2. Tie shoelaces
3. Roller skate
4. Jump rope

7. 1. At age 3, gross motor development and refinement in hand-eye coordination enable a child to ride a tricycle. The fine motor skills required to tie shoelaces and the gross motor skills required for roller-skating and jumping rope develop around age 5.

CN: Health promotion and maintenance; CNS: None; CL: Application

8. A 6-month-old infant is admitted to the pediatric unit for a 2-week course of antibiotics. His parents can visit only on weekends. Which action indicates that the nurse understands the infant's emotional needs?

1. The nurse places the infant in a four-bed unit.
2. The nurse places the infant in a room away from other children.
3. The nurse assigns the infant to a different nurse each day.
4. The nurse assigns the infant to the same nurse as often as possible.

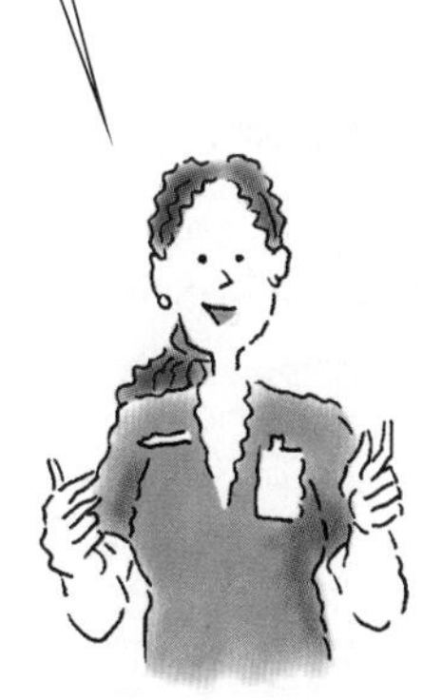
Which action indicates that the nurse understands?

8. 4. Building a sense of trust is crucial with an infant at this stage of growth and development. Consistent caregivers will promote a sense of trust. Placing him in a four-bed unit isn't the best choice because a 6-month-old child doesn't play with other children. Placing him in a room away from other children would isolate him from others, which is neither necessary nor helpful.

CN: Health promotion and maintenance; CNS: None; CL: Application

9. A term neonate weighs 7½ lb (3 kg) at birth. When he's 1 year old, approximately how much should he weigh?

1. 16 lb (7.3 kg)
2. 22 lb (10 kg)
3. 28 lb (12.7 kg)
4. 32 lb (14.5 kg)

9. 2. A term neonate who weighs 7½ lb at birth should triple his birth weight by age 1 year; therefore, he should weigh approximately 22 to 23 pounds. A weight of 16 pounds is roughly a doubling of birth weight, which should occur by 6 months. A weight of 28 or 32 pounds indicates a gain that exceeds three times the birth weight.

CN: Health promotion and maintenance; CNS: None; CL: Analysis

10. Which behavior by a preschool child indicates that the child is in the appropriate stage of growth and development?

1. He cries in protest when his mother leaves.
2. He asks for a bandage after having blood drawn.
3. He's upset about having a scar after surgery.
4. He wants to know why his friends don't visit.

10. 2. A preschooler typically asks for a bandage after having blood drawn because he has poorly defined body boundaries and believes he will lose all of his blood from the hole the needle has made. A toddler cries in protest when the parent leaves. An adolescent might be upset about a surgical scar because he's concerned about body image. A school-age child might ask why his friends don't visit because peers become important by that age.

CN: Heath promotion and maintenance; CNS: None; CL: Analysis

11. A nurse observes parents playing with their 10-month-old daughter. Which behavior indicates that the infant is developing object permanence?

1. She looks for the toy that her parents hid under the blanket.
2. She returns the play blocks to the same spot on the table.
3. She recognizes that a ball of clay is the same object even when it's flattened out.
4. She bangs two cubes in her hands and throws them to the floor.

11. 1. Object permanence is exhibited by the infant looking for objects that have been hidden from sight. Returning the blocks to the same spot on the table is imitative behavior. Recognizing that a ball of clay is the same object even when flattened out is an example of the theory of conservation, which occurs in early-school-age children. Banging two cubes in her hands and throwing them to the floor is normal behavior for a 10-month old but doesn't indicate object permanence.

CN: Health promotion and maintenance; CNS: None; CL: Application

12. A nurse is teaching the parents of a 6-month-old infant about age-specific growth and development. Which statement is true regarding infant development? Select all that apply:

1. A 6-month-old infant has trouble holding objects.
2. A 6-month-old infant can usually roll from prone to supine and supine to prone positions.
3. A teething ring is appropriate for a 6-month-old infant.
4. Head lag is commonly noted in infants at age 6 months.
5. Lack of visual coordination usually resolves by age 6 months.

13. A nurse is conducting a physical examination on an infant. Identify the anatomical landmark she should use to measure chest circumference.

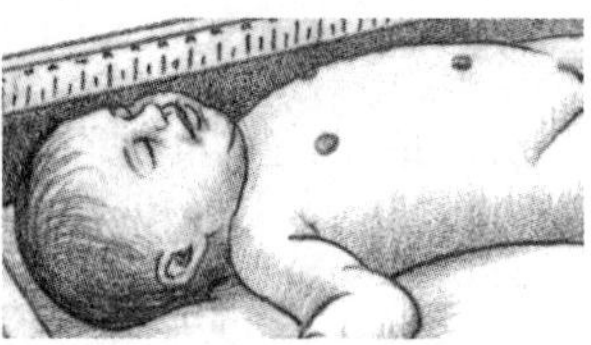

14. The nurse is examining the breasts of an adolescent girl. She classifies her sexual maturity as Tanner stage 3. Which graphic depicts this stage?

1. 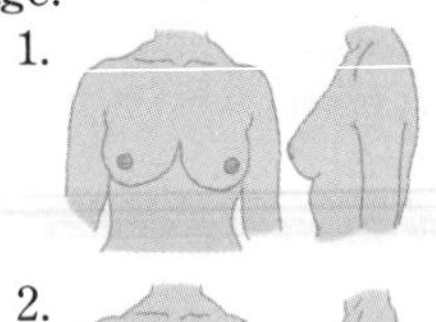
2. 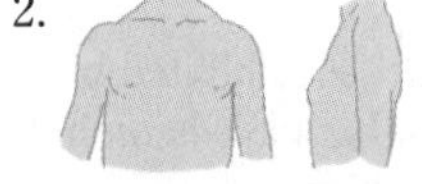
3. 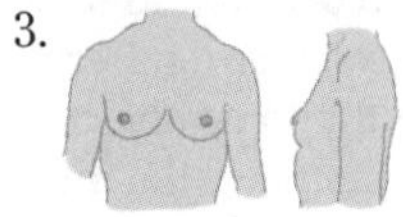
4. 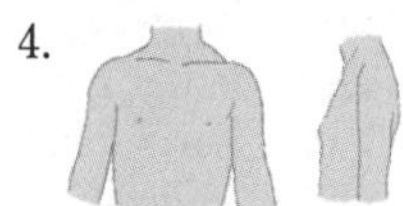

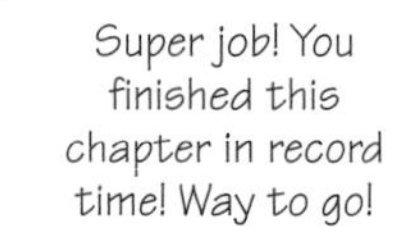

Super job! You finished this chapter in record time! Way to go!

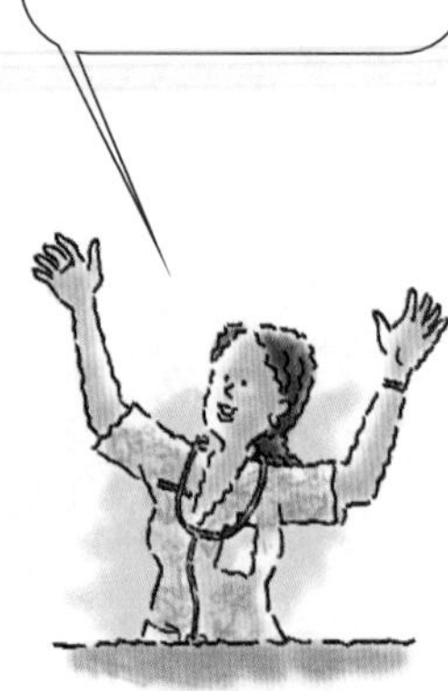

12. 2, 3, 5. Gross motor skills of the 6-month-old infant include rolling from front to back and back to front. Teething usually begins around age 6 months and, therefore, a teething ring is appropriate. Visual coordination is usually resolved by age 6 months. At age 6 months, fine motor skills include purposeful grasps. The 6-month-old infant should have good head control and should no longer display head lag when pulled up to a sitting position.

CN: Health promotion and maintenance; CNS: None; CL: Application

13. Chest circumference is most accurately measured by placing the measuring tape around the infant's chest with the tape covering the nipples. If measured above or below the nipples, a false measurement is obtained.

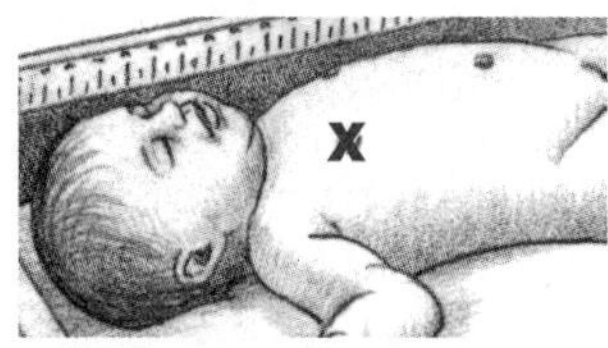

CN: Health promotion and maintenance; CNS: None; CL: Application

14. 2. In Tanner stage 3, the entire breast enlarges and the nipple doesn't protrude. Option 1 shows Tanner stage 5: an adult breast has developed, the nipple protrudes, and the areola no longer appears separate from the breast. Option 3 shows Tanner stage 4: the breast enlarges and the nipple and papilla protrude and appear as a secondary mound. Option 4 shows Tanner stage 2: breast buds appear and the areola is slightly widened and appears as a small mound.

CN: Physiological integrity; CNS: Reduction of risk potential; CL: Application

CN: Client needs category CNS: Client needs subcategory CL: Cognitive level

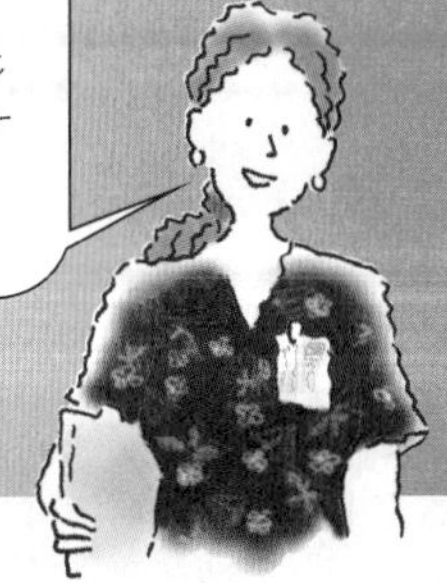

You've reached our test on cardiovascular disorders in children. Before taking this comprehensive test, why not bolster yourself with a heart-healthy snack of celery and low-fat cream cheese? Yum!

Chapter 27 Cardiovascular disorders

1. A nurse is performing a cardiac assessment on a 2-year-old. The first heart sound (S_1) can best be heard at which location?

1. Third or fourth intercostal space
2. The apex with the stethoscope bell
3. Second intercostal space, midclavicular line
4. Fifth intercostal space, left midclavicular line

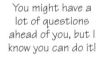

1. 4. The S_1 can best be heard at the fifth intercostal space, left midclavicular line. The fourth heart sound can be heard at the third or fourth intercostal space. The third heart sound is heard with the stethoscope bell at the apex of the heart. The second heart sound is heard at the second intercostal space.

CN: Health promotion and maintenance; CNS: None; CL: Application

2. The nurse auscultates the first heart sound, interpreting this sound as occurring:

1. late in diastole.
2. early in diastole.
3. with closure of the mitral and tricuspid valves.
4. with closure of the aortic and pulmonic valves.

2. 3. The S_1 occurs during systole with closure of the mitral and tricuspid valves. The fourth heart sound is heard late in diastole and may be a normal finding in children. The third heart sound is heard early in diastole. The second heart sound occurs during diastole with closure of the aortic and pulmonic valves.

CN: Health promotion and maintenance; CNS: None; CL: Analysis

3. A nurse is performing a cardiac assessment on a child. Which characteristic would indicate a diagnosis of a grade 1 heart murmur?

1. The murmur is equal to the heart sounds.
2. The murmur is softer than the heart sounds.
3. The murmur can be heard with the naked ear.
4. The murmur is associated with a precordial thrill.

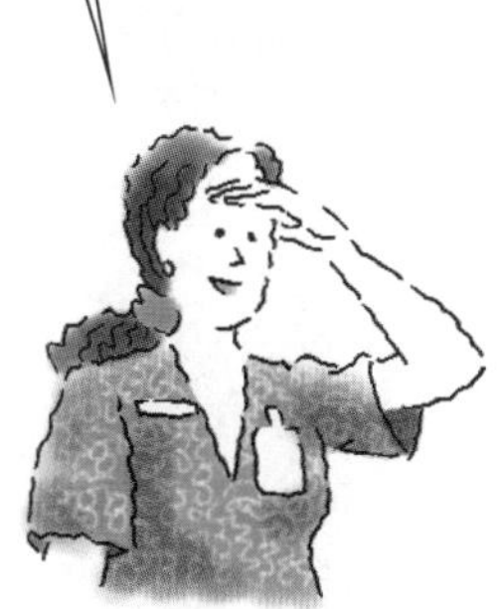

You might have a lot of questions ahead of you, but I know you can do it!

3. 2. A grade 1 heart murmur is commonly difficult to hear and softer than the heart sounds. A grade 2 murmur is usually equal to the heart sounds. A grade 6 murmur can be heard with the naked ear or with the stethoscope off the chest. A grade 4 murmur is associated with a precordial thrill. A thrill is a palpable manifestation associated with a loud murmur.

CN: Health promotion and maintenance; CNS: None; CL: Analysis

CN: Client needs category CNS: Client needs subcategory CL: Cognitive level

4. A graduate nurse has started working in a pediatric intensive care unit. She's measuring the client's cardiac output. To understand cardiac output, the nurse must know that stroke volume is the:

1. volume of blood returning to the heart.
2. ability of the cardiac muscle to act as an efficient pump.
3. resistance the ventricles pump against when ejecting blood.
4. amount of blood ejected by the heart in any one contraction.

4. 4. Stroke volume is the amount of blood ejected by the heart in any one contraction. It's influenced by preload, afterload, and contractility. Preload is the amount of blood returning to the heart. Contractility is the ability of the cardiac muscle to act as an efficient pump. Afterload is the resistance the ventricles pump against when ejecting blood.

CN: Physiological integrity; CNS: Physiological adaptation; CL: Application

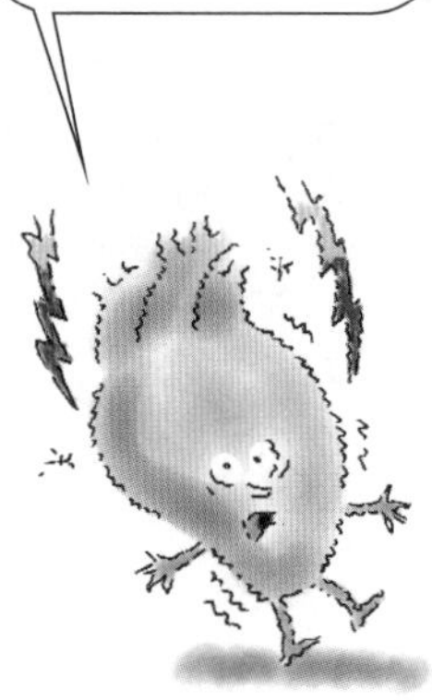

Yikes! Is this what they mean by cardiogenic shock?

5. A child is diagnosed with cardiogenic shock. Which condition would the nurse expect to occur with this child?

1. Decreased cardiac output
2. A reduction in circulating blood volume
3. Overwhelming sepsis and circulating bacterial toxins
4. Inflow or outflow obstruction of the main bloodstream

5. 1. *Cardiogenic shock* occurs when cardiac output is decreased and tissue oxygen needs aren't adequately met. *Hypovolemic shock* is a reduction in circulating blood volume. *Septic shock* is overwhelming sepsis and circulating bacterial toxins. *Obstructive shock* is an inflow or outflow obstruction of the main bloodstream.

CN: Physiological integrity; CNS: Physiological adaptation; CL: Application

6. Which sign is considered a late sign of shock in children?

1. Tachycardia
2. Hypotension
3. Delayed capillary refill
4. Pale, cool, mottled skin

6. 2. Hypotension is considered a late sign of shock in children. This represents a decompensated state and impending cardiopulmonary arrest. Tachycardia; delayed capillary refill; and pale, cool, mottled skin are earlier indicators of shock that may show compensation.

CN: Physiological integrity; CNS: Physiological adaptation; CL: Analysis

7. Which factor indicating a cardiac defect might be found when assessing a 1-month-old?

1. Weight gain
2. Hyperactivity
3. Poor nutritional intake
4. Pink mucous membranes

7. 3. Infants and children with heart defects tend to have poor nutritional intake and weight loss, indicating poor cardiac output, heart failure, or hypoxemia. The child appears lethargic or tired because of the heart failure or hypoxia. Pink, moist mucous membranes are normal.

CN: Health promotion and maintenance; CNS: None; CL: Analysis

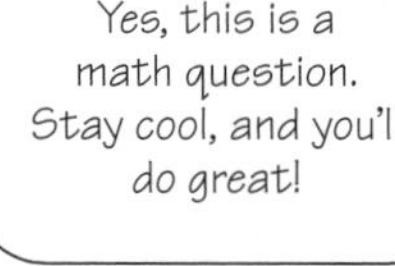

Yes, this is a math question. Stay cool, and you'll do great!

8. A 2-year-old child is showing signs of shock. A 10-ml/kg bolus of normal saline solution is ordered. The child weighs 20 kg. How many milliliters should be administered?

1. 20 ml
2. 100 ml
3. 200 ml
4. 2,000 ml

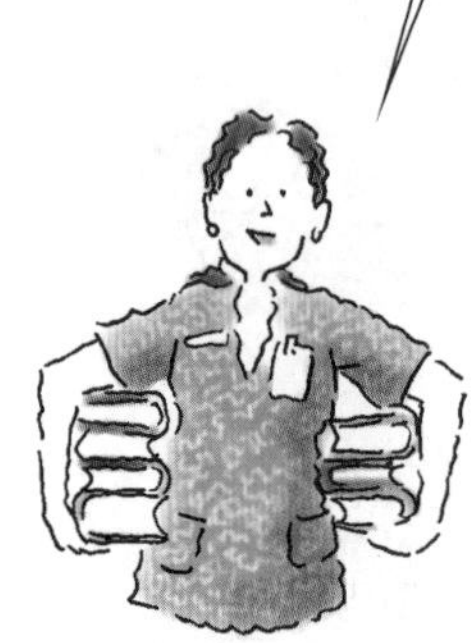

8. 3. The correct formula for this calculation is 10 ml/kg × 20 kg. The correct answer is 200 ml. The other options are incorrect.

CN: Physiological integrity; CNS: Pharmacological and parenteral therapies; CL: Analysis

9. Which of the following arrhythmias is commonly found in neonates and infants?
1. Atrial fibrillation
2. Bradyarrhythmias
3. Premature atrial contractions
4. Premature ventricular contractions

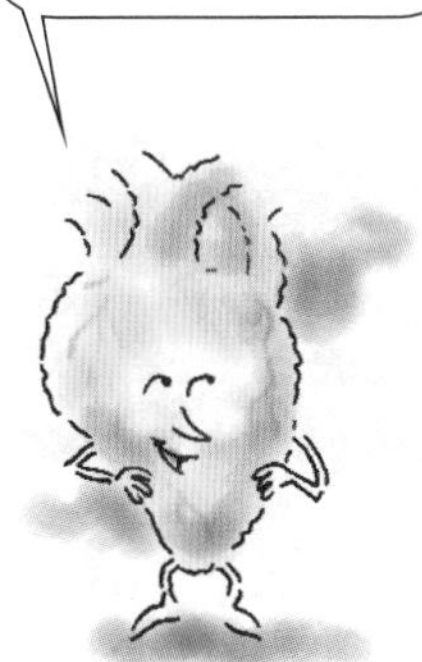
Pick an arrhythmia, any correct arrhythmia.

9. 3. Premature atrial contractions are common in fetuses, neonates, and children. They occur from increased automaticity of an atrial cell anywhere except the sinoatrial node. Atrial fibrillation is an uncommon arrhythmia in children occurring from a disorganized state of electrical activity in the atria. Bradyarrhythmias are usually congenital, surgically acquired, or caused by infection. Premature ventricular contractions are more common in adolescents.

CN: Physiological integrity; CNS: Physiological adaptation; CL: Analysis

10. A nurse is reviewing the waveforms of an electrocardiogram of an infant with a nursing student. The nurse will tell the student that which waveform indicates ventricular depolarization and contraction?
1. P wave
2. PR interval
3. QRS complex
4. T wave

10. 3. The QRS complex reflects ventricular depolarization and contraction. The P wave represents atrial depolarization and contraction. The PR interval represents the time it takes an impulse to trace from the atrioventricular node to the bundle of His. The T wave represents repolarization of the ventricles.

CN: Physiological integrity; CNS: Reduction of risk potential; CL: Application

11. Which evaluation of cardiovascular status is noninvasive?
1. Transthoracic echocardiogram
2. Cardiac enzyme levels
3. Cardiac catheterization
4. Transesophageal pacing

11. 1. A transthoracic echocardiogram is a noninvasive procedure to visualize the anatomy of the heart. Blood testing determines cardiac enzyme levels. Cardiac catheterization involves passing a catheter into the chambers of the heart for direct visualization of the heart and great vessels. Transesophageal pacing requires a probe to be placed in the esophagus for high-frequency ultrasound.

CN: Physiological integrity; CNS: Reduction of risk potential; CL: Analysis

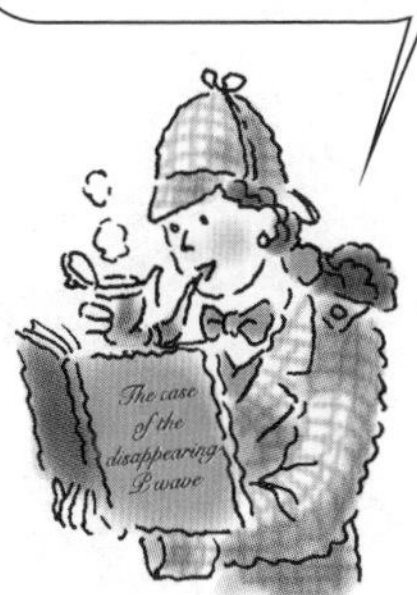
I think I detect the correct statement.
The case of the disappearing P wave

12. Which statement about using an echocardiogram to evaluate cardiac function in a child is the most correct?
1. The child must be sedated in order to get an accurate result.
2. It uses sound waves to measure and evaluate cardiac structures and function.
3. The transthoracic method of echocardiogram is an invasive procedure.
4. It is the most definitive method of evaluating cardiac function.

12. 2. Echocardiograms use sound waves to measure and evaluate cardiac structures and function. The transthoracic method is not an invasive procedure; however, the transesophageal method is considered invasive. The child does not have to be sedated, but lying quietly is preferred. While an echocardiogram gives the physician a good idea of cardiac function, a cardiac catheterization is the definitive method for a complete and accurate picture.

CN: Physiological integrity; CNS: Reduction of risk potential; CL: Application

13. Before a cardiac catheterization, which intervention is most appropriate for a child and his parents?

1. Supplying a map of the hospital
2. Limiting visitors to parents only
3. Offering a guided tour of the hospital and catheterization laboratory
4. Explaining that the child can't eat or drink for 1 to 2 days postoperatively

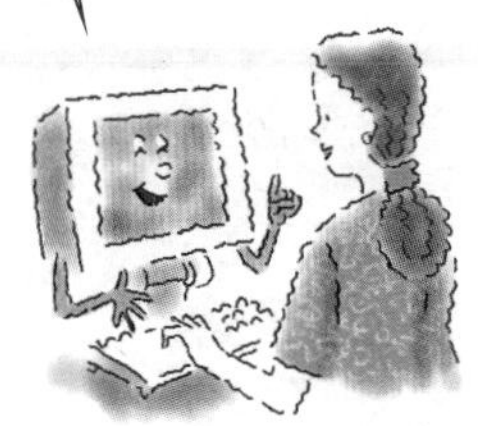

What can you do to ease the family's fears?

13. 3. A guided tour will help minimize fears and allay anxieties for the child and parents. It gives the opportunity for questions and teaching. A map of the hospital is helpful, but a tour provides the family with more information. Visitors should include all significant others and siblings as part of the preoperative teaching. The child will be able to start clear liquids and advance as tolerated after the procedure is completed and the child is fully awake.

CN: Physiological integrity; CNS: Physiological adaptation; CL: Analysis

14. The nurse is teaching the parents of a child who is scheduled for a cardiac catheterization. Which statement by the nurse is the most accurate regarding cardiac catheterization?

1. It's a noninvasive procedure.
2. General anesthesia is required.
3. It uses high-frequency sound waves to produce an image of the heart in motion.
4. It provides visualization of the heart and great vessels with radiopaque dye.

14. 4. Cardiac catheterization provides visualization of the heart and great vessels. It's an invasive procedure in which a thin catheter is passed into the chambers of the heart through a peripheral vein or artery. General anesthesia may be used for more complex catheterizations or procedures that place the child at greater risk. High-frequency sound waves describe ultrasound and echocardiography. Conscious sedation is usually given before cardiac catheterization.

CN: Physiological integrity; CNS: Reduction of risk potential; CL: Application

15. Which nursing intervention is most appropriate when caring for a child in the immediate postcatheterization phase?

1. Elevate the head of the bed 45 degrees.
2. Encourage the child to remain flat.
3. Assess vital signs every 2 to 4 hours.
4. Replace a bloody groin dressing with a new dressing.

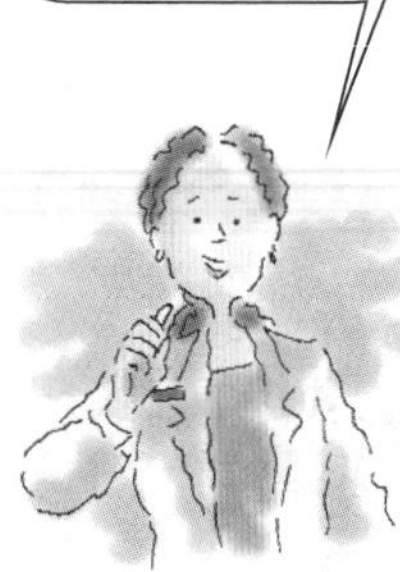

You've already answered 15 questions! See how time flies when you're taking a test?

15. 2. During recovery, the child should remain flat in bed, keeping the punctured leg straight for the prescribed time. The child should avoid raising the head, sitting, straining the abdomen, or coughing. Vital signs are taken every 15 minutes until the child is awake and stable, then every half hour, then hourly as ordered. If bleeding occurs at the insertion site, the nurse should mark the margins with a pen and monitor for changes.

CN: Physiological integrity; CNS: Physiological adaptation; CL: Analysis

16. Which home care instruction is included for a child postcatheterization?

1. The child should drink fluids and eat a regular diet.
2. The child may participate in sports once home.
3. The child can routinely bathe after returning home.
4. The child may return to school the next day.

16. 1. A regular diet and increased fluids are encouraged postcatheterization. Increased fluids may flush the injected dyes out of the system. Normal activities may be resumed, but strenuous physical activities or sports should be avoided for about 3 days. Prolonged bathing can be resumed in 3 days. A sponge bath is encouraged until then. The child may return to school 3 days after discharge.

CN: Physiological integrity; CNS: Physiological adaptation; CL: Analysis

17. A 2-year-old child is being monitored after cardiac surgery. Which sign represents a decrease in cardiac output?
1. Hypertension
2. Increased urine output
3. Weak peripheral pulses
4. Capillary refill less than 2 seconds

18. A 3-year-old child is experiencing distress after having cardiac surgery. Which sign indicates cardiac tamponade?
1. Hypertension
2. Muffled heart sounds
3. Widened pulse pressures
4. Increased chest tube drainage

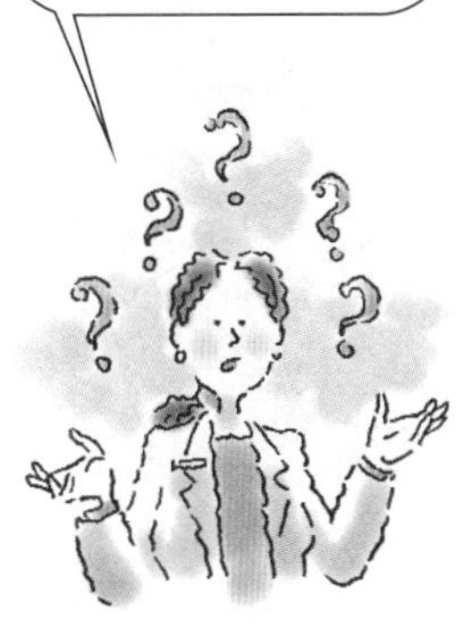

All of these signs may appear, but only one indicates cardiac tamponade. Which one?

19. A nurse is monitoring fluid and electrolyte balance in a child after cardiac surgery requiring cardiopulmonary bypass. Which finding is expected?
1. Increased urine output
2. Increased sodium level
3. Decreased sodium level
4. Increased potassium level

20. A nurse is teaching wound care to parents after cardiac surgery. Which statement is <u>most appropriate</u>?
1. Lotions and powders are acceptable.
2. Your child can take a complete bath tomorrow.
3. Tingling, itching, and numbness are normal sensations at the wound site.
4. If the sterile adhesive strips over the incision fall off, call the physician.

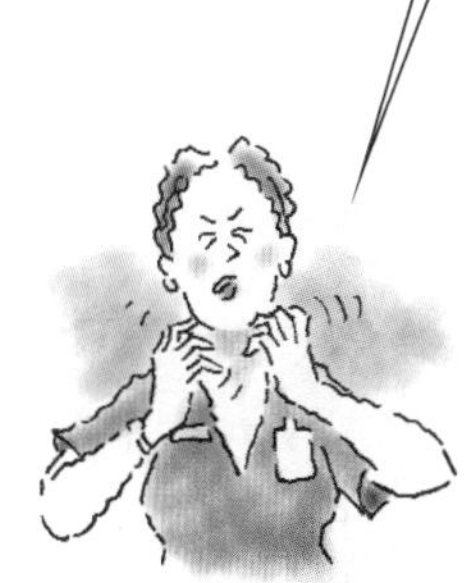

I'm itching to get question 20 correct.

21. Parents ask a nurse about their 8-year-old son's activity level after cardiac surgery. Which response would be best?
1. There are no exercise limitations.
2. The child may resume school in 3 days.
3. Encourage a balance of rest and exercise.
4. Climbing and contact sports are restricted for 1 week.

17. 3. Signs of decreased cardiac output include weak peripheral pulses, hypotension, low urine output, delayed capillary refill, and cool extremities.

CN: Physiological integrity; CNS: Physiological adaptation; CL: Analysis

18. 2. Symptoms of cardiac tamponade include muffled heart sounds, hypotension, a narrowing pulse pressure, and sudden cessation of chest tube drainage. Cardiac tamponade occurs when a large volume of fluid interferes with ventricular filling and pumping and collects in the pericardial sac, decreasing cardiac output.

CN: Physiological integrity; CNS: Physiological adaptation; CL: Analysis

19. 2. In response to surgery and cardiopulmonary bypass, the body secretes aldosterone and antidiuretic hormone. This in turn increases sodium levels, decreases potassium levels, increases water retention, and decreases urine output.

CN: Physiological integrity; CNS: Physiological adaptation; CL: Analysis

20. 3. As the area heals, tingling, itching, and numbness are normal sensations and will eventually go away. Lotions and powders should be avoided during the first 2 weeks after surgery. A complete bath should be delayed for the first week, although sponge baths are allowed. Adhesive strips may loosen or fall off on their own. This is a common and normal occurrence.

CN: Physiological integrity; CNS: Physiological adaptation; CL: Analysis

21. 3. Activity should be increased gradually each day, allowing for a sensible balance of rest and exercise. School and large crowds should be avoided for at least 2 weeks to prevent exposure to people with active infections. Sports and contact activities should be restricted for about 6 weeks, giving the sternum enough time to heal.

CN: Physiological integrity; CNS: Physiological adaptation; CL: Analysis

22. Which home care instruction is most appropriate for a child after cardiac surgery?
1. Don't stop giving the child the prescribed drugs until the physician says so.
2. Maintain a sodium-restricted diet.
3. Routine dental care can be resumed.
4. Immunizations are delayed indefinitely.

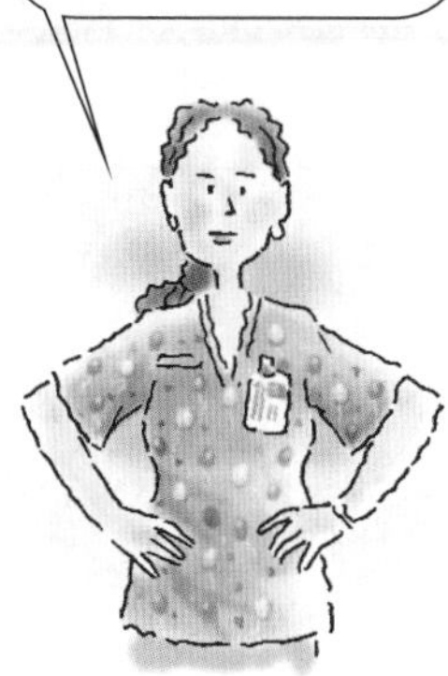

It's important that a child's family understands all home care instructions.

22. 1. Drugs, such as digoxin and furosemide, shouldn't be stopped abruptly. There are no diet restrictions, and the child may resume his regular diet. Routine dental care is usually delayed 6 months after surgery. Immunizations are delayed at least 6 weeks after surgery.

CN: Physiological integrity; CNS: Reduction of risk potential; CL: Analysis

23. A 4-year-old client with a chest tube is placed on water seal. Which statement is correct?
1. The water level rises with inhalation.
2. Bubbling is seen in the suction chamber.
3. Bubbling is seen in the water seal chamber.
4. Water seal is obtained by clamping the tube.

23. 1. The water seal chamber is functioning appropriately when the water level rises in the chamber with inhalation and falls with expiration. This shows that negative pressure required in the lung is being maintained. Bubbling in the suction chamber should be seen only when suction is being used. Bubbling in the water seal chamber generally indicates the presence of an air leak. The chest tube should never be clamped; a tension pneumothorax may occur. Water seal is activated when the suction is disconnected.

CN: Physiological integrity; CNS: Reduction of risk potential; CL: Application

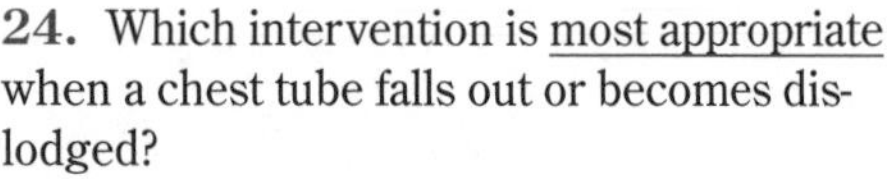

24. Which intervention is most appropriate when a chest tube falls out or becomes dislodged?
1. Place a dry gauze dressing over the insertion site.
2. Place a petroleum gauze dressing over the insertion site.
3. Wipe the tube with alcohol and reinsert it.
4. Call the physician immediately.

24. 2. Petroleum gauze should be placed over the site immediately to prevent a pneumothorax. The physician should be notified after this step. A dry gauze dressing will allow air to enter pleural space, leading to a pneumothorax. The tube is reinserted only by a physician using a sterile thoracotomy tray.

CN: Physiological integrity; CNS: Reduction of risk potential; CL: Application

25. When assessing a child with heart failure, which findings should the nurse expect to find?
1. Bradycardia
2. Decreased respiratory rate
3. Gallop murmur
4. Strong, bounding pulses

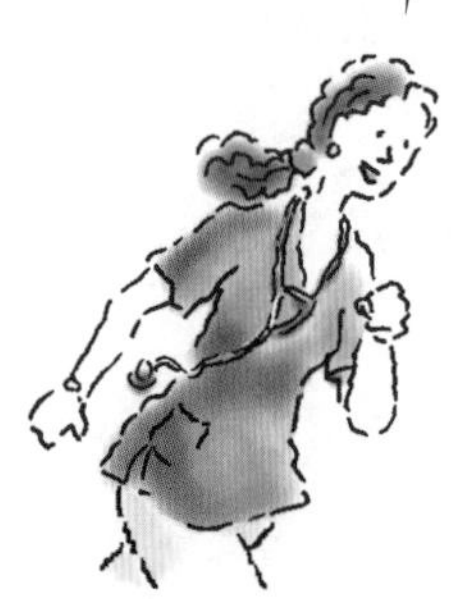

Question 25 is a milestone. Way to go!

25. 3. When the heart stretches beyond efficiency, an extra heart sound or S_3 gallop murmur may be audible. This is related to excessive preload and ventricular dilation. Tachycardia occurs as a compensatory mechanism to the decrease in cardiac output. It also attempts to increase the force and rate of myocardial contraction and increase oxygen consumption of the heart. The respiratory rate increases, not decreases, in an attempt to increase oxygenation. Pulses are usually weak and thready.

CN: Physiological integrity; CNS: Physiological adaptation; CL: Analysis

26. An emergency room nurse is caring for a pediatric client in heart failure. Which symptom is consistent with a diagnosis of left-sided heart failure?

1. Weight gain
2. Peripheral edema
3. Neck vein distention
4. Tachypnea and dyspnea

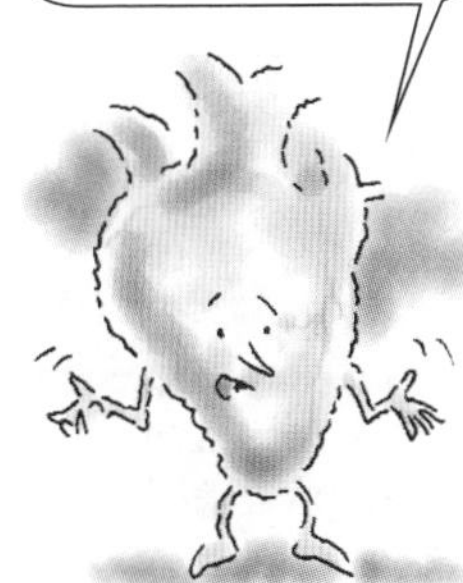

Do you know what happens when my left side isn't working properly?

26. 4. Respiratory symptoms, such as tachypnea and dyspnea, are seen as a result of pulmonary congestion. Peripheral edema, jugular vein distention, and weight gain are seen with systemic venous congestion or right-sided heart failure. Fluid accumulates in the interstitial spaces because of blood pooling in the venous circulation.

CN: Physiological integrity; CNS: Physiological adaptation; CL: Application

27. Which intervention is <u>most appropriate</u> when caring for an infant with heart failure?

1. Limit fluid intake.
2. Avoid using infant seats.
3. Cluster nursing activities.
4. Place the infant prone or supine.

27. 3. Energy expenditures need to be limited to reduce metabolic and oxygen needs. Nursing care should be clustered, followed by long periods of undisturbed rest. Fluid may be restricted in older children, but infants' nutritional requirements depend on fluid needs. Infants should be placed in the semi-Fowler or upright position. Infant seats help maintain an upright position. This facilitates lung expansion, provides less restrictive movement of the diaphragm, relieves pressure from abdominal organs, and decreases pulmonary congestion.

CN: Physiological integrity; CNS: Physiological adaptation; CL: Analysis

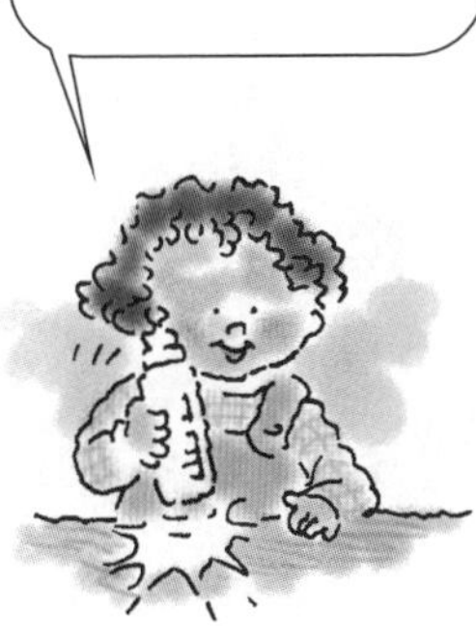

What's the diet plan?

28. Which diet plan is recommended for an infant with heart failure?

1. Restrict fluids.
2. Weigh once a week.
3. Use low-sodium formula.
4. Increase caloric content per ounce.

28. 4. Formulas with increased caloric content are given to meet the greater caloric requirements from the overworked heart and labored breathing. Fluid restriction and low-sodium formulas aren't recommended. An infant's nutritional needs depend on fluid. Daily weights at the same time of the day on the same scale before feedings are recommended to follow trends in nutritional stability and diuresis. Low-sodium formulas may cause hyponatremia.

CN: Physiological integrity; CNS: Basic care and comfort; CL: Application

29. A boy with patent ductus arteriosus was delivered 6 hours earlier and is being held by his mother. As the nurse enters the room to assess the neonate's vital signs, the mother says, "The physician says that my baby has a heart murmur. Does that mean he has a bad heart?" Which response by the nurse would be the most appropriate?

1. "He'll need more tests to determine his heart condition."
2. "He'll require oxygen therapy at home for a while."
3. "He'll be fine. Don't worry about him."
4. "The murmur is caused by the natural opening, which can take a day or two to close. It's a normal part of your baby's transition."

29. 4. Although the nurse may want to tell the client not to worry, the most appropriate response would be to explain the neonate's present condition, to relieve the mother and to acknowledge an awareness of the condition. A neonate's vascular system changes with birth; certain factors help to reverse the flow of blood through the ductus and ultimately favor its closure. This closure typically begins within the first 24 hours after birth and ends within a few days after birth. The other responses don't adequately address the mother's question.

CN: Health promotion and maintenance; CNS: None; CL: Analysis

30. A teenage client with heart failure is prescribed digoxin (Lanoxin) and asks the nurse, "What's the drug supposed to do?" The nurse teaches the teenager based on the understanding that this drug belongs to which classification?

1. Angiotensin-converting enzyme (ACE) inhibitor
2. Cardiac glycoside
3. Diuretic
4. Vasodilator

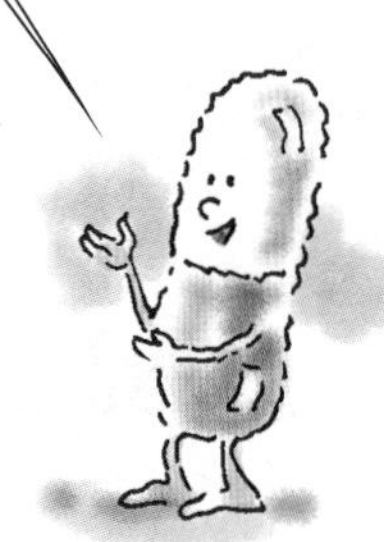

Knowing the classification of a drug can help you remember its actions.

30. 2. Digoxin is a cardiac glycoside. It decreases the workload of the heart and improves myocardial function. ACE inhibitors cause vasodilation and increase sodium excretion. Diuretics help remove excess fluid. Vasodilators enhance cardiac output by decreasing afterload.

CN: Physiological integrity; CNS: Pharmacological and parenteral therapies; CL: Application

31. Which assessment finding would lead the nurse to suspect a child has a digoxin level greater than 2 ng/ml?

1. Weight gain
2. Tachycardia
3. Nausea and vomiting
4. Seizures

31. 3. Digoxin toxicity in infants and children may present with nausea, vomiting, anorexia, or a slow, irregular apical heart rate. Weight gain, tachycardia, or seizures wouldn't be seen in digoxin toxicity.

CN: Physiological integrity; CNS: Pharmacological and parenteral therapies; CL: Analysis

32. An 11-month-old infant with heart failure weighs 10 kg. Digoxin is prescribed as 10 mcg/kg/day in divided doses every 12 hours. How much is given per dose?

1. 10 mcg
2. 50 mcg
3. 100 mcg
4. 500 mcg

32. 2. 10 kg × 10 mcg/kg/day = 100 mcg/day divided by 2 doses = 50 mcg/dose.

CN: Physiological integrity; CNS: Pharmacological and parenteral therapies; CL: Analysis

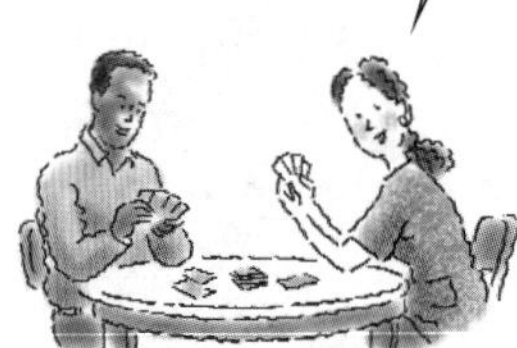

I don't think this ace will inhibit me.

33. A client with heart failure is given captopril (Capoten), an angiotensin-converting enzyme (ACE) inhibitor. Which action occurs with this type of drug?

1. Vasoconstriction
2. Increased sodium excretion
3. Decreased sodium excretion
4. Increased vascular resistance

33. 2. ACE inhibitors block the conversion of angiotensin I to angiotensin II in the kidney. This causes decreased aldosterone, vasodilation, and increased sodium excretion. As a vasodilator, it also acts to reduce vascular resistance by the manipulation of afterload.

CN: Physiological integrity; CNS: Pharmacological and parenteral therapies; CL: Application

34. The parents of a newborn child have just been told that he has a heart defect known as *patent ductus arteriosus.* Which statement made by the parents indicates that teaching has been effective?

1. "Heart failure is uncommon in this defect."
2. "The ductus normally closes completely by age 6 weeks."
3. "An open ductus arteriosus causes decreased blood flow to the lungs."
4. "It represents a cyanotic defect with decreased pulmonary blood flow."

34. 2. At birth, oxygenated blood normally causes the ductus to constrict, and the vessel closes completely by age 6 weeks. This defect is considered an acyanotic defect with increased pulmonary blood flow. The open ductus arteriosus can cause an excessive blood flow to the lungs because of the high pressure in the aorta. Heart failure is common in premature infants with a patent ductus arteriosus.

CN: Physiological integrity; CNS: Physiological adaptation; CL: Analysis

35. Which intervention or drug is recommended initially for preterm neonates to close a patent ductus arteriosus?
1. Indomethacin
2. Prostaglandin E_1
3. Surgical ligation
4. Cardiac catheterization

35. 1. Preterm neonates with good renal function may receive oral indomethacin, a prostaglandin inhibitor, to encourage ductal closure. If this isn't effective, surgery is suggested. Prostaglandin E_1 will ensure patency of a patent ductus arteriosus for infants dependent on an open ductus arteriosus. Surgical ligation and a cardiac catheterization procedure may also be performed in infants and children.

CN: Physiological integrity; CNS: Physiological adaptation; CL: Analysis

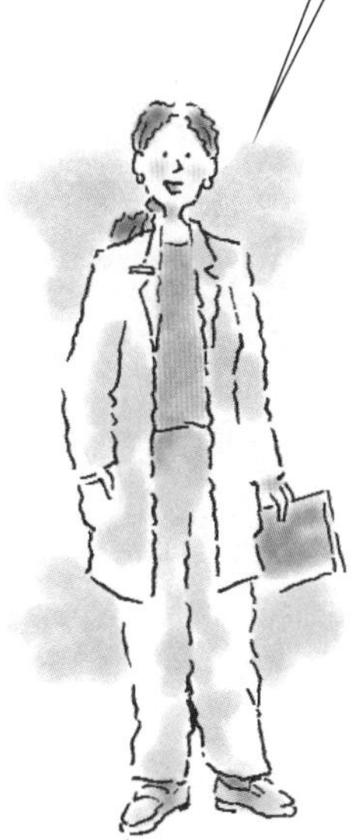

Question 36 asks which finding you expect, not necessarily one that may or may not occur.

36. A nurse is caring for a client with patent ductus arteriosus. Which assessment finding is consistent with this diagnosis?
1. Weak peripheral pulses
2. Machinelike murmur
3. Narrowed pulse pressure
4. Right ventricular hypertrophy

36. 2. The continuous, turbulent flow of blood from the aorta through the patent ductus arteriosus to the pulmonary artery produces a machinelike murmur. There's a widened pulse pressure and bounding peripheral pulses from the runoff of blood from the aorta to the pulmonary artery. Left ventricular hypertrophy created from the left to right shunting of blood can be seen on X-ray.

CN: Physiological integrity; CNS: Physiological adaptation; CL: Analysis

37. During observation of a child who has undergone cardiac catheterization, the nurse notes significant bleeding from the percutaneous femoral catheterization site. Which action should be taken first?
1. Apply direct, continuous pressure.
2. Assess the pulse and blood pressure.
3. Seek the assistance of another nurse.
4. Check the pulses in the affected leg.

37. 1. Bleeding from a major vessel must be stopped immediately to prevent massive hemorrhage. Vital signs would be taken after bleeding control measures are instituted. Calling for help is important, but pressure on the site must be applied and maintained while help is found. Pulses would be checked after bleeding is controlled.

CN: Physiological integrity; CNS: Reduction of risk potential; CL: Application

38. Which finding is expected during an assessment of a child with an acyanotic heart defect?
1. Overweight
2. Bradycardia
3. Hepatomegaly
4. Decreased respiratory rate

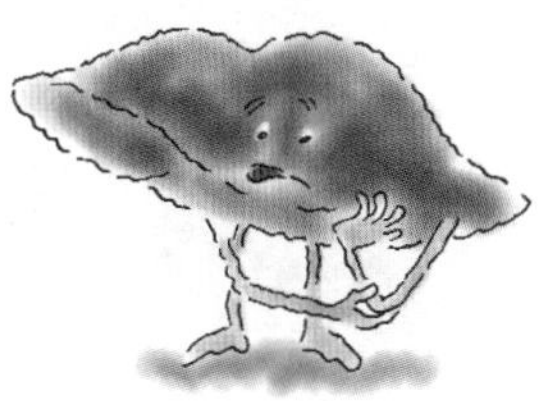

How did I get into a chapter on cardiovascular disorders?

38. 3. Hepatomegaly may result from blood backing up into the liver due to the difficulty of entering the right side of the heart. The increase in blood flow to the lungs may cause tachycardia (not bradycardia) and increased respiratory rates to compensate. Poor growth and development, not excess weight gain, may be seen because of the increased energy required for breathing.

CN: Physiological integrity; CNS: Physiological adaptation; CL: Analysis

39. Eisenmenger's complex consists of pulmonary vascular resistance exceeding systemic pressure. This can occur in which cardiac anomaly when untreated?

1. Aortic stenosis
2. Atrial septal defect
3. Pulmonary stenosis
4. Ventricular septal defect

39. 4. In moderate to large untreated ventricular septal defects, the constant excess flow will increase pulmonary vascular resistance. As time progresses, pressures in the right ventricle and left ventricle may change, causing higher pressures on the right side. A right-to-left shunt results, and pulmonary hypertension occurs.

CN: Physiological integrity; CNS: Physiological adaptation; CL: Analysis

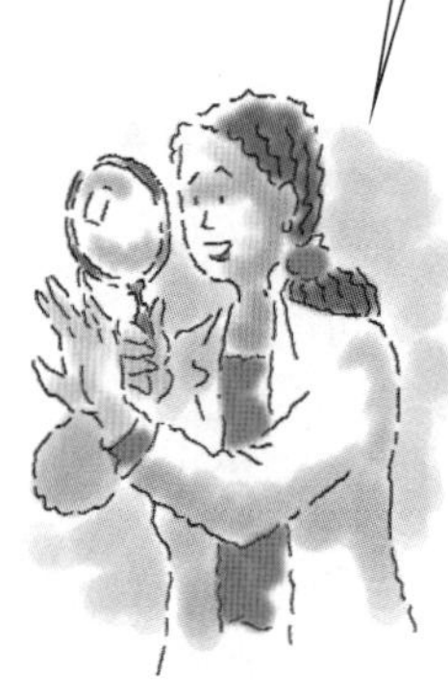

You can see this sign without a magnifying glass!

40. Which sign may be seen in a child with ventricular septal defect?

1. Cyanosis of the nailbeds
2. Above-average height on growth chart
3. Above-average weight gain on growth chart
4. Pink nailbeds with capillary refill less than 2 seconds

40. 1. Cyanotic nailbeds can be seen when pulmonary resistance increases and causes the left to right shunt to reverse and shunt right to left. This shift leads to signs of heart failure and cyanosis. Children with the defect usually present with symptoms of heart failure, poor growth and development, and failure to thrive.

CN: Physiological integrity; CNS: Physiological adaptation; CL: Analysis

41. When caring for a child diagnosed with a ventricular septal defect, which description would the nurse incorporate when teaching the parents about this condition?

1. It is a narrowing of the aortic arch.
2. It is a failure of a septum to develop completely between the atria.
3. It is a narrowing of the values at the entrance of the pulmonary artery.
4. It is a failure of a septum to develop completely between the ventricles.

41. 4. Failure of a septum to develop between the ventricles results in a left-to-right shunt, which is noted as a ventricular septal defect. The narrowing of the aortic arch describes coarctation of the aorta. Narrowing of the valves at the pulmonary artery describes pulmonic stenosis. When the septum fails to develop between the atria, it's considered an atrial septal defect.

CN: Physiological integrity; CNS: Physiological adaptation; CL: Application

42. Which curative surgical intervention is recommended for a child with ventricular septal defect?

1. Surgery with pulmonary artery banding
2. Defect repair through cardiac catheterization
3. Surgery with purse-string suture or Dacron patch repair
4. Surgery when severe pulmonary hypertension is noted

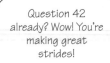

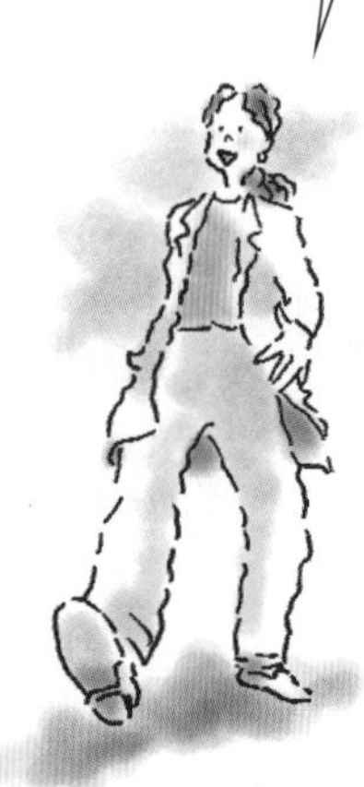

Question 42 already? Wow! You're making great strides!

42. 3. Surgery is recommended for children ages 1 to 4. A median sternotomy incision is placed with the heart on cardiopulmonary bypass. For small defects, a stitch closure is performed. For larger defects, a patch is sewn. Surgery with pulmonary artery banding is only a palliative procedure for children too small or too ill but in heart failure. Cardiac catheterization repairs have been performed for selective cases but aren't approved for general care. Severe pulmonary hypertension would lead to an inoperable condition. If repaired, the excess blood flow to the lungs by patching the defect may be fatal.

CN: Physiological integrity; CNS: Physiological adaptation; CL: Application

43. A child with a ventricular septal defect repair is receiving dopamine (Intropin) postoperatively. The nurse should teach the child's parents that this medication is most likely to be given for which action?

1. To decrease heart rate
2. To decrease urine output
3. To increase cardiac output
4. To decrease cardiac contractility

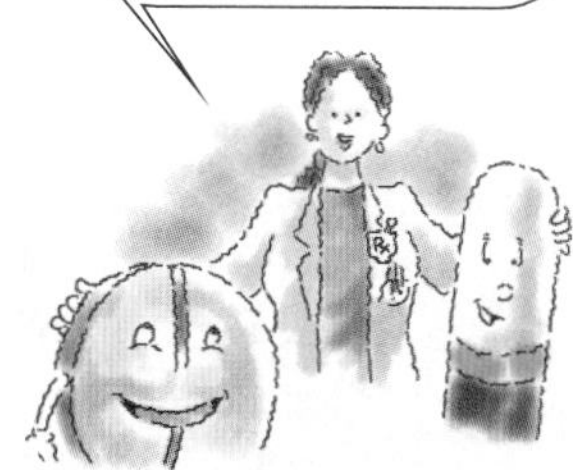

You know more about drugs than you realize!

43. 3. Dopamine stimulates $beta_1$- and $beta_2$-adrenergic receptors. It's a selective cardiac stimulant that will increase cardiac output, heart rate, and cardiac contractility. Urine output increases in response to dilation of the blood vessels to the mesentery and kidneys.

CN: Physiological integrity; CNS: Pharmacological and parenteral therapies; CL: Application

44. A child returns to his room after a cardiac catheterization. Which statement regarding mobility would be appropriate for the nurse to teach the child and his parents?

1. The child may sit in a chair with the affected extremity immobilized.
2. The child will be maintained on bed rest with no further activity restrictions.
3. The child will be maintained on bed rest with the affected extremity immobilized.
4. The child may get out of bed to go to the bathroom, if necessary.

44. 3. The child should be maintained on bed rest with the affected extremity immobilized after cardiac catheterization to prevent hemorrhage. Allowing the child to sit in a chair with the affected extremity immobilized, to move the affected extremity while on bed rest, or to have bathroom privileges places him at risk for hemorrhage.

CN: Physiological integrity; CNS: Reduction of risk potential; CL: Application

45. A client with Down syndrome (trisomy 21) comes to the pediatric clinic for a well visit. Which cardiac anomaly would this child be at risk for considering his health history?

1. Atrial septal defect
2. Pulmonic stenosis
3. Ventricular septal defect
4. Endocardial cushion defect

45. 4. Endocardial cushion defects are seen most in children with Down syndrome. Atrial septal defects account for about 10% of all cardiac anomalies. Pulmonic stenosis is responsible for about 8% of all cardiac anomalies. Ventricular septal defects are the most common cardiac anomaly.

CN: Health promotion and maintenance; CNS: None; CL: Application

46. Which finding would concern the nurse who's caring for an infant after a right femoral cardiac catheterization?

1. Weak right dorsalis pedis pulse
2. Elevated temperature
3. Decreased urine output
4. Slightly bloody drainage around catheterization site dressing

46. 1. The pulse below the catheterization site should be strong and equal to the unaffected extremity. A weakened pulse may indicate vessel obstruction or perfusion problems. Elevated temperature and decreased urine output are relatively normal findings after catheterization and may be the result of decreased oral fluids. A small amount of bloody drainage is normal; however, the site must be assessed frequently for increased bleeding.

CN: Physiological integrity; CNS: Reduction of risk potential; CL: Application

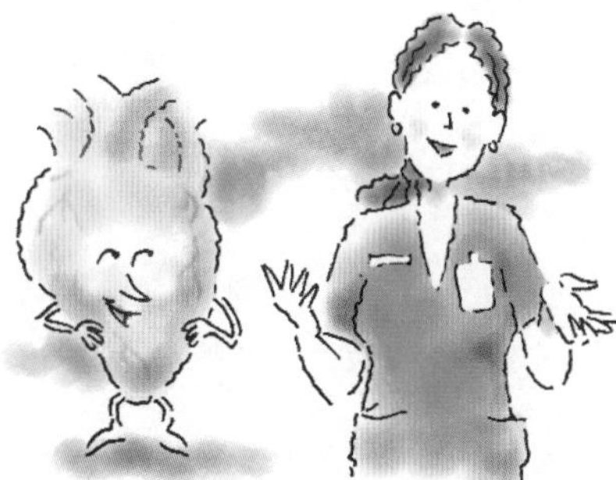

We both think you're doing great!

47. Which cardiac anomaly produces a left-to-right shunt?
1. Atrial septal defect
2. Pulmonic stenosis
3. Tetralogy of Fallot
4. Total anomalous pulmonary venous return

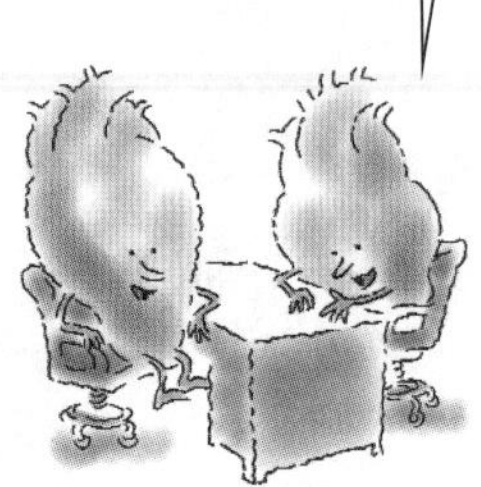

My shunt is left to right. How about yours?

47. 1. Atrial septal defects shunt from left to right because pressures are greater on the left side of the heart. Pulmonic stenosis, tetralogy of Fallot, and total anomalous pulmonary venous return will show a right-to-left shunting of blood.

CN: Health promotion and maintenance; CNS: None; CL: Analysis

48. A child with an atrial septal defect repair is entering postoperative day 3. Which intervention would be most appropriate?
1. Give the child nothing by mouth.
2. Maintain strict bed rest.
3. Take vital signs every 8 hours.
4. Administer an analgesic as needed.

48. 4. Pain management is always a priority and should be given on an as-needed basis. By day 3, the child should be advancing to a regular diet. Activity should include activity as able in the step-down unit, with coughing and deep breathing exercises. Vital signs should be performed routinely every 2 to 4 hours.

CN: Physiological integrity; CNS: Physiological adaptation; CL: Application

49. A 3-year-old child is on postoperative day 5 for an atrial septal defect repair. Which nursing diagnosis would be most appropriate?
1. *Activity intolerance*
2. *Chronic pain*
3. *Social isolation*
4. *Risk for imbalanced fluid volume*

49. 4. Diuretics may still be used as needed at this point. By day 5, the child's activity level will be normal and there will be little to no pain. The child isn't isolated from anyone and can usually attend the playroom on day 3 or 4.

CN: Physiological integrity; CNS: Physiological adaptation; CL: Analysis

50. A 6-month-old infant with uncorrected tetralogy of Fallot suddenly becomes increasingly cyanotic and diaphoretic, with weak peripheral pulses and an increased respiratory rate. What should the nurse do immediately?
1. Administer oxygen.
2. Administer morphine sulfate.
3. Place the infant in a knee-chest position.
4. Place the infant in Fowler's position.

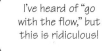

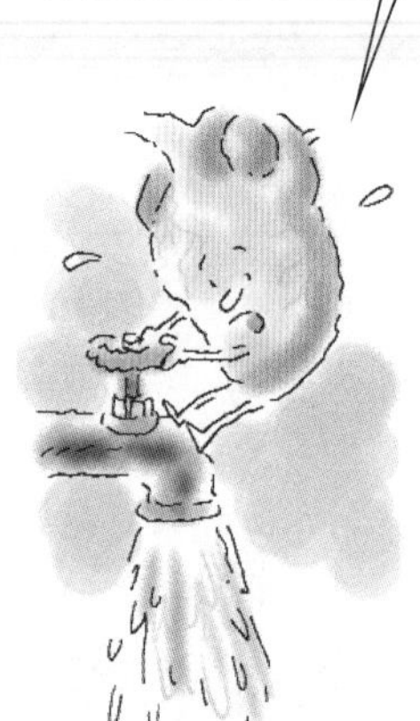

I've heard of "go with the flow," but this is ridiculous!

50. 3. The knee-chest position reduces the workload of the heart by increasing the blood return to the heart and keeping the blood flow more centralized. Oxygen should be administered quickly but only after placing the infant in the knee-chest position. Morphine should be administered after repositioning and oxygen administration are completed. Fowler's position wouldn't improve the situation.

CN: Safe, effective care environment; CNS: Management of care; CL: Application

51. A client is diagnosed with coarctation of the aorta. Which finding should the nurse expect during an assessment?
1. Normal blood pressure
2. Increased blood pressure in the upper extremities
3. Decreased blood pressure in the upper extremities
4. Decreased or absent pulses in the upper extremities

51. 2. As blood is pumped from the left ventricle to the aorta, some blood flows to the head and upper extremities while the rest meets obstruction and jets through the constricted area. Pressures and pulses are greater in the upper extremities. Decreased or absent pulses are found in the lower extremities.

CN: Physiological integrity; CNS: Physiological adaptation; CL: Analysis

52. A child with coarctation of the aorta experiences a postsurgical recoarctation. Which treatment should the nurse expect the physician to recommend?

1. Bypass graft repair
2. Patch aortoplasty
3. Balloon angioplasty
4. Left subclavian flap angioplasty

52. 3. Balloon angioplasty is the treatment of choice for postsurgical recoarctations. Bypass graft repair, patch angioplasty, and left subclavian flap angioplasty are surgical options to treat the original coarctation.

CN: Physiological integrity; CNS: Physiological adaptation; CL: Analysis

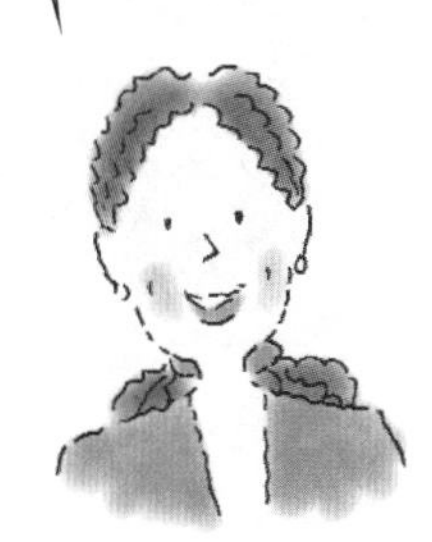

Hint: Cardiac anomalies can be extreme.

53. Which factor is a necessary part of assessment for a child with a possible cardiac anomaly?

1. Skin turgor
2. Temperature
3. Pupil size and reaction to light
4. Blood pressure in four extremities

53. 4. Measuring blood pressure in all four extremities is necessary to document hypertension and the blood pressure gradient between the upper and lower extremities. Temperature, skin turgor, and pupillary assessment are also important, but are not as specific for cardiac assessment as the blood pressure.

CN: Physiological integrity; CNS: Physiological adaptation; CL: Application

54. Which intervention is recommended postoperatively for a client with coarctation of the aorta repair?

1. Give a vasoconstrictor.
2. Maintain hypothermia.
3. Maintain a normal to low blood pressure.
4. Give a bolus of I.V. fluids.

54. 3. Blood pressure is tightly managed and kept low so there's no excessive pressure on the fresh suture lines. Vasoconstrictors would be contraindicated. Normothermia is maintained, and diuretics may be given to decrease fluid volume.

CN: Physiological integrity; CNS: Physiological adaptation; CL: Analysis

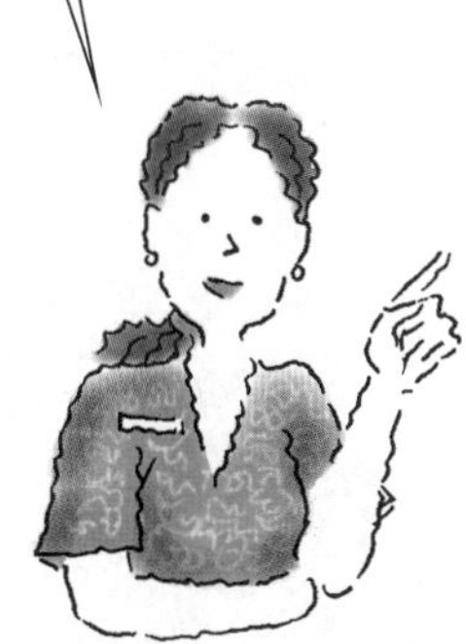

When it comes to assessment, practice makes perfect!

55. Which assessment is expected when assessing a child with tetralogy of Fallot?

1. Machinelike murmur
2. Eisenmenger's complex
3. Increasing cyanosis with crying or activity
4. Higher pressures in the upper extremities than with the lower extremities

55. 3. A child with tetralogy of Fallot will be mildly cyanotic at rest and have increasing cyanosis with crying, activity, or straining, as with a bowel movement. A machinelike murmur is a characteristic of patent ductus arteriosus. Eisenmenger's complex is a complication of pulmonary pressure exceeding systemic pressure. Higher pressures in the upper extremities are characteristic of coarctation of the aorta.

CN: Physiological integrity; CNS: Physiological adaptation; CL: Application

56. A child with tetralogy of Fallot has clubbing of the fingers and toes. Which condition is most likely to be causing this clubbing?

1. Polycythemia
2. Chronic hypoxia
3. Pansystolic murmur
4. Abnormal growth and development

56. 2. Chronic hypoxia longer than 6 months causes clubbing of the fingers and toes when untreated. Hypoxia varies with the degree of pulmonic stenosis. Polycythemia is an increased number of red blood cells as a result of the chronic hypoxemia. A pansystolic murmur is heard at the middle to lower left sternal border but has no impact on clubbing. Growth and development may appear normal.

CN: Physiological integrity; CNS: Physiological adaptation; CL: Analysis

57. A child with tetralogy of Fallot may assume which position of comfort during exercise?
1. Prone
2. Semi-Fowler's
3. Side-lying
4. Squat

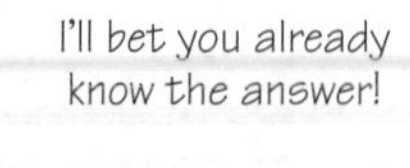

I'll bet you already know the answer!

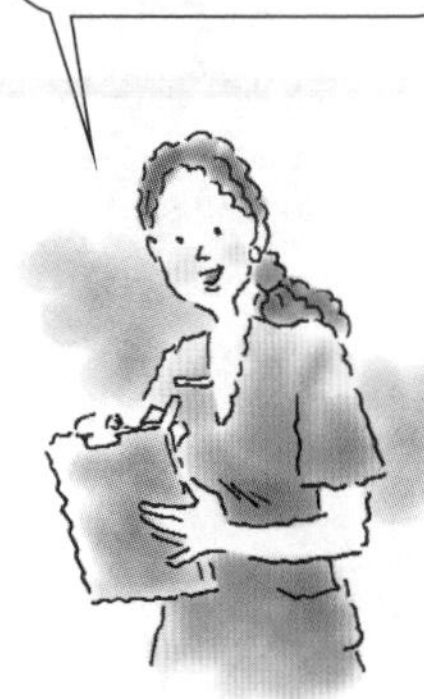

57. 4. A child may squat or assume a knee-chest position to reduce venous blood flow from the lower extremities and to increase systemic vascular resistance, which diverts more blood flow into the pulmonary artery. Prone, semi-Fowler's, and side-lying positions won't produce this effect.
CN: Physiological integrity; CNS: Physiological adaptation; CL: Analysis

58. A nurse is describing tetralogy of Fallot to a child's parents. Which statement by the parents demonstrates that the teaching has been effective?
1. "The condition is commonly referred to as 'blue tets.'"
2. "A child with this condition experiences hypercyanotic, or 'tet,' spells."
3. "A child with this condition experiences frequent respiratory infections."
4. "A child with this condition experiences decreased or absent pulses in the lower extremities."

58. 2. Hypercyanotic, or "tet," spells may occur as a result of increasing obstruction of right ventricular outflow, resulting in decreased pulmonary blood flow and increased right-to-left shunting. Infants with mild obstruction to blood flow have little or no right-to-left shunting and appear pink, or "pink tets." Frequent respiratory infections are seen in defects with increased pulmonary blood flow, such as a patent ductus arteriosus. Decreased or absent pulses in the lower extremities is a sign of Coarctation of the aorta.
CN: Physiological integrity; CNS: Physiological adaptation; CL: Analysis

59. A child diagnosed with tetralogy of Fallot has been ordered to undergo testing. Which test would indicate the direction and amount of shunting in this child?
1. Chest radiography
2. Echocardiography
3. Electrocardiography (ECG)
4. Cardiac catheterization

59. 4. Cardiac catheterization provides specific information about the direction and amount of shunting, coronary anatomy, and each portion of the heart defect. Chest radiographs will show right ventricular hypertrophy pushing the heart apex upward, resulting in a boot-shaped silhouette. Echocardiogram scans define such defects as large ventricular septal defects, pulmonic stenosis, and malposition of the aorta. ECG shows right ventricular hypertrophy with tall R waves.
CN: Physiological integrity; CNS: Reduction of risk potential; CL: Application

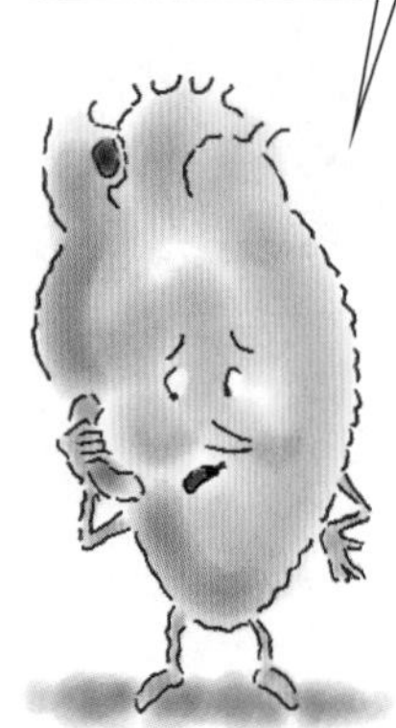

Hello? Is anybody there? I must have a bad connection.

60. A nurse is teaching parents about tricuspid atresia. Which statement indicates that the parents understand this disorder?
1. "There's a narrowing at the aortic outflow tract."
2. "The pulmonary veins don't return to the left atrium."
3. "There's a narrowing at the entrance of the pulmonary artery."
4. "There's no communication between the right atrium and right ventricle."

60. 4. Tricuspid atresia is failure of the tricuspid valve to develop, leaving no communication between the right atrium and right ventricle. Narrowing at the aortic outflow tract is aortic stenosis. Total anomalous pulmonary venous return is a defect in which the pulmonary veins don't return to the left atrium but abnormally return to the right side of the heart. The narrowing at the entrance of the pulmonary artery represents pulmonic stenosis.
CN: Physiological integrity; CNS: Physiological adaptation; CL: Analysis

61. Which characteristic can be noted during the assessment of a child with tricuspid atresia?

1. Cyanosis
2. Machinelike murmur
3. Decreased respiratory rate
4. Capillary refill more than 2 seconds

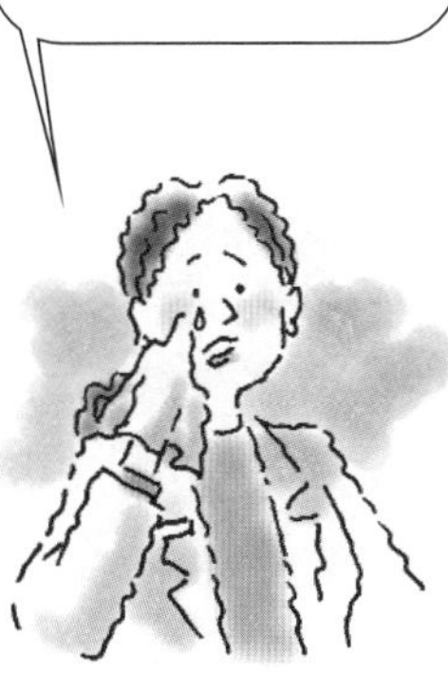

Tricuspid atresia always makes me blue.

61. 1. Cyanosis is the most consistent clinical sign of tricuspid atresia. Tachypnea and dyspnea are commonly present because of the decreased pulmonary blood flow and right-to-left shunting. Tricuspid atresia doesn't have a characteristic murmur. A machinelike murmur is characteristic of a patent ductus arteriosus. Decreased oxygenation would increase capillary refill time.

CN: Physiological integrity; CNS: Physiological adaptation; CL: Analysis

62. A child with tricuspid atresia develops polycythemia. Which statement is the most accurate concerning this manifestation?

1. The red blood cell count is normal.
2. There is an increased ability for the oxygen to carry blood.
3. There is little to no effect on the blood clotting system.
4. The viscosity of the blood is unchanged.

62. 2. Polycythemia is an increased number of red blood cells, thereby increasing the ability of the blood to carry oxygen to the cells. Due to this clinical manifestation, the viscosity of the blood increases, and there is not as much room for clotting factors. This leaves the child at risk for blood clotting disorders.

CN: Physiological integrity; CNS: Physiological adaptation; CL: Application

63. A child has been diagnosed with tricuspid atresia. Which operation should a nurse expect the physician to recommend?

1. Blalock-Taussig operation
2. Fontan procedure
3. Jatene procedure
4. Patch closure

63. 2. The Fontan procedure is used to correct tricuspid atresia. It separates the systemic and pulmonary circulations by closing septal defects and previous shunts and connecting the systemic venous structures with the pulmonary arteries. The Blalock-Taussig operation is used to palliate children with tricuspid atresia. The Jatene procedure is used to correct a mixed defect such as transposition of the great arteries. Patch closures are used for defects such as a ventricular or atrial septal defect.

CN: Physiological integrity; CNS: Physiological adaptation; CL: Application

64. Which guideline should the nurse follow when administering digoxin (Lanoxin) to an infant?

1. Mix the digoxin with the infant's food.
2. Double the subsequent dose if a dose is missed.
3. Give the digoxin with antacids when possible.
4. Withhold the dose if the apical pulse rate is less than 90 beats/minute.

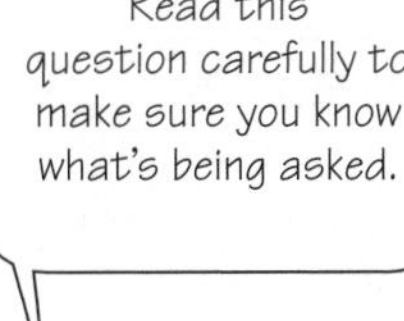

Read this question carefully to make sure you know what's being asked.

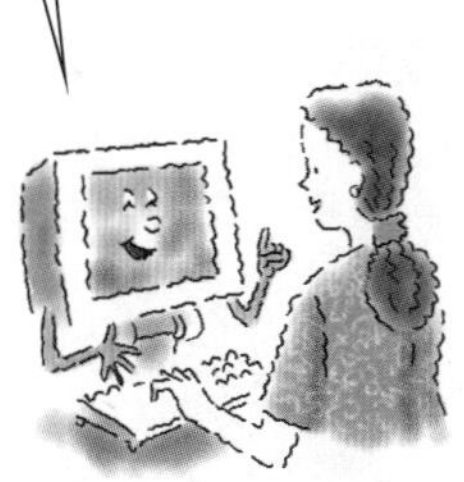

64. 4. Digoxin is used to decrease heart rate; however, the apical pulse must be carefully monitored to detect a severe reduction. Administering digoxin to an infant with a heart rate of less than 90 beats/minute could further reduce the rate and compromise cardiac output. Mixing digoxin with food may interfere with accurate dosing. Double-dosing should never be done. Antacids may decrease drug absorption.

CN: Physiological integrity; CNS: Pharmacological and parenteral therapies; CL: Application

65. What part of the assessment of a child who has undergone complete repair of total anomalous pulmonary venous connection would lead the nurse to suspect that the complication of pulmonary venous obstruction has occurred?

1. Decreased work of breathing
2. Decreasing respiratory rate
3. Decreasing oxygenation saturation levels
4. Increasing urine output

65. 3. A child who has pulmonary venous obstruction will exhibit signs of increasing respiratory distress, such as increased respiratory rate, dyspnea, and shortness of breath. Oxygen saturation levels will decrease. Urine output will decrease as the heart fails.

CN: Physiological integrity; CNS: Physiological adaptation; CL: Application

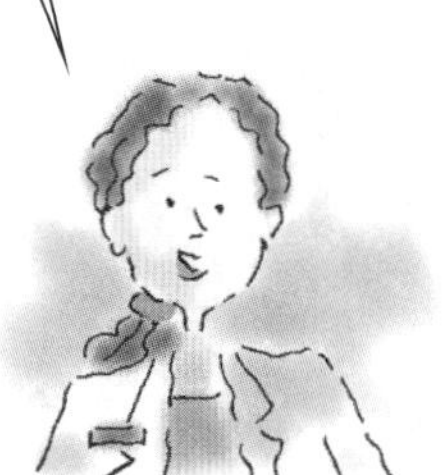
You're halfway there. Fantastic!

66. Which finding is <u>common</u> during an assessment of a child with a total anomalous pulmonary venous return defect?

1. Hypertension
2. Frequent respiratory infections
3. Normal growth and development
4. Above-average weight gain on the growth chart

66. 2. Children with total anomalous pulmonary venous return defects are prone to repeated respiratory infections due to increased pulmonary blood flow. Hypertension usually occurs with coarctation of the aorta, an acyanotic defect with obstructive flow. Poor feeding and failure to thrive are also signs. Infants look thin and malnourished.

CN: Physiological integrity; CNS: Physiological adaptation; CL: Application

67. Which complication may result <u>after</u> the repair of total anomalous pulmonary venous return?

1. Hypotension
2. Pulmonary hypertension
3. Ventricular arrhythmias
4. Pulmonary vein dilatation

67. 2. Pulmonary hypertension, atrial arrhythmias, and pulmonary vein obstruction are complications that may result postoperatively. The left atrium is small and sensitive to fluid volume loading. An increase in the pressure in the right atrium is required to ensure left atrial filling.

CN: Physiological integrity; CNS: Physiological adaptation; CL: Analysis

68. An infant has recently been diagnosed with tricuspid atresia and the parents have been told that their child will need a series of three, staged surgeries. Which statement indicates that the parents have an understanding of the procedures?

1. "My child will have this dusky color for the rest of his life."
2. "These procedures will make my child have a normal heart."
3. "Once fixed, my baby will not have to take any more medicine."
4. "My baby will be just like all of the other children once the surgeries are all done."

68. 1. The child will be dusky, particularly around mucus membranes and nail beds, for the rest of its life as a result of chronic hypoxemia. The surgeries do not make the child have a "normal" heart, as they do not fix the original defect. The child will more than likely be on medications for the rest of its life, and the child will more than likely be smaller in stature than other children.

CN: Physiological integrity; CNS: Physiological adaptation; CL: Analysis

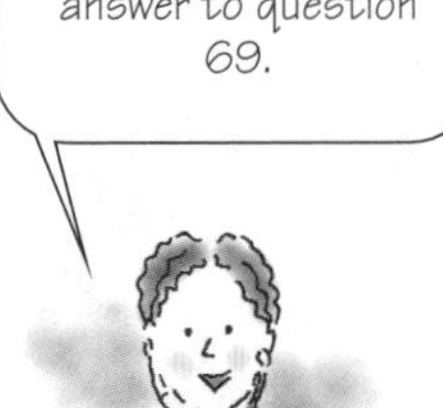
Listen closely and you'll hear the answer to question 69.

69. Which finding commonly occurs during an assessment of a child with truncus arteriosus?

1. Weak, thready pulses
2. Narrowed pulse pressure
3. Pink and moist mucous membranes
4. Harsh systolic regurgitant murmur

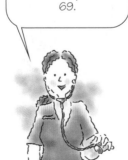

69. 4. As a result of the ventricular septal defect, a harsh systolic regurgitant murmur is heard along the left sternal border and is usually accompanied by a thrill. Increasing pulmonary blood flow causes bounding pulses and a widened pulse pressure. Systemic and pulmonary blood mixing leads to mild or moderate cyanosis, so mucous membranes may appear dull or gray.

CN: Physiological integrity; CNS: Physiological adaptation; CL: Analysis

70. Treatment for truncus arteriosus includes digoxin and diuretics. Which technique would be best for giving these drugs to an infant?

1. Use a measuring spoon.
2. Use a graduated dropper.
3. Mix the drug with baby food.
4. Mix the drug in a bottle with juice or milk.

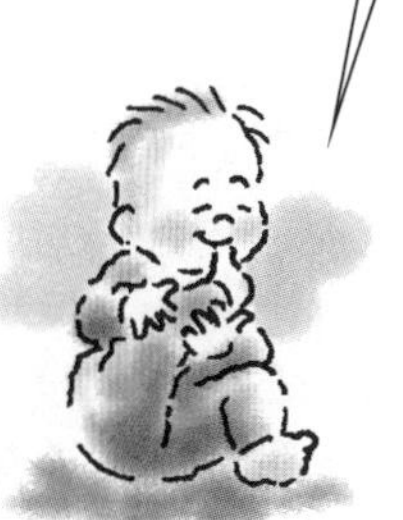

If it doesn't taste good, I don't want it.

70. 2. Using a dropper allows the exact dosage to be given. A measuring spoon isn't as exact as a dropper. Mixing drugs with juice, milk, or food may cause a problem if the child doesn't completely finish the meal because then how much the child received isn't definite. In addition, this may prevent the child from drinking or eating for fear of tasting the drug.

CN: Physiological integrity; CNS: Pharmacological and parenteral therapies; CL: Application

71. Which change would the nurse expect after administering oxygen to an infant with uncorrected tetralogy of Fallot?

1. Disappearance of the murmur
2. No evidence of cyanosis
3. Improvement of finger clubbing
4. Less agitation

71. 4. Supplemental oxygen will help the infant breathe more easily and feel less anxious or agitated. Disappearance of the murmur, no evidence of cyanosis, and improvement of finger clubbing would not occur as a result of supplemental oxygen administration.

CN: Physiological integrity; CNS: Physiological adaptation; CL: Application

72. Which statement about transposition of the great arteries is correct?

1. Electrocardiography will always show arrhythmias.
2. Diagnosis can be made in utero.
3. Chest X-ray can show an accurate view of the defect.
4. Heart failure isn't a related complication.

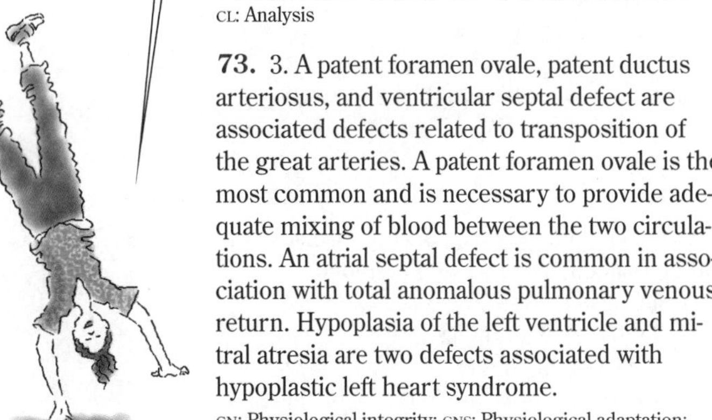

You're almost up to question 75! Way to go!

72. 2. Echocardiography done by a fetal cardiologist can diagnose transposition of the great arteries in utero. The other defects associated with this defect include a patent foramen ovale and a ventricular septal defect that contribute to developing heart failure. Electrocardiography may or may not reveal arrhythmias. Chest X-ray can show cardiomegaly and pulmonary vascular markings only. Echocardiography or cardiac catheterization may be required preoperatively to show the coronary artery anatomy before surgical repair.

CN: Physiological integrity; CNS: Physiological adaptation; CL: Analysis

73. A nurse is assessing a child with transposition of the great arteries. Which associated defect should the nurse expect to see in this client?

1. Mitral atresia
2. Atrial septal defect
3. Patent foramen ovale
4. Hypoplasia of the left ventricle

73. 3. A patent foramen ovale, patent ductus arteriosus, and ventricular septal defect are associated defects related to transposition of the great arteries. A patent foramen ovale is the most common and is necessary to provide adequate mixing of blood between the two circulations. An atrial septal defect is common in association with total anomalous pulmonary venous return. Hypoplasia of the left ventricle and mitral atresia are two defects associated with hypoplastic left heart syndrome.

CN: Physiological integrity; CNS: Physiological adaptation; CL: Analysis

74. Administration of which drug would be the <u>most important</u> in treating transposition of the great arteries?

1. Digoxin
2. Diuretics
3. Antibiotics
4. Prostaglandin E_1

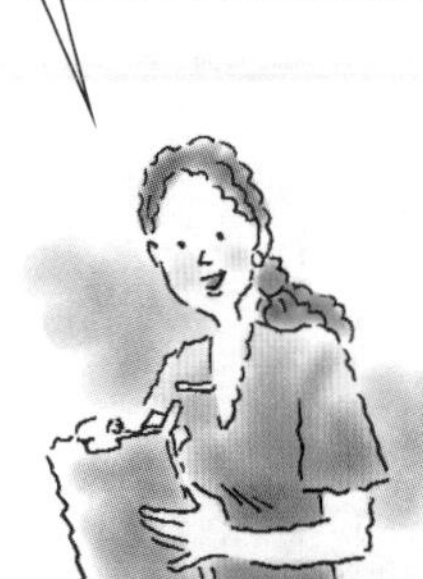

It's most important that you read each question carefully.

74. 4. Prostaglandin E_1 is necessary to maintain patency of the patent ductus arteriosus and improve systemic arterial flow in children with inadequate intracardiac mixing. Digoxin and diuretics will treat heart failure when present. Antibiotics are given in the immediate preoperative phase.

CN: Physiological integrity; CNS: Pharmacological and parenteral therapies; CL: Application

75. Which surgical procedure is recommended for repair of transposition of the great arteries?

1. Jatene procedure
2. Fontan procedure
3. Balloon atrial septostomy
4. Blalock-Taussig operation

75. 1. The Jatene procedure involves transposing the great arteries and mobilizing and reimplanting the coronary arteries. The Fontan procedure is recommended for repair of tricuspid atresia. Balloon atrial septostomy is a palliative procedure used during cardiac catheterization for those children without a coexisting lesion. Blalock-Taussig operation is used to palliate tricuspid atresia and pulmonic atresia.

CN: Physiological integrity; CNS: Physiological adaptation; CL: Application

76. Which statement best describes a characteristic of valvular pulmonic stenosis?

1. The valve is normal.
2. The right ventricle is hypoplastic.
3. Left ventricular hypertrophy develops.
4. Divisions between the cusps are fused.

76. 4. Blood flow through the valve is restricted by fusion of the divisions between the cusps. The valve may be normal or malformed. Right ventricular hypertrophy develops due to resistance to blood flow.

CN: Physiological integrity; CNS: Physiological adaptation; CL: Analysis

77. During the assessment of a child with pulmonic stenosis, which finding is <u>most common</u>?

1. Hyperactivity
2. Normal respiratory rate
3. Systolic ejection murmur
4. Capillary refill more than 2 seconds

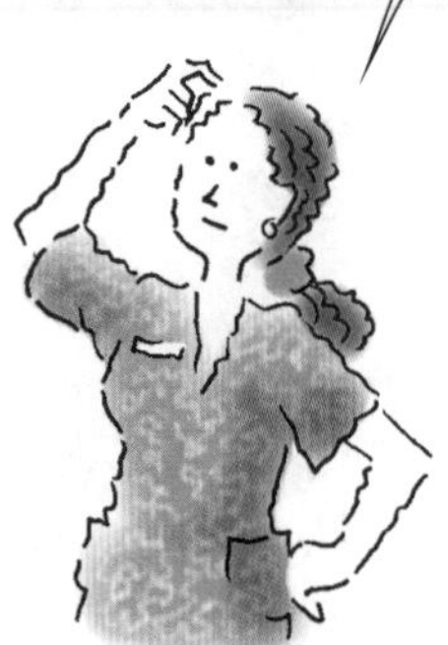

All of these conditions may occur, but which occurs most commonly?

77. 3. A systolic ejection murmur, which may be accompanied by a thrill, can be heard at the upper left sternal border. The decrease in pulmonary blood flow causes fatigue and dyspnea. Systemic cyanosis may result from right ventricular failure that increases the capillary refill time.

CN: Physiological integrity; CNS: Physiological adaptation; CL: Analysis

78. Which finding is seen during cardiac catheterization of a child with pulmonic stenosis?

1. Right-to-left shunting
2. Left-to-right shunting
3. Decreased pressure in the right side of the heart
4. Increased oxygenation in the left side of the heart

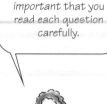

78. 1. Right-to-left shunting develops through a patent foramen ovale, an atrial septal defect, or a ventricular septal defect due to right ventricular failure and an increase in pressure in the right side of the heart. Decreased oxygenation in the left side of the heart is noted because of the right-to-left shunt and decreased pulmonary blood flow.

CN: Physiological integrity; CNS: Physiological adaptation; CL: Analysis

79. A nurse is caring for a 16-year-old client with aortic stenosis. Which finding is associated with aortic stenosis when the child is active?

1. Chest pain
2. Right ventricular failure
3. Increased cardiac output
4. Loud systolic regurgitant murmur with a thrill

Keep going!
You're doing great!

79. 1. Children with aortic stenosis may develop chest pain similar to angina when they're active. They're also at risk for tachycardia, syncope, hypotension, left ventricular failure, dyspnea, fatigue, and palpitations. Poor left ventricular ejection leads to a decreased cardiac output. Loud systolic regurgitant murmurs are heard with ventricular septal defects.

CN: Physiological integrity; CNS: Physiological adaptation; CL: Application

80. A nurse is teaching the parents of a child with congenital aortic stenosis. Which statement should the nurse include in her teaching about this disorder?

1. It can result from rheumatic fever (infection with group A streptococci).
2. It accounts for 25% of all congenital defects.
3. It causes an increase in cardiac output.
4. It's classified as an acyanotic defect with increased pulmonary blood flow.

80. 1. Aortic stenosis can result from rheumatic fever, which can damage the aortic valve in the first 8 weeks of pregnancy. It accounts for about 5% of all congenital defects. It causes a decrease in cardiac output. Aortic stenosis is classified as an acyanotic defect with obstructed flow from the ventricles.

CN: Physiological integrity; CNS: Physiological adaptation; CL: Analysis

81. Which instruction would be most appropriate for a child with aortic stenosis?

1. Restrict exercise.
2. Avoid prostaglandin E_1.
3. Avoid digoxin and diuretics.
4. Allow the child to exercise freely.

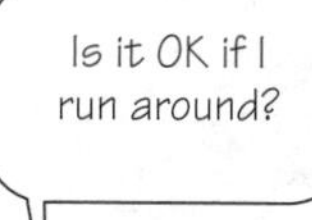
Is it OK if I
run around?

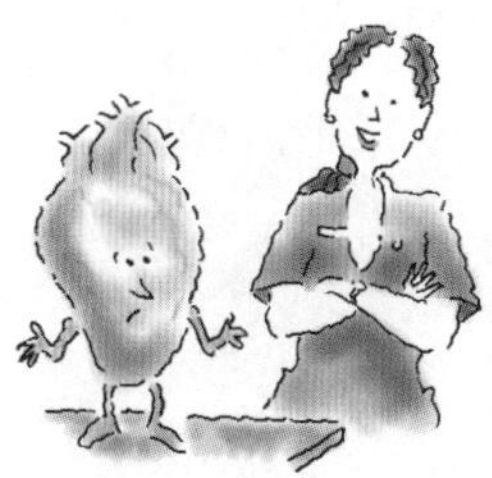

81. 1. Exercise should be restricted because of low cardiac output and left ventricular failure. Strenuous activity has been reported to result in sudden death from the development of myocardial ischemia. Prostaglandin E_1 is recommended to maintain the patency of the ductus arteriosus in the neonate with critical aortic stenosis. This allows for improved systemic blood flow. Digoxin and diuretics may be required for the critically ill infant experiencing heart failure as a result of severe aortic stenosis.

CN: Physiological integrity; CNS: Physiological adaptation; CL: Application

82. The nurse is planning care for a 9-year-old male child with heart failure. Which nursing diagnosis should receive priority?

1. *Risk for decreased cardiac tissue perfusion related to sympathetic response to heart failure*
2. *Imbalanced nutrition: Less than body requirement related to rapid tiring while feeding*
3. *Anxiety (parent) related to unknown nature of child's illness*
4. *Decreased cardiac output related to cardiac defect*

82. 4. The primary nursing diagnosis for a child with heart failure is *Decreased cardiac output related to cardiac defect.* The most common cause of heart failure in children is congenital heart defects. Some defects result from the blood being pumped from the left side of the heart to the right side of the heart. The heart can't manage the extra volume, resulting in the pulmonary system becoming overloaded. *Risk for decreased cardiac tissue perfusion, Imbalanced nutrition,* and *Anxiety* don't take priority over decreased cardiac output.

CN: Physiological integrity; CNS: Physiological adaptation; CL: Application

83. Which nursing diagnosis is the most appropriate when caring for an infant with hypoplastic left heart syndrome?

1. *Death anxiety*
2. *Delayed growth and development*
3. *Deficient diversional activity*
4. *Risk for activity intolerance*

83. 1. Without intervention, death usually occurs within the first few days of life as a result of progressive hypoxia, acidosis, and shock as the ductus closes and systemic perfusion diminishes. If the parents choose cardiac transplantation, the child may die waiting for a donor heart. For those who choose surgery, the child may not survive the three stages of the surgery. The other three choices don't apply to this type of defect because of the low survival rates.

CN: Physiological integrity; CNS: Physiological adaptation; CL: Analysis

84. A child receives prednisone after undergoing a heart transplant. What is the desired effect of this medication?

1. Stimulate appetite.
2. Suppress immune response.
3. Improve wound healing.
4. Prevent fluid retention.

84. 2. The goal of prednisone for this client is to suppress the immune system, thereby preventing organ rejection. Prednisone is often used in combination with other immunosuppressant medications in order to prevent rejection. While corticosteroids do stimulate appetites, that is not the desired effect for this child. Prednisone and other corticosteroids cause decreased ability of wounds to heal; fluid retention is one of the side effects.

CN: Physiological integrity; CNS: Pharmacological and parenteral therapies; CL: Application

85. Which adverse reaction to prednisone would a nurse expect to observe in a child who has received a heart transplant?

1. Weight loss
2. Hyperpyrexia
3. Anorexia
4. Poor wound healing

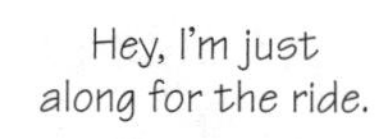
Hey, I'm just along for the ride.

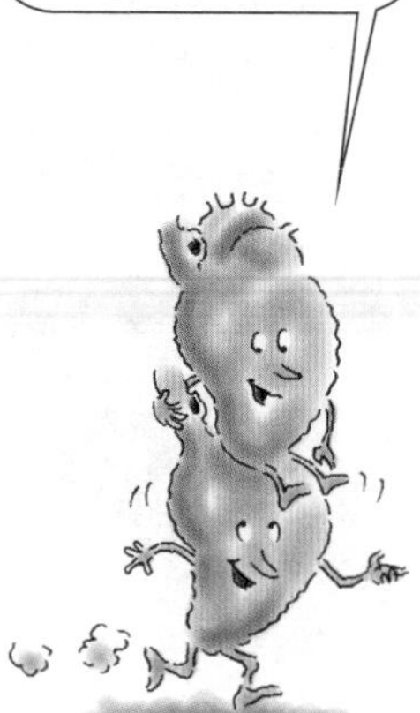

85. 4. Common adverse reactions to prednisone include poor wound healing, weight gain, delayed temperature response, increased appetite, delayed sexual maturation, growth impairment, and a cushingoid appearance. The school-age child who has received prednisone is usually overweight and has a moon-shaped face.

CN: Physiological integrity; CNS: Pharmacological and parenteral therapies; CL: Application

86. A child is given 0.5 mg/kg/day of prednisone divided into two doses. The child weighs 10 kg. How much is given in each dose?

1. 2.5 mg
2. 5 mg
3. 10 mg
4. 1.5 mg

86. 1. The child should receive 2.5 mg/dose. Use the following equations:

$0.5 \text{ mg/kg} \times 10 \text{ kg} = 5 \text{ mg};$

$5 \text{ mg}/2 \text{ doses} = 2.5 \text{ mg/dose}$

CN: Physiological integrity; CNS: Pharmacological and parenteral therapies; CL: Analysis

87. A 3-year-old client has a high red blood cell count and polycythemia. In planning care, the nurse would anticipate which goal to help prevent clot formation?

1. The child won't have signs of dehydration.
2. The child won't have signs of dyspnea.
3. The child will be pain free.
4. The child will attain the 40th percentile of weight for his age.

87. 1. When dehydration occurs, blood is thicker and more prone to clotting. Dyspnea would be a sign of hypoxia. Pain and weight gain would not be indicators of blood clot formation.

CN: Physiological integrity; CNS: Reduction of risk potential; CL: Application

88. Which statement about bacterial/infective endocarditis is the most accurate?

1. Bacteria invading only tissues of the heart
2. Infection of the valves and inner lining of the heart
3. Inappropriate fusion of the endocardial cushions in fetal life
4. Caused by alterations in cardiac preload, afterload, contractility, or heart rate

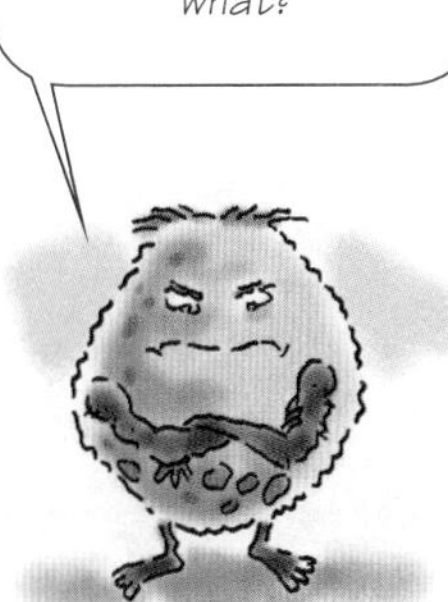

Are you blaming me for this, or what?

88. 2. Bacterial or infective endocarditis is an infection of the valves and inner lining of the heart. It's usually caused by the bacteria *Streptococcus viridans* and commonly affects children with acquired or congenital anomalies of the heart or great vessels. Bacteria may grow into adjacent tissues and may break off and embolize elsewhere, such as the spleen, kidney, lung, skin, and central nervous system. Endocardial cushion defects represent inappropriate fusion of the endocardial cushions in fetal life. Alterations in preload, afterload, contractility, or heart rate refer to heart failure.

CN: Physiological integrity; CNS: Physiological adaptation; CL: Application

89. A child with suspected bacterial endocarditis arrives at the emergency department. Which finding is expected during assessment?

1. Weight gain
2. Bradycardia
3. Low-grade fever
4. Increased hemoglobin level

89. 3. Symptoms may include a low-grade intermittent fever, decrease in hemoglobin level, tachycardia, anorexia, weight loss, and decreased activity level. Bacteremia leads to these signs of an infection.

CN: Physiological integrity; CNS: Physiological adaptation; CL: Application

90. Which factor may lead to bacterial endocarditis in a child with underlying heart disease?

1. History of a cold for 3 days
2. Dental work pretreated with antibiotics
3. Peripheral I.V. catheter in place for 1 day
4. Indwelling urinary catheter for 2 days leading to a urinary tract infection

90. 4. Bacterial organisms can enter the bloodstream from any site of infection such as a urinary tract infection. Gram-negative bacilli are common causative agents. Colds are usually viral, not bacterial. Dental work is a common portal of entry if not pretreated with antibiotics. A peripheral I.V. catheter is an entry site, but only if signs and symptoms of infection are present. Long-term indwelling catheters pose a higher risk for infection.

CN: Physiological integrity; CNS: Physiological adaptation; CL: Analysis

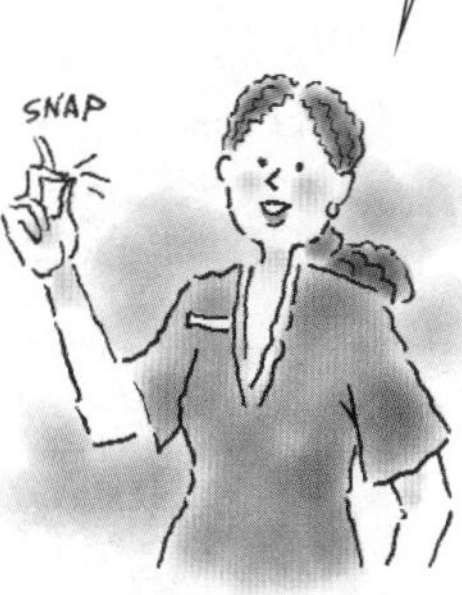

Wow! You finished question 90! The rest should be a snap!
SNAP

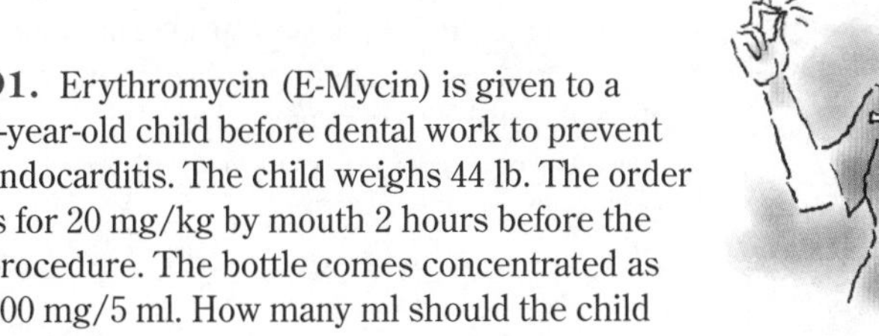

91. Erythromycin (E-Mycin) is given to a 6-year-old child before dental work to prevent endocarditis. The child weighs 44 lb. The order is for 20 mg/kg by mouth 2 hours before the procedure. The bottle comes concentrated as 400 mg/5 ml. How many ml should the child receive?

1. 2.5 ml
2. 5 ml
3. 5.5 ml
4. 10 ml

91. 2. The child should receive 5 ml. Use the following equations:

Convert pounds to kilograms:

44 lb/2.2 kg = 20 kg

Then, determine how many mg to give:

20 mg/kg × 20 kg = 400 mg

Next, determine how many ml to give:

400 mg/400 mg × 5 ml = 5 ml

(desired/have × amount on hand = amount to administer)

CN: Physiological integrity; CNS: Pharmacological and parenteral therapies; CL: Analysis

92. What would be the <u>most</u> common adverse reaction a nurse might observe after administering enteric-coated erythromycin (Ery-tab)?

1. Weight gain
2. Constipation
3. Increased appetite
4. Nausea and vomiting

93. A child is hospitalized with bacterial endocarditis. Which nursing diagnosis is most appropriate?

1. *Constipation*
2. *Excess fluid volume*
3. *Deficient diversional activity*
4. *Imbalanced nutrition: More than body requirements*

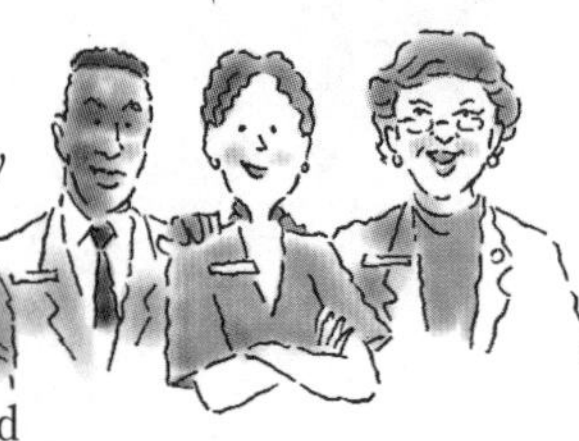

Nursing diagnoses: Share the knowledge!

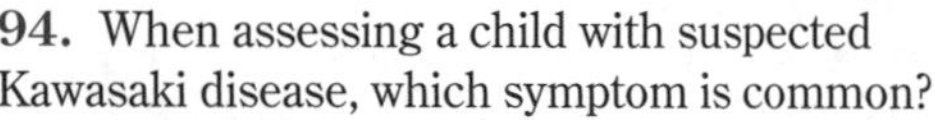

94. When assessing a child with suspected Kawasaki disease, which symptom is common?

1. Low-grade fever
2. "Strawberry" tongue
3. Pink, moist mucous membranes
4. Bilateral conjunctival infection with yellow exudate

95. A nurse is teaching the parents of a child with Kawasaki disease. Which statement should the nurse include in her teaching about this disorder?

1. It mostly occurs in the summer and fall.
2. Diagnosis can be made with laboratory testing.
3. It's an acute systemic vasculitis of unknown cause.
4. It manifests in two different stages: acute and subacute.

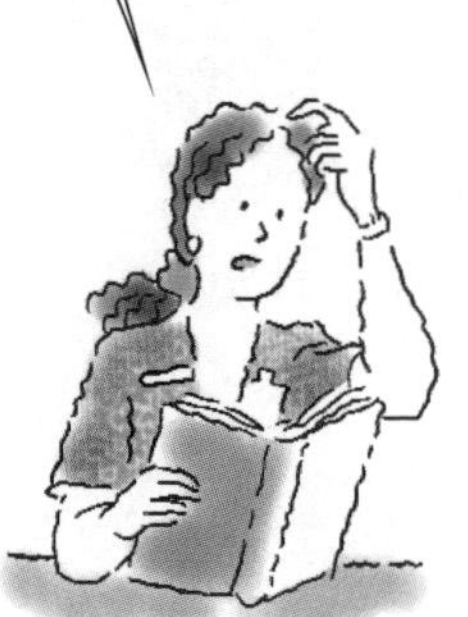

Which statement is most appropriate?

92. 4. Erythromycin is an antibiotic. Common adverse effects include nausea, vomiting, diarrhea, abdominal pain, and anorexia. It should be given with a full glass of water and after meals or with food to lessen GI symptoms.

CN: Physiological integrity; CNS: Pharmacological and parenteral therapies; CL: Application

93. 3. Treatment for bacterial endocarditis requires long-term hospitalization or home care for I.V. antibiotics. Children may be bored and depressed, needing age-appropriate activities. *Excess fluid volume, Constipation,* and *Imbalanced nutrition: More than body requirements* may be possible nursing diagnoses related to the adverse reactions of antibiotics, such as GI upset.

CN: Physiological integrity; CNS: Physiological adaptation; CL: Analysis

94. 2. Inflammation of the pharynx and oral mucosa develops, causing red, cracked lips and a "strawberry" tongue in which the normal coating of the tongue sloughs off. A high fever of 5 or more days unresponsive to antibiotics and antipyretics is also part of the diagnostic criteria. The eyes are generally dry without exudation.

CN: Physiological integrity; CNS: Physiological adaptation; CL: Application

95. 3. Kawasaki disease can best be described as an acute systemic vasculitis of unknown cause. Most cases are geographic and seasonal, with most occurring in the late winter and early spring. Diagnosis is based on clinical findings of five of the six diagnostic criteria and associated laboratory results. There's no specific laboratory test for diagnosis. There are three stages: acute, subacute, and convalescent.

CN: Physiological integrity; CNS: Physiological adaptation; CL: Application

96. Which characteristic indicates that a child with Kawasaki disease has entered the <u>subacute</u> phase?

1. Polymorphous rash
2. Normal blood values
3. Cervical lymphadenopathy
4. Desquamation of the hands and feet

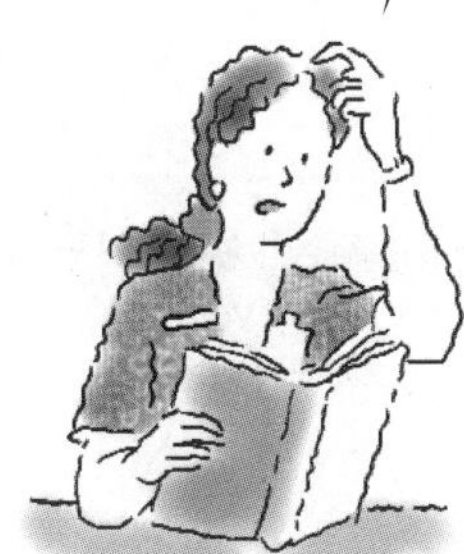

What happens during the subacute phase of this disease?

96. 4. The subacute phase shows characteristic desquamation of the hands and feet. Blood values return to normal at the end of the convalescent phase. Cervical lymphadenopathy and a polymorphous rash can be seen in the acute phase due to the onset of inflammation and fever.

CN: Physiological integrity; CNS: Physiological adaptation; CL: Analysis

97. A nurse is caring for a child with Kawasaki disease. Which symptom should concern the nurse the most?

1. Mild diarrhea
2. Pain in the joints
3. Abdominal pain with vomiting
4. Increased erythrocyte sedimentation rate (ESR)

97. 3. The most serious complication of this disease is cardiac involvement. Abdominal pain, vomiting, and restlessness are the main symptoms of an acute myocardial infarction in children. Mild diarrhea can be treated with oral fluids. Pain in the joints is an expected sign of arthritis that usually occurs in the subacute phase. An increased ESR is a reflection of the inflammatory process and may be seen for 2 to 4 weeks after the onset of symptoms.

CN: Physiological integrity; CNS: Physiological adaptation; CL: Analysis

98. A child is undergoing testing to rule out a diagnosis of Kawasaki disease. Which test result may lead to this diagnosis?

1. Hematuria
2. Elevated leukocyte count
3. Normal or decreased platelet count
4. Decreased erythrocyte sedimentation rate

98. 2. Inflammation of the small vessels, along with pancarditis, leads to an elevated leukocyte count, increased platelet count, and proteinuria or sterile pyuria. The capillaries, venules, and arterioles are affected first, then the medium-sized muscular arteries. These laboratory results contribute to the clinical presentation and diagnosis of Kawasaki disease.

CN: Physiological integrity; CNS: Physiological adaptation; CL: Analysis

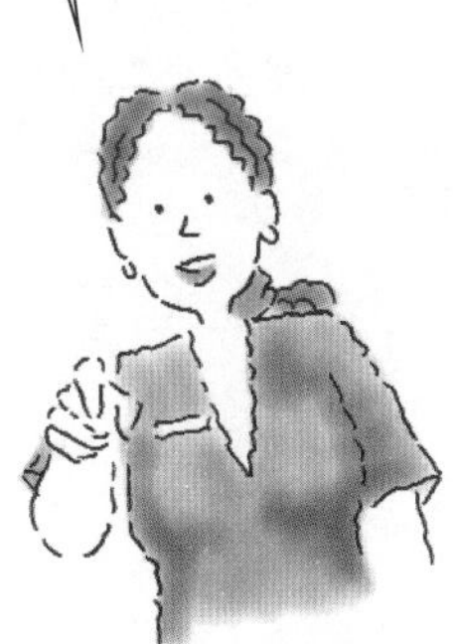

Here's another dosing question. You can do it!

99. Therapy for Kawasaki disease includes I.V. gamma globulin, prescribed at 400 mg/kg/day for 4 days. The child weighs 10 kg. How much is given per dose?

1. 200 mg
2. 400 mg
3. 2,000 mg
4. 4,000 mg

99. 4. The child should receive 4,000 mg. Use the following equation:

$400 \text{ mg/kg} \times 10 \text{ kg} = 4{,}000 \text{ mg or } 4 \text{ g}$

CN: Physiological integrity; CNS: Pharmacological and parenteral therapies; CL: Analysis

100. A child is receiving 8 g of I.V. gamma globulin for treatment of Kawasaki disease. The child weighs 20 kg. The order is for 8 g of gamma globulin over 12 hours. The concentration is 8 g in 300 ml of normal saline. How many milliliters per hour will this child receive?

1. 12 ml/hour
2. 25 ml/hour
3. 50 ml/hour
4. 40 ml/hour

100. 2. The child should receive 25 ml/hour. Use the following equation:
300 ml/12 hours = 25 ml/hour

CN: Physiological integrity; CNS: Pharmacological and parenteral therapies; CL: Analysis

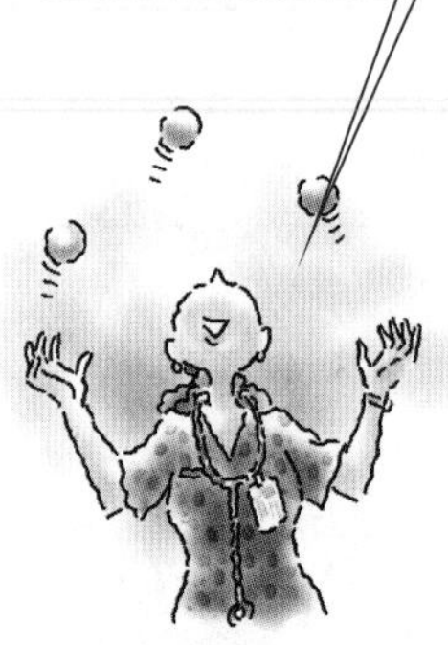

The numbers just keep coming!

101. A child is prescribed aspirin as part of the therapy for Kawasaki disease. The order is for 80 mg/kg/day orally in four divided doses until the child is afebrile. The child weighs 15 kg. How much is given in one dose?

1. 60 mg
2. 300 mg
3. 320 mg
4. 1,200 mg

101. 2. The child should receive 300 mg in one dose. Use the following equation:
First, determine how many mg should be given in one day:
80 mg/kg × 15 kg = 1,200 mg
Then, determine how many mg should be given in one dose:
1,200 mg/4 doses = 300 mg/dose

CN: Physiological integrity; CNS: Pharmacological and parenteral therapies; CL: Analysis

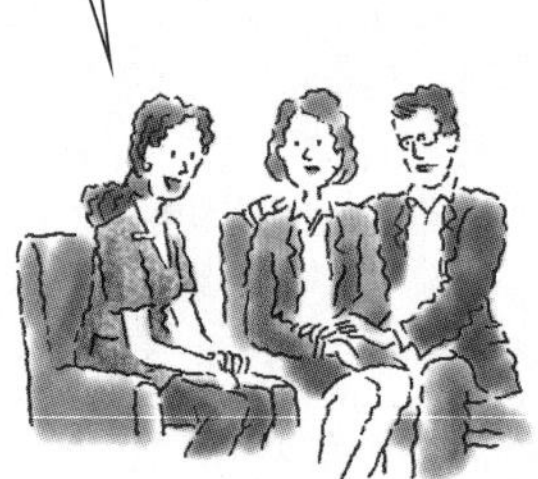

Listen for feedback to find out if your instructions were understood.

102. A nurse is giving discharge instructions to the parents of a child with Kawasaki disease. Which statement by the parents shows an understanding of the treatment plan?

1. "A regular diet can be resumed at home."
2. "Black, tarry stools are considered normal."
3. "My child should use a soft-bristled toothbrush."
4. "My child can return to playing football next week."

102. 3. Because of the anticoagulant effects of aspirin therapy, a soft-bristled toothbrush will prevent bleeding of the gums. A low-cholesterol diet should be followed until coronary artery involvement resolves. Black, tarry stools are abnormal and are signs of bleeding that should be reported to the physician immediately. Contact sports should be avoided because of the cardiac involvement and excessive bruising that may occur as a result of aspirin therapy.

CN: Physiological integrity; CNS: Physiological adaptation; CL: Analysis

103. A nurse is preparing the family of a client with Kawasaki disease for discharge. Which instruction is most appropriate?

1. Stop the aspirin when you return home.
2. Immunizations can be given in 2 weeks.
3. The child may return to school in 1 week.
4. Frequent echocardiography will be needed.

103. 4. Because of the risk of coronary artery involvement and possible aneurysm development, repeat echocardiography and electrocardiography will be required the first few weeks and at 6 months. Aspirin therapy may be continued for 2 weeks after the onset of symptoms. If signs of coronary artery involvement are present, aspirin therapy may be continued indefinitely. Live-virus vaccines should be avoided for 6 to 11 months after gamma globulin therapy because of an increased risk of a cross-sensitivity reaction to the antibodies found in the dose given. Returning to school should be avoided until cleared by the physician.

CN: Physiological integrity; CNS: Physiological adaptation; CL: Analysis

104. A nurse is teaching the parents of a child with acute rheumatic fever about the disorder. Which statement would be the most accurate concerning this condition?

1. A progressive inflammation of the small vessels
2. A mucocutaneous lymph node syndrome
3. A serious infection of the endocardial surface of the heart
4. A sequela of group A beta-hemolytic streptococcal infections

104. 4. Acute rheumatic fever is a multisystem disorder caused by group A beta-hemolytic streptococcal infections. It may involve the heart, joints, central nervous system, and skin. Kawasaki disease is also known as a mucocutaneous lymph node syndrome characterized by a progressive inflammation of the small vessels. Endocarditis describes a serious infection of the endocardial surface of the heart.

CN: Health promotion and maintenance; CNS: None; CL: Application

Read carefully. Question 104 asks about acute rheumatic fever, not chronic.

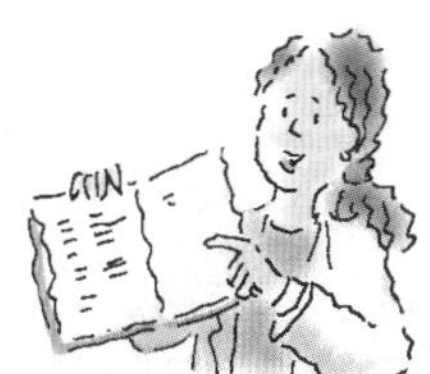

105. Which assessment finding is expected in a child with acute rheumatic fever?

1. Leukocytosis
2. Normal electrocardiogram
3. High fever for 5 or more days
4. Normal erythrocyte sedimentation rate

105. 1. Leukocytosis can be seen as an immune response triggered by colonization of the pharynx with group A streptococci. The electrocardiogram will show a prolonged PR interval as a result of carditis. The inflammatory response will cause an elevated erythrocyte sedimentation rate. A low-grade fever is a minor manifestation. A high fever of 5 or more days may represent Kawasaki disease.

CN: Physiological integrity; CNS: Physiological adaptation; CL: Application

106. Which criteria is required to establish a diagnosis of acute rheumatic fever?

1. Laboratory tests
2. Fever and four Jones criteria
3. Positive blood cultures for *Staphylococcus* organisms
4. Use of Jones criteria and presence of a streptococcal infection

106. 4. Two major or one major and two minor manifestations from Jones criteria and the presence of a streptococcal infection justify the diagnosis of rheumatic fever. There's no single laboratory test for diagnosis. Fever and four diagnostic criteria are required to diagnose Kawasaki disease. Blood cultures would be positive for *Streptococcus*, not *Staphylococcus*, organisms.

CN: Physiological integrity; CNS: Physiological adaptation; CL: Analysis

I was just trying to "keep up with the Jones."

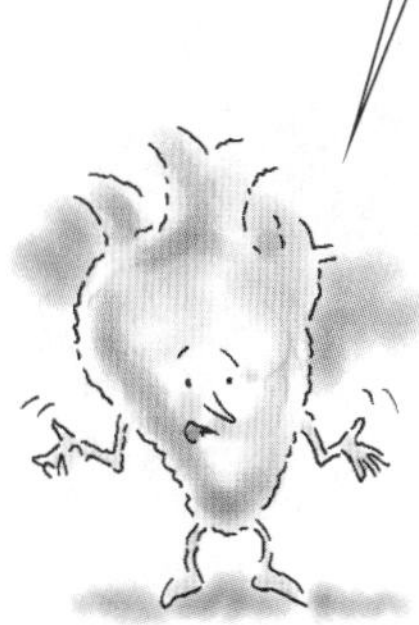

107. Which diagnostic criteria is considered major for Jones criteria for acute rheumatic fever?

1. Carditis
2. Prolonged PR interval
3. Low-grade fever
4. Previous heart disease

107. 1. Carditis is a major diagnostic criteria of acute rheumatic fever. It's the only manifestation that can lead to death or long-term sequelae. Prolonged PR interval, low-grade fever, and previous heart disease are considered minor diagnostic criteria for Jones criteria.

CN: Physiological integrity; CNS: Physiological adaptation; CL: Application

108. A nurse is caring for a child with acute rheumatic fever. Which symptom would indicate Sydenham's chorea, a major manifestation of acute rheumatic fever?

1. Cardiomegaly
2. Regurgitant murmur
3. Pericardial friction rubs
4. Involuntary muscle movements

108. 4. Sydenham's chorea is an involvement of the central nervous system by the rheumatic process. This is seen as muscular incoordination; purposeless, involuntary movements; and emotional lability. A regurgitant murmur, cardiomegaly, and a pericardial friction rub are clinical signs of rheumatic carditis.

CN: Physiological integrity; CNS: Physiological adaptation; CL: Application

109. Criteria for rheumatic fever are being discussed with parents. A nurse realizes that the parents understand chorea when they make which statement?

1. "My child may not be able to walk."
2. "Long movies may help for relaxation."
3. "My child might have difficulty in school."
4. "Many activities and visitors are recommended."

109. 3. Chorea may last 1 to 6 months. Central nervous system involvement contributes to a shortened attention span, so children might have difficulty learning in school. A quiet environment is required for treatment. Muscle incoordination may cause the child to be more clumsy than usual when walking.

CN: Physiological integrity; CNS: Physiological adaptation; CL: Analysis

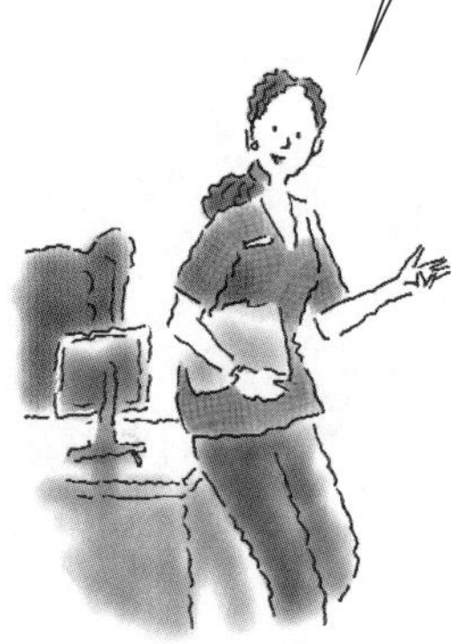

Question 110 is asking for the most appropriate intervention.

110. A 3-year-old child has a positive culture for *Streptococcus* organisms. Which intervention is most appropriate?

1. Give aspirin.
2. Give antibiotics.
3. Give corticosteroids.
4. Encourage fluid intake.

110. 2. Infection caused by *Streptococcus* organisms is treated with antibiotics, mainly penicillin. Antipyretics, such as acetaminophen, may be given for fever. Aspirin isn't recommended. Corticosteroids have no implication. Fluid intake is encouraged to prevent dehydration from decreased oral intake due to the sore throat or to replace fluids lost because of possible diarrhea from the antibiotics.

CN: Physiological integrity; CNS: Physiological adaptation; CL: Analysis

111. A nurse is preparing a child for discharge after being diagnosed with rheumatic fever without carditis. What instructions should the nurse give the parents?

1. Give aspirin for signs of chorea.
2. Give penicillin for 1 month total.
3. Only give penicillin for dental work.
4. It isn't necessary to give penicillin before dental procedures.

111. 4. Children who might benefit from prophylactic penicillin include those with unrepaired congenital heart defects, heart defects repaired with synthetic material, or prior infective endocarditis, and some children with heart transplants. Prophylactic antibiotic therapy isn't otherwise recommended.

CN: Physiological integrity; CNS: Pharmacological and parenteral therapies; CL: Application

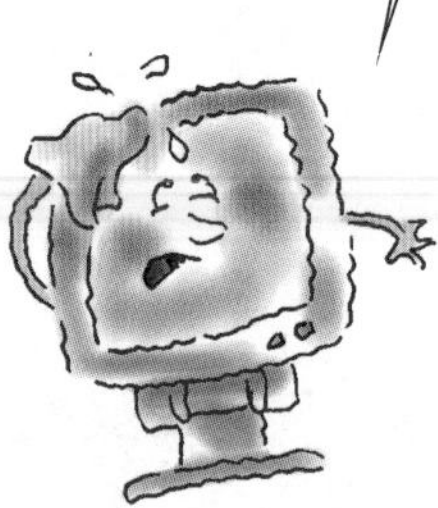

112. Which nursing diagnosis is most appropriate for a child with rheumatic fever?

1. *Imbalanced nutrition: More than body requirements*
2. *Risk for injury*
3. *Delayed growth and development*
4. *Impaired gas exchange*

112. 2. Because of symptoms of chorea, safety measures should be taken to prevent falls or injury. There may be *Imbalanced nutrition: Less than body requirements* due to a sore throat and dysphagia. Growth and development usually aren't delayed. *Impaired gas exchange* usually isn't an issue unless the condition worsens with carditis and heart failure is present.

CN: Physiological integrity; CNS: Physiological adaptation; CL: Analysis

CN: Client needs category CNS: Client needs subcategory CL: Cognitive level

113. The nurse is teaching the parents of a child with sinus bradycardia. Which statement about the condition is the most correct?

1. "It is a heart rate less than normal for age."
2. "It is a heart rate greater than normal for age."
3. "It is a variation of the normal cardiac rhythm."
4. "It is an increase in sinus node impulse formation."

113. 1. Sinus bradycardia can best be described as a heart rate less than normal for age. Sinus tachycardia refers to a heart rate greater than normal for age or an increase in sinus node impulse formation. A sinus arrhythmia is a variation of the normal cardiac rhythm.

CN: Physiological integrity; CNS: Physiological adaptation; CL: Application

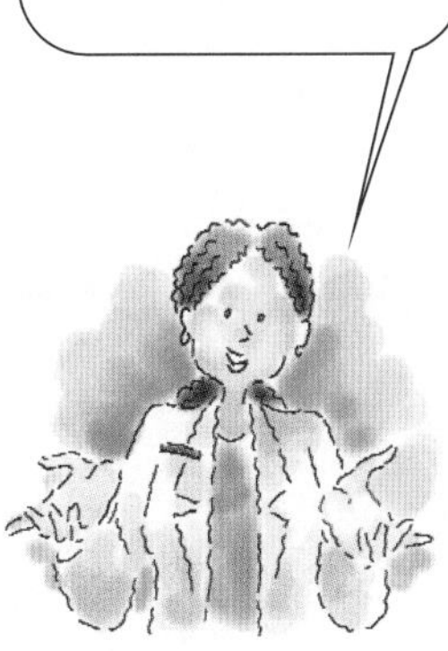

Sometimes abnormal is normal, and vice versa!

114. In which condition or group is sinus bradycardia a normal finding?

1. Hypoxia
2. Hypothermia
3. Growth-delayed adolescent
4. Physically conditioned adolescent

114. 4. A physically conditioned adolescent might have a lower than normal heart rate; this is of no significance. Hypoxia and hypothermia are pathologic states in which a slow heart rate may produce a compromised hemodynamic state. Growth-delayed adolescents won't have bradycardia as a normal finding.

CN: Physiological integrity; CNS: Physiological adaptation; CL: Analysis

115. Treatment for a child with sinus bradycardia includes atropine 0.02 mg/kg/dose. If the child weighs 20 kg, how much is given per dose?

1. 0.02 mg
2. 0.04 mg
3. 0.2 mg
4. 0.4 mg

115. 4. The child should receive 0.4 mg. Use the following equation:

$0.02 \text{ mg/kg} \times 20 \text{ kg} = 0.4 \text{ mg}$

CN: Physiological integrity; CNS: Pharmacological and parenteral therapies; CL: Analysis

116. Atropine, an anticholinergic agent, is being administered to a child with sinus bradycardia. Which statement is the most accurate about the administration of this medication?

1. It increases heart rate.
2. It raises blood pressure.
3. It dilates bronchial tubes.
4. It decreases heart rate.

116. 1. Atropine blocks vagal impulses to the myocardium and stimulates the cardio-inhibitory center in the medulla, thereby increasing heart rate and cardiac output. Atropine is not given to directly increase blood pressure or dilate the bronchial tubes.

CN: Physiological integrity; CNS: Pharmacological and parenteral therapies; CL: Application

117. A nurse has given atropine to treat sinus bradycardia in an 11-month-old infant. Which adverse reaction may be noted?

1. Lethargy
2. Diarrhea
3. No tears when crying
4. Increased urine output

117. 3. Atropine dries up secretions and also lessens the response of ciliary and iris sphincter muscles in the eye, causing mydriasis. It usually causes paradoxical excitement in children. Constipation and urinary retention can be seen due to a decrease in smooth-muscle contractions of the GI and genitourinary tracts.

CN: Physiological integrity; CNS: Pharmacological and parenteral therapies; CL: Application

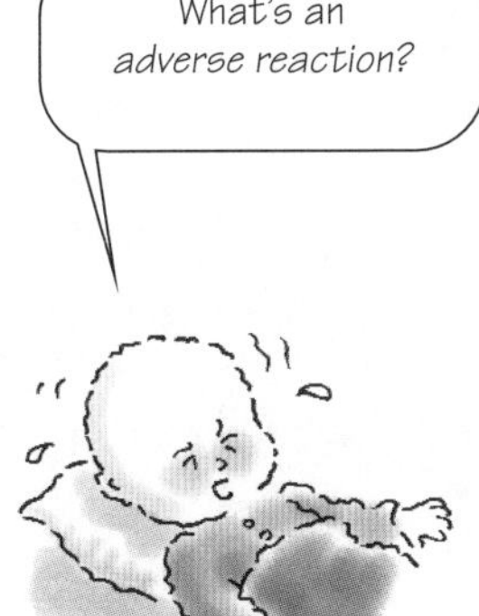

What's an adverse reaction?

118. Which condition could cause sinus tachycardia?
1. Fever
2. Hypothermia
3. Hypothyroidism
4. Hypoxia

118. 1. Sinus tachycardia is commonly seen in children with a fever. It's usually a result of a noncardiac cause. Hypothermia, hypothyroidism, and hypoxia will result in sinus bradycardia.
CN: Physiological integrity; CNS: Physiological adaptation; CL: Analysis

119. Which arrhythmia commonly seen in children involves heart rate changes related to respirations?
1. Sinus arrhythmia
2. Sinus block
3. Sinus bradycardia
4. Sinus tachycardia

119. 1. In sinus arrhythmia, heart rate increases with inhalation and decreases with exhalation in response to changes in intrathoracic pressure during respiration. Sinus arrhythmia is a common occurrence in childhood and adolescence. Sinus block, sinus bradycardia, and sinus tachycardia are respiration-independent arrhythmias.
CN: Physiological integrity; CNS: Physiological adaptation; CL: Analysis

120. Which condition may lead to sinus arrest or sinus pause in a child?
1. Hypokalemia
2. Hyperthermia
3. Valsalva's maneuver
4. Decreased intracranial pressure

120. 3. Sinus arrest may occur in children when vagal tone is increased such as during Valsalva's maneuver in vomiting, gagging, or straining during a bowel movement. This represents a failure of the sinoatrial node to generate an impulse. A straight line or pause occurs, indicating the absence of electrical activity. After the pause, another impulse will be generated and a cardiac complex will appear. Hyperkalemia, hypothermia, and increased intracranial pressure are pathologic conditions that may also produce sinus arrest.
CN: Physiological integrity; CNS: Physiological adaptation; CL: Analysis

121. Which statement is the most correct regarding the use of amiodarone (Cordarone)?
1. It is used to treat atrial dysrhythmias.
2. It is used to treat ventricular dysrhythmias.
3. It is used to treat both atrial and ventricular dysrhythmias.
4. It is used to treat heart failure.

121. 3. Amiodarone is used to treat both atrial and ventricular dysrhythmias. It is not used in the treatment of heart failure.
CN: Physiological integrity; CNS: Pharmacological and parenteral therapies; CL: Application

122. To which classification does isoproterenol belong?
1. Adrenergic agonist
2. Anticholinergic
3. Beta-adrenergic blocker
4. Vasopressor

122. 3. Isoproterenol acts as a beta-adrenergic blocker to reduce peripheral resistance and increase the force of cardiac contraction without producing vasoconstriction. It also acts as a bronchodilator, relaxing bronchial smooth muscle and creating peripheral vasodilation.

CN: Physiological integrity; CNS: Pharmacological and parenteral therapies; CL: Analysis

123. Which finding may be seen in a 1-year-old child with supraventricular tachycardia?
1. Heart rate of 100 beats/minute
2. Heart rate of 180 beats/minute
3. Heart rate less than 80 beats/minute
4. Heart rate more than 240 beats/minute

123. 4. Supraventricular tachycardia may be related to increased automaticity of an atrial cell other than the sinoatrial node, or as a reentry mechanism. The rhythm is regular and can occur at rates of 240 beats/minute or more. A heart rate of 100 beats/minute is a normal finding for a 1-year-old child. A heart rate around 180 beats/minute may represent sinus tachycardia. A heart rate of less than 80 beats/minute can be characterized as sinus bradycardia.

CN: Physiological integrity; CNS: Physiological adaptation; CL: Analysis

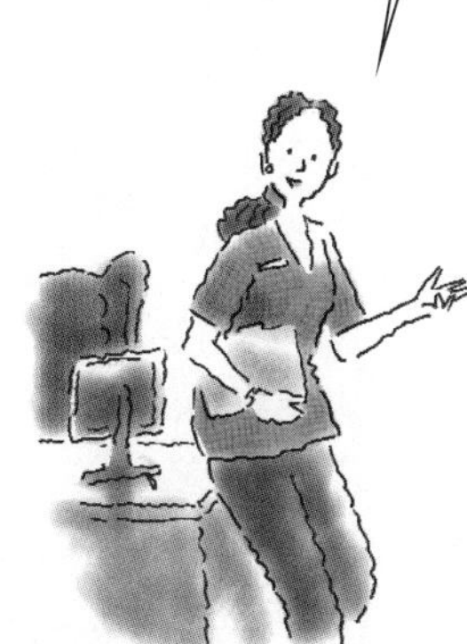

In question 124, the word first is your clue to the right answer.

124. A 2-year-old child is experiencing supraventricular tachycardia. Which intervention should be attempted first?
1. Administration of digoxin
2. Administration of verapamil
3. Synchronized cardioversion
4. Immersion of the child's hands in cold water

124. 4. Vagal maneuvers such as immersion of the hands in cold water are commonly tried first as a mechanism to decrease the heart rate. Other vagal maneuvers include breath-holding, carotid massage, gagging, and placing the head lower than the rest of the body. Synchronized cardioversion may be required if vagal maneuvers and drugs are ineffective. If a child has low cardiac output, cardioversion may be used instead of drugs. Verapamil isn't recommended. Digoxin is one of the most common drugs given to help decrease heart rate by increasing myocardial contractility and automaticity and reducing excitability.

CN: Physiological integrity; CNS: Reduction of risk potential; CL: Application

125. A 2-month-old infant arrives in the emergency department with a heart rate of 180 beats/minute and a temperature of 103.1° F (39.5° C) rectally. Which intervention is most appropriate?
1. Give acetaminophen (Tylenol).
2. Encourage fluid intake.
3. Apply carotid massage.
4. Place the infant's hands in cold water.

125. 1. Acetaminophen should be given first to decrease the temperature. A heart rate of 180 beats/minute is normal in an infant with a fever. A tepid sponge bath may be given to help decrease the temperature and calm the infant. Carotid massage is an attempt to decrease the heart rate as a vagal maneuver. This won't work in this infant because the source of the increased heart rate is fever. Fluid intake is encouraged after the acetaminophen is given to help replace insensible fluid losses.

CN: Physiological integrity; CNS: Physiological adaptation; CL: Application

126. A critically ill 4-year-old is in the pediatric intensive care unit. Telemetry monitoring reveals junctional tachycardia. Identify where this arrhythmia originates.

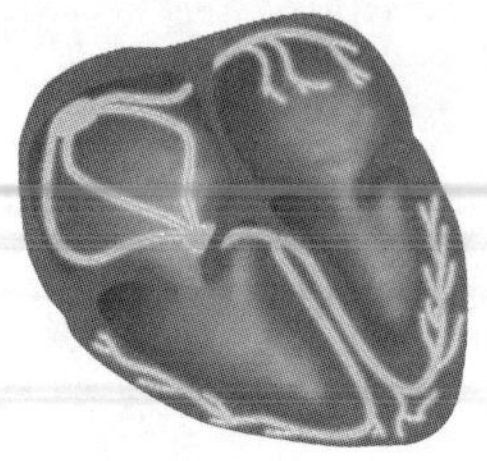

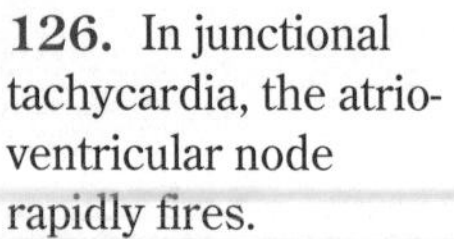

126. In junctional tachycardia, the atrioventricular node rapidly fires.

CN: Physiological integrity; CNS: Physiological adaptation; CL: Analysis

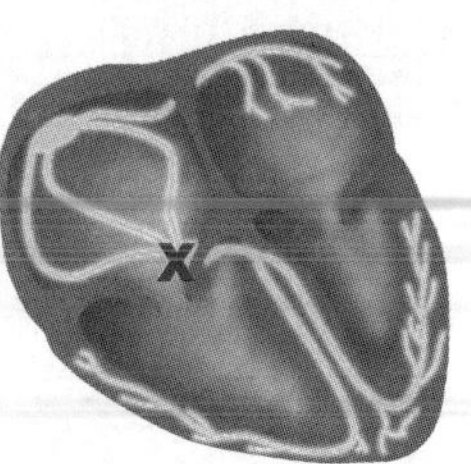

127. An infant who weighs 8 kg is to receive ampicillin 25 mg/kg I.V. every 6 hours. How many milligrams should the nurse administer per dose? Record your answer using a whole number.

______________________ milligrams

127. 200. The nurse should calculate the correct dose using the following equation:

$25 \text{ mg/kg} \times 8 \text{ kg} = 200 \text{ mg}$.

CN: Physiological integrity; CNS: Pharmacological and parenteral therapies; CL: Application

128. The nurse is caring for an infant with a heart defect that involves increased pulmonary blood flow. Which illustration shows a congenital heart disorder with increased pulmonary blood flow?

1.

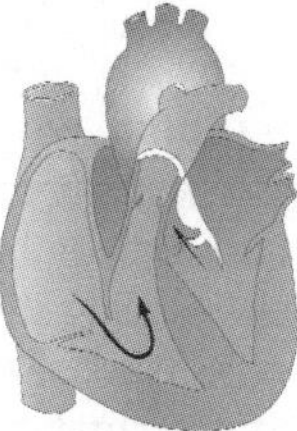

2.

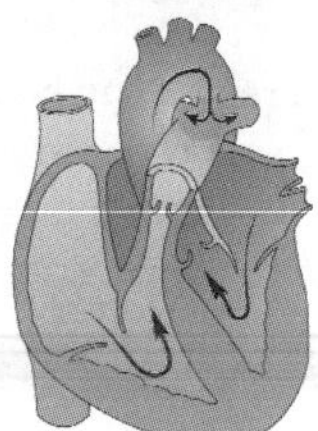

3.

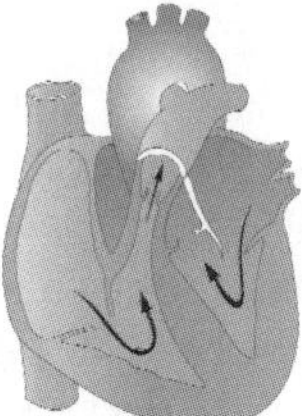

4.

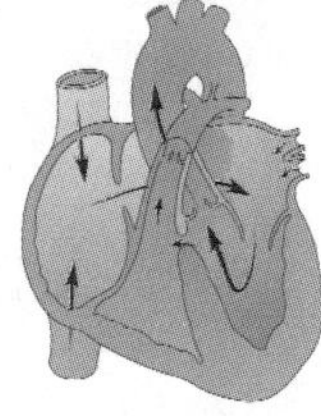

128. 2. In patent ductus arteriosus, an accessory fetal structure that connects the pulmonary artery to the aorta fails to close at birth. This allows blood to shunt from the aorta to the pulmonary artery. Option 1 depicts aortic stenosis (narrowed aortic valve) and option 3 shows pulmonic stenosis (narrowed pulmonic valve); both are obstruction to blood flow disorders. Option 4 shows tricuspid atresia (failure of the tricuspid valve to develop), a decreased pulmonary blood flow disorder.

CN: Physiological integrity; CNS: Physiological adaptation; CL: Analysis

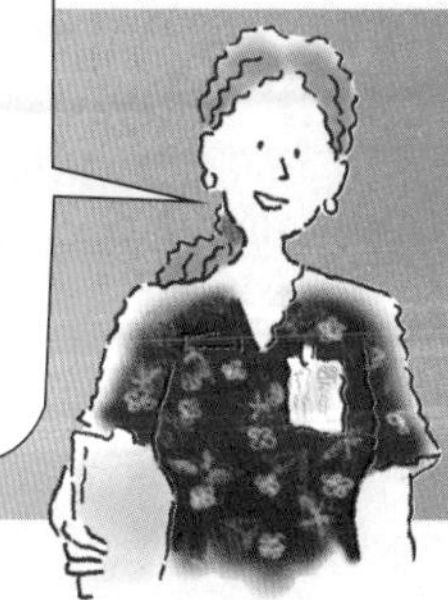

This chapter covers sickle cell disease, varicella, Rocky Mountain spotted fever, leukemia, and many other blood and immune system disorders in kids. It's a whopper of a chapter on a critically important area. If you're ready, let's begin!

Chapter 28
Hematologic & immune disorders

1. A child comes to the emergency department feeling feverish and lethargic. Which assessment finding suggests Reye's syndrome?

1. Fever, profoundly impaired consciousness, and hepatomegaly
2. Fever, splenomegaly, and hyperactive reflexes
3. Afebrile, intractable vomiting, and rhinorrhea
4. Malaise, cough, and sore throat

1. 1. Reye's syndrome is defined as toxic encephalopathy, characterized by fever, profoundly impaired consciousness, and disordered hepatic function. Intractable vomiting occurs during the first stage of Reye's syndrome, but rhinorrhea usually precedes the onset of the illness. Reye's syndrome doesn't affect the spleen but causes fatty degeneration of the liver. Hyperactive reflexes occur with central nervous system involvement. Malaise, cough, and sore throat are viral symptoms that commonly precede the illness.

CN: Physiological integrity; CNS: Physiological adaptation; CL: Analysis

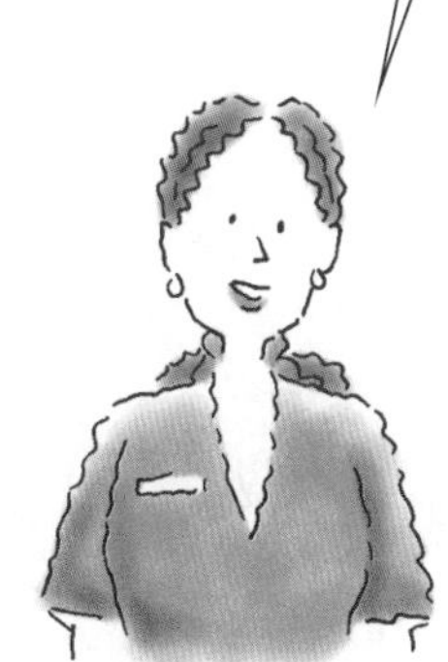

Early diagnosis is crucial to treating Reye's syndrome.

2. Which aspect is most important for successful management of the child with Reye's syndrome?

1. Early diagnosis
2. Initiation of antibiotics
3. Isolation of the child
4. Staging of the illness

2. 1. Early diagnosis and therapy are essential because of the rapid clinical course of the disease and its high mortality. Reye's syndrome is associated with a viral illness, and antibiotic therapy isn't crucial to preventing the initial progression of the illness. Isolation isn't necessary because the disease isn't communicable. Staging, although important to therapy, occurs after a differential diagnosis is made.

CN: Physiological integrity; CNS: Reduction of risk potential; CL: Application

3. A child with Reye's syndrome is in stage I of the illness. Which measure can be taken to prevent further progression of the illness?

1. Invasive monitoring
2. Endotracheal intubation
3. Hypertonic glucose solution
4. Pancuronium bromide (Pavulon)

3. 3. For children in stage I of Reye's syndrome, treatment is primarily supportive and directed toward restoring blood glucose levels and correcting acid-base imbalances. I.V. administration of dextrose solutions with added insulin helps to replace glycogen stores. Noninvasive monitoring is adequate to assess status at this stage. Endotracheal intubation may be necessary later. Pancuronium bromide is used as an adjunct to endotracheal intubation and wouldn't be used in this stage of Reye's syndrome.

CN: Physiological integrity; CNS: Reduction of risk potential; CL: Application

4. Which group of laboratory results, along with the clinical manifestations, establishes a diagnosis of Reye's syndrome?

1. Elevated liver enzymes and prolonged prothrombin and partial thromboplastin times
2. Increased serum glucose and insulin levels
3. Increased bilirubin and alkaline phosphatase levels
4. Decreased serum glucose and ammonia levels

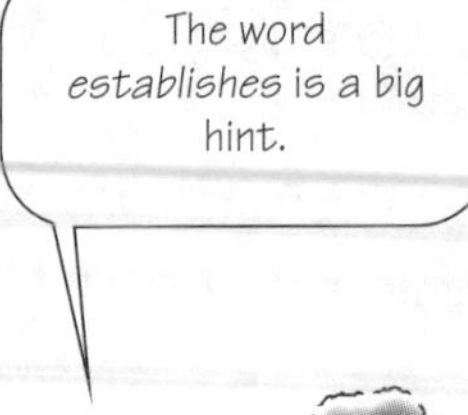
The word establishes is a big hint.

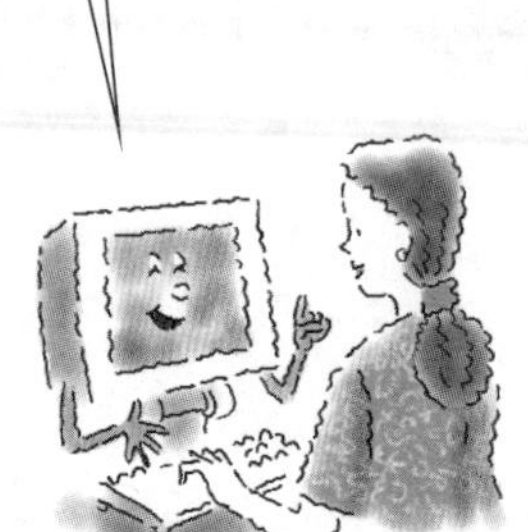

4. 1. Reye's syndrome causes fatty degeneration of the liver, altering results of liver function studies. Decreased serum glucose levels, with reduced insulin levels, occur secondary to dehydration caused by intractable vomiting. Serum bilirubin and alkaline phosphatase usually aren't affected.

CN: Physiological integrity; CNS: Physiological adaptation; CL: Analysis

5. In the latter stages of Reye's syndrome, which major intervention is directed toward preventing or reducing cerebral edema?

1. Noninvasive pressure monitoring
2. Paralysis and sedation
3. Liberal fluid replacement
4. Nonassisted ventilation

5. 2. Skeletal muscles are paralyzed with the administration of pancuronium (Pavulon). This prevents activity, especially coughing, that might increase intracranial pressure (ICP). Invasive monitoring is essential to detect increased ICP. Liberal fluid replacement may increase cerebral edema and should be strictly monitored. Tracheal intubation is performed as soon as possible to prevent hypoventilation and increased carbon dioxide levels.

CN: Physiological integrity; CNS: Reduction of risk potential; CL: Analysis

6. Which assessment change would indicate increased intracranial pressure (ICP) in a child acutely ill with Reye's syndrome?

1. Irritability and quick pupil response
2. Increased blood pressure and decreased heart rate
3. Decreased blood pressure and increased heart rate
4. Sluggish pupil response and decreased blood pressure

6. 2. A marked increase in ICP will trigger the pressure response; increased ICP produces an elevation in blood pressure with a reflex slowing of the heart rate. Irritability is commonly an early sign, but pupillary response becomes more sluggish in response to increased ICP.

CN: Physiological integrity; CNS: Physiological adaptation; CL: Application

7. A client with Reye's syndrome is exhibiting increased intracranial pressure (ICP). Which nursing intervention would be the most appropriate for this client?

1. Position the child with the head elevated and the neck in a neutral position.
2. Maintain the child in the prone position.
3. Cluster together interventions that may be perceived as noxious.
4. Position the child in the supine position, with the child's head turned to the side.

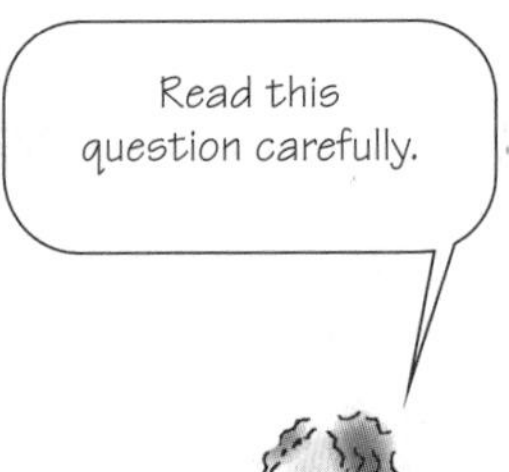
Read this question carefully.

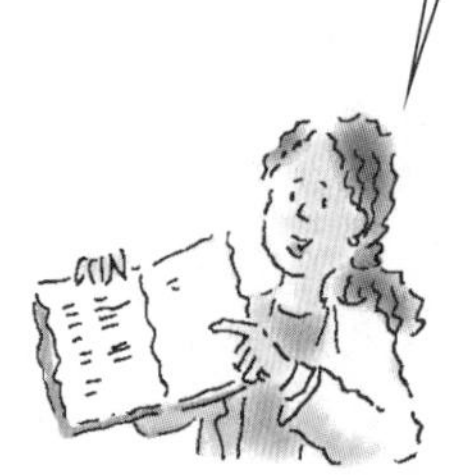

7. 1. Positioning the child with the head elevated and neck in the neutral position helps decrease ICP. The prone and supine positions cause increased ICP. Interventions that may be perceived as noxious should be spaced over time because, if clustered together, they may have a cumulative effect in increasing ICP. Turning the head to the side may impede venous return from the head and increase ICP.

CN: Physiological integrity; CNS: Physiological adaptation; CL: Application

8. The goal of nursing care for a client with Reye's syndrome is to minimize intracranial pressure (ICP). Which nursing intervention helps to meet this goal?

1. Keeping the head of bed flat
2. Frequent position changes
3. Positioning to avoid neck flexion
4. Suctioning and chest physiotherapy

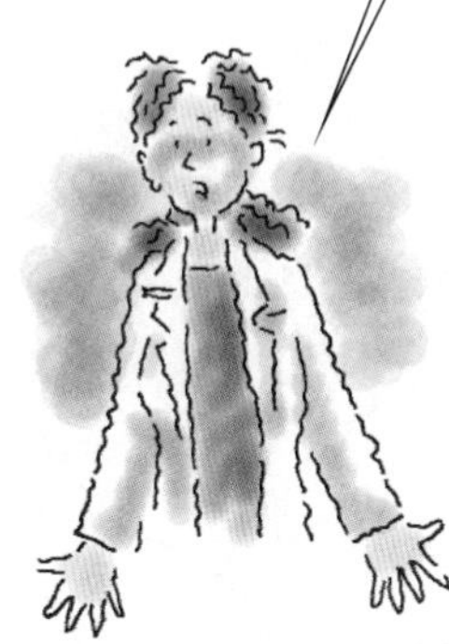

Stay calm when encountering NCLEX questions you're unsure about. That's what I do.

8. 3. Jugular vein compression can increase ICP by interfering with venous return. The head of the bed should be elevated to help promote venous return. Nursing procedures such as frequent positioning tend to cause overstimulation; therefore, care should be taken to avoid such procedures to prevent increased ICP. Suctioning and percussion are poorly tolerated and are contraindicated, unless concurrent respiratory problems are present.
CN: Physiological integrity; CNS: Physiological adaptation; CL: Application

9. Which nursing intervention should be included in the care of an unconscious child with Reye's syndrome?

1. Keeping the arms and legs flexed
2. Placing the child on a sheepskin
3. Avoiding the use of lotions on the skin
4. Placing the client in a supine position

9. 2. Placing the child on a sheepskin helps to prevent pressure on prominent areas of the body. Keeping extremities in a flexed position can lead to contractures. Rubbing the extremities with lotion stimulates circulation and helps prevent drying of the skin. Placing the child supine would be contraindicated because of the risk of aspiration and increasing intracranial pressure. The supine position puts undue pressure on the sacral and occipital areas.
CN: Physiological integrity; CNS: Physiological adaptation; CL: Application

10. Which medication has been connected to the development of Reye's syndrome?

1. Acetaminophen (Tylenol)
2. Aspirin
3. Ibuprofen (Motrin)
4. Guaifenesin (Robitussin)

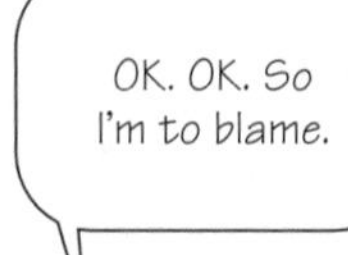

OK. OK. So I'm to blame.

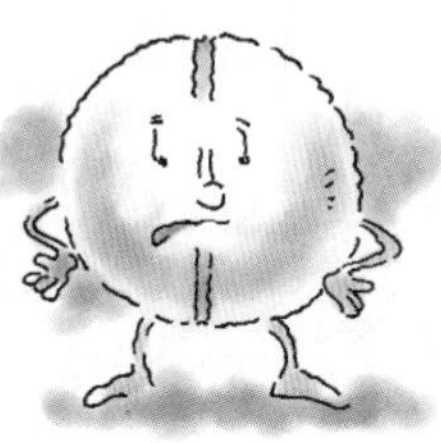

10. 2. Aspirin administration is associated with the development of Reye's syndrome. Acetaminophen, ibuprofen, and guaifenesin haven't been associated with the development of Reye's syndrome. In fact, there has been a decreased incidence of Reye's syndrome with the increased use of acetaminophen and ibuprofen for management of fevers in children.
CN: Physiological integrity; CNS: Pharmacological and parenteral therapies; CL: Application

11. Parents should be told to stop acetylsalicylic acid (aspirin) administration and notify a physician if their child is exposed to which condition?

1. Stress
2. Scabies
3. Influenza
4. Environmental allergies

11. 3. A strong association exists between influenza and aspirin administration and the development of Reye's syndrome. There's no contraindication with the other conditions.
CN: Physiological integrity; CNS: Pharmacological and parenteral therapies; CL: Application

12. Which nursing intervention should be included in the care of a client with Reye's syndrome who's receiving pancuronium (Pavulon)?

1. Applying artificial tears as needed
2. Providing regular tactile stimulation
3. Performing active range-of-motion (ROM) exercises
4. Placing the client in a supine position

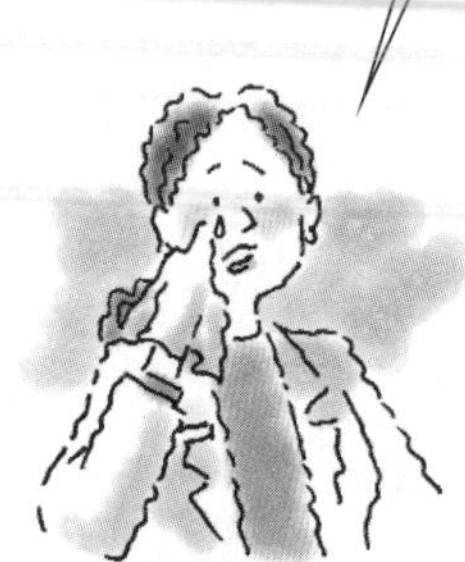

You're doing so well I'm going to cry.

12. 1. Pancuronium suppresses the corneal reflex, making the eyes prone to irritation. Artificial tears prevent drying. Tactile stimulation isn't appropriate because it may elicit a pressure response. Active ROM exercises may cause an increase in pressure. The head of the bed should be elevated slightly, with the paralyzed client in a side-lying or semiprone position to prevent aspiration and minimize intracranial pressure.

CN: Physiological integrity; CNS: Pharmacological and parenteral therapies; CL: Application

13. Which goal should be achieved by performing a craniotomy on a client with Reye's syndrome?

1. Decreasing carbon dioxide levels
2. Determining the extent of brain injury
3. Reducing pressure from an edematous brain
4. Allowing continuous monitoring of intracranial pressure (ICP)

13. 3. In severe cases of cerebral edema, creating bilateral bone flaps (craniotomy) is most effective in decreasing ICP. Carbon dioxide levels can be decreased through mechanical ventilation. Most clients with Reye's syndrome recover without any resulting brain injury. Continuous monitoring of ICP is implemented through central venous pressure lines.

CN: Physiological integrity; CNS: Reduction of risk potential; CL: Analysis

14. Parents of a child with Reye's syndrome need a great deal of emotional support. Which nursing intervention should be included to reduce stress and alleviate fears?

1. Not accepting aggressive behavior from the parents
2. Encouraging the parents not to overreact and to hope for the best
3. Letting the parents interpret the child's behaviors and responses
4. Explaining therapies and clarifying or reinforcing the information given

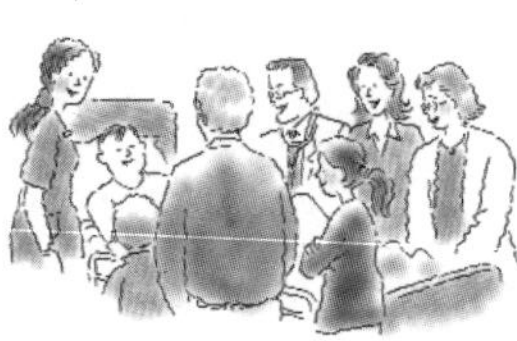

Be sensitive not only to your client's needs, but to the family's needs as well.

14. 4. Explaining treatments and therapies will help to alleviate undue stress in the parents. An awareness of the potential for aggressive behaviors provides nurses with the understanding that helps them support the parents in their grief. Being too quick to reassure may block a parent's expression of fears. Parents may need help interpreting their child's behavior to avoid assigning erroneous meanings to the many signs their child exhibits.

CN: Psychosocial integrity; CNS: None; CL: Application

15. Which clinical manifestation should you expect to see in a client in stage V of Reye's syndrome?

1. Vomiting, lethargy, and drowsiness
2. Seizures, flaccidity, and respiratory arrest
3. Hyperventilation and coma
4. Disorientation, aggressiveness, and combativeness

15. 2. Staging criteria were developed to help evaluate the client's progress and to evaluate the efficacy of therapies. The clinical manifestations of stage V include seizures, loss of deep tendon reflexes, flaccidity, and respiratory arrest. Vomiting, lethargy, and drowsiness occur in stage I. Hyperventilation and coma occur in stage III. Disorientation and aggressive behavior occur in stage II.

CN: Physiological integrity; CNS: Physiological adaptation; CL: Analysis

16. A nurse is administering an immunization to a 2-month-old child. Which immunity will the child form?

1. Acquired immunity
2. Active immunity
3. Natural immunity
4. Passive immunity

16. 2. Active immunity occurs when the individual forms immune bodies against certain diseases, either by having the disease or by the introduction of a vaccine into the individual. Acquired immunity results from exposure to the bacteria, virus, or toxins. Natural immunity is resistance to infection or toxicity. Passive immunity is a temporary immunity caused by transfusion of immune plasma proteins.

CN: Health promotion and maintenance; CNS: None; CL: Application

17. The parent of a neonate asks the nurse what is the recommended age for beginning hepatitis B immunization. Which response is the most accurate?

1. Birth
2. 4 months
3. 6 months
4. 1 year

17. 1. According to the American Academy of Pediatrics, birth to age 2 months is the recommended time for beginning hepatitis B immunizations.

CN: Health promotion and maintenance; CNS: None; CL: Application

18. It would be most appropriate for which infant to begin receiving the measles vaccine?

1. A 6-month-old
2. A 12-month-old
3. An 18-month-old
4. A 24-month-old

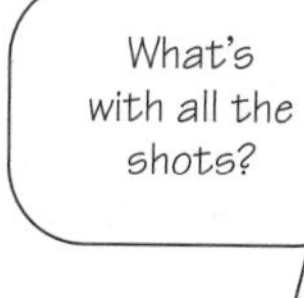

What's with all the shots?

18. 2. According to the American Academy of Pediatrics, the first dose of the measles vaccine should be administered at age 12 to 15 months.

CN: Health promotion and maintenance; CNS: None; CL: Application

19. Which immunization should a healthy 2-month-old infant receive?

1. Measles, mumps, rubella (MMR), and inactivated polio (IPV)
2. Measles, mumps, and rubella (MMR), and varicella
3. Diphtheria, tetanus, and pertussis (DTP), and influenza nasal mist
4. DTP and IPV

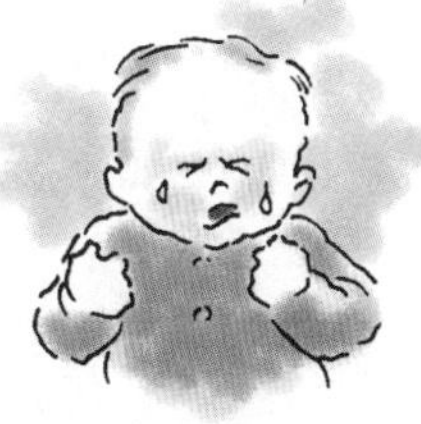

19. 4. At age 2 months, DTP and IPV are the recommended immunizations. DTP and IPV are given again at 4 months, and DTP is given again alone at 6 months. MMR is given at age 12 months. Influenza nasal mist is a weakened live vaccine which should be given to health individuals over 2 years of age.

CN: Health promotion and maintenance; CNS: None; CL: Application

20. The child who's diagnosed with thalassemia major (Cooley's anemia) typically suffers complications from the disease and from the treatment. This child is at risk for which condition?

1. Hypertrophy of the thyroid
2. Hypertrophy of the thymus
3. Polycythemia vera and thrombosis
4. Chronic hypoxia and iron overload

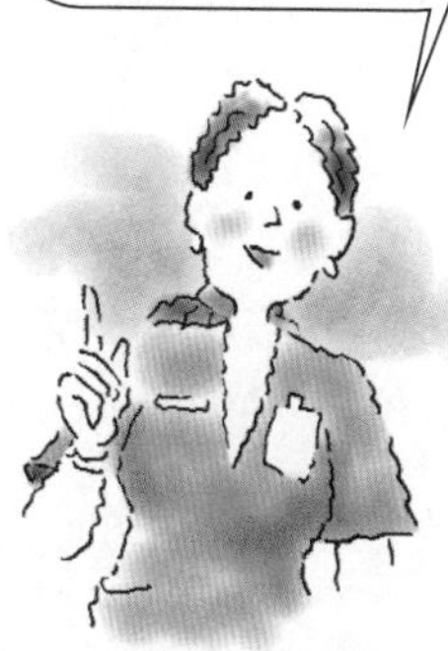

Test-taking tip: Read every question and all the options carefully before selecting your answer.

20. 4. In thalassemia major, increased destruction of red blood cells (RBCs) causes anemia. RBCs also have a shortened life span. The body responds by increasing the production of RBCs, but it can't adequately produce enough mature cells to meet the body's demands. This process results in chronic hypoxia. Children with the disorder are given multiple transfusions of packed RBCs. The combination of excessive RBC destruction and multiple transfusions causes too much iron to be deposited in organs and tissues and results in damage to the involved organs. The thymus and thyroid aren't involved. Polycythemia vera refers to excessive RBC production, which can result in thrombosis.

CN: Physiological integrity; CNS: Reduction of risk potential; CL: Analysis

21. Which is the treatment of choice for severe aplastic anemia?

1. Liver transplantation
2. Exchange transfusion
3. Bone marrow transplantation
4. Administration of intravenous immunoglobulins

21. 3. Aplastic anemia refers to either a congenital or an acquired condition in which severe pancytopenia, or decrease in cellular components of the blood, occurs. Children with the condition have profound anemia, are susceptible to infections, and risk bleeding. When a good match of donor bone marrow is available, transplantation is the treatment of choice. Liver transplantation, exchange transfusion, and the administration of intravenous immunoglobulins aren't treatments for aplastic anemia.

CN: Physiological integrity; CNS: Physiological adaptation; CL: Application

22. Which type of transfusion is most likely to be given to a child with sickle cell anemia?

1. Plasma
2. Platelets
3. Whole blood
4. Packed red blood cells (RBCs)

22. 4. Packed RBCs are given to children when their hemoglobin is dangerously low. Severe anemia decreases oxygen perfusion and leads to increased sickling of cells. Packed cells are RBCs with plasma removed. If enough whole blood were given to reach the desired hemoglobin level, fluid overload could occur. Thus, the plasma is removed and packed RBCs are infused. The RBCs are needed to transport oxygen. Platelets are given to children with low platelets, not anemia.

CN: Physiological integrity; CNS: Pharmacological and parenteral therapies; CL: Analysis

23. Which direction is <u>most important</u> when administering immunizations?

1. Properly store the vaccine, and follow the recommended procedure for injection.
2. Monitor clients for approximately 1 hour after administration for adverse reactions.
3. Take the vaccine out of refrigeration 1 hour before administration.
4. Inject multiple vaccines at the same injection site.

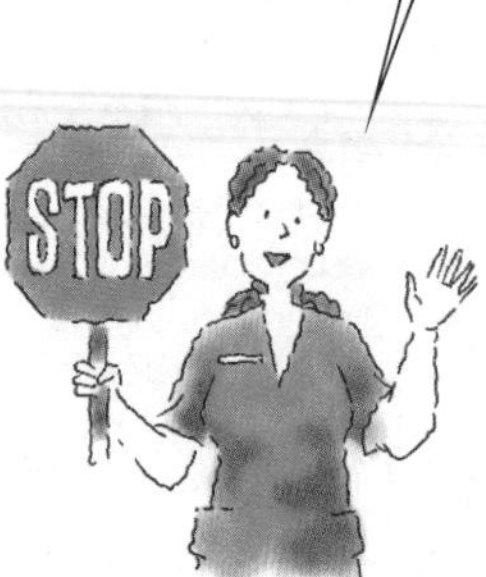

Stop and think: Which direction would be of primary importance?
STOP

23. 1. Vaccines must be properly stored to ensure their potency. The nurse must be familiar with the manufacturer's directions for storage and reconstitution of the vaccine. Faulty refrigeration is a major cause of primary vaccine failure. It isn't necessary to monitor the clients, but the nurse should teach parents to call the physician and report any adverse effects. Taking the vaccine out of refrigeration too early can affect its potency. If more than one vaccine is to be administered, different injection sites should be used. The nurse should note which vaccine is given and at what site in case of a local reaction.

CN: Health promotion and maintenance; CNS: None; CL: Application

24. Which symptom is the most common manifestation of severe combined immunodeficiency disease (SCID)?
1. Bruising
2. Failure to thrive
3. Prolonged bleeding
4. Susceptibility to infection

24. 4. SCID is characterized by absence of both humoral and cell-mediated immunity. The most common manifestation is susceptibility to infection early in life, most often by age 3 months. SCID is characterized by chronic infection, failure to completely recover from an infection, and frequent reinfection. The history reveals no logical source for infection. Failure to thrive is a consequence of persistent illnesses. Prolonged bleeding and bruising indicate abnormalities in the clotting system.

CN: Physiological integrity; CNS: Physiological adaptation; CL: Analysis

25. A child is admitted to the hospital for an asthma exacerbation. The nursing history reveals this client was exposed to chickenpox 1 week ago. When would this client require isolation, if he were to remain hospitalized?
1. Isolation isn't required.
2. Immediate isolation is required.
3. Isolation would be required 10 days after exposure.
4. Isolation would be required 12 days after exposure.

25. 2. The incubation period for chickenpox is 2 to 3 weeks, commonly 13 to 17 days. A client is commonly isolated 1 week after exposure to avoid the risk of an earlier breakout. A person is infectious from 1 day before eruption of lesions to 6 days after the vesicles have formed crusts.

CN: Safe, effective care environment; CNS: Safety and infection control; CL: Application

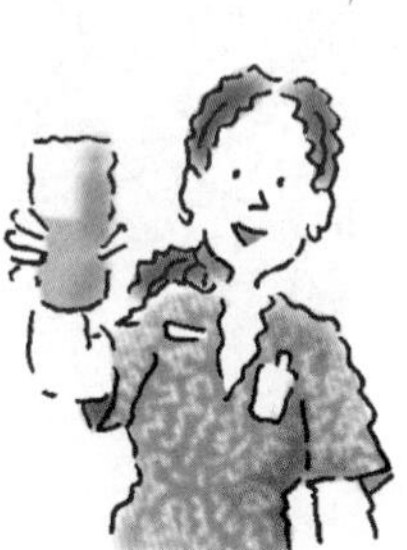

Here's to you! Twenty-five questions, and you're doing great.

26. On assessment of a child's skin, the nurse notes a papular pruritic rash with some vesicles. The rash is profuse on the trunk and sparse on the distal limbs. Based on this assessment, which illness does the client have?
1. Measles
2. Mumps
3. Roseola
4. Chickenpox

26. 4. Chickenpox rash is highly pruritic. The rash begins as a macule, rapidly progresses to a papule, then becomes a vesicle. All three stages are present in varying degrees at one time. Measles begins as an erythematous maculopapular eruption on the face; the eruption gradually spreads downward. Mumps isn't associated with a skin rash. Roseola rash is nonpruritic and is described as discrete rose-pink macules, appearing first on the trunk and then spreading to the neck, face, and extremities.

CN: Health promotion and maintenance; CNS: None; CL: Analysis

27. Which response would be appropriate to a parent inquiring about when her child with chickenpox can return to school?

1. When the child is afebrile
2. When all vesicles have dried
3. When vesicles begin to crust over
4. When lesions and vesicles are gone

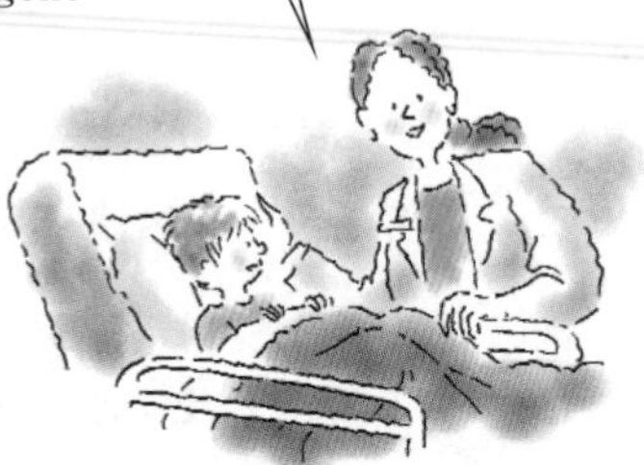

Chickenpox is highly contagious. Teach parents how to assess when it's safe to send kids back to school.

27. 2. Chickenpox is contagious. It's transmitted through direct contact, droplet spread, and contact with contaminated objects. Vesicles break open; therefore, a person is potentially contagious until all vesicles have dried. It isn't necessary to wait until dried lesions have disappeared. Some vesicles may be crusted over, and new ones may have formed. Macules, papules, vesicles, and crusting are present in varying degrees at one time. A child may be free from fever but continue to have vesicles. Isolation is usually necessary only for about 1 week after the onset of the disease.
CN: Health promotion and maintenance; CNS: None; CL: Analysis

28. Which symptoms are clinical manifestations associated with roseola?

1. Apparent sickness, fever, and rash
2. Fever for 3 to 4 days, followed by rash
3. Rash, without history of fever or illness
4. Rash for 3 to 4 days, followed by high fevers

28. 2. Roseola is manifested by persistent high fever for 3 to 4 days in a child who appears well. Fever precedes the rash. When the rash appears, a precipitous drop in fever occurs and the temperature returns to normal.
CN: Health promotion and maintenance; CNS: None; CL: Analysis

29. Which assessment finding is consistent with a roseola rash?

1. Maculopapular red spots
2. Macular and pruritic, with papules and vesicles
3. Rose-pink macules that fade on pressure
4. Red maculopapular eruption, beginning on the face

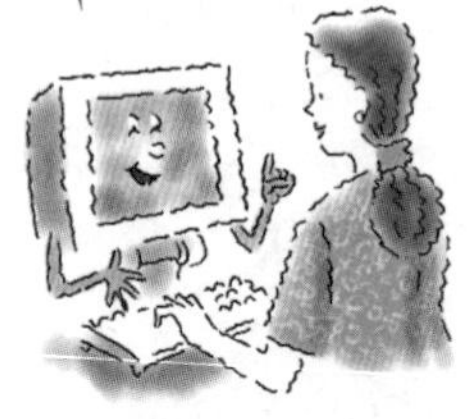

Read each question carefully, and don't do anything rash.

29. 3. Roseola rashes are discrete, rose-pink macules or maculopapules that fade on pressure and usually last 1 to 2 days. Maculopapular red spots may indicate fifth disease. Chickenpox rash is macular, with papules and vesicles. Roseola isn't pruritic. Measles begin as a maculopapular eruption on the face.
CN: Health promotion and maintenance; CNS: None; CL: Application

30. Which complication can be caused by a child with chickenpox scratching open and severely irritating the vesicles on his abdomen?

1. Myocarditis
2. Neuritis
3. Obstructive laryngitis
4. Secondary bacterial infection

30. 4. Secondary bacterial infections can occur as a complication of chickenpox. Irritation of skin lesions can lead to cellulitis or even an abscess. Myocarditis isn't considered a complication of chickenpox but has been noted as a complication of mumps. Neuritis has been associated with diphtheria. Obstructive laryngitis occurs as a complication of measles.
CN: Physiological integrity; CNS: Reduction of risk potential; CL: Application

31. Which characteristic best describes the cough of an infant who was admitted to the hospital with suspected pertussis?

1. Dry, hacking, more frequent on awakening
2. Loose and nonproductive
3. Occurring more frequently during the day
4. Harsh, associated with a high-pitched crowing sound

31. 4. The cough associated with pertussis is a harsh series of short, rapid coughs, followed by a sudden inspiration and a high-pitched crowing sound. Cheeks become flushed or cyanotic, eyes bulge, and the tongue protrudes. Paroxysm may continue until a thick mucus plug is dislodged. This cough occurs most commonly at night.

CN: Physiological integrity; CNS: Physiological adaptation; CL: Analysis

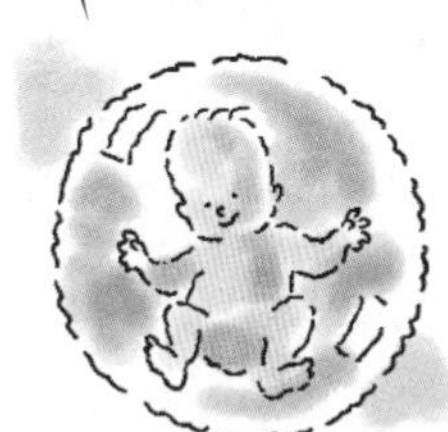
Think before you respond: Can I contract rubella?

32. Which communicable disease requires isolating an infected child from pregnant women?

1. Pertussis
2. Roseola
3. Rubella
4. Scarlet fever

32. 3. Rubella (German measles) has a teratogenic effect on the fetus. An infected child must be isolated from pregnant women. Pertussis, roseola, and scarlet fever don't have any teratogenic effects on a fetus.

CN: Safe, effective care environment; CNS: Safety and infection control; CL: Application

33. The nurse would expect the physician to order which medication as the treatment of choice for scarlet fever?

1. Acyclovir (Zovirax)
2. Amphotericin B
3. Ibuprofen (Motrin)
4. Penicillin

33. 4. The causative agent of scarlet fever is group A beta-hemolytic streptococci, which is susceptible to penicillin. Erythromycin is used for penicillin-sensitive children. Anti-inflammatory drugs, such as ibuprofen, aren't indicated for these clients. Acyclovir is used in the treatment of herpes infections. Amphotericin B is used to treat fungal infections.

CN: Physiological integrity; CNS: Pharmacological and parenteral therapies; CL: Application

34. Which period of isolation is indicated for a child with scarlet fever?

1. Until the associated rash disappears
2. Until completion of antibiotic therapy
3. Until the client is fever-free for 24 hours
4. Until 24 hours after initiation of treatment

34. 4. A child requires respiratory isolation until 24 hours after initiation of treatment. Rash may persist for 3 weeks. It isn't necessary to wait until the end of treatment. Fever usually breaks 24 hours after therapy has begun. It isn't necessary to maintain isolation for an additional 24 hours.

CN: Safe, effective care environment; CNS: Safety and infection control; CL: Application

35. Which instruction should be included in the teaching about care of a child with chickenpox?

1. Administer penicillin or erythromycin as ordered.
2. Administer local or systemic antipruritics as ordered.
3. Offer periods of interaction with other children to provide distraction.
4. Avoid administering varicella-zoster immune globulin to children receiving long-term salicylate therapy.

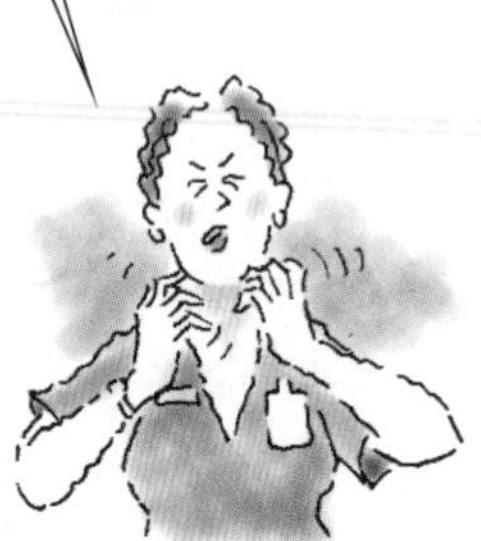

So this is what they mean by "highly pruritic."

35. 2. Chickenpox is highly pruritic. Preventing the child from scratching is necessary to prevent scarring and secondary infection caused by irritation of lesions. Penicillin and erythromycin aren't usually used in the treatment of chickenpox. Interaction with other children would be contraindicated because of the risk of communication, unless the other children previously have had chickenpox or been immunized. Varicella-zoster immune globulin *should* be administered to exposed children who are on long-term aspirin therapy because of the possible risk of Reye's syndrome.

CN: Physiological integrity; CNS: Pharmacological and parenteral therapies; CL: Application

36. A child is admitted with scarlet fever. Which causative agent does the nurse identify as a contributor to this infection?

1. Roseola
2. Staphylococcal parotitis
3. Streptococcal pharyngitis
4. Chickenpox

36. 3. The causative agent of scarlet fever is group A beta-hemolytic streptococci; therefore, scarlet fever may follow a strep throat infection. Roseola, parotitis, and chickenpox aren't strep infections and don't contribute to scarlet fever.

CN: Physiological integrity; CNS: Reduction of risk potential; CL: Analysis

37. A mother infected with human immunodeficiency virus (HIV) inquires about the possibility of breast-feeding her newborn. Which statement would be a correct response?

1. Breast-feeding isn't an option.
2. Breast-feeding would be best for your baby.
3. Breast-feeding is only an option if the mother is taking zidovudine (Retrovir).
4. Breast-feeding is an option if milk is expressed and fed by a bottle.

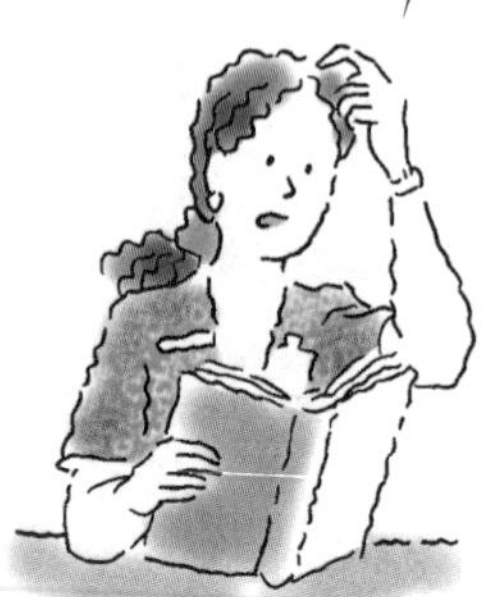

In which body fluids has HIV been isolated?

37. 1. Mothers infected with HIV are unable to breast-feed because HIV has been isolated in breast milk and could be transmitted to the infant. Taking zidovudine doesn't prevent transmission. The risk of breast-feeding isn't associated with direct contact with the breast but with the possibility of HIV contained in the breast milk.

CN: Health promotion and maintenance; CNS: None; CL: Application

38. Which subjective assessment finding helps diagnose human immunodeficiency virus (HIV) infection in children?

1. Excessive weight gain
2. Arrhythmia
3. Intermittent diarrhea
4. Tolerance of feedings

38. 3. A differential diagnosis may be based on the presence of an underlying cellular immunodeficiency-related disease; symptoms include intermittent episodes of diarrhea, repeated respiratory infections, and the inability to tolerate feedings. Poor weight gain and failure to thrive are objective assessment findings that result from intolerance of feedings and frequent infections. Arrhythmia isn't associated with HIV.

CN: Physiological integrity; CNS: Physiological adaptation; CL: Analysis

39. Which approach should be included in the diagnostic workup for a 12-month-old infant who's suspected of having acquired immunodeficiency syndrome (AIDS)?

1. Sputum culture
2. Esophageal biopsy
3. Parental counseling prior to testing
4. Human immunodeficiency syndrome (HIV) enzyme-linked immunosorbent assay (ELISA)

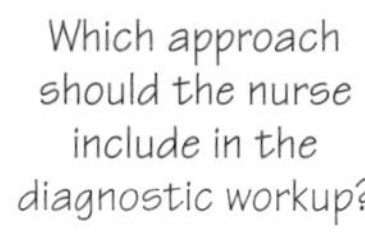

Which approach
should the nurse
include in the
diagnostic workup?

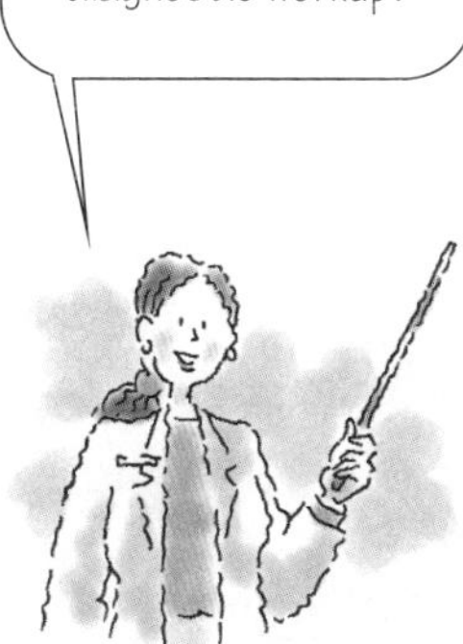

39. 3. AIDS and HIV are devastating diagnoses. Before testing, parents should be counseled regarding the disease, reasons for the tests, confidentiality, and benefits of early treatment. Sputum culture might help diagnose an upper respiratory infection associated with AIDS but isn't a diagnostic test for AIDS. Esophageal biopsy isn't indicated. ELISA isn't used diagnostically for children younger than 18 months because of the maternal antibodies in the child's blood.

CN: Psychosocial integrity; CNS: None; CL: Application

40. Parents of a child with Kawasaki disease should be taught the importance of keeping follow-up appointments to monitor and prevent which complication?

1. Encephalitis
2. Glomerulonephritis
3. Myocardial infarction (MI)
4. Idiopathic thrombocytopenia

40. 3. In Kawasaki disease, inflammation of small and medium blood vessels can result in weakening of the vessels and aneurysm formation, especially in the heart. Blood flow through damaged vessels can cause thrombus formation and MI. Encephalitis, glomerulonephritis, and idiopathic thrombocytopenia aren't associated with Kawasaki disease.

CN: Health promotion and maintenance; CNS: None; CL: Application

41. The nurse is working overnight in the emergency department when a client is admitted with sickle cell crisis. Which intervention should the nurse expect to perform?

1. Giving blood transfusions
2. Giving antibiotics
3. Increasing fluid intake and giving analgesics
4. Preparing the client for a splenectomy

41. 3. The primary therapy for sickle cell crisis is to increase fluid intake according to age and to give analgesics. Blood transfusions are only given conservatively to avoid iron overload. Antibiotics are given to clients with fever. Routine splenectomy isn't recommended. Splenectomy in clients with sickle cell anemia is controversial.

CN: Physiological integrity; CNS: Physiological adaptation; CL: Application

42. A child comes to the emergency department suspected of being in vaso-occlusive crisis. Which assessment findings would indicate that the client is having a <u>vaso-occlusive crisis</u>?

1. Hypotension and thready pulse
2. Pallor and poor capillary refill
3. Anemia, jaundice, and reticulocytosis
4. Acute leg pain and hand-foot syndrome

Question 42 is testing your knowledge of the four types of episodic crisis.

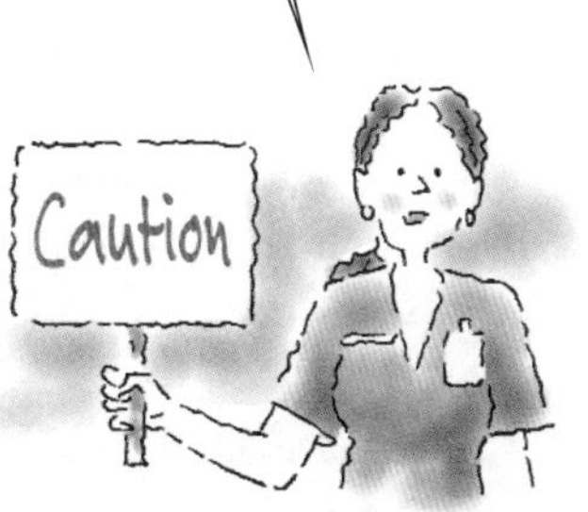

42. 4. Vaso-occlusive crises are the result of sickled cells obstructing the blood vessels. The major symptoms are fever, acute pain from visceral hypoxia, hand-foot syndrome, and arthralgia. A precipitous drop in blood volume is indicative of a splenic sequestration crisis and is exhibited by hypotension and a thready pulse. Aplastic crisis exhibits pallor and poor capillary refill and may result in symptoms of shock. Hyperhemolytic crisis is characterized by anemia, jaundice, and reticulocytosis and may also produce symptoms of shock.

CN: Physiological integrity; CNS: Physiological adaptation; CL: Analysis

43. Which response would be appropriate to give to a parent inquiring about a child who tests positive for sickle cell trait?

1. "Your child has sickle cell anemia."
2. "Your child is a carrier of the disorder but doesn't have sickle cell anemia."
3. "Your child is a carrier of the disease and will pass the disease to any offspring."
4. "Your child doesn't have the disease at present but may show evidence of the disease as he gets older."

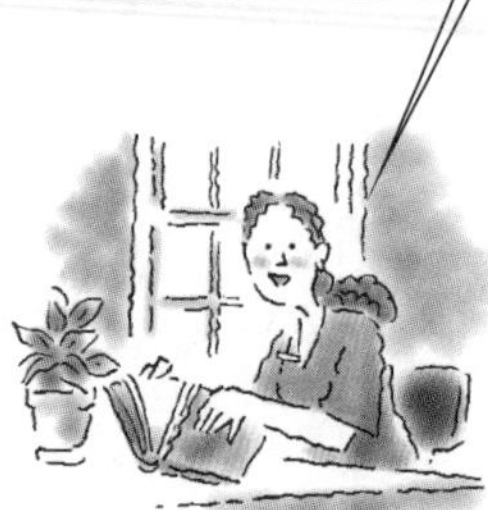

43. 2. A child with sickle cell trait is only a carrier and may never show any symptoms, except under special hypoxic conditions. A child with sickle cell trait doesn't have the disease and will never test positive for sickle cell anemia. Sickle cell anemia would be transmitted to offspring only as the result of a union between two individuals who are positive for the trait.

CN: Health promotion and maintenance; CNS: None; CL: Application

44. What is the primary nursing objective in caring for a child with sickle cell anemia in vaso-occlusive crisis?

1. Managing pain
2. Providing a cool environment
3. Immobilizing the affected part
4. Restricting fluids

44. 1. Pain management is an important aspect in the care of a client with sickle cell anemia in vaso-occlusive crisis. The goal is to prevent sickling. This can be accomplished by promoting tissue oxygenation, hydration, and rest, which minimize energy expenditure and oxygen utilization. A cool environment can cause vasoconstriction and thus more sickling and pain. Immobilization can promote stasis and increase sickling.

CN: Physiological integrity; CNS: Basic care and comfort; CL: Analysis

45. The nurse avoids palpating the abdomen of a child in vaso-occlusive crisis to prevent which complication?

1. Risk of splenic rupture
2. Risk of inducing vomiting
3. Increase in abdominal pain
4. Risk of blood cell destruction

45. 1. Palpating a child's abdomen in vaso-occlusive crisis should be avoided because sequestered red blood cells may precipitate splenic rupture. Abdominal pain alone wouldn't be a reason to avoid palpation. Vomiting or blood cell destruction wouldn't occur from palpation of the abdomen.

CN: Physiological integrity; CNS: Reduction of risk potential; CL: Application

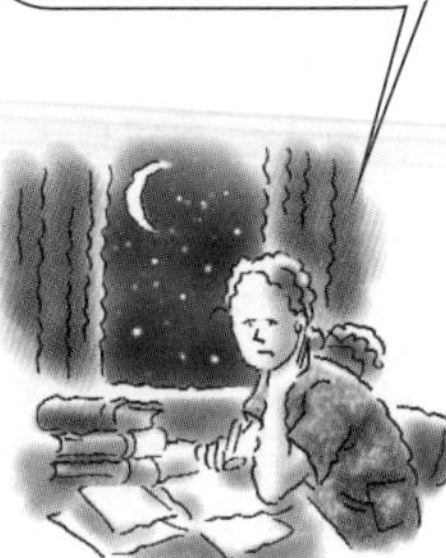

Which nursing intervention will help me keep going?

46. Which intervention is the most effective in maximizing tissue perfusion for a child in vaso-occlusive crisis?

1. Administering analgesics
2. Monitoring fluid restrictions
3. Encouraging activity as tolerated
4. Administering oxygen as prescribed

46. 4. Administering oxygen is the most effective way to maximize tissue perfusion. Short-term oxygen therapy helps to prevent hypoxia, which leads to metabolic acidosis, causing sickling. Long-term oxygen therapy will depress erythropoiesis. Analgesics are used to control pain. Hydration is essential to promote hemodilution and maintain electrolyte balance. Bed rest should be promoted to reduce oxygen utilization.

CN: Physiological integrity; CNS: Reduction of risk potential; CL: Application

CN: Client needs category CNS: Client needs subcategory CL: Cognitive level

47. Which nursing measure is most important to decrease the postoperative complications of a client with sickle cell anemia?

1. Increasing fluids
2. Preparing the child psychologically
3. Discouraging coughing
4. Limiting the use of analgesics

47. 1. The main surgical risk of anesthesia is hypoxia; however, emotional stress, demands of wound healing, and the potential for infection can each increase the sickling phenomenon. Increased fluids are encouraged because keeping the child well-hydrated is important for hemodilution to prevent sickling. Preparing the child psychologically to decrease fear will minimize undue emotional stress. Deep coughing is encouraged to promote pulmonary hygiene and prevent respiratory tract infection. Analgesics are used to control wound pain and to prevent abdominal splinting and decreased ventilation.

CN: Physiological integrity; CNS: Reduction of risk potential; CL: Application

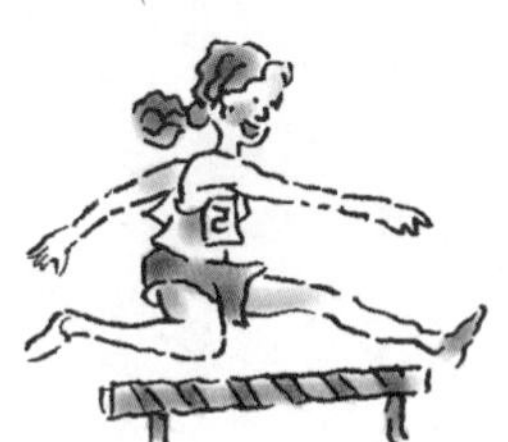

Don't let question 48 trip you up! It's asking you to prioritize.

48. Which factor should be included as a priority in teaching parents about prevention of infection in children with sickle cell anemia?

1. Providing adequate nutrition
2. Avoiding emotional stress
3. Visiting the physician when sick
4. Avoiding strenuous physical exertion

48. 1. The nurse must stress adequate nutrition. Avoiding strenuous physical exertion and emotional stress are important aspects to prevent sickling, but adequate nutrition remains a priority. Frequent medical supervision is imperative to prevention because infection is commonly a predisposing factor toward development of a crisis.

CN: Health promotion and maintenance; CNS: None; CL: Application

49. Which schedule is recommended for the immunization of normal infants and children in the first year of life?

1. Birth, 2 months, 4 months, 6 months, 12 months
2. 1 month, 3 months, 5 months, 9 months, 18 months
3. 2 months, 6 months, 9 months, 12 months, 14 months
4. 2 months, 4 months, 6 months, 12 to 15 months

49. 1. The nurse needs to be aware of the schedule for immunizations, as well as the latest recommendations for their use. According to the American Academy of Pediatrics, the recommended age for beginning primary immunizations of normal infants is at birth.

CN: Health promotion and maintenance; CNS: None; CL: Application

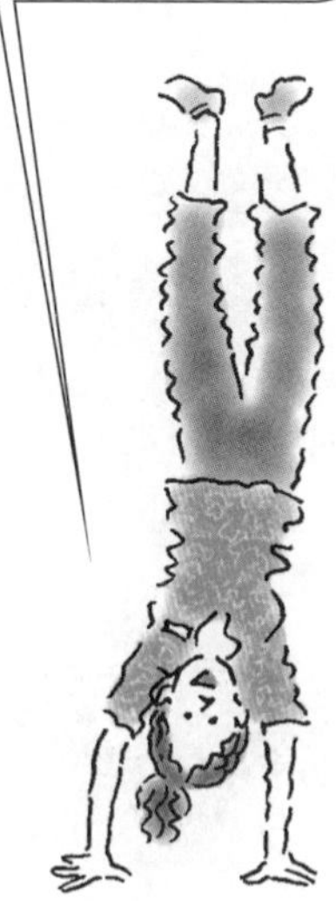

You've reached question 50! You're doing great!

50. Which assessment findings would indicate vaso-occlusive crisis in a child with sickle cell anemia?

1. Painful urination
2. Pain with ambulation
3. Complaints of throat pain
4. Fever with associated rash

50. 2. Bone pain is one of the major symptoms of vaso-occlusive crisis in clients with sickle cell anemia. Hand-foot syndrome, characterized by edematous painful extremities, is usually exhibited in the refusal of the child to bear weight and ambulate. Painful urination doesn't occur, but sickle cell anemia can cause kidney abnormalities. Throat pain isn't a symptom of vaso-occlusive crisis. Fever commonly accompanies vaso-occlusive crisis but isn't associated with rash.

CN: Physiological integrity; CNS: Physiological adaptation; CL: Analysis

51. The nurse is assessing a child with sickle cell anemia. Which bone-related complications would the nurse be alert for during assessment?
1. Arthritis
2. Osteoporosis
3. Osteogenic sarcoma
4. Spontaneous fractures

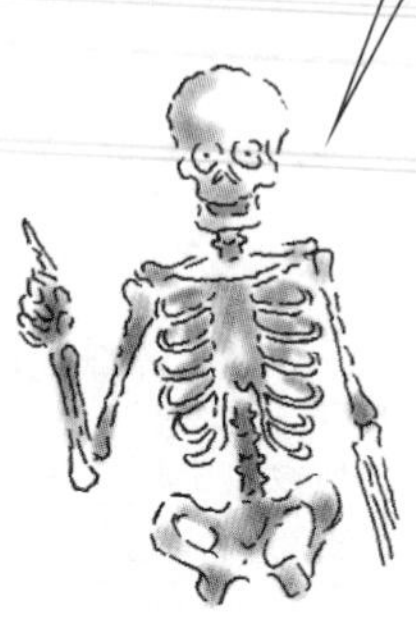

I was minding my own business when things got really complicated.

51. 2. Sickle cell anemia causes hyperplasia and congestion of the bone marrow, resulting in osteoporosis. Arthritis doesn't occur secondary to sickle cell anemia; however, a crisis can cause localized swelling over joints, resulting in arthralgia. Bones do become weakened, but spontaneous fractures don't occur as a result. Osteogenic sarcoma is bone cancer; sickle cell anemia isn't a contributing factor to bone cancer.

CN: Physiological integrity; CNS: Physiological adaptation; CL: Application

52. What is a nurse's role with the parents of a child who has been diagnosed with sickle cell anemia?
1. Encouraging selective birth methods or abortion
2. Referring only sickle cell–positive parents for counseling
3. Rendering support to parents of newly diagnosed children
4. Reinforcing the idea that transmission is unlikely in subsequent pregnancies

52. 3. The nurse can be instrumental in providing genetic counseling. She can give parents correct information about the disease and render support to parents of newly diagnosed children. Alternative birth methods are discussed, but parents make their own decisions. All heterozygous, or trait-positive, parents should be referred for genetic counseling. The risk of transmission in subsequent pregnancies remains the same.

CN: Health promotion and maintenance; CNS: None; CL: Application

53. A 14-year-old girl is admitted for sickle cell crisis. Which nursing intervention would be the most important?
1. Gathering information about the child's ability to cope with this condition
2. Monitoring the child's temperature every 2 hours
3. Providing adequate oxygenation, hydrations, and pain management
4. Making sure the family is involved in every step of the child's care

53. 3. The most critical need of a client in sickle cell crisis is to provide adequate oxygenation, hydrations, and pain management until the crisis passes. Obtaining a temperature every 2 hours would not be the priority intervention. While assessing the client's ability to cope and involving the family in the child's care are important, they aren't the priority interventions during a sickle cell crisis.

CN: Safe, effective care environment; CNS: Management of care; CL: Analysis

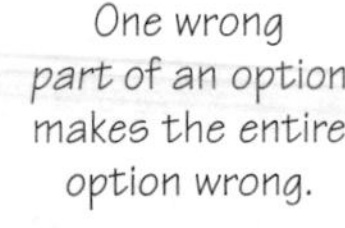

One wrong part of an option makes the entire option wrong.

54. A nurse is administering a blood transfusion to a client with sickle cell anemia. Which assessment findings would indicate that the client is having a transfusion reaction?
1. Diaphoresis and hot flashes
2. Urticaria, flushing, and wheezing
3. Fever, urticaria, and red raised rash
4. Fever, disorientation, and abdominal pain

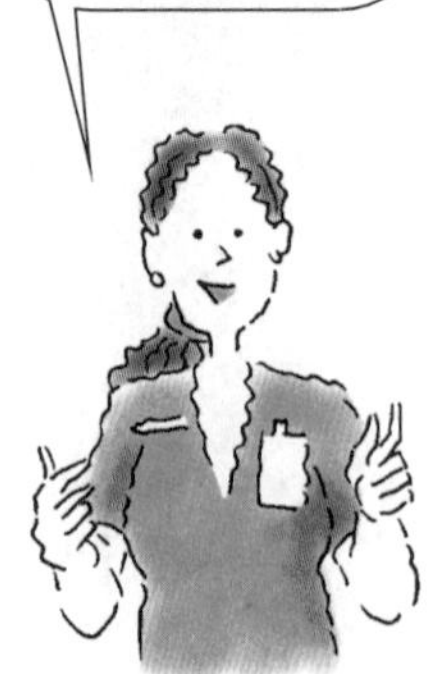

54. 2. Allergic reactions may occur when the recipient reacts to allergens in the donor's blood; this reaction causes urticaria, flushing, and wheezing. A febrile reaction can occur, causing fever and urticaria, but it isn't accompanied by rash. Diaphoresis, hot flashes, disorientation, and abdominal pain aren't symptoms of a transfusion reaction.

CN: Physiological integrity; CNS: Reduction of risk potential; CL: Analysis

CN: Client needs category CNS: Client needs subcategory CL: Cognitive level

55. A mother brings her 5-year-old child to the clinic and asks the nurse how often a child should receive the influenza virus vaccine. Which response would be the most accurate?

1. Annually
2. Twice a year
3. Never; contraindicated in children
4. Only with the outbreak of illness

55. 1. The influenza virus vaccine is usually administered annually. The vaccine isn't contraindicated in children but is targeted at clients with chronic cardiac, pulmonary, hematologic, and neurologic problems. The vaccine is given to prevent the onset of illness before an outbreak occurs.

CN: Health promotion and maintenance; CNS: None; CL: Application

56. A 3-year-old sister of a neonate is diagnosed with pertussis. The mother has a history of having been immunized as a child. Which information should be included in teaching the mother about possible infection of her neonate?

1. The baby will inevitably contract pertussis.
2. Immune globulin is effective in protecting the infant.
3. The risk to the infant depends on the mother's immune status.
4. Erythromycin should be administered prophylactically to the infant.

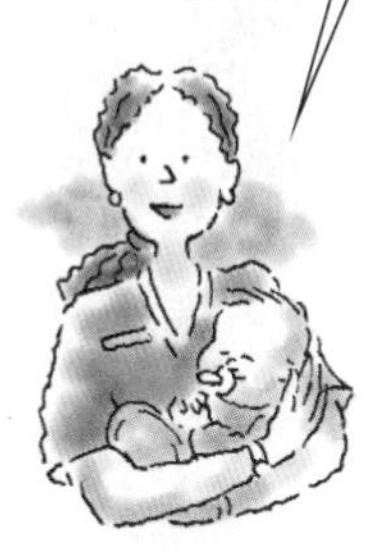
Prevention is
commonly the
best medicine!

56. 4. In exposed, high-risk persons such as neonates, erythromycin may be effective in preventing or lessening severity of the disease if administered during the preparoxysmal stage. Immune globulin isn't indicated because it's used as an immunization against hepatitis A. Neonates exposed to pertussis are at considerable risk for infections, regardless of the mother's immune status; however, infection isn't inevitable.

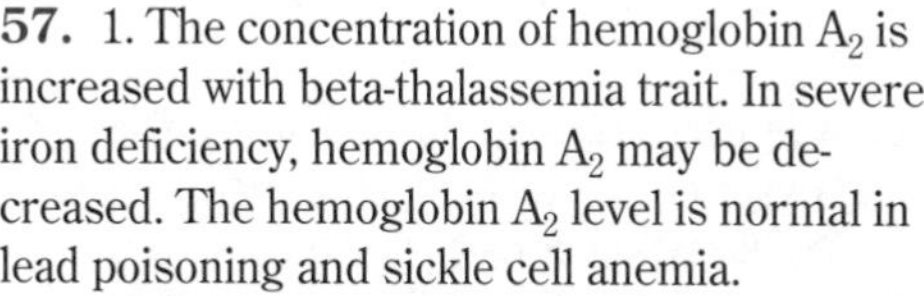

CN: Health promotion and maintenance; CNS: None; CL: Application

57. A child has recently been admitted to the pediatric unit with laboratory values indicating an increase in hemoglobin A_2. Based on this finding, the nurse should expect to follow a care plan based on which condition?

1. Beta-thalassemia trait
2. Iron deficiency
3. Lead poisoning
4. Sickle cell anemia

57. 1. The concentration of hemoglobin A_2 is increased with beta-thalassemia trait. In severe iron deficiency, hemoglobin A_2 may be decreased. The hemoglobin A_2 level is normal in lead poisoning and sickle cell anemia.

CN: Physiological integrity; CNS: Reduction of risk potential; CL: Application

58. A 4-year-old child has a petechial rash but is otherwise well. The platelet count is 20,000/µl, and the hemoglobin level and white blood cell (WBC) count are normal. Which diagnosis is most likely?

1. Acute lymphoblastic leukemia (ALL)
2. Disseminated intravascular coagulation (DIC)
3. Idiopathic thrombocytopenic purpura (ITP)
4. Systemic lupus erythematosus (SLE)

58. 3. The onset of ITP typically occurs between ages 1 and 6. Clients look well, except for a petechial rash. ALL is associated with a low platelet count but an *abnormal* hemoglobin level and WBC count. DIC is secondary to a severe underlying disease. SLE is rare in a 4-year-old child.

CN: Physiological integrity; CNS: Physiological adaptation; CL: Analysis

59. Which instruction should be included in a nurse's discharge teaching for the parents of a newborn diagnosed with sickle cell anemia?

1. Stressing the importance of iron supplementation
2. Stressing the importance of monthly vitamin B_{12} injections
3. Reviewing signs of abdominal pain in infants and demonstrating how to take a temperature
4. Explaining that immunizations are contraindicated

59. 3. Acute splenic sequestration is a serious complication of sickle cell anemia. Early detection of splenomegaly by parents is an important aspect of client management. Parents should be able to take the temperature and identify abdominal pain. A temperature of 101.3° F to 102.2° F (38.5° C to 39° C) calls for emergency evaluation, even if the child appears well. Folic acid requirement is increased; therefore, supplementation may be indicated. Vitamin B_{12} supplementation and iron supplementation aren't necessary. Parents should be encouraged to keep immunizations up to date.

CN: Health promotion and maintenance; CNS: None; CL: Application

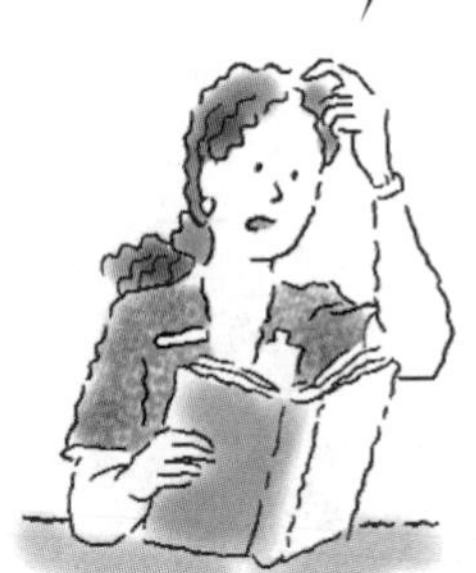

Question 60 asks about a prognosis, not a diagnosis.

60. Which finding yields a poor prognosis for a child with leukemia?

1. Presence of a mediastinal mass
2. Late central nervous system (CNS) leukemia
3. Normal white blood cell (WBC) count at diagnosis
4. Disease presents between ages 2 and 10

60. 1. The presence of a mediastinal mass indicates a poor prognosis for children with leukemia. The prognosis is poorer if age at onset is younger than 2 years or older than 10 years. A WBC count of 100,000/µl or higher and early CNS leukemia also indicate a poor prognosis for a child with leukemia.

CN: Physiological integrity; CNS: Physiological adaptation; CL: Analysis

61. A 1-year-old boy in the pediatrician's office for an examination is noted to be pale. He's in the 75th percentile for weight and the 25th percentile for length. His physical examination is normal, but his hematocrit is 24%. Which question would be <u>most helpful</u> in establishing a diagnosis of anemia?

1. Is the child on any medications?
2. What's the child's usual daily diet?
3. Did the child receive phototherapy for jaundice?
4. What's the pattern and appearance of bowel movements?

61. 2. Iron deficiency anemia is the most common nutritional deficiency in children between ages 9 months and 15 months. Anemia in a 1-year-old child is mostly nutritional in origin, and its cause will be suggested by a detailed nutritional history. None of the other selections would be helpful in diagnosing anemia.

CN: Health promotion and maintenance; CNS: None; CL: Analysis

62. A nurse is teaching the parents of a child newly diagnosed with Hodgkin's disease. Which statement should the nurse include in her teaching?

1. Staging laparotomy is mandatory for every client.
2. Excessive weight gain can be a symptom.
3. Hodgkin's disease is rare before age 5.
4. Incidence of Hodgkin's disease peaks between ages 11 and 15.

62. 3. Hodgkin's disease is rare before age 5. Staging laparotomy is *not* recommended for clients who have obvious intra-abdominal disease by noninvasive studies. Systemic symptoms of Hodgkin's disease include fever, night sweats, malaise, weight loss, and pruritus. The peak incidence of Hodgkin's disease occurs in late adolescence and young adulthood (ages 15 to 34).

CN: Physiological integrity; CNS: Physiological adaptation; CL: Analysis

63. The nurse is caring for a child with perinatally acquired human immunodeficiency virus. At which age do children usually demonstrate symptoms of acquired immunodeficiency syndrome (AIDS)?

1. Within the first month of life
2. At 1 to 3 months of age
3. At 18 to 24 months of age
4. At 3 to 5 years of age

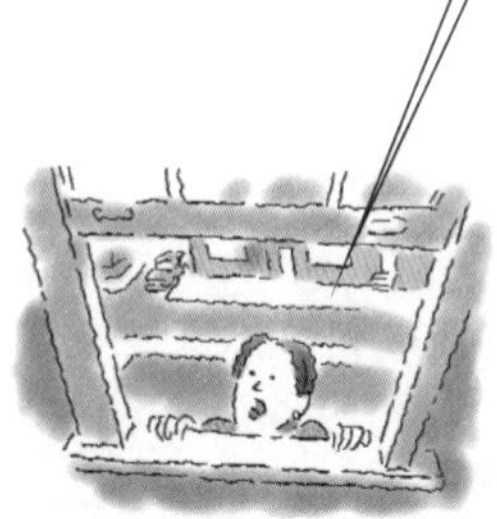
These questions are tough! Hang in there!

63. 3. The majority of children with perinatally transmitted AIDS appear normal in early infancy. Symptoms usually develop at 18 to 24 months of age.

CN: Physiological integrity; CNS: Physiological adaptation; CL: Application

64. Which factors may make adolescent girls at risk for iron deficiency anemia?

1. Menses
2. Vegetarian diet
3. Weight-loss diets
4. All of the above

64. 4. All the options make adolescent girls, who are still growing, at risk for iron deficiency anemia. That's because these girls lose blood monthly with menstrual periods, and they typically consume inadequate amounts of nutrients because of their eating patterns, which include hurried meals, vegetarian diets, and weight-loss diets.

CN: Health promotion and maintenance; CNS: None; CL: Analysis

65. Which treatment would be most appropriate for a child diagnosed with iron deficiency anemia?

1. Blood transfusion
2. Oral ferrous sulfate
3. An iron-fortified cereal
4. Intramuscular iron dextran

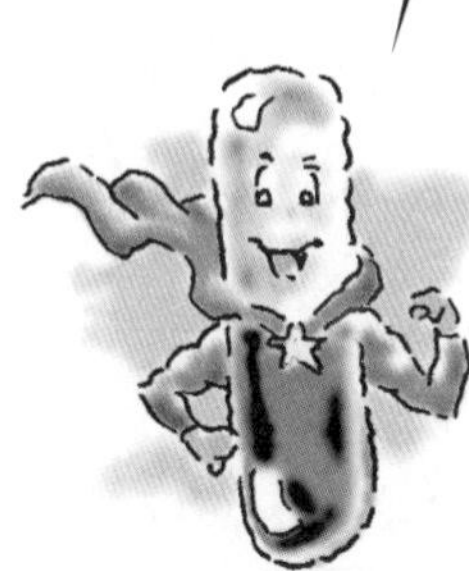
I can help with iron deficiency anemia.

65. 2. A prompt rise in hemoglobin level and hematocrit follows the administration of oral ferrous sulfate. Blood transfusion is rarely indicated unless a child becomes symptomatic or is further compromised by a superimposed infection. Dietary modifications are appropriate long-term measures, but they won't make enough iron available to replenish iron stores. Intramuscular dextran is reserved for situations in which compliance can't be achieved because it's expensive, painful, and no more effective than oral iron.

CN: Physiological integrity; CNS: Physiological adaptation; CL: Application

66. A child is admitted to the hospital with flu-like symptoms. Diagnostic testing reveals the IgM antibody parvovirus B19 is present. The nurse interprets this finding as being indicative of which condition?

1. Roseola
2. Fifth disease
3. Varicella
4. Mumps

66. 2. Fifth disease is known to be caused by human parvovirus B19. Roseola is thought to be caused by the human herpes virus 6. Varicella is caused by the varicella-zoster virus. Mumps is caused by the paramyxovirus.

CN: Physiological integrity; CNS: Reduction of risk potential; CL: Application

67. A 6-year-old child has been diagnosed with Rocky Mountain spotted fever. In teaching the parents about the cause of the illness, a nurse would be correct in telling them that a bite by which animal or insect caused the illness?
1. Cat
2. Mosquito
3. Spider
4. Tick

67. 4. Rocky Mountain spotted fever is caused by *Rickettsia rickettsii*, which is transmitted by the bite of a tick. Mosquito, spider, and cat bites haven't been known to transmit *R. rickettsii*.
CN: Safe, effective care environment; CNS: Safety and infection control; CL: Application

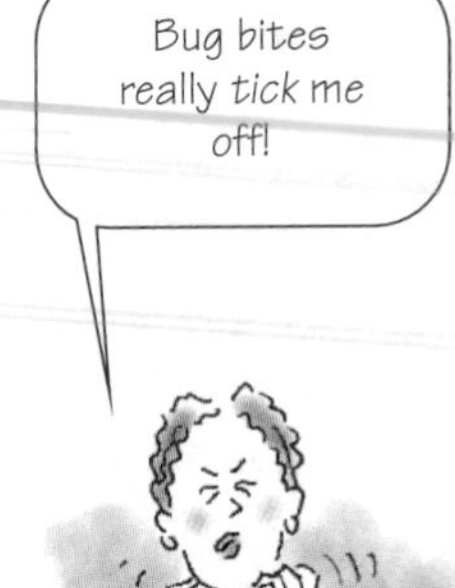

Bug bites really tick me off!

68. An iron dextran (InFeD) injection has been ordered for an 8-month-old child with iron deficiency anemia whose parents haven't been compliant with oral supplements. What is the correct method of injection for InFeD?
1. Intradermal
2. Subcutaneous
3. Intramuscular
4. Intramuscular using the Z-track method

68. 4. If iron dextran is ordered, it must be injected deeply into a large muscle mass, using the Z-track method to minimize skin staining and irritation. Neither a subcutaneous nor an intradermal injection would inject the dextran into the muscle. The Z-track method is preferred over a normal intramuscular injection.
CN: Physiological integrity; CNS: Pharmacological and parenteral therapies; CL: Application

69. Which food is an appropriate source of dietary iron for the prevention of nutritional anemia?
1. Citrus fruits
2. Fish
3. Green vegetables
4. Milk products

69. 3. Green vegetables are good sources of iron. Citrus foods aren't sources of iron but help with the absorption of iron. Fish isn't a good source of dietary iron. Milk is deficient in iron and should be limited in cases of nutritional anemia.
CN: Physiological integrity; CNS: Basic care and comfort; CL: Application

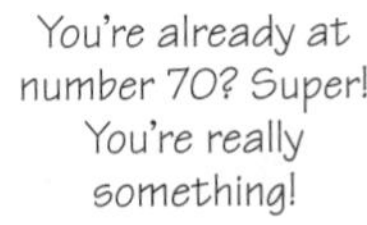

You're already at number 70? Super! You're really something!

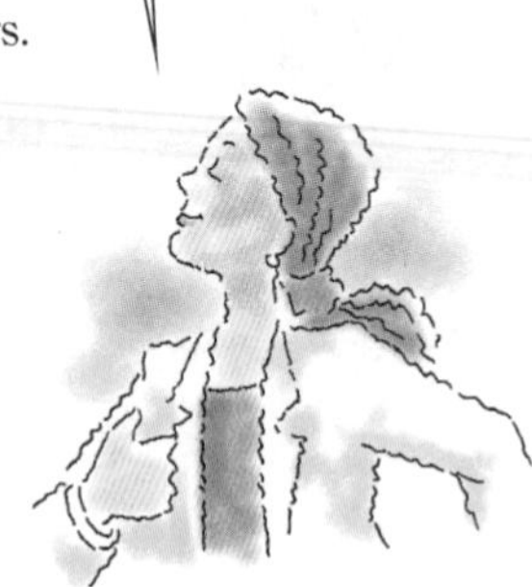

70. Which instruction should a nurse provide when teaching parents the proper administration of liquid oral iron supplements?
1. Give the supplements with food.
2. Stop the medication if vomiting occurs.
3. Decrease the dose if constipation occurs.
4. Give the medicine via a dropper or through a straw.

70. 4. Liquid iron preparations may temporarily stain the teeth; therefore, the drug should be given by dropper or through a straw. Supplements should be given between meals, when the presence of free hydrochloric acid is greatest. If vomiting occurs, supplementation shouldn't be stopped; instead, it should be administered with food. Constipation can be decreased by increasing intake of fruits and vegetables.
CN: Physiological integrity; CNS: Pharmacological and parenteral therapies; CL: Application

71. Which symptom is the primary clinical manifestation of hemophilia?
1. Petechiae
2. Prolonged bleeding
3. Decreased clotting time
4. Decreased white blood cell (WBC) count

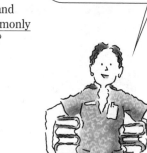

71. 2. The effect of hemophilia is prolonged bleeding, anywhere from or within the body. With severe deficiencies, hemorrhage can occur as a result of minor trauma. Petechiae are uncommon in persons with hemophilia because repair of small hemorrhages depends on platelet function, not on blood clotting mechanisms. Clotting time is increased in a client with hemophilia. A decrease in WBCs is *not* indicative of hemophilia.

CN: Physiological integrity; CNS: Physiological adaptation; CL: Analysis

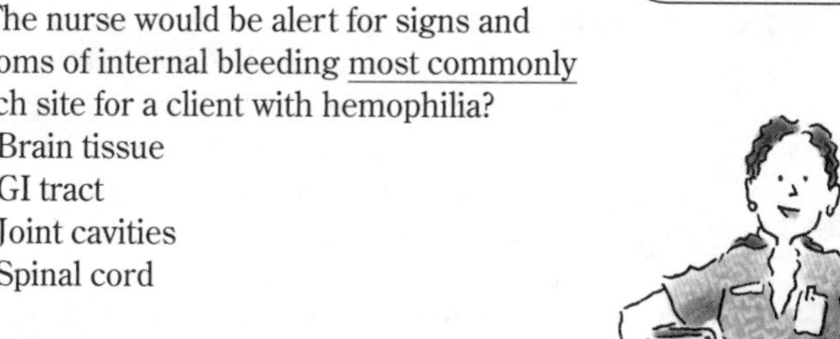

Careful! All of these answers may be accurate, but this question is asking for the most common site.

72. The nurse would be alert for signs and symptoms of internal bleeding most commonly at which site for a client with hemophilia?
1. Brain tissue
2. GI tract
3. Joint cavities
4. Spinal cord

72. 3. The joint cavities, especially the knees, ankles, and elbows, are the most common site of internal bleeding. This bleeding typically results in bone changes and crippling, disabling deformities. Intracranial hemorrhage occurs less commonly than expected because the brain tissue has a high concentration of thromboplastin. Hemorrhage along the GI tract and spinal cord can occur but are less common.

CN: Physiological integrity; CNS: Physiological adaptation; CL: Application

73. Which measure should parents of a hemophilic child be taught to prepare them to initiate immediate treatment before blood loss is excessive?
1. Apply heat to the area.
2. Withhold factor replacement.
3. Apply pressure for at least 5 minutes.
4. Immobilize and elevate the affected area.

73. 4. Elevating the area above the level of the heart will decrease blood flow. Cold, not heat, should be applied to promote vasoconstriction. Factor replacement should *not* be delayed. Pressure should be applied to the area for at least 10 to 15 minutes to allow clot formation.

CN: Physiological integrity; CNS: Physiological adaptation; CL: Application

74. A 2-year-old child with hemophilia who sustains a joint injury is best treated promptly in which location?
1. Home
2. Clinic
3. Hospital unit
4. Emergency department

74. 1. Prompt treatment to prevent joint injury and other complications is best delivered in the home. After the child reaches age 2 or 3 years, parents can learn venipuncture techniques so treatment can be done at home and further injury avoided. The life of the child and family is also less disrupted. The child may be transfused on a regular basis to prevent bleeding and will be given additional doses of the missing factor when an injury occurs. By mid- to late-school age, children can learn to administer their own treatment.

CN: Physiological integrity; CNS: Reduction of risk potential; CL: Application

75. Which nursing measure is an important aid in prevention of the crippling effects of joint degeneration caused by hemophilia?
1. Avoiding the use of analgesics
2. Using aspirin for pain relief
3. Administering replacement factor
4. Using active range-of-motion (ROM) exercises

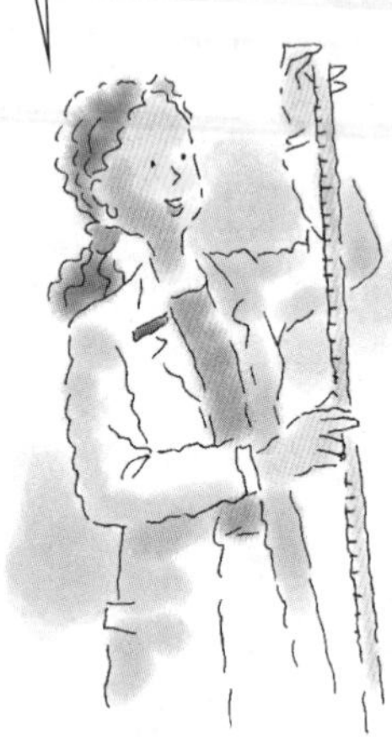

Read carefully. This question is looking for a preventive measure.

75. 3. Prevention of bleeding is the goal and is achieved by factor replacement therapy. Active ROM exercises are contraindicated after a bleeding episode because the joint capsule can be stretched, causing bleeding. Acetaminophen should be used for pain relief because aspirin has anticoagulant effects. Analgesics should be administered before physical therapy to control pain and provide the maximum benefit.
CN: Physiological integrity; CNS: Physiological adaptation; CL: Application

76. When comparing bleeding disorders, an increased tendency to bleed in which area differentiates von Willebrand's disease from hemophilia?
1. Brain tissue
2. GI tract
3. Mucous membranes
4. Spinal cord

76. 3. The most characteristic clinical feature of von Willebrand's disease is an increased tendency to bleed from mucous membranes, which may be seen as frequent nosebleeds or menorrhagia. In hemophilia, the joint cavities are the most common site of internal bleeding. Bleeding into the GI tract, spinal cord, and brain tissue can occur, but these are *not* the most common sites for bleeding.
CN: Physiological integrity; CNS: Physiological adaptation; CL: Application

77. Which nursing measure should be implemented for a client with von Willebrand's disease who's having epistaxis?
1. Lying the child supine
2. Avoiding packing of the nostrils
3. Avoiding pressure to the nose
4. Applying pressure to the nose

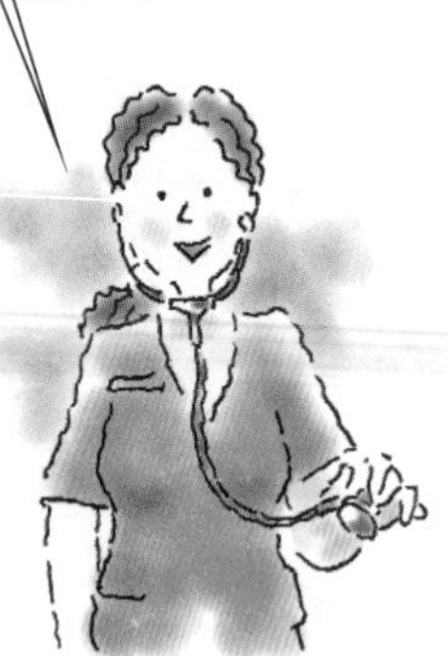

Epistaxis is a term from early in your program. Remember?

77. 4. Applying pressure to the nose may stop bleeding because most bleeds occur in the anterior part of the nasal septum. Encourage mouth breathing at this time. The child should be instructed to sit up and lean forward to avoid aspiration of blood. Packing with tissue or cotton may be used to help stop bleeding, although care must be taken in removing packing to avoid dislodging the clot. Pressure should be maintained for at least 10 minutes to allow clotting to occur.
CN: Physiological integrity; CNS: Physiological adaptation; CL: Application

78. A nurse is teaching the parents of a child with acute lymphoblastic leukemia. The parents ask for information about what helps determine long-term survival. The nurse discusses which of the following as the three most important prognostic factors?
1. Histologic type of disease, initial platelet count, and type of treatment
2. Type of treatment, stage at diagnosis, and child's age at diagnosis
3. Histologic type of disease, initial white blood cell (WBC) count, and client's age at diagnosis
4. Progression of illness, WBC count at time of diagnosis, and client's age at diagnosis

78. 3. Histologic type of leukemia is the factor whose prognostic value is considered to be of greatest significance in determining long-range outcome. Children with a normal or low WBC count appear to have a much better prognosis than those with a high WBC count. Children diagnosed between ages 2 and 10 have consistently demonstrated a better prognosis than those diagnosed before age 2 or after age 10.
CN: Physiological integrity; CNS: Physiological adaptation; CL: Analysis

79. Which complications are the three main consequences of leukemia?

1. Bone deformities, spherocytosis, and infection
2. Anemia, infection, and bleeding tendencies
3. Lymphocytopoiesis, growth delays, and hirsutism
4. Polycythemia, decreased clotting time, and infection

79. 2. The three main consequences of leukemia are anemia, caused by decreased erythrocyte production; infection secondary to neutropenia; and bleeding tendencies, from decreased platelet production. Bone deformities don't occur with leukemia, although bones may become painful because of the proliferation of cells in the bone marrow. Spherocytosis refers to erythrocytes taking on a spheroid shape and isn't a feature in leukemia. Lymphocytopoesis is production of lymphocytes with leukemia. Mature cells aren't produced in adequate numbers. Hirsutism and growth delay can be a result of large doses of steroids but aren't common in leukemia. Anemia, not polycythemia, occurs. Clotting times would be prolonged.

CN: Physiological integrity; CNS: Physiological adaptation; CL: Application

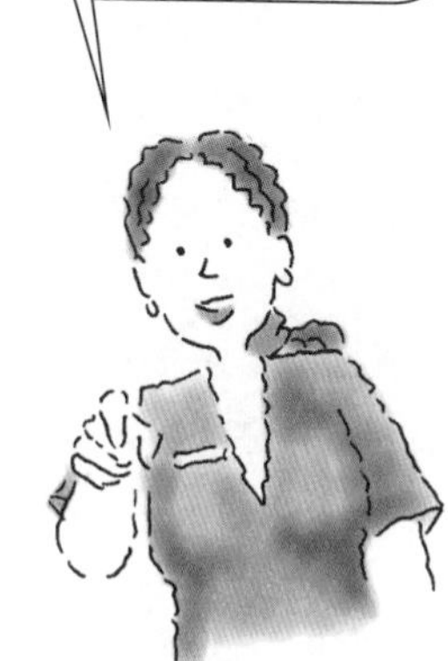

You, my friend, are doing extraordinarily well. Keep up the good work!

80. A child is seen in the pediatrician's office for complaints of bone and joint pain. Which other assessment finding may suggest leukemia?

1. Abdominal pain
2. Increased activity level
3. Increased appetite
4. Petechiae

80. 4. The most common signs and symptoms of leukemia are a result of infiltration of the bone marrow. These include fever, pallor, fatigue, anorexia, and petechiae, along with bone and joint pain. Abdominal pain may be caused by areas of inflammation from normal flora within the GI tract or any number of other causes. Increased appetite can occur, but it usually isn't a presenting symptom.

CN: Physiological integrity; CNS: Physiological adaptation; CL: Application

81. Which assessment finding in a client with leukemia would indicate that the cancer has invaded the brain?

1. Headache and vomiting
2. Restlessness and tachycardia
3. Hypervigilant and anxious behavior
4. Increased heart rate and decreased blood pressure

81. 1. The usual effect of leukemic infiltration of the brain is increased intracranial pressure. The proliferation of cells interferes with the flow of cerebrospinal fluid in the subarachnoid space and at the base of the brain. The increased fluid pressure causes dilation of the ventricles, which creates symptoms of severe headache, vomiting, irritability, lethargy, increased blood pressure, decreased heart rate and, eventually, coma. Children with a variety of illnesses are typically hypervigilant and anxious when hospitalized.

CN: Physiological integrity; CNS: Physiological adaptation; CL: Analysis

82. A student nurse asks the nurse on the hematology unit which type of leukemia has the best prognosis. Which response would be the most accurate?
1. Acute lymphoblastic leukemia
2. Acute myelogenous leukemia
3. Basophilic leukemia
4. Eosinophilic leukemia

82. 1. Acute lymphoblastic leukemia, which accounts for more than 80% of all childhood cases, carries the best prognosis. Acute myelogenous leukemia, with several subtypes, accounts for most of the other leukemias affecting children. Basophilic and eosinophilic leukemia are named for the specific cells involved. These are much rarer and carry a poorer prognosis.

CN: Physiological integrity; CNS: Physiological adaptation; CL: Application

83. Which finding is the reason to perform a spinal tap on a client newly diagnosed with leukemia?
1. To rule out meningitis
2. To decrease intracranial pressure (ICP)
3. To aid in classification of the leukemia
4. To assess for central nervous system (CNS) infiltration

83. 4. A spinal tap is performed to assess for CNS infiltration. A spinal tap can be done to rule out meningitis, but this isn't the indication for the test on a leukemic client. It wouldn't be done to decrease ICP, nor does it aid in the classification of the leukemia. Spinal taps can result in brain stem herniation in cases of increased ICP.

CN: Physiological integrity; CNS: Physiological adaptation; CL: Application

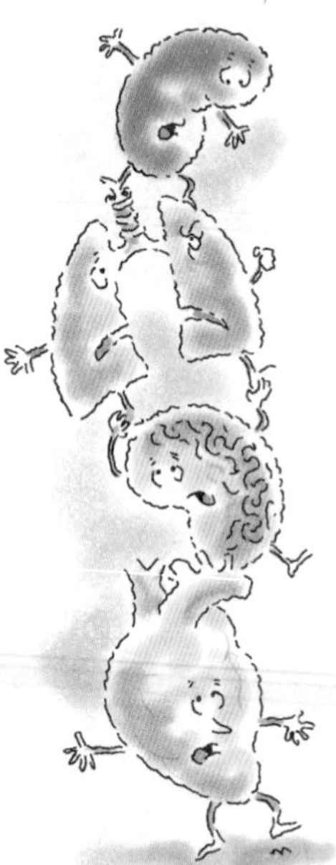

Think back to basic physiology. Which organs metabolize drugs?

84. Which test is performed on a client with leukemia before initiation of therapy to evaluate the child's ability to metabolize chemotherapeutic agents?
1. Lumbar puncture
2. Liver function studies
3. Complete blood count (CBC)
4. Peripheral blood smear

84. 2. Liver and kidney function studies are done before initiation of chemotherapy to evaluate the child's ability to metabolize the chemotherapeutic agents. A lumbar puncture is performed to assess for central nervous system infiltration. A CBC is performed to assess for anemia and white blood cell count. A peripheral blood smear is done to assess the maturity and morphology of red blood cells.

CN: Physiological integrity; CNS: Pharmacological and parenteral therapies; CL: Analysis

85. Which statement by the nurse most accurately explains the need for a child with pauciarticular juvenile rheumatoid arthritis (JRA) to have an annual eye exam?
1. "Detached retinas are commonly associated with the disease."
2. "Painless iritis (inflammation of the iris) is commonly seen with the disease."
3. "Glaucoma is commonly seen with the disease."
4. "Strabismus is commonly seen with the disease."

85. 2. Painless iritis may be found in 75% of children with pauciarticular JRA. If it's not detected and is left untreated, permanent scarring in the anterior chamber of the eye may occur, with loss of vision. Children should have annual slit lamp examinations by an ophthalmologist. Detached retinas, glaucoma, and strabismus aren't commonly associated with the disease.

CN: Health promotion and maintenance; CNS: None; CL: Application

86. Which medication would the nurse expect the physician to order most commonly for a client with leukemia as prophylaxis against *Pneumocystic carinii* pneumonia?

1. Co-trimoxazole (Bactrim)
2. Oral nystatin suspension
3. Prednisone
4. Vincristine

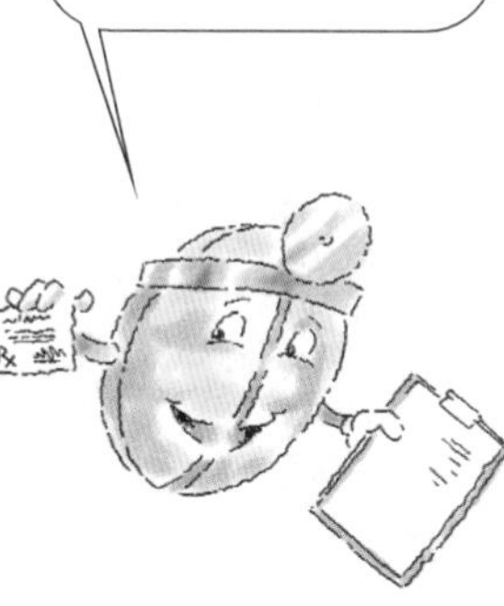

Here's a prescription for the drug of choice. Do you know which one it is?

86. 1. The most common cause of death from leukemia is overwhelming infection. *P. carinii* infection is lethal to a child with leukemia. As prophylaxis against *P. carinii* pneumonia, continuous low dosages of co-trimoxazole are typically prescribed. Oral nystatin suspension would be indicated for the treatment of thrush. Prednisone isn't an antibiotic and increases susceptibility to infection. Vincristine is an antineoplastic agent.

CN: Physiological integrity; CNS: Pharmacological and parenteral therapies; CL: Application

87. A 4-year-old child is diagnosed as having acute lymphocytic leukemia. His white blood cell (WBC) count, especially the neutrophil count, is low. Which intervention should the nurse teach the parents?

1. Protect the child from falls because of his increased risk of bleeding.
2. Protect the child from infections because his resistance to infection is decreased.
3. Provide rest periods because the oxygen-carrying capacity of the child's blood is diminished.
4. Treat constipation, which frequently accompanies a decrease in WBC.

87. 2. One of the complications of both acute lymphocytic leukemia and its treatment is a decreased WBC count, especially a decreased absolute neutrophil count. Because neutrophils are the body's first line of defense against infection, the child must be protected from infection. Bleeding is a risk factor if platelets or other coagulation factors are decreased. A decreased hemoglobin level, hematocrit, or both would reduce the oxygen-carrying capacity of the child's blood. Constipation isn't related to the WBC count.

CN: Safe, effective care environment; CNS: Safety and infection control; CL: Application

88. Which treatment measure should be implemented for a child with leukemia who has been exposed to chickenpox?

1. No treatment is indicated.
2. Acyclovir (Zovirax) should be started on exposure.
3. Varicella-zoster immune globulin (VZIG) should be given with evidence of the disease.
4. VZIG should be given within 72 hours of exposure.

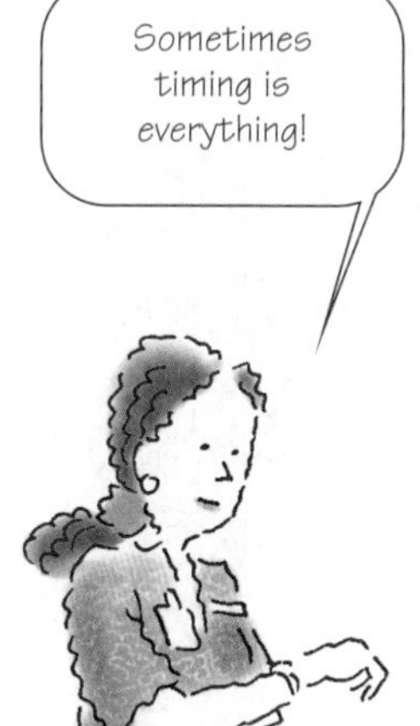

88. 4. Varicella is a lethal organism to a child with leukemia. VZIG, given within 72 hours, may favorably alter the course of the disease. Giving the vaccine at the onset of symptoms wouldn't likely decrease the severity of the illness. Acyclovir may be given if the child develops the disease but not if the child has just been exposed.

CN: Health promotion and maintenance; CNS: None; CL: Analysis

89. Nausea and vomiting are common adverse effects of radiation and chemotherapy. When should a nurse administer antiemetics?

1. 30 minutes before initiation of therapy
2. With the administration of therapy
3. Immediately after nausea begins
4. When therapy is completed

89. 1. Antiemetics are most beneficial if given before the onset of nausea and vomiting. To calculate the optimum time for administration, the first dose is given 30 minutes to 1 hour before nausea is expected, and then every 2, 4, or 6 hours for approximately 24 hours after chemotherapy. If the antiemetic was given with the medication or after the medication, it could lose its maximum effectiveness when needed.

CN: Physiological integrity; CNS: Pharmacological and parenteral therapies; CL: Application

90. A child is admitted to the pediatric unit with an unknown mass in her lower left abdomen. Which action should be the nurse's priority?

1. Obtain the history of the illness.
2. Place a "Do not palpate abdomen" sign over the child's bed.
3. Obtain a complete set of vital signs.
4. Schedule a hemoglobin and hematocrit test for early morning.

90. 2. The nurse must take measures to prevent palpation of the mass, if possible. If the mass is a malignant tumor, a do-not-palpate warning will help prevent trauma and rupture of the suspected tumor capsule. Rupture of the tumor capsule may cause seeding of cancer cells throughout the abdomen. Obtaining the history and vital signs and scheduling laboratory work are important, but not the priority.

CN: Physiological integrity; CNS: Physiological adaptation; CL: Analysis

91. Which nursing measure is helpful when mouth ulcers develop as an adverse effect of chemotherapy?

1. Using lemon glycerin swabs
2. Administering milk of magnesia
3. Providing a bland, moist, soft diet
4. Frequently washing the mouth with full-strength hydrogen peroxide

91. 3. Oral ulcers are red, eroded, and painful. Providing a bland, moist, soft diet will make chewing and swallowing less painful. The use of lemon glycerin swabs and milk of magnesia should be avoided. Glycerin, a trihydric alcohol, absorbs water and dries the membranes. Milk of magnesia also has a drying effect because unabsorbed magnesium salts exert an osmotic pressure on tissue fluids. Many children also find the taste unpleasant. Frequent mouthwashes without alcohol are indicated. Peroxide shouldn't be used because it's irritating to tissues.

CN: Physiological integrity; CNS: Basic care and comfort; CL: Application

Don't stop now! You're doing a great job!

92. The parents of a child undergoing irradiation are taught about post-irradiation somnolence. Which statement, if made by the parents, indicates that the teaching has been effective?

1. "This neurologic syndrome will occur immediately."
2. "This neurologic syndrome usually occurs within 1 to 2 weeks."
3. "This neurologic syndrome usually occurs within 5 to 8 weeks."
4. "This neurologic syndrome usually occurs within 3 to 6 months."

92. 3. Postirradiation somnolence may develop 5 to 8 weeks after CNS irradiation and may last 3 to 15 days. It's characterized by somnolence with or without fever, anorexia, nausea, and vomiting. Although the syndrome isn't thought to be clinically significant, parents should be prepared to expect such symptoms and encouraged to allow the child needed rest.

CN: Physiological integrity; CNS: Physiological adaptation; CL: Application

93. Which intervention can prevent hemorrhagic cystitis caused by bladder irritation from chemotherapeutic medications?

1. Giving antacids
2. Giving antibiotics
3. Restricting fluid intake
4. Increasing fluid intake

93. 4. Sterile hemorrhagic cystitis is an adverse effect of chemical irritation of the bladder from cyclophosphamide. It can be prevented by liberal fluid intake (at least 1½ times the recommended daily fluid requirement). Antibiotics don't aid in the prevention of sterile hemorrhagic cystitis. Restricting fluids would only increase the risk of developing cystitis. Antacids wouldn't be indicated for treatment.

CN: Physiological integrity; CNS: Reduction of risk potential; CL: Application

94. The parents of a child diagnosed with leukemia have stated that they'll give aspirin to their child for pain relief. Which statement about aspirin by the nurse would be the most accurate?

1. "It's contraindicated because it decreases platelet production."
2. "It's contraindicated because it promotes bleeding tendencies."
3. "It's not a strong enough analgesic."
4. "It decreases the effects of methotrexate (Trexall)."

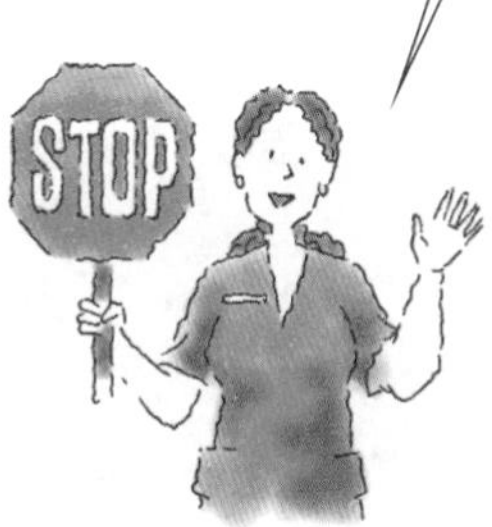

What other conditions is aspirin used for?
STOP

94. 2. Aspirin would be contraindicated because it promotes bleeding. Aspirin use has also been associated with Reye's syndrome in children. For home use, acetaminophen (Tylenol) is recommended for mild to moderate pain. Aspirin enhances the effects of methotrexate and has no effect on platelet production. Nonopioid analgesia has been effective for mild to moderate pain in clients with leukemia.

CN: Physiological integrity; CNS: Pharmacological and parenteral therapies; CL: Application

95. Which nursing measure helps prepare the parent and child for alopecia, a common adverse effect of several chemotherapeutic agents?

1. Introducing the idea of a wig after hair loss occurs
2. Explaining that hair typically begins to regrow in 6 to 9 months
3. Stressing that hair loss during a second treatment with the same medication will be more severe
4. Explaining that, as hair thins, keeping it clean, short, and fluffy may camouflage partial baldness

95. 4. The nurse must prepare parents and children for possible hair loss. Cutting the hair short lessens the impact of seeing large quantities of hair on bed linens and clothing. Sometimes, keeping the hair short and fuller can make a wig unnecessary. Hair usually regrows in 6 months, depending on the treatment protocol. A child should be encouraged to pick out a wig similar to his own hair style and color before the hair falls out to foster adjustment to hair loss. Hair loss during a second treatment with the same medication is usually less severe.

CN: Psychosocial integrity; CNS: None; CL: Application

96. A nurse is discussing childhood cancer with the parents of a child in an oncology unit. Which statement by the nurse would be the most accurate?

1. "The most common site for children's cancer is the bone marrow."
2. "All childhood cancers have a high mortality rate."
3. "Children with leukemia have a higher survival rate if they're older than 11 when diagnosed."
4. "The prognosis for children with cancer isn't affected by treatment strategies."

96. 1. Childhood cancers occur most commonly in rapidly growing tissue, especially in the bone marrow. Mortality depends on the time of diagnosis, the type of cancer, and the age at which the child was diagnosed. Children who are diagnosed between the ages of 2 and 9 consistently demonstrate a better prognosis. Treatment strategies are tailored to produce the most favorable prognosis.

CN: Physiological integrity; CNS: Physiological adaptation; CL: Application

97. Which condition assessed by the nurse would be an early warning sign of childhood cancer?

1. Difficult in swallowing
2. Nagging cough or hoarseness
3. Slight change in bowel and bladder habits
4. Swellings, lumps, or masses anywhere on the body

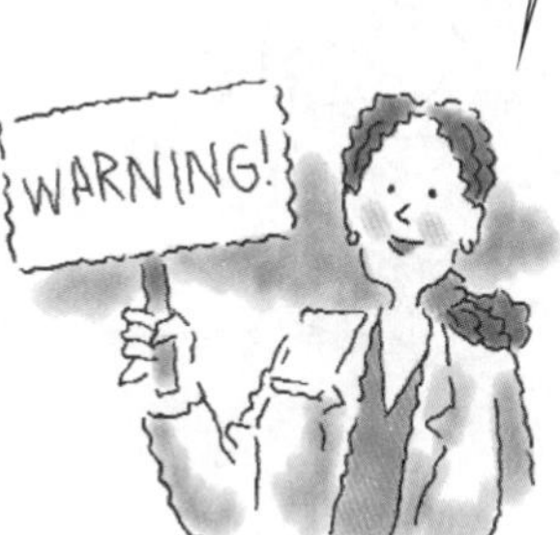

97. 4. By being aware of early signs of childhood cancer, nurses can refer children for further evaluation. Swellings, lumps, or masses anywhere on the body are early warning signals of childhood cancer. Difficulty swallowing, cough, and hoarseness are early signs of cancer in adults. Usually there's also a marked change in bowel or bladder habits, not associated with dietary intake.

CN: Health promotion and maintenance; CNS: None; CL: Application

98. Which nursing intervention helps to decrease the adverse effects of radiation therapy on the GI tract?

1. Avoiding the use of antispasmodics
2. Encouraging fluids and a soft diet
3. Giving antiemetics when nausea or vomiting occurs
4. Avoiding mouthwashes to prevent irritation of mouth ulcers

98. 2. Radiation therapy can cause adverse effects such as nausea and vomiting, anorexia, mucosal ulceration, and diarrhea. Antispasmodics are used to help reduce diarrhea. Encouraging fluids and a soft diet will help with anorexia. Antiemetics should be given before the onset of nausea. Frequent mouthwashes are indicated to prevent mycosis.

CN: Physiological integrity; CNS: Physiological adaptation; CL: Application

99. Short-term steroid therapy is used in clients with leukemia to promote which reaction?

1. Increased appetite
2. Altered body image
3. Increased platelet production
4. Decreased susceptibility to infection

99. 1. Short-term steroid therapy produces no acute toxicities and results in two beneficial reactions: increased appetite and a sense of well-being. Physical changes, such as "moon face," a result of steroid use, can cause alterations in body image and can be extremely distressing to children. Prednisone (steroid therapy) has no effect on platelet production but may increase susceptibility to infection.

CN: Physiological integrity; CNS: Pharmacological and parenteral therapies; CL: Application

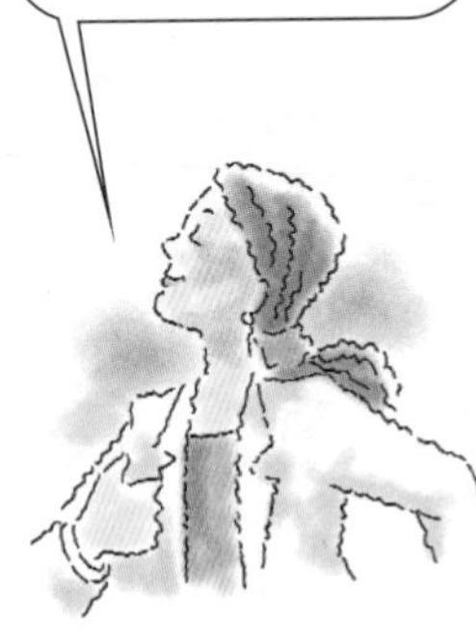

One hundred questions! You must be proud!

100. Teaching children with leukemia and their families should include potential adverse effects of treatments. Which of the following is an adverse effect of prednisone?

1. Decreased appetite
2. Increased blood glucose
3. Decreased risk of infection
4. Decreased hair growth

100. 2. Prednisone may cause an increase in blood glucose requiring doses of insulin, especially when other factors are involved. Increased appetite, increased risk of infection, and increased hair growth are also adverse effects of prednisone.

CN: Physiological integrity; CNS: Pharmacological and parenteral therapies; CL: Application

101. Which intervention is a priority for a hemophilic child who has fallen and badly bruised his leg?

1. Appropriate dose of aspirin and rest
2. Immobilization of the leg and a dose of ibuprofen
3. Heating pad and administration of factor VIII concentrate
4. Pressure on the site and administration of the required clotting factor

101. 4. With any bleeding injury in a client with hemophilia, the first line of treatment is always to replace the clotting factor. Pressure is applied along with cool compresses, and the extremity is immobilized. Aspirin isn't used because of its anticoagulant properties and the risk of Reye's syndrome in children. Immobilizing the leg and giving ibuprofen would be done after applying pressure and administering the necessary clotting factor. Heat isn't used because it increases bleeding.

CN: Safe, effective care environment; CNS: Management of care; CL: Application

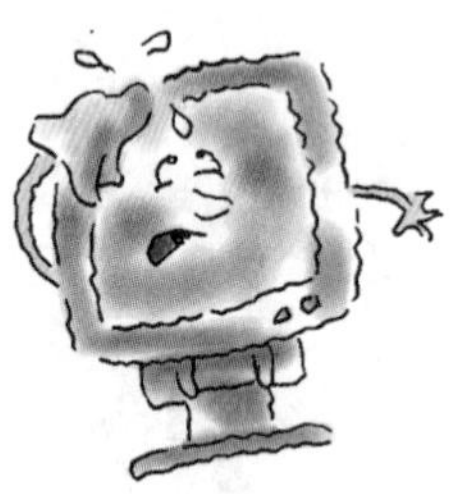

The pressure is really on to prioritize.

102. When teaching an adolescent with iron deficiency anemia about diet choices, which menu selection would indicate that more instruction is necessary?

1. Caesar salad and pretzels
2. Cheeseburger with milkshake
3. Red beans and rice with sausage
4. Egg sandwich and snack peanuts

102. 1. Caesar salad and pretzels aren't foods high in iron and protein. Meats (especially organ meats), eggs, and nuts have high protein and iron.

CN: Physiological integrity; CNS: Basic care and comfort; CL: Analysis

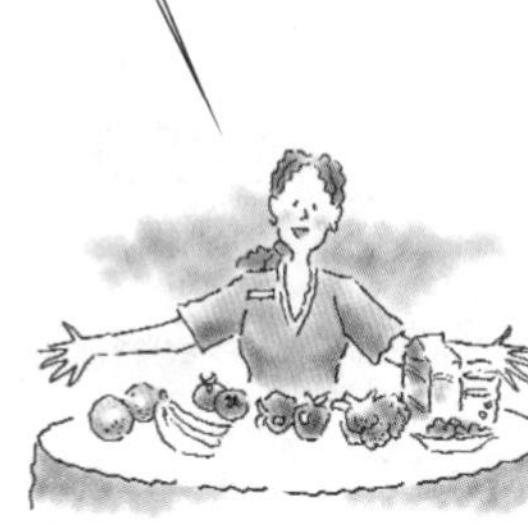

Good diet choices are important for clients of all ages.

103. A nurse is speaking to the mother of a child with leukemia who wants to know why her child is so susceptible to infection if he has too many white blood cells (WBCs). Which response would be most accurate?

1. This is an adverse effect of the medication he has to take.
2. He hasn't been able to eat a proper diet since he's been sick.
3. Leukemia is a problem of tumors in the internal organs that prevent his ability to fight infection.
4. Leukemia causes production of too many immature WBCs, which can't fight infection very well.

103. 4. Leukemia is an unrestricted proliferation of immature WBCs, which don't function properly and are a poor defense against infection. Diet contributes to overall health but doesn't cause the overproduction of WBCs. There are no solid tumors in the internal organs in leukemia. Medications such as chemotherapy can diminish the immune system's effectiveness; however, they don't cause the overproduction of immature WBCs and the poor resistance to infection that the mother asked about.

CN: Physiological integrity; CNS: Physiological adaptation; CL: Application

104. A nurse is developing a teaching plan for parents of a toddler who was just diagnosed with sickle cell anemia. Which statement is important to emphasize in the teaching plan?

1. If they have any more children, those children will also have sickle cell anemia.
2. Knowing how to prevent vaso-occlusive crisis is an important part of the parent's role.
3. The child will have a greater tendency to bleed and should avoid contact sports.
4. Vaso-occlusive crisis will occur eventually, requiring medical care.

104. 2. Prevention is the key to teaching a family of a child with sickle cell anemia. The nurse should emphasize the daily use of prescribed oral antibiotics and avoidance of dehydration, high altitudes, and cold. These interventions can dramatically reduce the incidence of crisis. The disease is autosomal recessive, so each pregnancy has a 1 in 4 chance of the child having the disease, a 1 in 4 chance of not having the disease, and a 2 in 4 chance of carrying the trait. Abnormal bleeding and the need to avoid contact sports are associated with hemophilia.

CN: Health promotion and maintenance; CNS: None; CL: Application

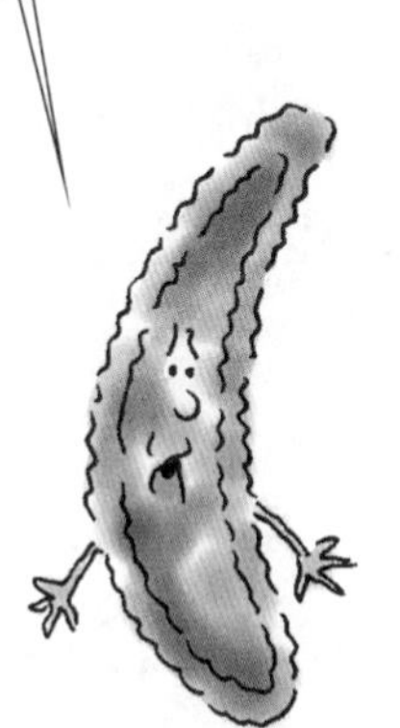

105. A grandmother calls the pediatric children's clinic to find out whether her 3-year-old grandson can get shingles from her. Which response would be appropriate?

1. No, shingles don't occur in small children.
2. Yes, the grandson can get shingles from her. Shingles are caused by the herpes zoster virus.
3. The grandson could develop shingles if the lesions are on exposed skin areas and are weeping.
4. No, but the grandson would be exposed to the varicella-zoster virus, which could lead to the development of chickenpox.

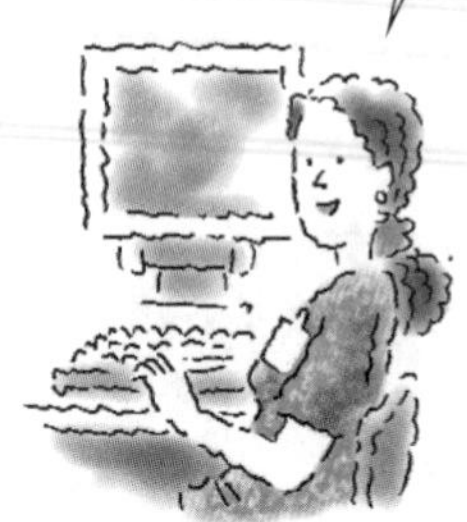

105. 4. Shingles occur when a dormant varicella-zoster virus in a nerve becomes inflamed. The vesicles of shingles contain the virus and would expose others to it. The grandson couldn't develop shingles from such exposure. A herpes virus doesn't cause shingles. Shingles can occur in children, but only if they have previously had chickenpox. The impetus for the inflammation is internal, not external.

CN: Safe, effective care environment; CNS: Safety and infection control; CL: Analysis

106. A child with idiopathic thrombocytopenic purpura is admitted to the hospital with a platelet count of 20,000/mm^3. He should be closely monitored for which condition?

1. Hyperactivity
2. Proteinuria
3. Hand-foot syndrome
4. Change in level of consciousness (LOC)

106. 4. When the platelet count drops to 20,000/mm^3, the child is at risk for spontaneous bleeding, including intracranially. A change in LOC is an important sign of increased intracranial pressure. This child is likely to become somnolent and difficult to arouse—not hyperactive. Proteinuria is more common in glomerulonephritis. With blood in the urine, protein also increases—but this isn't the primary concern. Hand-foot syndrome occurs in a child with sickle cell disease.

CN: Physiological integrity; CNS: Reduction of risk potential; CL: Application

107. Infants must be monitored closely because they can't report changes in their condition. In a 1-month-old infant, which are the signs of increased intracranial pressure (ICP)?

1. Bulging fontanels, a high-pitched cry, vomiting
2. Frequent crying, sunken fontanel, pulse rate above 120 beats/minute
3. Blood-tinged vomitus, legs flexed to the abdomen, frequent crying
4. Falling asleep during feeding, pulse rate above 120 beats/minute when fussing, irregular arm and leg movements

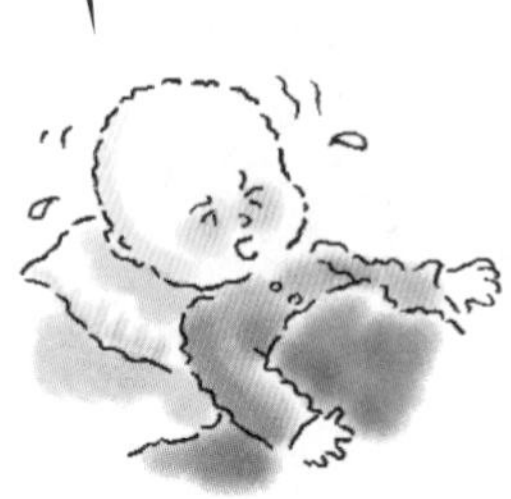

I can't tell you what's wrong, so look for the signs.

107. 1. Because fontanels haven't closed by the age of 1 month, they bulge with increasing ICP. A high-pitched cry and vomiting also signal increased ICP. Quality of the cry is an important sign in an infant. Vomiting should be distinguished from a small amount of formula regurgitation, which is normal. Frequent crying may result from various stressors, and quality of the cry should be assessed. Blood-tinged vomitus, flexed legs, and crying indicate an abdominal disorder and pain. Infants normally have irregular arm and leg movements. A pulse rate of 120 beats/minute is normal for a 1-month-old infant at rest; in fact, the pulse may increase to 200 beats/minute during stress.

CN: Physiological integrity; CNS: Reduction of risk potential; CL: Analysis

CN: Client needs category CNS: Client needs subcategory CL: Cognitive level

108. Discharge teaching for the family of a school-age child with idiopathic thrombocytopenia should include restriction of which activity?
1. Swimming
2. Bicycle riding
3. Computer games
4. Exposure to large crowds

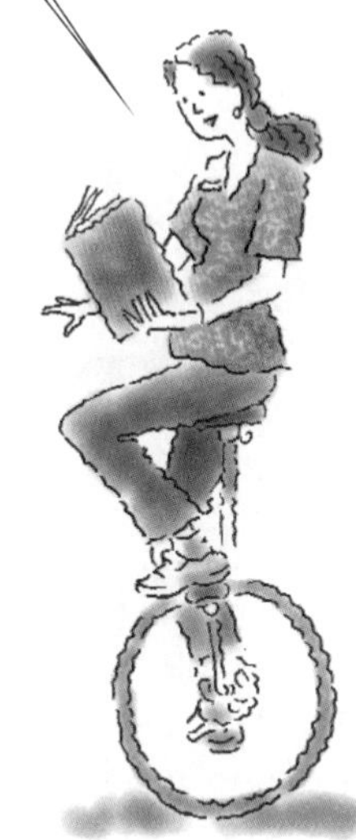

Let' see. Which activity should be restricted?

108. 2. When routine blood counts reveal the platelet level is 100,000/mm^3 or less, the child shouldn't engage in contact sports, bicycle or scooter riding, climbing, or other activities that could lead to injury (especially to the head). Swimming releases energy, builds muscle, and allows the child to compete without risking injury, as long as she follows normal safety precautions. Computer games don't cause physical injury. This child need not avoid large crowds because idiopathic thrombocytopenia doesn't suppress the immune system.

CN: Safe, effective care environment; CNS: Safety and infection control; CL: Application

109. A 17-year-old boy with classic hemophilia (hemophilia A) is admitted to the hospital for surgery. His preoperative preparation should include which treatment?
1. Bed rest
2. Transfusion of clotting factor 8
3. I.V. analgesics given around the clock
4. Hydration at 50% above the normal fluid requirement

109. 2. In classic hemophilia or hemophilia A, clotting factor 8 is deficient. This factor must be transfused before surgery and at intervals afterward to prevent bleeding during and after surgery. Analgesics would be indicated if the child experienced bleeding, especially into the joints. Hydration above the normal requirement isn't needed. Because the child wasn't admitted for bleeding, bed rest isn't necessary.

CN: Physiological integrity; CNS: Reduction of risk potential; CL: Application

110. A child with hemophilia is hospitalized with bleeding into the knee. Which action should the nurse take first?
1. Prepare to administer a whole blood transfusion.
2. Prepare to administer a plasma transfusion.
3. Perform active range-of-motion (ROM) exercise on the affected part.
4. Elevate the affected part.

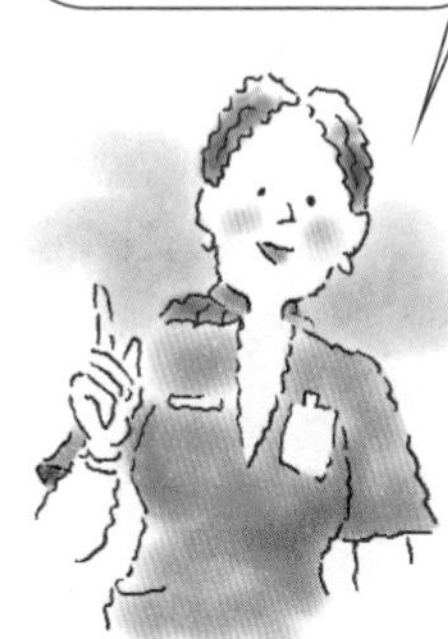

Hint! It's the first action the nurse should take.

110. 4. Bleeding into the joints is the most common type of bleeding episode in the more severe hemophilia forms. Elevating the affected part and applying pressure and cold are indicated. The nurse should anticipate transfusing the missing clotting factor—not whole blood or plasma, which won't stop the bleeding promptly and may pose a risk of fluid overload. Active ROM exercises are contraindicated because they may cause more bleeding, injury, and pain.

CN: Physiological integrity; CNS: Reduction of risk potential; CL: Application

111. Which measure is indicated for a child in sickle cell vaso-occlusive crisis?
1. Immobilizing the affected part
2. Applying warm packs to the affected part
3. Applying cool packs to the affected part
4. Performing active range-of-motion (ROM) exercises to the affected part

111. 2. Applying warm packs promotes vasodilation and perfusion and provides pain relief and comfort. Immobilization leads to stasis, which promotes sickling. Cool packs are contraindicated because they cause vasoconstriction and may precipitate red blood cell sickling. A child in vaso-occlusive crisis experiences acute pain and limits movement of the affected part. After the acute crisis passes, the child should be encouraged to ambulate. Active ROM exercises increase pain in the affected part.

CN: Physiological integrity; CNS: Basic care and comfort; CL: Application

112. A 4-year-old child has recently been diagnosed with acute lymphocytic leukemia (ALL). What information about ALL should the nurse provide when educating the client's parents? Select all that apply:

1. Leukemia is a rare form of childhood cancer.
2. ALL affects all blood-forming organs and systems throughout the body.
3. The child shouldn't brush his teeth because of the increased risk of bleeding.
4. Adverse effects of treatment include sleepiness, alopecia, and stomatitis.
5. There's a 95% chance of remission with treatment.
6. The child shouldn't be disciplined during this difficult time.

112. 2, 4, 5. In ALL, abnormal white blood cells proliferate, but they don't mature past the blast stage. These blast cells crowd out the healthy white blood cells, red blood cells, and platelets in the bone marrow, leading to bone marrow depression. The blast cells also infiltrate the liver, spleen, kidneys, and lymph tissue. Common adverse effects of chemotherapy and radiation include nausea, vomiting, diarrhea, sleepiness, alopecia, anemia, stomatitis, mucositis, pain, reddened skin, and increased susceptibility to infection. There's a 95% chance of obtaining remission with treatment. Leukemia is the most common form of childhood cancer. The child still needs appropriate discipline and limits. A lack of consistent parenting may lead to negative behaviors and fear.

CN: Physiological integrity; CNS: Reduction of risk potential; CL: Application

113. A child with sickle cell anemia is being treated for a crisis. The physician orders morphine sulfate (Duramorph) 2 mg I.V. The concentration of the vial is 10 mg/1 ml of solution. How many milliliters of solution should the nurse administer? Record your answer using one decimal point.

________________ milliliters

113. 0.2. The nurse should calculate the volume to be given using this equation: $2 \text{ mg}/X \text{ ml} = 10 \text{ mg}/1 \text{ ml}$; $10X = 2$; $X = 0.2$ ml.

CN: Physiological integrity; CNS: Pharmacological and parenteral therapies; CL: Application

114. A child with sickle cell anemia is being discharged after treatment for a crisis. Which instructions for avoiding future crises should the nurse provide to the client and his family? Select all that apply:

1. Avoid foods high in folic acid.
2. Drink plenty of fluids.
3. Use cold packs to relieve joint pain.
4. Report a sore throat to an adult immediately.
5. Restrict activity to quiet board games.
6. Wash hands before meals and after playing.

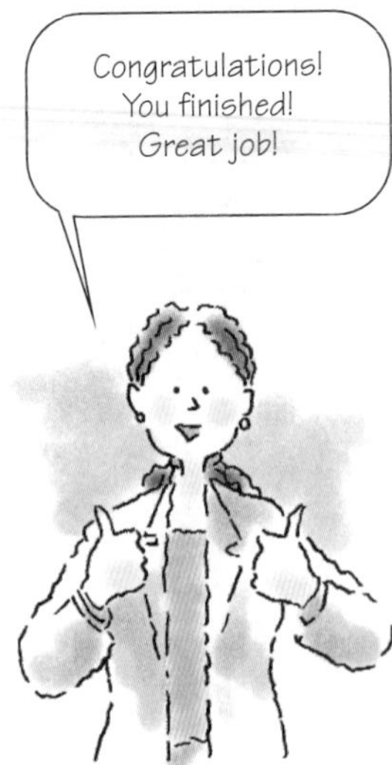
Congratulations!
You finished!
Great job!

114. 2, 4, 6. Fluids should be encouraged to prevent stasis in the bloodstream, which can lead to sickling. Sore throats, and any other cold symptoms, should be reported because they may indicate the presence of an infection, which can precipitate a crisis (red blood cells sickle and obstruct blood flow to tissues). Children with sickle cell anemia should learn appropriate measures to prevent infection, such as proper hand-washing techniques and good nutrition practices. Folic acid intake should be encouraged to help support new cell growth because new cells replace fragile, sickled cells. Warm packs should be applied to provide comfort and relieve pain; cold packs cause vasoconstriction. The child should maintain an active, normal life. When the child experiences a pain crisis, he limits his own activity according to his pain level.

CN: Physiological integrity; CNS: Reduction of risk potential; CL: Application

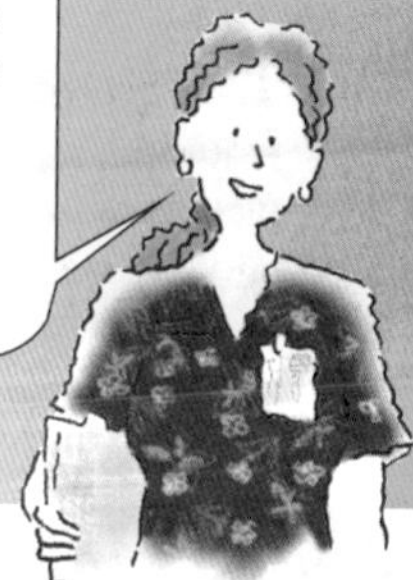

From the simple otitis media to the uncommon and dangerous epiglottiditis, this chapter covers a wide variety of respiratory disorders in children. So, take a deep breath and go for it!

Chapter 29 Respiratory disorders

1. Following the death of an infant from sudden infant death syndrome (SIDS), which response by a nurse to the grieving parents is most appropriate?

1. "You didn't cause your infant's death."
2. "An autopsy will confirm the cause of your infant's death."
3. "Don't worry, you'll have more children."
4. "Be sure to place your next infant on his back to sleep."

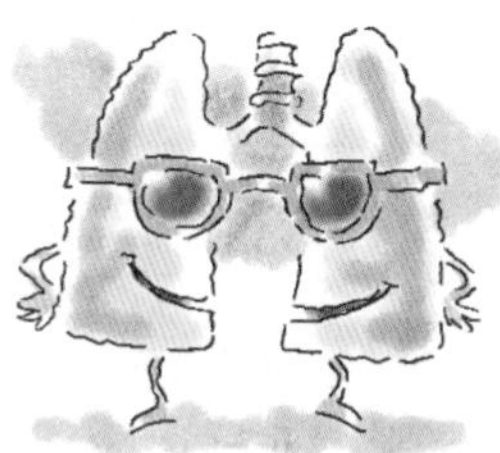

Cool! You made it to chapter 29. Keep up the good work!

1. 1. The nurse can best support grieving parents by correcting the common falsehood that they could have prevented the infant's death. While an autopsy may need to be performed, it isn't a supportive response to grieving parents. Telling the parents that they will have more children minimizes the death of this infant and belittles the parent's feelings of grief. Instructing the parents to position future infants on their back suggests that the parents could have prevented this child's death.

CN: Psychosocial integrity; CNS: None; CL: Analysis

2. Which child has an increased risk of sudden infant death syndrome (SIDS)?

1. A neonate born at 32 weeks' gestation weighing 4 lb (1.8 kg)
2. A 2-year-old with a broken arm
3. An infant hospitalized with a temperature of 103.4° F (39.7° C)
4. A first-born child

2. 1. Premature infants, especially those with low birth weight, have an increased risk for SIDS. Infants with apnea, central nervous system disorders, or respiratory disorders have a higher risk of SIDS. Peak age for SIDS is 2 to 4 months. Hospitalization for fever is insignificant. There's an increased risk of SIDS in subsequent siblings of two or more SIDS victims.

CN: Physiological integrity; CNS: Reduction of risk potential; CL: Analysis

3. A 6-week-old infant is brought to the emergency department not breathing; a preliminary finding of sudden infant death syndrome (SIDS) is made to the parents. Which intervention should the nurse take <u>initially</u>?

1. Call their spiritual advisor.
2. Explain the etiology of SIDS.
3. Allow them to see their infant.
4. Collect the infant's belongings and give them to the parents.

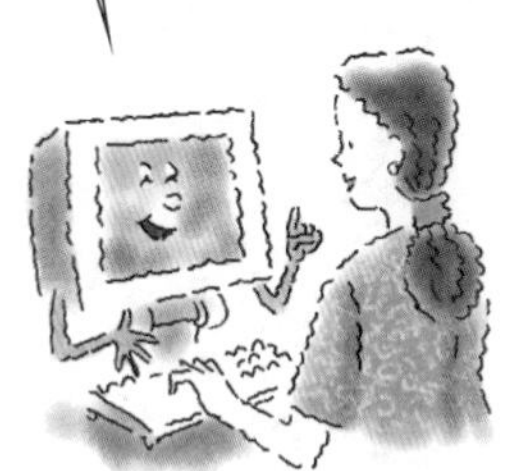

3. 3. The parents need time with their infant to assist with the grieving process. Calling their pastor and collecting the infant's belongings are also important steps in the plan of care but aren't priorities. The parents will be too upset to understand an explanation of SIDS at this time.

CN: Psychosocial integrity; CNS: None; CL: Application

4. The family of an infant that died from sudden infant death syndrome (SIDS) asks the nurse what risk factors could have predisposed their child to SIDS. Which response would be the most accurate?

1. Breast feeding the infant
2. Gestational age of 42 weeks
3. Immunizations
4. Low birth weight

4. 4. Prematurity, low birth weight, maternal smoking, and multiple births are important risk factors associated with SIDS. Breast feeding and a gestational age of 42 weeks aren't significant. Immunizations have been disproved to be associated with the disorder.

CN: Physiological integrity; CNS: Reduction of risk potential; CL: Application

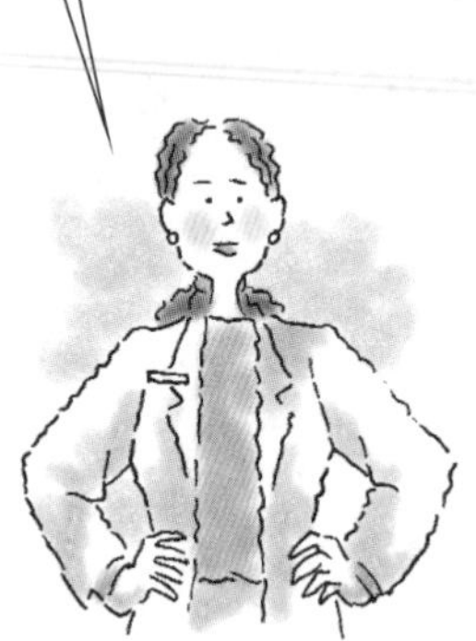

It's important to be sensitive to a family's feelings when they've lost a child to SIDS.

5. An infant is brought to the emergency department (ED) and pronounced dead with the preliminary finding of sudden infant death syndrome (SIDS). Which question to the parents is appropriate?

1. Did you hear the infant cry out?
2. Was the infant's head buried in a blanket?
3. Were any of the siblings jealous of the new baby?
4. How did the infant look when you found him?

5. 4. Only factual questions should be asked during the initial history in the ED. The other questions imply blame, guilt, or neglect.

CN: Physiological integrity; CNS: Physiological adaptation; CL: Application

6. Which diagnostic test should be included in the care plan for children with an increased risk of sudden infant death syndrome (SIDS)?

1. Pulmonary function tests at regular intervals
2. Home apnea monitor
3. Pulse oximetry while sleeping
4. Chest X-ray at age 1 month

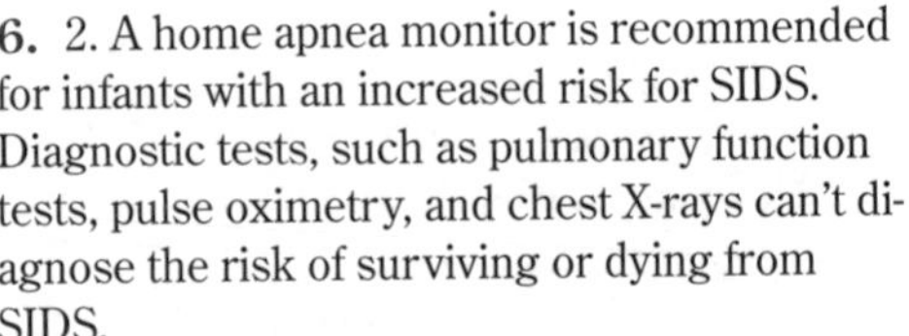

6. 2. A home apnea monitor is recommended for infants with an increased risk for SIDS. Diagnostic tests, such as pulmonary function tests, pulse oximetry, and chest X-rays can't diagnose the risk of surviving or dying from SIDS.

CN: Physiological integrity; CNS: Reduction of risk potential; CL: Application

7. Which reaction is usually exhibited by the family of an infant who has died from sudden infant death syndrome (SIDS)?

1. Feelings of blame or guilt
2. Acceptance of the diagnosis
3. Requests for the infant's belongings
4. Questions regarding the etiology of the diagnosis

7. 1. During the first few moments, the parents often are in shock and have overwhelming feelings of blame or guilt. Acceptance of the diagnosis and questions regarding the etiology may not occur until the parents have had time to see the child. The infant's belongings are usually packaged for the family to take home but some parents may see this as a painful reminder.

CN: Psychosocial integrity; CNS: None; CL: Application

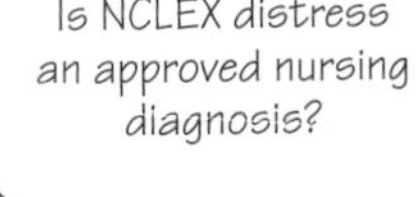

Is NCLEX distress an approved nursing diagnosis?

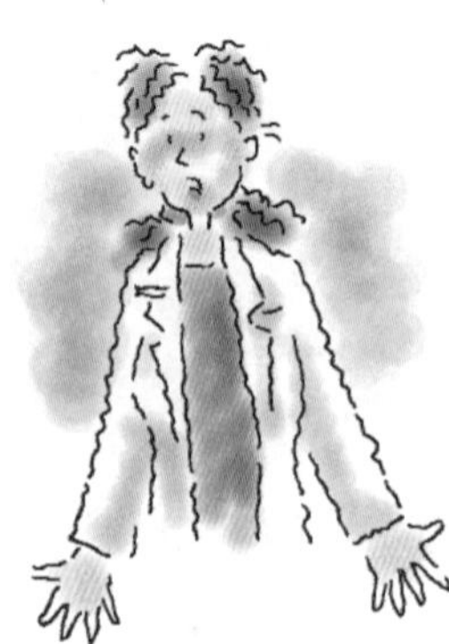

8. The parents of an infant who just died from sudden infant death syndrome (SIDS) are angry at God and refuse to see any member of the clergy. Which nursing diagnosis is most appropriate?

1. *Ineffective coping*
2. *Spiritual distress*
3. *Complicated grieving*
4. *Chronic sorrow*

8. 2. The defining characteristics of *Spiritual distress* include anger and refusing to interact with spiritual leaders. While anger is part of the grieving process, there's no indication that the parents aren't coping effectively or are experiencing *Complicated grieving*. Since *Chronic sorrow,* as the name implies, occurs over a period of time and may be cyclical, this isn't an appropriate nursing diagnosis since the death has just occurred.

CN: Psychosocial integrity; CNS: None; CL: Analysis

CN: Client needs category CNS: Client needs subcategory CL: Cognitive level

9. Which plan is most appropriate for a nurse scheduling a home visit to parents who lost an infant to sudden infant death syndrome (SIDS)?
1. One visit in 2 weeks
2. No visit is necessary
3. As soon after death as possible
4. One visit with parents only, no siblings

9. 3. When parents return home, a visit is necessary as soon after the death as possible. The nurse should assess what the parents have been told, what they think happened, and how they've explained this to the other siblings. Not all of these issues will be resolved in one visit. The number of visits and plan for intervention must be flexible. The needs of the siblings must always be considered.
CN: Psychosocial integrity; CNS: None; CL: Application

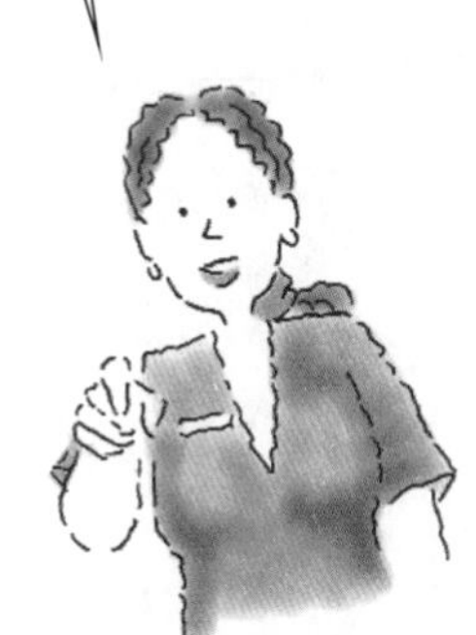

Make sure you understand the grieving process necessary for SIDS parents.

10. About 1 week after the death of an infant from sudden infant death syndrome (SIDS), which behavior should a nurse expect to observe in a parent?
1. Disorganized thinking
2. Feelings of guilt
3. Repressed thoughts
4. Structured thinking

10. 4. About 1 week after the death, the parent of the infant would most likely be in the turmoil phase. In the turmoil phase, structured thinking is common. Almost immediately, at the time of death, parents may have repressed thoughts and feelings of guilt or blame. Within a day or two, the parents enter the impact phase of crisis. This consists of disorganized thoughts in which they can't deal with the crisis in concrete terms.
CN: Psychosocial integrity; CNS: None; CL: Application

11. Which position is recommended for placing an infant to sleep?
1. Prone position
2. Supine position
3. Side-lying position
4. With head of bed elevated 30 degrees

11. 2. The American Academy of Pediatrics endorses placing infants face-up in their cribs as a way to reduce sudden infant death syndrome (SIDS). Placing infants on their stomach is thought to make an attack of apnea harder to fight off but how exactly the sleeping position predisposes a child to SIDS is still unclear. The side-lying position promotes gastric emptying. Raising the head of the bed 30 degrees is recommended for infants with gastroesophageal reflux.
CN: Health promotion and maintenance; CNS: None; CL: Application

12. Which activity should be recommended for <u>long-term</u> support of parents with an infant who has died of sudden infant death syndrome (SIDS)?
1. Attending support groups
2. Attending church regularly
3. Attending counseling sessions
4. Discussing feelings with family and friends

12. 1. The best support will come from parents who have had the same experience. Attending church and discussing feelings with family and friends can offer support but they may not understand the experience. Counseling sessions are usually a short-term support.
CN: Psychosocial integrity; CNS: None; CL: Application

13. Which intervention is best to help a 2-year-old child adapt to hospitalization?

1. Allow the child to have favorite toys.
2. Allow the child to play with equipment used on him.
3. Explain procedures in simple terms.
4. Ask one or both parents to stay with the child.

13. 4. The most important factor in helping a child cope with new and strange surroundings is to have the security of the parents being present. This is the hallmark of family-centered care. Placing the child's favorite toys in the room provides distraction and allows the child to have something of his own with him but may *not* alleviate fears. Allowing the child to play with the equipment may pose a safety hazard and isn't appropriate. Explaining procedures in simple terms is important but a 2-year-old has limited understanding.

CN: Psychosocial integrity; CNS: None; CL: Application

14. A 2-year-old child comes to the emergency department with inspiratory stridor and a barking cough. A preliminary diagnosis of croup has been made. Which action should be an initial intervention?

1. Administer I.V. antibiotics.
2. Provide oxygen by facemask.
3. Establish and maintain the airway.
4. Ask the mother to go to the waiting room.

14. 3. The initial priority is to establish and maintain the airway. Edema and accumulation of secretions may contribute to airway obstruction. Antibiotics aren't indicated for viral illnesses. Oxygen should be administered by tent as soon as possible to decrease the child's distress. Allowing the child to stay with the mother reduces anxiety and distress.

CN: Physiological integrity; CNS: Physiological adaptation; CL: Application

Congratulations! You've finished the first 15 questions! Good job!

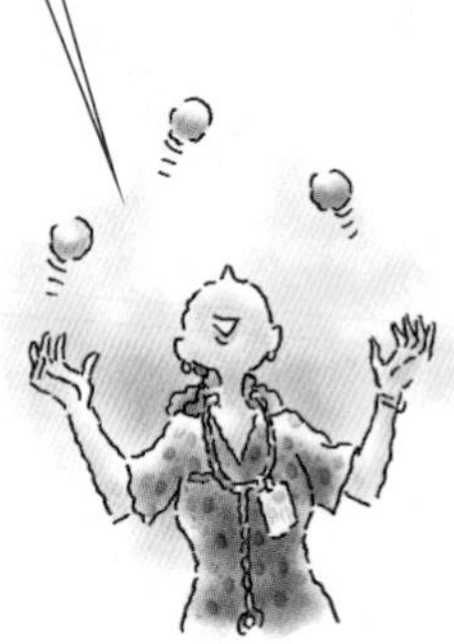

15. Which action is the best intervention for parents to take if their child is experiencing an episode of "midnight croup," or acute spasmodic laryngitis?

1. Give warm liquids.
2. Raise the heat on the thermostat.
3. Provide humidified air with cool mist.
4. Take the child into the bathroom with a warm running shower.

15. 3. High humidity with cool mist provides the most relief. Raising the heat on the thermostat will result in dry, warm air, which may cause secretions to adhere to the airway wall. A warm, running shower provides a mist that may be helpful to moisten and decrease the viscosity of airway secretions and may also decrease laryngeal spasm, but cool liquids would be best for the child. If unable to take liquid, the child needs to be in the emergency department.

CN: Physiological integrity; CNS: Physiological adaptation; CL: Application

This question is asking for the symptom most commonly associated with croup.

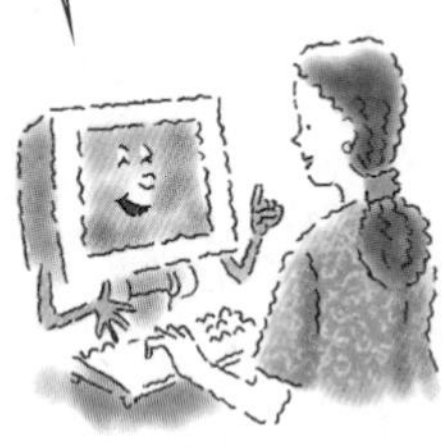

16. Which sign is most characteristic of a child with croup?

1. Barking cough
2. Fever
3. High heart rate
4. Respiratory distress

16. 1. A resonant cough described as "barking" is the most characteristic sign of croup. The child may present with a low-grade or high fever depending on whether the etiologic agent is viral or bacterial. While the child with croup may have a rapid heart rate, it isn't a characteristic sign of croup. The child may have varying degrees of respiratory distress related to swelling or obstruction.

CN: Physiological integrity; CNS: Physiological adaptation; CL: Analysis

17. Which sign should alert a nurse that an 18-month-old child with croup is experiencing increased respiratory distress?
1. A barking cough
2. Intercostal retractions
3. Clubbing of the fingers
4. Increased anterior-posterior chest diameter

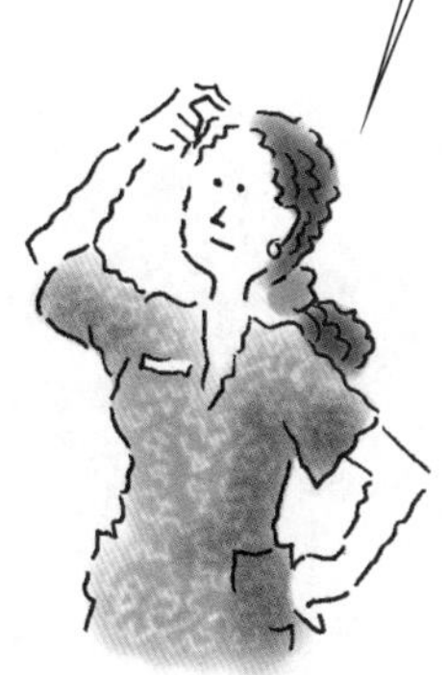

I know what's important, but what's the most important?

17. 2. Intercostal retractions occur as the child's breathing becomes more labored and the use of other muscles is necessary to draw air into the lungs. A barking cough occurs in a child with croup and itself isn't a sign that the condition is worsening. Clubbing of the fingers and a change in chest diameter occur with chronic respiratory conditions.
CN: Physiological integrity; CNS: Physiological adaptation; CL: Analysis

18. Which intervention is the most important goal for a child with ineffective airway clearance?
1. Reducing the child's anxiety
2. Maintaining a patent airway
3. Providing adequate oral fluids
4. Administering medications as ordered

18. 2. The most important goal is to maintain a patent airway. Reducing anxiety and administering medications will follow after the airway is secure. The child shouldn't be allowed to eat or drink anything to prevent the risk of aspiration.
CN: Physiological integrity; CNS: Physiological adaptation; CL: Application

19. A 19-month-old child with croup is crying as a nurse tries to auscultate breath sounds. Which intervention by the nurse would be most appropriate?
1. Ignore the crying and listen to breaths sounds as best as possible.
2. Tell the parents that they are upsetting the child and to wait outside the room.
3. Tell the child, in a loud and firm voice, that he must sit still and cooperate.
4. Hand the stethoscope to the child to examine before auscultating his lungs.

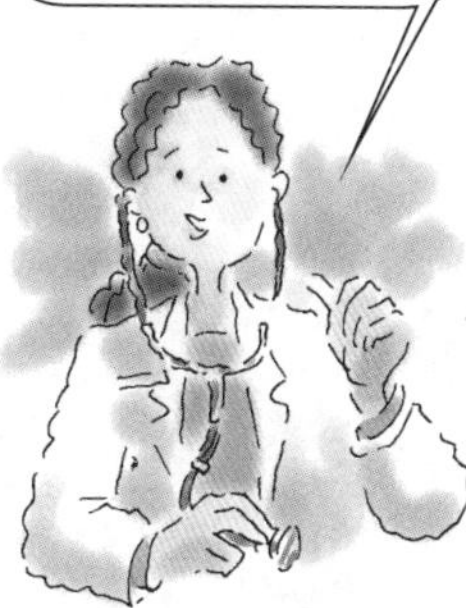

It's important to gain the child's trust.

19. 4. Developmentally, children at this age are curious. Therefore, encouraging the child to play with the stethoscope will distract him and help gain trust so that the nurse will be able to auscultate the lungs. Ignoring the child's crying may only get him more upset and won't help the nurse gain his trust. The nurse should use the parents to help quiet and comfort the child. Asking the parents to leave may only upset the child more. The nurse should speak to the child in a soft, comforting tone of voice.
CN: Health promotion and maintenance; CNS: None; CL: Analysis

20. Which precaution is recommended when caring for children with respiratory infections such as croup?
1. Enforce hand washing.
2. Place the child in isolation.
3. Teach children to use tissues.
4. Keep siblings in the same room.

20. 1. Hand washing helps prevent the spread of infections. Ill children should be placed in separate bedrooms if possible but don't need to be isolated. Teaching children to use tissues properly is important, but the key is disposal and hand washing after use.
CN: Health promotion and maintenance; CNS: None; CL: Application

21. What is the best time to administer a nebulizer treatment to a child with croup?
1. During naptime
2. During playtime
3. After the child eats
4. After the parents leave

21. 1. The nurse should administer nebulizer treatments at prescribed intervals. During naptime allows for as little disruption as possible. Administering treatment during playtime will disrupt the child's daily pattern. A child should be given a treatment before eating so the airway will be open and the work of eating will be decreased. Parents are usually helpful when administering treatments. The child can sit on the parents' lap to help decrease anxiety or fear.
CN: Physiological integrity; CNS: Pharmacological and parenteral therapies; CL: Application

22. During the recovery stages of croup, a nurse should explain which intervention to parents?

1. Limiting oral fluid intake
2. Recognizing signs of respiratory distress
3. Providing three nutritious meals per day
4. Allowing the child to go to the playground

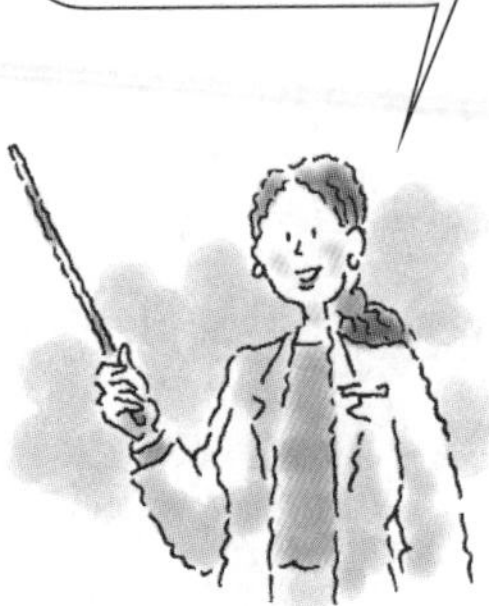

Adequate parent teaching is essential for managing a child with croup.

22. 2. Although most children recover without complications, the parents should be able to recognize signs and symptoms of respiratory distress and know how to access emergency services. Oral fluids should be encouraged because fluids help to thin secretions. Although nutrition is important, frequent small nutritious snacks are usually more appealing than an entire meal. Children should have optimal rest and engage in quiet play. A comfortable environment free from noxious stimuli lessens respiratory distress.

CN: Physiological integrity; CNS: Physiological adaptation; CL: Application

23. Which instruction should a nurse give the parents of a 2-year-old child who wakes in the night with a barking cough?

1. Provide humidified air for the child to breath.
2. Call for an ambulance immediately.
3. Place the child in a warm, dry room.
4. Begin rescue breathing at once.

23. 1. Humidified air reduces laryngeal irritation and spasm and helps liquefy secretions. The child doesn't need emergency care at this time; however, if the child develops respiratory distress, the parents should be instructed to call emergency medical services and not to drive the child to the hospital themselves. The child shouldn't be placed in a warm, dry room as cool, humidified air is used to reduce laryngospasm. The child doesn't require rescue breathing at the time. Rescue breathing is necessary if the child stops breathing.

CN: Physiological integrity; CNS: Reduction of risk potential; CL: Application

24. The nurse is assessing a child recently brought to the emergency department. Which observations would cause the nurse to suspect epiglottitis?

1. Decreased secretions
2. Drooling
3. Low-grade fever
4. Spontaneous cough

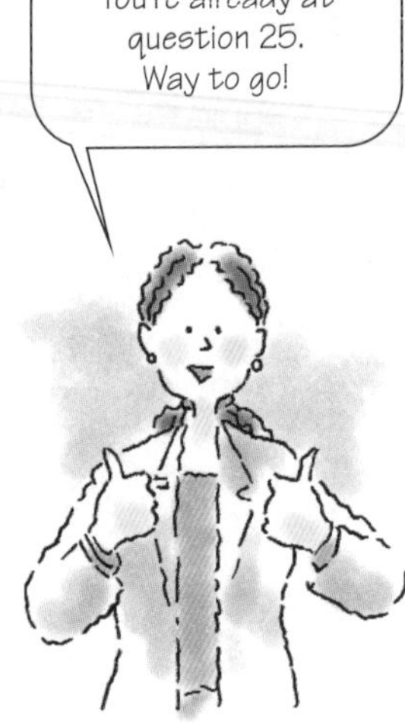

You're already at question 25. Way to go!

24. 2. Drooling of saliva is common due to the pain of swallowing, excessive secretions, and sore throat. The child usually has a high fever and the absence of a spontaneous cough. The classic picture is the child in a tripod position with mouth open and tongue protruding.

CN: Physiological integrity; CNS: Physiological adaptation; CL: Application

25. Which strategy is the best plan of care for a child with acute epiglottitis?

1. Encourage oral fluids for hydration.
2. Maintain the client in semi-Fowler's position.
3. Administer I.V. antibiotic therapy.
4. Maintain respiratory isolation for 48 hours.

25. 3. The etiologic agent for epiglottitis is usually bacterial; therefore, the treatment consists of I.V. antibiotic therapy. The client shouldn't be allowed anything by mouth during the initial phases of the infection to prevent aspiration. The client should be placed in Fowler's position or any position that provides the most comfort and security. Respiratory isolation isn't required.

CN: Physiological integrity; CNS: Physiological adaptation; CL: Application

26. A 2-year-old child is found on the floor next to his toy chest. After first determining unresponsiveness and calling for help, which step should be taken next?

1. Start mouth-to-mouth resuscitation.
2. Begin chest compressions.
3. Check for a pulse.
4. Open the airway.

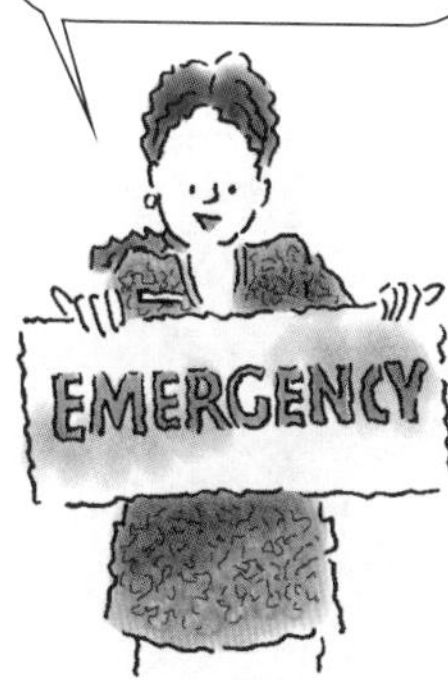

It's important to prioritize in an emergency situation.
EMERGENCY

26. 4. The airway should be opened by using the chin thrust and breathlessness should be determined at the start of cardiopulmonary resuscitation. The sequence of airway, breathing, and circulation needs to be followed.

CN: Physiological integrity; CNS: Physiological adaptation; CL: Application

27. A 10-month-old infant is found in respiratory arrest and cardiopulmonary resuscitation is started. Which site is best to check for a pulse?

1. Brachial
2. Carotid
3. Femoral
4. Radial

27. 1. Palpation of the brachial artery is recommended. The short, chubby neck of infants makes rapid location of the carotid artery difficult. After age 1, the carotid would be used. The femoral pulse, often palpated in a hospital setting, may be difficult to assess because of the infant's position, fat folds, and clothing. The radial pulse isn't a good indicator of central artery perfusion.

CN: Physiological integrity; CNS: Physiological adaptation; CL: Application

28. When giving rescue breathing to an infant under age 1, what is the ratio of breaths per second?

1. 1 breath every 2 to 3 seconds
2. 1 breath every 3 to 5 seconds
3. 1 breath every 4 to 6 seconds
4. 1 breath every 5 to 7 seconds

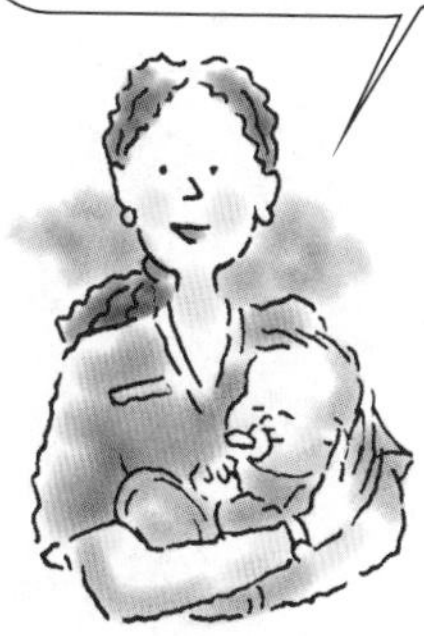

The procedure for rescue breathing for infants is different from that for adults.

28. 2. Rescue breathing should be performed once every 3 to 5 seconds until spontaneous breathing resumes. This provides approximately 20 breaths/minute. One breath every 2 to 3 seconds may cause gastric distention. One breath every 5 to 6 seconds is recommended for adults.

CN: Physiological integrity; CNS: Physiological adaptation; CL: Application

29. When performing chest compressions on a 2-year-old child, which depth is correct?

1. ½″ to 1″ (1 to 2.5 cm)
2. 1″ to 1½″ (2.5 to 3.5 cm)
3. 1½″ to 2″ (3.5 to 5 cm)
4. 2″ to 2½″ (5 to 6.5 cm)

29. 2. The chest compressions should equal approximately one-third to one-half the total depth of the chest. This corresponds to about 1 to 1½″ in a child age 1 to 8, ½″ to 1″ for an infant younger than age 1, and 1½″ to 2″ for an adult.

CN: Physiological integrity; CNS: Physiological adaptation; CL: Application

30. A nurse rescuer knows that chest compressions must be coordinated with ventilations. Which ratio should the nurse rescuer use for a 3-year-old child?

1. 15 compressions to 1 ventilation
2. 15 compressions to 2 ventilations
3. 30 compressions to 1 ventilation
4. 30 compressions to 2 ventilations

30. 4. A single health care provider rescuer should use a ratio of 30 chest compressions to 2 ventilations for children ages 1 year to the onset of adolescence. Ratios of 15:1, 15:2, and 30:1 won't provide optimal compression and ventilation.

CN: Physiological integrity; CNS: Physiological adaptation; CL: Application

31. A 10-month-old child is found choking and soon becomes unconscious. Which intervention should a nurse attempt <u>first</u> after opening the airway?

1. Look inside the child's mouth for a foreign object.
2. Give five back blows and five chest thrusts.
3. Attempt a blind finger sweep.
4. Attempt rescue breathing.

31. 1. After the airway is open, the nurse should check for a foreign object and remove it with a finger sweep if it can be seen. After this step, rescue breathing should be attempted. If ventilation is unsuccessful, the nurse should then give five back blows and five chest thrusts in an attempt to dislodge the object. Blind finger sweeps should never be performed because this may push the object further back into the airway.

CN: Physiological integrity; CNS: Physiological adaptation; CL: Application

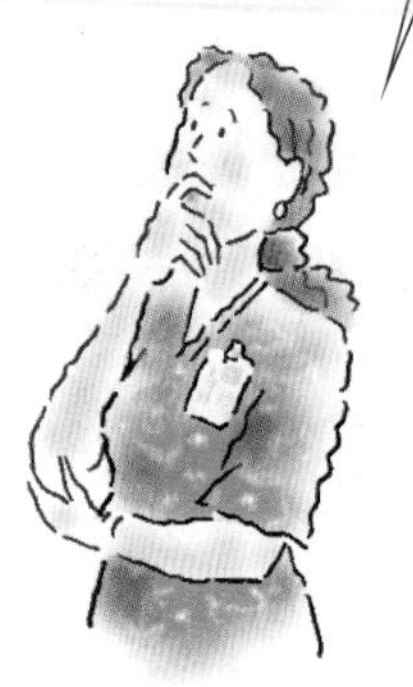

I am going to feel like a real heel if I get this answer wrong.

32. Using which part of the hands is appropriate when performing chest compressions on a child between ages 1 and 8?

1. Heels of both hands
2. Heel of one hand
3. Index and middle fingers
4. Thumbs of both hands

32. 2. The heel of one hand is recommended for performing chest compressions on children between ages 1 and 8. Two hands are used for adult cardiopulmonary resuscitation. Chest thrusts administered with the middle and third fingers, and in some cases the thumbs of each hand, are used on infants younger than age 1.

CN: Physiological integrity; CNS: Physiological adaptation; CL: Application

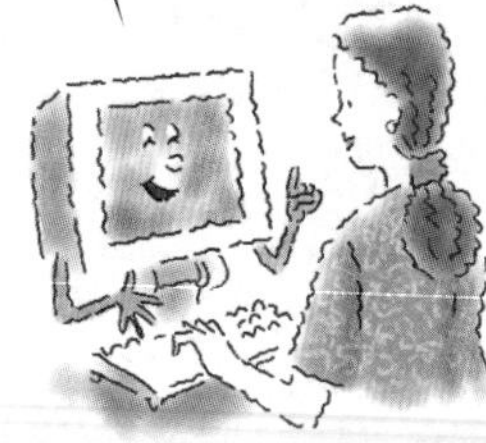

Again, you're being asked to prioritize.

33. A 3-year-old child is brought to the emergency department not breathing, cyanotic, and lethargic. The mother states that she thinks he swallowed a penny. Which intervention should the nurse take <u>first</u>?

1. Give 100% oxygen.
2. Administer five back blows.
3. Attempt a blind finger sweep.
4. Administer abdominal thrusts.

33. 4. A child between ages 1 and 8 should receive abdominal thrusts to help dislodge the object. Administering 100% oxygen won't help if the airway is occluded. Infants younger than age 1 should receive back blows before chest thrusts. Blind finger sweeps should never be performed because this could push the object further back into the airway.

CN: Physiological integrity; CNS: Physiological adaptation; CL: Application

34. Which statement by the parent of a 4-year-old boy who just had a tonsillectomy indicates that a nurse's discharge instruction has been successful?

1. "I will keep him flat on his back in bed."
2. "I will sit him in bed at a 45-degree angle."
3. "I will place him on his stomach with his head to the side."
4. "I will place him on his back with his head on a pillow."

34. 3. Laying the child on his stomach with the head turned to the side allows blood and other secretions to drain from the mouth and pharynx, reducing the risk of aspiration. Placing the child flat on his back, on his back with a pillow, or at a 45-degree angle doesn't promote drainage and increases the likelihood of aspiration.

CN: Physiological integrity; CNS: Reduction of risk potential; CL: Application

35. A 7-month-old child is diagnosed with otitis media; the physician orders amoxicillin 40 mg/kg/day to be administered three times per day. The child weighs 9 kg. How much amoxicillin should the child receive per dose?
1. 120 mg
2. 180 mg
3. 200 mg
4. 360 mg

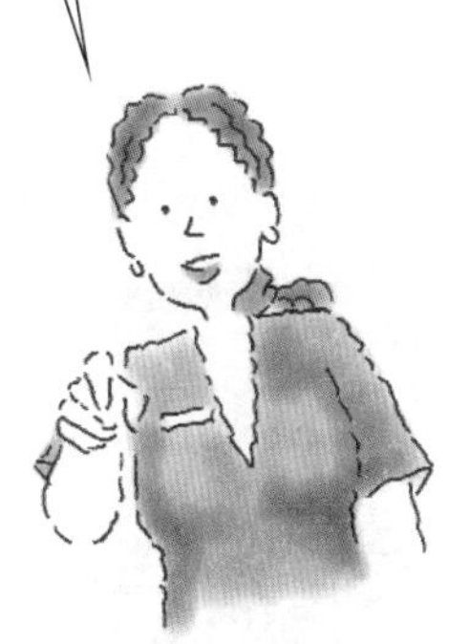

Make sure you understand this formula. You'll use it again later in this chapter.

35. 1. The child should receive 120 mg per dose. Here are the calculations: 40 mg × 9 kg = 360 mg/day; 360 mg/3 doses = 120 mg/dose.
CN: Physiological integrity; CNS: Pharmacological and parenteral therapies; CL: Application

36. Children with chronic otitis media commonly require surgery for a myringotomy and ear tube placement. Which management strategy explains the purpose of the ear tubes?
1. To administer antibiotics
2. To flush the middle ear
3. To increase pressure
4. To drain fluid

36. 4. Ear tubes allow normal fluid to drain (not flush) from the middle ear. They also allow ventilation. The purpose isn't to administer medication. The tubes also allow pressure to equalize in the middle ear.
CN: Physiological integrity; CNS: Physiological adaptation; CL: Application

37. A nurse is discharging a 10-month-old client with eardrops. Which information should she give the parent about how to administer the drops?
1. Pull the earlobe upward.
2. Pull the earlobe up and back.
3. Pull the earlobe down and back.
4. Pull the earlobe down and forward.

37. 3. For infants, the parent should be told to gently pull the earlobe down and back to visualize the external auditory canal. For children over age 3 and for adults, the earlobe is gently pulled slightly up and back.
CN: Physiological integrity; CNS: Pharmacological and parenteral therapies; CL: Application

38. A child is diagnosed with right chronic otitis media. After the child returns from surgery for myringotomy and placement of ear tubes, which intervention is appropriate?
1. Apply gauze dressings.
2. Position the child on the left side.
3. Position the child on the right side.
4. Apply warm compresses to both ears.

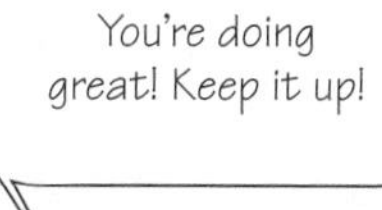

You're doing great! Keep it up!

38. 3. The child should be positioned on the right side to facilitate drainage. Gauze dressings aren't necessary after surgery. Some physicians may prefer a loose cotton wick. The left side isn't an area of concern for drainage. Warm compresses may help to facilitate drainage only when used on the affected ear.
CN: Physiological integrity; CNS: Physiological adaptation; CL: Application

39. To reduce the risk of an infant developing otitis media, a nurse should instruct the parents to:
1. treat all cold symptoms with antibiotics.
2. place the infant in an upright position when feeding from a bottle.
3. avoid washing the ears to keep them dry.
4. swab the outer ear with a cotton-tipped swab.

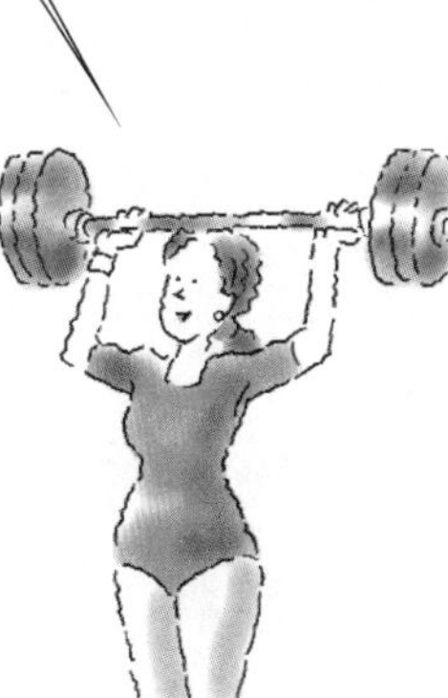

39. 2. The risk of otitis media can be reduced by bottle feeding an infant in the upright position. Formula that pools in the nasopharynx is a good medium for bacterial growth which can move through the shortened, horizontal eustachian tube of the infant. Administering antibiotics with cold symptoms won't reduce the risk of otitis media since colds are due to viral causes. Washing the ears, getting them wet or swabbing the outer ear doesn't contribute to otitis media.
CN: Health promotion and maintenance; CNS: None; CL: Application

40. The nurse is assessing with an otoscope a child suspected of acute otitis media. Which assessment would be indicative of this condition?

1. Pearl-gray tympanic membrane
2. Bright red, bulging tympanic membrane
3. Dull gray membrane with fluid behind the eardrum
4. Bright red or yellow, bulging or retracted, tympanic membrane

40. 4. With acute otitis media, the tympanic membrane may present as bright red or yellow, bulging or retracted. A pearl-gray tympanic membrane is a normal finding. Dull gray membrane fluid is consistent with subacute or chronic otitis media.

CN: Physiological integrity; CNS: Physiological adaptation; CL: Application

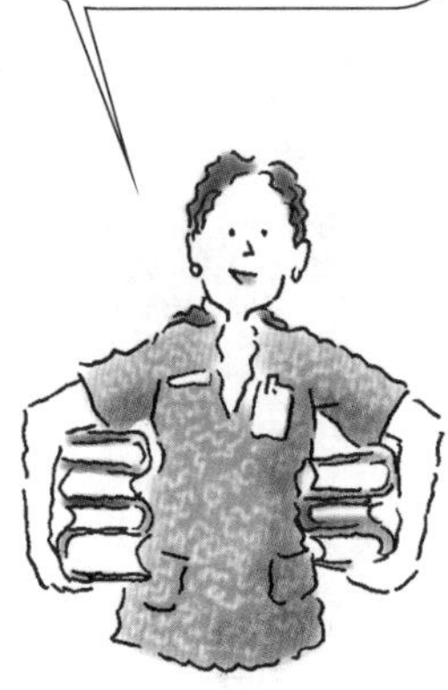

Question 41 is asking about a proximate cause of otitis media.

41. A nurse is teaching the parents of a 1-year-old infant with otitis media. Which statement regarding predisposing factors for otitis media would be the most accurate for the nurse to make?

1. The cartilage lining is overdeveloped.
2. When infants sit up, it favors the pooling of fluid.
3. Humoral defense mechanisms decrease the risk of infection.
4. Eustachian tubes are short, wide, and straight and lie in a horizontal plane.

41. 4. In an infant or child, the eustachian tubes are short, wide, and straight, and lie in a horizontal plane, allowing them to be more easily blocked by conditions such as large adenoids and infections. Until the eustachian tubes change in size and angle, children are more susceptible to otitis media. Cartilage lining is underdeveloped, making the tubes more distensible and more likely to open inappropriately. The usual lying-down position of infants favors the pooling of fluid such as formula in the pharyngeal cavity. Immature humoral defense mechanisms increase the risk of infection.

CN: Physiological integrity; CNS: Physiological adaptation; CL: Analysis

42. Which complication is most commonly related to acute otitis media?

1. Eardrum perforation
2. Hearing loss
3. Meningitis
4. Tympanosclerosis

42. 1. Eardrum perforation is the most common complication as the exudate accumulates and pressure increases. Hearing loss in most cases is conductive in nature and mild in severity but is less common than eardrum perforation. Hearing tests aren't usually performed during episodes of otitis media. Tympanosclerosis and meningitis are possible but uncommon when adequate antibiotic therapy is implemented.

CN: Physiological integrity; CNS: Physiological adaptation; CL: Application

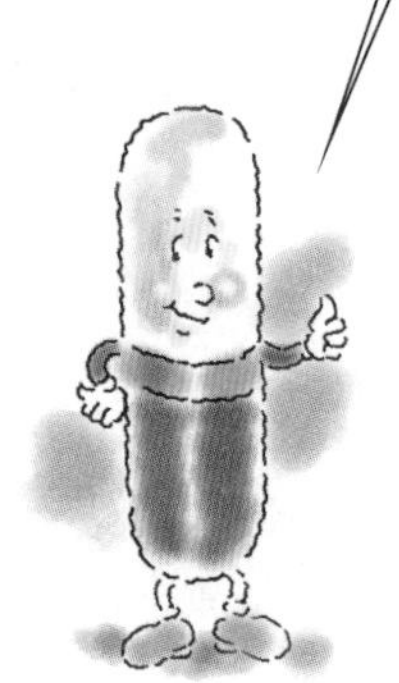

It's important that I stay the course.

43. Which statement by the parent of a child with otitis media indicates an understanding of a nurse's discharge instruction on the use of antibiotics?

1. "I will give my child the full course of antibiotics."
2. "I will stop the antibiotics when my child no longer has ear pain."
3. "I will give the antibiotics whenever my child has ear pain."
4. "I will put antibiotics in the affected ear."

43. 1. Antibiotics should be given for the full prescribed course of therapy regardless of whether the child has symptoms. Antibiotics are taken at prescribed intervals and not for episodes of ear pain. Oral antibiotics are used to treat otitis media.

CN: Physiological integrity; CNS: Pharmacological and parental therapies; CL: Application

44. A 2-year-old child is diagnosed with epiglottitis. Ampicillin is ordered 50 mg/kg/day in 6 divided doses. The client weighs 12 kg. How much ampicillin is given per dose?

1. 50 mg
2. 100 mg
3. 200 mg
4. 300 mg

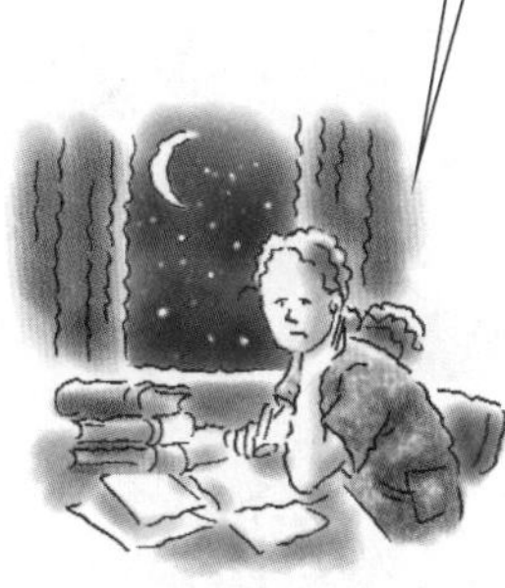

What did I tell you? Here's that formula again!

44. 2. The child should receive 100 mg per dose. Here are the calculations:

50 mg × 12 kg = 600 mg/day;
600 mg/6 doses = 100 mg/dose.

CN: Physiological integrity; CNS: Pharmacological and parenteral therapies; CL: Application

45. A 3-year-old child is receiving ampicillin for acute epiglottitis. Which of the following would lead the nurse to suspect an adverse effect to ampicillin?

1. Constipation
2. Generalized rash
3. Increased appetite
4. Low-grade temperature

45. 2. Some clients may develop an erythematous or maculopapular rash after 3 to 14 days of therapy; however, this complication doesn't necessitate discontinuing the drug. Nausea, vomiting, epigastric pain, and diarrhea are adverse effects that may necessitate discontinuation of the drug.

CN: Physiological integrity; CNS: Pharmacological and parenteral therapies; CL: Application

46. A 3-year-old child is given a preliminary diagnosis of acute epiglottitis. Which nursing intervention is appropriate?

1. Obtain a throat culture immediately.
2. Place the child in a side-lying position.
3. Don't attempt to visualize the epiglottis.
4. Use a tongue blade to look inside the throat.

46. 3. The nurse shouldn't attempt to visualize the epiglottis. The use of tongue blades or throat culture swabs may cause the epiglottis to spasm and totally occlude the airway. Throat inspection should be attempted only when immediate intubation or tracheostomy can be performed in the event of further or complete obstruction. The child should always remain in the position that provides the most comfort and security and ease of breathing.

CN: Physiological integrity; CNS: Physiological adaptation; CL: Application

47. An infant is brought to the clinic for her 6-month vaccines. The nurse tells the mother that administration of which vaccine is an appropriate step for prevention of epiglottitis?

1. Diphtheria vaccine
2. *Haemophilus influenzae* type B (Hib) vaccine
3. Measles vaccine
4. Oral poliovirus vaccine (OPV)

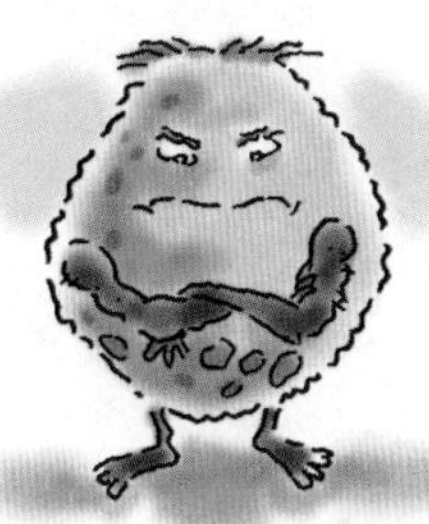

Vaccines. Who needs them?

47. 2. Epiglottitis is caused by the bacterial agent *H. influenzae*. The American Academy of Pediatrics recommends that, beginning at age 2 months, children receive the Hib conjugate vaccine. A decline in the incidence of epiglottitis has been seen as a result of this vaccination regimen. The OPV, measles, mumps, and rubella vaccine, and diphtheria vaccine are preventive for those diseases.

CN: Health promotion and maintenance; CNS: None; CL: Application

48. Which sign in a 3-year-old child with acute epiglottitis indicates that the client's respiratory distress is increasing?

1. Progressive barking cough
2. Increasing irritability
3. Increasing heart rate
4. Productive cough

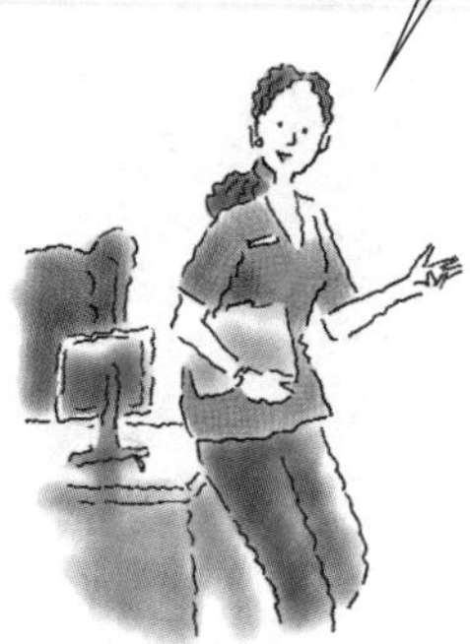

This question is asking about an increase—not just a presence—of symptoms.

48. 3. Increasing heart rate is an early sign of hypoxia. A progressive barking cough is characteristic of spasmodic croup. A child in respiratory distress will be irritable and restless. As distress increases, the child will become lethargic related to the work of breathing and impending respiratory failure. A productive cough shows that secretions are moving and the child can effectively clear them.

CN: Physiological integrity; CNS: Physiological adaptation; CL: Application

49. While examining a child with acute epiglottitis, a nurse should have which item available?

1. Cool mist tent
2. Intubation equipment
3. Tongue blades
4. Viral culture medium

49. 2. Emergency intubation equipment should be at the bedside to secure the airway if examination precipitates further or complete obstruction. Viral culture medium and cool mist tents are recommended for the diagnosis and treatment of croup. Tongue blades are contraindicated and may cause the epiglottis to spasm.

CN: Physiological integrity; CNS: Physiological adaptation; CL: Application

50. A 2-year-old child is brought to the emergency department in respiratory distress. The child is drooling, sitting upright and leaning forward with chin thrust out, mouth open, and tongue protruding. Which nursing intervention is most appropriate?

1. Check the child's gag reflex with a tongue blade.
2. Allow the child to cry to keep the lungs expanded.
3. Check the airway for a foreign body obstruction.
4. Support the child in an upright position on the parent's lap.

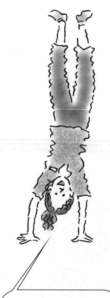

50. 4. The classic signs of epiglottitis are drooling, sitting upright, and leaning forward with chin thrust out, mouth open, and tongue protruding. The child with epiglottitis should be kept in an upright position to ease the work of breathing and to avoid aspiration of secretions and obstruction of the airway by the swollen epiglottis. Placing the child on the lap of a parent may help reduce the child's anxiety. The gag reflex of a child with epiglottitis should never be checked unless emergency personnel and equipment are immediately available to perform a tracheotomy if the airway should become obstructed by the swollen epiglottis. Likewise, crying and inspecting the airway for a foreign body may also cause entrapment of the epiglottis and obstruction of the airway.

CN: Physiological integrity; CNS: Reduction of risk potential; CL: Application

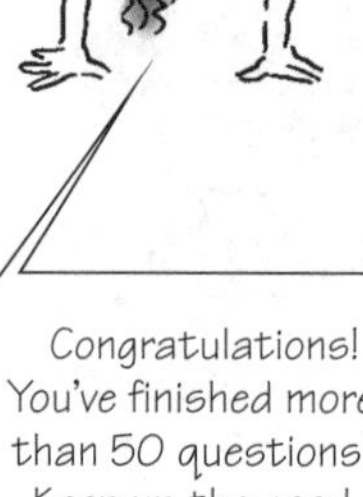

Congratulations! You've finished more than 50 questions! Keep up the good work!

51. What is the best position for a nurse to place a 3-year-old child with right lower lobe pneumonia?

1. On the right side
2. On the left side
3. Supine
4. Prone

51. 2. The child with right lower lobe pneumonia should be placed on his left side. This places the unaffected left lung in a position so that gravity will promote blood flow to the healthy lung tissue, improving gas exchange. Placing the child on the right side, his back, or his stomach doesn't promote circulation to the unaffected lung.

CN: Physiological integrity; CNS: Physiological adaptation; CL: Application

52. The arterial blood gas analysis of a child with asthma shows a pH of 7.30, P_{CO_2} of 56 mm Hg, and HCO_3^- of 25 mEq/L. The nurse determines that the child has which condition?

1. Metabolic acidosis
2. Metabolic alkalosis
3. Respiratory acidosis
4. Respiratory alkalosis

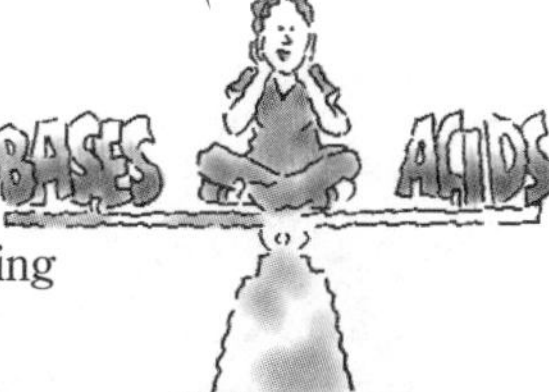
I think I sense an acid-base disturbance coming on.
BASES
ACIDS

52. 3. Respiratory acidosis is an acid-base disturbance characterized by excess CO_2 in the blood, indicated by a P_{CO_2} greater than 45 mm Hg. The pH level is usually below the normal range of 7.36 to 7.45. The HCO_3^- level is normal in the acute stage and elevated in the chronic stage.

CN: Physiological integrity; CNS: Physiological adaptation; CL: Analysis

53. Which neonate is at high risk for developing bronchopulmonary dysplasia?

1. A neonate born at 38 weeks' gestation receiving 1 to 4 L oxygen during feedings
2. A premature neonate born at 36 weeks' gestation receiving supplemental oxygen
3. A premature neonate born at 28 weeks' gestation on a high-pressure ventilator
4. A neonate born at 42 weeks' gestation who requires treatments for respiratory syncytial virus

53. 3. Premature neonates with low birth weight on high-pressure ventilators are at highest risk for developing bronchopulmonary dysplasia. Supplemental oxygen, respiratory treatments, and 1 to 4 L oxygen for feedings are *not* high risk factors for bronchopulmonary dysplasia.

CN: Physiological integrity; CNS: Reduction of risk potential; CL: Application

54. Which nursing diagnosis is the priority for an infant with bronchopulmonary dysplasia?

1. *Imbalanced nutrition: Less than body requirements*
2. *Effective breast-feeding*
3. *Impaired gas exchange*
4. *Risk for imbalanced fluid volume*

54. 3. The infant will have *Impaired gas exchange* related to retention of carbon dioxide and borderline oxygenation secondary to fibrosis of the lungs. Although the infant may require increased caloric intake and may have excess fluid volume, *Imbalanced nutrition: Less than body requirements, Effective breast-feeding,* and *Risk for imbalanced fluid volume* aren't priority nursing diagnoses.

CN: Physiological integrity; CNS: Physiological adaptation; CL: Analysis

55. Which management strategy is recommended when caring for an infant with bronchopulmonary dysplasia?

1. Provide frequent playful stimuli.
2. Decrease oxygen during feedings.
3. Place the infant on a set schedule.
4. Place the infant in an open crib.

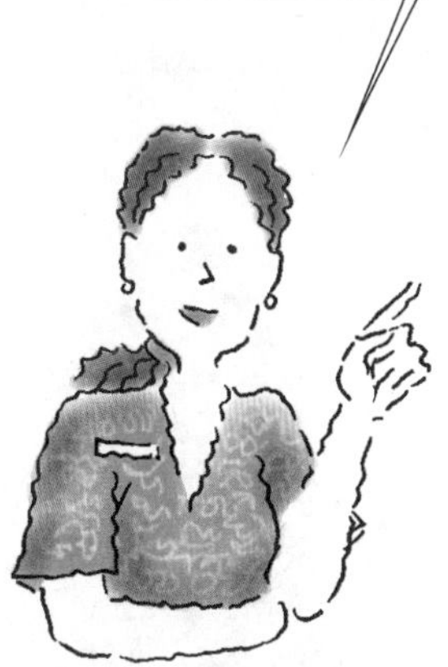
Which management strategy is recommended in question 55?

55. 3. Timing care activities with rest periods to avoid fatigue and to decrease respiratory effort is essential. Early stimulation activities are recommended but the infant will have limited tolerance for them because of the illness. Oxygen is usually increased during feedings to help decrease respiratory and energy requirements. Thermoregulation is important because both hypothermia and hyperthermia will increase oxygen consumption and may increase oxygen requirements. These infants are usually maintained on warmer beds or inside Isolettes.

CN: Safe, effective care environment; CNS: Management of care; CL: Application

56. The nurse is planning care for a child admitted to the pediatric unit with bronchopulmonary dysplasia. Which symptom is the nurse most likely to assess?

1. Minimal work of breathing
2. Tachypnea and dyspnea
3. Easily consolable
4. Hypotension

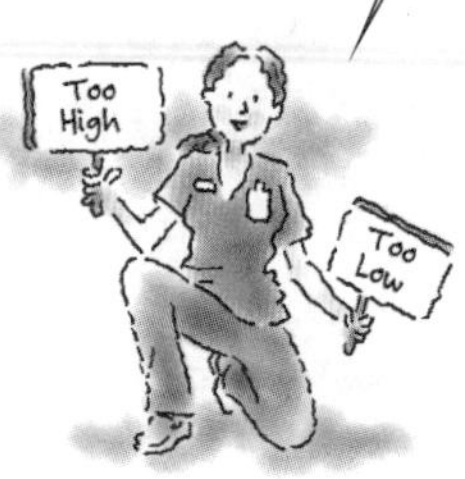
Be sure not to confuse the prefixes hyper and hypo!
Too High
Too Low

56. 2. Tachypnea, dyspnea, and wheezing are intermittently or chronically present secondary to airway obstruction and increased airway resistance. These infants usually show increased work of breathing and increased use of accessory muscles. They're frequently described as irritable and difficult to comfort. Pulmonary hypertension is a common finding resulting from fibrosis and chronic hypoxia.

CN: Physiological integrity; CNS: Physiological adaptation; CL: Application

57. Which intervention is most appropriate for helping parents to cope with a child newly diagnosed with bronchopulmonary dysplasia?

1. Teach cardiopulmonary resuscitation.
2. Refer them to support groups.
3. Help parents identify necessary lifestyle changes.
4. Evaluate and assess parents' stress and anxiety levels.

57. 4. The emotional impact of bronchopulmonary dysplasia is clearly a crisis situation. The parents are experiencing grief and sorrow over the loss of a "healthy" child. The other strategies are more appropriate for long-term intervention.

CN: Psychosocial integrity; CNS: None; CL: Application

58. The nursing care plan for an infant with bronchopulmonary dysplasia includes the nursing diagnosis of *Impaired gas exchange.* Which nursing action would be most appropriate for a nurse to include?

1. Provide chest physiotherapy.
2. Provide enteral feedings.
3. Provide appropriate age-related activities.
4. Promote bonding between parent and child.

58. 1. All these activities are appropriate to include in the care of a child with bronchopulmonary dysplasia; however, providing chest physiotherapy addresses the nursing diagnosis of *Impaired gas exchange.*

CN: Physiological integrity; CNS: Basic care and comfort; CL: Analysis

59. Theophylline is ordered for a 1-year-old client with bronchopulmonary dysplasia. The recommended dosage is 24 mg/kg/day. The client weighs 10 kg. How much is given per dose when administered 4 times per day?

1. 60 mg/dose
2. 80 mg/dose
3. 120 mg/dose
4. 240 mg/dose

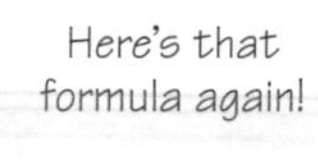

59. 1. The child should receive 60 mg/dose. Here are the calculations:

$$24 \text{ mg/kg} \times 10 \text{ kg} = 240 \text{ mg/day};$$
$$240 \text{ mg/4 doses} = 60 \text{ mg/dose}.$$

CN: Physiological integrity; CNS: Pharmacological and parenteral therapies; CL: Application

60. Infants with bronchopulmonary dysplasia require frequent, prolonged rest periods. Which sign indicates overstimulation?

1. Increased alertness
2. Good eye contact
3. Cyanosis
4. Lethargy

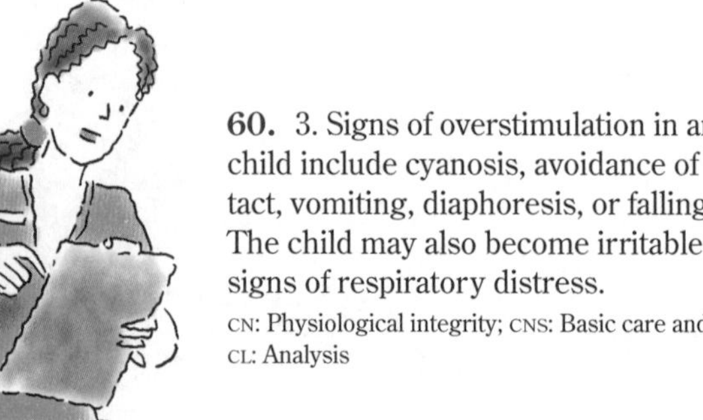

60. 3. Signs of overstimulation in an immature child include cyanosis, avoidance of eye contact, vomiting, diaphoresis, or falling asleep. The child may also become irritable and show signs of respiratory distress.

CN: Physiological integrity; CNS: Basic care and comfort; CL: Analysis

61. Which outcome should be anticipated of parental care of a child with bronchopulmonary dysplasia?
1. Reports increased levels of stress
2. Makes safe decisions with professional assistance only
3. Participates in routine, but not complex, caretaking activities
4. Verbalizes the causes, risks, therapy options, and nursing care

61. 4. The parents should understand the causes, risks, and care of their infant by the time of discharge. Having the parents verbalize this information is the only way to assess their understanding. The parents should report decreased levels of stress, be capable of making decisions independently, and participate in routine and complex care.
CN: Physiological integrity; CNS: Basic care and comfort; CL: Analysis

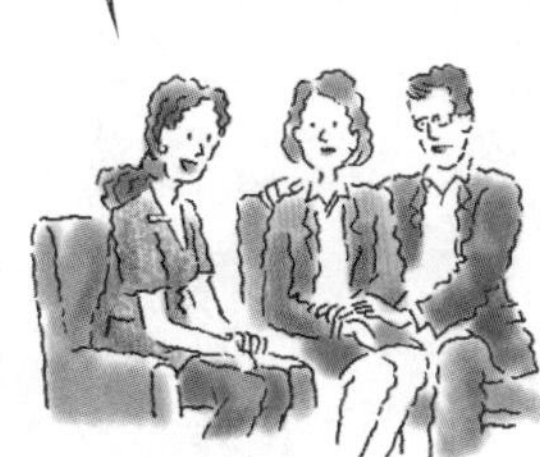

Encourage parents to verbalize their understanding of their infant's disorder.

62. Bronchopulmonary dysplasia can be classified into four categories. Which characteristic is noted during the early or <u>first</u> stage of the disease?
1. Interstitial fibrosis
2. Signs of emphysema
3. Hyperexpansion on chest X-ray
4. Resemblance to respiratory distress syndrome

62. 4. Stage I can be characterized by early interstitial changes and resembles respiratory distress syndrome. Stage IV shows interstitial fibrosis and hyperexpansion on chest X-ray. Stage III shows signs of the beginning of chronic disease with interstitial edema, signs of emphysema, and pulmonary hypertension.
CN: Physiological integrity; CNS: Physiological adaptation; CL: Analysis

63. Bronchopulmonary dysplasia can cause increased fluid in the lungs due to disruption of the alveolar-capillary membrane, and the client may begin receiving furosemide (Lasix). Which adverse effect is possible?
1. Hypercalcemia
2. Hyperkalemia
3. Hypernatremia
4. Irregular heart rhythm

63. 4. An irregular heart rhythm and muscle cramps are adverse effects related to hypokalemia and hypocalcemia and not hypercalcemia or hyperkalemia. Diuretics cause volume depletion by inhibiting reabsorption of sodium and chloride. Hypocalcemia is related to the urinary excretion of calcium. Hypokalemia can occur with excessive fluid loss or as part of contraction alkalosis.
CN: Physiological integrity; CNS: Pharmacological and parenteral therapies; CL: Application

64. A pediatric client is to receive furosemide (Lasix) 4 mg/kg/day in one daily dose. The client weighs 20 kg. How many milligrams should be administered in each dose?
1. 20
2. 40
3. 80
4. 160

64. 3. The child should receive 80 mg per dose. Here are the calculations:

$4 \text{ mg/kg} \times 20 \text{ kg} = 80 \text{ mg}.$

CN: Physiological integrity; CNS: Pharmacological and parenteral therapies; CL: Application

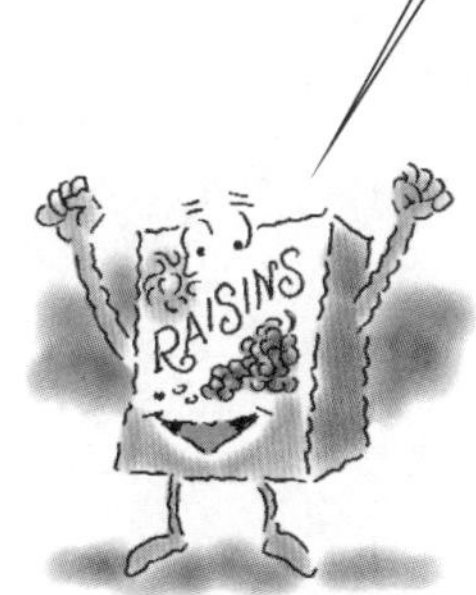

We're raising awareness about our potassium content.
RAISINS

65. A 2-year-old child with bronchopulmonary dysplasia is placed on furosemide (Lasix) once per day. The parents are being educated on foods that are rich in potassium. Which food should the nurse recommend?
1. Apples
2. Oranges
3. Peaches
4. Raisins

65. 4. Raisins, dates, figs, and prunes are among the highest potassium-rich foods. They average 17 to 20 mEq of potassium. Apples, oranges, and peaches have very low amounts of potassium. They average 3 to 4 mEq.
CN: Physiological integrity; CNS: Pharmacological and parenteral therapies; CL: Application

66. Which reason necessitates tracheostomy tube placement in long-term care of infants with bronchopulmonary dysplasia?

1. Increased risk of tracheomalacia
2. Inability to wean from the ventilator
3. Need to allow for gastrostomy tube feedings
4. Increased signs of respiratory distress

66. 2. Tracheostomy may be required after a child has been ventilator dependent for 6 to 8 weeks and is unable to wean from the ventilator. This will allow for oral feedings and reduce the risks of tracheomalacia and bronchomalacia.

CN: Physiological integrity; CNS: Physiological adaptation; CL: Analysis

Ask yourself what you would need if the worst occurred.
STOP

67. A 1-year-old infant with bronchopulmonary dysplasia has just received a tracheostomy. Which intervention is appropriate?

1. Keep extra tracheostomy tubes at the bedside.
2. Secure ties at the side of the neck for easy access.
3. Change the tracheostomy tube 2 weeks after surgery.
4. Secure the tracheostomy ties tightly to prevent dislodgment of the tube.

67. 1. Extra tracheostomy tubes should be kept at the bedside in case of an emergency, including one size smaller in case the appropriate size doesn't fit due to edema or lack of a tract formation. Ties are usually placed at the back of the neck. The ties should be placed securely but allow the width of a little finger for room to prevent excessive pressure or skin breakdown. The first tracheostomy tube change is usually performed by the physician after 7 days.

CN: Physiological integrity; CNS: Reduction of risk potential; CL: Application

68. An 11-month-old infant with bronchopulmonary dysplasia and a tracheostomy experiences a decline in oxygen saturation from 97% to 88%. He appears anxious and his heart rate is 180 beats/minute. Which intervention is most appropriate?

1. Change the tracheostomy tube.
2. Suction the tracheostomy tube.
3. Obtain an arterial blood gas (ABG) level.
4. Increase the oxygen flow rate.

68. 2. Tracheostomy tubes, particularly in small children, require frequent suctioning to remove mucus plugs and excessive secretions. The tracheostomy tube can be changed if suctioning is unsuccessful. Obtaining an ABG level may be beneficial if oxygen saturation remains low and the child appears to be in respiratory distress. Increasing the oxygen flow rate will only help if the airway is patent.

CN: Physiological integrity; CNS: Reduction of risk potential; CL: Analysis

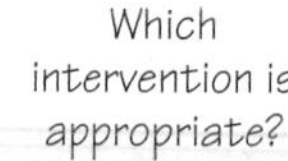

69. Which intervention is appropriate when suctioning a tracheostomy tube?

1. Hypoventilate the child before suctioning.
2. Repeat the suctioning process for two intervals.
3. Insert the catheter 1 to 2 cm below the tracheostomy tube.
4. Inject a small amount of normal saline solution into the tube before suctioning.

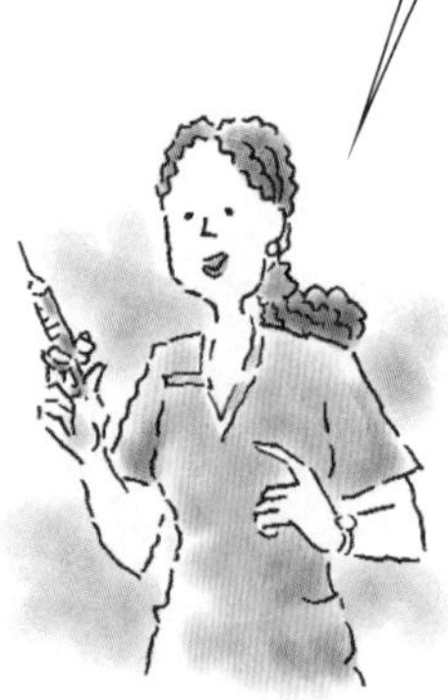

69. 4. Injecting a small amount (1–2 drops) of normal saline solution helps to loosen secretions for easier aspiration. Preservative-free normal saline solution should be used. The child should be hyperventilated before and after suctioning to prevent hypoxia. The suctioning process should be repeated until the trachea is clear. If the catheter is inserted too far, it will irritate the carina and may cause blood-tinged secretions. The catheter should be inserted *0.5 cm beyond* the tracheostomy tube.

CN: Physiological integrity; CNS: Reduction of risk potential; CL: Application

70. Which characteristic distinguishes allergies from colds?

1. Skin tests can diagnose a cold.
2. Allergies are accompanied by fever.
3. Colds cause itching of the eyes and nose.
4. Allergies trigger constant and consistent bouts of sneezing.

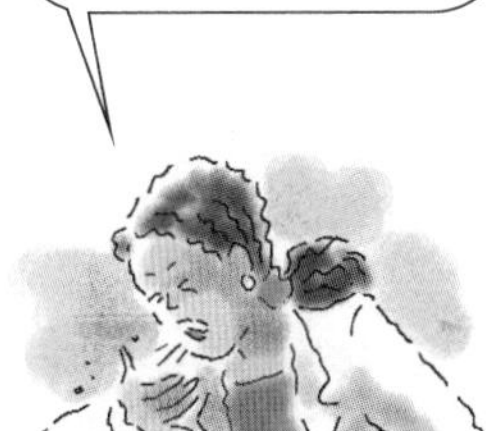

Cold or allergies? That is the (Ah-choo) question!

70. 4. Allergies elicit consistent bouts of sneezing, are seldom accompanied by fever, and tend to cause itching of the eyes and nose. Skin testing is performed to determine the client's sensitivity to specific allergens. Colds are accompanied by fever and are characterized by sporadic sneezing.

CN: Health promotion and maintenance; CNS: None; CL: Analysis

71. A 2-year-old with pneumonia is placed in an oxygen tent with mist. Which nursing action is a priority?

1. Change the child's bed linens and pajamas frequently.
2. Maintain a steady body temperature.
3. Avoid the use of equipment or toys that can produce sparks.
4. Keep the plastic sides of the tent tucked in.

71. 3. While all the interventions are appropriate for caring for a child in an oxygen tent with mist, sparks in the presence of oxygen can cause a fire. Therefore, all equipment and toys that may produce a spark should be avoided. Bed linens and pajamas may become damp due to the cool mist and should be changed when needed, but only after the risk of fire has been addressed. Keeping the child dry will help promote a steady body temperature which is important since shivering increases oxygen intake. The sides of the tent should be tucked in since oxygen is heavier than air, making oxygen loss greater at the bottom of the tent.

CN: Safe, effective care environment; CNS: Management of care; CL: Analysis

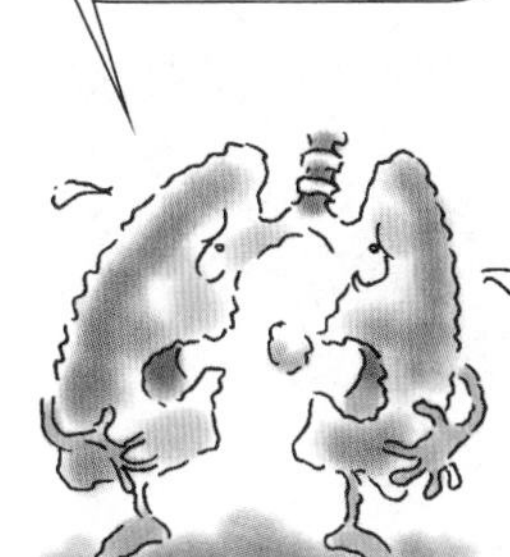

We really need to watch out for those triggers.

72. A 2-year-old child has been diagnosed with asthma. The parents ask about the most common asthma triggers. What is the nurse's response?

1. Weather
2. Peanut butter
3. The cat next door
4. One parent with asthma

72. 1. Excessively cold air, wet or humid changes in weather and seasons, and air pollution are some of the most common asthma triggers. Household pets are also a trigger. Evidence suggests that asthma is partly hereditary in nature. Food allergens are rarely responsible for airway reactions in children.

CN: Physiological integrity; CNS: Physiological adaptation; CL: Application

73. The nurse is assessing breath sounds of a child admitted with asthma. Which breath sound is the <u>most</u> common in asthma?

1. Stridor
2. Rhonchi
3. Rales
4. Wheezing

73. 4. Asthma frequently presents with wheezing and coughing. Airway inflammation and edema increase mucus production. Other signs include dyspnea, tachycardia, and tachypnea. Stridor is heard in croup. Rhonchi and rales are not as common in asthma as wheezing.

CN: Physiological integrity; CNS: Physiological adaptation; CL: Application

74. The presence of which factor would place a child at increased risk for an asthma-related death?

1. Use of an inhaler at home
2. One admission for asthma last year
3. Prior admission to the general pediatric floor
4. Prior admission to an intensive care unit for asthma

74. 4. Asthma results in varying degrees of respiratory distress. A prior admission to an intensive care unit marks an increased severity and need of immediate therapy. Two or more hospitalizations for asthma, a recent hospitalization or emergency department visit in the past month, or three or more emergency department visits in the past year puts a child at high risk for asthma-related death. Current use of systemic steroids would also be a risk factor.

CN: Physiological integrity; CNS: Reduction of risk potential; CL: Analysis

75. Which characteristic distinguishes status asthmaticus from asthma?

1. Several attacks per month
2. Less than six attacks per year
3. Little or no response to bronchodilators
4. Constant and unrelieved by bronchodilators

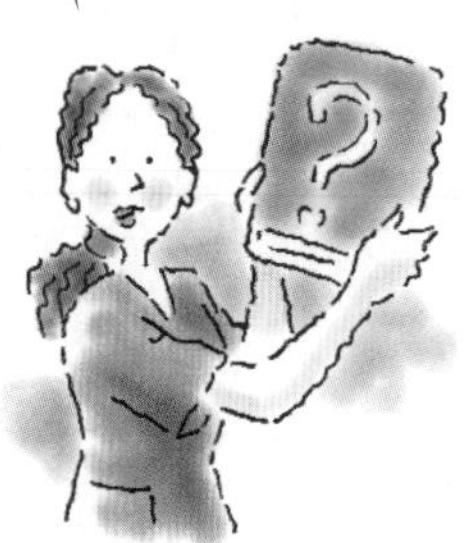

This question is asking you to distinguish between varying degrees of asthma.

75. 4. Status asthmaticus can best be described as constant and unrelieved by bronchodilators. Moderate asthma is characterized by several attacks per month. Mild asthma is less than 6 attacks per year. Little or no response to bronchodilators would describe severe asthma.

CN: Physiological integrity; CNS: Physiological adaptation; CL: Application

76. A 2-year-old child with status asthmaticus is admitted to the pediatric unit and begins to receive continuous treatment with albuterol (Proventil), given by nebulizer. The nurse should observe for which adverse reaction?

1. Bradycardia
2. Lethargy
3. Tachycardia
4. Tachypnea

76. 3. Albuterol is a rapid-acting bronchodilator. Common adverse effects include tachycardia, nervousness, tremors, insomnia, irritability, and headache.

CN: Physiological integrity; CNS: Pharmacological and parenteral therapies; CL: Application

77. A 10-year-old child is admitted with asthma. The physician orders an aminophylline infusion. A loading dose of 6 mg/kg is ordered. The client weighs 30 kg. How much aminophylline is contained in the loading dose?

1. 60 mg
2. 90 mg
3. 120 mg
4. 180 mg

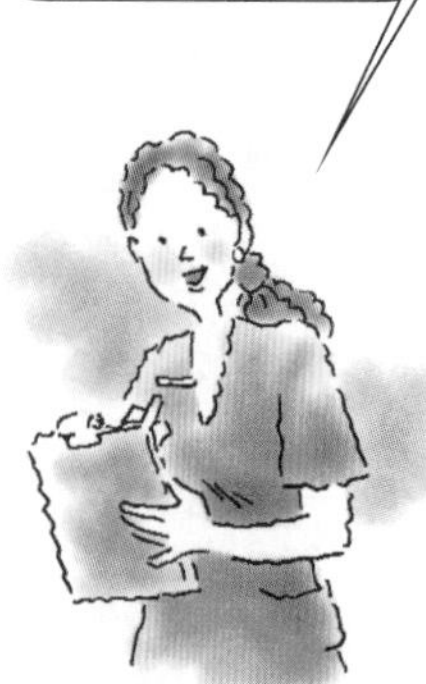

Do you know why it's called a loading dose?

77. 4. The child should receive 180 mg per dose. Here are the calculations:

$6 \text{ mg/kg} \times 30 \text{ kg} = 180 \text{ mg}$.

CN: Physiological integrity; CNS: Pharmacological and parenteral therapies; CL: Application

78. A 10-year-old client with asthma has recently started receiving I.V. aminophylline. He begins to vomit and complains of his stomach hurting. Which nursing intervention is appropriate?

1. Check the theophylline level.
2. Increase the infusion rate.
3. Take no action; aminophylline can cause nausea.
4. Stop the infusion and call the physician.

78. 1. Although nausea and GI upset are adverse effects of aminophylline, they can also represent signs of toxicity. The theophylline level should be checked to make sure the blood level is in the therapeutic range of 10 to 20 mcg/ml. The aminophylline drip may need to be decreased based on the blood level. The infusion shouldn't be stopped until a theophylline level is obtained.

CN: Physiological integrity; CNS: Pharmacological and parenteral therapies; CL: Analysis

79. Which finding should a nurse expect on a typical X-ray of a child with asthma?

1. Atelectasis
2. Hemothorax
3. Infiltrates
4. Pneumothoraces

79. 1. Hyperexpansion, atelectasis, and a flattened diaphragm are typical X-ray findings for a child with asthma. Air becomes trapped behind the narrowed airways and the residual capacity rises, leading to hyperinflation. Hypoxemia results from areas of the lung not being well perfused. A hemothorax isn't a finding related to asthma. Infiltrates and pneumothoraces are uncommon.

CN: Physiological integrity; CNS: Physiological adaptation; CL: Analysis

80. Which intervention is most appropriate for a client with atelectasis?

1. Perform chest physiotherapy.
2. Give increased I.V. fluids.
3. Administer oxygen.
4. Obtain arterial blood gas (ABG) levels.

80. 1. Chest physiotherapy and incentive spirometry help to enhance the clearance of mucus and open the alveoli. I.V. and oral fluids are recommended to help liquefy and thin secretions. Administration of oxygen will *not* give enough pressure to open the alveoli. Obtaining ABG levels isn't necessary.

CN: Physiological integrity; CNS: Physiological adaptation; CL: Application

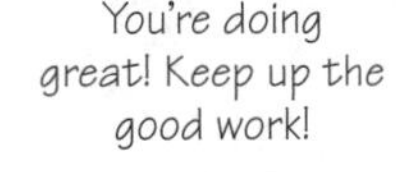
You're doing great! Keep up the good work!

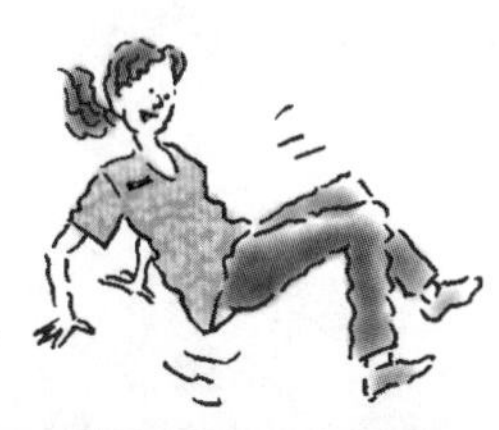

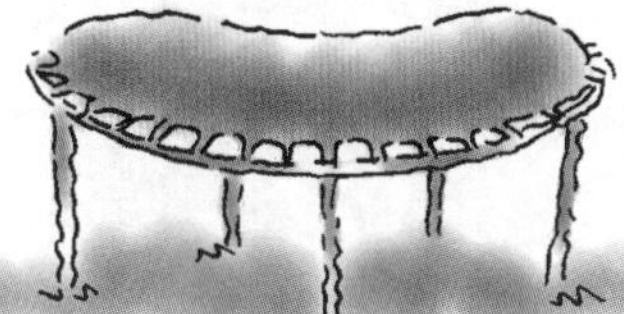

81. The parents of a 10-year-old child recently diagnosed with asthma ask if the child can continue to play sports. Which response is most appropriate?

1. Sports don't cause asthma attacks.
2. You should limit activities to quiet play.
3. It's okay to play some sports but swimming isn't recommended.
4. Physical activity and sports are encouraged, provided the asthma is under control.

81. 4. Participation in sports is encouraged but should be evaluated on an individual basis provided the asthma is under control. Exercise-induced asthma is an example of the airway hyperactivity common to asthmatics. Swimming is well-tolerated related to the type of breathing and the moisture in the air. Exclusion from sports or activities may hamper peer interaction.

CN: Physiological integrity; CNS: Physiological adaptation; CL: Analysis

82. The nurse is caring for a child with asthma who is being treated with aminophylline. The child's aminophylline level is returned as normal. Which level falls within the normal range?

1. 2 to 4 mcg/ml
2. 5 to 15 mcg/ml
3. 10 to 20 mcg/ml
4. 20 to 30 mcg/ml

82. 3. The normal therapeutic range of aminophylline is considered to be 10 to 20 mcg/ml. Levels below 10 mcg/ml are considered to be less than therapeutic. Symptoms of toxicity such as nausea, tachycardia, and irritability can appear when levels exceed 20 mcg/ml. Levels greater than 30 mcg/ml can cause seizures and arrhythmias.

CN: Physiological integrity; CNS: Pharmacological and parenteral therapies; CL: Application

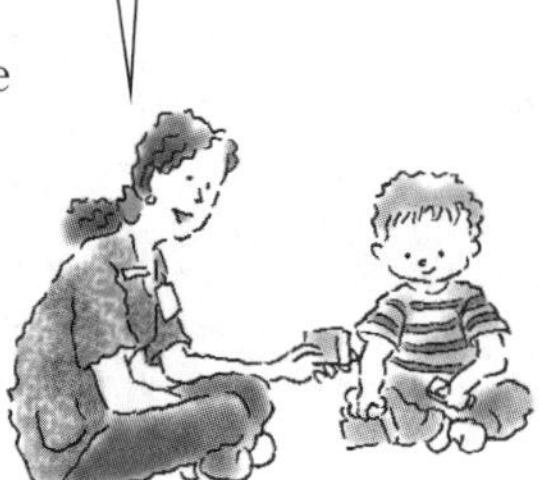

Keep this client's age in mind when answering question 83.

83. Which nursing intervention is appropriate to correct dehydration for a 2-year-old client with asthma?

1. Give warm liquids.
2. Give cold juice or ice pops.
3. Provide three meals and three snacks.
4. Give I.V. fluid boluses.

83. 1. Liquids are best tolerated if they're warm. Cold liquids may cause bronchospasm and should be avoided. Dehydration should be corrected slowly. Small, frequent meals should be provided to avoid abdominal distention that may interfere with diaphragm excursion. Overhydration may increase interstitial pulmonary fluid and exacerbate small airway obstruction.

CN: Physiological integrity; CNS: Physiological adaptation; CL: Application

84. Which intervention by the parents is appropriate to "allergy proof" the home?

1. Cover floors with carpeting.
2. Designate the basement as the play area.
3. Dust and clean the house thoroughly twice a month.
4. Use foam rubber pillows and synthetic blankets.

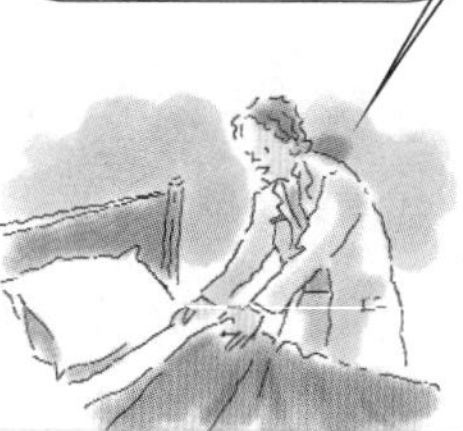

"Allergy proofing" a home can be just as important as "kid proofing" it.

84. 4. Bedding should be free from allergens with hypoallergenic covers. Unnecessary rugs should be removed and floors should be bare and mopped a few times a week to reduce dust. Basements or cellars should be avoided to lessen the child's exposure to molds and mildew. Dusting and cleaning should occur daily or at least weekly.

CN: Physiological integrity; CNS: Physiological adaptation; CL: Application

85. Which nursing diagnosis is appropriate for a client with acute asthma?

1. *Imbalanced nutrition: More than body requirements*
2. *Excess fluid volume*
3. *Activity intolerance*
4. *Constipation*

85. 3. Ineffective oxygen supply and demand may lead to activity intolerance. The nurse should promote rest and encourage developmentally appropriate activities. Nutrition may be decreased due to respiratory distress and GI upset. Dehydration is common due to diaphoresis, insensible water loss, and hyperventilation. Medications given to treat asthma may cause nausea, vomiting, and diarrhea, *not* constipation.

CN: Physiological integrity; CNS: Physiological adaptation; CL: Analysis

86. A nurse is explaining bronchiolitis to the parents of an infant admitted with the condition. Which explanation by the nurse would be the most accurate?

1. Acute inflammation and obstruction of the bronchioles
2. Airway obstruction from aspiration of a solid object
3. Inflammation of the pulmonary parenchyma
4. Acute highly contagious crouplike syndrome

86. 1. Bronchiolitis is an infection of the bronchioles, causing the mucosa to become edematous, inflamed, and full of mucus. Lower airway obstruction from a solid object is a form of a foreign body aspiration. Pneumonia is characterized by inflammation of the pulmonary parenchyma. Crouplike syndromes are generally upper airway infections or obstructions.

CN: Physiological integrity; CNS: Physiological adaptation; CL: Application

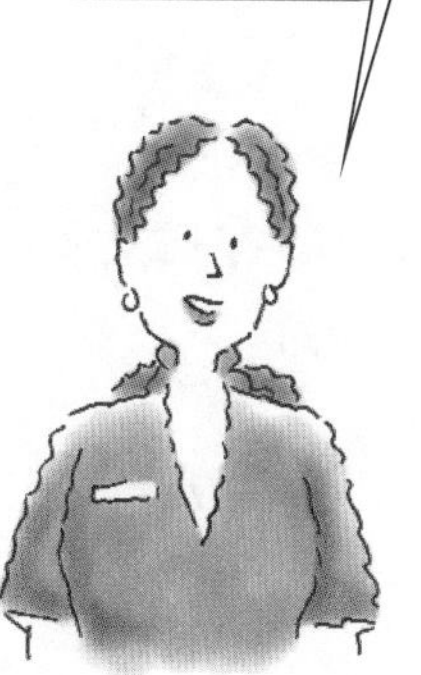

Consider the pathology of bronchiolitis when answering question 87.

87. A 2-month-old infant is brought to the emergency department and a preliminary diagnosis of bronchiolitis is given. Which symptom should a nurse expect to find on assessment?

1. Bradycardia
2. Increased appetite
3. Wheezing on auscultation
4. No signs of an upper respiratory infection

87. 3. In bronchiolitis, the bronchioles become narrowed and edematous. This can cause wheezing. These infants typically have a 2- to 3-day history of an upper respiratory infection and feeding difficulties with loss of appetite due to nasal congestion and increased work of breathing. This combination leads to respiratory distress with tachypnea and tachycardia.

CN: Physiological integrity; CNS: Physiological adaptation; CL: Application

88. In most cases, bronchiolitis is caused by a viral agent, most commonly respiratory syncytial virus (RSV). The nurse should keep in mind which statement regarding RSV infections?

1. It's more prevalent in the summer and fall months.
2. It's most likely to attack the respiratory tract mucosa.
3. It's more commonly seen in children older than age 5.
4. It's not particularly contagious.

88. 2. RSV attacks the respiratory tract mucosa. The virus is most prevalent in the winter and early spring months. Most children develop the infection between ages 2 and 6 months, and RSV generally occurs during the first 3 years of life. RSV is a highly contagious respiratory virus.

CN: Physiological integrity; CNS: Physiological adaptation; CL: Application

89. Which precaution should a nurse caring for a 2-month-old infant with respiratory syncytial virus (RSV) take to prevent the spread of infection?

1. Gloves only
2. Gown, gloves, and mask
3. No precautions required; the virus isn't contagious
4. Proper hand washing between clients

89. 2. RSV is highly contagious and is spread through direct contact with infectious secretions via hands, droplets, and fomites. Gowns, gloves, and masks should be worn for client care to prevent the spread of infection.

CN: Safe, effective care environment; CNS: Safety and infection control; CL: Application

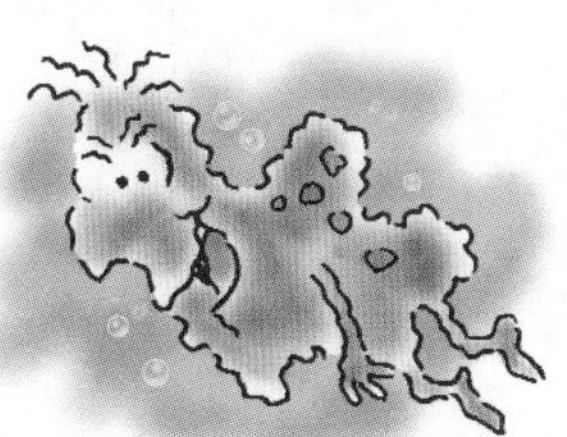

You better take precautions if you want to avoid the likes of me.

90. The nurse teaches parents that the test used to diagnose respiratory syncytial virus (RSV) is:

1. Blood test
2. Nasopharyngeal washings
3. Sputum culture
4. Throat culture

90. 2. RSV can only be diagnosed with direct aspiration of nasal secretions or nasopharyngeal washings. Positive identification is accomplished using the enzyme-linked immunosorbent assay. Blood, throat, and sputum cultures can't definitively diagnose RSV.

CN: Physiological integrity; CNS: Physiological adaptation; CL: Application

91. Which child would be at increased risk for a respiratory syncytial virus (RSV) infection?

1. A 2-month-old child managed at home
2. A 2-month-old child with bronchopulmonary dysplasia
3. A 3-month-old child requiring low-flow oxygen
4. A 2-year-old child

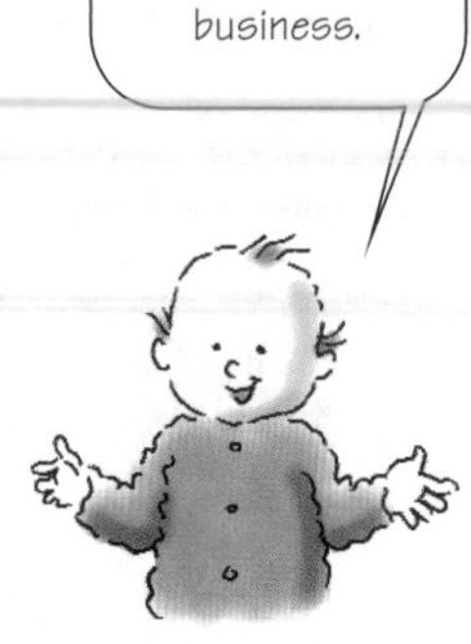

RSV is risky business.

91. 2. Infants with cardiac or pulmonary conditions are at highest risk for RSV. Because of their underlying conditions, they usually require mechanical ventilation. Many infants can be managed at home; few require hospitalization. A 3-month-old on low-flow oxygen has some risks of progression but is *not* at a high risk. A 2-year-old child has built up the immune system and can tolerate the infection without major problems.

CN: Physiological integrity; CNS: Reduction of risk potential; CL: Analysis

92. Which medication can help to prevent respiratory syncytial virus (RSV)?

1. Aminophylline
2. Bronchodilators
3. Corticosteroids
4. Respigam

92. 4. Respigam is I.V. RSV immune globulin. It can help to prevent serious lower respiratory tract infections caused by RSV. The first dose is given before RSV season, with monthly doses given throughout the season for protection. This agent is indicated for children younger than age 24 months with bronchopulmonary dysplasia or a history of prematurity. Bronchodilators, aminophylline, and corticosteroids are sometimes used for treatment.

CN: Health promotion and maintenance; CNS: None; CL: Analysis

93. Which medication is an antiviral agent used to treat bronchiolitis caused by respiratory syncytial virus (RSV)?

1. Albuterol
2. Aminophylline
3. Cromolyn sodium
4. Ribavirin (Virazole)

93. 4. Ribavirin is an antiviral agent sometimes used to reduce the severity of bronchiolitis caused by RSV. Aminophylline and albuterol are bronchodilators and haven't been proven effective in viral bronchiolitis. Cromolyn sodium is an inhaled anti-inflammatory agent.

CN: Physiological integrity; CNS: Pharmacological and parenteral therapies; CL: Analysis

94. Which intervention is most important when monitoring dehydration in an infant with bronchiolitis?

1. Measurement of intake and output
2. Blood levels every 4 hours
3. Urinalysis every 8 hours
4. Weighing each diaper

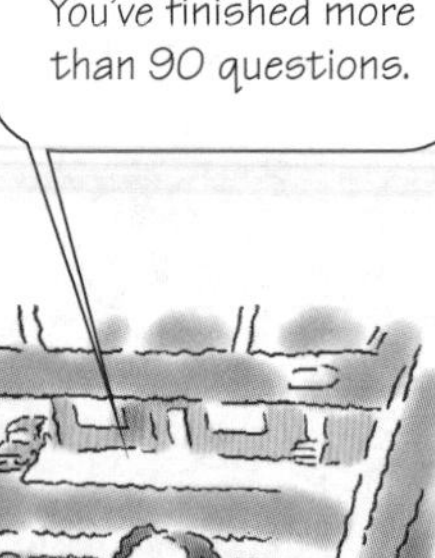

Hang in there!
You've finished more than 90 questions.

94. 1. Accurate measurement of intake and output is essential to assess for dehydration. Blood levels may be obtained daily or every other day. A urinalysis every 8 hours isn't necessary. Urine specific gravities are recommended but can be obtained with diaper changes. Weighing diapers is a way of measuring output only.

CN: Physiological integrity; CNS: Physiological adaptation; CL: Application

CN: Client needs category CNS: Client needs subcategory CL: Cognitive level

95. Which nursing diagnosis is the priority for an infant with bronchiolitis?

1. *Imbalanced nutrition: More than body requirements*
2. *Deficient diversional activity*
3. *Impaired gas exchange*
4. *Social isolation*

95. 3. Infants with bronchiolitis will have impaired gas exchange related to bronchiolar obstruction, atelectasis, and hyperinflation. Nutrition may be seen as less than body requirements. If respiratory distress is present, these infants should have nothing by mouth and fluids given I.V. only. *Deficient diversional activity* and *Social isolation* usually aren't priorities. These infants are too uncomfortable to respond to social stimuli and need quiet, soothing activities that minimize energy.

CN: Physiological integrity; CNS: Physiological adaptation; CL: Analysis

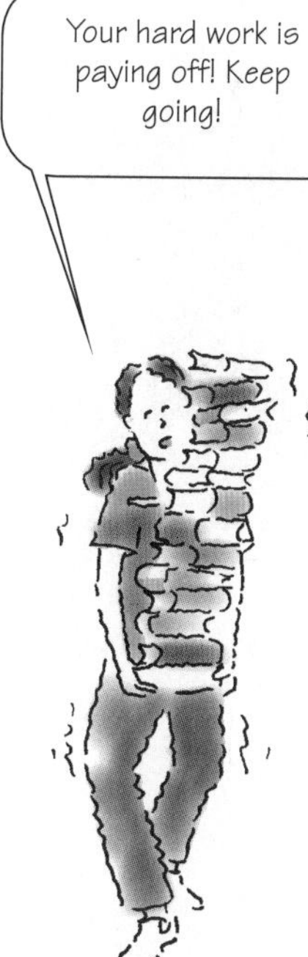

Your hard work is paying off! Keep going!

96. Which teaching point is essential for parents caring for a child with bronchiolitis at home?

1. Place the child in a prone position for comfort.
2. Use warm mist to replace insensible fluid loss.
3. Recognize signs of increasing respiratory distress.
4. Engage the child in many activities to prevent developmental delay.

96. 3. It's essential for parents to be able to recognize signs of increasing respiratory distress and know how to count the respiratory rate. The child should be positioned with the head of the bed elevated for comfort and to facilitate removal of secretions. Use of cool mist may help to replace insensible fluid loss. Quiet play activities are required only as the child's energy level permits. These infants show clinical improvement in 3 to 4 days; therefore, developmental delay isn't an issue.

CN: Physiological integrity; CNS: Physiological adaptation; CL: Analysis

97. The nurse is teaching the parents of a child with pneumonia about the condition. Which description is correct?

1. Inflammation of the large airways
2. Severe infection of the bronchioles
3. Inflammation of the pulmonary parenchyma
4. Acute viral infection with maximum effect at the bronchiolar level

97. 3. Pneumonia is an inflammation of the pulmonary parenchyma. Bronchitis is inflammation of the large airways. Bronchiolitis is a severe infection of the bronchioles. Bronchiolitis and respiratory syncytial virus are terms for an acute viral infection with maximum effect at the bronchiolar level.

CN: Physiological integrity; CNS: Physiological adaptation; CL: Application

98. Which organism is the most common causative agent for bacterial pneumonia?

1. Mycoplasma
2. Parainfluenza virus
3. Pneumococci
4. Respiratory syncytial virus (RSV)

98. 3. Pneumococcal pneumonia is the most common causative agent, accounting for about 90% of bacterial pneumonia. Mycoplasma is a causative agent for primary atypical pneumonia. Parainfluenza virus and RSV account for viral pneumonia.

CN: Physiological integrity; CNS: Physiological adaptation; CL: Application

99. The nurse is caring for an 8-year-old child admitted with pneumonia. Based on the child's age, which type of pneumonia would the nurse suspect?

1. Enteric bacilli
2. Mycoplasma pneumonia
3. Staphylococcal pneumonia
4. Streptococcal pneumonia

99. 2. Mycoplasma pneumonia is a primary atypical pneumonia seen in children between ages 5 and 12. Enteric bacilli, staphylococcal pneumonia, and streptococcal pneumonia are mostly seen in children in the 3 month to 5 year age-group.

CN: Physiological integrity; CNS: Physiological adaptation; CL: Application

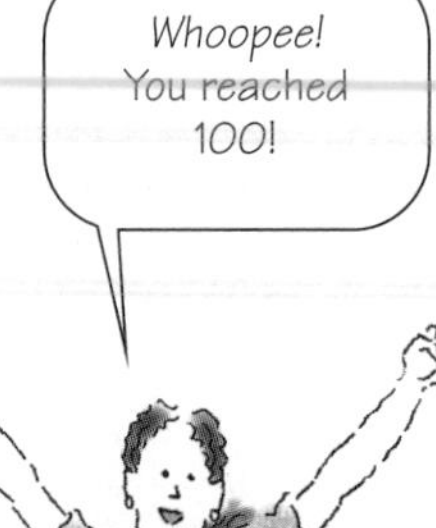

Whoopee! You reached 100!

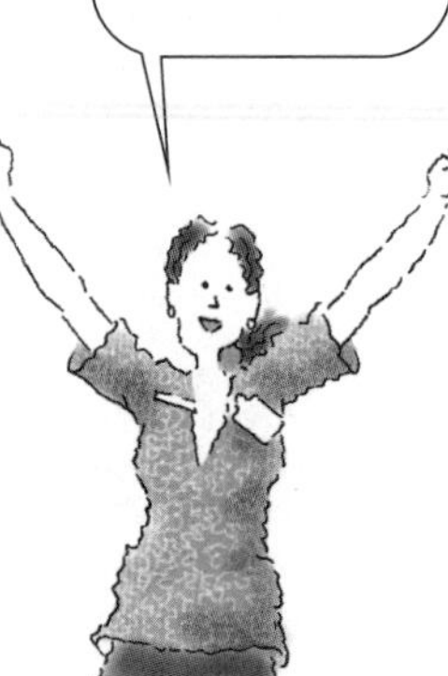

100. The nurse knows to monitor a child with a diagnosis of pertussis for the development of which sign or symptom?

1. Barking cough
2. Whooping cough
3. Abrupt high fever
4. Inspiratory stridor

100. 2. Pertussis is characterized by consistent short, rapid coughs followed by a sudden inspiration with a high-pitched whooping sound. A barking cough and inspiratory stridor are noted with croup. Pertussis is usually accompanied by a low-grade fever.

CN: Physiological integrity; CNS: Physiological adaptation; CL: Application

101. Which test is the definitive means of diagnosing tuberculosis (TB)?

1. Chest X-ray
2. Sputum sample
3. Tuberculin test
4. Urine culture

101. 2. A sputum culture is the definitive test. X-rays usually appear normal in children with TB. The tuberculin test isn't necessarily the most reliable test for TB in children. Stool cultures and gastric washings will show positive results on acid-fast smears but aren't specific for *Mycobacterium tuberculosis.* Sputum samples are difficult to obtain from children, so gastric washings commonly replace them.

CN: Physiological integrity; CNS: Physiological adaptation; CL: Analysis

102. The nurse is assessing a child who has been admitted to the emergency department with a diagnosis of tuberculosis. Which symptom would the nurse expect to observe?

1. Chills
2. Hyperactivity
3. Lymphadenitis
4. Weight gain

102. 3. Children are usually asymptomatic and typically don't manifest the usual pulmonary symptoms, but lymphadenitis is more likely in infants and children than in adults. Weight loss, anorexia, night sweats, fatigue, and malaise are general responses to the disease.

CN: Physiological integrity; CNS: Physiological adaptation; CL: Application

103. Which adverse effect can be expected by the parents of a 2-year-old child who has been started on rifampin (Rifadin) after testing positive for tuberculosis?

1. Hyperactivity
2. Orange body secretions
3. Decreased bilirubin levels
4. Decreased levels of liver enzymes

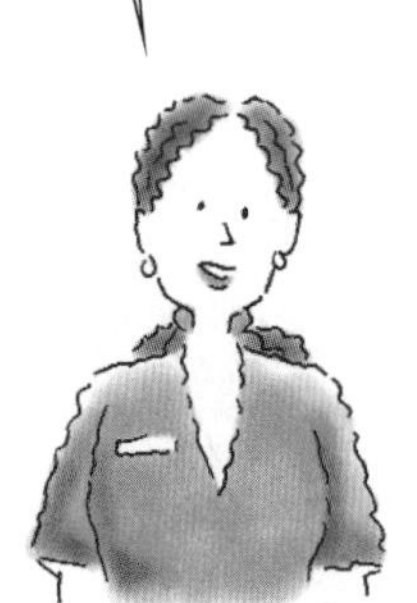

Not all adverse effects are serious.

103. 2. Rifampin and its metabolites will turn urine, feces, sputum, tears, and sweat an orange color. This isn't a serious adverse effect. Rifampin may also cause GI upset, headache, drowsiness, dizziness, visual disturbances, and fever. Liver enzyme and bilirubin levels increase because of hepatic metabolism of the drug. Parents should be taught the signs and symptoms of hepatitis and hyperbilirubinemia such as jaundice of the sclera or skin.

CN: Physiological integrity; CNS: Pharmacological and parenteral therapies; CL: Application

CN: Client needs category CNS: Client needs subcategory CL: Cognitive level

104. Children younger than age 3 are prone to aspirating foreign bodies. Which action is recommended to prevent aspiration?

1. Cut hot dogs in half.
2. Limit popcorn and peanuts.
3. Cut grapes into small pieces.
4. Limit hard candy to special occasions.

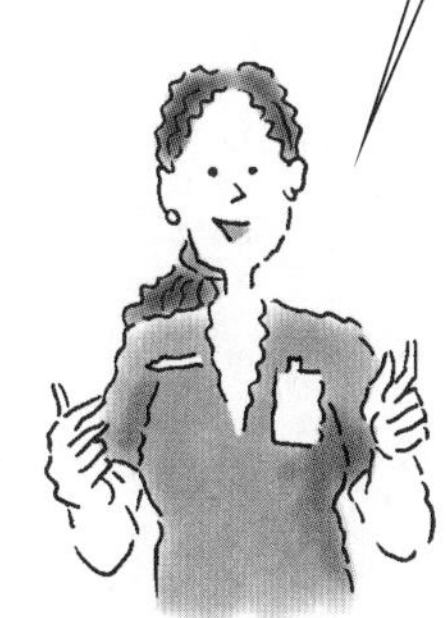

The next four questions address foreign body aspiration.

104. 3. Grapes, hotdogs, and sausage should be cut into many small pieces. Hard candy, raisins, popcorn, and peanuts should be avoided for children age 4 and younger.

CN: Physiological integrity; CNS: Reduction of risk potential; CL: Application

105. A child is admitted with a possible tracheal foreign body. Which findings would most likely indicate a foreign body in the trachea?

1. Cough, dyspnea, and drooling
2. Cough, stridor, and changes in phonation
3. Expiratory wheeze and inspiratory stridor
4. Cough, asymmetrical breath sounds, and wheeze

105. 3. Expiratory and inspiratory noise indicates that the foreign body is in the trachea. Cough, dyspnea, drooling, and gagging indicate supraglottic obstruction. A cough with stridor and changes in phonation would occur if the foreign body were in the larynx. Asymmetrical breath sounds indicate that the object may be located in the bronchi.

CN: Physiological integrity; CNS: Physiological adaptation; CL: Application

106. Which activity is recommended to prevent foreign body aspiration during meals?

1. Insist that children are seated.
2. Give children toys to play with.
3. Allow children to watch television.
4. Allow children to eat in a separate room.

106. 1. Children should remain seated while eating. The risk of aspiration increases if the child is running, jumping, or talking with food in their mouth. Television and toys are a dangerous distraction to toddlers and young children and should be avoided. Children need constant supervision and should be monitored while eating snacks and meals.

CN: Safe, effective care environment; CNS: Safety and infection control; CL: Application

107. The nurse is preparing a child for testing for a foreign body aspiration. The nurse explains to the child's parents that the best diagnostic tool for diagnosis of foreign body aspiration is:

1. Bronchoscopy
2. Chest X-ray
3. Fluoroscopy
4. Lateral neck X-ray

107. 1. Bronchoscopy can give a definitive diagnosis of the presence of foreign bodies and is also the best choice for removal of the object with direct visualization. Chest X-ray and lateral neck X-ray may also be used but findings vary. Some films may appear normal or show changes such as inflammation related to the presence of the foreign body. Fluoroscopy is valuable in detecting and localizing foreign bodies in the bronchi.

CN: Physiological integrity; CNS: Physiological adaptation; CL: Application

108. Which intervention is <u>most</u> appropriate for a child with cystic fibrosis who is having difficulty clearing secretions?

1. Perform chest physiotherapy four times per day.
2. Administer pancreatic enzymes with meals.
3. Provide oxygen by nasal cannula at all times.
4. Provide a high-calorie, high-protein diet at each meal.

108. 1. Chest physiotherapy should be performed to mobilize secretions so they can be more easily cleared. Pancreatic enzymes should be administered with meals to aid in digestion. Administering oxygen may improve oxygenation but won't help clear secretions. A high-calorie, high-protein diet is important for normal growth and development, but won't aid in clearing secretions.

CN: Physiological integrity; CNS: Reduction of risk potential; CL: Application

109. Which statement by the parent of a 16-month-old child with cystic fibrosis should alert a nurse to investigate further?

1. "My child is not walking yet."
2. "My child is saying a few words and short phrases."
3. "My child doesn't interact with other 16-month-olds."
4. "My child cries when I leave the room."

109. 1. A toddler should be walking by 15 months. At 10 months, an infant holds on to furniture while walking, walks with support at 11 months, and takes his first steps at 12 months. By 12 months, a child can say a few words, with more words and short phrases being added each month. A child at 16 months engages in solitary play and has little interaction with other children. Separation anxiety is common in toddlers.

CN: Psychosocial integrity; CNS: None; CL: Analysis

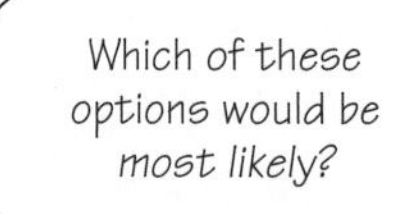

Which of these options would be most likely?

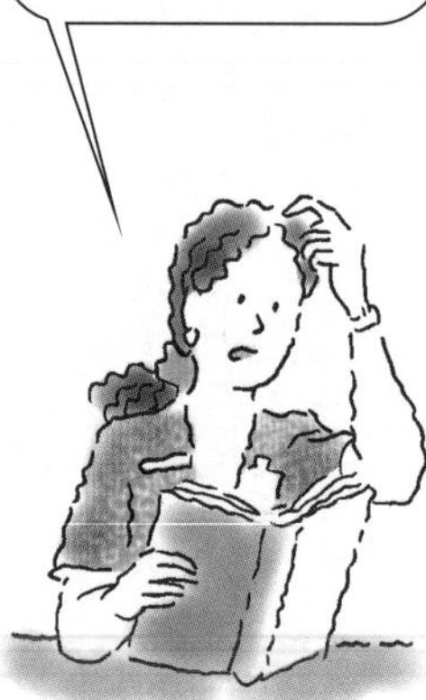

110. A nurse is performing an assessment on a newborn with a possible diagnosis of cystic fibrosis. Which of the following is an early sign of the disease?

1. Constipation
2. Decreased appetite
3. Hyperalbuminemia
4. Meconium ileus

110. 4. Meconium ileus is commonly a presenting sign of cystic fibrosis. Thick, mucilaginous meconium blocks the lumen of the small intestine, causing intestinal obstruction, abdominal distention, and vomiting. Large-volume, loose, frequent, foul-smelling stools are common. These infants may have an increased appetite related to poor absorption from the intestine. The undigested food is excreted, increasing the bulk of feces. Hypoalbuminemia is a common result from the decreased absorption of protein.

CN: Physiological integrity; CNS: Physiological adaptation; CL: Application

111. Which intervention would be most appropriate for a nurse to perform when the parents of a child with cystic fibrosis tell her they are having difficulty coping?

1. Tell the parents they shouldn't expect to have a normal family life.
2. Refer the parents to a cystic fibrosis support group.
3. Show the parents how to perform chest physiotherapy at home.
4. Tell the parents that with good medical care their child can live into adulthood.

111. 2. Support groups can provide the parents with the support they need to cope with their child's condition as well as provide them with accurate information on the disorder. The family shouldn't be discouraged from having as normal a life as possible. Showing the parents how to perform chest physiotherapy is an important intervention, but won't help them cope with their child's condition. With good medical care, children with cystic fibrosis can live into adulthood, but telling the parent this doesn't promote the coping skills the parents need.
CN: Physiological integrity; CNS: None; CL: Application

112. A toddler with suspected cystic fibrosis is admitted for testing. The nurse explains that the diagnostic criteria for chloride levels is:

1. Below 20 mEq/L
2. Below 40 mEq/L
3. 40 to 60 mEq/L
4. Above 60 mEq/L

112. 4. A chloride concentration greater than 60 mEq/L is diagnostic of cystic fibrosis. Normal sweat chloride content is less than 40 mEq/L, with the average being 18 mEq/L. Levels between 40 and 60 mEq/L are highly suggestive of cystic fibrosis.
CN: Physiological integrity; CNS: Physiological adaptation; CL: Application

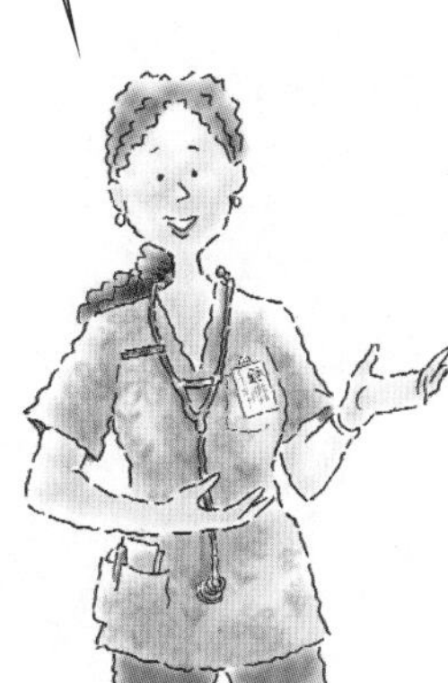
In light of the pathology of cystic fibrosis, which is the only diet that makes sense?

113. The parents ask which diet is recommended for their child, who has cystic fibrosis. What is the nurse's response?

1. Fat-restricted
2. High-calorie
3. Low-protein
4. Sodium-restricted

113. 2. A well-balanced high-calorie, high-protein diet is recommended for a child with cystic fibrosis due to the impaired intestinal absorption. Fat restriction isn't required because digestion and absorption of fat in the intestine are impaired. The child usually increases enzyme intake when high-fat foods are eaten. Low-sodium foods can lead to hyponatremia; therefore, high-sodium foods are recommended, especially during hot weather or when the child has a fever.
CN: Physiological integrity; CNS: Basic care and comfort; CL: Application

114. Which statement concerning pancreatic enzymes for a cystic fibrosis client is correct?

1. Capsules may not be opened.
2. Microcapsules can be crushed.
3. Encourage eating throughout the day.
4. Administer enzymes at each meal and with snacks.

114. 4. Enzymes are administered with each feeding, meal, and snack to optimize absorption of the nutrients consumed. Regular capsules may be opened and the contents mixed with a small amount of applesauce or other nonalkaline food. Microcapsules can't be crushed due to the enteric coating. Eating throughout the day should be discouraged. Three meals and two or three snacks per day are recommended.
CN: Physiological integrity; CNS: Physiological adaptation; CL: Application

115. A nurse should include which information on nutrition when teaching the family of a child with cystic fibrosis?

1. Provide a high-calorie, high-protein diet.
2. Place the child on a daily 1,200 ml fluid restriction.
3. Restrict daily intake of sodium to 1.5 g/day.
4. Provide adequate amounts of fat-soluble vitamins.

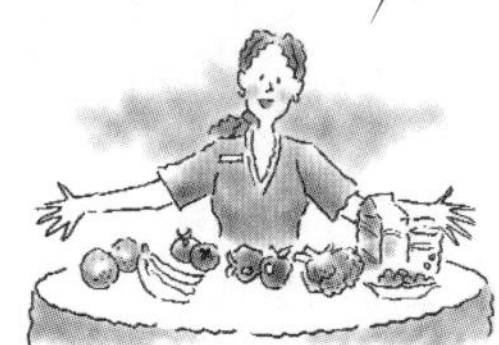
Teach the family about proper nutrition.

115. 1. To promote growth and development, the child should eat a high-calorie, high-protein diet. The child with cystic fibrosis should also be encouraged to consume higher than usual amounts of fluids and sodium. The child should be given water-soluble forms of fat-soluble vitamins.

CN: Physiological integrity; CNS: Basic care and comfort; CL: Application

116. A nurse is caring for a client with cystic fibrosis. Ranitidine (Zantac) 4 mg/kg/day every 12 hours is ordered. The child weighs 20 kg. How many milligrams are given per dose?

1. 16
2. 20
3. 40
4. 80

116. 3. The child should receive 40 mg per dose. Here are the calculations:

$20 \text{ kg} \times 4 \text{ mg/kg} = 80 \text{ mg};$

$24 \text{ hr}/12 \text{ hr} = 2 \text{ doses};$

$80 \text{ mg}/2 \text{ doses} = 40 \text{ mg}.$

CN: Physiological integrity; CNS: Pharmacological and parenteral therapies; CL: Application

117. Which intervention is appropriate for care of the child with cystic fibrosis?

1. Decrease exercise and limit physical activity.
2. Administer cough suppressants and antihistamines.
3. Administer chest physiotherapy two to four times per day.
4. Administer bronchodilator or nebulizer treatments after chest physiotherapy.

117. 3. Chest physiotherapy is recommended two to four times per day to help loosen and move secretions to facilitate expectoration. Exercise and physical activity is recommended to stimulate mucus secretion and to establish a good habitual breathing pattern. Cough suppressants and antihistamines are contraindicated. The goal is for the child to be able to cough and expectorate mucus secretions. Bronchodilator or nebulizer treatments are given before chest physiotherapy to help open the bronchi for easier expectoration.

CN: Safe, effective care environment; CNS: Management of care; CL: Application

118. Which statement is appropriate for a nurse to address to the parents of a child with cystic fibrosis who are planning to have a second child?

1. Genetic counseling is recommended.
2. There's a 50% chance the child will be normal.
3. There's a 50% chance of the child being affected.
4. There's a 25% chance the child will only be a carrier.

118. 1. Genetic counseling should be recommended. Cystic fibrosis is an autosomal-recessive disease. Therefore, there's a 25% chance of the child having the disease, a 25% chance of the child being normal, and a 50% chance of the child being a carrier.

CN: Health promotion and maintenance; CNS: None; CL: Application

119. Parents ask the nurse about the cause of their child's cystic fibrosis. Which statement best describes this autosomal-recessive disorder?

1. The genetic disorder is carried on the X chromosome.
2. Both parents must pass the defective gene or set of genes.
3. Only one defective gene or set of genes is passed by one parent.
4. The child has an extra chromosome, resulting in an XXY karyotype.

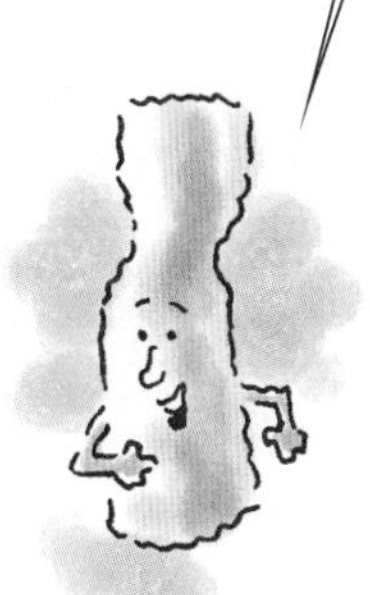
They just
keep passing
me along.

119. 2. In recessive disorders such as cystic fibrosis, both parents must pass the defective gene or set of genes to the child. Sex-linked genetic disorders are carried on the X chromosome. Dominant disorders are characterized by only one defective gene or set of genes passed by one parent. A child with an XXY karyotype would have Klinefelter's syndrome.
CN: Health promotion and maintenance; CNS: None; CL: Application

120. When a nurse enters the room to give an antibiotic elixir to a 3-year-old child, the child says the medication is "yucky" and refuses to take it. Which response by the nurse is best?

1. "Do you want to take the medicine with vanilla ice cream or chocolate ice cream?"
2. "If you don't take the medicine I will tell your mother."
3. "The doctor says you must take the medicine."
4. "You need to take this medicine to get better."

120. 1. Offering the child a choice of how he wants to take the medication provides the child with some control. Threatening to tell the child's mother won't help and erodes any trust between the child and nurse. Telling the child that the doctor says he must take the medication also isn't helpful. At age 3, trying to reason with the child about why he needs to take the medication won't work because his thinking is still concrete.
CN: Psychosocial integrity; CNS: None; CL: Analysis

121. Ceftazidime (Fortaz) has been ordered for a client with cystic fibrosis. The order states to give 40 mg/kg every 8 hours. The child is 2 years old and weighs 38.5 lb. How many milligrams of the ceftazidime is given in one dose?

1. 116
2. 233
3. 260
4. 466

121. 2. The child should receive 233 mg per dose. Here are the calculations: 38.5 lb/2.2 kg = 17.5 kg (1 lb equals 2.2 kg); 40 mg/kg × 17.5 kg = 700 mg; 24 hours/8 hours = 3 doses; 700 mg/3 doses = 233 mg.
CN: Physiological integrity; CNS: Pharmacological and parenteral therapies; CL: Application

122. A child with cystic fibrosis is placed on an oral antibiotic to be given in four equally divided doses per day for 14 days. Which time schedule is most appropriate?

1. 8 a.m., 12 p.m., 4 p.m., 8 p.m.
2. 8 a.m., 2 p.m., 8 p.m., 2 a.m.
3. 9 a.m., 1 p.m., 5 p.m., 9 p.m.
4. 10 a.m., 2 p.m., 6 p.m., 10 p.m.

122. 2. The doses should be given routinely every 6 hours. This helps maintain a therapeutic blood level of the antibiotic. The other answers have doses only every 4 hours during the day and then no doses for 12 hours at night.
CN: Physiological integrity; CNS: Pharmacological and parenteral therapies; CL: Analysis

123. Which complication of cystic fibrosis may eventually lead to death?

1. Rectal prolapse
2. Pulmonary obstruction
3. Gastroesophageal reflux
4. Reproductive system obstruction

123. 2. Pulmonary obstruction related to thickened mucus secretions can lead to a progressive pulmonary disturbance and secondary infections that can lead to death. Rectal prolapse is managed with enzyme replacement therapy and manipulation of the rectum back into place. Gastroesophageal reflux can be managed with medications and proper reflux precautions. Obstruction of the reproductive system can lead to infertility due to increased mucus blocking sperm entry in the female or blockage of the vas deferens in the male.

CN: Physiological integrity; CNS: Physiological adaptation; CL: Analysis

124. Which method is best for evaluation of a 6-year-old child with cystic fibrosis who has been placed on an aerosol inhaler?

1. Ask if the parents have any questions.
2. Ask if the child can explain the procedure.
3. Ask the parents if they understand the usage.
4. Ask the client to perform a return demonstration.

124. 4. A return demonstration is the best evaluation. It will show if the client can repeat the steps shown and appropriately use the inhaler. The parents should understand how the inhaler should be used and ask questions, but the child must be able to correctly demonstrate usage first. The child may have difficulty explaining the procedure at age 6.

CN: Physiological integrity; CNS: Pharmacological and parenteral therapies; CL: Application

125. Which intervention is appropriate for a 2-year-old client with chest trauma who has a left lower chest tube in place?

1. Stripping or milking the tubing
2. Requiring routine dressing changes
3. Clamping the chest tube during transport
4. Inspecting tubing for kinks or obstructions

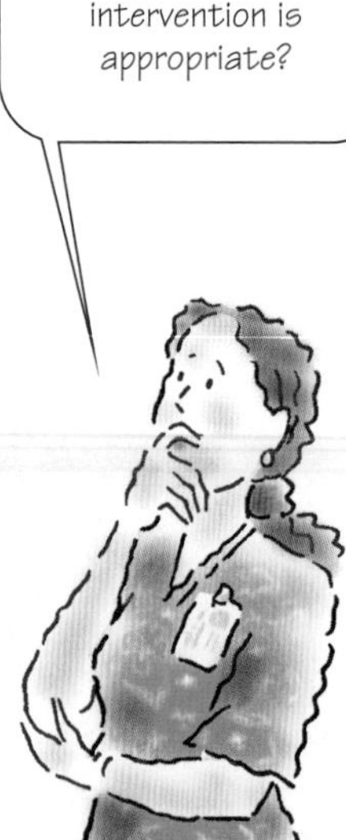
Which intervention is appropriate?

125. 4. Tubing should be inspected for kinks or obstructions so that drainage can flow freely. Manipulation of the tubing should be avoided. The pressure created from stripping can damage the pleural space or mediastinum. There's no need for routine dressing changes if the dressing isn't soiled and there's no evidence of infection. Inspect and palpate around the dressing routinely. The chest tube should never be clamped because it may lead to a tension pneumothorax. Waterseal will protect the client during transit.

CN: Physiological integrity; CNS: Physiological adaptation; CL: Application

126. A toddler in respiratory distress is admitted to the pediatric intensive care unit. When he refuses to keep his oxygen face mask on, his mother tries to help. Which action by a nurse is most appropriate?

1. Giving the child his favorite toy to play with
2. Having the mother read the child's favorite book to him
3. Administering a strong sedative so the child will sleep
4. Telling the child that the face mask will help him breathe better

126. 2. Having the mother read the child's favorite book will ease his anxiety and provide comfort to the child. Although giving the child a favorite toy is also appropriate, the child needs his mother's comfort because the face mask is frightening. Sedation is contraindicated because it can mask signs of respiratory distress. A toddler is too young to understand that something will make him feel better.

CN: Safe, effective care environment; CNS: Management of care; CL: Application

I know this is one of your favorite books.

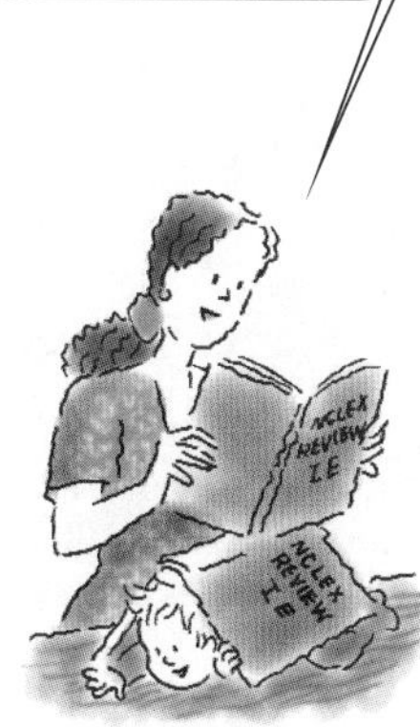

127. A 12-year-old boy is discharged from the hospital after an acute asthma attack with a prescription for budesonide (Pulmicort Turbuhaler). Which signs and symptoms should the nurse instruct him and his parents to report to the physician immediately?

1. Diarrhea
2. Bradycardia
3. Weight loss
4. Oral candidiasis

127. 4. One of the adverse reactions to budesonide is oral candidiasis and parents should be instructed to monitor the child's mouth for this. Diarrhea, bradycardia, and weight loss are not adverse reactions to this corticosteroid.

CN: Physiological integrity; CNS: Pharmacological and parenteral therapies; CL: Analysis

128. A 6-year-old with a history of asthma is being evaluated by an allergist who orders skin testing to be done at the next visit. Which action by a nurse will help ensure accurate skin testing results?

1. Making sure the child doesn't have a runny nose
2. Making sure the child hasn't received antihistamines in the past 7 days
3. Using the child's posterior legs for testing
4. Limiting testing to environmental allergens

128. 2. Antihistamines may alter results of skin testing and should be withheld at least 1 week before testing. A runny nose won't alter test results. The forearm and upper back are the best sites for allergy testing. Testing only for environmental allergens precludes diagnosis of allergies to other substances.

CN: Physiological integrity; CNS: Pharmacological and parenteral therapies; CL: Application

Moving along nicely! Keep it up!

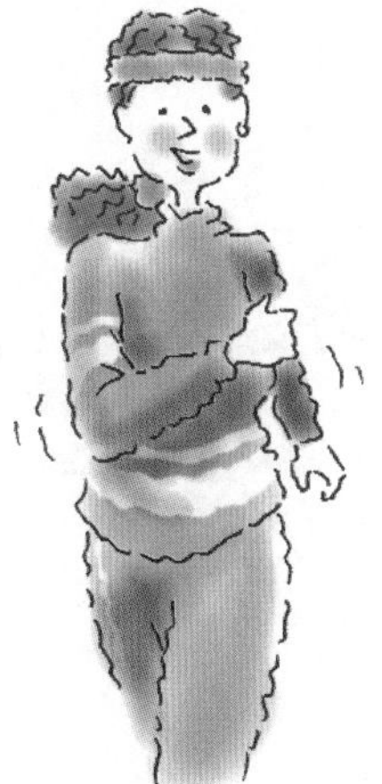

129. Which sign should alert a nurse to a potentially life-threatening complication in a child who received an allergy shot 30 minutes earlier?

1. Urinary output less than 30 ml/hour
2. Heart rate of 58 beats per minute
3. Blood pressure of 82/48 mm Hg
4. Rash

129. 3. Anaphylaxis can cause hypotension and tachycardia (not bradycardia). Urinary urgency and incontinence, not anuria, may also be reported. A rash may signal an allergic reaction, but not a severe one such as anaphylaxis.

CN: Physiological integrity; CNS: Physiological adaptation; CL: Analysis

130. The nurse is caring for a 17-year-old female client with cystic fibrosis who has been admitted to the hospital to receive I.V. antibiotic and respiratory treatment for exacerbation of a lung infection. The client has many questions about her future and the consequences of the disease. Which statements about the course of cystic fibrosis are true? Select all that apply:

1. Breast development is frequently delayed.
2. The client is at risk for developing diabetes.
3. Pregnancy and childbearing aren't affected.
4. Normal sexual relationships can be expected.
5. Only males carry the gene for the disease.
6. By age 20, the client should be able to decrease the frequency of respiratory treatment.

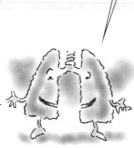

130. 1, 2, 4. Cystic fibrosis delays growth and the onset of puberty. Children with cystic fibrosis tend to be smaller than average size and develop secondary sex characteristics later in life. In addition, clients with cystic fibrosis are at risk for developing diabetes mellitus because the pancreatic duct becomes obstructed as pancreatic tissues are destroyed. Clients with cystis fibrosis can expect to have normal sexual relationships, but fertility becomes difficult because thick secretions obstruct the cervix and block sperm entry. Both men and women carry the gene for cystic fibrosis. Pulmonary disease commonly progresses as the client ages, requiring additional respiratory treatment, not less.

CN: Physiological integrity; CNS: Physiological adaptation; CL: Analysis

131. A nurse is preparing to administer the first dose of tobramycin (Nebcin) to an adolescent with cystic fibrosis. The order is for 3 mg/kg I.V. daily in three divided doses. The client weighs 110 lb. How many milligrams should the nurse administer per dose? Record your answer using a whole number.

______________________ milligrams

131. 50. To perform this dosage calculation, the nurse should first convert the client's weight to kilograms using this formula: 1 kg/2.2 lb = X kg/110 lb; 2.2X = 110; X = 50 kg. Then, she should calculate the client's daily dose using this formula: 50 kg × 3 mg/kg = 150 mg. Finally, the nurse should calculate the divided dose: 150 mg ÷ 3 doses = 50 mg/dose.

CN: Physiological integrity; CNS: Pharmacological and parenteral therapies; CL: Application

You finished chapter 29! Now you can breathe easier.

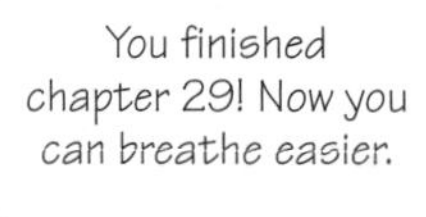

132. A parent is planning to enroll her 9-month-old infant in a daycare facility. She asks the nurse what to look for as indicators that the daycare facility is adhering to good infection control measures. How should the nurse reply? Select all that apply:

1. The facility keeps boxes of gloves in the director's office.
2. Diapers are discarded into covered receptacles.
3. Toys are kept on the floor for the children to share.
4. Disposable papers are used on the diaper-changing surfaces.
5. Facilities for hand hygiene are located in every classroom.
6. Soiled clothing and cloth diapers are sent home in labeled paper bags.

132. 2, 4, 5. A parent can assess infection control measures by appraising steps taken by the facility to prevent the spread of potential diseases. Placing diapers in covered receptacles, covering the diaper-changing surfaces with disposable papers, and ensuring that there are hand sanitizers and sinks available for personnel to wash their hands after activities are all indicators that infection control measures are being followed. Gloves should be readily available to personnel and, therefore, should be kept in every room, not in an office. Typically, toys are shared by numerous children; however, this contributes to the spread of germs and infections. All soiled clothing and cloth diapers should be placed in a sealed plastic bag prior to being sent home.

CN: Safe, effective care environment; CNS: Safety and infection control; CL: Application

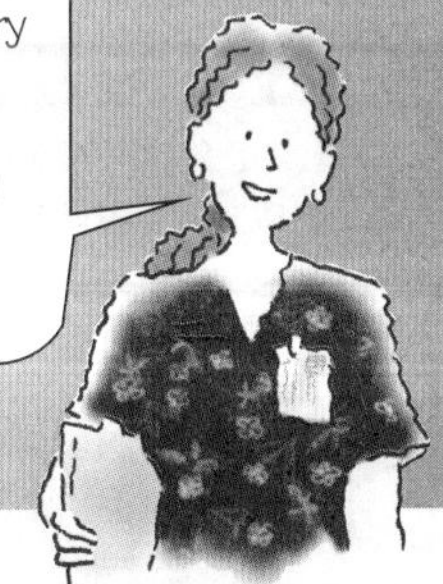
Here are two Web sites you can check for more information about neurosensory disorders in children: www.adhd.org (Attention Deficit Disorder Association) and www.ndss.org (National Down Syndrome Society).

Chapter 30
Neurosensory disorders

1. A mother of a 3-year-old with a myelomeningocele is thinking about having another baby. A nurse should inform the woman that she should increase her intake of which acid?

1. Folic acid to 0.4 mg/day
2. Folic acid to 4 mg/day
3. Ascorbic acid to 0.4 mg/day
4. Ascorbic acid to 4 mg/day

1. 2. The American Academy of Pediatrics recommends that a woman who has had a child with a neural tube defect increase her intake of folic acid to 4 mg per day one month before becoming pregnant and continue this regimen through the first trimester. A woman who has no family history of neural tube defects should take 0.4 mg. All women of childbearing age should be encouraged to take a folic acid supplement because the majority of pregnancies in the United States are unplanned. Ascorbic acid hasn't been shown to have any effect on preventing neural tube defects.

CN: Health promotion and maintenance; CNS: None; CL: Application

2. Which nursing diagnosis is <u>most relevant</u> in the first 12 hours of life for a neonate born with a myelomeningocele?

1. *Risk for infection*
2. *Constipation*
3. *Impaired physical mobility*
4. *Delayed growth and development*

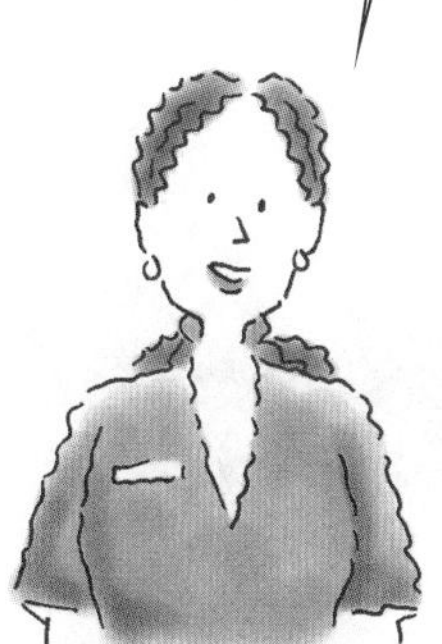
Most relevant—that's the key phrase for question 2.

2. 1. All of these diagnoses are important for a child with a myelomeningocele. However, during the first 12 hours of life, the most life-threatening event would be an infection. The other diagnoses will be addressed as the child develops.

CN: Physiological integrity; CNS: Reduction of risk potential; CL: Application

3. A neonate has been brought to the emergency room by its mother. The nurse suspects that the child may have hydrocephalus. Which observations would indicate this condition?

1. Bulging fontanel, low-pitched cry
2. Depressed fontanel, low-pitched cry
3. Bulging fontanel, eyes rotated downward
4. Depressed fontanel, eyes rotated downward

3. 3. Hydrocephalus is caused from the alteration in circulation of the cerebrospinal fluid (CSF). The amount of CSF increases, causing the fontanel to bulge. This also causes an increase in intracranial pressure. This increase in pressure causes the neonate's eyes to deviate downward (the "setting sun sign"), and the neonate's cry becomes high-pitched.

CN: Health promotion and maintenance; CNS: None; CL: Analysis

CN: Client needs category   CNS: Client needs subcategory   CL: Cognitive level

4. Which nursing action should be included in the care plan for a child following shunt insertion on the right side of the head to relieve hydrocephalus?

1. Place the child flat in bed on the right side.
2. Place the child flat in bed on the left side.
3. Place the child in a semi-Fowler's position.
4. Place the child in an upright position.

4. 2. The child should be flat in bed to avoid rapid decompression of cerebrospinal fluid (CSF) and on the left side or on his back to avoid occlusion of the shunt and blockage of the drainage of CSF. Placing the child in a semi-Fowler's or upright position may promote too rapid decompression of CSF.

CN: Physiological integrity; CNS: Reduction of risk potential; CL: Application

Remember, in emergency situations, your first priority is to ensure the client's safety.

5. Which nursing action is <u>appropriate</u> when a child has a seizure?

1. Inserting a nasogastric tube to prevent emesis
2. Restraining the extremities with a pillow or blanket
3. Inserting a tongue blade to prevent injury to the tongue
4. Padding the side rails of the bed to protect the child from injury

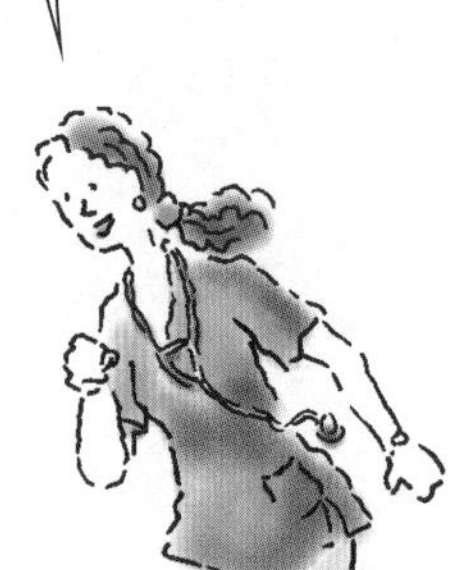

5. 4. A child having a seizure could fall out of bed or injure himself on anything, including the side rails of the bed. Attempts to insert anything into the child's mouth may injure the child. Attempting to restrain the child won't stop seizures. In fact, tactile stimulation may increase the seizure activity; therefore, it must be limited as much as possible.

CN: Safe, effective care environment; CNS: Safety and infection control; CL: Application

6. A mother brings her infant to the emergency department and says he had a seizure. While a nurse is obtaining a history, the mother says she was running out of formula so she stretched the formula by adding three times the normal amount of water. Electrolytes and blood glucose levels are drawn on the infant. The nurse should expect which laboratory value?

1. Blood glucose: 120 mg/dl
2. Chloride: 104 mmol/L
3. Potassium: 4 mmol/L
4. Sodium: 125 mmol/L

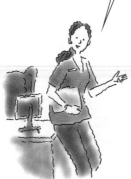

For the NCLEX, you need to be familiar with normal lab values.

6. 4. Diluting formula in a different manner than is recommended alters the infant's electrolyte levels. Normal serum sodium for an infant is 135 to 145 mmol/L. When formula is diluted, the infant's sodium is also diluted and will decrease. Hyponatremia is one of the causes of seizures in infants. The other values are all within normal limits.

CN: Physiological integrity; CNS: Reduction of risk potential; CL: Analysis

7. For which symptom should a nurse assess a neonate diagnosed with bacterial meningitis?

1. Hypothermia, irritability, and poor feeding
2. Positive Babinski's reflex, mottling, and pallor
3. Headache, nuchal rigidity, and developmental delays
4. Positive Moro's embrace reflex, hyperthermia, and sunken fontanel

7. 1. The clinical appearance of a neonate with meningitis is different from that of a child or an adult. Neonates may be either hypothermic or hyperthermic. The irritation to the meninges causes the neonates to be irritable and to have a decreased appetite. They may be pale and mottled with a bulging, full fontanel. Older children and adults with meningitis have headaches, nuchal rigidity, and hyperthermia as clinical manifestations. Normal neonates have positive Moro's embrace and Babinski's reflexes. Developmental delays, if present, would appear when the child was older.

CN: Physiological integrity; CNS: Physiological adaptation; CL: Application

8. Which type of behavior demonstrated by a 6-year-old should help a school nurse differentiate between attention deficit hyperactivity disorder (ADHD) and learning disability?
1. The child reverses letters and words while reading.
2. The child is easily distracted and reacts impulsively.
3. The child is always getting into fights during recess.
4. The child has a difficult time reading a chapter book.

8. 2. Two of the most common characteristics of children with ADHD include inattention and impulsiveness. Children who reverse letters and words while reading have dyslexia. Although aggressiveness may be common in children with ADHD, it isn't a characteristic that will help diagnose this disorder. Six-year-old children aren't usually cognitively ready to read a chapter book.
CN: Health promotion and maintenance; CNS: None;
CL: Analysis

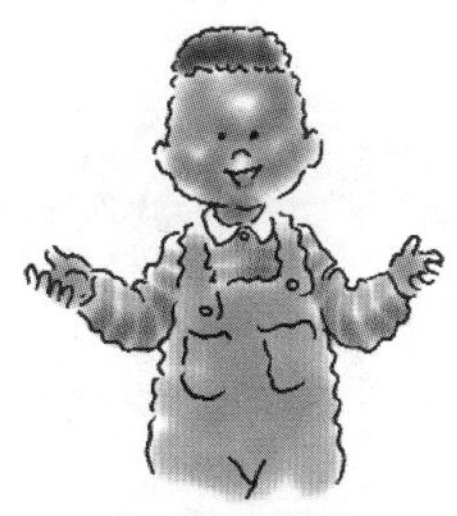
I'm trying to
pay attention.
Really I am.

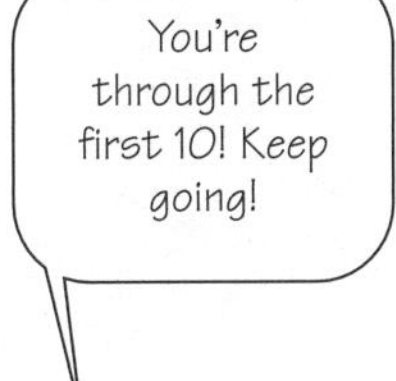

9. Which statement by the parent of a child with cerebral palsy indicates that a nurse's teaching has been successful?
1. "My child's muscles will get stronger over time."
2. "My child's condition will get progressively worse."
3. "My child will have low intelligence."
4. "My child will need continual therapy to maintain functioning."

9. 4. The child with cerebral palsy needs continual treatment and therapy to maintain or improve functioning. Without therapy, muscles will get progressively weaker and more spastic. Although some children with cerebral palsy are mentally retarded, many have normal intelligence.
CN: Health promotion and maintenance; CNS: None;
CL: Analysis

10. While assessing a full-term neonate, which symptom should cause the nurse to suspect a neurologic impairment?
1. A weak sucking reflex
2. A positive rooting reflex
3. A positive Babinski's reflex
4. Startle reflex in response to a loud noise

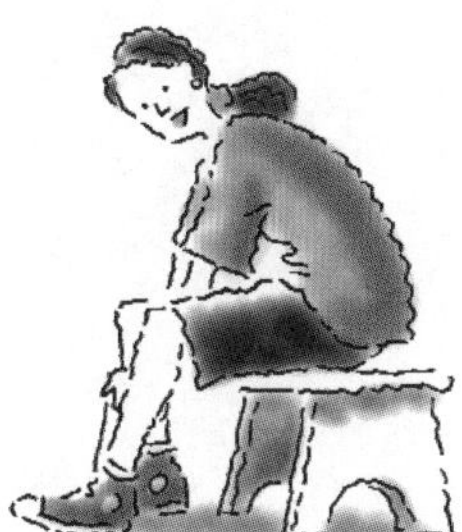
You're
through the
first 10! Keep
going!

10. 1. Normal neonates have a strong, vigorous sucking reflex. The rooting reflex is present at birth and disappears when the infant is between ages 3 and 4 months. A positive Babinski's reflex is present at birth and disappears by the time the infant is age 2 years. The startle reflex is present at birth and disappears when the infant is about age 4 months.
CN: Health promotion and maintenance; CNS: None;
CL: Application

11. A mother reports that her school-age child has been reprimanded for daydreaming during class. This is a new behavior, and the child's grades are dropping. The nurse should suspect which problem?
1. The child may have a hearing problem and needs to have his hearing checked.
2. The child may have a learning disability and needs referral to the special education department.
3. The child may have attention deficit hyperactivity disorder (ADHD) and needs medication.
4. The child may be having absence seizures and needs to see his primary health care provider for evaluation.

11. 4. Absence seizures are commonly misinterpreted as daydreaming. The child loses awareness but no alteration in motor activity is exhibited. A mild hearing problem is usually exhibited as leaning forward, talking louder, listening to louder TV and music than usual, and a repetitive "what?" from the child. There isn't enough information to indicate a learning disability. ADHD isn't characterized by episodes of quietness.
CN: Physiological integrity; CNS: Physiological adaptation;
CL: Analysis

12. A 2-month-old infant is brought to the well-baby clinic for his first check-up. On initial assessment, the nurse notes the infant's head circumference is at the 95th percentile. Which action should the nurse take <u>initially</u>?

1. Assess vital signs.
2. Measure the head again.
3. Assess neurologic signs.
4. Notify the primary health care provider.

12. 2. Whenever there's a question about vital signs or assessment data, the first logical step would be to reassess to determine if an error had been made initially. Notifying the primary health care provider and assessing neurologic and vital signs are important and would follow the reassessment.

CN: Health promotion and maintenance; CNS: None; CL: Analysis

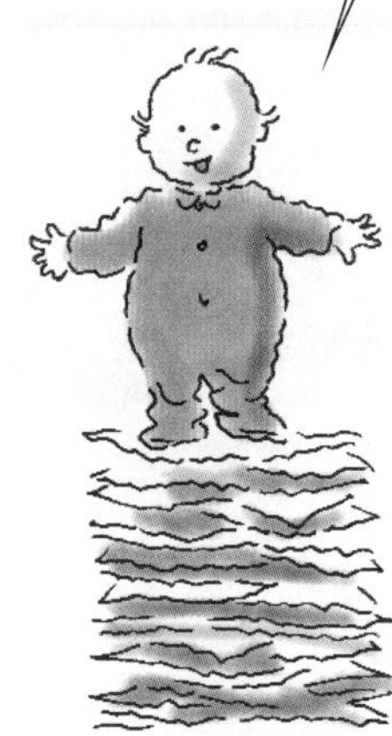
Now I should be in the 1000th percentile.

13. Which observation indicates to a nurse that the mother of a child with cerebral palsy needs further instruction?

1. The mother gives the child assistive devices for eating.
2. The mother fusses over the mess the child is making.
3. The mother provides adequate time for the child to finish eating.
4. The mother provides finger foods.

13. 2. Parents should encourage the child with cerebral palsy to be as independent as possible even if a mess is made while attempting to eat. Assistive devices can help the child with weak or spastic muscles eat independently. The child with cerebral palsy requires more time to bring food to the mouth and to chew and shouldn't be rushed. The parents should provide a calm and stress-free environment for eating. Providing the child with finger foods helps him eat independently.

CN: Physiological integrity; CNS: Basic care and comfort; CL: Analysis

14. A 2-year-old child is admitted to the pediatric unit with the diagnosis of bacterial meningitis. Which measure would be appropriate for a nurse to perform first?

1. Obtain a urine specimen.
2. Draw ordered laboratory tests.
3. Place the toddler in respiratory isolation.
4. Explain the treatment plan to the parents.

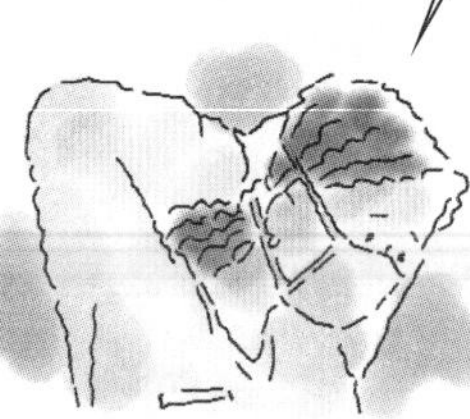
Take the necessary precautions to protect yourself and others from possible infection.

14. 3. Nurses should take necessary precautions to protect themselves and others from possible infection from the bacterial organism causing meningitis. The affected child should immediately be placed in respiratory isolation; then the parents can be informed about the treatment plan. This should be done before laboratory tests are performed.

CN: Safe, effective care environment; CNS: Safety and infection control; CL: Application

15. Which sign or symptom should a nurse expect to be present in a 12-year-old child admitted to the pediatric unit with a diagnosis of possible brain tumor?

1. Bulging fontanel
2. High-pitched cry
3. Behavioral changes
4. Change in vital signs

15. 3. In a school-age child with a closed cranium, a common symptom of a brain tumor is behavior change due to the increased cranial pressure. A bulging fontanel and high-pitched cry are typical signs in an infant. A change in vital signs is a later sign of increased intracranial pressure.

CN: Physiological integrity; CNS: Physiological adaptation; CL: Application

16. A preschool-age child has just been admitted to the pediatric unit with a diagnosis of bacterial meningitis. A nurse should include which recommendation in the nursing plan?

1. Take vital signs every 4 hours.
2. Monitor temperature every 4 hours.
3. Decrease environmental stimulation.
4. Encourage the parents to hold the child.

16. 3. A child with the diagnosis of meningitis is much more comfortable with decreased environmental stimuli. Noise and bright lights stimulate the child and can be irritating, causing the child to cry, in turn increasing intracranial pressure. Vital signs would be taken initially every hour and temperature monitored every two hours. Children are usually much more comfortable if allowed to lie flat because this position doesn't cause increased meningeal irritation.

CN: Physiological integrity; CNS: Physiological adaptation; CL: Application

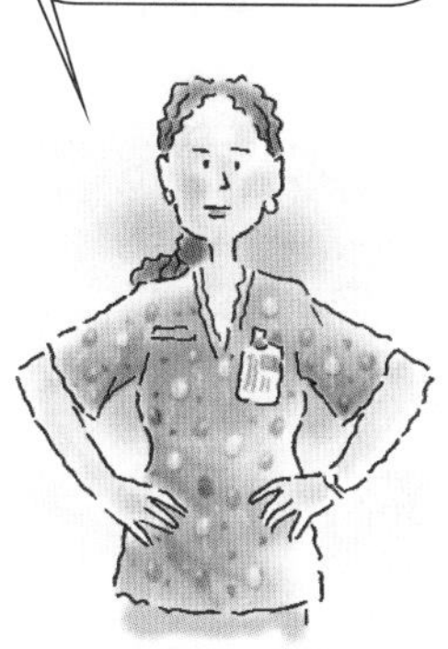

The important word in the question is first!

17. A child has just returned to the pediatric unit following ventriculoperitoneal shunt placement for hydrocephalus. Which intervention should a nurse perform first?

1. Assess intake and output.
2. Place the child on the side opposite the shunt.
3. Offer fluids because the child has a dry mouth.
4. Administer pain medication by mouth as ordered.

17. 2. Following shunt placement surgery, the child should be placed on the side opposite of the surgical site to prevent pressure on the shunt valve. Intake and output will be assessed, but that isn't the priority nursing intervention. The child is usually on nothing-by-mouth status until the nasogastric tube is removed and bowel sounds return. Pain medication should be administered by an I.V. route initially postoperatively.

CN: Physiological integrity; CNS: Basic care and comfort; CL: Application

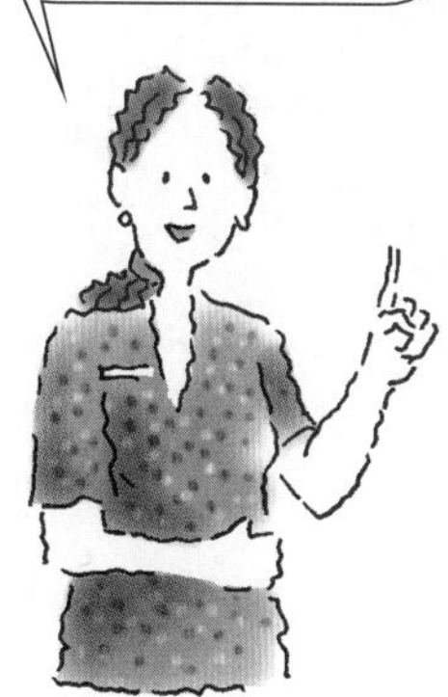

18. An otherwise healthy 18-month-old child has a history of febrile seizures and is in the well-child clinic today. Which statement by the father would indicate to the nurse that additional teaching needs to be done?

1. "I have ibuprofen available in case it's needed."
2. "My child will outgrow these seizures by age 5."
3. "I always keep phenobarbital with me in case of a fever."
4. "The most likely time for a seizure is when the fever is rising."

18. 3. Anticonvulsant drugs, such as phenobarbital, are administered to children with prolonged seizures or neurologic abnormalities. Ibuprofen, not phenobarbital, is given for fever. Febrile seizures usually occur after age 6 months and are unusual after age 5 years. Treatment is to decrease the temperature because seizures occur as the temperature rises.

CN: Health promotion and maintenance; CNS: None; CL: Application

19. When assessing a 5-month-old infant, which symptom should alert a nurse that the infant needs further follow-up?

1. Absent grasp reflex
2. Rolls from back to side
3. Balances head when sitting
4. Moro's embrace reflex present

19. 4. Moro's embrace reflex should be absent at 4 months. Grasp reflex begins to fade at 2 months and should be absent at 3 months. A 4-month-old infant should be able to roll from back to side and balance his head when sitting.

CN: Health promotion and maintenance; CNS: None; CL: Application

20. An adolescent is started on valproic acid (Depakene) to treat seizures. Which statement should be included when educating the adolescent?

1. This medication has no adverse effects.
2. A common adverse effect is weight gain.
3. Drowsiness and irritability commonly occur.
4. Early morning dosing is recommended to decrease insomnia.

20. 2. Weight gain is a common adverse effect of valproic acid. Drowsiness and irritability are adverse effects more commonly associated with phenobarbital. Felbamate (Felbatol) more commonly causes insomnia.

CN: Physiological integrity; CNS: Pharmacological and parenteral therapies; CL: Application

21. Which statement about cerebral palsy is accurate?

1. Cerebral palsy is a condition that runs in families.
2. Cerebral palsy means there will be many disabilities.
3. Cerebral palsy is a condition that doesn't get worse.
4. Cerebral palsy occurs because of too much oxygen to the brain.

21. 3. By definition, cerebral palsy is a nonprogressive neuromuscular disorder. It can be mild or quite severe and is believed to be the result of a hypoxia event during the pregnancy or the birth process.

CN: Physiological integrity; CNS: Physiological adaptation; CL: Application

22. An older child has a craniotomy for removal of a brain tumor. Which statement would be appropriate for a nurse to say to the parents?

1. "Your child really had a close call."
2. "I'm sure your child will be back to normal soon."
3. "I'm so glad to hear your child doesn't have cancer."
4. "What has the physician told you about the tumor?"

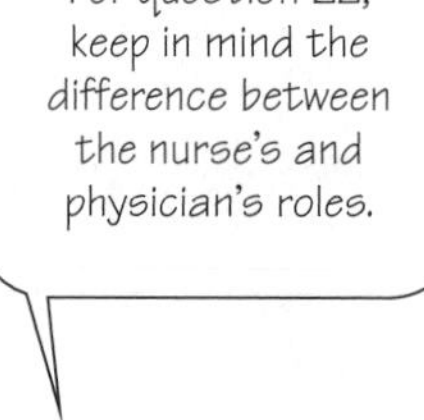

For question 22, keep in mind the difference between the nurse's and physician's roles.

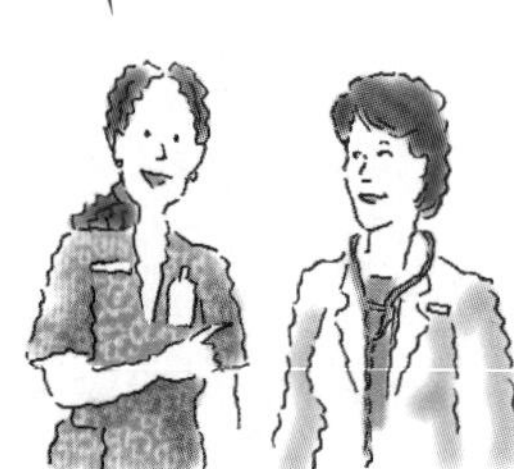

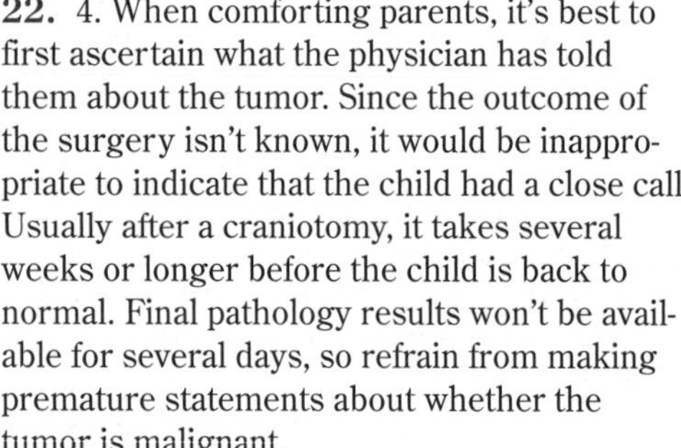

22. 4. When comforting parents, it's best to first ascertain what the physician has told them about the tumor. Since the outcome of the surgery isn't known, it would be inappropriate to indicate that the child had a close call. Usually after a craniotomy, it takes several weeks or longer before the child is back to normal. Final pathology results won't be available for several days, so refrain from making premature statements about whether the tumor is malignant.

CN: Psychosocial integrity; CNS: None; CL: Application

23. A 6-month-old infant is being admitted with a diagnosis of bacterial meningitis. A nurse should place the infant in which room?

1. A room with a 12-month-old infant with urinary tract infection
2. A room with an 8-month-old infant with failure to thrive
3. An isolation room near the nurses' station
4. A two-bed room in the middle of the hall

23. 3. A child who has the diagnosis of bacterial meningitis will need to be placed in isolation near the nurses' station until that child has received I.V. antibiotics for 24 hours. The child is considered contagious. Additionally, bacterial meningitis can be quite serious; therefore, the child should be placed near the nurse's station for close monitoring and easier access in case of a crisis.

CN: Safe, effective care environment; CNS: Safety and infection control; CL: Application

24. In caring for a 9-year-old child immediately after a head injury, a nurse notes a blood pressure of 110/60, a heart rate of 78, dilated and nonreactive pupils, minimal response to pain, and slow response to name. Which symptom should cause the nurse the most concern?

1. Vital signs
2. Nonreactive pupils
3. Slow response to name
4. Minimal response to pain

24. 2. Dilated and nonreactive pupils indicate that anoxia or ischemia of the brain has occurred. If the pupils are also fixed (don't move), then herniation of the brain stem has occurred. The vital signs are normal. Slow response to name can be normal after a head injury. Minimal response to pain is an indication of the child's level of consciousness.

CN: Physiological integrity; CNS: Physiological adaptation; CL: Application

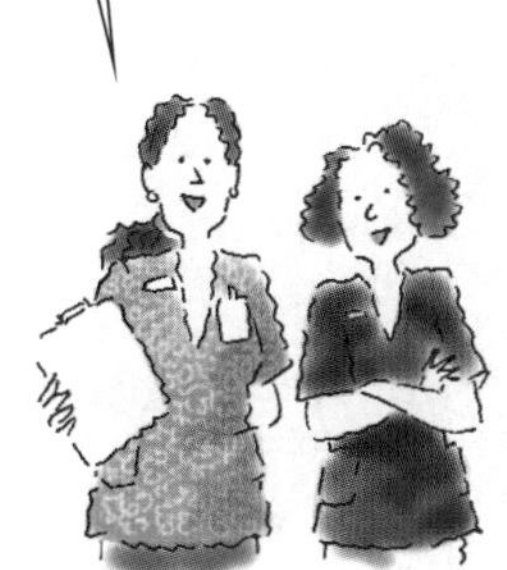

The ability to delegate responsibly is often tested on the NCLEX.

25. Which assignment made by a charge nurse would be appropriate?

1. A registered nurse (RN) to an infant newly diagnosed with bacterial meningitis
2. A student nurse to an adolescent with cystic fibrosis and many medications
3. A licensed practical nurse (LPN) or a licensed vocational nurse (LVN) to a newly admitted child with acute leukemia, receiving blood
4. A nursing assistant to a transfer client with a head injury and frequent seizures

25. 1. An RN would be appropriately assigned to care for an infant with meningitis. The RN would make frequent assessments and provide a high level of care. Student nurses may not be allowed to give medications without supervision and it may be easier for the RN or LPN to provide care to this client. In many institutions, LPNs (or LVNs) aren't allowed to monitor clients receiving blood or blood products. A transfer client with a head injury would need frequent assessments that only an RN or an LPN would be able to provide.

CN: Safe, effective care environment; CNS: Management of care; CL: Application

26. An infant has returned to the pediatric unit after repair of a myelomeningocele. A nurse notices that the infant has had no urine output in the past 2 hours. Which nursing intervention would be most appropriate?

1. Perform Credé's maneuver on the infant's bladder.
2. Catheterize the infant's bladder.
3. Ask the mother to breast-feed the infant.
4. Increase the I.V. fluid rate.

26. 2. Swelling around the surgical site may cause transient urinary retention and catheterization is required to empty the bladder. Credé's maneuver isn't recommended because it can cause renal rupture. Breast-feeding the infant would be inappropriate in this situation. The fluid rate wouldn't be increased because there's no indication that the infant is dehydrated.

CN: Physiological integrity; CNS: Reduction of risk potential; CL: Application

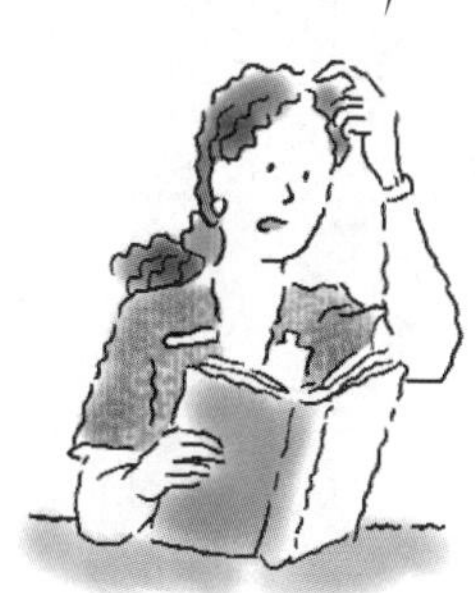

Is this mother doing the correct thing or not?

27. A 2-month-old infant who had an L4-L5 myelomeningocele repair comes to the clinic for a well-baby checkup. The mother reports that she catheterizes the infant every 2 to 3 hours. Which aspect of care should a nurse discuss with the mother?

1. Changing to a special diet
2. Scheduled immunizations
3. Normal gross motor function
4. Possibility of developing a latex allergy

27. 4. Children who are exposed repeatedly to latex products, such as during bladder catheterizations, are at high risk for developing a latex allergy. There's no need for a special diet unless another problem indicates that it would be necessary. This infant would receive the regularly scheduled immunizations. Gross motor function will be abnormal in an infant with an L4-L5 repair.

CN: Health promotion and maintenance; CNS: None; CL: Application

28. Which intervention prevents a 17-month-old child with spastic cerebral palsy from going into a scissoring position?

1. Keep the child in leg braces 23 hours per day.
2. Let the child lay down as much as possible.
3. Try to keep the child as quiet as possible.
4. Place the child on your hip.

28. 4. To interrupt the scissoring position, flex the knees and hips. Placing the child on the hip is an easy way to stop this common spastic positioning. Wearing leg braces 23 hours per day is inappropriate and doesn't allow the child to move freely. Trying to keep the child quiet and flat are inappropriate. This child needs stimulation and movement to reach the goal of development to the fullest potential.

CN: Physiological integrity; CNS: Basic care and comfort; CL: Application

29. The mother of a child with a ventriculoperitoneal shunt says her child has a temperature of 101.2° F (38.4° C), a blood pressure of 108/68 mm Hg, and a pulse of 100. The child is lethargic and vomited the night before. Other children in the family have had similar symptoms. Which nursing intervention is most appropriate?

1. Provide symptomatic treatment.
2. Advise the mother this is a viral infection.
3. Consult the primary health care provider.
4. Have the mother bring the child to the primary health care provider's office.

29. 4. One of the complications of a ventriculoperitoneal shunt is a shunt infection. Shunt infections can have similar symptoms as a viral infection, so it's best to have the child examined. These symptoms may be due to the same viral infection that the siblings have, but it's better to have the child examined to rule out a shunt infection because infection can progress quickly to a very serious illness.

CN: Physiological integrity; CNS: Reduction of risk potential; CL: Application

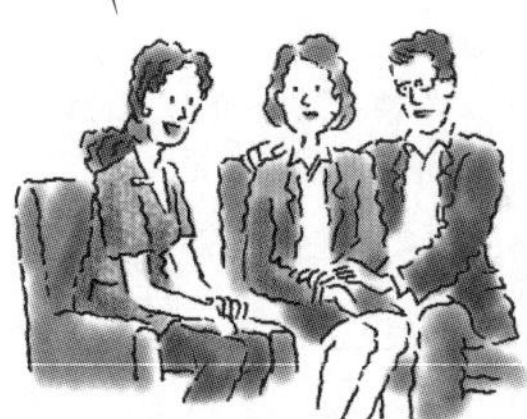

Make sure both parents understand the rationale for treatment of a sick child.

30. The mother of a 10-year-old child with attention deficit hyperactivity disorder says her husband won't allow their child to take more than 5 mg of methylphenidate (Ritalin) every morning. The child isn't doing better in school. Which recommendation should a nurse make to the mother?

1. Sneak the medication to the child anyway.
2. Put the child in charge of administering the medication.
3. Bring the child's father to the clinic to discuss the medication.
4. Have the school nurse give the child the rest of the medication.

30. 3. Bringing the father to the clinic for a teaching session about the medication should assist him in understanding why it's necessary for the child to receive the full dose. A nurse shouldn't advise dishonesty to a client or family. The father should be included in the treatment as much as possible.

CN: Physiological integrity; CNS: Pharmacological and parenteral therapies; CL: Application

31. A hospitalized child is to receive 75 mg of acetaminophen (Tylenol) for fever control. How much will the nurse administer if the acetaminophen is 40 mg per 0.4 ml?

1. 0.37 ml
2. 0.75 ml
3. 1.12 ml
4. 1.5 ml

31. 2. The nurse will administer 0.75 ml. Because 10 mg equals 0.1 ml, then 75 mg equals 0.75 ml.

CN: Physiological integrity; CNS: Pharmacological and parenteral therapies; CL: Application

32. The nurse is preparing a toddler for a lumbar puncture. For this procedure, the nurse should place the child in which position?

1. Lying prone, with the neck flexed
2. Sitting up, with the back straight
3. Lying on one side, with the back curved
4. Lying prone, with the feet higher than the head

32. 3. Lumbar puncture involves placing a needle between the lumbar vertebrae into the subarachnoid space. For this procedure, the nurse should position the client on one side, with the back curved, because curving the back maximizes the space between the lumbar vertebrae, facilitating needle insertion. Prone and seated positions don't achieve separation of the vertebrae.

CN: Physiological integrity; CNS: Reduction of risk potential; CL: Application

33. When caring for a school-age child who has had a brain tumor removed, a nurse makes the following assessment: pupils equal and reactive to light; motor strength equal; knows name, date, but not location; and complains of a headache. Which nursing intervention would be most appropriate?

1. Provide medication for the headache.
2. Immediately notify the primary health care provider.
3. Check what the child's level of consciousness (LOC) has been.
4. Call the child's parents to come and sit at the child's bedside.

33. 3. When there's an abnormality in current assessment data, it's vital to determine what the client's previous status was. Determine whether the status has changed or remained the same. Providing medication for the headache would be done after ascertaining the previous LOC. Contacting the primary health care provider and the child's parents isn't necessary before a final assessment has been made.

CN: Physiological integrity; CNS: Physiological adaptation; CL: Application

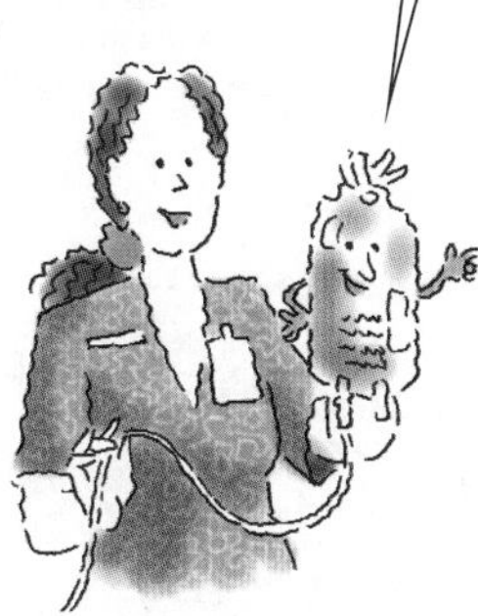

I'm happy to accommodate any drip rate that is needed.

34. Following a craniotomy on a child, I.V. fluids are ordered to run at 27 ml/hour. The tubing delivers 60 ml/hour. How many drops per minute should the nurse set the pump for?

1. 14 drops/minute
2. 27 drops/minute
3. 54 drops/minute
4. 60 drops/minute

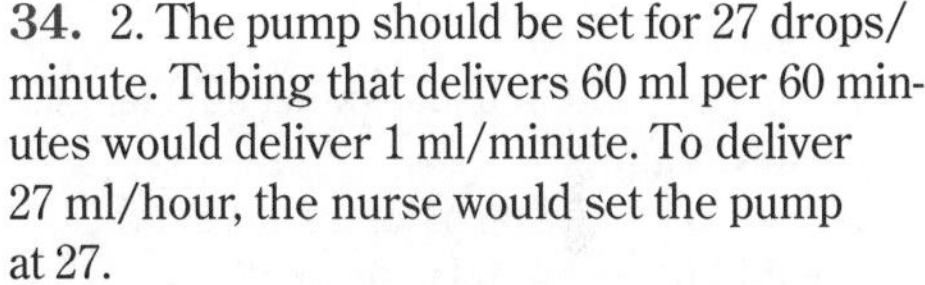

34. 2. The pump should be set for 27 drops/minute. Tubing that delivers 60 ml per 60 minutes would deliver 1 ml/minute. To deliver 27 ml/hour, the nurse would set the pump at 27.

CN: Physiological integrity; CNS: Pharmacological and parenteral therapies; CL: Application

35. The parents of a 19-month-old child bring their toddler to the clinic for a regular checkup. When palpating the toddler's fontanels, what should the nurse expect to find?

1. Closed anterior fontanel and open posterior fontanel
2. Open anterior fontanel and closed posterior fontanel
3. Closed anterior and posterior fontanels
4. Open anterior and posterior fontanels

35. 3. By age 18 months, the anterior and posterior fontanels should be closed. The diamond-shaped anterior fontanel normally closes between ages 9 and 18 months. The triangular posterior fontanel normally closes between ages 2 and 3 months.

CN: Health promotion and maintenance; CNS: None; CL: Application

36. A 10-year-old child with a concussion is admitted to the pediatric unit. A nurse should place this child in a room with which roommate?

1. A 6-year-old child with osteomyelitis
2. An 8-year-old child with gastroenteritis
3. A 10-year-old child with rheumatic fever
4. A 12-year-old child with a fractured femur

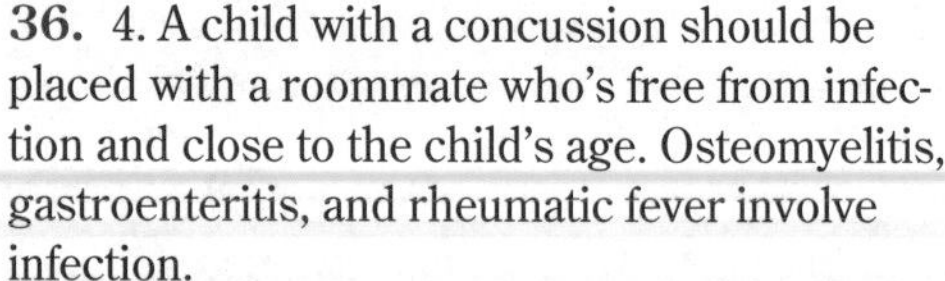

36. 4. A child with a concussion should be placed with a roommate who's free from infection and close to the child's age. Osteomyelitis, gastroenteritis, and rheumatic fever involve infection.

CN: Safe, effective care environment; CNS: Management of care; CL: Application

37. A nurse notes that a 4-year-old child with cerebral palsy has a weight at the 30th percentile and a height at the 60th percentile. Which requirement should a nurse advise the family about the child?

1. He should eat fewer calories per day.
2. His height and weight are within the normal range.
3. He needs to increase his number of calories per day.
4. He is small for a 4-year-old child and will never be average.

37. 2. The height and weight are between the 25th and 75th percentile, so the child is considered normal.

CN: Health promotion and maintenance; CNS: None; CL: Application

38. After a pathogen compromises the blood-brain and blood-cerebrospinal fluid (CSF) barriers, infection will spread to the meninges for which reason?

1. The spinal fluid has a rich erythrocyte content.
2. Glucose content of the spinal fluid is relatively high.
3. There's a build-up of infectious exudate within the ventricular system.
4. CSF is devoid of the body's major defense systems.

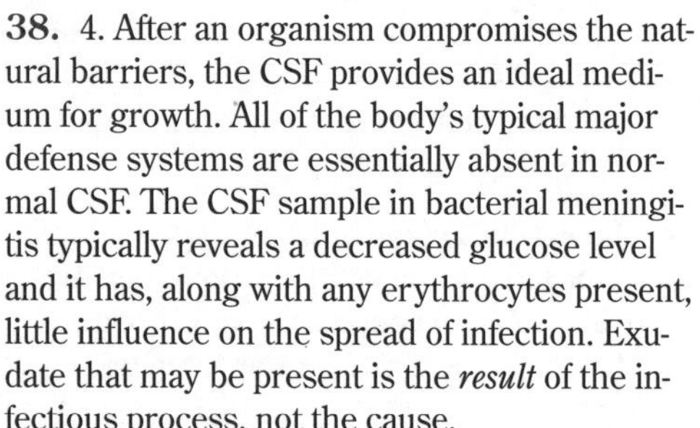

38. 4. After an organism compromises the natural barriers, the CSF provides an ideal medium for growth. All of the body's typical major defense systems are essentially absent in normal CSF. The CSF sample in bacterial meningitis typically reveals a decreased glucose level and it has, along with any erythrocytes present, little influence on the spread of infection. Exudate that may be present is the ***result*** of the infectious process, not the cause.

CN: Physiological integrity; CNS: Physiological adaptation; CL: Analysis

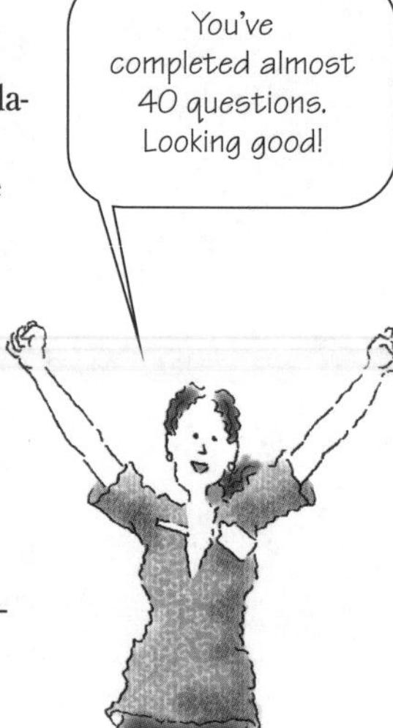

You've completed almost 40 questions. Looking good!

39. Which mechanism causes the severe headache that accompanies an increase in intracranial pressure (ICP)?

1. Cervical hyperextension
2. Stretching of the meninges
3. Cerebral ischemia related to altered circulation
4. Reflex spasm of the neck extensors to splint the neck against cervical flexion

39. 2. The mechanism producing the headache that accompanies increased ICP may be the stretching of the meninges and pain fibers associated with blood vessels. With nuchal rigidity, cervical flexion is painful due to the stretching of the inflamed meninges, and the pain triggers a reflex spasm of the neck extensors to splint the area against further cervical flexion. It occurs in response to the pain; it doesn't cause it. Cerebral ischemia occurs because of vascular obstruction and decreased perfusion of the brain tissue.

CN: Physiological integrity; CNS: Physiological adaptation; CL: Analysis

40. While assessing the breath sounds of a child admitted with fever, seizures, and vomiting, the nurse notes petechiae on the child's back. What is the most appropriate initial action by the nurse?

1. Cover the petechiae with dry sterile dressings.
2. Initiate seizure precautions.
3. Suspect that the child has been abused.
4. Assess the child's neurologic status.

40. 4. Since fever, seizures, vomiting, and petechiae are signs of meningitis, the nurse should promptly assess the child's neurologic status and report the findings to the physician. Petechiae are tiny purple or red spots within the dermal or submucosal layers of the skin and do not require dry sterile dressings nor are they signs of abuse. While the nurse should already have initiated seizure precautions, the finding of petechiae wouldn't be a reason to initiate seizure precautions.

CN: Physiological integrity; CNS: Physiological adaptation; CL: Analysis

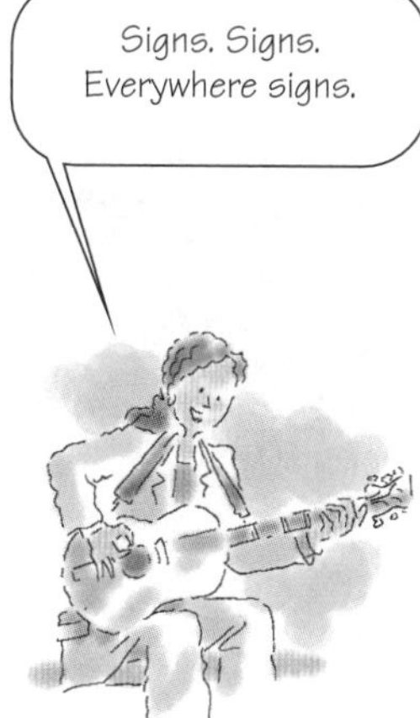
Signs. Signs. Everywhere signs.

41. A nurse is assessing a 3-year-old child with suspected nuchal rigidity. Which assessment data indicates nuchal rigidity?

1. Positive Kernig's sign
2. Negative Brudzinski's sign
3. Positive Homans' sign
4. Negative Kernig's sign

41. 1. A positive Kernig's sign indicates nuchal rigidity, caused by an irritative lesion of the subarachnoid space. Brudzinski's sign is also indicative of the condition. Homans' sign indicates venous inflammation of the lower leg, not nuchal rigidity.

CN: Physiological integrity; CNS: Physiological adaptation; CL: Application

42. A nurse is caring for a child with spina bifida. The child's mother asks the nurse what she did to cause the birth defect. Which statement would be the nurse's <u>best</u> response?

1. "Older age at conception is one of the major causes of the defect."
2. "It's a common complication of amniocentesis."
3. "It has been linked to maternal alcohol consumption during pregnancy."
4. "The cause is unknown and there are many environmental factors that may contribute to it."

42. 4. There is no known cause of spina bifida, but scientists believe that it's linked to hereditary and environmental factors; neural tube defects, including spina bifida, have been strongly linked to low dietary intake of folic acid. Maternal age doesn't have an impact on spina bifida. An amniocentesis is performed to help diagnose spina bifida in utero but doesn't cause the disorder. Maternal alcohol intake during pregnancy has been linked to mental retardation, craniofacial defects, and cardiac abnormalities, not spina bifida.

CN: Physiological integrity; CNS: Physiological adaptation; CL: Application

Check these signs carefully. They're critical for answering question 43.

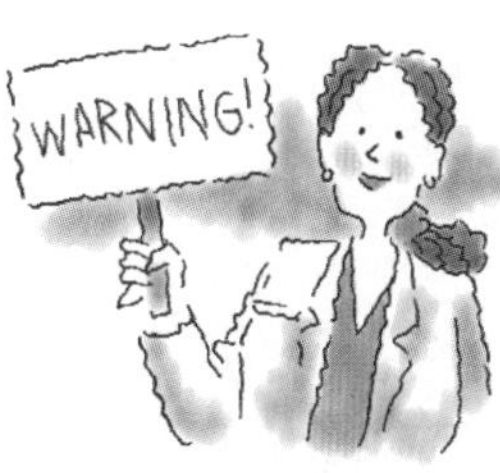
WARNING!

43. A child with a diagnosis of meningococcal meningitis develops signs of sepsis and a purpuric rash over both lower extremities. The primary health care provider should be notified immediately because these signs could be indicative of which complication?

1. A severe allergic reaction to the antibiotic regimen with impending anaphylaxis
2. Onset of the syndrome of inappropriate antidiuretic hormone (SIADH)
3. Fulminant (Waterhouse–Friderichsen syndrome) meningococcemia
4. Adhesive arachnoiditis

43. 3. Meningococcemia is a serious complication usually associated with meningococcal infection. When onset is severe, sudden, and rapid (fulminant), it's known as Waterhouse–Friderichsen syndrome. Anaphylactic shock would need to be differentiated from septic shock. SIADH can be an acute complication, but it wouldn't be accompanied by the purpuric rash. Adhesive arachnoiditis occurs in the chronic phase of the disease and leads to obstruction of the flow of cerebrospinal fluid.

CN: Physiological integrity; CNS: Reduction of risk potential; CL: Application

44. A 1-month-old infant is admitted to the pediatric unit and diagnosed with bacterial meningitis. Which assessment findings by the nurse support the diagnosis?

1. Hemorrhagic rash, first appearing as petechiae
2. Photophobia
3. Fever, change in feeding pattern, vomiting, or diarrhea
4. Fever, lethargy, and purpura or large necrotic patches

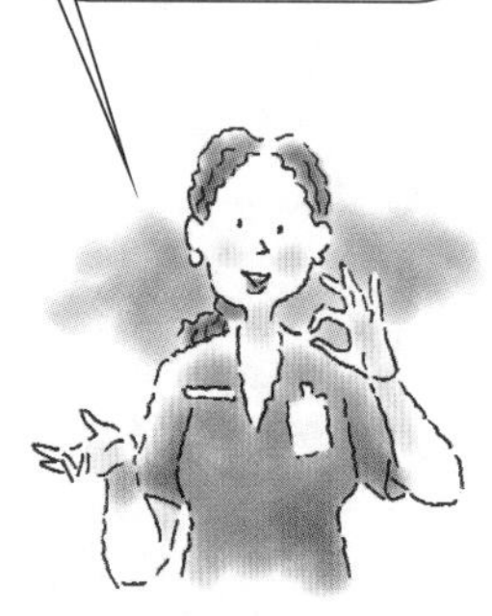

I see you've finished 44 questions. Super! Are you at least having "a little bit" of fun?

44. 3. Fever, change in feeding patterns, vomiting, and diarrhea are commonly observed in children with bacterial meningitis. Hemorrhagic rashes, petechiae, photophobia, fever, lethargy, and purpura are common manifestations in older children with meningitis.

CN: Physiological integrity; CNS: Physiological adaptation; CL: Application

45. To alleviate the child's pain and fear of lumbar puncture, which intervention should a nurse perform?

1. Sedate the child with fentanyl (Sublimaze).
2. Apply a topical anesthetic to the skin 5 to 10 minutes prepuncture.
3. Have a parent hold the child in their lap during the tap procedure.
4. Have the child inhale small amounts of nitrous oxide gas prepuncture.

45. 1. Sedation with fentanyl or other drugs can alleviate the pain and fear associated with a lumbar puncture. A topical anesthetic can be applied, but it should be done 1 hour before the procedure to be fully effective. Parents holding a child in their lap increases the risk of neurologic injury due to the inability to assume and maintain the proper anatomic position required for a safe lumbar puncture. Use of nitrous oxide gas isn't recommended.

CN: Physiological integrity; CNS: Basic care and comfort; CL: Application

46. Antimicrobial therapy to treat meningitis should be instituted <u>immediately after</u> which event?

1. Admission to the nursing unit
2. Initiation of I.V. therapy
3. Identification of the causative organism
4. Collection of cerebrospinal fluid (CSF) and blood for culture

46. 4. Antibiotics are always begun immediately after the collection of CSF and blood cultures. Admission and initiation of I.V. therapy aren't, by themselves, appropriate times to begin antimicrobial therapy. After the specific organism is identified, bacteria-specific antibiotics can be administered if the organism isn't covered by the initial choice of antibiotic therapy.

CN: Physiological integrity; CNS: Pharmacological and parenteral therapies; CL: Analysis

47. A nurse is teaching the parents of a child diagnosed with meningitis about the child's medications. Which statement by the nurse is the most accurate with respect to the use of steroid therapy (dexamethasone) in conjunction with antimicrobial therapy?

1. "It's the treatment of choice in aseptic meningitis."
2. "It's used for the prevention of GI hemorrhage."
3. "It's used for the management of problems related to blood pressure."
4. "It's used for the prevention of deafness with *Haemophilus influenzae* meningitis."

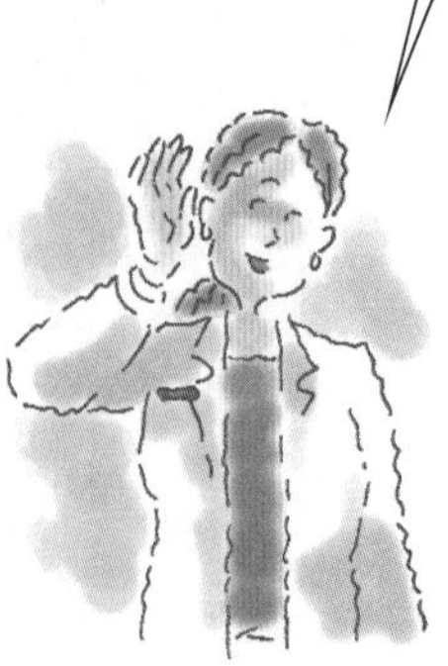

If you listen carefully, you can almost hear the answer to this question.

47. 4. Dexamethasone may play a role in the prevention of bilateral deafness in children with *H. influenzae* type b meningitis, and its use is recommended by the American Academy of Pediatrics. Treatment of aseptic meningitis is primarily symptomatic with acetaminophen for headache and muscle pain and positioning for comfort. Use of dexamethasone could complicate rather than prevent GI bleeding and problems related to blood pressure.

CN: Physiological integrity; CNS: Pharmacological and parenteral therapies; CL: Application

CN: Client needs category CNS: Client needs subcategory CL: Cognitive level

48. Which description is accurate about the incidence of sequelae in a client with bacterial meningitis?
1. Occur during the first 2 months of life
2. Occur in children with meningococcal meningitis
3. Primarily involve the fourth ventricle of the brain
4. Tend to affect the ocular nerves, leading to retinal damage

48. 1. In infants younger than age 2 months with bacterial meningitis, communicating hydrocephalus and the effects of cerebritis on the immature brain leads to the frequent occurrence of sequelae. Sequelae are least commonly seen in children experiencing meningococcal meningitis. Meningitis primarily affects the nerves for hearing rather than vision.
CN: Physiological integrity; CNS: Physiological adaptation; CL: Application

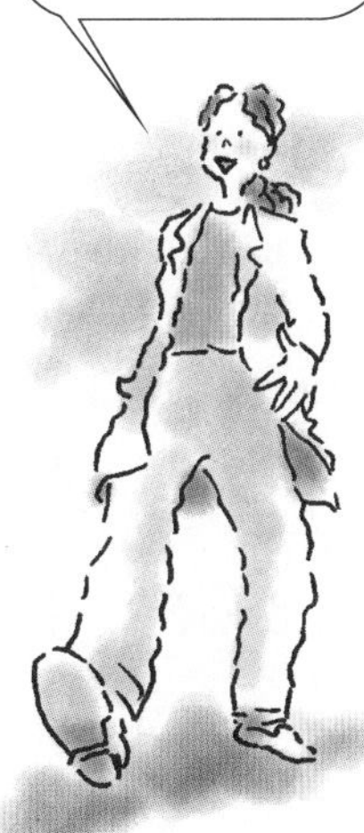

49. Which goal of nursing care is the most difficult to accomplish in caring for a child with meningitis?
1. Protecting self and others from possible infection
2. Avoiding actions that increase discomfort such as lifting the head
3. Keeping environmental stimuli to a minimum such as reduced light and noise
4. Maintaining I.V. infusion to administer adequate antimicrobial therapy

49. 4. One of the most difficult problems in the nursing care of children with meningitis is maintaining the I.V. infusion for the length of time needed to provide adequate therapy. All of the other options are important aspects in the provision of care to the child with meningitis, but they're secondary to antimicrobial therapy.
CN: Physiological integrity; CNS: Basic care and comfort; CL: Application

50. Which nursing assessment data should be given the <u>highest priority</u> for a child with clinical findings related to tubercular meningitis?
1. Onset and character of fever
2. Degree and extent of nuchal rigidity
3. Signs of increased intracranial pressure (ICP)
4. Occurrence of urine and fecal incontinence

50. 3. Assessment of fever and evaluation of nuchal rigidity are important aspects of care, but assessment for signs of increasing ICP should be the highest priority due to the life-threatening implications. Urinary and fecal incontinence can occur in a child who's ill from nearly any cause but don't pose a great danger to life.
CN: Physiological integrity; CNS: Reduction of risk potential; CL: Analysis

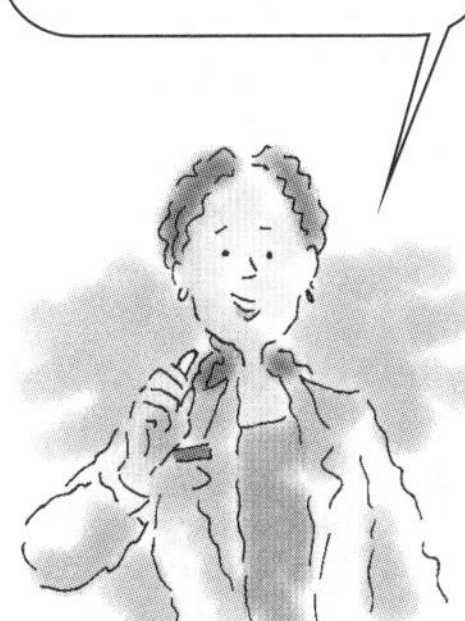

All of the choices in question 50 may be correct. So you need to prioritize.

51. The clinical manifestations of acute bacterial meningitis are dependent on which factor?
1. Age of the child
2. Length of the prodromal period
3. Time span from bacterial invasion to onset of symptoms
4. Degree of elevation of cerebrospinal fluid (CSF) glucose compared to serum glucose level

51. 1. Clinical manifestations of acute bacterial meningitis depend largely on the age of the child. Clinical manifestations aren't dependent on the prodromal or initial period of the disease nor the time from invasion of the host to the onset of the symptoms. The glucose level of the CSF is reduced, not elevated. A serum glucose level is drawn one-half hour before lumbar puncture so that the relationship between the CSF glucose and the serum glucose levels can be determined.
CN: Physiological integrity; CNS: Physiological adaptation; CL: Application

52. The mother of a child with a history of closed head injury asks the nurse why her son would begin having seizures without warning. Which response by the nurse is the most accurate?

1. "Clonic seizure activity is usually interpreted as falling."
2. "It's not unusual to develop seizures after a head injury because of brain trauma."
3. "Focal discharge in the brain may lead to absence seizures that go unnoticed."
4. "The epileptogenic focus in the brain needs multiple stimuli because it will discharge to cause a seizure."

52. 2. Stimuli from an earlier injury may eventually elicit seizure activity, a process known as kindling. Atonic seizures, not clonic, are frequently accompanied by falling. Focal seizures are partial seizures; absence seizures are generalized seizures. Focal seizures don't lead to absence seizures. The epileptogenic focus consists of a group of hyperexcitable neurons responsible for initiating synchronous, high-frequency discharges leading to a seizure rather than needing multiple stimuli.

CN: Physiological integrity; CNS: Physiological adaptation; CL: Application

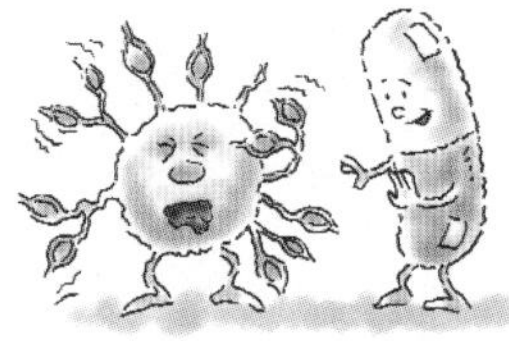

I'm sorry! I didn't mean to steal your thunder.

53. A student nurse asks the nurse how anticonvulsant drugs work. Which statement by the nurse would be the most accurate?

1. Suppression of sodium influx through the gated pores in the cell membrane
2. Enhancement of calcium influx through the gated pores in the cell membrane
3. Potentiation of dopamine, facilitating passage across the neuronal cell membrane
4. Suppression of potassium removal from the neuronal intracellular compartment

53. 1. Anticonvulsant drugs, such as phenytoin (Dilantin), suppress the influx of sodium, thereby decreasing the ability of the neurons to fire. Some anticonvulsant drugs, such as valproate sodium (Depakene) used for absence seizures, suppress the influx of calcium. The role of potassium and dopamine in the generation of seizure activity hasn't been identified.

CN: Physiological integrity; CNS: Pharmacological and parenteral therapies; CL: Application

54. During the trial period to determine the efficacy of an anticonvulsant drug, which caution should be explained to the parents?

1. Plasma levels of the drug will be monitored on a daily basis.
2. Drug dosage will be adjusted depending on the frequency of seizure activity.
3. The drug must be discontinued immediately if even the slightest problem occurs.
4. The child shouldn't participate in activities that could be hazardous if a seizure occurs.

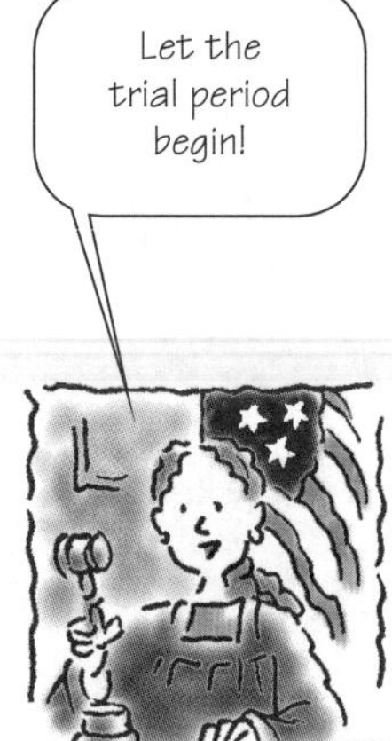

Let the trial period begin!

54. 4. Until seizure control is certain, clients shouldn't participate in activities (such as riding a bicycle) that could be hazardous if a seizure were to occur. Plasma levels need to be monitored periodically over the course of drug therapy; daily monitoring isn't necessary. Dosage changes are usually based on plasma drug levels as well as seizure control. Anticonvulsant drugs should be withdrawn over a period of 6 weeks to several months, never immediately, as this could precipitate status epilepticus.

CN: Physiological integrity; CNS: Pharmacological and parenteral therapies; CL: Analysis

55. Which nursing action should be included in the care plan to promote comfort in a 4-year-old child hospitalized with meningitis?

1. Avoid making noise when in the child's room.
2. Rock the child frequently.
3. Have the child's 2-year-old brother stay in the room.
4. Keep the lights on brightly so that he can see his mother.

55. 1. Meningeal irritation may cause seizures and heightens a child's sensitivity to all stimuli, including noise, lights, movement, and touch. Frequent rocking, presence of a younger sibling, and bright lights would increase stimulation.

CN: Physiological integrity; CNS: Basic care and comfort; CL: Application

CN: Client needs category CNS: Client needs subcategory CL: Cognitive level

56. The parents of a child with a history of seizures who has been taking phenytoin (Dilantin) ask the nurse why it's difficult to maintain therapeutic levels of this medication. Which statement by the nurse would be the most accurate?

1. "A drop in the plasma drug level will lead to a toxic state."
2. "The capacity to metabolize the drug becomes overwhelmed in time."
3. "Small increments in dosage lead to sharp increases in plasma drug levels."
4. "Large increases in dosage lead to more rapid stabilizing therapeutic effect."

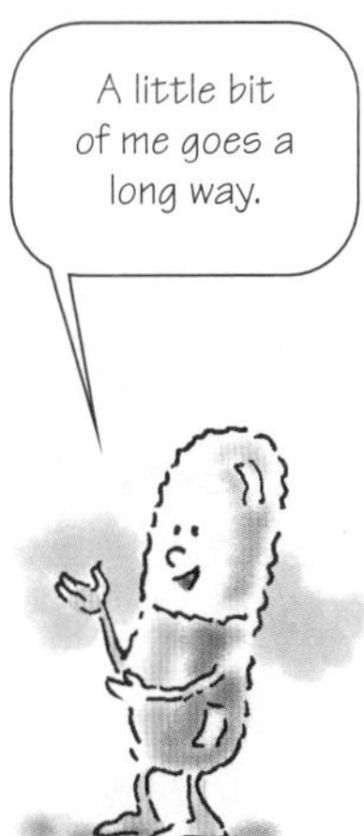

A little bit of me goes a long way.

57. Client teaching should stress which rule in relation to the differences in bioavailability of different forms of phenytoin?

1. Use the cheapest formulation the pharmacy has on hand at the time of refill.
2. Shop around to get the least expensive formulation.
3. There's no difference in one formulation from another, regardless of price.
4. Avoid switching formulations without the primary health care provider's approval.

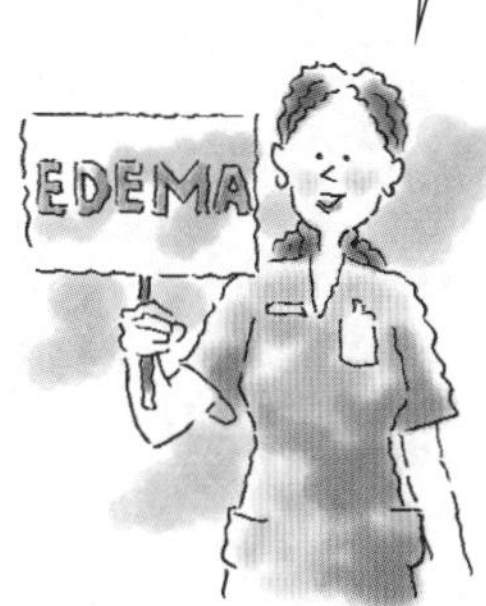

I'll give you this one... just because you've worked so hard.
EDEMA

58. To detect complications as early as possible in a child with meningitis who's receiving I.V. fluids, monitoring for which condition should be the nurse's *priority*?

1. Cerebral edema
2. Renal failure
3. Left-sided heart failure
4. Cardiogenic shock

59. Which instruction should be included in client teaching specifically related to anticonvulsant drug efficacy?

1. Wear a medical identification bracelet.
2. Maintain a seizure frequency chart.
3. Avoid potentially hazardous activities.
4. Discontinue the drug immediately if adverse effects are suspected.

56. 3. Within the therapeutic range for phenytoin, small increments in dosage produce sharp increases in plasma drug levels. The capacity of the liver to metabolize phenytoin is affected by slight changes in the dosage of the drug, not necessarily the length of time the client has been taking the drug. Large increments in dosage will greatly increase plasma levels leading to drug toxicity.

CN: Physiological integrity; CNS: Pharmacological and parenteral therapies; CL: Application

57. 4. Differences in bioavailability exist among different formulations (tablets and capsules) and among the same formulations produced by different manufacturers. Clients shouldn't switch from one formulation to another or from one brand to another without primary health care provider approval and supervision.

CN: Physiological integrity; CNS: Pharmacological and parenteral therapies; CL: Application

58. 1. Because the child with meningitis is already at increased risk of cerebral edema and increased intracranial pressure due to inflammation of the meningeal membranes, the nurse should monitor fluid intake and output to avoid fluid volume overload. Renal failure and cardiogenic shock aren't complications of I.V. therapy. The child with a healthy heart wouldn't be expected to develop left-sided heart failure.

CN: Physiological integrity; CNS: Pharmacological and parenteral therapies; CL: Application

59. 2. Ongoing evaluation of the therapeutic effects can be accomplished by maintaining a seizure frequency chart that indicates the date, time, and nature of all seizure activity. These data may be helpful in making dosage alterations and specific drug selection. Avoidance of hazardous activities and wearing a medical identification bracelet are ways to minimize danger related to seizure activity, but these factors don't affect drug efficacy. Anticonvulsant drugs should never be discontinued abruptly due to the potential for the development of status epilepticus.

CN: Physiological integrity; CNS: Pharmacological and parenteral therapies; CL: Application

60. I.V. administration of phenytoin would be contraindicated if which condition was identified in the preadmission assessment?
1. Episodic nosebleeds
2. History of Stokes-Adams syndrome
3. History of bone marrow depression
4. Attention deficit hyperactivity disorder (ADHD)

60. 2. I.V. administration of phenytoin can lead to arrhythmia and hypotension and is contraindicated in a history of sinus bradycardia, sinoatrial block, second- or third-degree heart block, or Stokes-Adams syndrome. Phenytoin would be administered cautiously in clients with episodic nosebleeds or bone marrow depression due to its adverse effects of leukopenia, anemia, and thrombocytopenia. Phenytoin has no known effect on ADHD but can interfere with cognitive function in excessive doses.

CN: Physiological integrity; CNS: Pharmacological and parenteral therapies; CL: Analysis

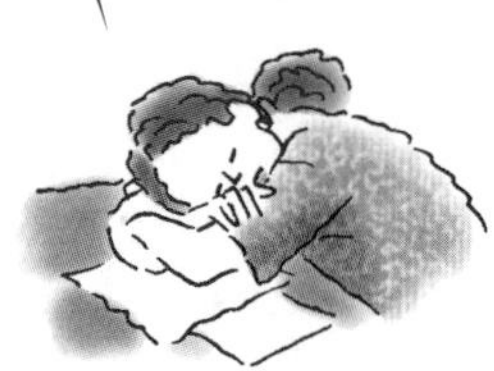

You should be able to answer this question with your eyes closed.

61. The parents of a child newly diagnosed with seizures ask the nurse at what time is seizure activity most likely to occur. Which response by the nurse would be the most accurate?
1. During the rapid eye movement (REM) stage of sleep
2. During long periods of excitement
3. While falling asleep and on awakening
4. While eating, particularly if the client is hurried

61. 3. Falling asleep or awakening from sleep are periods of functional instability of the brain; seizure activity is more likely to occur during these times. Eating quickly, excitement without undue fatigue, and REM sleep haven't been identified as contributing factors.

CN: Physiological integrity; CNS: Physiological adaptation; CL: Application

62. When educating the family of a child with seizures, it's appropriate to tell them to call emergency medical services in the event of a seizure if which complication occurs?
1. Continuous vomiting for 30 minutes after the seizure
2. Stereotypic or automatous body movements during the onset
3. Lack of expression, pallor, or flushing of the face during the seizure
4. Unilateral or bilateral posturing of one or more extremities during the onset

62. 1. Continuous vomiting after a seizure has ended can be a sign of an acute problem and indicates that the child requires an immediate medical evaluation. All of the other manifestations are normally present in various types of seizure activity and don't indicate a need for immediate medical evaluation.

CN: Physiological integrity; CNS: Reduction of risk potential; CL: Analysis

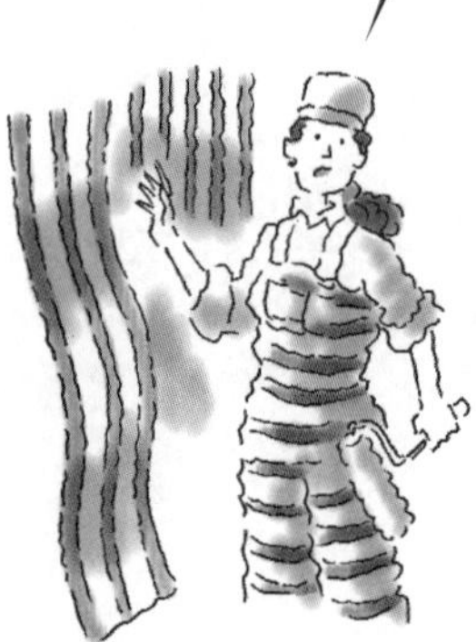

I'm afraid no one will like this pattern or am I being too sensitive?

63. Identifying factors that trigger seizure activity could lead to which alteration in the child's environment or activities of daily living?
1. Avoiding striped wallpaper and ceiling fans
2. Having the child sleep alone to prevent sleep interruption
3. Including extended periods of intense physical activity daily
4. Allowing the child to drink soda only between noon and 5 p.m.

63. 1. Striped wallpaper, ceiling fans, and blinking lights on a Christmas tree can all be triggers to seizure activity if the child is photosensitive. Sleep interruption hasn't been identified as a triggering factor. Avoidance of fatigue can reduce seizure activity; therefore, intense physical activity for extended periods should be avoided. Restricting caffeine intake by using caffeine-free soda is a dietary modification that may prevent seizures.

CN: Physiological integrity; CNS: Physiological adaptation; CL: Application

64. Which nursing intervention should be included to support the goal of avoiding injury, respiratory distress, or aspiration during a seizure?

1. Positioning the child with the head hyperextended
2. Placing a hand under the child's head for support
3. Using pillows to prop the child into the sitting position
4. Working a padded tongue blade or small plastic airway between the teeth

64. 2. Placing a hand or a small cushion or blanket under the child's head will help prevent injury. Position the child with the head in midline, not hyperextended, to promote a good airway and adequate ventilation. Don't attempt to prop the child up into a sitting position, but ease him to the floor to prevent falling and unnecessary injury. Don't put *anything* in the child's mouth because it could cause infection or obstruct the airway.

CN: Physiological integrity; CNS: Reduction of risk potential; CL: Application

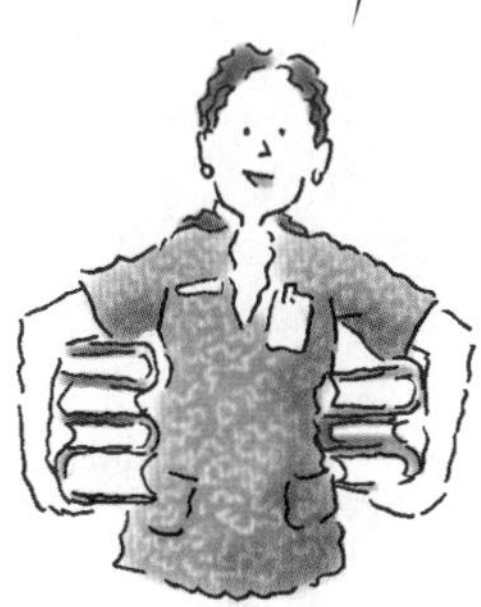
Hang on!
You've reached
question 65!

65. Which diagnostic measure is the most accurate in detecting neural tube defects?

1. Flat plate of the lower abdomen after the 23rd week of gestation
2. Significant level of alpha-fetoprotein present in the amniotic fluid
3. Amniocentesis for lecithin-sphingomyelin (L/S) ratio
4. Presence of high maternal levels of albumin after 12th week of gestation

65. 2. Significant levels of alpha-fetoprotein have been effective in detecting neural tube defects. Prenatal screening includes a combination of maternal serum and amniotic fluid levels, amniocentesis, amniography, and ultrasonography and has been relatively successful in diagnosing the defect. Flat plate X-rays of the abdomen, L/S ratio, and maternal serum albumin levels aren't diagnostic for the defect.

CN: Health promotion and maintenance; CNS: None; CL: Application

66. A nurse is teaching the parents of a child who has been diagnosed with spina bifida. Which statement by the nurse would be the most accurate description of spina bifida?

1. "It has little influence on the intellectual and perceptual abilities of the child."
2. "It's a simple neurologic defect that's completely corrected surgically within 1 to 2 days after birth."
3. "Its presence predisposes that many areas of the central nervous system (CNS) may not develop or function adequately."
4. "It's a complex neurologic disability that involves a collaborative health care team effort for the entire first year of life."

66. 3. When a spinal cord lesion exists at birth, it commonly leads to altered development or function of other areas of the CNS. Spina bifida is a complex neurologic defect that heavily impacts the physical, cognitive, and psychosocial development of the child and involves a collaborative, life-long management due to the chronicity and multiplicity of the problems involved.

CN: Physiological integrity; CNS: Physiological adaptation; CL: Application

67. Common deformities occurring in the child with spina bifida are related to the muscles of the lower extremities that are active or inactive. These may include which complication?

1. Club feet
2. Hip extension
3. Ankylosis of the knee
4. Abduction and external rotation of the hip

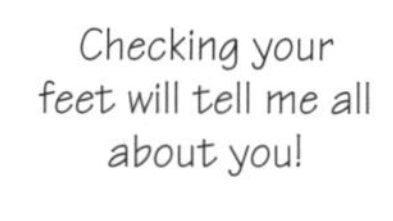
Checking your
feet will tell me all
about you!

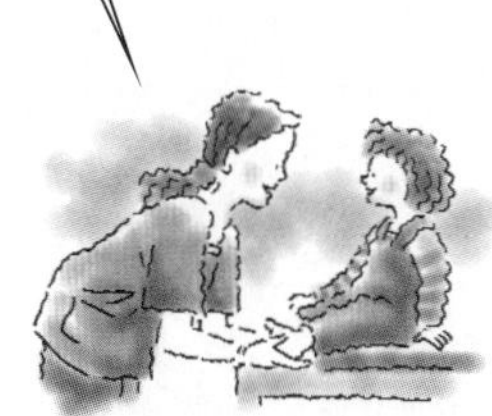

67. 1. The type and extent of deformity in the lower extremities depends on the muscles that are active or inactive. Passive positioning *in utero* may result in deformities of the feet such as equinovarus (club foot), knee flexion and extension contractures, hip flexion with adduction and internal rotation leading to subluxation or dislocation of the hip.

CN: Physiological integrity; CNS: Physiological adaptation; CL: Analysis

68. What's the nurse's priority when caring for a 10-month-old infant with meningitis?

1. Maintaining an adequate airway
2. Maintaining fluid and electrolyte balance
3. Controlling seizures
4. Controlling hyperthermia

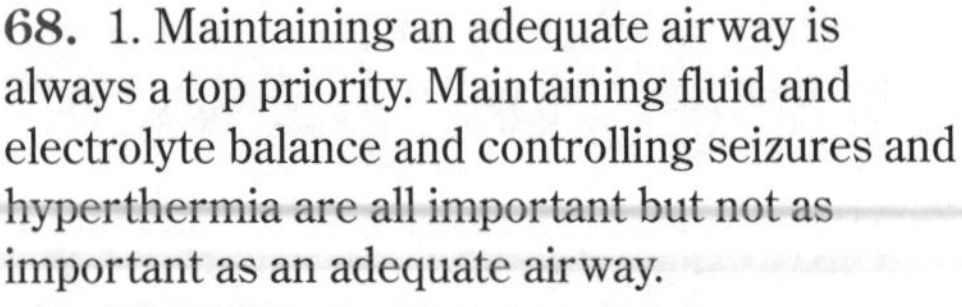

68. 1. Maintaining an adequate airway is always a top priority. Maintaining fluid and electrolyte balance and controlling seizures and hyperthermia are all important but not as important as an adequate airway.

CN: Physiological integrity; CNS: Reduction of risk potential; CL: Application

69. The nurse is caring for an infant with myelomeningocele and notices a change in the assessment which may indicate the infant has a chiari II malformation. Which change was noted in the assessment?

1. Rapidly progressing scoliosis
2. Changes in urologic functioning
3. Back pain below the site of the sac closure
4. Respiratory stridor

69. 4. Children with a myelomeningocele have a 90% chance of having a Chiari II malformation. This may lead to a possibility of respiratory function problems, such as respiratory stridor associated with paralysis of the vocal cords, apneic episodes of unknown cause, difficulty swallowing, and an abnormal gag reflex. Urologic function changes and scoliosis occur with myelomeningocele, but these complications aren't specifically related to Chiari II malformation. Lower back pain doesn't occur due to the loss of sensory function related to the cord defect.

CN: Physiological integrity; CNS: Reduction of risk potential; CL: Analysis

70. A child with myelomeningocele and hydrocephalus may demonstrate problems related to damage of the white matter caused by ventricular enlargement. This damage may manifest itself in which condition?

1. Inability to speak
2. Early hand dominance
3. Impaired intellectual functions
4. Flaccid paralysis of the lower extremities

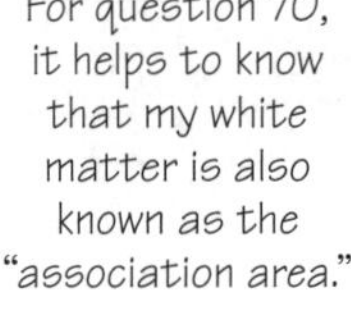

For question 70, it helps to know that my white matter is also known as the "association area."

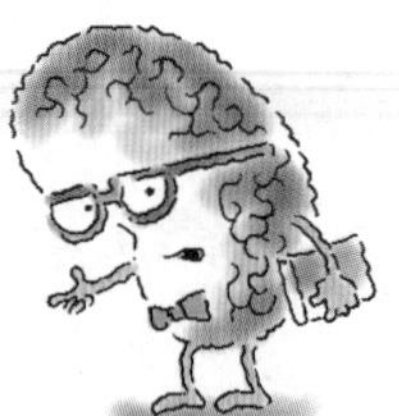

70. 3. Damage to the white matter (association area) caused by ventricular enlargement has been linked to impairment of intellectual and perceptual abilities often seen in children with spina bifida. It hasn't been related to hand dominance development, flaccid paralysis of the lower extremities, or the ability to speak, though it may affect the semantics of speech dependent upon the association areas.

CN: Physiological integrity; CNS: Physiological adaptation; CL: Analysis

71. The parents of a child newly diagnosed with myelomeningocele ask the nurse why surgical repair needs to be done immediately. Which response would be the most accurate?

1. "It's done for rapid restoration of the neural pathways to the legs."
2. "It's done to decrease the possibility of infection and further cord damage."
3. "It's done to expose the spinal cord defect to individualize the therapeutic strategy."
4. "It's done for removal of excess nerve tissue from the vertebral canal to decrease pressure on the cord."

71. 2. The myelomeningocele sac presents a dynamic disability and is treated as a life-threatening situation with sac closure taking place within the first 24 to 48 hours after birth. This early management decreases the possibility of infection and further injury to the exposed neural cord. There's complete loss of nervous function below the level of the spinal cord lesion. The aim of surgery is to replace the nerve tissue into the vertebral canal, cover the spinal defect, and achieve a watertight sac closure.

CN: Physiological integrity; CNS: Reduction of risk potential; CL: Application

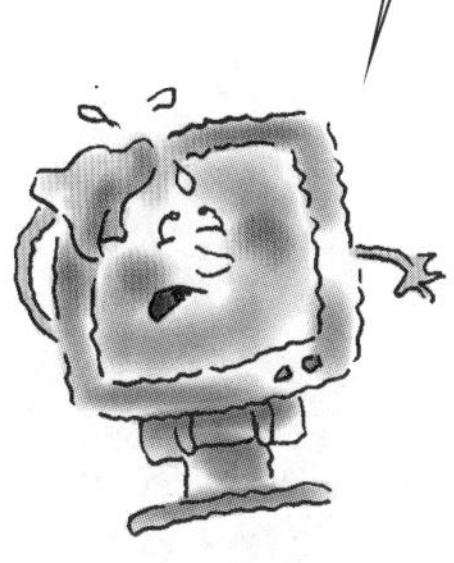

Don't sweat it! Just choose the most appropriate response.

72. One of the most important aspects of preoperative care with myelomeningocele is the positioning of the infant. Which position is the most appropriate?

1. Prone position with head turned to the side for feeding
2. Side-lying position with the head at a 30-degree angle to the feet
3. Prone position with a nasogastric (NG) tube inserted for feedings
4. Supported by diaper rolls, both anterior and posterior, in the side-lying position

72. 1. Prone position is used preoperatively because it minimizes tension on the sac and the risk of trauma. The head is turned to one side for feeding. There's no advantage to positioning the body with a 30-degree head elevation. Although feeding can be a problem in the prone position, it can be accomplished without the need for an NG tube. Side-lying or partial side-lying positions are better used *after* the repair has been accomplished unless it permits undesirable hip flexion.

CN: Physiological integrity; CNS: Reduction of risk potential; CL: Application

73. Large body areas of sensory and motor impairment associated with myelomeningocele necessitate which nursing intervention?

1. Gentle stretching of contractures
2. Vigorous active range-of-motion exercises
3. Frequent turning side-to-side and prone-to-supine
4. Keeping skin dry and avoiding the use of emollients and lubricants

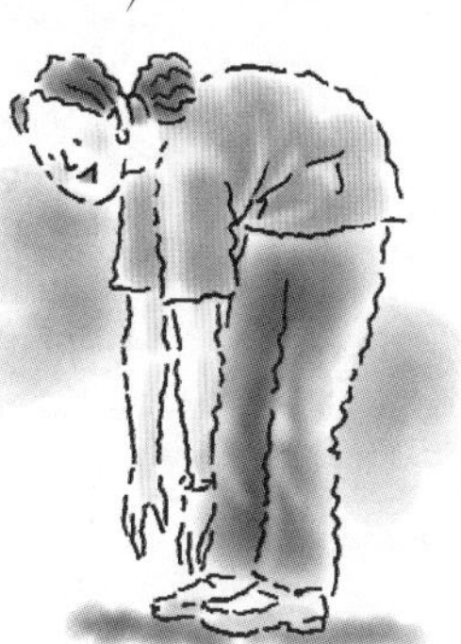

Sometimes it helps to stretch.

73. 1. Areas of sensory and motor impairment require meticulous care, including gentle range-of-motion exercises to prevent contractures as well as stretching of contractures when indicated. Vigorous exercise is avoided in contrast to the gentle range of motion that is recommended. Frequent turning is indicated in order to maintain skin integrity, but the supine position shouldn't be used to avoid pressure on the surgical site. Skin should be kept clean and dry, but lubrication can be used to facilitate massage, which increases circulation to the areas involved.

CN: Physiological integrity; CNS: Basic care and comfort; CL: Application

74. Children with spina bifida are at high risk for developing intraoperative anaphylaxis linked to an allergic response to latex. Which risk factor leads to this allergic response?

1. Weakened immune response
2. Need for life-long steroid therapy
3. Need for numerous bladder catheterizations
4. Use of large amounts of adhesive tape to attach sac dressings

74. 3. Children with spina bifida are at high risk for developing a latex allergy because of repeated exposure to latex products during multiple surgeries and from numerous bladder catheterizations related to lack of bladder function. A weakened immune response wouldn't elicit an anaphylactic reaction due to the reduced functioning of the immune response. Steroid therapy isn't indicated in the management of spina bifida and also wouldn't support an anaphylactic reaction. Sac removal is accomplished as quickly as possible after birth, and the sac usually isn't covered with any type of dressing because it may contribute to trauma to the sac.

CN: Physiological integrity; CNS: Reduction of risk potential; CL: Application

Taking folic acid before conception reduces certain risks in infants.

75. Which explanation about how to avoid the incidence of a second child with spina bifida is most accurate?

1. There's no known way to avoid it; adoption is recommended.
2. A previous pregnancy affected by a neural tube defect isn't a factor.
3. Prepregnancy intake of 4 mg of folic acid daily reduces the recurrence rate.
4. Aerobic exercise in the first trimester to decrease the chances of a positive alpha-fetoprotein (AFP).

75. 3. Studies have shown that women at high risk for having an infant with a neural tube defect, demonstrated by a previously delivered infant or fetus with spina bifida, significantly reduced the recurrence rate by taking supplements of folic acid before conception. The chances of having a second affected child are low (between 1% and 2%), but still greater than the chances of the general population. Aerobic exercise won't decrease the chances of a positive AFP.

CN: Health promotion and maintenance; CNS: None; CL: Analysis

76. A school-age child with a diagnosis of epilepsy is admitted to the pediatric unit of a local hospital for evaluation of his anticonvulsant medications. As a nurse enters the child's room, the child begins to have a seizure. Which nursing action should the nurse do <u>first</u>?

1. Push the call bell and ask for help.
2. Hold the child down so he doesn't injure himself.
3. Loosen any restrictive clothing.
4. Force the jaw open to maintain an open airway.

76. 3. The primary nursing goal during a seizure is to protect the client from physical injury and maintain a patent airway. Loosening clothing will allow free movement and aid in keeping the airway open. After making sure the client is safe from injury, the nurse should push the call bell only if further assistance is needed. The nurse should never forcibly hold a client down and shouldn't force the jaw open; the jaw could be injured or break.

CN: Physiological integrity; CNS: Reduction of risk potential; CL: Application

77. When planning care for a 9-year-old boy with Down syndrome, which statement should a nurse keep in mind?

1. Nursing interventions should be planned at a 9-year-old developmental level.
2. Nursing interventions should be planned at a 7-year-old developmental level.
3. The nurse should assess the child's developmental level before planning interventions.
4. The developmental level of the child is not important in planning care.

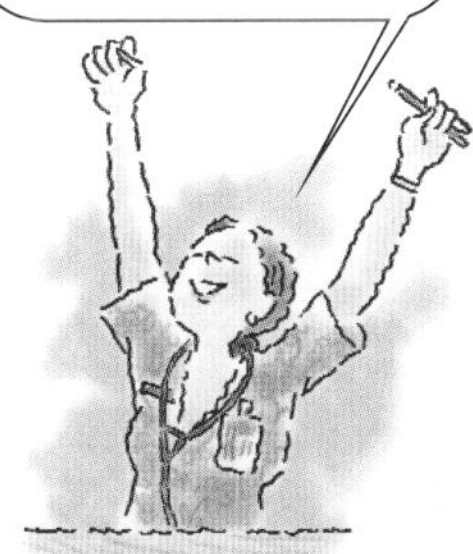

You're almost there and you've done a great job.

77. 3. Before developing a care plan, the nurse should assess the child's developmental level and plan care at that level. The nurse shouldn't plan care geared towards the child's chronological age without first assessing the child. The nurse also shouldn't assume that the child is at a lower developmental level without assessing the child. The child's developmental age is important in planning age-appropriate care and teaching.

CN: Health promotion and maintenance; CNS: None; CL: Application

78. A 6-year-old child is unconscious with a head injury from a bicycle accident. A nurse is assessing him for increased intracranial pressure (ICP). His baseline vital signs are respirations 20 breaths/minute; blood pressure 100/56 mm Hg; pulse 100 beats/minute. Which set of vital signs would indicate increased ICP?

1. Respirations 12 breaths/minute; blood pressure 90/45 mm Hg; pulse 80 beats/minute
2. Respirations 14 breaths/minute; blood pressure 130/40 mm Hg; pulse 70 beats/minute
3. Respirations 30 breaths/minute; blood pressure 80/45 mm Hg; pulse 130 beats/minute
4. Respirations 14 breaths/minute; blood pressure 70/58 mm Hg; pulse 102 beats/minute

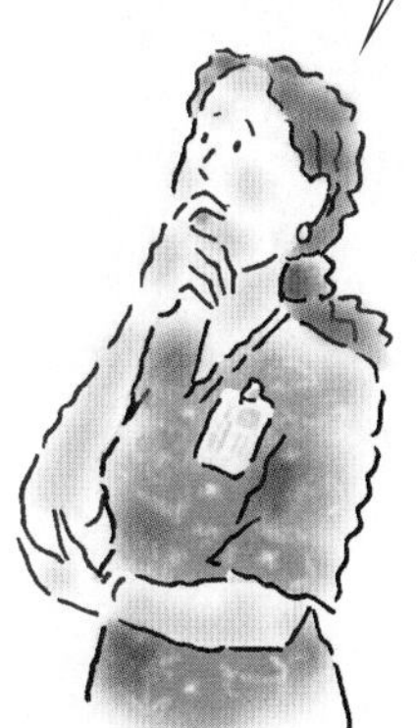

78. 2. Classic signs of increased ICP are a decrease in respirations, an increase in blood pressure, and a decrease in pulse rate. Option 1 may indicate normal vital signs. Options 3 and 4 may indicate shock.

CN: Physiological integrity; CNS: Physiological adaptation; CL: Analysis

79. When assessing an infant for changes in intracranial pressure (ICP), it's important to palpate the fontanels. Identify the area where a nurse should palpate to assess the anterior fontanel.

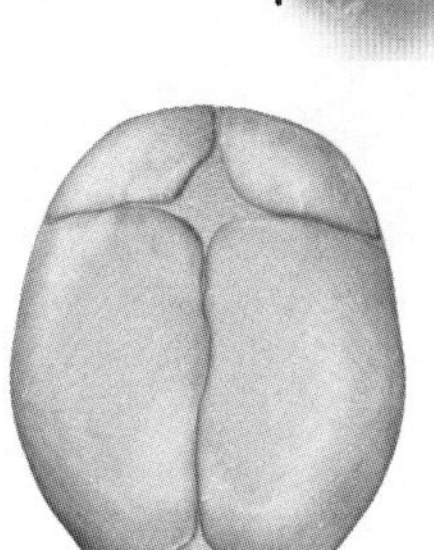

79. The anterior fontanel is formed by the junction of the sagittal, frontal, and coronal sutures. It's shaped like a diamond and normally measures 4 to 5 cm at its widest point. A widened, bulging fontanel is a sign of increased ICP.

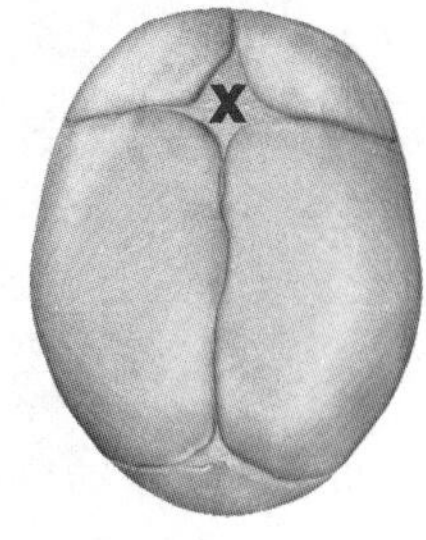

CN: Health promotion and maintenance; CNS: None; CL: Application

80. A nurse is preparing a dose of amoxicillin for a 3-year-old with acute otitis media. The child weighs 33 lb. The dosage prescribed is 50 mg/kg/day in divided doses every 8 hours. The concentration of the drug is 250 mg/5 ml. How many milliliters should the nurse administer? Record your answer using a whole number.

____________________ milliliters

81. A nurse is caring for a 3-year-old with viral meningitis. Which signs and symptoms should the nurse expect to find during the initial assessment? Select all that apply:

1. Bulging anterior fontanel
2. Fever
3. Nuchal rigidity
4. Petechiae
5. Irritability
6. Photophobia
7. Hypothermia

82. The nurse is assessing the primitive reflexes of a one-month-old infant. Which of the reflexes shown in the photos below should not be present after the age of 2 months?

1. 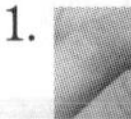 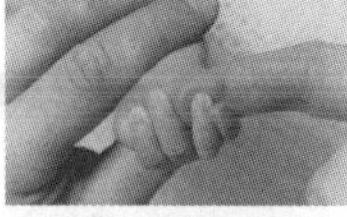
2. 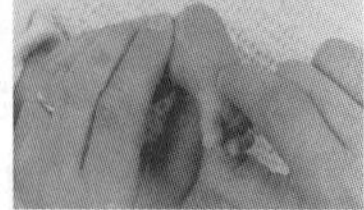
3. 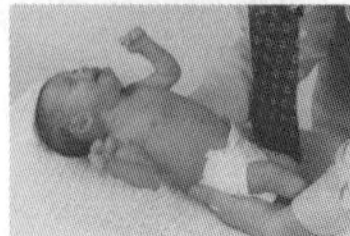
4. 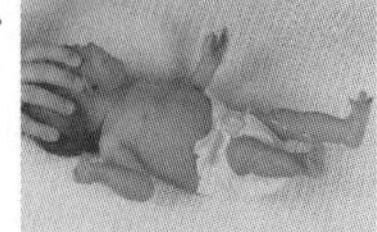

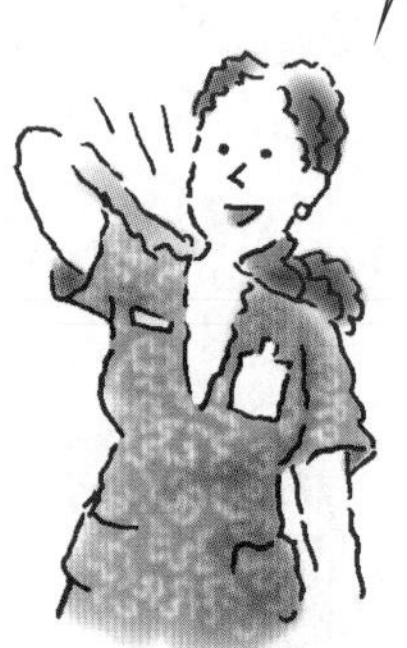

Congratulations! You finished! Give yourself a pat on the back.

80. 5. To calculate the child's weight in kilograms, the nurse should use the following formula: 1 kg/2.2 lb = X kg/33 lb; 2.2X = 33; X = 15 kg. Next, the nurse should calculate the daily dosage for the child: 50 mg/kg/day × 15 kg = 750 mg/day. To determine divided daily dosage, the nurse should know that "every 8 hours" means 3 times per day. So, she should perform the calculation in this way: Total daily dosage ÷ 3 times per day = divided daily dosage; 750 mg/day ÷ 3 = 250 mg. The drug's concentration is 250 mg/5 ml, so the nurse should administer 5 ml.

CN: Physiological integrity; CNS: Pharmacological and parenteral therapies; CL: Application

81. 2, 3, 5, 6. Common signs and symptoms of viral meningitis include fever, nuchal rigidity, irritability, and photophobia. A bulging anterior fontanel is a sign of hydrocephalus, which isn't likely to occur in a toddler because the anterior fontanel typically closes by age 18 months. A petechial, purpuric rash may be seen with bacterial meningitis. Hypothermia is a common sign of bacterial meningitis in an infant younger than age 3 months.

CN: Physiological integrity; CNS: Physiological adaptation; CL: Application

82. 4. Option 4 shows the tonic neck reflex. Persistence of this reflex beyond 2 months suggests asymmetric central nervous system development. Option 1 shows the palmer grasp reflex. This reflex disappears around age three to four months. Option 2 shows the plantar grasp reflex. This reflex disappears at age six to eight months. Option 3 shows the Moro reflex. This reflex disappears around age four months.

CN: Physiological integrity; CNS: Reduction of risk potential; CL: Analysis

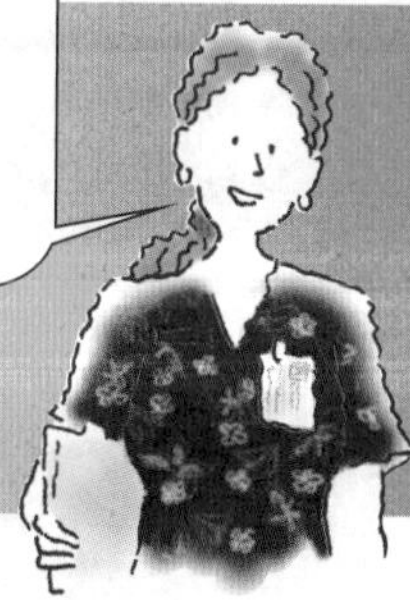

Challenge yourself with these sample questions on musculoskeletal system disorders in children. I'm betting you'll have a blast!

Chapter 31 Musculoskeletal disorders

1. A nurse is caring for a 10-year-old in Buck's traction for a fractured femur following a bicycle accident. Which intervention should the nurse do first when the child complains of increasing pain 1 hour after receiving an I.V. opioid analgesic?

1. Tell the child that he needs to give the analgesic time to work.
2. Perform a neurovascular assessment.
3. Make sure the weights are hanging freely.
4. Administer more analgesics.

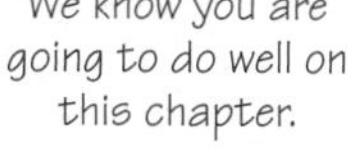

We know you are going to do well on this chapter.

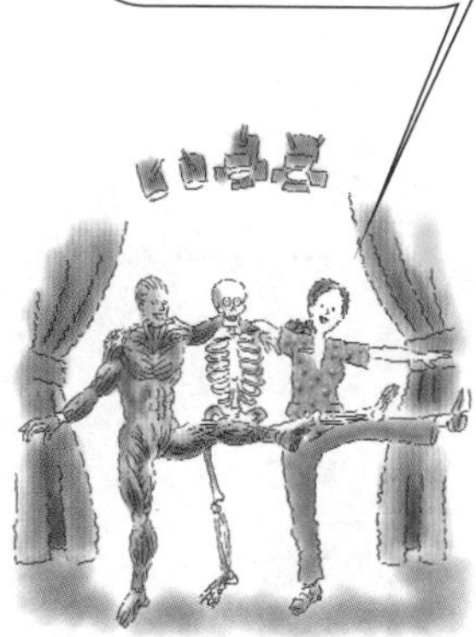

1. 2. Pain, unrelieved by analgesics, in a client with a dressing or cast may be a sign of compartment syndrome if pressure develops within the muscle and its surrounding structures due to the constrictive ace wrap dressing used in Buck's traction. The nurse should immediately perform a neurovascular assessment to detect signs of impaired circulation and nerve function. The findings should then immediately be reported to the physician and the pressure dressing loosened or removed. The child who has received an I.V. opioid should have had pain relief 1 hour after administration. While the weights in Buck's traction should hang freely, the child should be assessed first. More analgesics may be administered as ordered, but only after the neurovascular status is assessed.

CN: Physiological integrity; CNS: Reduction of risk potential; CL: Analysis

2. Which observation by a nurse indicates that an 18-month-old in Bryant's traction is properly positioned?

1. The hips are resting on the bed.
2. The hips are slightly elevated off the bed.
3. The hips are elevated above the level of the heart.
4. The hips are resting on a pillow.

2. 2. In Bryant's traction, the child's hips should be slightly elevated off the bed at a 15-degree angle. They shouldn't be resting on the bed or a pillow and shouldn't be elevated above the level of the heart.

CN: Physiological integrity; CNS: Basic care and comfort; CL: Application

3. A mother of a neonate with clubfoot feels guilty because she believes she did something to cause the condition. The nurse should explain that which factor causes clubfoot in neonates?

1. Unknown
2. Hereditary
3. Restricted movement in utero
4. Anomalous embryonic development

3. 1. The definitive cause of clubfoot is unknown. In some families, there's an increased incidence. Some postulate that anomalous embryonic development or restricted fetal movement are the reasons. Currently, there's no way to predict the occurrence of clubfoot.

CN: Psychosocial integrity; CNS: None; CL: Application

4. Which nursing diagnosis has the highest priority in a 6-year-old child who had a plaster cast applied 6 hours ago to the left leg for a fracture of the tibia?

1. *Deficient knowledge*
2. *Impaired physical mobility*
3. *Risk for peripheral neurovascular dysfunction*
4. *Dressing self-care deficit*

4. 3. The highest priority in a client with a newly applied cast is to assess for and prevent circulatory complications, which can lead to loss of function. The other nursing diagnoses are important for a client in a cast, but only after adequate circulation has been assured.
CN: Safe, effective care environment; CNS: Management of care; CL: Analysis

5. Which statement by the father of an 8-year-old boy with Duchenne's muscular dystrophy indicates that he has realistic expectations about the course of the disease?

1. "My son will gradually lose his ability to walk."
2. "Corticosteroids will help prevent muscle degeneration."
3. "Surgery will help my son walk."
4. "My son will have a normal lifespan."

5. 1. Duchenne's muscular dystrophy is a progressive muscular degenerative disorder in which children lose their ability to walk independently by age 12. Corticosteroids may slow muscle degeneration, but won't stop its progression. Surgery may be done to correct contractures but it doesn't change the course of the disease. Death occurs by early adulthood, usually from respiratory failure.
CN: Physiological integrity; CNS: Physiological adaptation; CL: Application

I've heard of muscle strengthening, but what's muscle lengthening?

6. A nurse is teaching the parents of a 3-month-old infant with severe torticollis who has presented with the head rotated to the left and the side bent to the right. Which statement by the parents about which muscle is shortened indicates that the teaching has been effective?

1. "It involves shortening of the left upper trapezius."
2. "It involves shortening of the right middle trapezius."
3. "It involves shortening of the left sternocleidomastoid."
4. "It involves shortening of the right sternocleidomastoid."

6. 4. The right sternocleidomastoid is shortened with the head in this position. The left upper trapezius isn't shortened; the right one is. The middle trapezius isn't affected, and the left sternocleidomastoid is in a lengthened position.
CN: Physiological integrity; CNS: Physiological adaptation; CL: Application

7. A 9-month-old infant has torticollis with rotation of the head to the left and side bending to the right. Placing the infant in which position would be most effective for developing muscle lengthening?

1. Prone
2. Supine
3. Left side-lying
4. Right side-lying

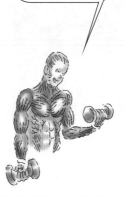

7. 3. The left side-lying position will help assist with lengthening of the muscles because this position will make it easier to stretch the sternocleidomastoid and upper trapezius. No other positions will assist in increasing muscle length.
CN: Physiological integrity; CNS: Reduction of risk potential; CL: Application

8. A nurse is teaching a 13-year-old girl diagnosed with scoliosis and her parents how to apply a Milwaukee brace. Which action should the nurse do first?
1. Refer them to a scoliosis support group.
2. Ask them to read the brochure that comes with the brace and then answer their questions.
3. Ask them what they already know about the brace and answer their questions.
4. Develop learning objectives and then explain them to the parents and teen.

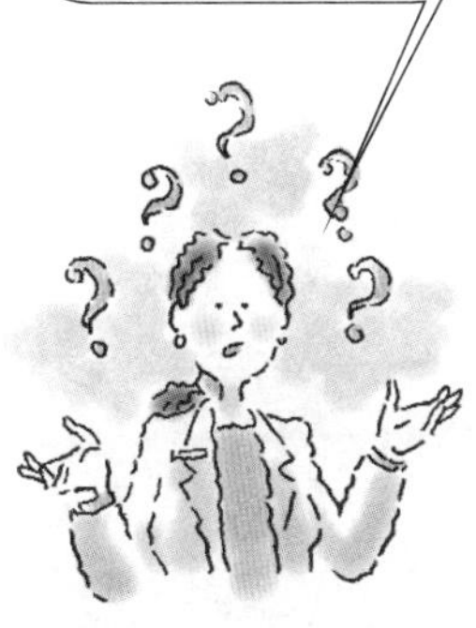

Does this mean
the brace was made
in Milwaukee?

8. 3. The first step in teaching this teen and her parents is to assess what they already know about the brace and answer their questions. This allows the nurse to clear up misconceptions and address their concerns. A support group is helpful but isn't the initial step the nurse should take. Written instructions should reinforce the teaching done by the nurse, not take the place of the nurse's teaching. Learning objectives should be developed with the teen and her parents.

CN: Health promotion and maintenance; CNS: None; CL: Application

9. A nurse is caring for a child who received a hip-spica cast 24 hours ago for hip dysplasia. Which nursing diagnoses should the nurse give the highest priority?
1. *Impaired gas exchange*
2. *Risk for peripheral neurovascular dysfunction*
3. *Risk for impaired skin integrity*
4. *Urinary retention*

9. 2. After cast application, a client is at risk for peripheral neurovascular dysfunction due to swelling within the confined space of the cast. Impaired gas exchange isn't a high risk since the cast was applied for hip dysplasia and not a fracture of a long bone, which would increase the risk of pulmonary embolism. Risk for impaired skin integrity and urinary retention is important, but neurovascular impairment is a higher priority.

CN: Safe, effective care environment; CNS: Management of care; CL: Analysis

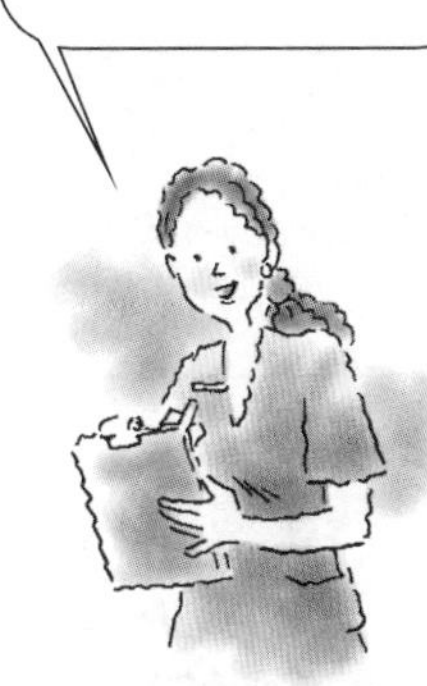

Congratulations!
You've finished the
first 10 questions!

10. Which intervention is appropriate for a child with a newly applied wet hip-spica cast?
1. Use the abductor bar to help move the child.
2. Cover the cast in plastic to keep it clean.
3. Reposition the child every 1 to 2 hours.
4. Use the fingertips when handling the cast.

10. 3. The child in a wet hip-spica cast should be turned every 1 to 2 hours to help dry all sides of the cast and prevent skin breakdown. The abductor bar shouldn't be used for turning the child, even with a dry cast. A wet cast shouldn't be covered with plastic because this impairs the drying of the cast. A wet cast should be handled using the palms because fingers may cause indentations and pressure points.

CN: Physiological integrity; CNS: Basic care and comfort; CL: Application

11. The parents of an infant born with clubfoot express feelings of guilt and anxiety about their child's condition. Which intervention should a nurse do first?
1. Teach them about their child's condition.
2. Introduce them to other parents whose children have the same condition.
3. Ask if they would like to speak with the chaplain.
4. Encourage discussion of their feelings.

11. 4. While all the options are appropriate interventions for the nurse to implement, the first step is to encourage the parents to verbalize their concerns and feelings about their child's condition. This helps alleviate anxiety and to develop a trusting therapeutic relationship.

CN: Physiological integrity; CNS: None; CL: Analysis

12. The Milwaukee brace is commonly used in the treatment of scoliosis. Which position best describes the placement of the pressure rods?
1. Laterally on convex portion of the curve
2. Laterally on concave portion of the curve
3. Posteriorly on convex portion of the curve
4. Posteriorly along the spinal column at the exact level of the curve

12. 1. Lateral pressure applied to the convex portion of the curve will help best in reducing the curvature. Pressure pads applied posteriorly will help maintain erect posture. Pressure applied to the concave portion of the curve will increase the lordosis.

CN: Physiological integrity; CNS: Reduction of risk potential; CL: Application

13. Strengthening of which muscle group is important in a client diagnosed with talipes equinovarus?

1. Evertors
2. Invertors
3. Plantar flexors
4. Plantar fascia musculature

13. 1. Because the foot is held in inversion, it's important to strengthen the evertors to counter the inversion present in the foot. Inversion is incorrect because the foot is already held in this position. Plantar musculature and plantar flexors aren't important because the foot is already in a plantar flexed position.

CN: Physiological integrity; CNS: Reduction of risk potential; CL: Analysis

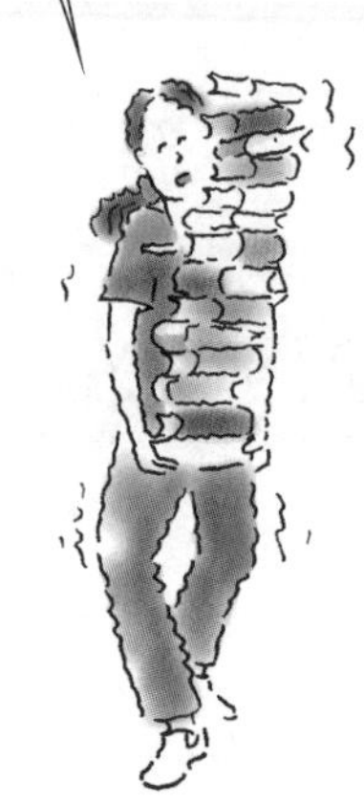

All this studying is strengthening my muscle groups. Oh, goody.

14. A nurse is caring for a 15-year-old who sustained a fracture of the femur 24 hours ago. Which finding should alert the nurse to an early complication?

1. Pain
2. Local swelling
3. Loss of function
4. Dyspnea

14. 4. After the fracture of a long bone, such as the femur, the client is at risk for fat embolism. Clinical manifestations include dyspnea, hypoxia, tachypnea, tachycardia, and chest pain. Pain, local swelling, and loss of function are all typical findings after a fracture.

CN: Physiological integrity; CNS: Reduction of risk potential; CL: Analysis

15. Which statement made by an adolescent girl with scoliosis indicates that she understands its treatment?

1. "I will have to wear a brace for several years."
2. "I can put on the brace after I get home from school."
3. "I should avoid any exercise that will stretch my spine."
4. "I can remove the brace at night."

15. 1. A brace worn to correct scoliosis must be worn for several years to correct the spinal deformity. The child must wear the brace all day, even during school and sleep. Exercises are commonly prescribed to be performed several times per day to stretch and strengthen back muscles. It should only be removed for 1 hour each day while bathing.

CN: Physiological integrity; CNS: Basic care and comfort; CL: Analysis

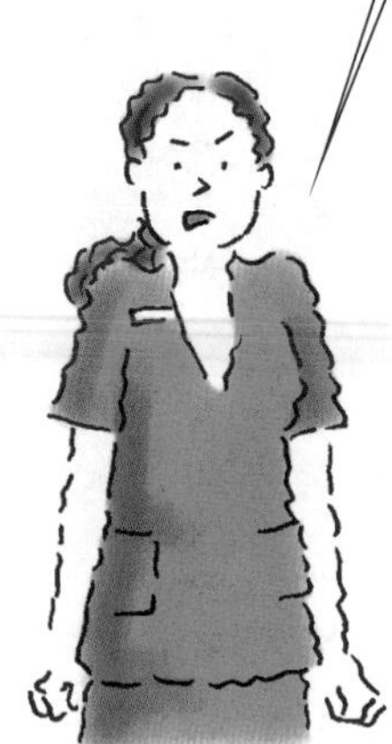

Brace yourself. Question 15 requires a long-term solution.

16. A child has just returned to his room with a cast on his leg after open reduction of a fractured femur. What's the most appropriate action for a nurse to take when a 6 cm by 10 cm area of blood is noted on the cast?

1. Tape gauze pads over the bloody area.
2. Mark the bloody drainage and monitor hourly.
3. Assess vital signs.
4. Call the physician.

16. 3. The most appropriate action for the nurse is to assess the client's vital signs for evidence of hemorrhage, such as tachycardia and hypotension. After the nurse has assessed the client, the physician should be notified with the findings. Gauze pads may be placed over the bloody drainage after the client is assessed and the physician notified. The size of the bloody drainage should be monitored after the client is assessed and the physician notified.

CN: Physiological integrity; CNS: Reduction of risk potential; CL: Application

17. Which observation by a nurse indicates proper fit of crutches in a 9-year-old boy?

1. The crutches fit snugly under the axilla.
2. The crutches end 2″ (5 cm) below the axilla.
3. The elbow is flexed 60 degrees.
4. The elbow is flexed 90 degrees.

17. 2. The crutches should end 2″ below the axilla and the elbow should be flexed 20 to 30 degrees.

CN: Physiological integrity; CNS: Basic care and comfort; CL: Application

18. Which technique may assist a 3-month-old client diagnosed with torticollis?

1. Lying supine
2. Gentle massage
3. Range-of-motion (ROM) exercises
4. Lying on the side

18. 4. Side-lying opposite the affected side may help elongate shortened muscles. Lying supine won't assist with elongation of muscles. Gentle massage won't assist with elongation of muscles. ROM exercises won't assist with shortened muscles unless in specific patterns and with stretching.

CN: Health promotion and maintenance; CNS: None; CL: Application

19. A physical therapist has instructed the nursing staff in range-of-motion (ROM) exercises for an infant with torticollis. Which intervention should a nurse perform if she feels uncomfortable performing the stretches that result in crying and grimacing of the client?

1. Check the primary health care provider's orders.
2. Call the primary health care provider.
3. Call the physical therapist.
4. Discontinue the exercises.

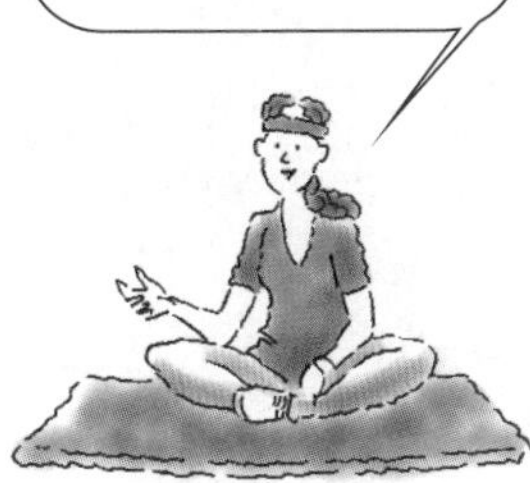

Do you think there's any truth to no pain, no gain?

19. 3. The only cure for the torticollis is exercise or surgery. The therapist is the expert in exercise and should be called for assistance in this situation. The primary health care provider would be called only if there was concern over the orders written or an abnormal development in the child.

CN: Physiological integrity; CNS: Physiological adaptation; CL: Analysis

20. A client has developed a right torticollis with side-bending to the right and rotation to the left. Which exercises may assist in reduction of the torticollis?

1. Rotation exercises to the right
2. Rotation exercises to the left
3. Cervical extension exercises
4. Cervical flexion exercises

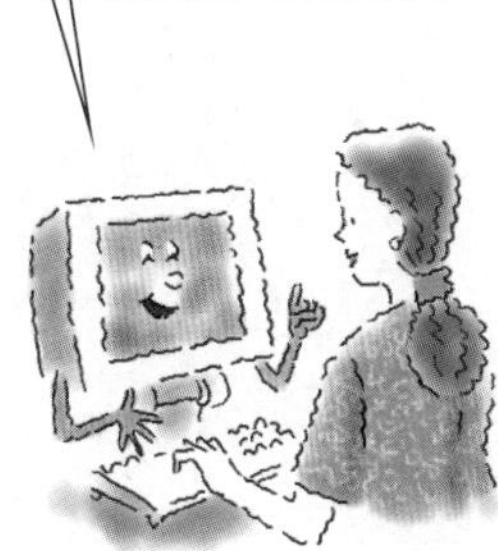

You've done 20 questions already. Great job!!

20. 1. Performing rotation exercises to the right will help increase the length of the shortened right sternocleidomastoid. Rotation to the left will just add to the torticollis because the head is already rotated in that direction. Cervical extension exercises won't lengthen tightened muscles. Cervical flexion will add to shortening of the muscles.

CN: Physiological integrity; CNS: Reduction of risk potential; CL: Application

21. Which complication may occur due to severe scoliosis?

1. Increased vital capacity
2. Increased oxygen uptake
3. Diminished vital capacity
4. Decreased residual volume

21. 3. Scoliosis of greater than 60 degrees can cause shifting of organs and decreased ability for the ribs to expand, thus decreasing vital capacity. An increase in vital capacity also won't occur secondary to a decrease in chest expansion. An increase in oxygen uptake won't occur secondary to a decrease in chest expansion. Residual volume will increase secondary to decreased ability of the lungs to expel air.

CN: Physiological integrity; CNS: Physiological adaptation; CL: Analysis

22. A 4-year-old child is diagnosed with cerebral palsy and resultant thoracic scoliosis. Which condition may be the cause of the scoliosis?

1. Hypotonia
2. Mental retardation
3. Autonomic dysreflexia
4. Increased thoracic kyphosis

22. 1. Cerebral palsy is usually associated with some degree of hypotonia or hypertonia. Poor muscle tone may result in scoliosis. Mental retardation isn't a cause of scoliosis. Autonomic dysreflexia is described in spinal cord injury and involves abnormal muscle spasms secondary to abnormal inhibitory neurons present during stretch reflexes. Increased thoracic kyphosis won't result in scoliosis.

CN: Physiological integrity; CNS: Physiological adaptation; CL: Application

23. Which statement by the parents of a child with crutches indicates understanding of how to safely walk down stairs?

1. "First place the crutches on the lower step."
2. "Advance the fractured leg first."
3. "Advance the strong leg first."
4. "First place the crutch on the fractured side on the lower step."

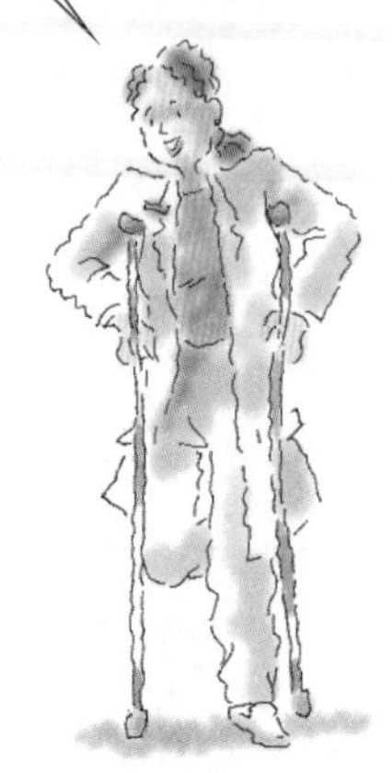

Read question 23 carefully and take it one step at a time.

23. 1. To walk down the stairs with crutches, the crutches are first placed on the lower step. Then the fractured or weaker leg is lowered, followed by the unaffected or stronger leg. This way the arms and unaffected leg share the work of carrying the body weight.

CN: Safe, effective care environment; CNS: Safety and infection control; CL: Application

24. During a scoliosis screening, a school nurse notices a raised iliac crest height. She should suspect which condition?

1. Forward head posture
2. Leg length discrepancy
3. Increased lumbar lordosis
4. Increased thoracic kyphosis

24. 2. A raised iliac crest may be indicative of a leg length discrepancy or a curvature in the lumbar spine. It isn't indicative of forward head posture, lumbar lordosis, or thoracic kyphosis.

CN: Health promotion and maintenance; CNS: None; CL: Application

25. A school nurse is performing a scoliosis screening on a group of students. Which student would most commonly develop this condition?

1. A 7-year-old girl
2. A 7-year-old boy
3. A 13-year-old girl
4. A 13-year old boy

25. 3. Scoliosis is eight times more prominent in adolescent girls than boys. Peak incidence is between ages 8 and 15. Therefore, a 13-year-old girl is at the highest risk. Seven-year-old boys and girls are at lower risk.

CN: Health promotion and maintenance; CNS: None; CL: Analysis

26. In caring for a child with a Harrington instrumentation rod placement, which symptom should be of <u>greatest concern</u> 2 days post-operatively?

1. Fever of 99.5° F (37.5° C)
2. Pain along the incision
3. Decreased urinary output
4. Hypoactive bowel sounds

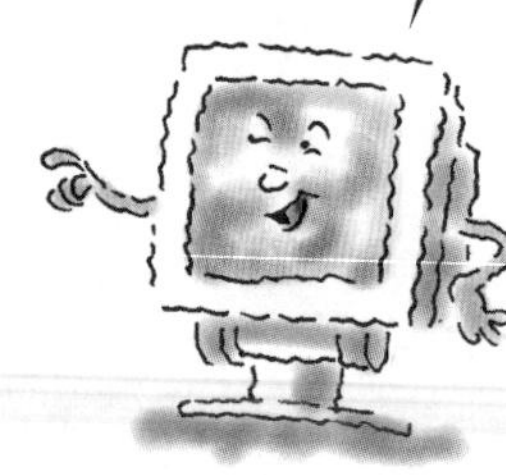

In question 26, you've got to determine the symptom that causes the most concern.

26. 3. Because of extensive blood loss during surgery and possible renal hypoperfusion, decreased urinary output could indicate decreased renal function. A fever of 99.5° F is of concern, but it may be due to decreased chest expansion secondary to anesthesia, surgery, and pain. Pain along the incision site is expected. A paralytic ileus is common after this surgery, and the client may have a nasogastric tube for the first 48 hours.

CN: Physiological integrity; CNS: Reduction of risk potential; CL: Analysis

27. Observing which structure will serve a nurse best when screening a child for scoliosis?

1. Iliac crests
2. Spinous processes
3. Acromion processes
4. Posterior superior iliac spines

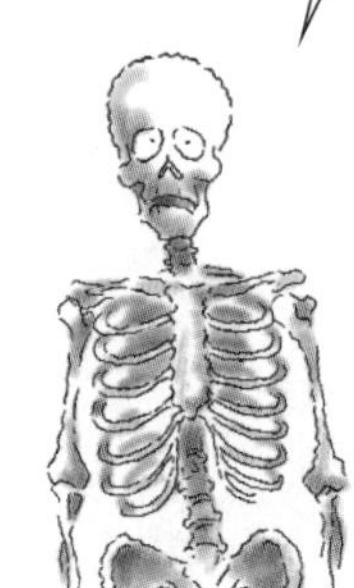

No bones about it. You're doing great!

27. 2. Spinous processes are the best bony landmark to identify when attempting to screen for scoliosis because this will show lateral deviation of the column. Abnormalities in the acromion process, iliac crests, and posterior superior iliac spines may not be indicative of scoliosis.

CN: Health promotion and maintenance; CNS: None; CL: Application

28. Which intervention may be a possible treatment choice for talipes equinovarus?

1. Traction
2. Serial casting
3. Short leg braces
4. Inversion range-of-motion exercises

28. 2. Serial casting is a treatment choice in attempts to change the length of soft tissue. Traction isn't an option. Corrective shoes are used instead of short leg braces. Inversion exercises won't help; eversion exercise will.

CN: Physiological integrity; CNS: Reduction of risk potential; CL: Application

29. When performing stretches with a child who has scoliosis, which technique should be used?

1. Slow and sustained
2. Until a change in muscle length is seen
3. Quick movements to the end range of pain
4. Slow movements for brief, 3- to 4-second periods

29. 1. Stretches should be slow and sustained. It's difficult to see changes in muscle length. Stretches shouldn't be performed with quick movements. Stretches should be performed for longer than a few seconds.

CN: Health promotion and maintenance; CNS: None; CL: Application

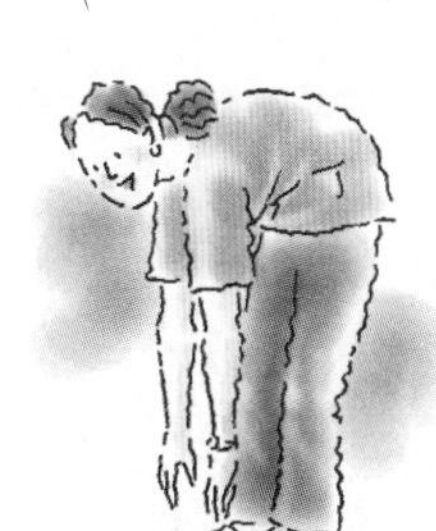

You might need a stretch right now. Why not take a brief one and then get right back to work?

30. Which observation by a nurse indicates that the parent of a neonate with developmental dysplasia of the hip understands the discharge teaching?

1. A folded towel is placed between the infant's legs.
2. The infant is wearing three diapers.
3. The infant is tightly swaddled in a blanket.
4. The infant is placed in a prone position to sleep.

30. 2. Placing several diapers on the infant will keep the hips and knees flexed and the hips abducted. A towel placed between the legs is not enough to keep the hips abducted. Swaddling the infant tightly straightens the legs and doesn't allow the hips to be abducted. Placing the infant in a prone position won't keep the hips abducted and isn't recommended due to the increased risk of sudden infant death syndrome.

CN: Physiological integrity; CNS: Basic care and comfort; CL: Application

31. A nurse is caring for an infant with suspected developmental dysplasia of the hip (DDH). Which information should the nurse give the parents about diagnostic testing?

1. A diagnosis can't be confirmed until the child begins to walk.
2. Diagnostic testing is performed at 6 months if the dysplasia hasn't resolved by then.
3. A radiopaque dye will be injected into the subarachnoid space of the spine.
4. An X-ray confirms the diagnosis.

31. 4. X-rays show the location of the femur head and a shallow acetabulum, confirming the diagnosis DDH. The diagnosis can be made in the neonate and should be made as soon as possible since it becomes more difficult to correct as the child ages. Myelography is an invasive procedure used to evaluate abnormalities of the spinal canal and cord. It isn't used in the diagnosis of congenital hip dysplasia.

CN: Physiological integrity; CNS: Physiological adaptation; CL: Application

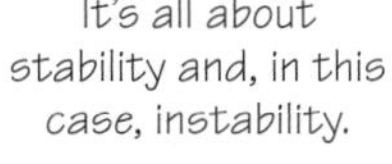

It's all about stability and, in this case, instability.

32. Which hip position should be avoided in an 8-month-old infant who has been diagnosed with developmental dysplasia of the hip?

1. Extension
2. Abduction
3. Internal rotation
4. External rotation

32. 3. Internal rotation of the hip is an unstable position and should be avoided in infants with hip instability. Hip extension is a relatively stable position. Typically, the child is placed in slight abduction while in a hip-spica cast. External rotation isn't necessarily an unstable position, as long as it isn't externally rotated too far.

CN: Physiological integrity; CNS: Reduction of risk potential; CL: Application

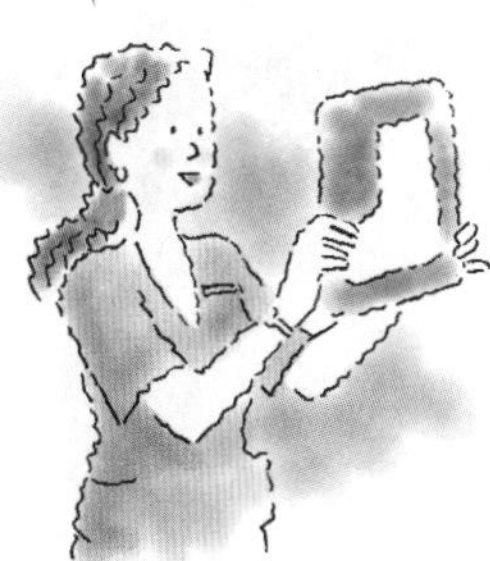

33. Which activity in a client with muscular dystrophy should a nurse anticipate the client having difficulty with <u>first</u>?

1. Breathing
2. Sitting
3. Standing
4. Swallowing

33. 3. Muscular dystrophy usually affects postural muscles of the hip and shoulder first. Sitting may be affected, but a client would have difficulty standing before having difficulty sitting. Swallowing and breathing are usually affected last.

CN: Physiological integrity; CNS: Physiological adaptation; CL: Application

34. The nurse would expect her client's suspected developmental dysplasia of the hip (DDH) to be confirmed by which diagnostic technique?

1. X-ray
2. Positive Ortolani's signs
3. Positive Trendelenburg gait
4. Audible clicking with adduction

34. 1. X-ray will confirm the diagnosis of DDH. All of the options are positive signs of DDH, but only the X-ray will confirm the diagnosis.
CN: Physiological integrity; CNS: Physiological adaptation; CL: Application

35. Which finding should a nurse expect when assessing a neonate with a positive Galeazzi sign?

1. Raised iliac crest
2. Pelvic downward tilt on weight bearing
3. Knees are flexed to 90 degrees, one knee higher
4. Involved leg flexed to 90 degrees, audible click with external rotation

35. 3. A positive Galeazzi sign is used to help diagnose hip dislocation. It's exhibited as one knee being higher than the other. Raised iliac crest isn't indicative of specific hip pathology. A downward pelvic tilt with weight bearing is Trendelenburg gait. External rotation of the hip with audible click is Ortolani-Barlow test.
CN: Health promotion and maintenance; CNS: None; CL: Application

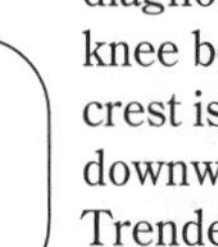

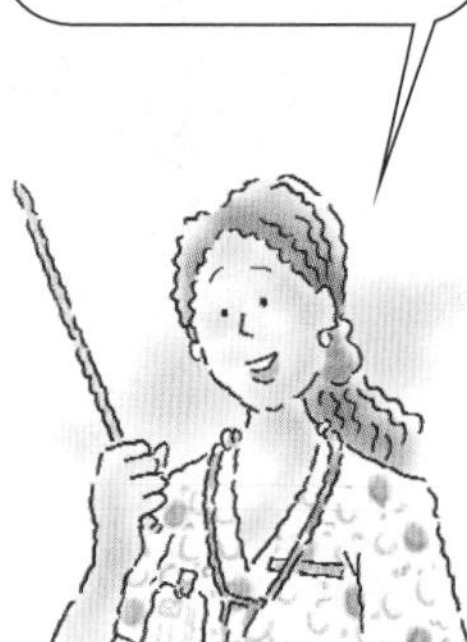

Question 36? Another chance to prioritize.

36. A young child sustains a dislocated hip as well as a subcapital fracture. Which complication is of <u>greatest concern</u>?

1. Avascular necrosis
2. Postsurgical infection
3. Hemorrhage during surgery
4. Poor postsurgical ambulation

36. 1. Avascular necrosis is common with fractures to the subcapital region secondary to possible compromise of blood supply to the femoral head. Postsurgical infection is always a concern but not a priority at first. Hemorrhage shouldn't occur. Poor postsurgical ambulation is of concern but not as much as the possibility of avascular necrosis.
CN: Physiological integrity; CNS: Reduction of risk potential; CL: Application

37. Which position of the femur is accurate in relation to the acetabulum in a child with developmental dysplasia of the hip (DDH)?

1. Anterior
2. Inferior
3. Posterior
4. Superior

37. 1. The head of the femur is anterior to the acetabulum in developmental dysplasia of the hip. All other positions are inaccurate.
CN: Physiological integrity; CNS: Physiological adaptation; CL: Application

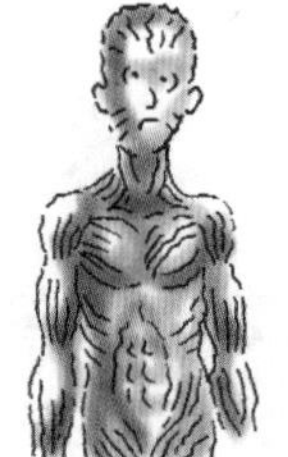

I'm not the muscle I used to be.

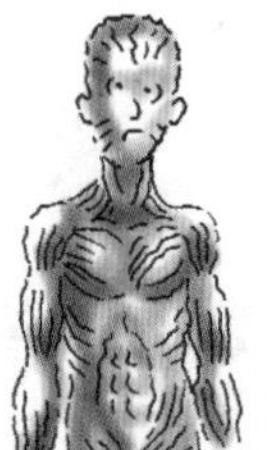

38. The nurse is planning to teach the parents of a child with newly diagnosed muscular dystrophy about the disease. Which description accurately describes this condition?

1. A demyelinating disease
2. Lesions of the brain cortex
3. Upper motor neuron lesions
4. Degeneration of muscle fibers

38. 4. Degeneration of muscle fibers with progressive weakness and wasting best describes muscular dystrophy. Demyelination of myelin sheaths is a description of multiple sclerosis. Lesions within the cortex and in upper motor neurons suggest a neurologic, not a muscular, disease.
CN: Physiological integrity; CNS: Physiological adaptation; CL: Application

39. When a child is suspected of having muscular dystrophy, a nurse should expect which muscles to be affected <u>first</u>?

1. Muscles of the hip
2. Muscles of the foot
3. Muscles of the hand
4. Muscles of respiration

39. 1. Positional muscles of the hip and shoulder are affected first. Progression advances to muscles of the foot and hand. Involuntary muscles, such as the muscles of respiration, are affected last.
CN: Physiological integrity; CNS: Physiological adaptation; CL: Application

CN: Client needs category CNS: Client needs subcategory CL: Cognitive level

40. Which information should a nurse provide to the parents of child undergoing testing for the diagnosis of muscular dystrophy?

1. The genitals will be covered by a lead apron.
2. A local anesthetic will be used for the test.
3. Electrode wires will be attached to the scalp.
4. A fiber-optic endoscope will be inserted into a joint.

40. 2. A muscle biopsy, used to confirm the diagnosis of muscular dystrophy, shows the degeneration of muscle fibers and infiltration of fatty tissue. It's typically performed using a local anesthetic. Genitals are covered by a lead apron during an X-ray examination which is used to detect osseous, not muscular, problems. Electrode wires are attached to the scalp during EEG to observe brain wave activity. It isn't used to diagnose muscular dystrophy. Arthroscopy involves the insertion of a fiber-optic scope into a joint and isn't used to diagnose muscular dystrophy.

CN: Physiological integrity; CNS: Basic care and comfort; CL: Application

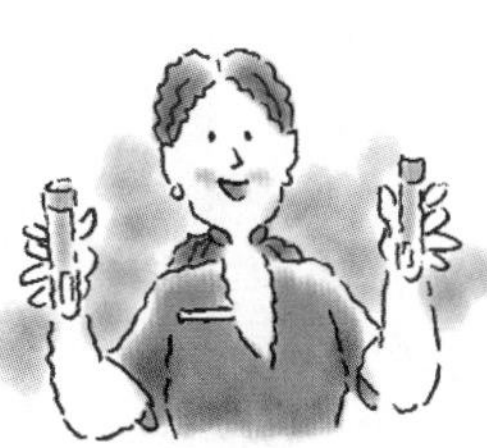

Question 41 asks which lab test helps in diagnosing the condition.

41. The nurse is reviewing the laboratory tests of a child diagnosed with muscular dystrophy. Which laboratory test would aid in the diagnosis of this condition?

1. Bilirubin
2. Creatinine
3. Serum potassium
4. Sodium

41. 2. Creatinine values would aid in the diagnosis of muscular dystrophy. Creatinine is a by-product of muscle metabolism as it hypertrophies. Bilirubin is a by-product of liver function. Potassium and sodium levels can change due to various factors and aren't indicators of muscular dystrophy.

CN: Health promotion and maintenance; CNS: None; CL: Application

42. The nurse is teaching the student nurse about muscular dystrophy. The student nurse asks which form of muscular dystrophy is most common. Which response is most accurate?

1. Duchenne's
2. Becker's
3. Limb girdle
4. Myotonic

42. 1. Duchenne's, also known as pseudohypertrophic, accounts for 50% of all cases of muscular dystrophy. It affects cardiac and respiratory muscles, as well as all voluntary muscles.

CN: Physiological integrity; CNS: Physiological adaptation; CL: Application

43. Which condition would alert the nurse that a child might be suffering from muscular dystrophy?

1. Hypertonia of extremities
2. Increased lumbar lordosis
3. Upper extremity spasticity
4. Hyperactive lower extremity reflexes

43. 2. An increased lumbar lordosis would be seen in a child suffering from muscular dystrophy secondary to paralysis of lower lumbar postural muscles; it also occurs to increase lower extremity support. Hypertonia isn't seen in this disease. Upper extremity spasticity isn't seen because this disease isn't due to upper motor neuron lesions. Hyperactive reflexes aren't indications of muscular dystrophy.

CN: Physiological integrity; CNS: Physiological adaptation; CL: Analysis

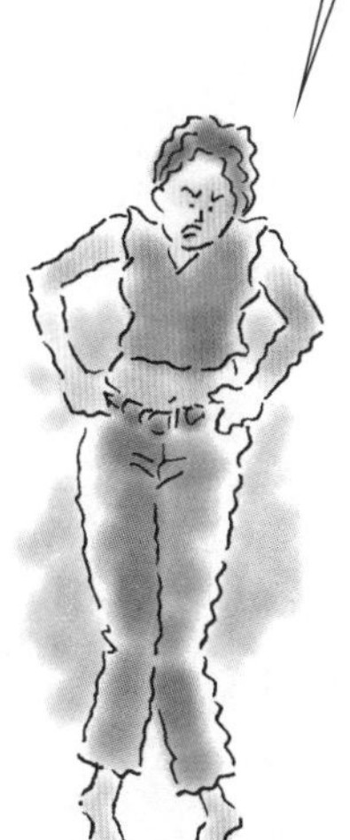

It's all in the jeans...I mean the genes.

44. The parents of a child with Duchenne's muscular dystrophy want to know how it is acquired. The most accurate response by the nurse would be which mechanism?

1. Virus
2. Hereditary
3. Autoimmune factors
4. Environmental toxins

44. 2. Muscular dystrophy is hereditary and acquired through a recessive sex-linked trait. Therefore, it isn't viral, autoimmune, or caused by toxins.

CN: Physiological integrity; CNS: Physiological adaptation; CL: Application

45. A client with muscular dystrophy has lost complete control of his lower extremities. He has some strength bilaterally in the upper extremities, but poor trunk control. Which mechanism would be the most important to have on the wheelchair?

1. Antitip device
2. Extended breaks
3. Headrest support
4. Wheelchair belt

45. 4. This client has poor trunk control; a belt will prevent him from falling out of the wheelchair. Antitip devices, head rest supports, and extended breaks are all important options but aren't the best choice in this situation.

CN: Safe, effective care environment; CNS: Safety and infection control; CL: Application

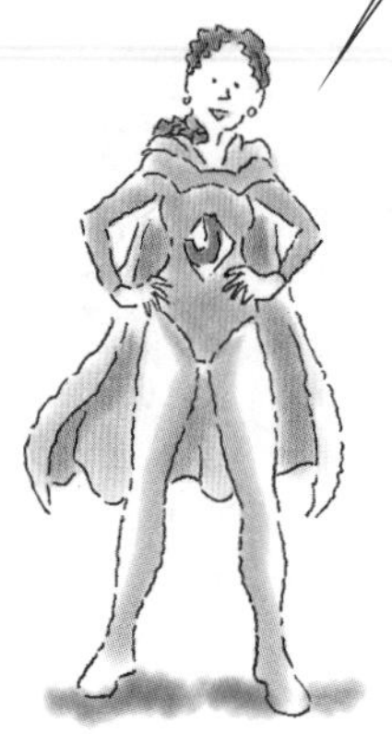
Question 45
tests your ability to
ensure the client's
safety.

46. A 2-year-old infant has muscular dystrophy. His legs are held together with the knees touching. Which muscles are contracted?

1. Hip abductors
2. Hip adductors
3. Hip extensors
4. Hip flexors

46. 2. The hip adductors are in a shortened position. The abductors are in a lengthened position. This position isn't indicative of hip flexor or hip extensor shortening.

CN: Health promotion and maintenance; CNS: None; CL: Application

47. A 12-year-old child diagnosed with muscular dystrophy is hospitalized secondary to a fall. Surgery is necessary as well as skeletal traction. Which complication should be of <u>greatest concern</u> to the nursing staff?

1. Skin integrity
2. Infection of pin sites
3. Respiratory infection
4. Nonunion healing of the fracture

47. 3. Respiratory infection can be fatal for clients with muscular dystrophy due to poor chest expansion and decreased ability to mobilize secretions. Skin integrity, infection of pin sites, and nonunion healing are important but not as important as prevention of respiratory infection.

CN: Physiological integrity; CNS: Reduction of risk potential; CL: Analysis

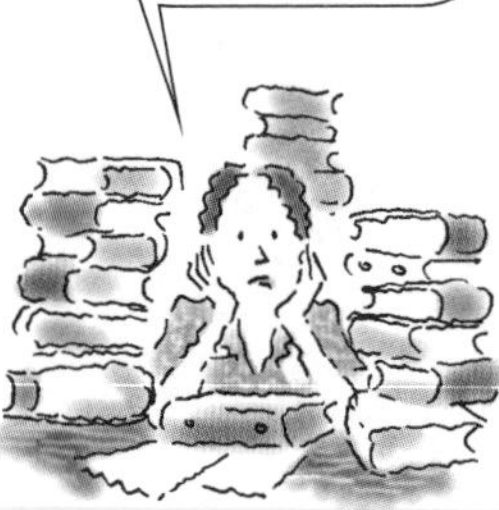
Prioritize?
What a
surprise!

48. A nurse is talking with a 12-year-old boy and his parents about his osteogenesis imperfecta. Which is the best response by the nurse when the boy reports that he likes to swim?

1. Tell him that he should also add a weight-bearing exercise.
2. Tell him that swimming isn't safe since he can slip on the wet area around the pool.
3. Tell him that he should restrict his exercise to only swimming.
4. Tell him that any form of exercises isn't safe.

48. 1. Swimming is a beneficial form of exercise for people with osteogenesis imperfecta, but since it does little to prevent bone loss, the client should add a weight-bearing exercise. Although wet areas around the pool are a risk for the person with osteogenesis imperfecta, the risk can be minimized by walking carefully and wearing nonskid footwear. In the past, clients with osteogenesis imperfecta were told that exercise increased the risk of bone fractures. Mild forms of exercise are encouraged to promote bone density, cardiovascular conditioning, and to maintain joint mobility.

CN: Health promotion and maintenance; CNS: None; CL: Application

49. Which problem is most commonly encountered by adolescent females with scoliosis?

1. Respiratory distress
2. Poor self-esteem
3. Poor appetite
4. Renal difficulty

49. 2. Poor self-esteem is a major issue with many adolescents. The use of orthopedic appliances, such as those used to treat scoliosis, make this issue much more significant for adolescents with scoliosis. Although respiratory distress and poor appetite may surface, they aren't as common as self-esteem problems. Renal problems aren't usually an issue in adolescents with scoliosis.

CN: Health promotion and maintenance; CNS: None; CL: Application

CN: Client needs category CNS: Client needs subcategory CL: Cognitive level

50. A child has developed difficulty ambulating and tends to walk on his toes. Which surgical technique may benefit the client?
1. Adductor release
2. Hamstring release
3. Plantar fascia release
4. Achilles tendon release

50. 4. A shortened Achilles tendon may cause a child to walk on his toes. A release of the tendon may assist the child in walking. An adductor release is commonly performed if the legs are held together. A plantar fascia release won't help, and a hamstring release is done only when there's a knee flexion contracture.
CN: Physiological integrity; CNS: Reduction of risk potential; CL: Application

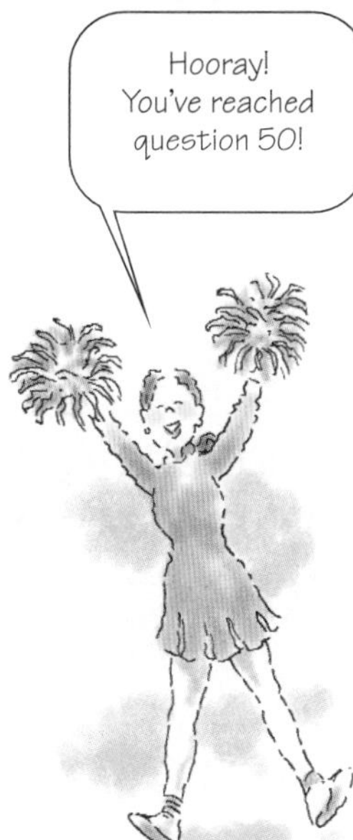

51. The parents of a child with muscular dystrophy ask the nurse what causes this condition. The nurse responds that muscular dystrophy is a result of:
1. gene mutation.
2. chromosomal aberration.
3. unknown nongenetic origin.
4. environmental factors.

51. 1. Muscular dystrophy is a result of a gene mutation. It isn't from a chromosome aberration or environmental factors. It's genetic, and there's a known origin of the disease.
CN: Physiological integrity; CNS: Physiological adaptation; CL: Application

52. The nurse is assessing a child suspected of having muscular dystrophy for muscle weakness. At what age would evidence of muscle weakness associated with muscular dystrophy appear?
1. Age 1
2. Age 2
3. Age 3
4. Age 4

52. 3. Studies have shown that children diagnosed with muscular dystrophy usually show some form of weakness around age 3.
CN: Health promotion and maintenance; CNS: None; CL: Application

53. To promote safe transfers in a client with muscular dystrophy, a nurse should teach exercises to maintain which muscles?
1. Gastrocnemius
2. Gluteus maximus
3. Hamstrings
4. Quadriceps

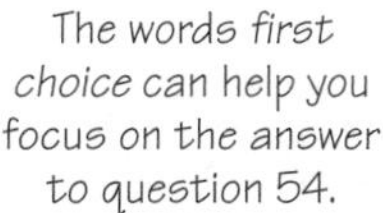

The words first choice can help you focus on the answer to question 54.

53. 2. Gluteus maximus is the strongest muscle in the body and is important for standing as well as for transfers. All of the named muscles are important, but the maintenance of the gluteus maximus will enable maximum function.
CN: Health promotion and maintenance; CNS: None; CL: Application

54. Which of the following strategies would be the <u>first choice</u> in attempting to maximize function in a child with muscular dystrophy?
1. Long leg braces
2. Motorized wheelchair
3. Manual wheelchair
4. Walker

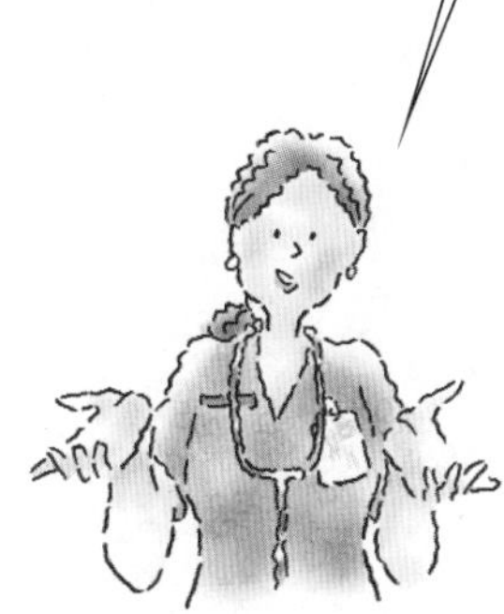

54. 1. Long leg braces are functional assistive devices that provide increased independence and increased use of upper and lower body strength. Wheelchairs, both motorized and manual, provide less independence and less use of upper and lower body strength. Walkers are functional assistive devices that provide less independence than braces.
CN: Physiological integrity; CNS: Basic care and comfort; CL: Application

55. A child is having increased difficulty getting out of his chair at school. Which recommendation should the nurse make to assist the child?
1. A seat cushion
2. Long leg braces
3. Powered wheelchair
4. Removable arm rests on wheelchair

55. 1. A seat cushion will put the hip extensors at an advantage and make it somewhat easier to get up. Long leg braces wouldn't be the first choice. A powered wheelchair wouldn't be important in assisting with the transfer. Removable armrests have no bearing on assisting the client.
CN: Physiological integrity; CNS: Basic care and comfort; CL: Application

56. What findings would be expected while palpating the muscles of a child with muscular dystrophy?

1. Soft on palpation
2. Firm or woody on palpation
3. Extremely hard on palpation
4. No muscle consistency on palpation

56. 2. Muscles will commonly be firm on palpation secondary to the infiltration of fatty tissue and connective tissue into the muscle. The muscles won't be soft secondary to the infiltration and won't be hard upon palpation. There's some consistency to the muscle although, in advanced stages, atrophy is present.

CN: Physiological integrity; CNS: Physiological adaptation; CL: Analysis

57. A nurse should instruct a wheelchair-bound client with muscular dystrophy in which exercise to best prevent skin breakdown?

1. Wheelchair push-ups
2. Leaning side-to-side
3. Leaning forward
4. Gluteal sets

57. 1. A wheelchair push-up will alleviate the most pressure off the buttocks. Leaning side-to-side and leaning forward will help but not as much as wheelchair push-ups. Gluteal sets won't help with pressure relief.

CN: Health promotion and maintenance; CNS: None; CL: Application

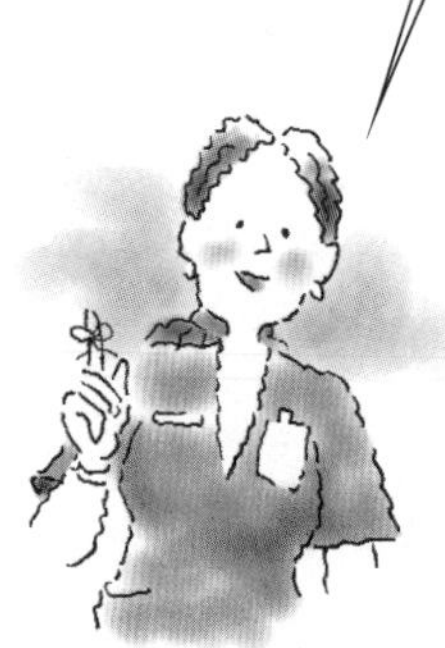

To remember Gower's sign, think going somewhere— that's a description of what the child is trying to do.

58. How would the nurse best describe Gower's sign to the parents of a child with muscular dystrophy?

1. A transfer technique
2. A waddling-type gait
3. The pelvis position during gait
4. Muscle twitching present during a quick stretch

58. 1. Gowers' sign is a description of a transfer technique present during some phases of muscular dystrophy. The child turns on the side or abdomen, extends the knees, and pushes on the torso to an upright position by walking his hands up the legs. Waddling-type gait doesn't describe Gowers' sign. The position of the pelvis during gait isn't described by Gowers' sign. Muscle twitching present after a quick stretch is described as *clonus*.

CN: Physiological integrity; CNS: Physiological adaptation; CL: Analysis

Focus on what response is best.

59. A 13-year-old boy admitted with a fractured femur had an open reduction and internal fixation 2 days ago and currently is in traction. He asks the nurse what would happen to him if a terrorist decided to bomb the hospital. What's the nurse's best response?

1. "I wouldn't worry about that. Spend your energy on getting well and going home."
2. "We have plans to call your parents and take care of you if there's a problem."
3. "What do you think might happen if terrorists attack?"
4. "That's silly thinking. Why would anyone bomb a hospital?"

59. 3. Something prompted the child to ask such a question, and the nurse needs to take advantage of this opportunity to further explore his concerns and fears. Option 1 discounts the boy's feelings and may actually increase his anxiety. Although option 2 may be technically correct, it doesn't provide reassurance or help build a therapeutic relationship that can promote health and wellness. Option 4 is dismissive and childes the boy for asking the question.

CN: Physiological integrity; CNS: None; CL: Analysis

60. A client with bilateral fractured femurs is scheduled for a double-hip-spica cast. She says to the nurse, "Only 3 more months and I can go home." Further investigation reveals that the client and her family believe she'll be hospitalized until the cast comes off. The nurse should explain to the client and her family that the client:

1. may be hospitalized 2 to 4 months.
2. will go home 2 to 4 days after casting.
3. will go home 1 week after casting.
4. will go home as soon as she can move.

60. 2. The cast will dry fairly rapidly with the use of fiberglass casting material. The time spent in the hospital after casting, typically 2 to 4 days, will be for teaching the client and her family how to care for her at home and evaluating the client's skin integrity and neurovascular status before discharge. The timeframes in the other options given are inaccurate for a double-hip-spica cast.

CN: Health promotion and maintenance; CNS: None; CL: Application

61. Which observation by a nurse indicates that an infant in a hip-spica cast is properly positioned?

1. The infant's upper body and cast are at a 180-degree angle.
2. The infant's hips are higher than the head.
3. The infant's upper body and the cast are at a 45-degree angle.
4. The infant is flat in bed.

61. 1. The infant's body and cast should be at a 180-degree angle. While the cast should be kept level with the body, it should be on a slant with the head of the bed elevated so that urine and stool can drain downward and not soil the cast.

CN: Physiological integrity; CNS: Basic care and comfort; CL: Application

62. The nurse receives a report on a child admitted with severe muscular dystrophy. The nurse suspects the child has been diagnosed with the most severe form of the disease, known as:

1. Duchenne's.
2. fascioscapulohumeral.
3. limb girdle.
4. myotonic.

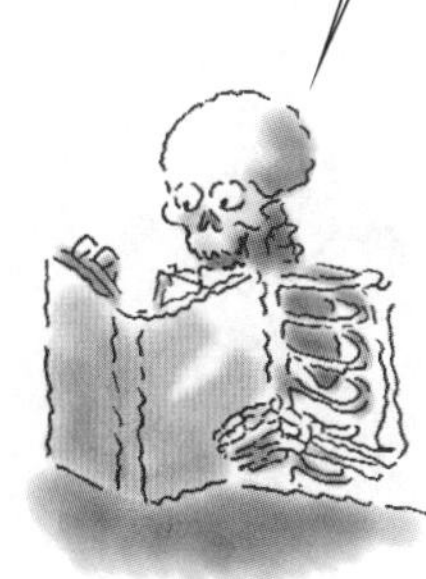
I know all about
pain over a bony
prominence.

62. 1. Studies have shown that Duchenne's is the most severe form of muscular dystrophy, affecting all voluntary muscles as well as cardiac and respiratory muscles.

CN: Physiological integrity; CNS: Physiological adaptation; CL: Analysis

63. Which finding should alert a nurse to a potential complication in a client with a cast following fracture of the radius?

1. Discomfort occurs at the site of the break.
2. Fingers are pink and warm.
3. Swelling is reduced with cast elevation.
4. Pain occurs over a bony prominence.

63. 4. Pain over a bony prominence, such as in the wrist or elbow, signals an impending pressure ulcer and requires prompt attention. Pain or discomfort at the site of the fracture is expected and is relieved by analgesics. Warm and pink fingers are an expected finding. Swelling may be relieved by elevation of the extremity. Swelling that isn't relieved by elevation of the affected limb should be reported to the physician.

CN: Physiological integrity; CNS: Reduction of risk potential; CL: Application

64. The parents of a child with newly diagnosed developmental dysplasia of the hip (DDH) ask the nurse how their child developed this condition. The nurse explains that the greatest number of cases is caused by which condition?

1. Dislocation
2. Subluxation
3. Acetabular dysplasia
4. Dislocation with fracture

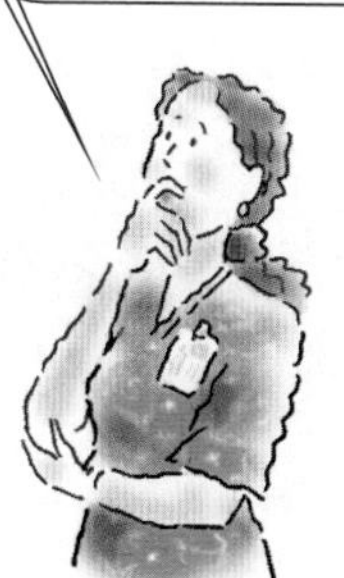
The greatest
number of cases?
This is getting
complicated.

64. 2. Studies show that subluxation accounts for the greatest number of cases of DDH.

CN: Physiological integrity; CNS: Physiological adaptation; CL: Application

65. Which finding would the nurse expect in a client with developmental dysplasia of the hip (DDH)?

1. Ligamentum teres is shortened.
2. Femoral head loses contact with acetabulum and is displaced inferiorly.
3. Femoral head loses contact with the acetabulum and is displaced posteriorly.
4. Femoral head maintains contact with acetabulum, but there's noted capsular rupture.

65. 3. In DDH, the femoral head loses contact with the acetabulum and is displaced posteriorly, not inferiorly. Ligamentum teres is lengthened.

CN: Physiological integrity; CNS: Physiological adaptation; CL: Application

66. A toddler is immobilized with traction to the legs. Which play activity would be appropriate for this child?

1. Pounding board
2. Tinker toys
3. Pull toy
4. Board games

66. 1. A pounding board is appropriate for an immobilized toddler because it promotes physical development and provides an acceptable energy outlet. Toys with small parts, such as tinker toys, aren't suitable because a toddler may swallow the parts. A pull toy is suitable for most toddlers, but not for one who is immobilized. Board games are usually too advanced for the developmental skills of a toddler.

CN: Health promotion and maintenance; CNS: None; CL: Application

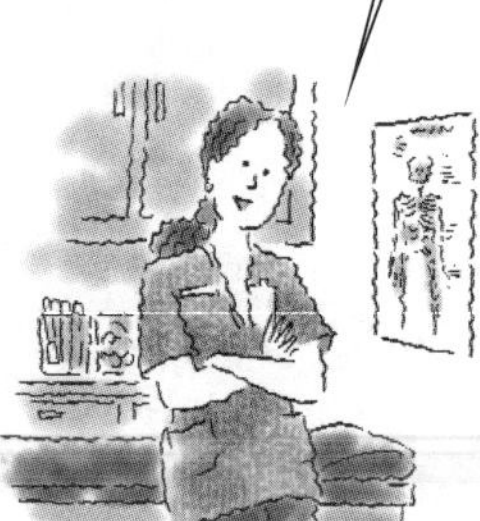

Knowing the shape of a hip-spica cast can help answer this question.

67. Which choice is best for handling a client's hip-spica cast that has been soiled?

1. Clean with damp cloth and dry cleanser.
2. Clean with soap and water.
3. Don't do anything.
4. Change the cast.

67. 1. A damp cloth is best to use rather than water. Water will break the cast down. If nothing is done, the cast will give off an odor. Changing the cast isn't an option.

CN: Physiological integrity; CNS: Basic care and comfort; CL: Application

68. Which position is best for a child in a hip-spica cast who needs to be toileted?

1. Supine
2. Sitting in a toilet chair
3. Shoulder lower than buttocks
4. Buttocks lower than shoulder

68. 4. The buttocks need to be lowered to toilet the child. This will keep the cast from being soiled. Supine will cause soiling of the cast. The child isn't able to use a toilet chair.

CN: Physiological integrity; CNS: Basic care and comfort; CL: Application

69. Which intervention should a nurse perform in a 4-year-old child in Buck's traction?

1. Provide daily pin site care.
2. Release weights for 1 hour each day.
3. Change the child's position every 4 hours.
4. Unwrap the elastic bandage every shift to assess the skin.

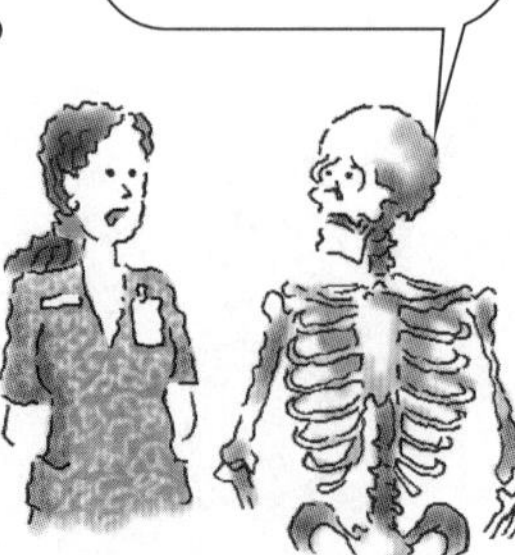

Pulling and pins? This doesn't sound like fun.

69. 1. Buck's traction is a form of skeletal traction which pulls directly on the skeleton using a pin placed into the bone. Pin site care involves cleaning the insertion sites to reduce the risk of infection and observing the site for signs and symptoms of infection. Weights should hang freely and shouldn't be released. The child's position should be changed every 2 hours to prevent skin breakdown. Elastic bandages are used in skin, not skeletal, traction.

CN: Physiological integrity; CNS: Basic care and comfort; CL: Application

70. The nurse observes a client who has a positive Trendelenburg gait. Which characteristic would indicate this gait?
1. Pelvis tilts downward upon weight bearing
2. Pelvis tilts upward upon weight bearing
3. Abnormal height of the iliac crests
4. Leg length discrepancy

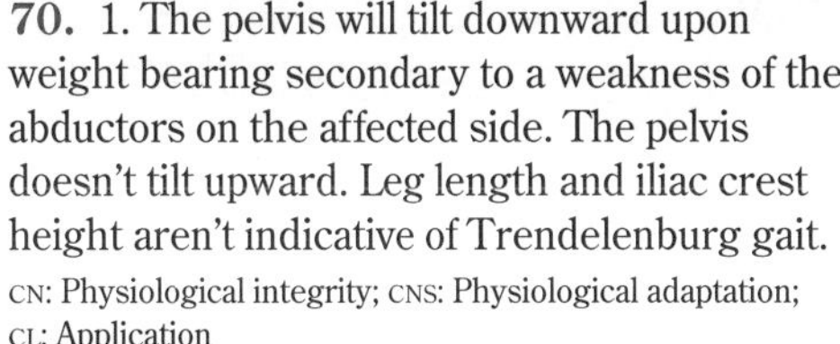

70. 1. The pelvis will tilt downward upon weight bearing secondary to a weakness of the abductors on the affected side. The pelvis doesn't tilt upward. Leg length and iliac crest height aren't indicative of Trendelenburg gait.
CN: Physiological integrity; CNS: Physiological adaptation; CL: Application

71. Which complication involving leg length should a nurse anticipate in a client with developmental dysplasia of the hip?
1. Increased hip abduction
2. Increased leg length on the affected side
3. Decreased leg length on the affected side
4. No change in muscle length or leg length

71. 3. The internal rotation with subsequent dislocation will cause the leg to be shorter, not longer. There's usually *decreased* abduction as well as muscle and leg length changes.
CN: Physiological integrity; CNS: Physiological adaptation; CL: Analysis

72. A nurse recognizes that the parent of a child with developmental hip dysplasia needs more teaching when the parent places the child in a position that encourages:
1. hip abduction.
2. knee extension.
3. external rotation.
4. internal rotation.

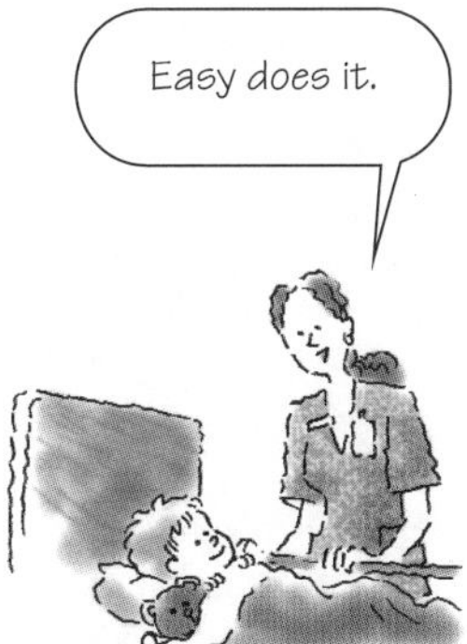

72. 4. Internal rotation increases the risk of hip dislocation. Abduction, external rotation, and knee extension won't increase the risk of dislocation.
CN: Health promotion and maintenance; CNS: None; CL: Application

73. Immediately after a spinal fusion, which restriction is usually put on the child's activity?
1. Supine bed rest
2. Non-weight bearing
3. No restriction
4. Limited weight bearing

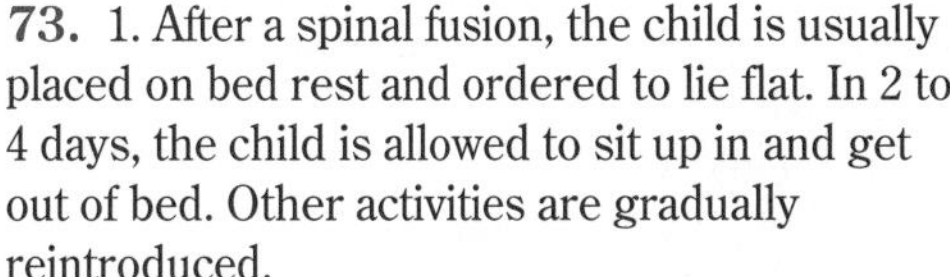

73. 1. After a spinal fusion, the child is usually placed on bed rest and ordered to lie flat. In 2 to 4 days, the child is allowed to sit up in and get out of bed. Other activities are gradually reintroduced.
CN: Physiological integrity; CNS: Basic care and comfort; CL: Application

74. Which intervention should a nurse expect to use to prevent venous stasis after skeletal traction application?
1. Bed rest only
2. Convoluted foam mattress
3. Vigorous pulmonary care
4. Antiembolism stockings or an intermittent compression device

74. 4. To prevent venous stasis after skeletal traction application, antiembolism stockings or an intermittent compression device is used on the unaffected leg. Bed rest can *cause* venous stasis. Convoluted foam mattresses and pulmonary care don't prevent venous stasis.
CN: Health promotion and maintenance; CNS: None; CL: Application

75. A 13-year-old girl is suspected of having structural scoliosis by her school nurse. What should the nurse ask the girl to do to help confirm her suspicion?
1. Bend over and touch her toes while the nurse observes from the back.
2. Stand sideways while the nurse observes her profile.
3. Assume a knee-chest position on the examination table.
4. Arch her back while the nurse observes her from the back.

75. 1. As the child bends over, the curvature of the spine is more apparent. The scapula on one side becomes more prominent, and the opposite side hollows. The knee-chest position is used for lumbar puncture. Scoliosis can't be properly assessed from the side or the front.
CN: Health promotion and maintenance; CNS: None; CL: Application

76. At the scene of a trauma, which nursing intervention is appropriate for a child with a suspected fracture?

1. Never move the child.
2. Sit the child up to facilitate breathing.
3. Move the child to a safe place immediately.
4. Immobilize the extremity and then move child to a safe place.

76. 4. At the scene of a trauma, the nurse should immobilize the extremity of a child with a suspected fracture and then move him to a safe place. If the child is already in a safe place, don't attempt to move him. Never try to sit the child up; this could make the fracture worse.
CN: Safe, effective care environment; CNS: Safety and infection control; CL: Application

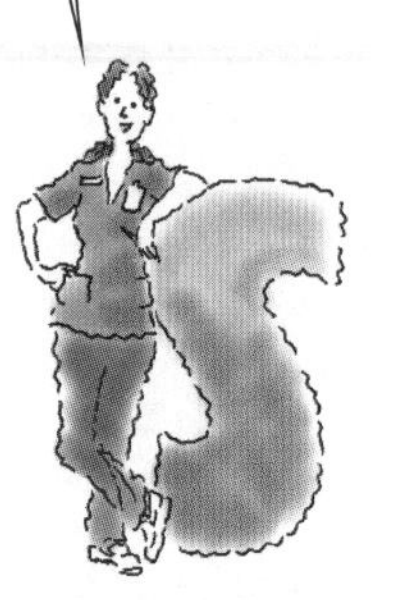

At a trauma scene, think safety first!

77. A nurse is assessing an 18-month-old infant who's in Bryant's traction for a fractured left femur. The infant is properly positioned when:

1. the left leg is extended 90 degrees off the bed.
2. the right leg is extended 90 degrees off the bed.
3. both legs are extended 90 degrees off the bed.
4. both legs are extended at 180 degrees with the upper body.

77. 3. Bryant's traction, a type of skin traction, is for lower extremity fractures in children younger than age 2 years. Both legs are suspended at 90 degrees off the bed, even though only one is fractured, with the child's body weight providing the countertraction.
CN: Physiological integrity; CNS: Basic care and comfort; CL: Application

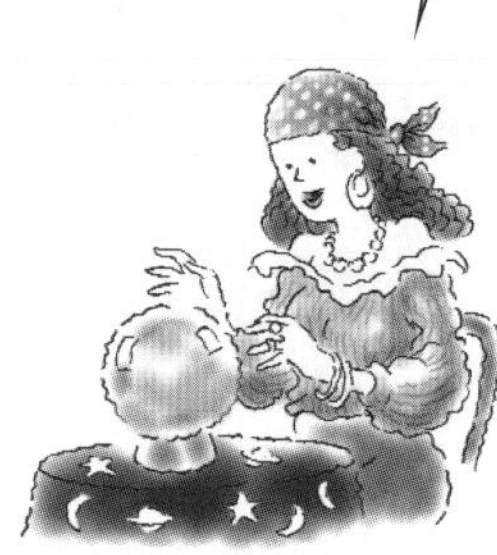

Is Homans' sign an astrological sign?

78. A child in skeletal traction for a fracture of the right femur exhibits a positive Homans' sign, complains of left-sided leg pain, and has edema in the left leg. A nurse should further assess the child for which condition?

1. A fat emboli
2. An infection
3. A pulmonary embolism
4. Deep vein thrombosis (DVT)

78. 4. Unilateral leg pain and edema with a positive Homans' sign (not always present) should lead you to suspect DVT. Symptoms of fat emboli include restlessness, tachypnea, and tachycardia and are more common in long bone injuries. It's unlikely that an infection would occur on the opposite side of the fracture without cause. Tachycardia, chest pain, and shortness of breath may be symptoms of a pulmonary embolism.
CN: Physiological integrity; CNS: Reduction of risk potential; CL: Analysis

79. Nursing care for a client in traction may include which intervention?

1. Assessing pin sites every shift and as needed
2. Ensuring that the rope knots catch on the pulley
3. Adding and removing weights per client's request
4. Placing all joints through range of motion (ROM) every shift

79. 1. Nursing care for a client in traction may include assessing pin sites every shift and as needed and ensuring that the knots in the rope don't catch on the pulley. Weights should be added and removed per the primary health care provider's order, and all joints, except those immediately proximal and distal to the fracture, should be placed through ROM every shift.
CN: Physiological integrity; CNS: Basic care and comfort; CL: Application

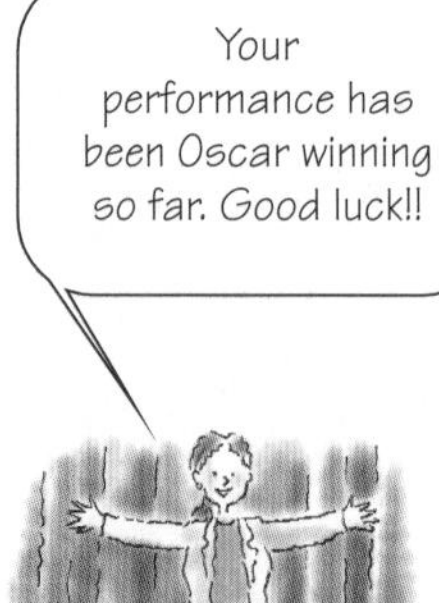

Your performance has been Oscar winning so far. Good luck!!

80. After assisting the primary health care provider in applying a cast, a nurse should include which intervention in the immediate cast care?

1. Rest the cast on the bedside table
2. Dispose of the plaster water in the sink
3. Support the cast with her palms
4. Wait until the cast dries before cleaning surrounding skin

80. 3. After a cast has been applied, it should be immediately supported with the palms of the nurse's hands. Later, the nurse should dispose of the plaster water in a sink with a plaster trap or in a garbage bag, clean the surrounding skin before the cast dries, and make sure that the cast isn't resting on a hard or sharp surface.
CN: Physiological integrity; CNS: Reduction of risk potential; CL: Application

CN: Client needs category CNS: Client needs subcategory CL: Cognitive level

81. A school-age child tells a nurse that he's experiencing intense itching from under his cast. What's the most appropriate response for the nurse to make?

1. "Toughen up, there's nothing that can be done."
2. "Place the eraser-end of a new pencil under the cast to scratch."
3. "Elevate the cast above the level of your heart."
4. "Aim cool air from a hair dryer under the cast."

81. 4. Cool air from a hair dryer may soothe the itchiness. Telling the child to toughen up isn't therapeutic, erodes the nurse-client relationship, and isn't true since cool air may relieve itchiness. Nothing should be placed under a cast because this can cause skin irritation and breakdown. Elevating the cast above the heart doesn't relieve itching. This position is used to reduce swelling.

CN: Physiological integrity; CNS: Basic care and comfort; CL: Application

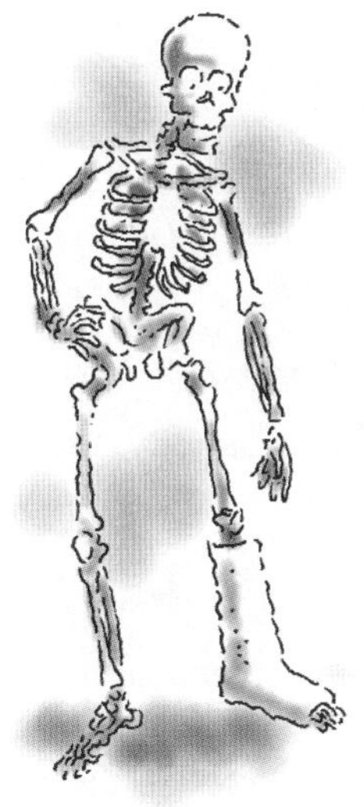

Can you help me prevent foot drop?

82. Which nursing intervention should be taken if, while a cast is drying, the client complains of heat from the cast?

1. Remove the cast immediately.
2. Notify the primary health care provider.
3. Assess the client for other signs of infection.
4. Explain to the client that this is a normal sensation.

82. 4. Normally, as the cast is drying, the client may complain of heat from the cast. The nurse should offer reassurance but doesn't need to notify the primary health care provider or remove the cast. Heat from the cast isn't a sign of infection.

CN: Physiological integrity; CNS: Reduction of risk potential; CL: Application

83. Which nursing intervention can be implemented to <u>prevent</u> foot drop in a casted leg?

1. Encourage bed rest.
2. Support the foot with 45 degrees of flexion.
3. Support the foot with 90 degrees of flexion.
4. Place a stocking on the foot to provide warmth.

83. 3. To prevent foot drop in a casted leg, the foot should be supported with 90 degrees of flexion. Bed rest can cause foot drop. Keeping the extremity warm won't prevent foot drop.

CN: Health promotion and maintenance; CNS: None; CL: Application

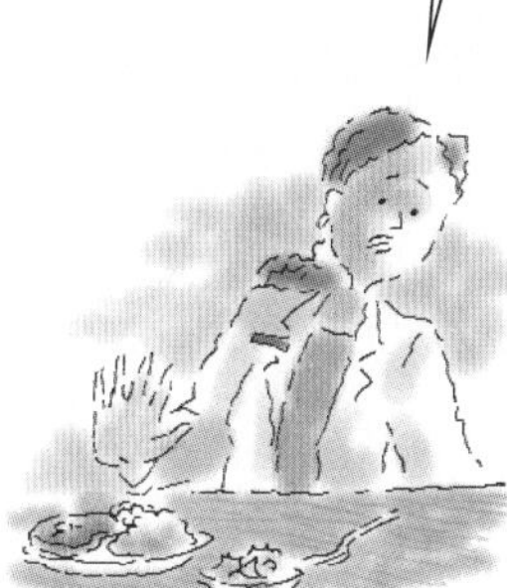

My eyes are bigger than my stomach...or not.

84. A client with a hip-spica cast should avoid gas-forming foods for which reason?

1. To prevent flatus
2. To prevent diarrhea
3. To prevent constipation
4. To prevent abdominal distention

84. 4. A client with a hip-spica cast should avoid gas-forming foods to prevent abdominal distention. Gas-forming foods may cause flatus, but that isn't a reason to avoid them. Gas-forming foods don't generally cause diarrhea or constipation.

CN: Physiological integrity; CNS: Reduction of risk potential; CL: Application

85. A nurse determines that a client with a fractured left femur understands the instructions for touch down weight bearing when he makes which statement?

1. "I will place full weight on my left leg."
2. "I will place about 30% to 50% of my weight on my left leg."
3. "I will keep my left leg off the floor."
4. "I will allow my left leg to touch the floor without placing weight on it."

85. 4. Touch-down weight bearing allows the client to put no weight on the extremity, but the client may touch the floor with the affected extremity. Full weight bearing allows for full weight bearing on the affected extremity. Partial weight bearing allows for only 30% to 50% weight bearing on the affected extremity. Non-weight bearing is no weight on the extremity, and the extremity must remain elevated.

CN: Physiological integrity; CNS: Basic care and comfort; CL: Application

86. Which strategy should a nurse teach an adolescent to prevent sports-related injuries?

1. Warming up
2. Pacing activity
3. Building strength
4. Moderating intensity

86. 1. To prevent sports-related injuries, instruct your client that the best prevention is warming up. Pacing activity, building strength, and using moderate intensity are also prevention measures.

CN: Health promotion and maintenance; CNS: None; CL: Application

87. Which activity may be most helpful for a child who's allowed full activity after repair of a clubfoot?

1. Playing catch
2. Standing
3. Swimming
4. Walking

87. 4. Walking will stimulate all of the involved muscles and help with strengthening. All of the options are good exercises, but walking is the best choice.

CN: Health promotion and maintenance; CNS: None; CL: Application

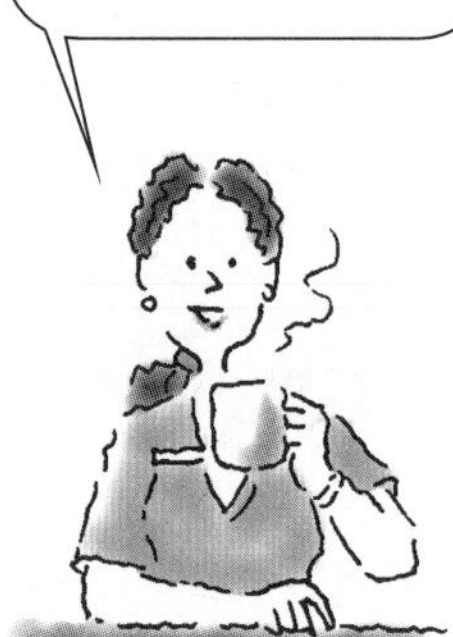

This warming-up activity should keep me awake for the rest of the test.

88. Which statement by the parent of an infant diagnosed with clubfoot indicates understanding of the casting treatment regimen?

1. "The cast will come off in 8 weeks."
2. "The cast will come off in 2 weeks."
3. "The cast will come off when my child starts to walk."
4. "The cast will come off when my child starts to crawl."

88. 2. Because an infant grows quickly, a series of casts will be needed as often as every 2 weeks to correct the deformity as the child grows. Eight weeks is too long to leave a cast on the rapidly growing child. Casting should be complete by the time the child is crawling and walking.

CN: Physiological integrity; CNS: Reduction of risk potential; CL: Analysis

89. The X-ray result for a child who experienced a fall on the basketball court indicates a greenstick fracture of the tibia. Which graphic represents a greenstick fracture?

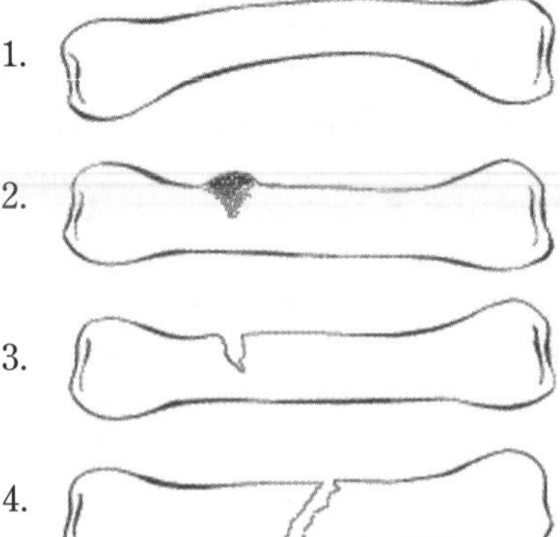

89. 3. A greenstick fracture occurs when the bone is bent beyond its limits, causing an incomplete fracture. The first graphic is a plastic deformation or bend, where there is a microscopic fracture line where the bone bends. The second graphic shows a buckle fracture which occurs due to compression of the porous bone, causing a raised area or bulge at the fracture site. The fourth graphic is of a complete fracture in which the bone is broken into separate pieces.

CN: Physiological integrity; CNS: Physiological adaptation; CL: Application

90. Which instruction should be included in the teaching plan for a 10-year-old with a fracture of the radial bone?

1. Report capillary refill less than 3 seconds.
2. Report warmth under the cast during the first 24 hours after application.
3. Report foul odors coming from the cast.
4. Report cool fingers that warm within 20 minutes of being covered.

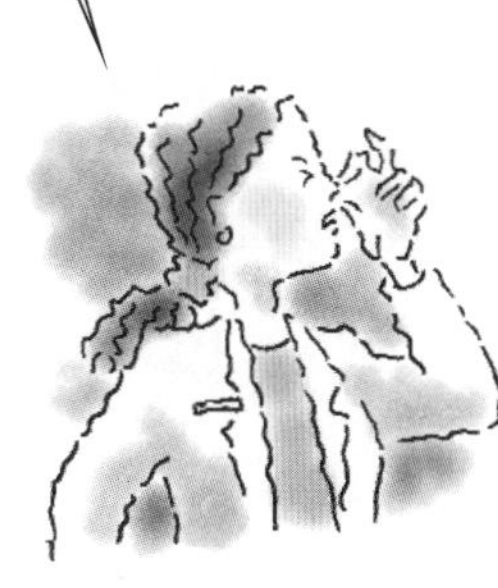

The nose knows the answer to this question.

90. 3. Foul odors from the cast may be a sign of infection and should be reported to the physician immediately. Capillary refill less than 3 seconds is a normal finding. During the first 24 hours, the client may feel warmth under the cast as it dries. After 24 hours, warmth may be a sign of infection and should be reported. Cool fingers that warm up within 20 minutes of being covered is normal; cool fingers that don't warm up after 20 minutes of being covered should be reported because the client may have circulatory impairment under the cast.

CN: Physiological integrity; CNS: Reduction of risk potential; CL: Application

91. Which history finding is the <u>most significant</u> related to developmental dysplasia of the hip (DDH)?

1. Mother's activity during the third trimester
2. Breech presentation at birth
3. Infant's serum calcium level at birth
4. Apgar score of 4 at 1 minute and 6 at 5 minutes

91. 2. Breech presentation is a factor commonly associated with DDH. The mother's activity during the third trimester, the infant's serum calcium level at birth, and Apgar scores have no bearing on DDH.

CN: Health promotion and maintenance; CNS: None; CL: Application

92. A 13-year-old with structural scoliosis has Harrington rods inserted. Which position would be best during the postoperative period?

1. Supine in bed
2. Side-lying
3. Semi-Fowler's
4. High Fowler's

92. 1. After placement of Harrington rods, the client must remain flat in bed. The gatch on a manual bed should be taped, and electric beds should be unplugged to prevent the client from raising the head or foot of the bed. Other positions, such as side-lying, semi-Fowler's, or high Fowler's, could prove damaging because the rods may not be able to maintain the spine in a straight position.

CN: Physiological integrity; CNS: Reduction of risk potential; CL: Application

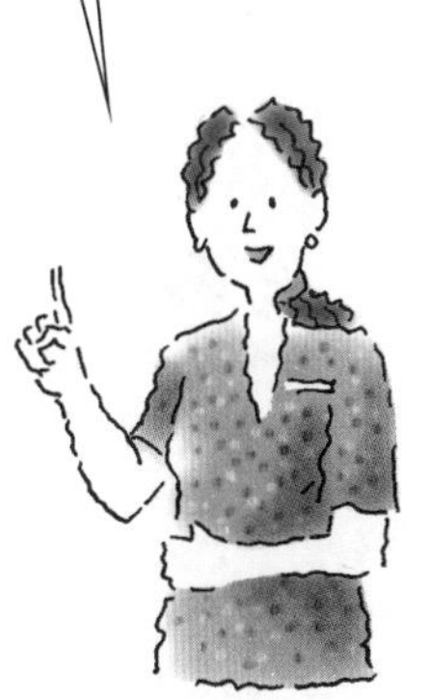

Remember you're looking for the nursing diagnosis with the highest priority.

93. A nurse notes dyspnea and calf pain in a 14-year-old client 48 hours after open reduction of a fractured femur. Which nursing diagnosis has the <u>highest priority</u>?

1. *Impaired gas exchange*
2. *Acute pain*
3. *Impaired physical mobility*
4. *Deficient knowledge*

93. 1. Immobility, a fractured femur, and orthopedic surgery all increase the risk of deep vein thrombosis (DVT). The client who complains of calf pain and dyspnea should be promptly assessed for a pulmonary embolism. While all these nursing diagnoses are appropriate, assessing for *Impaired gas exchange* has the highest priority.

CN: Physiological integrity; CNS: Reduction of risk potential; CL: Analysis

94. A 6-month-old male with developmental dysplasia of the hip has been treated for the past 6 weeks with a Frejka splint, which maintains abduction through padding of the diaper area. At his follow-up visit, the child's mother reports that she removes the splint when he gets too fussy and that he settles down and sleeps well for several hours after the padding is removed. Which response by the nurse would be most appropriate?

1. "I can tell you're concerned about his comfort, but he must wear the padded splint except during the three times per day when you perform range-of-motion exercises on his legs."
2. "I'm pleased that you recognize that the padding is too thick and have adjusted it so he can sleep comfortably."
3. "I realize that seeing him uncomfortable is difficult for you, but he needs to keep his splint on except when you bathe him or change his diaper."
4. "If he seems uncomfortable while wearing the splint, it's important that you call us immediately."

94. 3. Soft abduction devices, such as the Frejka splint, must be worn continually except for diaper changes and skin care. The abduction position must be maintained to establish a deep hip socket. Discomfort is anticipated; appropriate responses including changing position, holding, cuddling, and providing diversion.
CN: Physiological integrity; CNS: Physiological adaptation; CL: Application

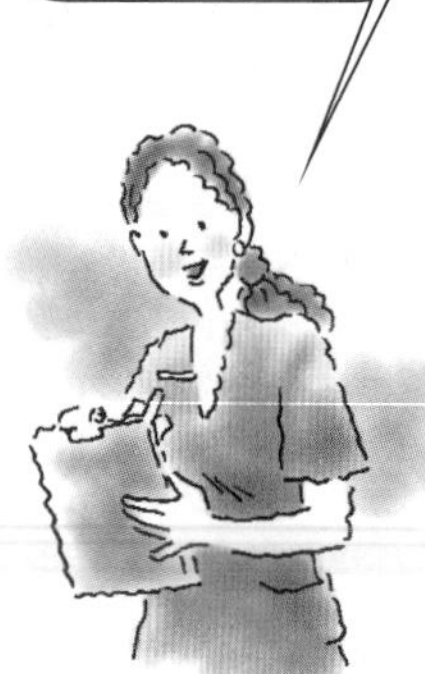

Questions 95 and 96 are asking you to prioritize!

95. A nurse is caring for a 2-year-old child who weighs 25 lb (11.3 kg) and has a simple fracture of his femur. For this client, which initial treatment is most likely?

1. Setting the fracture with a pin during surgery
2. Placing the child in skeletal traction
3. Immediately setting and casting the fractured leg
4. Putting the child in Bryant's traction

95. 4. Bryant's traction is the usual method for treating a child younger than age 3 and weighing less than 35 lb (15.9 kg). Surgery and pin placement is an invasive treatment that isn't usually needed. Skeletal traction is used for older children. For a femur fracture to heal properly, it usually requires traction before casting.
CN: Physiological integrity; CNS: Reduction of risk potential; CL: Application

96. A female client, age 15 months, has just had a hip-spica cast applied. Which nursing intervention is a priority for this client?

1. Limit fluids so she won't urinate often and won't risk getting the cast wet.
2. Instruct the parents on how to get their child home in the car.
3. Assess sensation, circulation, and motion of her feet and toes.
4. Avoid giving her pain medication so she won't become constipated.

96. 3. Assessing sensation, circulation, and motion is necessary in all children with a cast. Fluids should be encouraged; careful diapering and padding will keep the cast dry. Instructions about discharge can be shared with the parents at a later date. Children experiencing pain should receive medication as needed.
CN: Safe, effective care environment; CNS: Management of care; CL: Application

97. A male client, age 16, was injured in a motorcycle accident and fractured his left tibia and fibula. He's in a long leg cast and complains of deep pain unrelieved by analgesics. The physician must be notified immediately because the client may be exhibiting the signs and symptoms of which condition?

1. Volkmann's contracture
2. Dupuytren's contracture
3. Compartment syndrome
4. Peroneal nerve compression

97. 3. Deep pain unrelieved by analgesics is an important sign of compartment syndrome, which may occur with a crush injury or when a fracture is reduced. Compartment syndrome occurs when swelling associated with inflammation reduces blood flow to the affected areas; casting causes additional constriction of blood flow. Volkmann's contracture is a contraction of the fingers and sometimes the wrist that occurs after severe injury or improper use of a tourniquet or cast. Dupuytren's contracture is a flexion deformity of the fingers or toes caused by shortening, thickening, and fibrosis of the palmar or plantar fascia. Peroneal nerve compression is compression of the nerve that innervates the calf and foot.

CN: Physiological integrity; CNS: Physiological adaptation; CL: Analysis

98. A 6-year-old boy is admitted to a pediatric unit for treatment of osteomyelitis. The nurse knows that the peak incidence in children is between ages 1 and 12 and that boys are affected two to three times more commonly than girls. Which organism most commonly causes osteomyelitis?

1. *Staphylococcus epidermidis*
2. *Escherichia coli* O157.H7
3. *Pneumocystis carinii*
4. *Staphylococcus aureus*

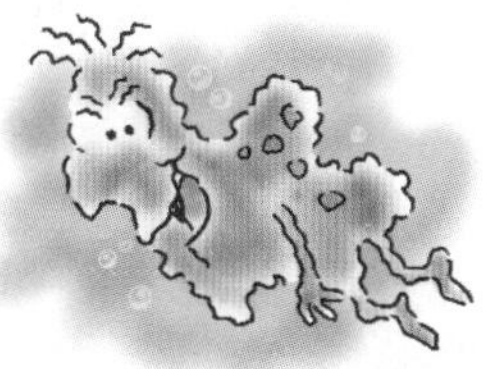
I admit it!
I'm the
common
cause.

98. 4. *S. aureus* is the most common causative pathogen of osteomyelitis; the usual source of the infection is an upper respiratory infection. *S. epidermidis* is a microorganism found on the skin of healthy individuals. *E. coli* O157.H7, which is in uncooked meat, can cause a severe case of diarrhea. *P. carinii* causes pneumonia in clients with human immunodeficiency virus or acquired immunodeficiency syndrome but doesn't normally cause healthy individuals to become ill.

CN: Physiological integrity; CNS: Physiological adaptation; CL: Application

99. A 14-year-old girl was recently fitted with a full back brace for scoliosis. Which response by the girl indicates she understands when she must wear the brace.

1. "I can leave the brace off for school parties."
2. "I have to wear the brace all the time, except when bathing."
3. "I can take the brace off for a couple of hours if my back starts to hurt."
4. "I only have to wear the brace for a couple of weeks."

99. 2. A brace must be worn at all times except for bathing. It can't be removed for other reasons including parties and discomfort. Most braces must be worn for several months to 1 year.

CN: Physiological integrity; CNS: Reduction of risk potential; CL: Analysis

100. A 16-year-old client had a full body cast applied 3 days ago. She's diaphoretic, tachycardic, and tachypneic. Which condition is the client most likely experiencing?

1. Pneumonia
2. Compartment syndrome
3. Anxiety
4. Decreased intestinal motility

100. 3. The client is exhibiting signs and symptoms of anxiety most likely caused by the feeling of being claustrophobic. Pneumonia usually presents with fever and coughing. A client with compartment syndrome would exhibit signs of intense pain unrelieved by analgesics. Compression of the mesenteric blood supply can cause constipation, but the symptoms don't indicate that constipation is the most likely condition.

CN: Psychological integrity; CNS: Psychological adaptation; CL: Analysis

101. A nurse is preparing to give an I.M. injection into the left leg of a 2-year-old client. Identify the area where the nurse would give the injection.

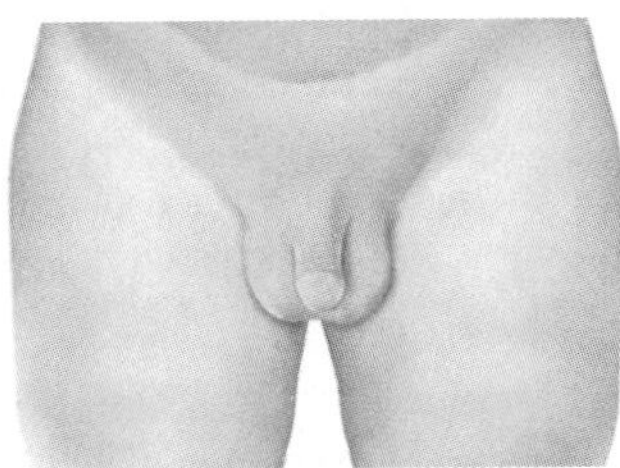

101. The vastus lateralis muscle, located in the thigh, is the muscle into which the nurse should administer an I.M. injection for a toddler. To give the injection, the nurse should first divide the distance between the greater trochanter and the knee joints into quadrants, then inject in the center of the upper quadrant.

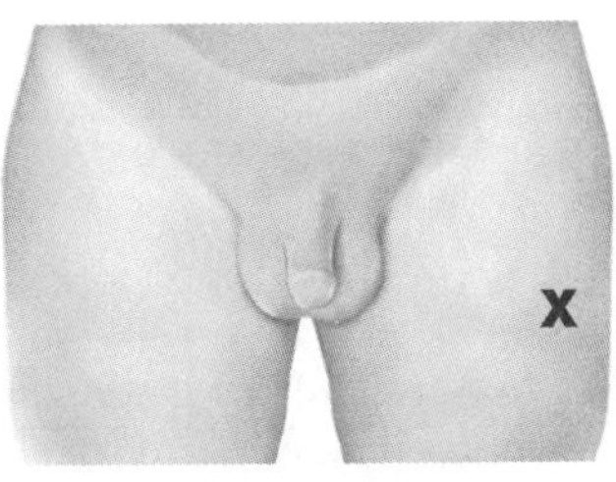
X

CN: Physiological integrity; CNS: Pharmacological and parenteral therapies; CL: Application

102. A nurse is caring for a 5-year-old client who's in the terminal stages of cancer. Which statements are true? Select all that apply:

1. The parents may be at different stages in dealing with the child's impending death.
2. The child is thinking about the future and knows he may not be able to participate.
3. The dying child may become clingy and act like a toddler.
4. Whispering in the child's room will help the child cope.
5. The death of a child may have long-term disruptive effects on the family.
6. The child doesn't fully understand the concept of death.

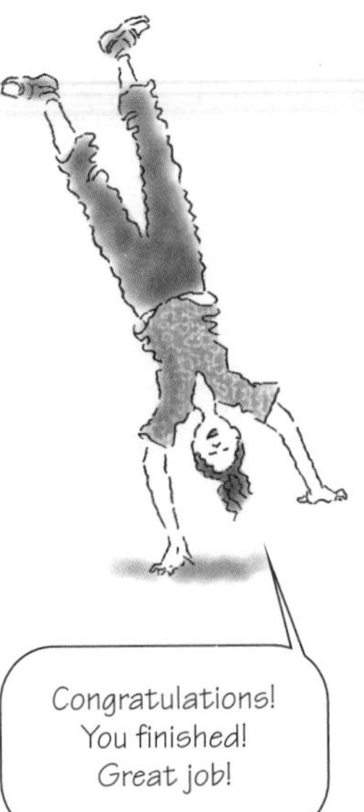
Congratulations!
You finished!
Great job!

102. 1, 3, 5, 6. When dealing with a dying child, parents may be at different stages of grief at different times. The child may regress in his behaviors. The stress of a child's death commonly results in divorce and behavioral problems in siblings. Preschoolers see death as temporary, a type of sleep or separation. They recognize the word "dead" but don't fully understand its meaning. Thinking about the future is typical of an adolescent facing death, not a preschooler. Whispering in front of the child only increases his fear of death.

CN: Psychosocial integrity; CNS: None; CL: Analysis

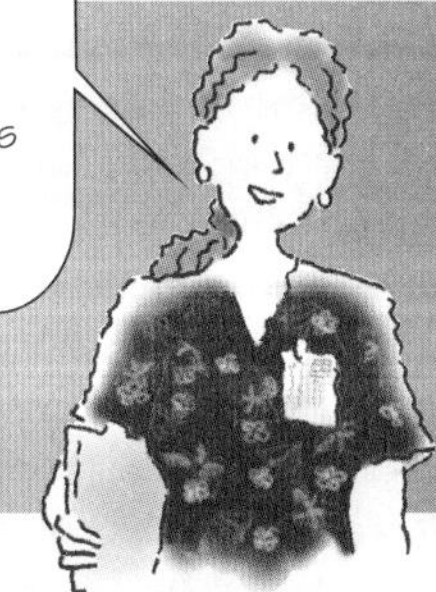

I'll bet that when you started nursing school, you had no idea kids could be subject to so many GI disorders. This chapter tests you on the most common ones. Good luck!

Chapter 32 Gastrointestinal disorders

1. Which statement by the mother of a child with celiac disease indicates an understanding of a nurse's dietary counseling?
1. "I won't serve wheat, rye, oats, or barley."
2. "I will provide a diet high in gluten."
3. "I won't serve potatoes, rice, or flour."
4. "I can safely serve any frozen or packaged food."

1. 1. The child with celiac disease should consume a gluten-free diet, thus eliminating foods containing wheat, rye, oats, and barley. Foods containing potatoes, rice, and flour are permissible. The mother should read the packages of all foods carefully to ensure that they're gluten-free.

CN: Physiological integrity; CNS: Basic care and comfort; CL: Application

2. Which goal is <u>most important</u> when teaching the parents of a child diagnosed with celiac disease?
1. Promote a normal life for the child.
2. Stress the importance of good health in preventing infection.
3. Introduce the parents and child to a peer with celiac disease.
4. Help the parents and child follow the prescribed dietary restrictions.

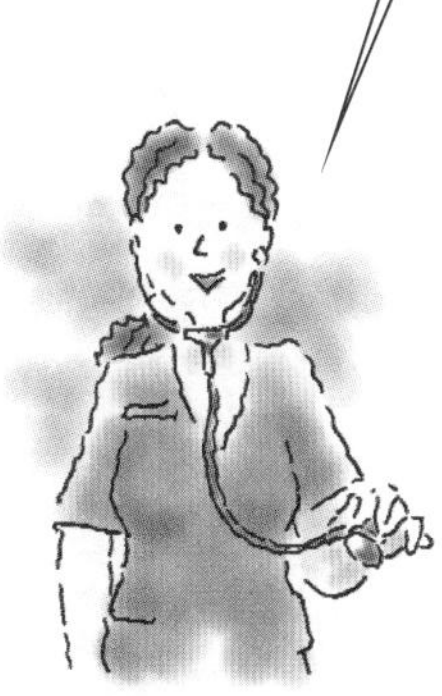

In question 2, the words most important guide you to the right answer.

2. 4. It takes a long time to describe the disease process, the specific role of gluten, and the foods that must be restricted. Gluten is added to many foods but is obscurely listed on labels. To avoid hidden sources of gluten, parents need to read labels carefully. Promoting a normal life for the child, stressing good health in preventing infection, and meeting a peer with celiac disease are also important nursing considerations, but they would come after the dietary means of dealing with this chronic disease.

CN: Physiological integrity; CNS: Reduction of risk potential; CL: Analysis

3. What characteristic stool would a nurse expect to find in a child diagnosed with celiac disease?
1. Constipated hard stool
2. Clay-colored stool
3. Red currant jelly stool
4. Foul-smelling, fatty, frothy stool

3. 4. Steatorrhea (fatty, foul-smelling frothy, bulky stools) is common because of the inability to absorb fat. Profuse and watery diarrhea, not constipated hard stool, is usually a sign or celiac crisis. Clay-colored stools are characteristic of a decrease or absence of conjugated bilirubin. Red currant jelly type stool is an indication of intussusception.

CN: Physiological integrity; CNS: Physiological adaptation; CL: Application

4. A client with celiac disease is being discharged from the hospital. Which food item should be included in his diet?
1. Oatmeal cereal
2. Sliced pepperoni
3. Cheese pizza
4. Rice

4. 4. Sources of gluten found in wheat, rye, barley, and oats should be avoided. Rice and corn are suitable substitutes because they don't contain gluten. Pizza, luncheon meat, and cereal contain gluten and, when broken down, can't be digested by people with celiac disease.

CN: Physiological integrity; CNS: Basic care and comfort; CL: Application

CN: Client needs category CNS: Client needs subcategory CL: Cognitive level

5. To help promote a normal life for a child with celiac disease, which intervention should his parents use?

1. Treat the child differently from other siblings.
2. Focus on restrictions that make him feel different.
3. Introduce the child to another peer with celiac disease.
4. Don't allow the child to express doubt in keeping with dietary restrictions.

5. 3. Introducing the child to another child with celiac disease will let him know he isn't alone. It will show him how other people live a normal life with similar restrictions. Treat the child no differently from other siblings, but stress appropriate limit setting. Instead of focusing on restrictions that make him feel different, the nurse should encourage the parents to focus on ways he can be normal. Allow the child with celiac disease to express his feelings about dietary restrictions.

CN: Psychosocial integrity; CNS: None; CL: Application

You'll be finished before you know it!

6. Which assessment should a nurse make to evaluate the effectiveness of nutritional therapy for a child with celiac disease?

1. Vital signs
2. Appearance, size, and number of stools
3. Blood urea nitrogen (BUN) and serum creatinine levels
4. Intake and output

6. 2. The fat, bulky, foul-smelling stools should be gone when a child with celiac disease follows a gluten-free diet. Vital signs, BUN and serum creatinine levels, and intake and output aren't affected by a gluten-free diet.

CN: Physiological integrity; CNS: Basic care and comfort; CL: Analysis

7. Within 1 or 2 days after starting their prescribed diet, most children with celiac disease show which characteristic?

1. Diarrhea
2. Foul-smelling stools
3. Improved appetite
4. Weight loss

7. 3. Within a day or two of starting their diet, most children with celiac disease show improved appetite, disappearance of diarrhea, and weight gain. It takes longer than 2 days for steatorrhea (fatty, oily, foul-smelling stools) to subside.

CN: Physiological integrity; CNS: Physiological adaptation; CL: Application

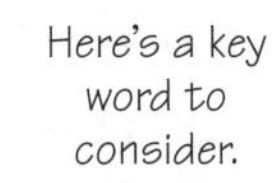

Here's a key word to consider.

8. In caring for a neonate with cleft lip and palate, which issue is <u>first</u> encountered by the nurse?

1. Feeding difficulties
2. Operative care
3. Pain management
4. Parental reaction

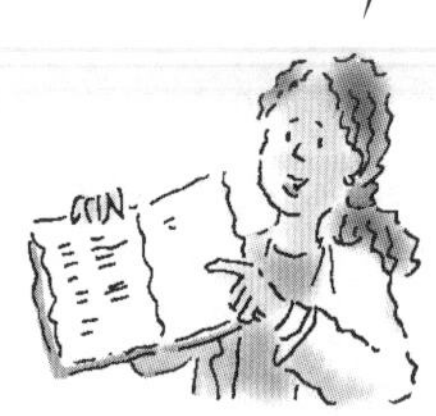

8. 4. Parents typically show strong negative responses to this deformity. They may mourn the loss of the perfect child. Helping the parents cope with their child's condition is the first step. Feeding issues are important, but parents must first cope with the reality of their neonate's condition. Surgical repair is usually delayed until 6 to 12 weeks of age. This deformity isn't painful.

CN: Psychosocial integrity; CNS: None; CL: Analysis

9. To prevent trauma to the suture line of an infant who underwent cleft lip repair, a nurse should perform which intervention?

1. Place mittens on the infant's hands.
2. Maintain arm restraints.
3. Not allow the parents to touch the infant.
4. Remove the lip device from the infant after surgery.

9. 2. Arm restraints are used to prevent the infant from rubbing the sutures. Placing mittens alone won't prevent the infant from rubbing the suture line. Parental contact will increase the infant's comfort. The lip device shouldn't be removed.

CN: Physiological integrity; CNS: Reduction of risk potential; CL: Analysis

10. To prevent tissue infection and breakdown after cleft palate or lip repair, a nurse should use which intervention?

1. Keep the suture line moist at all times.
2. Allow the infant to suck on his pacifier.
3. Rinse the infant's mouth with water after each feeding.
4. Follow orders from the physician to not feed the infant by mouth.

10. 3. To prevent formula buildup around the suture line, the mouth is usually rinsed. The sutures should be kept dry at all times. Placing objects in the mouth is generally avoided after surgery. Infants are fed by mouth using the syringe technique.

CN: Physiological integrity; CNS: Physiological adaptation; CL: Analysis

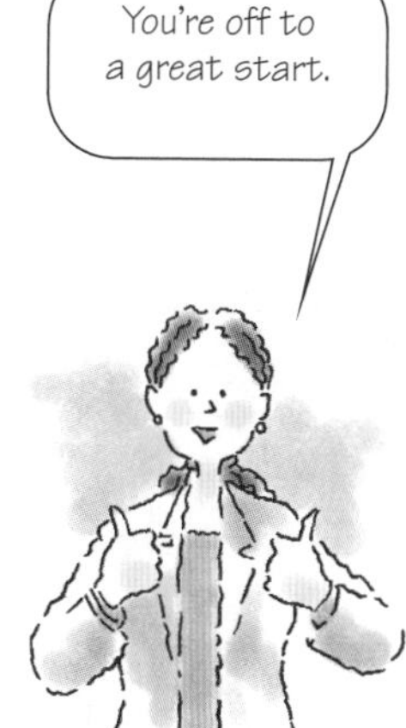
You're off to a great start.

11. Which nursing intervention has the highest priority in an infant during the first 24 hours after surgery for cleft lip repair?

1. Carefully clean the suture line using sterile technique after feedings to reduce the risk of infection.
2. Position the infant in the prone position after feedings to promote drainage.
3. Allow the infant to cry to promote lung expansion.
4. Encourage the infant to use a pacifier to satisfy the urge to suck.

11. 1. The suture line must be cleaned after each feeding to reduce the risk of infection, which could adversely affect the healing and cosmetic results. The incision should be cleaned carefully so the sutures are not disrupted. A sterile solution should be used to reduce the risk of infection. The infant shouldn't be placed on his abdomen in the prone position because this puts pressure on the incision and may affect healing. Anticipatory care should be provided to reduce the risk of the infant crying, which puts pressure on the incision. Pacifiers and other firm objects shouldn't be placed in the infant's mouth because they can disrupt the suture line.

CN: Physiological integrity; CNS: Reduction of risk potential; CL: Application

12. When bottle-feeding an infant with a cleft palate or lip, gentle steady pressure should be applied to the base of the bottle for which reason?

1. To reduce the risk of choking or coughing
2. To prevent further damage to the affected area
3. To decrease the amount of formula lost while eating
4. To decrease the amount of noise the infant makes when eating

12. 1. Children with cleft palate or lip have a greater risk of choking while eating, so all measures are used to reduce this risk. Steady pressure creates a seal when the nipple is against the cleft palate or lip, reducing the risk of aspiration. The nurse can't cause more damage to an infant's cleft lip or palate unless proper precautions aren't followed postoperatively. If the nipple is cut correctly and proper procedures are followed, the infant won't lose a lot of formula during a feeding. Infants with cleft palate or lip usually make more noise while eating.

CN: Physiological integrity; CNS: Reduction of risk potential; CL: Application

13. Which nursing intervention should be used when feeding an infant with cleft lip and palate?

1. Burp the infant often.
2. Limit the amount the infant eats.
3. Feed the infant at scheduled times.
4. Remove the nipple if the infant is making loud noises.

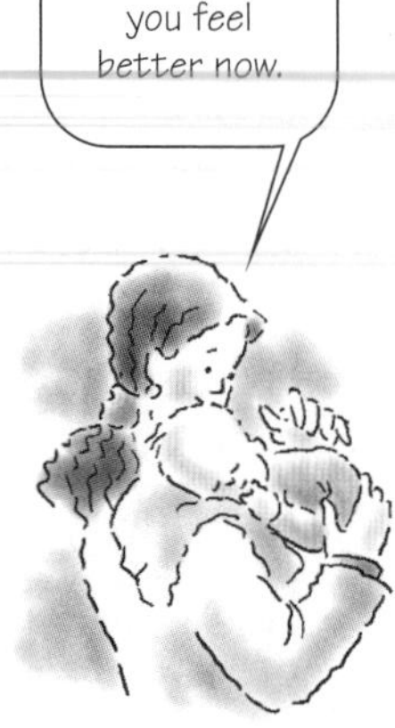

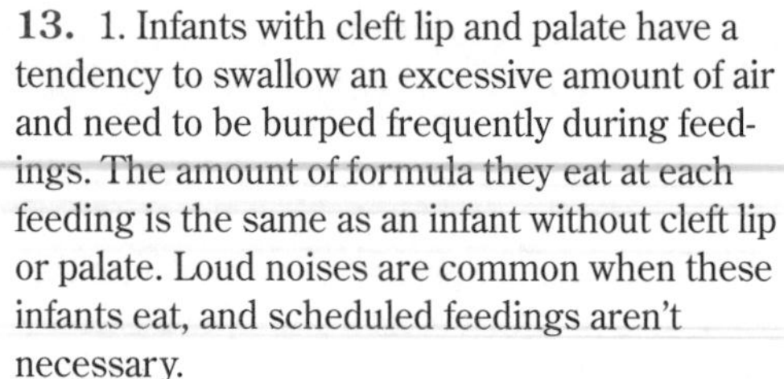

13. 1. Infants with cleft lip and palate have a tendency to swallow an excessive amount of air and need to be burped frequently during feedings. The amount of formula they eat at each feeding is the same as an infant without cleft lip or palate. Loud noises are common when these infants eat, and scheduled feedings aren't necessary.
CN: Physiological integrity; CNS: Physiological adaptation; CL: Application

14. Which intervention is essential in the nursing care of an infant with cleft lip or palate?

1. Discourage breast-feeding.
2. Hold the infant flat while feeding.
3. Involve the parents as soon as possible.
4. Use a normal nursery nipple for feedings.

14. 3. The sooner the parents become involved, the quicker they're able to determine the method of feeding best suited for them and the infant. Breast-feeding, like bottle-feeding, may be difficult but can be facilitated if the mother intends to breast-feed. Feedings are usually given in the upright position to prevent formula from coming through the nose. Various special nipples have been devised for infants with cleft lip or palate; a normal nursery nipple isn't effective. Sometimes, especially if the cleft isn't severe, breast-feeding may be easier because the human nipple conforms to the shape of the infant's mouth.
CN: Physiological integrity; CNS: Physiological adaptation; CL: Application

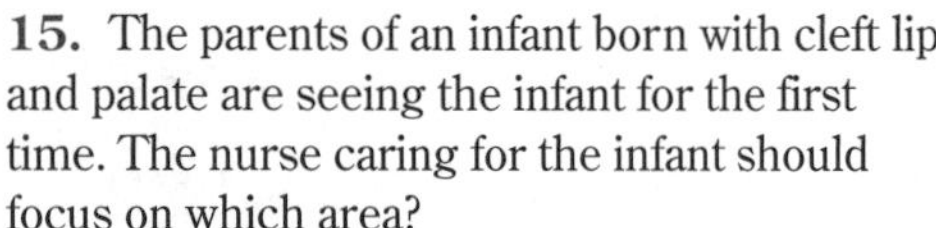

15. The parents of an infant born with cleft lip and palate are seeing the infant for the first time. The nurse caring for the infant should focus on which area?

1. The infant's positive features
2. Irritation with how the infant eats
3. Ambivalence in caring for an infant with this defect
4. Dissatisfaction with the infant's physical appearance

15. 1. To relieve the parents' anxiety, positive aspects of the infant's physical appearance need to be emphasized. Showing optimism toward surgical correction and showing a photograph of possible cosmetic improvements may be helpful. Because this is the parents' first encounter with the infant, there isn't any indication of irritation, ambivalence, or dissatisfaction.
CN: Psychosocial integrity; CNS: None; CL: Application

16. Following repair of a cleft lip in a 3-month-old, the mother asks the nurse what would be the most appropriate toy to bring the infant. Which toy should the nurse recommend?

1. A plastic teething ring
2. A stuffed animal
3. A mobile to hang over the crib
4. Children's books

16. 3. Given the infant's age, a mobile would be the most appropriate toy because he doesn't have the manual dexterity to play with a stuffed animal. The mobile would provide the infant with visual stimulation. A plastic teething ring and a stuffed animal should be avoided because they can disrupt the suture line if the infant sucks on them. The infant wouldn't be able to understand children's stories but may enjoy the sound of another person's voice. A mobile, however, could be used when no one was around to read.
CN: Physiological integrity; CNS: None; CL: Analysis

CN: Client needs category CNS: Client needs subcategory CL: Cognitive level

17. The mother of a neonate born with a cleft lip and palate is preparing to feed him for the first time. Which intervention should the nurse teach the mother first?

1. Burp the neonate.
2. Clean the mouth.
3. Hold the neonate in an upright position.
4. Prepare the bottle using a normal nursery nipple.

17. 3. When neonates are held in the upright position, the formula is less likely to leak out of the nose or mouth. Neonates need to be burped frequently but not before a feeding. There's no need to clean the mouth before eating. After surgical repair, the mouth is cleaned at the suture site to prevent infection. The bottle should be prepared using a special nipple or feeding device.
CN: Physiological integrity; CNS: Physiological adaptation; CL: Application

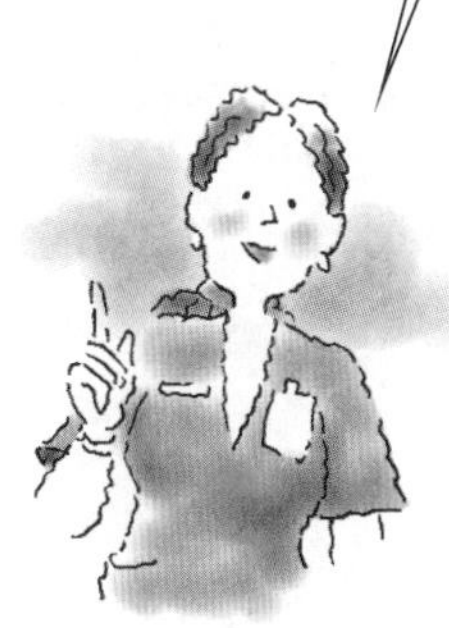

There are many things to teach this mother, so what do you teach her first?

18. An infant returns from surgery after repair of a cleft palate. Which nursing intervention should be done first?

1. Offer a pacifier for comfort.
2. Position the infant on his side.
3. Suction the mouth and nose of all secretions.
4. Remove the arm restraints placed on the infant after surgery.

18. 2. The infant should be positioned on his side to allow oral secretions to drain from the mouth and avoid suctioning. Pacifiers shouldn't be used because they can damage the suture line. Arm restraints should be kept on to protect the suture line. The restraints should be removed periodically to allow for full range of motion during this time. Only one restraint should be removed at a time, and the infant should be closely supervised.
CN: Physiological integrity; CNS: Reduction of risk potential; CL: Analysis

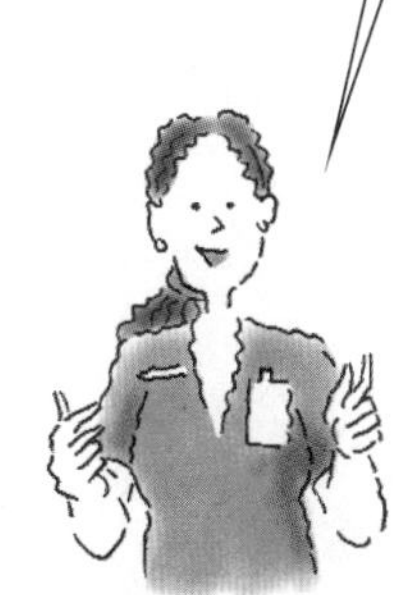

Client teaching includes the family.

19. A small child has just had surgical repair of a cleft palate. Which instruction should be included in the discharge teaching to his parents?

1. Continue a normal diet.
2. Continue using arm restraints at home.
3. Don't allow the child to drink from a cup.
4. Establish good mouth care and proper brushing.

19. 2. Arm restraints are also used at home to keep the child's hands away from the mouth until the palate is healed. A soft diet is recommended; no food harder than mashed potatoes can be eaten. Fluids are best taken from a cup. Proper mouth care is encouraged after the palate is healed.
CN: Physiological integrity; CNS: Physiological adaptation; CL: Application

20. In which position should a nurse place an infant following cleft lip and palate repair to irrigate the mouth after feeding?

1. Supine with the head to the side
2. Fowler's position with the head to the side
3. Upright with the head tilted forward
4. Prone with the head over the side of the bed

20. 3. Following repair of a cleft palate, the nurse should irrigate the infant's mouth with the infant in an upright position and head tilted forward to prevent aspiration. A supine or Fowler's position with the head to the side won't prevent aspiration. The prone position isn't appropriate following cleft lip repair because this may put pressure on the suture line.
CN: Physiological integrity; CNS: Reduction of risk potential; CL: Application

21. After an infant with a cleft lip has surgical repair and heals, the nurse would instruct the parents that they may see:

1. a large scar on the lip.
2. an abnormally large upper lip.
3. a distorted jaw.
4. minimal scarring.

21. 4. If there's no trauma or infection to the site, healing occurs with little scar formation. There may be some inflammation right after surgery, but after healing, the lip is a normal size. No jaw malformation occurs with cleft lip repair.
CN: Physiological integrity; CNS: Physiological adaptation; CL: Application

22. The nurse would explain to the parents of a newborn with a cleft lip and palate that they will need to schedule an appointment with which specialist?

1. Cardiologist
2. Neurologist
3. Nutritionist
4. Otolaryngologist

22. 4. An otolaryngologist is used because ear infections are common, along with hearing loss. Cardiac and brain function is usually normal. A nutritionist isn't needed unless the neonate becomes malnourished.

CN: Safe, effective care environment; CNS: Management of care; CL: Application

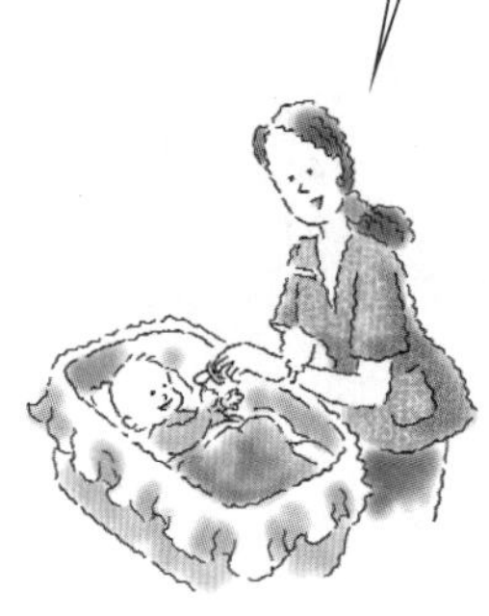

This will help satisfy the infant's need to suck.

23. Which sign should alert a nurse to dehydration in a neonate with esophageal atresia and tracheoesophageal fistula?

1. Bulging eyeballs
2. Sunken anterior fontanelle
3. Skin that returns briskly when pinched
4. Weight gain

23. 2. A sunken anterior fontanelle is a sign of dehydration in the neonate whose fontanelle hasn't yet closed. Bulging eyeballs and weight gain are signs of overhydration. Skin that returns quickly when pinched is a sign of adequate hydration.

CN: Physiological integrity; CNS: Reduction of risk potential; CL: Application

24. Feedings are being withheld in a neonate with esophageal atresia and tracheoesophageal fistula until a gastrostomy tube can be placed. Which nursing action would be most appropriate when the neonate is irritable and crying?

1. Offer him a pacifier.
2. Encourage his parents to talk to him.
3. Encourage his parents to hold him.
4. Distract him by placing a mobile over the crib.

24. 1. A neonate who's unable to suck to obtain nutrition may be comforted if given a pacifier to satisfy his need to suck. Encouraging his parents to hold and talk to him and placing a mobile over the crib are appropriate interventions but won't satisfy a newborn as much as a pacifier.

CN: Physiological integrity; CNS: Basic care and comfort; CL: Analysis

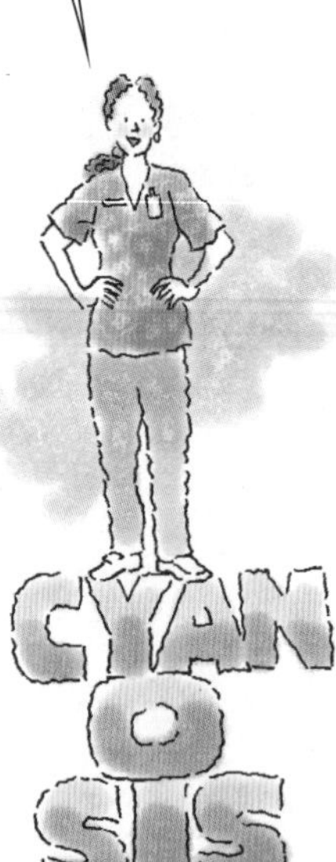

25. Which finding indicates to a nurse that a neonate born with esophageal atresia needs suctioning?

1. Cyanosis
2. Decreased production of saliva
3. Inability to cough
4. Inadequate swallow

25. 1. Cyanosis occurs when fluid from the blind pouch is aspirated into the trachea, requiring suctioning. Increased saliva production is common, along with choking, coughing, and sneezing. The ability to swallow isn't affected by this disorder.

CN: Physiological integrity; CNS: Physiological adaptation; CL: Analysis

26. For a neonate suspected of having esophageal atresia, a definitive diagnostic evaluation would include which factor?

1. Decreased breath sounds
2. Absence of bowel sounds
3. How the neonate tolerates eating
4. Ability to pass a catheter down the esophagus

26. 4. A moderately stiff catheter will meet resistance if the esophagus is blocked and will pass unobstructed if the esophagus is patent. Breath sounds are normal unless aspiration occurs. The intestinal tract isn't affected with this anomaly, so bowel sounds are present. If a neonate doesn't tolerate eating, it doesn't mean he has an esophageal atresia.

CN: Physiological integrity; CNS: Physiological adaptation; CL: Analysis

27. For a neonate diagnosed with a tracheoesophageal fistula, which intervention would be needed?

1. Start antibiotic therapy.
2. Keep the neonate lying flat.
3. Continue feedings.
4. Remove the diagnostic catheter from the esophagus.

27. 1. Antibiotic therapy is started because aspiration pneumonia is inevitable and appears early. The neonate's head is usually kept in an upright position to prevent aspiration. I.V. fluids are started, and the neonate isn't allowed oral intake. The catheter is left in the upper esophageal pouch to easily remove fluid that collects there.

CN: Physiological integrity; CNS: Pharmacological and parenteral therapies; CL: Analysis

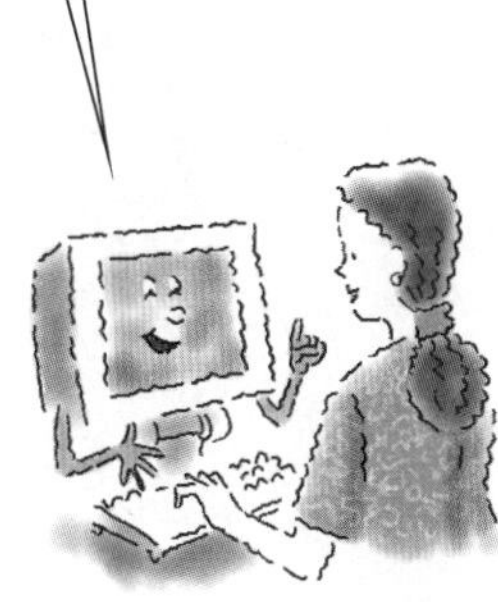

Question 28 asks you to prioritize your care.

28. When tracheoesophageal fistula or esophageal atresia is suspected, which nursing intervention should be done first?

1. Give oxygen.
2. Tell the parents.
3. Put the neonate in an Isolette or on a radiant warmer.
4. Report the suspicion to the physician.

28. 4. The physician needs to be told so that immediate diagnostic tests can be done for a definitive diagnosis and surgical correction. Oxygen should be given only after notifying the physician, except in the case of an emergency. It isn't the nurse's responsibility to inform the parents of the suspected finding. By the time tracheoesophageal fistula or esophageal atresia is suspected, the neonate would have already been placed in an Isolette or a radiant warmer.

CN: Physiological integrity; CNS: Physiological adaptation; CL: Analysis

29. Which complication may follow the surgical repair of a tracheoesophageal fistula?

1. Atelectasis
2. Choking during feeding attempts
3. Damaged vocal cords
4. Infection

29. 1. Respiratory complications (atelectasis) are a threat to the neonate's life preoperatively and postoperatively because of the continual risk of aspiration. Choking is more likely to occur preoperatively, although careful attention is paid postoperatively when neonates begin to eat to make sure they can swallow without choking. Vocal cord damage isn't common after this repair. The neonate is generally given antibiotics preoperatively to prevent infection.

CN: Physiological integrity; CNS: Physiological adaptation; CL: Analysis

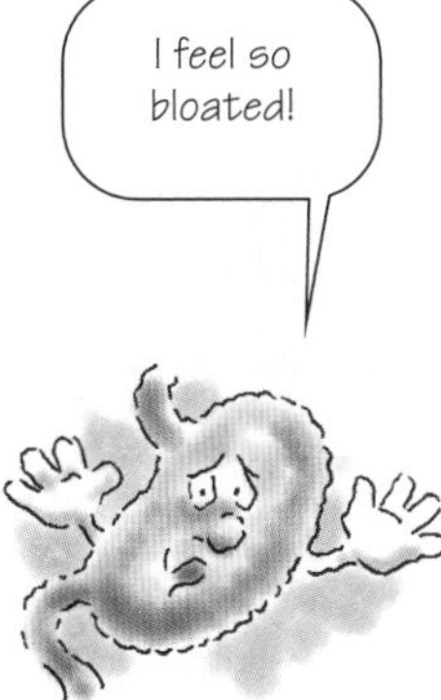

I feel so bloated!

30. The nurse is caring for an infant suspected of having esophageal atresia and tracheoesophageal fistula. Which sign would the nurse initially observe?

1. Abdominal distention
2. Decreased oral secretions
3. Normal respiratory effort
4. Scaphoid abdomen

30. 1. Crying may force air into the stomach, causing distention. Secretions in a client with this condition may be more visible, though normal in quantity, because of the client's inability to swallow effectively. Respiratory effort is usually more difficult. When no distal fistula is present, the abdomen will appear scaphoid.

CN: Physiological integrity; CNS: Physiological adaptation; CL: Application

31. Dietary management in a child diagnosed with ulcerative colitis should include which diet?

1. High-calorie diet
2. High-residue diet
3. Low-protein diet
4. Low-salt diet

31. 1. A high-calorie diet is given to combat weight loss and restore nitrogen balance. A low-residue or residue-free diet is encouraged to decrease bowel irritation. A high-protein diet is also encouraged. Salt reduction isn't a factor in this disease.

CN: Physiological integrity; CNS: Basic care and comfort; CL: Analysis

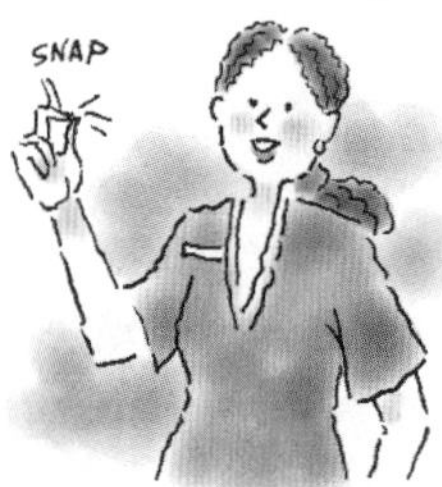
Immediately means, you know, right away!
SNAP

32. A neonate comes back from the operating room after surgical repair of a tracheoesophageal fistula and esophageal atresia. Which intervention is done <u>immediately</u>?

1. Maintain a patent airway.
2. Start feedings right away.
3. Let the parents hold the neonate right away.
4. Suction the endotracheal tube, stopping when resistance is met.

32. 1. Maintaining a patent airway is essential until sedation from surgery wears off. Feedings usually aren't started for at least 48 hours after surgery. Parents are encouraged to participate in the neonate's care, but not immediately after surgery. The catheter should be measured before suctioning so the tube doesn't meet resistance, which could cause damage.

CN: Safe, effective care environment; CNS: Management of care; CL: Application

33. Which discharge instruction should a nurse give the parents following repair of tracheoesophageal fistula and esophageal atresia in a neonate?

1. Give antibiotics through the feeding tube.
2. Maintain proper care of a chest tube.
3. Maintain proper positioning for feedings.
4. Utilize tips for preventing crying.

33. 3. The neonate should be kept in an upright position after feeding to reduce the risk of refluxed stomach contents and aspiration pneumonia. Although antibiotics are given after surgery, they're discontinued before discharge. Because the chest cavity is entered during surgery, the neonate may have a chest tube inserted that's removed prior to discharge. Because lung expansion is important following chest surgery, vigorous crying helps expand the lungs and shouldn't be discouraged.

CN: Physiological integrity; CNS: Basic care and comfort; CL: Application

34. Which nursing intervention should be done postoperatively for a neonate after repair of tracheoesophageal fistula and esophageal atresia?

1. Withhold mouth care.
2. Offer a pacifier frequently.
3. Decrease tactile stimulation.
4. Use restraints to prevent injury to the repair.

34. 2. Meeting the neonate's oral needs, such as by offering him a pacifier, is important because he can't drink from a bottle. The nurse should give mouth care to this neonate. The nurse should provide tactile stimulation. Restraints should be avoided, if possible.

CN: Physiological integrity; CNS: Physiological adaptation; CL: Application

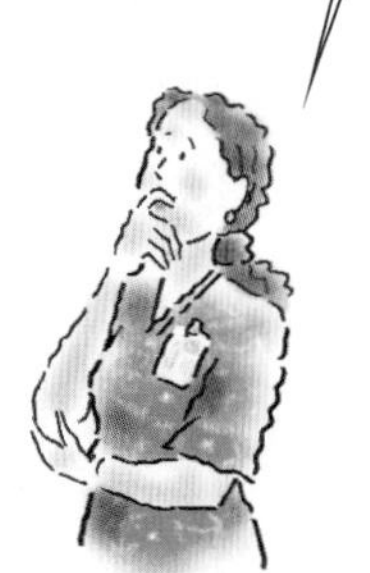
Hmmm. Now I have to think long term.

35. A client is admitted with a history of tracheoesophageal fistula and esophageal atresia repair. The nurse should evaluate this client for which potential <u>long-term</u> postoperative complication?

1. Oral aversion
2. Gastroesophageal reflux
3. Inability to tolerate feedings
4. Strictures

35. 4. Strictures of the anastomosis occur in 40% to 50% of the cases. Oral aversion can be a problem, but it occurs quickly after surgery. Reflux is a common complication but appears when feedings are started. If the neonate is having problems tolerating feedings, it's quickly noted.

CN: Physiological integrity; CNS: Physiological adaptation; CL: Application

36. The nurse would suspect which structural defect if she observes that a neonate has excessive salivation and drooling, accompanied by coughing, choking, and sneezing?

1. Cleft lip
2. Cleft palate
3. Gastroschisis
4. Tracheoesophageal fistula and esophageal atresia

36. 4. Because tracheoesophageal fistula and esophageal atresia cause an ineffective swallow, saliva and secretions appear in the mouth and around the lips. Coughing, choking, and sneezing occur for the same reason and usually after an attempt at eating. Cleft lip and palate don't produce excessive salivation. None of these symptoms occurs with gastroschisis.

CN: Physiological integrity; CNS: Physiological adaptation; CL: Application

37. Which nursing diagnosis takes the highest priority during the first 24 hours following surgical repair of esophageal atresia and tracheoesophageal fistula?

1. *Ineffective airway clearance*
2. *Imbalanced nutrition: Less than body requirements*
3. *Risk for impaired parenting*
4. *Ineffective infant feeding pattern*

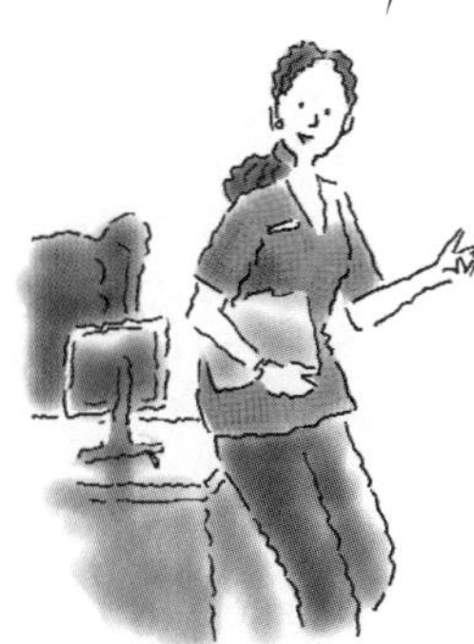

Think surgery for an esophageal disorder, and then prioritize.

37. 1. The priority nursing diagnosis for the first postoperative day is *Ineffective airway clearance.* The nurse must assess the infant's airway for the buildup of mucus and other secretions. The nurse must also perform a respiratory assessment and keep suction equipment, a laryngoscope, and endotracheal suction equipment immediately available. The other nursing diagnoses are all important in the infant in the immediate postoperative period, but assessing and maintaining a patent airway is the greatest priority.

CN: Physiological integrity; CNS: Reduction or risk potential; CL: Analysis

38. An infant was born with a portion of an organ protruding through an abnormal opening. The nurse would explain to the parents that this structural defect is which condition?

1. Cleft lip
2. Cleft palate
3. Gastroschisis
4. Tracheoesophageal fistula

38. 3. Gastroschisis is a herniation of the bowel through an abnormal opening in the abdominal wall. Cleft lip and palate are facial malformations, not herniations. Tracheoesophageal fistula is a malformation of the trachea and esophagus.

CN: Physiological integrity; CNS: Physiological adaptation; CL: Application

39. When an infant is diagnosed with a diaphragmatic hernia on the left side, which abdominal organ may be found in the thorax?

1. Appendix
2. Descending colon
3. Right kidney
4. Spleen

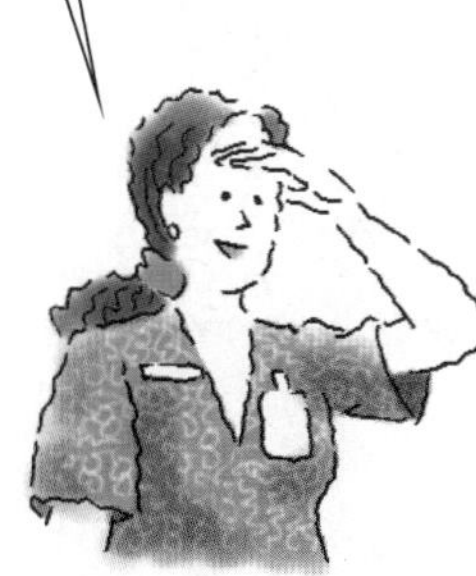

39. 4. The spleen has commonly been seen in the thorax of infants with this defect. The appendix and descending colon usually don't protrude into the thorax because of limited space from the other organs present. The right kidney wouldn't be seen with a left-sided defect.

CN: Physiological integrity; CNS: Physiological adaptation; CL: Analysis

40. In which direction does the mediastinum shift in an infant diagnosed with a diaphragmatic hernia?

1. No shift
2. Shifts to the affected side
3. Shifts to the unaffected side
4. Partial shifts to the affected or unaffected sides

40. 3. The increased volume in the chest cavity from the abdominal organs causes the mediastinum to shift to the unaffected side, which causes a partial collapse of that lung. Because of the increased volume on the affected side, the mediastinum can't shift that way.

CN: Physiological integrity; CNS: Physiological adaptation; CL: Analysis

41. Which is the best way to position an infant with a diaphragmatic hernia before surgery?
1. On the affected side
2. On the unaffected side
3. Supine
4. Trendelenburg's position

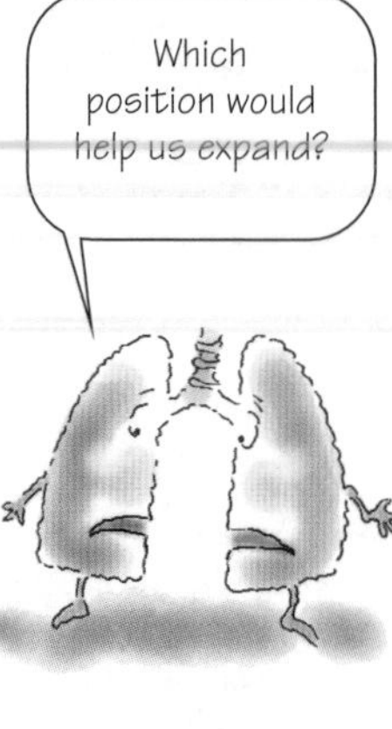

Which position would help us expand?

41. 1. Positioning the infant on the affected side lets the lung on the unaffected side expand, making breathing easier. Positioning the infant on the unaffected side or in Trendelenburg's position would further diminish respiration and would increase pressure in the chest cavity, compromising respirations. Supine position doesn't facilitate lung expansion.
CN: Physiological integrity; CNS: Basic care and comfort; CL: Analysis

42. Before surgery, which intervention should be used for an infant with a diaphragmatic hernia?
1. Feed the infant.
2. Provide tactile stimulation.
3. Prevent the infant from crying.
4. Place the infant on the unaffected side.

42. 3. To prevent the intestines from being pulled into the chest cavity by the negative pressure caused by crying, it should be avoided. The stomach and intestine in the chest cavity may also become distended with swallowed air from crying. The infant usually isn't fed until after surgery. Tactile stimulation is limited because it may disturb the infant's fragile condition. The infant is always placed on the affected side.
CN: Physiological integrity; CNS: Physiological adaptation; CL: Application

43. Which action by the nurse is essential when caring for a neonate with an omphalocele?
1. Keep the omphalocele dry.
2. Don't let the parents see the omphalocele.
3. Carefully position and handle the omphalocele.
4. Touch the omphalocele often to assess any changes.

43. 3. Careful positioning and handling prevent infection and rupture of the omphalocele. The omphalocele is kept moist until the neonate is taken to the operating room. The parents can see the defect if they so choose. Touching it often increases the risk of infection.
CN: Physiological integrity; CNS: Physiological adaptation; CL: Application

44. Which toy would be most appropriate for a nurse to give to an 8-month-old admitted for repair of a diaphragmatic hernia?
1. Large crayons and a coloring book
2. Colorful, plastic, multitextured rattle
3. Black-and-white mobile
4. Colorful pull toys

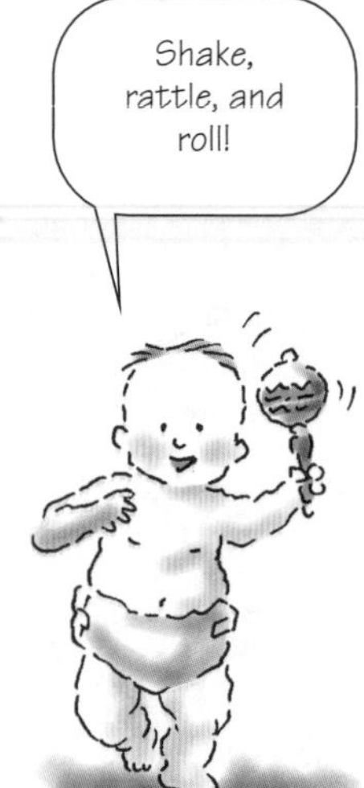

Shake, rattle, and roll!

44. 2. By 8 months old, an infant can transfer toys and enjoys different textures, making a colorful plastic rattle with different textures an age-appropriate toy. Because infants at this age still put objects in their mouths, crayons wouldn't be appropriate. Newborns enjoy the visual stimulation of black-and-white mobiles. Pull toys are appropriate for the toddler who's walking.
CN: Health promotion and maintenance; CNS: None; CL: Analysis

CN: Client needs category CNS: Client needs subcategory CL: Cognitive level

45. Which nursing intervention is most appropriate when an adolescent with a nasogastric (NG) tube in place following surgery for a ruptured appendix reports feeling nauseated?
1. Provide oral hygiene.
2. Measure the gastric drainage.
3. Assess serum electrolytes.
4. Irrigate the tube.

45. 4. When a client with an NG tube complains of nausea, the nurse should first determine the position of the tube and then irrigate it to check for patency. A clogged tube allows contents to accumulate in the stomach, contributing to nausea. Oral hygiene is important to promote comfort but isn't the most appropriate intervention here. Measuring the gastric drainage is important but won't relieve nausea. Serum electrolytes should be monitored in the client with an NG tube. Although an electrolyte imbalance may cause nausea, the tube should first be checked for patency.
CN: Physiological integrity; CNS: Reduction of risk potential; CL: Application

46. Which nursing intervention is most appropriate for a 1-month-old infant with pyloric stenosis who's vomiting?
1. Place the infant in a supine position to sleep.
2. Weigh the infant every 8 hours.
3. Assess for signs of dehydration.
4. Assess vital signs every 8 hours.

46. 3. Because the infant is vomiting, the nurse should assess for signs and symptoms of dehydration. The infant should be placed on the right side to sleep to prevent aspiration of vomitus. The infant should be weighed daily, not every 8 hours. Vital signs should be assessed every 4 hours until stable.
CN: Physiological integrity; CNS: Reduction of risk potential; CL: Application

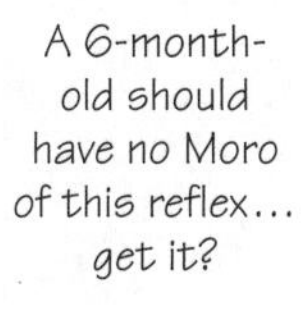

A 6-month-old should have no Moro of this reflex… get it?

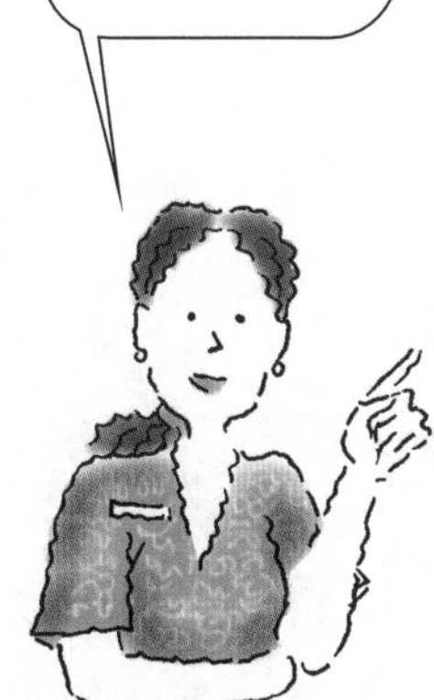

47. Which sign noted during an admission assessment of a 6-month-old infant admitted for intestinal obstruction should alert the nurse to a potential problem?
1. Moro reflex
2. Playing with feet
3. Eruption of the first tooth
4. Rolling from stomach to back

47. 1. By 6 months of age, the Moro reflex should no longer be observed. Playing with the feet, eruption of the first tooth, and rolling from stomach to back are all normal for a 6-month-old infant.
CN: Health promotion and maintenance; CNS: None; CL: Analysis

48. The nurse explains to an infant's parents that the pyloric canal narrows in clients with pyloric stenosis at:
1. the stomach and esophagus.
2. the stomach and duodenum.
3. both the stomach and esophagus and the stomach and duodenum.
4. neither the stomach and esophagus nor the stomach and duodenum.

48. 2. The narrowing of the pyloric canal occurs between the stomach and duodenum, where the pyloric sphincter is located. Hyperplasia and hypertrophy cause narrowing and, possibly, obstruction of the circular muscle of the pylorus.
CN: Physiological integrity; CNS: Physiological adaptation; CL: Application

49. The nurse caring for an infant with pyloric stenosis should be alert for which classic sign or symptom?
1. Loss of appetite
2. Chronic diarrhea
3. Projectile vomiting
4. Occasional nonprojectile vomiting

49. 3. The obstruction doesn't allow food to pass through to the duodenum. When the stomach becomes full, the infant vomits for relief. Chronic hunger is commonly seen. There's no diarrhea because food doesn't pass the stomach. Occasional nonprojectile vomiting may occur initially if the obstruction is only partial.
CN: Physiological integrity; CNS: Physiological adaptation; CL: Analysis

50. When assessing a neonate, the nurse notes visible peristaltic waves across the epigastrium. This characteristic is indicative of which disorder?

1. Hypertrophic pyloric stenosis
2. Imperforate anus
3. Intussusception
4. Short-gut syndrome

50. 1. The diagnosis of pyloric stenosis can be established from a finding of hypertrophic pyloric stenosis. Imperforate anus, intussusception, and short-gut syndrome are each diagnosed by other characteristics.
CN: Physiological integrity; CNS: Physiological adaptation; CL: Analysis

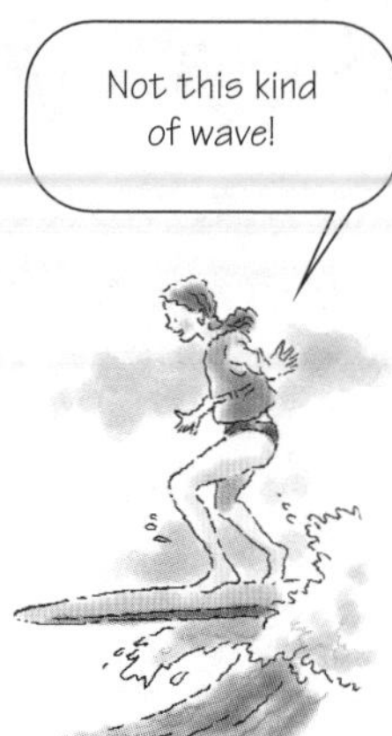

Not this kind of wave!

51. After surgical repair of pyloric stenosis, the nurse should expect an infant's <u>normal</u> feeding regimen to resume after what time frame?

1. 4 to 6 hours after surgery
2. 24 hours after surgery
3. 48 hours after surgery
4. 1 week after surgery

51. 3. Small frequent feedings of clear fluids are usually started 4 to 6 hours after surgery. If clear fluids are tolerated, formula feedings are started 24 hours after surgery, in gradually increasing amounts. It usually takes 48 hours to reach a normal full feeding regimen in this manner. The infant usually goes home on the fourth postoperative day.
CN: Physiological integrity; CNS: Physiological adaptation; CL: Application

52. A nurse admits an infant diagnosed with pyloric stenosis. Which nursing intervention would most likely be done <u>first</u>?

1. Weigh the infant.
2. Check urine specific gravity.
3. Place an I.V. catheter.
4. Change the infant and weigh the diaper.

52. 1. Weighing the infant would be done first so a baseline weight can be established and weight changes can be assessed. After a baseline weight is obtained, an I.V. catheter can be placed because oral feedings generally aren't given. These infants are usually dehydrated, so although specific gravity and checking the diaper are important tools to help assess their status, they aren't the first priority.
CN: Physiological integrity; CNS: Physiological adaptation; CL: Analysis

53. A nurse is caring for an infant with pyloric stenosis. After feeding the infant, the nurse should place him in which position?

1. Prone in Fowler's position
2. On his back without elevation
3. On the left side in Fowler's position
4. Slightly on the right side in high semi-Fowler's position

53. 4. Positioning the infant slightly on the right side in high semi-Fowler's position will help facilitate gastric emptying. The other positions won't facilitate gastric emptying and may cause the infant to vomit.
CN: Physiological integrity; CNS: Physiological adaptation; CL: Application

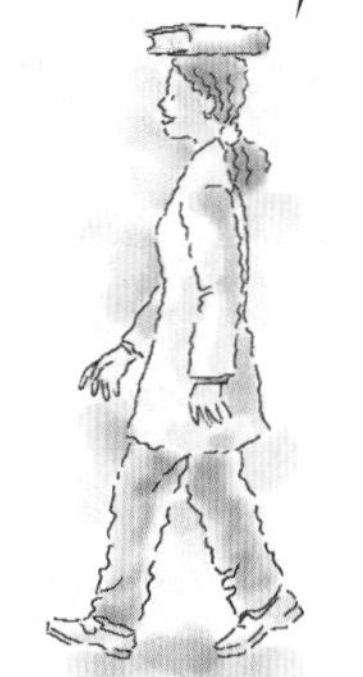

Here's that important positioning again!

54. When preparing to feed an infant with pyloric stenosis before surgical repair, which intervention is important?

1. Give feedings quickly.
2. Burp the infant frequently.
3. Discourage parental participation.
4. Don't give more feedings if the infant vomits.

54. 2. These infants usually swallow a lot of air from sucking on their hands and fingers because of their intensive hunger (feedings aren't easily tolerated). Burping frequently will lessen gastric distention and increase the likelihood that the infant will retain the feeding. Feedings are given slowly with the infant lying in a semiupright position. Parental participation should be encouraged and allowed to the extent possible. Record the type, amount, and character of the vomit as well as its relation to the feeding. The amount of feeding volume lost is usually refed to the infant.
CN: Physiological adaptation; CNS: Physiological adaptation; CL: Application

55. A nurse should expect which finding up to 48 hours after the surgical repair of pyloric stenosis?

1. Dysuria
2. Oral aversion
3. Scaphoid abdomen
4. Vomiting

55. 4. Even with successful surgery, most infants have some vomiting during the first 24 to 48 hours afterward. Dysuria isn't a complication with this surgical procedure. Oral aversion doesn't occur because these infants may be fed up until surgery. Scaphoid abdomen isn't characteristic of this condition; the abdomen may appear distended, not scaphoid.

CN: Physiological integrity; CNS: Physiological adaptation; CL: Application

56. Which intervention will help prevent vomiting in an infant diagnosed with pyloric stenosis?

1. Hold the infant for 1 hour after feeding.
2. Handle the infant minimally after feedings.
3. Space the feedings out, and give them in large amounts.
4. Lay the infant prone with the head of the bed elevated.

56. 2. Minimal handling, especially after a feeding, will help prevent vomiting. Holding the infant would provide too much stimulation, which might increase the risk of vomiting. Feedings are given frequently and slowly in small amounts. An infant should be positioned in a semi-Fowler's position and slightly on the right side after a feeding.

CN: Physiological integrity; CNS: Physiological adaptation; CL: Application

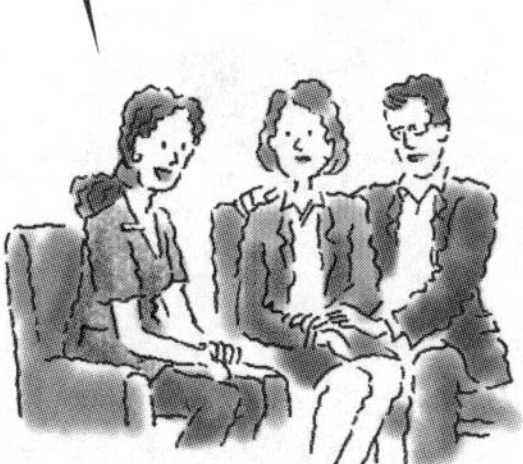

57. It's an important nursing function to give support to the parents of an infant diagnosed with pyloric stenosis. Which nursing intervention best serves that purpose?

1. Keep the parents informed of the infant's progress.
2. Provide all care for the infant, even when the parents visit.
3. Tell the parents to minimize handling of the infant at all times.
4. Tell the physician to keep the parents informed of the infant's progress.

57. 1. Keeping the parents informed will decrease their anxiety. The nurse should encourage the parents to be involved with the infant's care. Telling the parents to minimize handling of the infant isn't appropriate because parent-child contact is important. The physician is responsible for updating the parents on the infant's medical condition, and the nurse is responsible for updating the parents on the day-to-day activities of the infant and his improvement with the day's activities.

CN: Psychosocial integrity; CNS: None; CL: Analysis

58. Which symptom would be likely in an infant diagnosed with pyloric stenosis?

1. Apathy
2. Arrhythmia
3. Dry lips and skin
4. Hypothermia

58. 3. Dry lips and skin are signs of dehydration, which is common in infants with pyloric stenosis. These infants are constantly hungry because of their inability to retain feedings. Apathy, arrhythmias, and hypothermia aren't clinical findings with pyloric stenosis.

CN: Physiological integrity; CNS: Physiological adaptation; CL: Application

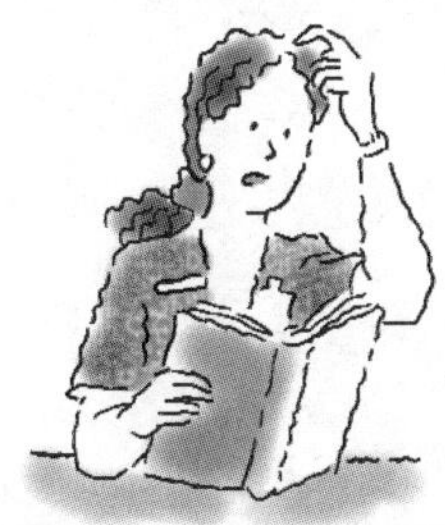

Question 59 asks what's normally found with a disease, not what's normal in a healthy infant.

59. When assessing an infant diagnosed with pyloric stenosis, which finding would the nurse consider normal?

1. Decreased or diminished bowel sounds
2. Heart murmur
3. Normal respiratory effort
4. Positive bowel sounds

59. 1. Bowel sounds decrease because food can't pass into the intestines. Heart murmurs may be present but aren't directly associated with pyloric stenosis. Normal respiratory effort is affected by the abdominal distention that pushes the diaphragm up into the pleural cavity.

CN: Physiological integrity; CNS: Physiological adaptation; CL: Analysis

60. The nurse explains to the parents of a child with hypertrophied pylorus that the defect is located between:

1. the colon and rectum.
2. the stomach and duodenum.
3. the stomach and esophagus.
4. the liver and bile ducts.

60. 2. This defect occurs at the pyloric sphincter, which is located between the stomach and duodenum. The colon, rectum, esophagus, liver, and bile ducts aren't affected by this obstructive disorder.

CN: Physiological integrity; CNS: Physiological adaptation; CL: Application

61. Which nursing intervention is the most important in dealing with a child who has been poisoned?

1. Stabilize the child.
2. Notify the parents.
3. Identify the poison.
4. Determine when the poisoning took place.

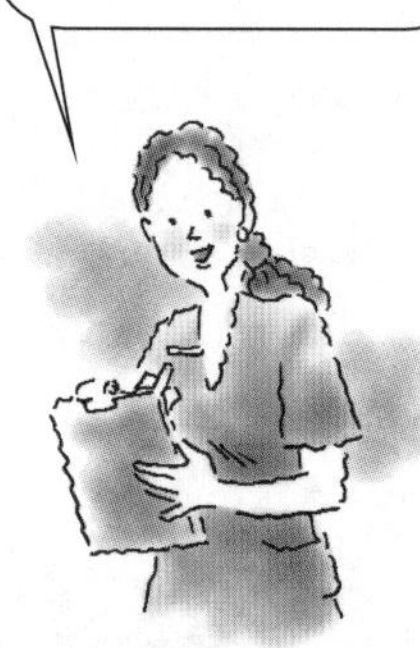

Practice setting priorities because it's part of nursing practice.

61. 1. Stabilization and the initial emergency treatment of the child (such as respiratory assistance, circulatory support, or control of seizures) will prevent further damage to the body from the poison. If the parents didn't bring the child in, they can be notified as soon as the child is stabilized or treated. Identification of the poison is crucial and should begin at the same time as the stabilization of the child, although the initial ABCs (airway, breathing, and circulation) should be assessed first. Determining when the poisoning took place is an important consideration, but emergency stabilization and treatment are priorities.

CN: Physiological integrity; CNS: Physiological adaptation; CL: Analysis

62. For a child who has ingested a poisonous substance, the initial step in emergency treatment is to stop the exposure to the substance. Which method would best achieve this?

1. Make the child vomit.
2. Call 911 as soon as possible.
3. Give large amounts of water to flush the system.
4. Empty the mouth of pills, plant parts, or other material.

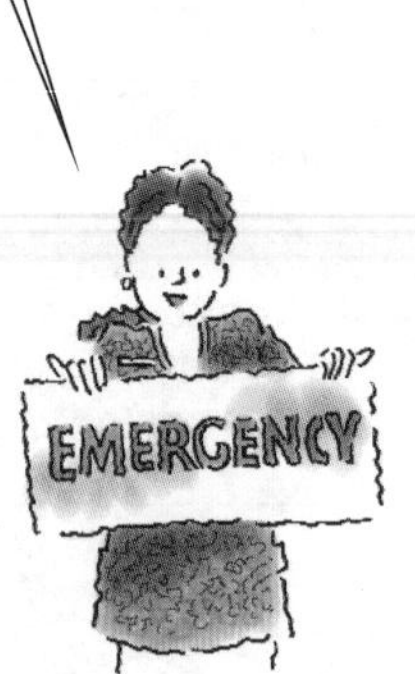

Would you know what to do first in this emergency situation?
EMERGENCY

62. 4. Emptying the mouth of pills, plant parts, or other material will stop exposure to the poison. Making the child vomit won't remove exposure to the substance; it's also contraindicated with some poisons. Calling 911 is important, but removing any further sources of the poison would come first. Only small amounts of water are recommended so the poison is confined to the smallest volume. Large amounts of water will let the poison pass the pylorus. The small intestines will then absorb fluid rapidly, increasing the potential toxicity.

CN: Physiological integrity; CNS: Physiological adaptation; CL: Analysis

63. In the recovery phase following an ingesion of drain cleaner by a child, the nurse should be alert for the development of which likely complication?

1. Esophageal strictures
2. Esophageal diverticula
3. Tracheal stenosis
4. Tracheal varices

63. 1. Scar tissue develops as the burn from the drain cleaner ingestion heals, leading to esophageal strictures. The formation of esophageal diverticula is rare. Tracheal stenosis may occur but only if the child vomited and aspirated. Tracheal varices don't commonly occur after drain cleaner ingestion.

CN: Physiological integrity; CNS: Physiological adaptation; CL: Analysis

CN: Client needs category CNS: Client needs subcategory CL: Cognitive level

64. A preschooler is brought to the emergency department after ingesting kerosene. The nurse should be alert for which complication?

1. Pneumonitis
2. Carditis
3. Uremia
4. Hepatitis

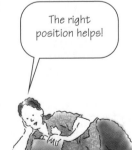

64. 1. Chemical pneumonitis is the most common complication following ingestion of a hydrocarbon, such as kerosene. The pneumonitis is caused by irritation from the hydrocarbon aspirated into the lungs. The other options aren't complications of kerosene ingestion.
CN: Physiological integrity; CNS: Physiological adaptation; CL: Analysis

65. Which action should a nurse instruct parents to perform first if their child ingests a poison?

1. Administer syrup of ipecac.
2. Call the poison control center.
3. Transport the child to the emergency department.
4. Watch the child for adverse effects.

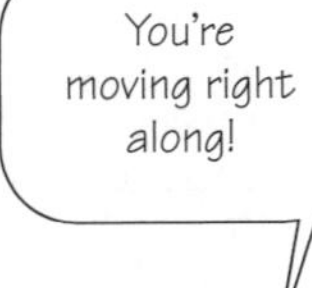

You're moving right along!

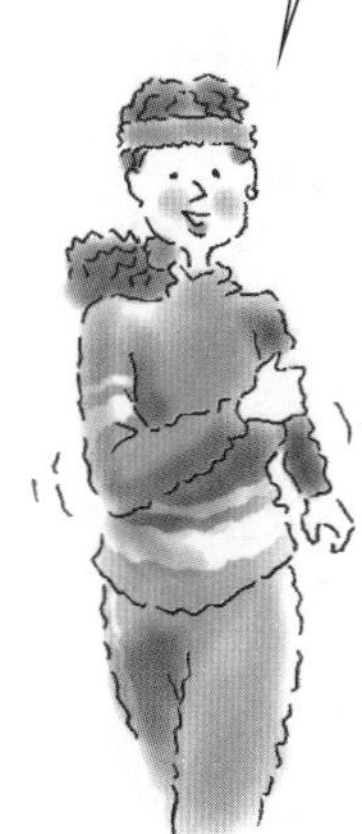

65. 2. The first step parents should take if their child has ingested a poisonous substance is to call the poison control center for instructions. Home administration of syrup of ipecac is no longer recommended by the American Academy of Pediatrics. The parents should contact poison control before transporting their child since valuable time may be lost if poison control recommends a specific action to take to remove the poisonous substance from the body. If the child needs to be taken to the emergency department, the parents should call emergency services to transport the child. Poison control may recommend watching the child for adverse effects, but parents shouldn't make this decision without consulting with poison control.
CN: Physiological integrity; CNS: Reduction of risk potential; CL: Analysis

66. If a child ingests poisonous hydrocarbons, an important nursing intervention would include which action?

1. Induce vomiting.
2. Keep the child calm and relaxed.
3. Scold the child for the wrongdoing.
4. Keep the parents away from the child.

66. 2. Keeping the child calm and relaxed will help prevent vomiting. If vomiting is induced, there's a strong chance the esophagus will be damaged from regurgitation of the gastric poison. Additionally, the risk of chemical pneumonitis exists if vomiting occurs. Scolding the child may upset him. The parents should remain with the child to help keep him calm.
CN: Physiological integrity; CNS: Physiological adaptation; CL: Analysis

67. Shock is a complication of several types of poisoning. Which measure would help reduce the risk of shock?

1. Keep the child on his right side.
2. Let the child maintain normal activity as possible.
3. Elevate the head and legs to the level of the heart.
4. Keep the head flat, and raise the legs to the level of the heart.

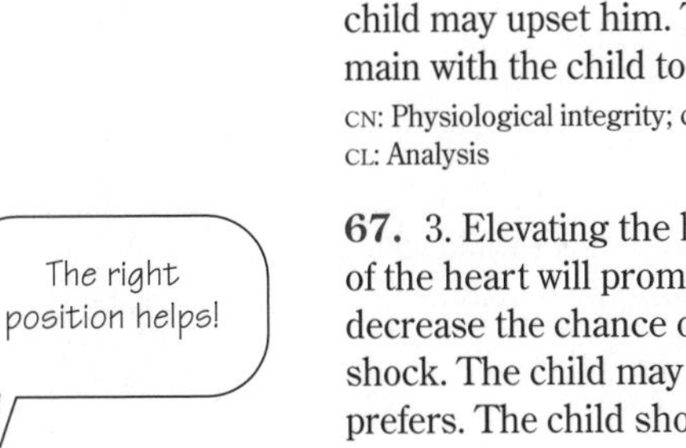

The right position helps!

67. 3. Elevating the head and legs to the level of the heart will promote venous drainage and decrease the chance of the child going into shock. The child may safely lie on the side he prefers. The child should be encouraged to get plenty of rest.
CN: Physiological integrity; CNS: Physiological adaptation; CL: Application

68. A 7-year-old child ingested several leaves of a poinsettia plant. After arrival in the emergency department, which intervention should be the main nursing function for this client?
1. Begin teaching accident prevention.
2. Provide emotional support to the child.
3. Be prepared for immediate intervention.
4. Provide emotional support to the parents.

68. 3. Time and speed are critical factors in recovery from poisonings. The remaining three answers are important nursing functions but don't require the immediate attention that first stabilizing the child does.
CN: Health promotion and maintenance; CNS: None; CL: Analysis

69. A child is being admitted through the emergency department with a diagnosis of suspected accidental poisoning by medication. The nurse is aware that which class of medication is the most common cause of accidental poisoning in children?
1. Pain medications
2. Vitamins
3. Laxatives
4. Antibiotics

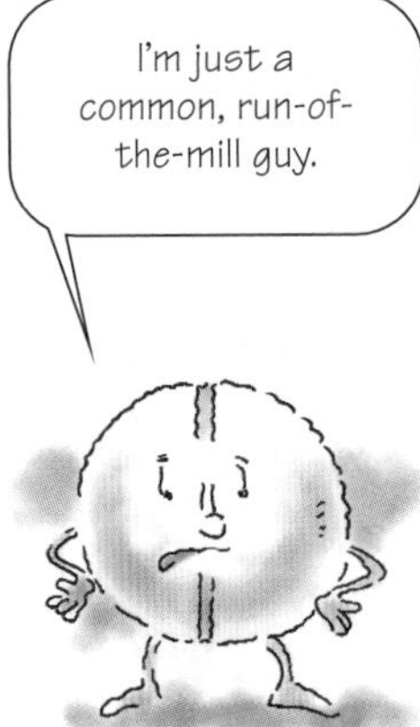
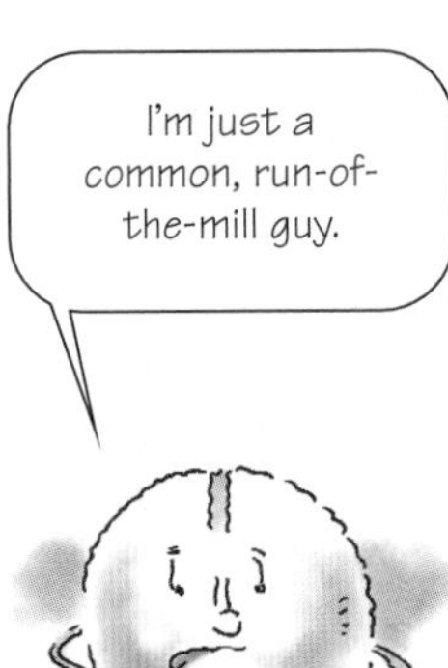

I'm just a common, run-of-the-mill guy.

69. 1. According to the Centers for Disease Control and Prevention, the most common accidentally ingested class of drugs is pain medications. The most common pain medications ingested are acetaminophen-containing (Tylenol-containing) drugs, non-steroidal anti-inflammatory drugs, and opioids. The other classes of drugs are less commonly ingested.
CN: Health promotion and maintenance; CNS: None; CL: Analysis

70. A client is undergoing testing for a diagnosis of ulcerative colitis. Which symptom would the nurse most likely identify during this initial diagnosis?
1. Constipation
2. Diarrhea
3. Vomiting
4. Weight loss

70. 2. Recurrent or persistent diarrhea is a common feature of ulcerative colitis. Constipation doesn't occur because the bowel becomes smooth and inflexible. Vomiting isn't common in this disease. Weight loss will occur after or during the episode, but not initially.
CN: Physiological integrity; CNS: Physiological adaptation; CL: Analysis

71. A child arrives in the emergency department after ingesting poisonous amounts of salicylates. How soon after ingestion should the nurse look for obvious signs of toxicity?
1. Immediately
2. 2 to 4 hours after ingestion
3. 6 hours after ingestion
4. 18 hours after ingestion

71. 3. There's usually a delay of 6 hours before evidence of toxicity is noted. Toxic evidence is rarely immediate. Aspirin will exert its peak effect in 2 to 4 hours. The effect of aspirin may last as long as 18 hours.
CN: Health promotion and maintenance; CNS: None; CL: Application

72. The nurse caring for a client with an extreme case of salicylate poisoning should anticipate, or prepare the client for, which treatment?
1. Gastric lavage
2. Hypothermia blankets
3. Peritoneal dialysis
4. Vitamin K injection

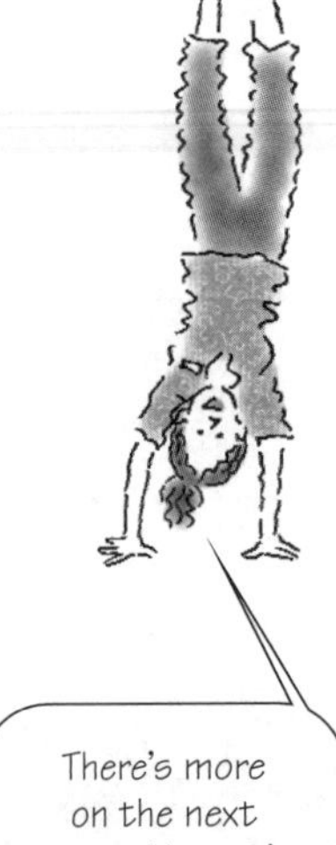

There's more on the next page. Hooray!

72. 3. Peritoneal dialysis is usually reserved for cases of life-threatening salicylism. Gastric lavage is used in the immediate treatment for salicylate poisoning because the stomach contents and salicylates will move from the stomach to the remainder of the GI tract, where vomiting will no longer result in the removal of the poison. Hyperthermia blankets may be used to reduce the possibility of seizures. Vitamin K may be used to decrease bleeding tendencies, but only if evidence of this exists.
CN: Physiological integrity; CNS: Physiological adaptation; CL: Analysis

CN: Client needs category CNS: Client needs subcategory CL: Cognitive level

73. When a child has been poisoned, identifying the ingested poison is an important treatment goal. Which action would help determine which poison was ingested?

1. Call the local poison control center.
2. Ask the child.
3. Ask the parents.
4. Save all evidence of poison.

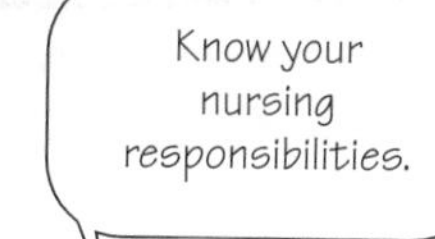

Know your nursing responsibilities.

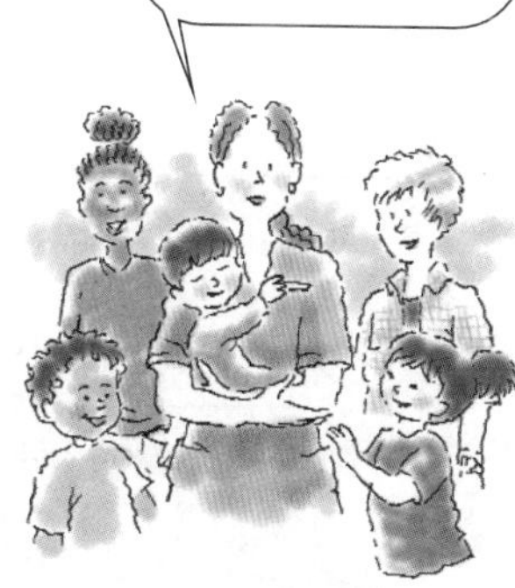

73. 4. Saving all evidence of poison (container, vomitus, urine) will help determine which drug was ingested and how much. Calling the local poison control center may help get information on specific poisons or if a certain household placed a call, although rarely can they help determine which poison has been ingested. Asking the child may help, but the child may fear punishment and may not be honest about the incident. The parent may be helpful in some instances, although the parent may not have been home or with the child when the ingestion occurred.

CN: Health promotion and maintenance; CNS: None; CL: Analysis

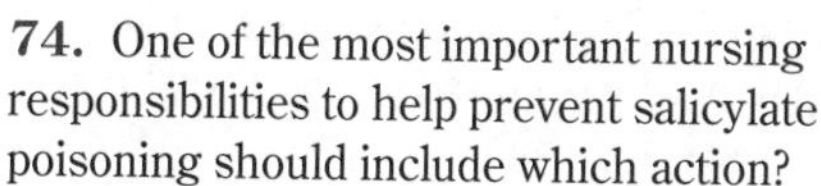

74. One of the most important nursing responsibilities to help prevent salicylate poisoning should include which action?

1. Identify salicylate overdose.
2. Teach children the hazards of ingesting nonfood items.
3. Decrease curiosity; teach parents to keep aspirin and drugs in clear view.
4. Teach parents to keep large amounts of drugs on hand but out of reach of children.

74. 2. Teaching children the hazards of ingesting nonfood items will help prevent ingestion of poisonous substances. Identifying the overdose won't prevent it from occurring. Aspirin and drugs should be kept out of the sight of children. Parents should be warned about keeping large amounts of drugs on hand.

CN: Health promotion and maintenance; CNS: None; CL: Application

75. In evaluating the effectiveness of therapy with acetylcysteine (Mucomyst) in a child with acetaminophen poisoning, which laboratory value would be the most important for the nurse to monitor?

1. Serum alanine aminotransferase and aspartate aminotransferase
2. Serum calcium levels
3. Prothrombin time (PT)
4. Serum glucose levels

75. 1. Acetaminophen poisoning damages the liver, leading to elevated serum alanine aminotransferase and aspartate aminotransferase levels. After therapy with acetylcysteine is started, these liver enzymes should begin to fall. Serum calcium levels may fall following chelation therapy in clients with lead poisoning. Because PT is elevated and blood glucose levels are reduced with salicylate poisoning, after treatment is initiated the nurse should observe the PT and blood glucose levels return to normal.

CN: Physiological integrity; CNS: Reduction of risk potential; CL: Analysis

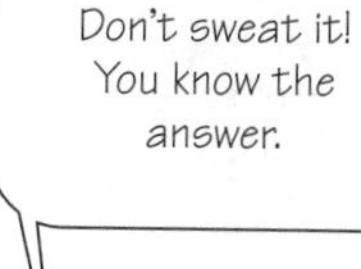

Don't sweat it! You know the answer.

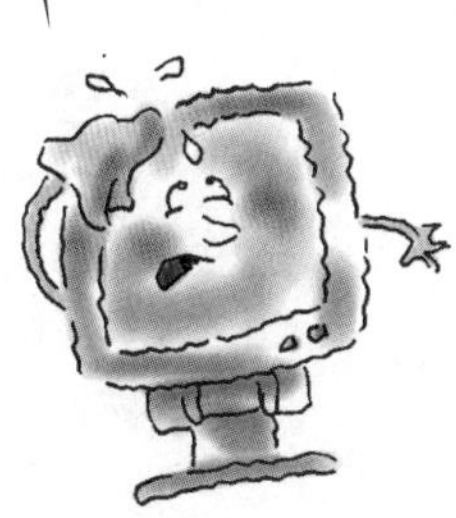

76. A client is diagnosed with acetaminophen poisoning. Which sign would the nurse expect when assessing the client 12 to 24 hours after ingestion?

1. Hyperthermia
2. Increased urine output
3. Profuse sweating
4. Rapid pulse

76. 3. During the first 12 to 24 hours, profuse sweating is a significant sign of acetaminophen poisoning. Weak pulse, hypothermia, and decreased urine output are also common findings.

CN: Physiological integrity; CNS: Physiological adaptation; CL: Analysis

77. For a client diagnosed with acetaminophen poisoning who comes to the emergency department 3 hours after ingestion, the most important therapeutic action is to:
1. perform gastric lavage.
2. obtain blood work.
3. give I.V. fluid.
4. use activated charcoal.

77. 4. If the client is seen within 4 hours, activated charcoal should be given to prevent absorption of acetominophen. Gastric lavage is recommended only if the client is seen within 1 hour of ingestion. Blood work would be obtained but wouldn't be the first priority. I.V. fluids would also be administered, but administering activated charcoal is the priority.
CN: Physiological integrity; CNS: Physiological adaptation; CL: Analysis

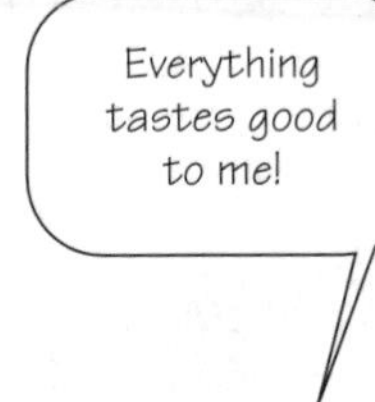
Everything tastes good to me!

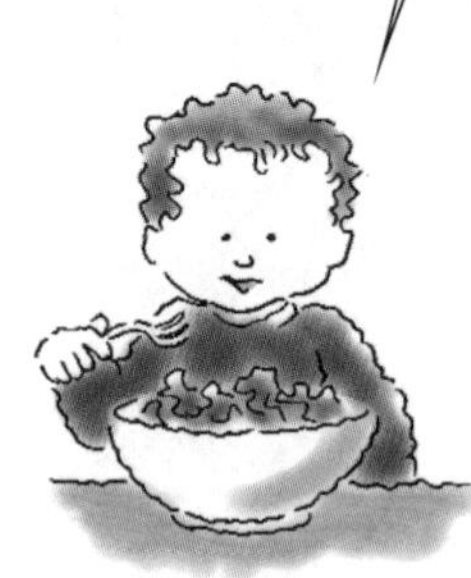

78. Which response by a nurse is most appropriate when the mother of a child admitted for ingesting a caustic cleaning product states she feels guilty?
1. "Now you'll know to keep all cleaning products locked up."
2. "Luckily, your child is going to be fine."
3. "You'll need to watch your child more carefully."
4. "Tell me more about your guilty feelings."

78. 4. Encouraging the mother to talk about her feelings shows the nurse accepts the mother's feelings and that she's prepared to listen. This also helps establish a trusting nurse-client relationship. Telling the mother she should keep all cleaning products locked up and that she needs to watch her child more carefully acknowledges that the mother was at fault and may block further communication. Telling the mother that the child will be fine dismisses the mother's feelings and may be giving false reassurances.
CN: Psychosocial integrity; CNS: None; CL: Analysis

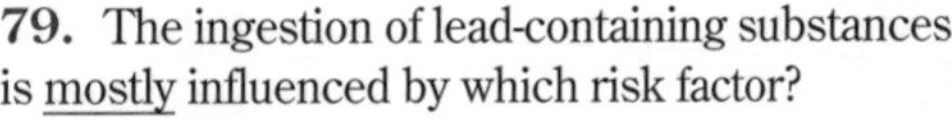

79. The ingestion of lead-containing substances is mostly influenced by which risk factor?
1. Child's age
2. Child's gender
3. Child's race
4. A parent with the same habit

79. 1. The highest risk of lead poisoning occurs in young children who have a tendency to put things in their mouth. In older homes that contain lead-based paint, paint chips may be eaten directly by the child or they may cling to toys or hands that are then put into the child's mouth. Poisoning isn't gender-related. African Americans have a higher incidence of lead poisoning, but it can happen in any race. Most parents don't eat lead-based paint on purpose.
CN: Health promotion and maintenance; CNS: None; CL: Application

80. The nurse explains to the mother of a child with lead poisoning that X-rays are necessary, as lead retained in the body is initially stored in the:
1. bone.
2. brain.
3. kidney.
4. liver.

80. 1. Ingested lead is initially absorbed by bone; X-rays reveal a characteristic "lead line" at the epiphyseal line. If chronic ingestion occurs, then the central nervous, renal, and hematologic systems are affected.
CN: Physiological integrity; CNS: Physiological adaptation; CL: Application

Be aware of the initial signs of lead poisoning.

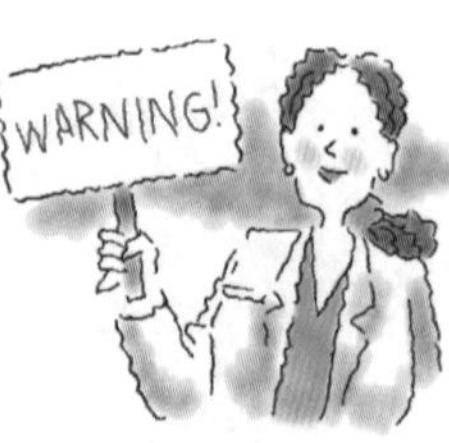
WARNING!

81. Which condition is one of the initial signs of lead poisoning?
1. Anemia
2. Constipation
3. Anorexia
4. Paralysis

81. 1. Lead is dangerously toxic to the biosynthesis of heme, and the reduced heme molecule in red blood cells causes anemia. Constipation and anorexia are vague, nonspecific symptoms. Paralysis may occur as toxic damage to the brain progresses.
CN: Physiological integrity; CNS: Physiological adaptation; CL: Analysis

82. The most serious and irreversible adverse effects of lead intoxication affect which system?
1. Central nervous system (CNS)
2. Hematologic system
3. Renal system
4. Respiratory system

82. 1. Damage that occurs to the CNS is difficult to repair. Damage to the hematologic and renal systems can be reversed if treated early. The respiratory system isn't affected until coma and death occur.
CN: Physiological integrity; CNS: Physiological adaptation; CL: Analysis

83. A mother of a recently admitted child asks the nurse about the black lines along her child's gums. The nurse would respond that the black lines indicate which of the following types of poisoning?
1. Acetaminophen
2. Lead
3. Plants
4. Salicylates

83. 2. One diagnostic characteristic of lead poisoning is black lines along the gums. Black lines don't occur along the gums with acetaminophen, plant, or salicylate poisoning.
CN: Physiological integrity; CNS: Physiological adaptation; CL: Application

84. The parents of a child with lead poisoning ask the nurse which procedure is the main treatment for lead poisoning. Which treatment would the nurse describe?
1. Exchange transfusion
2. Bone marrow transplant
3. Chelation therapy
4. Dialysis

84. 3. Chelation therapy is the main treatment for lead poisoning and involves the removal of metal by combining it with another substance. Sometimes exchange transfusions are used to rid the blood of lead quickly. Bone marrow transplants usually aren't needed. Dialysis usually isn't part of the treatment.
CN: Physiological integrity; CNS: Physiological adaptation; CL: Application

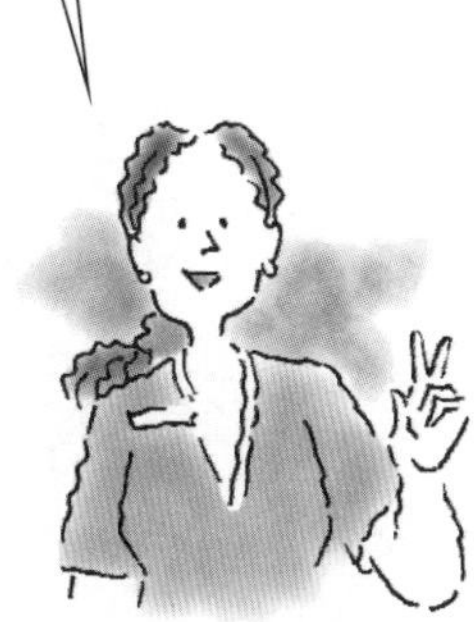
Watch for these two words—most important.

85. Which nursing objective should be the <u>most important</u> for a child with lead poisoning who must undergo chelation therapy?
1. Prepare the child for complete bed rest.
2. Prepare the child for I.V. fluid therapy.
3. Prepare the child for an extended hospital stay.
4. Prepare the child for a large number of injections.

85. 4. Chelation therapy involves getting a large number of injections in a relatively short period of time. It's traumatic to the majority of children, and they need some preparation for the treatment. The other components of the treatment plan are important but aren't as likely to cause the same anxiety as multiple injections. Allowing adequate rest to not aggravate the painful injection sites is important. Receiving I.V. fluid isn't as traumatizing as multiple injections. Physical activity is usually limited.
CN: Physiological integrity; CNS: Physiological adaptation; CL: Analysis

86. Which condition may occur during chelation therapy in a child with lead poisoning?
1. Hypercalcemia
2. Hypocalcemia
3. Hyperglycemia
4. Hypoglycemia

86. 2. A calcium chelating agent is used for the treatment of lead poisoning, so calcium is removed from the body with the lead. Hypocalcemia, not hypercalcemia, occurs. Hyperglycemia and hypoglycemia don't occur as a result of this therapy.
CN: Physiological integrity; CNS: Physiological adaptation; CL: Analysis

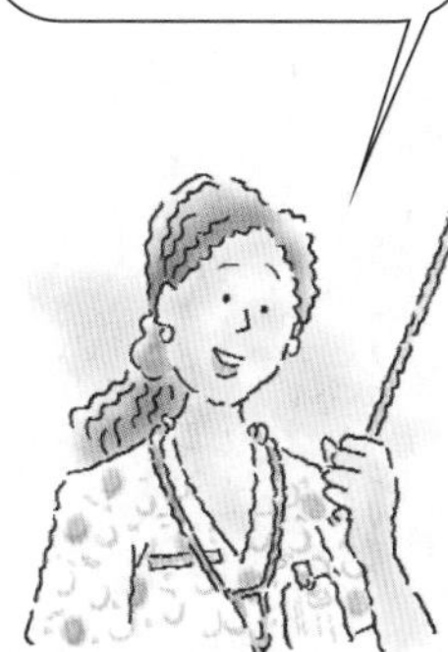
You know the routine; keep on teachin'.

87. Which intervention is the best way to prevent lead poisoning in children?
1. Educate the child.
2. Educate the public.
3. Identify high-risk groups.
4. Provide home chelation kits.

87. 2. By educating others about lead poisoning, including the danger signs, symptoms, and treatment, identification can be determined quickly. Very young children may not understand the dangers of lead poisoning. Identifying high-risk groups will help but won't prevent the poisoning. Home chelation kits currently aren't available.
CN: Health promotion and maintenance; CNS: None; CL: Analysis

88. When planning care for a 14-year-old client following surgical repair of a ruptured appendix, the nurse should plan interventions that:
1. reduce conflict between the client and his parents.
2. promote the development of an identity and independence.
3. encourage the development of trust.
4. confirm plans for the future.

88. 2. Since adolescents are in Erikson's stage of identity versus role confusion, the nursing care plan should include interventions that promote a sense of identity and independence. During adolescence, conflict is usually intensified, not reduced. Trust is a developmental task of infancy. Plans for the future aren't confirmed at age 14.
CN: Health promotion and maintenance; CNS: None; CL: Analysis

89. Certain forms of pica are caused by a deficiency. Which nutrient is most commonly deficient?
1. Minerals
2. Vitamin B complex
3. Vitamin C
4. Vitamin D

89. 1. Eating clay is related to zinc deficiency; eating chalk, to calcium deficiency. Vitamin deficiencies aren't related to pica.
CN: Health promotion and maintenance; CNS: None; CL: Analysis

90. Which action should a nurse take when a child with appendicitis reports a sudden cessation of abdominal pain?
1. Prepare the child and parents for discharge.
2. Begin feeding the child, as tolerated.
3. Prepare the child for emergency surgery.
4. Begin ambulation, as tolerated.

90. 3. The sudden cessation of abdominal pain in the client with appendicitis may indicate perforation or infarction of the appendix requiring emergency surgery. Therefore, the child shouldn't be prepared for discharge or given oral feedings. The child with a ruptured appendix should be on complete bed rest and be prepared for surgery.
CN: Physiological integrity; CNS: Reduction of risk potential; CL: Application

91. Which advice should a nurse give over the telephone to the mother of a 7-year-old child with abdominal pain, a low-grade fever, and vomiting?
1. Give prune juice to relieve constipation.
2. Test for rebound tenderness in the left lower quadrant of the abdomen.
3. Encourage fluids to prevent dehydration.
4. Seek immediate emergency medical care.

91. 4. The client with abdominal pain, fever, and vomiting (the cardinal signs of appendicitis) should seek immediate emergency care to reduce the risk of complications if the appendix should rupture. Prune juice has laxative effects and shouldn't be given because laxatives increase the risk of rupture of the appendix. The nurse shouldn't rely on the mother's findings when testing for rebound tenderness. The client should be given nothing by mouth in case surgery is needed.
CN: Physiological integrity; CNS: Reduction of risk potential; CL: Application

92. Which symptom is the most common for acute appendicitis?
1. Bradycardia
2. Fever
3. Pain descending to the lower left quadrant
4. Pain radiating down the legs

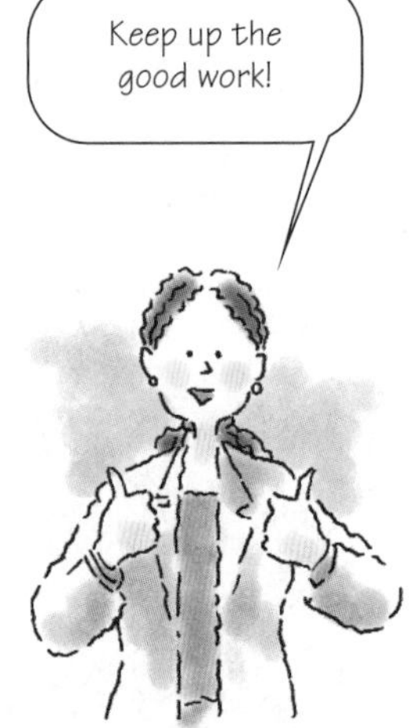

92. 2. Fever, abdominal pain, and tenderness are the first signs of appendicitis. Tachycardia, not bradycardia, is seen. Pain can be generalized or periumbilical. It usually descends to the lower right quadrant, not the left.
CN: Physiological integrity; CNS: Physiological adaptation; CL: Analysis

93. Which nursing intervention would be important to preoperatively perform in a child with appendicitis?

1. Give clear fluids.
2. Apply heat to the abdomen.
3. Maintain complete bed rest.
4. Administer an enema, if ordered.

93. 3. Bed rest will prevent aggravating the condition. Clients with appendicitis aren't allowed anything by mouth. Cold applications are placed on the abdomen because heat would increase blood flow to the area and possibly spread any infectious disease. Enemas may aggravate the condition.

CN: Physiological integrity; CNS: Reduction of risk potential; CL: Analysis

94. Postoperative care of a child with a ruptured appendix should include which treatment or intervention?

1. Liquid diet
2. Oral antibiotics for 7 to 10 days
3. Positioning the child on the left side
4. Parenteral antibiotics for 7 to 10 days

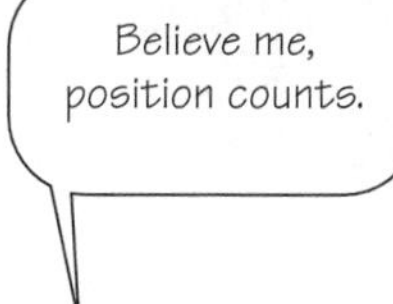
Believe me,
position counts.

94. 4. Parenteral antibiotics are used for 7 to 10 days postoperatively to help prevent the spread of infection. The child is kept on I.V. fluids and isn't allowed anything by mouth. Oral antibiotics may continue after the parenteral antibiotics are discontinued. The child is positioned on the right side after surgery.

CN: Physiological integrity; CNS: Reduction of risk potential; CL: Analysis

95. After surgical repair of a ruptured appendix, which position would be the <u>most appropriate</u>?

1. High Fowler's position
2. Left side
3. Semi-Fowler's position
4. Supine

95. 3. Using the semi-Fowler's or right side-lying positions will facilitate drainage from the peritoneal cavity and prevent the formation of a subdiaphragmatic abscess. High Fowler's, left side, and prone positions won't facilitate drainage from the peritoneal cavity.

CN: Physiological integrity; CNS: Physiological adaptation; CL: Analysis

96. Which statement by the parent of a child being treated for pinworms indicates that more teaching is necessary?

1. "I will make my child wash his hands well before meals."
2. "I will tell my child not to share hairbrushes or hats."
3. "I will give my child only one dose of medication."
4. "I will keep my child's nails short."

96. 2. Sharing hairbrushes and hats reduces the spread of lice, not pinworms. Hands should be washed well before food preparation and eating to avoid ingesting eggs that may be under the fingernails from scratching the itchy, infested perianal area. Only a single dose of medication, such as mebendazole, is needed to treat pinworms. Keeping the fingernails short reduces the risk of carrying the eggs under the nails.

CN: Safe, effective care environment; CNS: Safety and infection control; CL: Application

97. During an initial nursing assessment, a nurse determines that an 8-year-old child has right lower quadrant pain, a low-grade fever, nausea, rebound tenderness, and a positive psoas sign. The nurse suspects that the client has which condition?

1. Appendicitis
2. Gastroenteritis
3. Pancreatitis
4. Cholecystitis

97. 1. Right lower quadrant pain, a low-grade fever, nausea, rebound tenderness, and a positive psoas sign are all consistent with appendicitis. Gastroenteritis is characterized by generalized abdominal tenderness. Pancreatitis is characterized by pain in the left abdonimal quadrant. Cholecystitis is characterized by pain in the right upper abdominal quadrant.

CN: Physiological integrity; CNS: Physiological adaptation; CL: Analysis

98. A neonate has been diagnosed with a unilateral complete cleft lip and cleft palate. The nurse formulating the care plan for this neonate will have which nursing diagnosis as a priority?

1. *Risk for infection*
2. *Impaired skin integrity*
3. *Risk for aspiration*
4. *Delayed growth and development*

98. 3. Although all of these diagnoses are important for the neonate with a cleft lip and cleft palate, the most important diagnosis relates to the airway. Neonates with a cleft lip and a cleft palate may have an excessive amount of saliva and usually have a difficult time with feedings. Special feeding techniques, such as using a flanged nipple, may be necessary to prevent aspiration.

CN: Physiological integrity; CNS: Reduction of risk potential; CL: Analysis

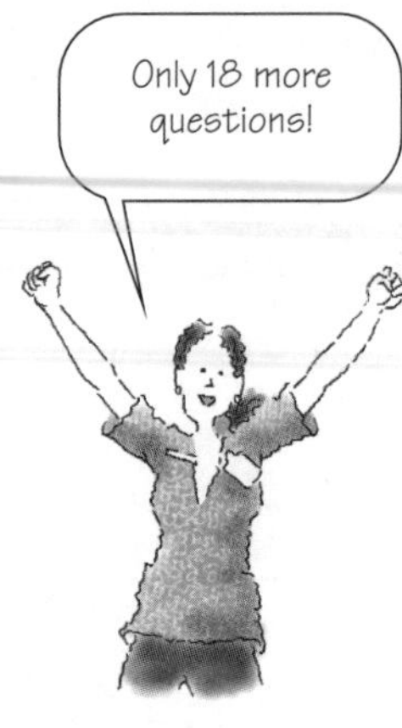

Only 18 more questions!

99. A neonate is suspected of having a tracheoesophageal fistula (type III/C). Which symptom would be seen on the <u>initial</u> assessment?

1. Excessive drooling
2. Excessive vomiting
3. Mottling
4. Polyhydramnios

99. 1. In type III/C tracheoesophageal fistula, the proximal end of the esophagus ends in a blind pouch and a fistula connects the distal end of the esophagus to the trachea. Saliva will pool in this pouch and cause the child to drool. Because the distal end of the esophagus is connected to the trachea, the neonate can't vomit, but he can aspirate and stomach acid may go into the lungs through this fistula, causing pneumonitis. Mottling is a netlike, reddish blue discoloration of the skin usually due to vascular contraction in response to hypothermia. The mother of a neonate with tracheoesophageal fistula may have had polyhydramnios.

CN: Physiological integrity; CNS: Reduction of risk potential; CL: Analysis

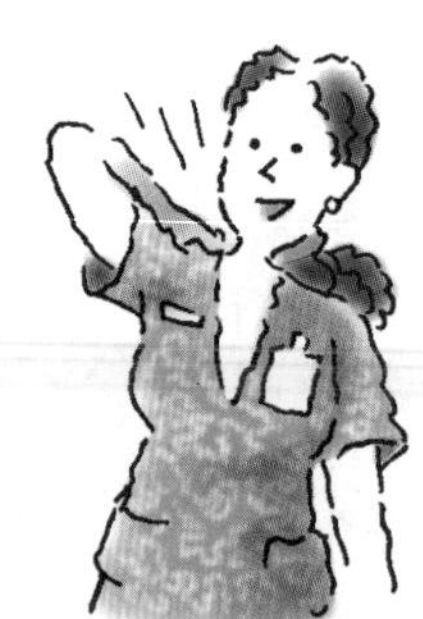

You made it to question 100. Good for you!

100. When assessing a client suspected of having pyloric stenosis, which finding should the nurse expect?

1. An "olive" mass in the right upper quadrant
2. An "olive" mass in the left upper quadrant
3. A "sausage" mass in the right upper quadrant
4. A "sausage" mass in the left upper quadrant

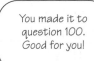

100. 1. Pyloric stenosis involves hypertrophy of the circular (or olive-shaped) muscle fibers of the pylorus. This hypertrophy is palpable in the right upper quadrant of the abdomen. A "sausage" mass is palpable in the right upper quadrant in children with intussusception. A "sausage" mass in the left upper quadrant wouldn't indicate pyloric stenosis.

CN: Physiological integrity; CNS: Physiological adaptation; CL: Analysis

101. A nurse caring for an infant with pyloric stenosis should expect to observe which laboratory values?

1. pH, 7.30; chloride, 120 mEq/L
2. pH, 7.38; chloride, 110 mEq/L
3. pH, 7.43; chloride, 100 mEq/L
4. pH, 7.49; chloride, 90 mEq/L

101. 4. Infants with pyloric stenosis vomit hydrochloric acid. This causes them to become alkalotic and hypochloremic. Normal serum pH is 7.35 to 7.45; levels above 7.45 represent alkalosis. The normal serum chloride level is 99 to 111 mEq/L; levels below 99 mEq/L represent hypochloremia.

CN: Physiological integrity; CNS: Physiological adaptation; CL: Analysis

102. Which nursing diagnosis has the highest priority in a 1-month-old infant admitted with projectile vomiting after feeding?

1. *Deficient fluid volume*
2. *Risk for impaired parenting*
3. *Interrupted breast-feeding*
4. *Risk for infection*

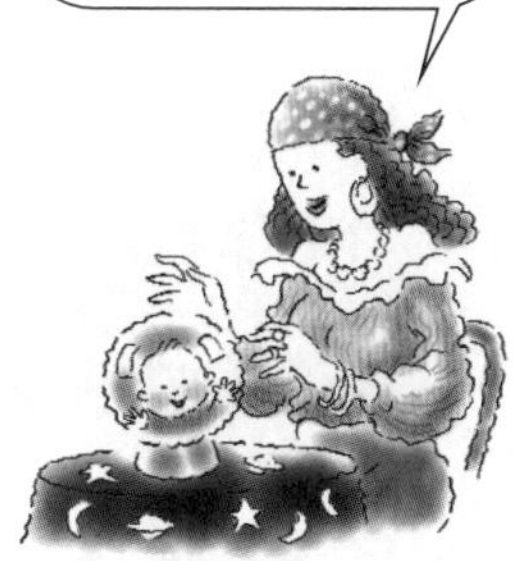
I see the highest priority nursing diagnosis for this infant.

102. 1. Projectile vomiting in an infant is a sign of pyloric stenosis, a condition that requires surgical intervention to correct. Because the infant has been vomiting, he is at risk for fluid and electrolyte imbalances that must be corrected before surgery. Whenever an infant is hospitalized, there's the *Risk for impaired parenting* and *Interrupted breast-feeding;* however, correcting fluid and electrolyte imbalances is a priority. Following surgery, the infant is at *Risk for infection* because the incision is near the diaper area.

CN: Physiological integrity; CNS: Reduction of risk potential; CL: Analysis

103. Which findings would the nurse assess in a premature neonate who may have necrotizing enterocolitis?

1. Abdominal distention and gastric retention
2. Gastric retention and guaiac-negative stools
3. Metabolic alkalosis and abdominal distention
4. Guaiac-negative stools and metabolic alkalosis

103. 1. Necrotizing enterocolitis is an ischemic disorder of the gut. The cause is unknown, but it's more common in premature neonates who had a hypoxic episode. The neonate's intestines become dilated and necrotic, and the abdomen becomes very distended. Paralytic ileus develops, causing the neonate to have gastric retention. These retained gastric contents, along with any passed stool, will be guaiac-positive. The neonate also develops metabolic acidosis.

CN: Physiological integrity; CNS: Physiological adaptation; CL: Analysis

104. An infant has been admitted to the hospital with gastroenteritis. The nursing care plan for this infant will consider which nursing diagnosis first?

1. *Acute pain*
2. *Diarrhea*
3. *Deficient fluid volume*
4. *Imbalanced nutrition: Less than body requirements*

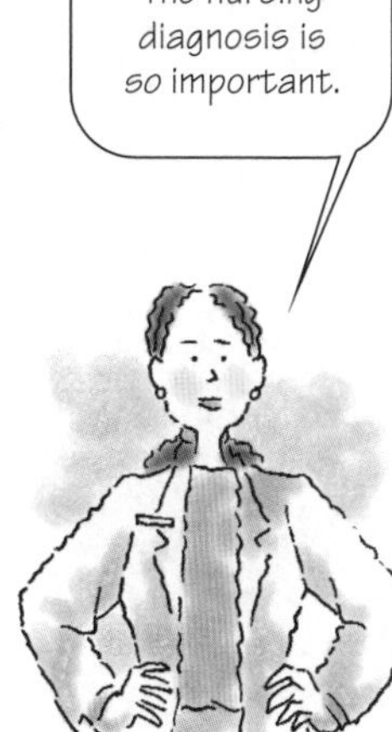
The nursing diagnosis is so important.

104. 3. Young children with gastroenteritis are at high risk for developing a fluid volume deficit. Their intestinal mucosa allows for more fluid and electrolytes to be lost when they have gastroenteritis. The main goal of the health care team should be to rehydrate the infant. The other nursing diagnoses are important, but deficient fluid volume is more life-threatening.

CN: Physiological integrity; CNS: Physiological adaptation; CL: Application

105. Nursing assessments in an infant with gastroenteritis should be directed toward detecting which potential problem?

1. Urinary retention
2. Heart failure
3. Electrolyte imbalance
4. Hyperactive reflexes

105. 3. Diarrhea in infants can rapidly lead to dehydration and electrolyte imbalances, especially hyponatremia and hypokalemia. Urinary retention isn't a sign of dehydration; however, it should be distinguished from kidney failure, which may occur with severe dehydration. Heart failure occurs with fluid volume overload, not fluid volume deficit. Reflexes are typically diminished or absent with hypokalemia.

CN: Physiological integrity; CNS: Reduction of risk potential; CL: Application

106. A mother calls the children's clinic, saying that she found her toddler with an open and empty bottle of acetaminophen (Tylenol), and wanting to know what to do. What's the priority intervention for this situation?

1. Ask the mother whether she has any syrup of ipecac.
2. Ask the mother to give the child a large glass of milk.
3. Ask the mother to bring the child to the emergency department (ED).
4. Ask the mother whether she knows cardiopulmonary resuscitation (CPR).

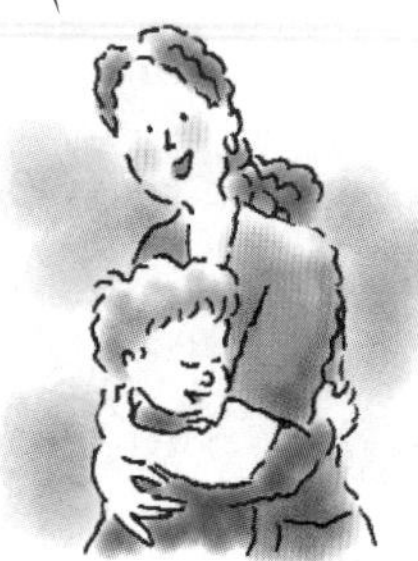
Do you know the priority intervention for this toddler?

106. 3. The child should be brought to the ED for evaluation and possible acetyleysteine administration. Home administration of syrup of ipecac is no longer recommended. Milk isn't an antidote for acetaminophen toxicity. Asking about CPR isn't appropriate as the priority intervention; it would distract from the immediate interventions needed.

CN: Safe, effective care environment; CNS: Safety and infection control; CL: Analysis

107. Which fact should be emphasized in the teaching plan for the parents of a child with celiac disease?

1. The gluten-free diet alterations must be continued for a lifetime.
2. The diet needs to be free of lactose because the child is intolerant.
3. Diet alterations are necessary when the child reports cramping and bloating.
4. The diet needs to be low in fats because of the malabsorption problem in the intestines.

107. 1. Celiac disease is the inability to digest gluten. The treatment is a gluten-free diet for life. It's important the diet is continued to avoid symptoms and the associated risk of colon cancer. The disease isn't caused by lactose intolerance or a problem digesting fats.

CN: Health promotion and maintenance; CNS: None; CL: Application

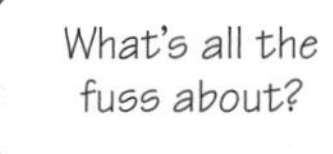
What's all the fuss about?

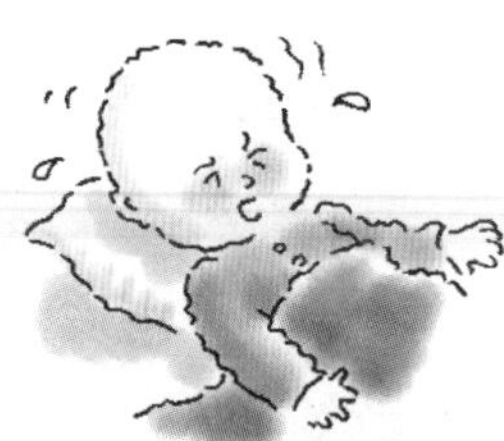

108. A pediatrician suspects that a child has pinworms and instructs the nurse to assess the child for their presence. Which is the most reliable method of assessing for pinworms?

1. A history of itching at the anal area and of restlessness at night
2. A blood culture
3. Eggs retrieved from the anal edge on a piece of cellophane tape
4. A stool culture

108. 3. Cellophane tape placed near the anal edge will capture the eggs. A history of itching and of restlessness aren't enough to definitely diagnosis pinworms. Neither a blood culture nor a stool culture would be helpful.

CN: Physiological integrity; CNS: Reduction of risk potential; CL: Application

109. An infant age 1 month is brought to the pediatrician's office. His mother states that he's fussy and cries as if in pain. He's tolerating normal amounts of formula, gaining weight, and having episodes of paroxysmal abdominal cramping after feedings. These signs and symptoms indicate that the infant most likely has which condition?

1. Intussusception
2. Meconium ileus
3. Colic
4. Pyloric stenosis

109. 3. An infant with colic exhibits symptoms of abdominal cramping after feedings, cries as if in pain, and is fussy. An intussusception begins suddenly and leads to bloody stools and vomiting. A meconium ileus is nonpassage of meconium by 24 hours of age. Signs of pyloric stenosis include projectile vomiting and weight loss.

CN: Physiological integrity; CNS: Physiological adaptation; CL: Analysis

110. A 16-year-old African-American student visits a school nurse with complaints of nausea and fatigue. The nurse determines a need to check for jaundice. Which area of the body should the nurse examine?

1. Sclera of the eye
2. Overall skin color
3. Outer ears and back of the neck
4. Tongue and inside the cheek area

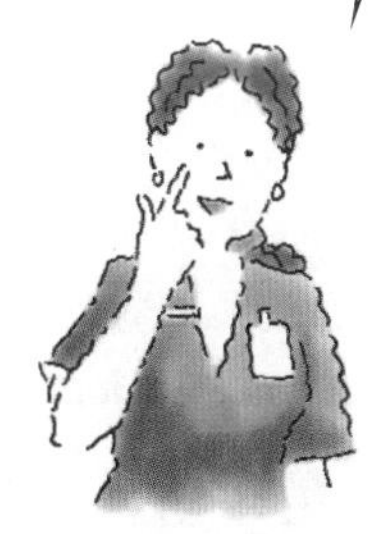

"Eye" think you know the answer to this one.

110. 1. The sclera is the best place to check for jaundice, especially in a person of darker color. The outer ears and back of the neck as well as the tongue and inside of the cheek aren't appropriate places to check for jaundice.
CN: Physiological integrity; CNS: Physiological adaptation; CL: Application

111. A mother brings her 4-week-old child to the clinic. She states that he hasn't been eating well and is lethargic when she holds and cuddles him. He has lost 7 oz (198.5 g) since birth. He's otherwise healthy and has no congenital defects. Which condition is the pediatrician most likely to diagnose?

1. Celiac disease
2. Failure to thrive
3. Hirschsprung's disease
4. Imperforate anus

111. 2. These signs and symptoms are classic of the condition failure to thrive. Celiac disease presents with steatorrhea, weight loss, and inability to digest gluten foods. Hirschsprung's disease and imperforate anus present with abdominal distention and absence of stool; no anal opening is present in imperforate anus.
CN: Physiological integrity; CNS: Physiological adaptation; CL: Application

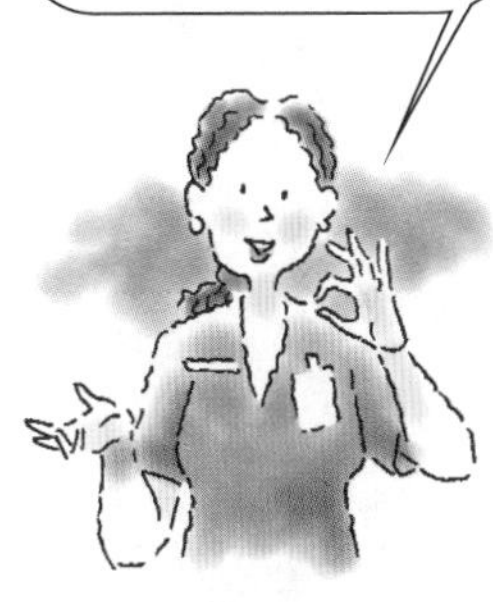

Just a little more to go and you're done with this chapter.

112. A 15-year-old client needs a nasogastric tube inserted because of peritonitis caused by a ruptured appendix. The client is afraid that the procedure will hurt. Which statement would most help decrease the client's anxiety?

1. "Breathe deeply through your mouth and relax. It will be over soon."
2. "This is a simple procedure, and it won't hurt."
3. "You'll feel pressure and be uncomfortable for a few minutes, but it shouldn't be painful."
4. "You're a man now and need to be able to handle pain."

112. 3. Discussing the procedure will help the client understand the extent of discomfort. Breathing deeply will help relieve discomfort, but the statement may also imply that the procedure will be painful and will, thus, increase the client's anxiety. By saying the procedure is simple, the nurse isn't acknowledging the client's concerns. Calling the client a man and telling him that he should be able to handle pain is condescending, No matter what the client's age, he has a right to express his fears and to have those fears acknowledged.
CN: Psychosocial integrity; CNS: None; CL: Analysis

113. A mother brings her 18-month-old child to the emergency department and tells a nurse that he has been ill for the past 2 days. He has a fever of 104° F (40° C), is irritable, has had diarrhea, and hasn't been wetting his diaper much in the past 24 hours. The child is admitted to the pediatric unit for treatment of moderate dehydration and gastroenteritis. I.V. therapy and strict intake and output are ordered. As rehydration occurs, the child is started on oral feedings of a rehydration fluid. When caring for this child during the later stage of rehydration, the nurse should take which action?

1. Force fluids.
2. Allow the client to drink as much as he wants.
3. Monitor the client's intake and output.
4. Monitor the client's ability to retain fluids.

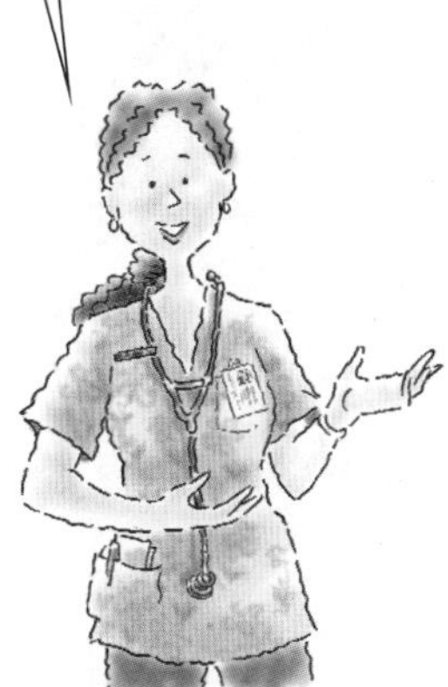

You're being asked for the *later stage* in question 113.

113. 4. The GI tract may not tolerate a full liquid diet immediately. Allowing only clear liquids gives the intestine time to heal, but the fluids should be reintroduced slowly to determine the child's ability to tolerate and retain them. The GI tract won't tolerate forcing fluids. Don't allow the client to drink as much as he wants; instead, offer small amounts of fluid every couple of hours. Monitoring intake and output is important and was *initially* ordered; it will continue until discharge.
CN: Physiological integrity; CNS: Basic care and comfort; CL: Analysis

114. A nurse is conducting an infant nutrition class for parents. Which foods should the nurse tell the parents it's OK to introduce during the first year of life? Select all that apply:

1. Sliced beef
2. Pureed fruits
3. Whole milk
4. Rice cereal
5. Strained vegetables
6. Fruit juice

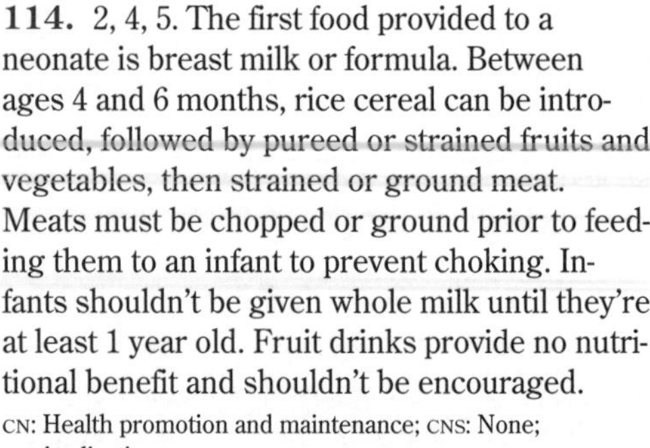

114. 2, 4, 5. The first food provided to a neonate is breast milk or formula. Between ages 4 and 6 months, rice cereal can be introduced, followed by pureed or strained fruits and vegetables, then strained or ground meat. Meats must be chopped or ground prior to feeding them to an infant to prevent choking. Infants shouldn't be given whole milk until they're at least 1 year old. Fruit drinks provide no nutritional benefit and shouldn't be encouraged.

CN: Health promotion and maintenance; CNS: None; CL: Application

115. A nurse is teaching a female adolescent with inflammatory bowel disease about treatment with corticosteroids. Which adverse effects are concerns for this client? Select all that apply:

1. Acne
2. Hirsutism
3. Mood swings
4. Osteoporosis
5. Growth spurts
6. Adrenal suppression

115. 1, 2, 3, 4, 6. Adverse effects of corticosteroids include acne, hirsutism, mood swings, osteoporosis, and adrenal suppression. Steroid use in children and adolescents may cause delayed growth, not growth spurts.

CN: Physiological integrity; CNS: Pharmacological and parenteral therapies; CL: Application

116. A mother brings her child to the pediatrician's office for evaluation of chronic stomach pain. The mother states that the pain seems to go away when she tells the child he can stay home from school. The physician diagnoses school phobia. Which other behaviors or symptoms may be present in the child with school phobia? Select all that apply:

1. Nausea
2. Headaches
3. Weight loss
4. Dizziness
5. Fever

116. 1, 2, 4. Children with school phobia commonly complain of vague symptoms, such as stomachaches, nausea, headaches, and dizziness, to avoid going to school. Typically, these symptoms don't occur on weekends. A careful history must be taken to identify a pattern of school avoidance. Such signs as weight loss and fever are more likely to have a physiologic cause and are uncommon in the child with school phobia.

CN: Psychosocial integrity; CNS: None; CL: Analysis

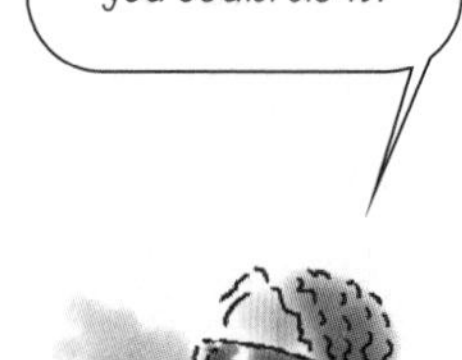

You're done with all those questions? I knew you could do it!

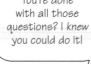

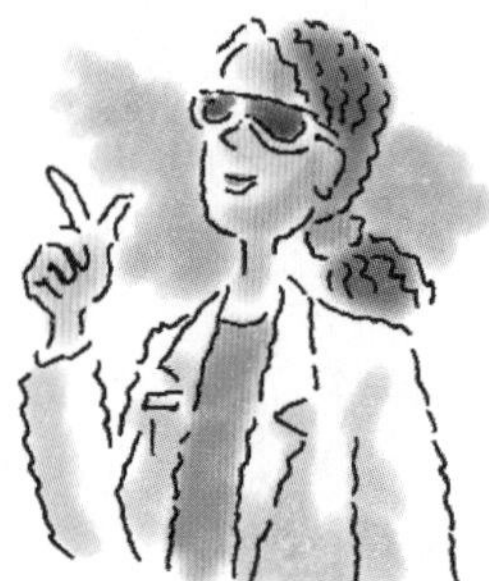

CN: Client needs category CNS: Client needs subcategory CL: Cognitive level

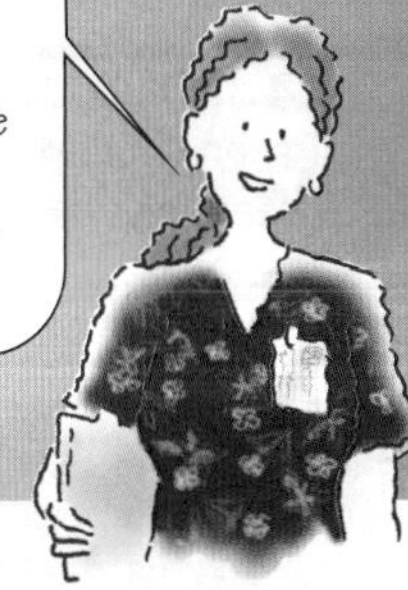

Caring for a child with an endocrine system disorder can be overwhelming. To get started on the right track, check out the Web site of the Juvenile Diabetes Research Foundation International at www.jdrf.org. Go for it!

Chapter 33 Endocrine disorders

1. When explaining the causes of hypothyroidism to the parents of a newly diagnosed infant, a nurse should recognize that further education is needed when the parents ask which question?

1. "Hypothyroidism can be only temporary, right?"
2. "Are you saying that hypothyroidism is caused by a problem in the way the thyroid gland develops?"
3. "Do you mean that hypothyroidism may be caused by a problem in the way the body makes thyroxine?"
4. "Hypothyroidism can be treated by exposing our baby to a special light, right?"

1. 4. Congenital hypothyroidism can be permanent or transient and may result from a defective thyroid gland or an enzymatic defect in thyroxine synthesis. Only the last question, which refers to phototherapy for physiologic jaundice, indicates that the parents need more information.

CN: Health promotion and maintenance; CNS: None; CL: Application

You're off to a good start.

2. An infant with hypothyroidism is receiving oral thyroid hormone. Which assessment findings should alert a nurse to a potential overdose?

1. Tachycardia, irritability, and diaphoresis
2. Bradycardia, excessive sleepiness, and dry scaly skin
3. Bradycardia, irritability, and cool extremities
4. Tachycardia, cool extremities, and irritability

2. 1. Clinical manifestations of thyroid hormone overdose in an infant include tachycardia, irritability, and diaphoresis. Bradycardia, excessive sleepiness, dry scaly skin, and cool extremities are manifestations of hypothyroidism.

CN: Physiological integrity; CNS: Pharmacological and parenteral therapies; CL: Application

3. When a nurse is teaching the parents of a neonate newly diagnosed with hypothyroidism, which statement should be included?

1. "A large goiter in a neonate doesn't present a problem."
2. "Preterm neonates usually aren't affected by hypothyroidism."
3. "Usually the neonate exhibits obvious signs of hypothyroidism."
4. "The severity of the disorder depends on the amount of thyroid tissue present."

3. 4. The severity of the disorder depends on the amount of thyroid tissue present. The more thyroid tissue is present, the less severe the disorder. A large goiter in a neonate could possibly occlude the airway and lead to obstruction. Preterm neonates are usually affected by hypothyroidism due to hypothalamic and pituitary immaturity. Usually the neonate doesn't exhibit obvious signs of the disorder because of maternal circulation.

CN: Health promotion and maintenance; CNS: None; CL: Application

CN: Client needs category CNS: Client needs subcategory CL: Cognitive level

4. Which condition is a subtle sign of hypothyroidism?

1. Diarrhea
2. Lethargy
3. Severe jaundice
4. Tachycardia

4. 2. Subtle signs of this disorder that may be seen shortly after birth include lethargy, poor feeding, prolonged jaundice, respiratory difficulty, cyanosis, constipation, and bradycardia. Diarrhea in the neonate isn't normal and isn't associated with this disorder. Severe jaundice needs immediate attention by the primary health care provider and isn't a subtle sign. Tachycardia typically occurs in hyperthyroidism, not hypothyroidism.

CN: Health promotion and maintenance; CNS: None; CL: Application

5. A nurse is assessing a toddler with hypothyroidism. Which signs should alert the nurse to the most serious complication of this condition?

1. Low hemoglobin and hematocrit
2. Cyanosis
3. Bone and muscle dystrophy
4. Mental retardation

5. 4. The most serious consequence of congenital hypothyroidism is delayed development of the central nervous system, which leads to severe mental retardation. The other choices occur but aren't the most serious consequences.

CN: Physiological integrity; CNS: Physiological adaptation; CL: Analysis

6. When counseling the parents of a neonate with congenital hypothyroidism, the nurse understands that the severity of the intellectual deficit is related to which parameter?

1. Duration of condition before treatment
2. Degree of hypothermia
3. Cranial malformations
4. Thyroxine (T_4) level at diagnosis

6. 1. The severity of the intellectual deficit is related to the degree of hypothyroidism and the duration of the condition before treatment. Cranial malformations don't affect the severity of the intellectual deficit nor does the degree of hypothermia as it relates to hypothyroidism. It isn't the specific T_4 level at diagnosis that affects the intellect but how long the client has been hospitalized.

CN: Health promotion and maintenance; CNS: None; CL: Application

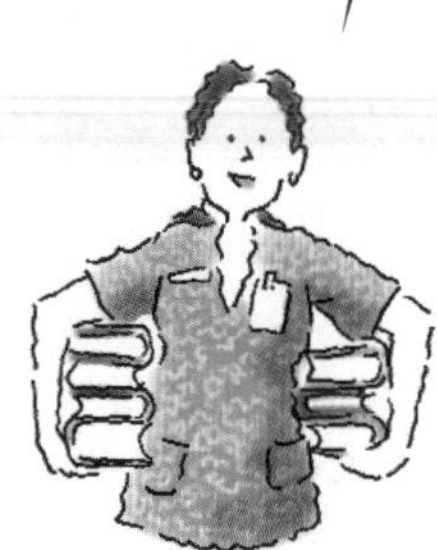
The diagnostic evaluation of a neonate may include tests that are mandated by the state.

7. Which statement should be included in an explanation of the diagnostic evaluation of neonates for congenital hypothyroidism?

1. Tests are mandatory in all states.
2. An arterial blood test is preferred.
3. Tests shouldn't be performed until after discharge.
4. Blood tests should be done after the first month of life.

7. 1. Heelstick blood tests are mandatory in all states and are usually performed on neonates between 2 and 6 days of age. Typically, specimens are taken before the neonate is discharged from the hospital; the test is included with other tests that screen the neonate for errors of metabolism.

CN: Health promotion and maintenance; CNS: None; CL: Application

8. Which result would indicate to a nurse the possibility that a neonate has congenital hypothyroidism?

1. High level thyroxine (T_4) and low level thyroid-stimulating hormone (TSH)
2. Low level T_4 and high level TSH
3. Normal TSH and high level T_4
4. Normal T_4 and low level TSH

8. 2. Screening results that show a low level of T_4 and a high level of TSH indicate congenital hypothyroidism and the need for further tests to determine the cause of the disease.
CN: Physiological integrity; CNS: Reduction of risk potential; CL: Application

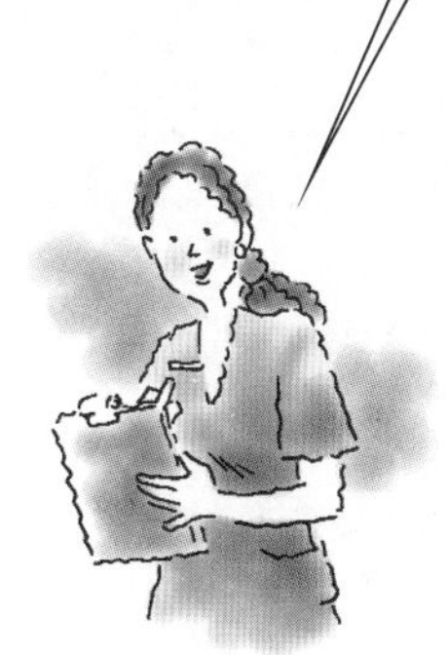

In question 9, the phrase *further teaching* indicates that you're looking for an *incorrect* statement.

9. A nurse is teaching parents about therapeutic management of their neonate diagnosed with congenital hypothyroidism. Which response by a parent would indicate the need for <u>further teaching</u>?

1. "My baby will need regular measurements of his thyroxine (T_4) levels."
2. "Treatment involves lifelong thyroid hormone replacement therapy."
3. "Treatment should begin as soon as possible after diagnosis is made."
4. "As my baby grows, his thyroid gland will mature and he won't need medications."

9. 4. Treatment involves lifelong thyroid hormone replacement therapy that begins as soon as possible after diagnosis to abolish all signs of hypothyroidism and to reestablish normal physical and mental development. The drug of choice is synthetic levothyroxine (Synthroid or Levothroid). Regular measurements of T_4 levels are important in ensuring optimum treatment.
CN: Health promotion and maintenance; CNS: None; CL: Application

10. Which comment made by the mother of a neonate at her 2-week office visit should alert the nurse to suspect congenital hypothyroidism?

1. "My baby is unusually quiet and good."
2. "My baby seems to be a yellowish color."
3. "After feedings, my baby pulls her legs up and cries."
4. "My baby seems to really look at my face during feeding time."

10. 1. Parental remarks about an unusually "quiet and good" neonate together with any of the early physical manifestations should lead to a suspicion of hypothyroidism, which requires a referral for specific tests. If a neonate begins to look yellow in color, hyperbilirubinemia may be the cause. If the neonate is pulling her legs up and crying after feedings, she might be showing signs of colic. The neonate likes looking at the human face and should show interest in this at age 2 weeks.
CN: Health promotion and maintenance; CNS: None; CL: Application

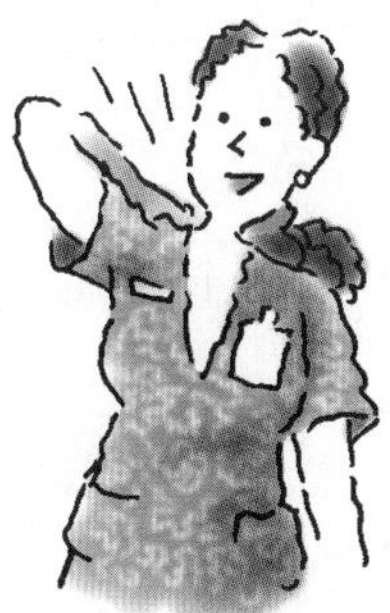

You've finished 10 questions already! Congratulations!

11. Which statement should be included when educating a mother about giving levothyroxine (Synthroid) to her neonate after a diagnosis of hypothyroidism is made?

1. The drug has a bitter taste.
2. The pill shouldn't be crushed.
3. Never put the medication in formula or juice.
4. If a dose is missed, double the dose the next day.

11. 4. If a dose is missed, twice the dose should be given the next day. The importance of compliance with the drug regimen for the neonate to achieve normal growth and development must be stressed. Because the drug is tasteless, it can be crushed and added to a small amount of water.
CN: Physiological integrity; CNS: Pharmacological and parenteral therapies; CL: Application

12. When teaching parents about signs that indicate levothyroxine (Synthroid) overdose, which comment from a parent indicates the need for <u>further teaching</u>?

1. "Irritability is a sign of overdose."
2. "If my baby's heartbeat is fast, I should count it."
3. "If my baby loses weight, I should be concerned."
4. "I shouldn't worry if my baby doesn't sleep very much."

12. 4. Parents need to be aware of signs indicating overdose, such as rapid pulse, dyspnea, irritability, insomnia, fever, sweating, and weight loss. The parents would be given acceptable parameters for the heart rate and weight loss or gain. If the baby is experiencing a heart rate or weight loss outside of the acceptable parameters, the physician should be called.

CN: Physiological integrity; CNS: Pharmacological and parenteral therapies; CL: Analysis

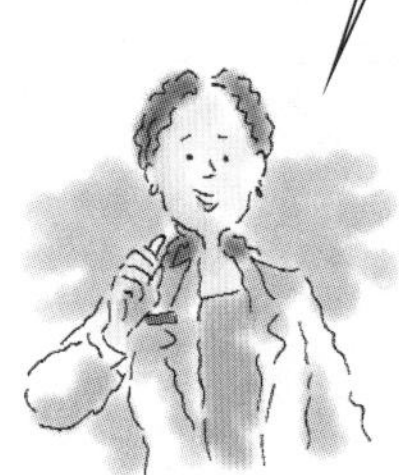

Watch out! Question 12 is another further teaching question.

13. A nurse should recognize that exophthalmos (protruding eyeballs) may occur in children with which condition?

1. Hypothyroidism
2. Hyperthyroidism
3. Hypoparathyroidism
4. Hyperparathyroidism

13. 2. Exophthalmos occurs when there's an overproduction of thyroid hormone, or hyperthyroidism. This sign should alert the physician to follow up with further testing.

CN: Health promotion and maintenance; CNS: None; CL: Application

14. A nurse is assessing a child with juvenile hypothyroidism. Which common clinical finding would most likely be observed?

1. Accelerated growth
2. Diarrhea
3. Dry skin
4. Insomnia

14. 3. Children with hypothyroidism will have dry skin. The other choices aren't evident in children with juvenile hypothyroidism.

CN: Health promotion and maintenance; CNS: None; CL: Application

15. A nurse is observing an infant with thyroid hormone deficiency. Which signs would the nurse <u>commonly</u> observe?

1. Tachycardia, profuse perspiration, and diarrhea
2. Lethargy, feeding difficulties, and constipation
3. Hypertonia, small fontanels, and moist skin
4. Dermatitis, dry skin, and round face

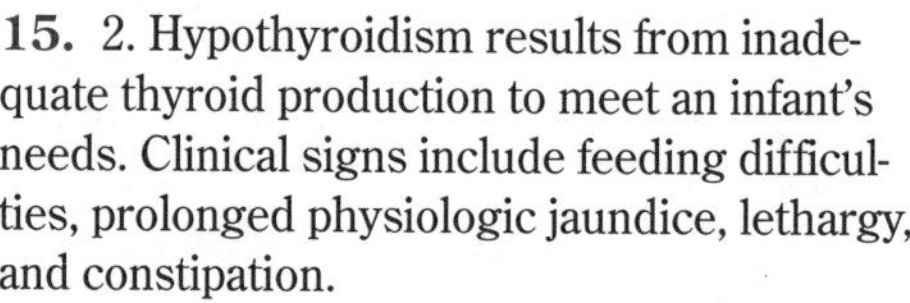
15. 2. Hypothyroidism results from inadequate thyroid production to meet an infant's needs. Clinical signs include feeding difficulties, prolonged physiologic jaundice, lethargy, and constipation.

CN: Health promotion and maintenance; CNS: None; CL: Analysis

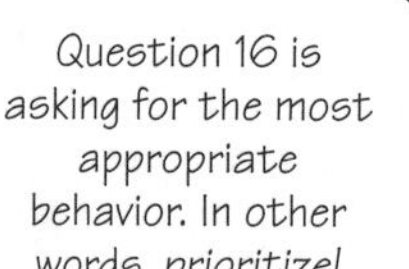

Question 16 is asking for the most appropriate behavior. In other words, prioritize!

16. When counseling parents of a neonate with congenital hypothyroidism, the nurse should encourage which behavior?

1. Seeking professional genetic counseling
2. Retracing the family tree for others born with this condition
3. Talking to relatives who have gone through a similar experience
4. Seeking alternative therapies for this condition

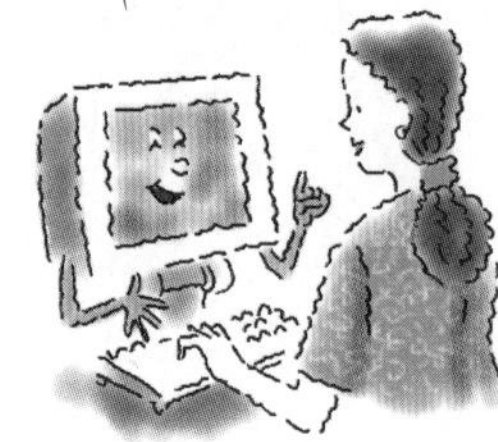

16. 1. Seeking professional genetic counseling is the best option for parents who have a neonate with a genetic disorder. Education about the disorder should occur as soon as the parents are ready, so they'll understand the genetic implications for future children. Retracing the family tree and talking to relatives won't help the parents to become better educated about the disorder. Seeking alternative therapies should be discouraged to prevent possible complications.

CN: Health promotion and maintenance; CNS: None; CL: Application

17. While receiving teaching about giving insulin injections, an adolescent questions the nurse about the reuse of disposable needles and syringes. Which response from the nurse is most appropriate?

1. "This is an unsafe practice."
2. "This is acceptable for up to 7 days."
3. "This is acceptable for only 48 hours."
4. "This is acceptable only if the family has very limited resources."

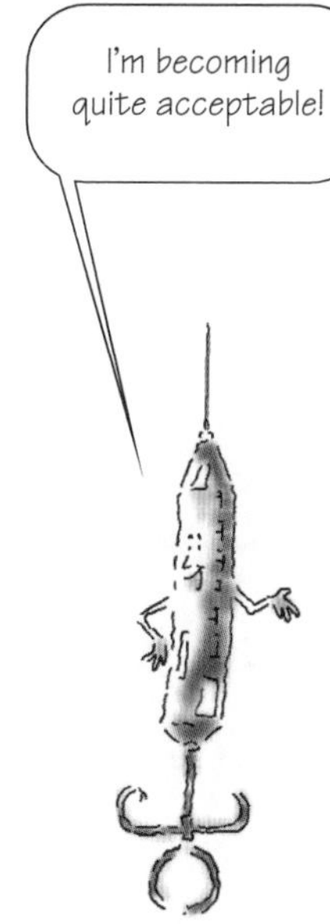
I'm becoming
quite acceptable!

17. 2. It has become acceptable practice for clients to reuse their own disposable needles and syringes for up to 7 days. Bacteria counts are unaffected, and there are considerable cost savings. If this method is approved, it's imperative to stress the importance of vigorous hand washing before handling equipment as well as capping the syringe immediately after use and storing it in the refrigerator to decrease the growth of organisms.

CN: Safe, effective care environment; CNS: Safety and infection control; CL: Application

18. When children are more physically active, which change in the management of the child with diabetes should the nurse expect?

1. Increased food intake
2. Decreased food intake
3. Decreased risk of insulin shock
4. Increased risk of hyperglycemia

18. 1. If a child is more active at one time of the day than another, food or insulin can be altered to meet the activity pattern of the individual. Food should be increased when children are more physically active. The child has an increased risk of insulin shock and a decreased risk of hyperglycemia when he's more physically active.

CN: Physiological integrity; CNS: Reduction of risk potential; CL: Application

19. When a nurse is helping an adolescent deal with diabetes, which characteristic of adolescence should be considered?

1. Wanting to be an individual
2. Needing to be like peers
3. Being preoccupied with future plans
4. Teaching peers that this is a serious disease

19. 2. Adolescents appear to have the most difficulty in adjusting to diabetes. Adolescence is a time when there's much stress on being "perfect" and being like one's peers and, to adolescents, having diabetes is being different.

CN: Health promotion and maintenance; CNS: None; CL: Application

20. An adolescent with diabetes tells the community nurse that he has recently started drinking alcohol on the weekends. Which action would initially be most appropriate for the nurse to take?

1. Recommend referral to counseling.
2. Make the adolescent promise to stop drinking.
3. Discuss with the adolescent why he has started drinking.
4. Teach the adolescent about the effects of alcohol on diabetes.

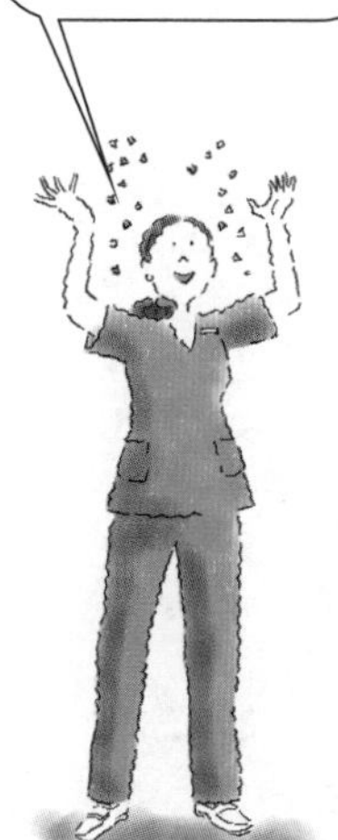
20 questions
completed?
That's cause for
celebration!

20. 4. Confusion about the effects of alcohol on blood glucose is common. Teenagers may believe that alcohol will increase blood glucose levels, when in fact the opposite occurs. Ingestion of alcohol inhibits the release of glycogen from the liver, resulting in hypoglycemia. Teens who drink alcohol may become hypoglycemic, but they are then treated as if they were intoxicated. Behaviors may be similar, such as shakiness, combativeness, slurred speech, and loss of consciousness. Finding out why the adolescent has started drinking and recommending counseling may be appropriate, but only after education is provided. An adolescent may promise to stop drinking but not follow through.

CN: Health promotion and maintenance; CNS: None; CL: Application

21. A child has experienced symptoms of hypoglycemia and has eaten sugar cubes. A nurse should follow this rapid-releasing sugar with which food?

1. Fruit juices
2. Six glasses of water
3. Foods that are high in protein
4. Complex carbohydrates and protein

21. 4. When a child exhibits signs of hypoglycemia, the majority of cases can be treated with a simple concentrated sugar, such as honey, that can be held in the mouth for a short time. A complex carbohydrate and protein, such as a slice of bread or a cracker spread with peanut butter, should follow the rapid-releasing sugar or the client may become hypoglycemic again.

CN: Health promotion and maintenance; CNS: None; CL: Application

22. The nurse is teaching the parents of a child newly diagnosed with diabetes to identify the signs and symptoms of hypoglycemia. Which response by the parents indicates the teaching has been effective?

1. “Irritability, shakiness, hunger, headache, and dizziness are signs to look for.”
2. “Drowsiness, lethargy, and decreased urine output need to be reported.”
3. “Abdominal pain, nausea and vomiting, and constipation are the most common findings.”
4. “We will report immediately any signs of urinary frequency.”

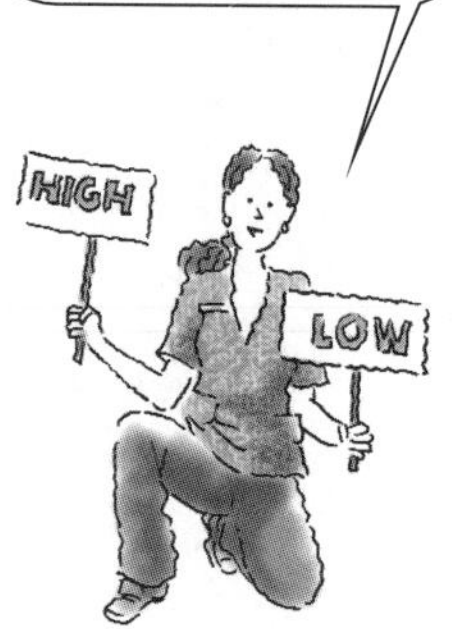

If you know the definitions of hypo and hyper, it can help you with a bunch of questions.
HIGH
LOW

22. 1. Signs of hypoglycemia include irritabi lity, shaky feeling, hunger, headache, and dizziness. Drowsiness, abdominal pain, polyuria, nausea, and vomiting are signs of ***hyper***glycemia.

CN: Physiological integrity; CNS: Physiological adaptation; CL: Application

23. The nurse is assessing a child recently admitted with diabetes who has developed ketoacidosis. Which statement is the most accurate?

1. This is a normal outcome of diabetes.
2. This is a life-threatening situation.
3. This is a situation that can easily be treated at home.
4. This is a situation best treated in the pediatrician’s office.

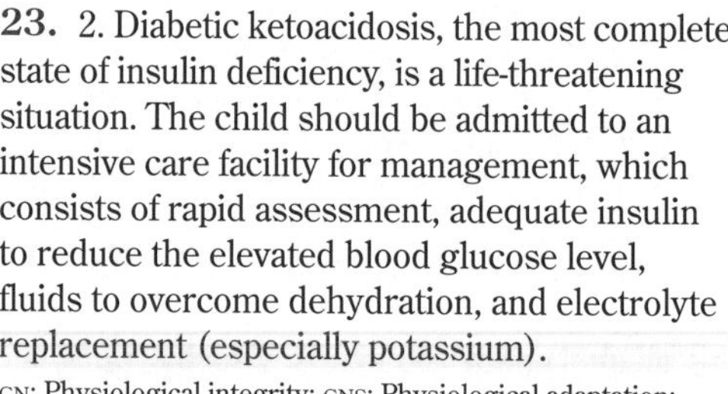

23. 2. Diabetic ketoacidosis, the most complete state of insulin deficiency, is a life-threatening situation. The child should be admitted to an intensive care facility for management, which consists of rapid assessment, adequate insulin to reduce the elevated blood glucose level, fluids to overcome dehydration, and electrolyte replacement (especially potassium).

CN: Physiological integrity; CNS: Physiological adaptation; CL: Application

24. Which guideline is appropriate when teaching an 11-year-old child who was recently diagnosed with diabetes about insulin injections?

1. The parents don’t need to be involved in learning this procedure.
2. Self-injection techniques aren’t usually taught until the child reaches age 16.
3. At age 11, the child should be old enough to give most of his own injections.
4. Self-injection techniques should be taught only when the child can reach all injection sites.

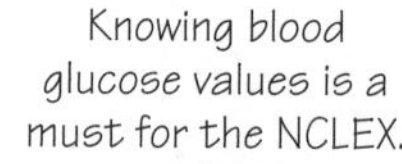

Knowing blood glucose values is a must for the NCLEX.

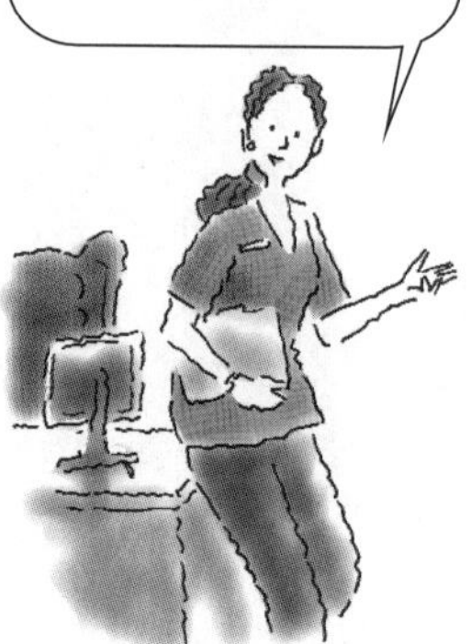

24. 3. The parents must supervise and manage the child’s therapeutic program, but the child should assume responsibility for self-management as soon as he’s capable. Children can learn to collect their own blood for glucose testing at a relatively young age (4 to 5 years), and most are able to check their blood glucose level and administer insulin at about age 9. Some children may be able to do it earlier.

CN: Health promotion and maintenance; CNS: None; CL: Application

25. The nurse suspects a client of having diabetic ketoacidosis. Which blood glucose value would be observed with this condition?
1. 50 mg/dl
2. 90 mg/dl
3. 150 mg/dl
4. 300 mg/dl

25. 4. Diabetic ketoacidosis is determined by the presence of hyperglycemia (blood glucose measurement of 300 mg/dl or higher), accompanied by acetone breath, dehydration, weak and rapid pulse, and a decreased level of consciousness.
CN: Physiological integrity; CNS: Physiological adaptation; CL: Analysis

26. A 2-year-old child has been admitted with a diagnosis of diabetes mellitus. Which cardinal sign would support this diagnosis?
1. Nausea
2. Seizure
3. Hyperactivity
4. Frequent urination

26. 4. Polyphagia, polyuria (frequent urination), polydipsia, and weight loss are cardinal signs of diabetes mellitus. Other signs include irritability, shortened attention span, lowered frustration tolerance, fatigue, dry skin, blurred vision, sores that are slow to heal, and flushed skin.
CN: Health promotion and maintenance; CNS: None; CL: Application

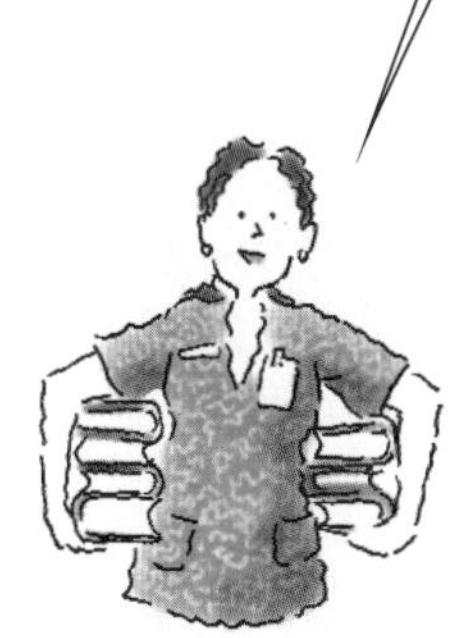

Teaching clients how to help manage their own conditions is a common subject on the NCLEX.

27. The parent of a child with diabetes asks a nurse why blood glucose monitoring is needed. The nurse should base her reply on which premise?
1. This is an easier method of testing.
2. This is a less expensive method of testing.
3. This allows children the ability to better manage their diabetes.
4. This gives children a greater sense of control over their diabetes.

27. 3. Blood glucose monitoring improves diabetes management and is used successfully by children from the onset of their diabetes. By testing their own blood, children are able to change their insulin regimen to maintain their glucose level in the normoglycemic range of 80 to 120 mg/dl. This allows them to better manage their diabetes.
CN: Health promotion and maintenance; CNS: None; CL: Application

28. To increase an adolescent's compliance with treatment for diabetes mellitus, the nurse should attempt which strategy?
1. Provide for a special diet in the high school cafeteria.
2. Clarify the adolescent's values to promote involvement in care.
3. Identify energy requirements for participation in sports activities.
4. Educate the adolescent about long-term consequences of poor metabolic control.

28. 2. Adolescent compliance with diabetes management may be hampered by dependence versus independence conflicts and ego development. Attempts to have the adolescent clarify personal values promotes involvement in his care and fosters compliance.
CN: Health promotion and maintenance; CNS: None; CL: Application

29. A child with diabetes type 1 tells the nurse he feels shaky. The nurse assesses the child's skin color to be pale and sweaty. Which action should the nurse initiate immediately?

1. Give supplemental insulin.
2. Have the child eat a glucose tablet.
3. Administer glucagon subcutaneously.
4. Offer the child a complex carbohydrate snack.

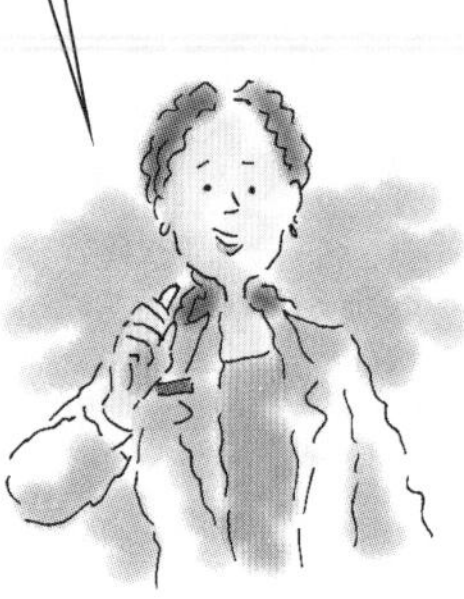

The word *immediately* signals a need for you to prioritize.

29. 2. These are symptoms of hypoglycemia. Rapid treatment involves giving the alert child a glucose tablet (4 mg of dextrose) or, if unavailable, a glass of glucose-containing liquid. It would be followed by a complex carbohydrate snack and protein. Giving supplemental insulin would be contraindicated because that would lower the blood glucose even more. Glucagon would be given only if there was a risk of aspiration with oral glucose, such as if the child was semiconscious.

CN: Safe, effective care environment; CNS: Management of care; CL: Application

30. The parents of a child diagnosed with diabetes ask the nurse about maintaining metabolic control during a minor illness with loss of appetite. Which nursing response is appropriate?

1. "Decrease the child's insulin by half the usual dose during the course of the illness."
2. "Call your physician to arrange hospitalization."
3. "Give increased amounts of clear liquids to prevent dehydration."
4. "Substitute calorie-containing liquids for uneaten solid food."

30. 4. Calorie-containing liquids can help to maintain more normal blood sugar levels as well as decrease the danger of dehydration. The child with diabetes should always take *at least* the usual dose of insulin during an illness based on more frequent blood sugar checks. During an illness where there's vomiting or loss of appetite, NPH insulin may be lowered by 25% to 30% to avoid hyperglycemia, and regular insulin is given according to home glucose monitoring results.

CN: Safe, effective care environment; CNS: Management of care; CL: Application

31. Which criteria should a nurse use to measure good metabolic control in a child with diabetes mellitus?

1. Fewer than eight episodes of severe hyperglycemia in a month
2. Infrequent occurrences of mild hypoglycemic reactions
3. Hemoglobin A values less than 12%
4. Growth below the 15th percentile

31. 2. Criteria for good metabolic control generally includes few episodes of hypoglycemia or hyperglycemia, hemoglobin A values less than 8%, and normal growth and development.

CN: Health promotion and maintenance; CNS: None; CL: Application

32. The nurse is assessing the neonate of a poorly controlled diabetic mother in the NICU. Which congenital anomaly would likely be observed?

1. Cataracts
2. Low-set ears
3. Cardiac malformations
4. Cleft lip and palate deformities

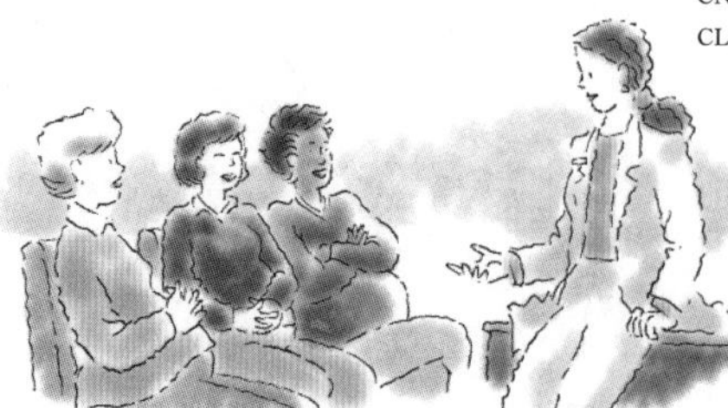

It's important for your baby's sake to control your diabetes.

32. 3. Cardiac and central nervous system anomalies, along with neural tube defects and skeletal and GI anomalies, are most likely to occur in uncontrolled maternal diabetes.

CN: Health promotion and maintenance; CNS: None; CL: Application

CN: Client needs category CNS: Client needs subcategory CL: Cognitive level

33. Which condition could possibly cause hypoglycemia?

1. Too little insulin
2. Mild illness with fever
3. Excessive exercise without a carbohydrate snack
4. Eating ice cream and cake to celebrate a birthday

33. 3. Excessive exercise without a carbohydrate snack could cause hypoglycemia. The other options describe situations that cause *hyper*glycemia.

CN: Health promotion and maintenance; CNS: None; CL: Application

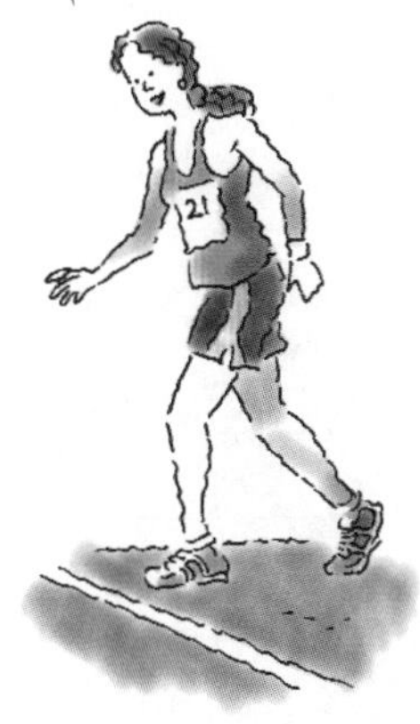

I'm glad I had a snack before I started to race.
21

34. Which assessment factor is the best indicator of a client's diabetic control during the preceding 2 to 3 months?

1. Fasting glucose level
2. Oral glucose tolerance level
3. Glycosylated hemoglobin test
4. A client's record of glucose monitoring

34. 3. A glycosylated hemoglobin level provides an overview of a person's blood glucose level over the previous 2 to 3 months. Glycosylated hemoglobin values are reported as a percentage of the total hemoglobin within an erythrocyte. The time frame is based on the fact that the usual life span of an erythrocyte is 2 to 3 months; a random blood sample, therefore, will theoretically give samples of erythrocytes for this same period. The other options won't indicate a true picture of the person's blood glucose level over the previous 2 to 3 months.

CN: Health promotion and maintenance; CNS: None; CL: Application

35. A client has received diet instruction as part of his treatment plan for diabetes type 1. Which statement by the client indicates to the nurse that he needs additional instructions?

1. "I'll need a bedtime snack because I take an evening dose of NPH insulin."
2. "I can eat whatever I want as long as I cover the calories with sufficient insulin."
3. "I can have an occasional low-calorie drink as long as I include it in my meal plan."
4. "I should eat meals as scheduled, even if I'm not hungry, to prevent hypoglycemia."

35. 2. The goal of diet therapy in diabetes mellitus is to attain and maintain ideal body weight. Each client will be prescribed a specific caloric intake and insulin regimen to help accomplish this goal.

CN: Physiological integrity; CNS: Basic care and comfort; CL: Analysis

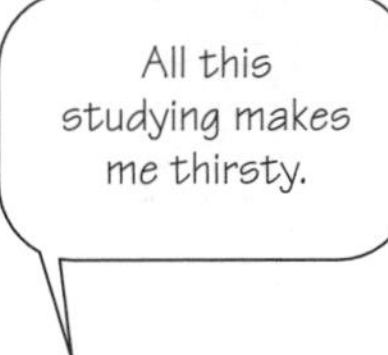

All this studying makes me thirsty.

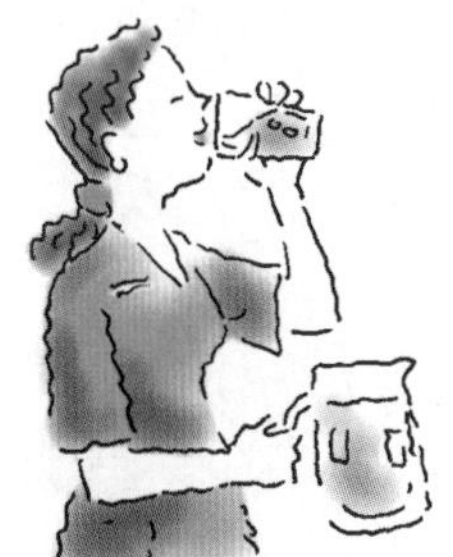

36. The nurse suspects a 10-year-old client with diabetes is hyperglycemic. Which symptom would indicate this condition?

1. Rapid heart rate
2. Headache
3. Hunger
4. Thirst

36. 4. Thirst (polydipsia) is one of the symptoms of hyperglycemia. Rapid heart rate, headache, and hunger are signs and symptoms of *hypo*glycemia.

CN: Physiological integrity; CNS: Physiological adaptation; CL: Application

37. A client is learning to mix regular insulin and NPH insulin in the same syringe. Which action, if performed by the client, would indicate the need for further teaching?

1. Withdrawing the NPH insulin first
2. Injecting air into the NPH insulin bottle first
3. After drawing up first insulin, removing air bubbles
4. Injecting an amount of air equal to the desired dose of insulin

37. 1. Regular insulin is *always* withdrawn first so it won't become contaminated with NPH insulin. The client is instructed to inject air into the NPH insulin bottle equal to the amount of insulin to be withdrawn, because there will be regular insulin in the syringe and he won't be able to inject air when he needs to withdraw the NPH. It's necessary to remove the air bubbles to ensure a correct dosage before drawing up the second insulin.

CN: Physiological integrity; CNS: Pharmacological and parenteral therapies; CL: Application

38. A client is diagnosed with diabetes type 1. The primary health care provider prescribes an insulin regimen of regular insulin and NPH insulin administered subcutaneously each morning. How soon after administration will the onset of regular insulin begin?

1. Within 5 minutes
2. ½ to 1 hour
3. 1 to 1½ hours
4. 4 to 8 hours

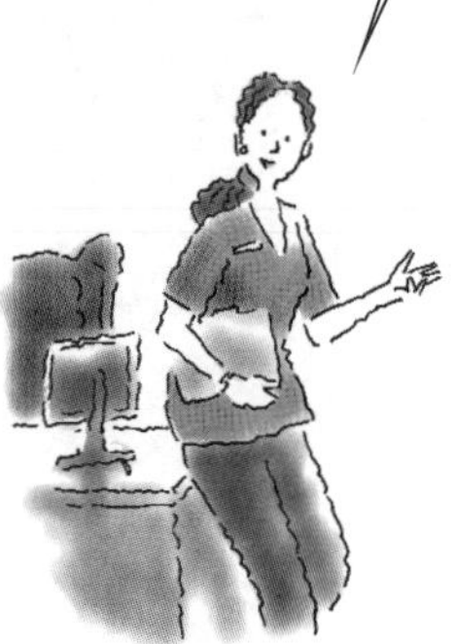

It's important to know how and when different types of insulin react.

38. 2. Regular insulin's onset is ½ to 1 hour, peak is 2 to 4 hours, and duration is 3 to 6 hours. Lispro insulin has an onset within 5 minutes. NPH insulin has an onset within 2 to 4 hours, and Ultralente insulin is the longest acting, with an onset of 6 to 10 hours.

CN: Physiological integrity; CNS: Pharmacological and parenteral therapies; CL: Application

39. When assessing a neonate for signs of diabetes insipidus, a nurse should recognize which symptom as a sign of this disorder?

1. Hyponatremia
2. Jaundice
3. Polyuria
4. Hypochloremia

39. 3. The cardinal sign of diabetes insipidus is polyuria, along with polydipsia. Hypernatremia, not hyponatremia, occurs with diabetes insipidus. Jaundice occurs because of abnormal bilirubin metabolism, not diabetes insipidus. Hyperchloremia, not hypochloremia, occurs with diabetes insipidus.

CN: Physiological integrity; CNS: Physiological adaptation; CL: Application

40. Which is an initial symptom of diabetes insipidus in an infant?

1. Dehydration
2. Inability to be aroused
3. Extreme hunger relieved by frequent feedings of milk
4. Irritability relieved with feedings of water but not milk

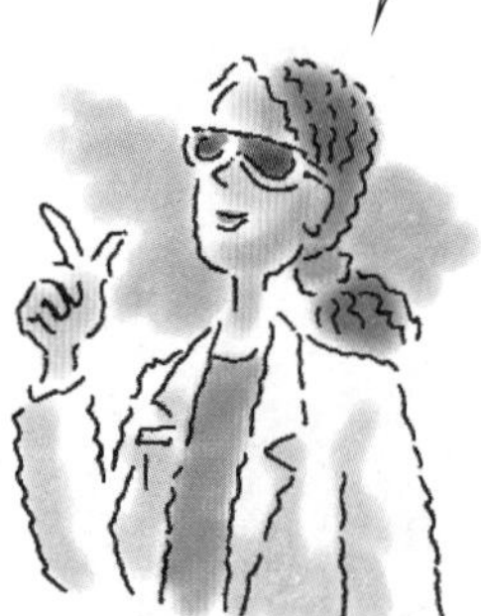

You've reached question 40. How cool is that?

40. 4. One initial symptom of diabetes insipidus in an infant is irritability relieved with feedings of water but not milk. Dehydration and the inability to be aroused are late symptoms.

CN: Health promotion and maintenance; CNS: None; CL: Application

41. A nurse is helping parents understand when treatments of growth hormone replacement will end. Which statement should be included?

1. The dosage of growth hormone will decrease as the child's age increases.
2. The dosage of growth hormone will increase as the time of epiphyseal closure nears.
3. After giving growth hormone replacement for 1 year, the dose will be tapered down.
4. Growth hormone replacement can't be abruptly stopped; it must be spread out over several months.

41. 2. Dosage of growth hormone is increased as the time of epiphyseal closure nears, to gain the best advantage of the growth hormone. The medication is then stopped. There's no tapering off of the dose.

CN: Physiological integrity; CNS: Pharmacological and parenteral therapies; CL: Application

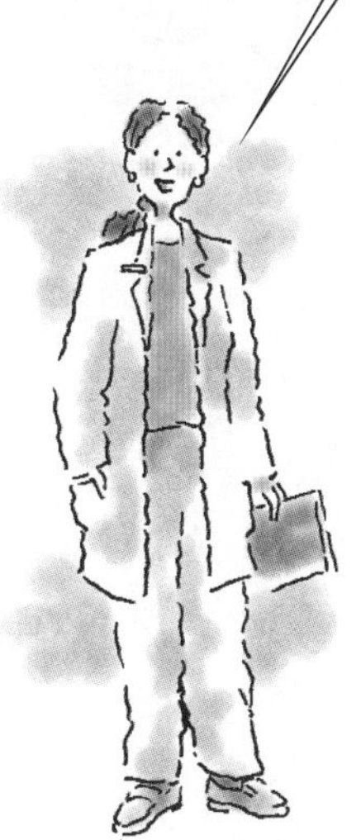

Question 42 asks you to identify a *knowledgeable* response.

42. A nurse is explaining diabetes insipidus to the parents of an infant with the disease. When explaining the diagnostic test that's used, which comment by a parent would indicate an understanding of the diagnostic test?

1. "Fluids will be offered every 2 hours."
2. "My infant's fluid intake will be restricted."
3. "I won't change anything about my infant's intake."
4. "Formula will be restricted, but glucose water is OK."

42. 2. The simplest test used to diagnose diabetes insipidus is restriction of oral fluids and observation of consequent changes in urine volume and concentration. A weight loss of 3% to 5% indicates severe dehydration, and the test should be terminated at this point. This is done in the hospital, and the infant is watched closely.

CN: Health promotion and maintenance; CNS: None; CL: Application

43. A nurse should anticipate which physiologic response in an infant being tested for diabetes insipidus?

1. Increase in urine output
2. Decrease in urine output
3. No effect on urine output
4. Increase in urine specific gravity

43. 3. In diabetes insipidus, fluid restriction for diagnostic testing has little or no effect on urine formation but causes weight loss from dehydration.

CN: Physiological integrity; CNS: Physiological adaptation; CL: Application

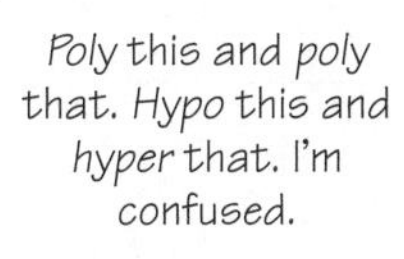

Poly this and *poly* that. *Hypo* this and *hyper* that. I'm confused.

44. An infant has a positive test result for diabetes insipidus. The nurse should anticipate the physician ordering a test dose of which medication?

1. Antidiuretic hormone
2. Biosynthetic growth hormone
3. Adrenocorticotropic hormone
4. Aqueous vasopressin (Pitressin Synthetic)

44. 4. If the fluid restriction test is positive, the child should be given a test dose of injected aqueous vasopressin, which should alleviate the polyuria and polydipsia. Unresponsiveness to exogenous vasopressin usually indicates nephrogenic diabetes insipidus. The other choices are used to determine other types of endocrine disorders.

CN: Physiological integrity; CNS: Pharmacological and parenteral therapies; CL: Application

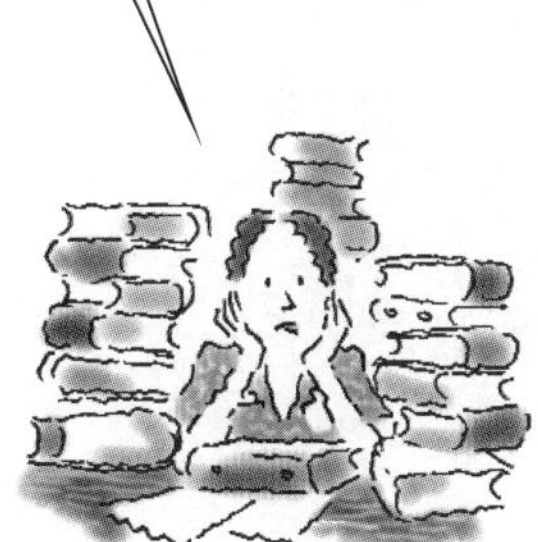

45. The nurse is teaching the parents of an infant diagnosed with diabetes insipidus. Which treatment would the nurse include in the teaching?

1. Antihypertensive medications
2. The need for blood products
3. Hormone replacement
4. Fluid restrictions

46. When providing information about treatments for diabetes insipidus to parents, a nurse explains the use of nasal spray and injections. Which indication might deter a parent from choosing nasal spray treatment?

1. Applications must be repeated every 8 to 12 hours.
2. Applications must be repeated every 2 to 4 hours.
3. Nasal sprays can't be used in infants.
4. Measurements are too difficult.

47. A nurse is teaching the parents of an infant with diabetes insipidus about an injectable drug used to treat the disorder. Which statement made by a parent would indicate the need for further teaching?

1. "I must hold the medication under warm running water for 10 to 15 minutes before administering it."
2. "The medication must be shaken vigorously before being drawn up into the syringe."
3. "Small brown particles must be seen in the suspension."
4. "I will store this medication in the refrigerator."

48. When teaching parents of an infant newly diagnosed with diabetes insipidus, which statement by a parent indicates a good understanding of this condition?

1. "When my infant stabilizes, I won't have to worry about giving hormone medication."
2. "I don't have to measure the amount of fluid intake that I give my infant."
3. "I realize that treatment for diabetes insipidus is lifelong."
4. "My infant will outgrow this condition."

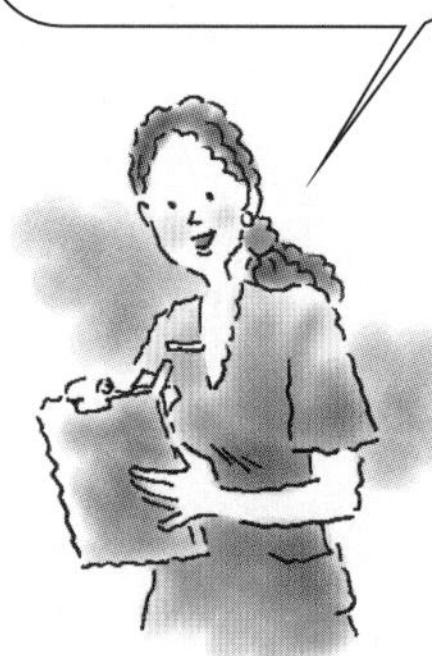

Although the word *deter* sounds like a negative, question 46 actually asks you to identify a true characteristic of nasal sprays.

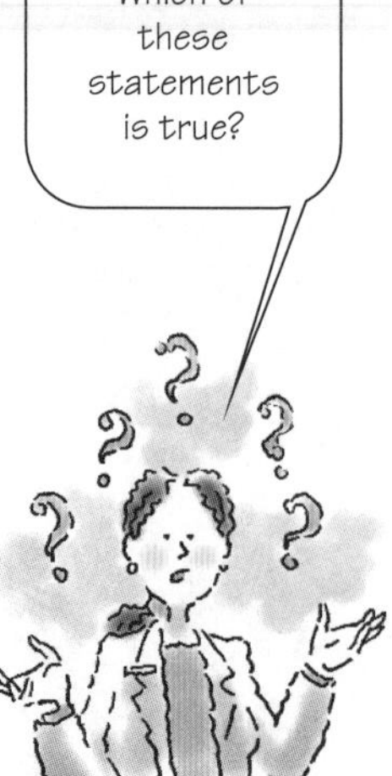

Which of these statements is true?

45. 3. The usual treatment for diabetes insipidus is hormone replacement with vasopressin or desmopressin acetate (DDAVP). No problem with hypertension is associated with this condition, and fluids shouldn't be restricted. Blood products shouldn't be needed.

CN: Health promotion and maintenance; CNS: None; CL: Application

46. 1. Applications of nasal spray used to treat diabetes insipidus must be repeated every 8 to 12 hours; injections last for 48 to 72 hours. The nasal spray must be timed for adequate night sleep. However, the injections are oil-based and quite painful. Nasal sprays have been used in infants with diabetes insipidus and are dispensed in premeasured intranasal inhalers, eliminating the need for measuring doses.

CN: Physiological integrity; CNS: Pharmacological and parenteral therapies CL: Analysis

47. 4. The medication should be stored at room temperature. When giving injectable vasopressin, it must be thoroughly resuspended in the oil by being held under warm running water for 10 to 15 minutes and shaken vigorously before being drawn into the syringe. If this isn't done, the oil may be injected minus the drug. Small brown particles, which indicate drug dispersion, must be seen in the suspension.

CN: Physiological integrity; CNS: Pharmacological and parenteral therapies; CL: Application

48. 3. Diabetes insipidus is a condition that will need lifelong treatment. The amount of fluid intake is very important and must be measured with the infant's output to monitor the medication regime. The infant won't outgrow this condition.

CN: Safe, effective care environment; CNS: Management of care; CL: Application

49. A child is admitted with diabetes insipidus. The nurse asks the parents if they know about this condition. Which statement tells the nurse that the parents understand the condition?

1. "We know that our child's thyroid is working too much."
2. "We know that our child's pituitary gland is not working hard enough."
3. "Our child's pituitary gland is working overtime."
4. "Our child's parathyroid gland is not doing a good job. It is acting very lazy."

49. 2. The principal disorder of posterior pituitary hypofunction is diabetes insipidus. The disorder results form hyposecretion of antidiuretic hormone, producing a state of uncontrolled diuresis. It is not caused by the thyroid gland or parathyroid gland.

CN: Health promotion and maintenance; CNS: None; CL: Application

50. After a nurse has explained the causes of diabetes insipidus to the parents, which statement made by a parent indicates the need for further teaching?

1. "This condition could be familial or congenital."
2. "Drinking alcohol during my pregnancy caused this condition."
3. "My child might have a tumor that's causing these symptoms."
4. "An infection such as meningitis may be the reason my child has diabetes insipidus."

50. 2. Drinking alcohol during pregnancy can lead to a neonate born with fetal alcohol syndrome but has no known correlation to diabetes insipidus. The other options are possible causes of diabetes insipidus.

CN: Health promotion and maintenance; CNS: None; CL: Application

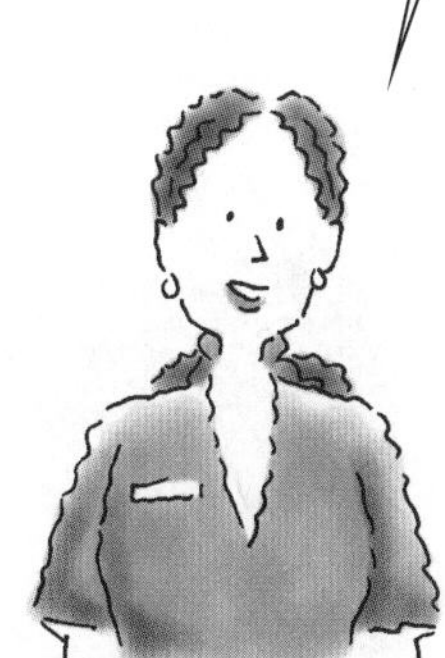

Question 51 asks for a common adverse effect of vasopressin administration.

51. Which assessment finding would alert a nurse to change the intranasal route for vasopressin administration?

1. Mucous membrane irritation
2. Severe coughing
3. Nosebleeds
4. Pneumonia

51. 1. Mucous membrane irritation caused by a cold or allergy renders the intranasal route unreliable. Severe coughing, pneumonia, or nosebleeds shouldn't interfere with the intranasal route.

CN: Physiological integrity; CNS: Pharmacological and parenteral therapies; CL: Application

52. A nurse should include which in-home management instruction for a child who's receiving desmopressin acetate (DDAVP) for symptomatic control of diabetes insipidus?

1. Give DDAVP only when urine output begins to decrease.
2. Cleanse skin with alcohol before application of the DDAVP dermal patch.
3. Increase the DDAVP dose if polyuria occurs just before the next scheduled dose.
4. Call the physician for an alternate route of DDAVP when the child has an upper respiratory infection (URI) or allergic rhinitis.

52. 4. Excessive nasal mucus associated with URI or allergic rhinitis may interfere with DDAVP absorption because it's given intranasally. Parents should be instructed to contact the physician for advice in altering the hormone dose during times when nasal mucus may be increased. The DDAVP dose should remain unchanged, even if there's polyuria just before the next dose. This is to avoid overmedicating the child.

CN: Safe, effective care environment; CNS: Management of care; CL: Application

53. A nurse is assessing a client with suspected hypopituitarism. Which sign or symptom of this condition would the nurse most commonly observe?
1. Sleep disturbance
2. Polyuria
3. Polydipsia
4. Short stature

53. 4. The most common sign in most instances of hypopituitarism is short stature. Sleep disturbance may indicate thyrotoxicosis. Polydipsia and polyuria may be indications of diabetes mellitus or diabetes insipidus.
CN: Physiological integrity; CNS: Physiological adaptation; CL: Application

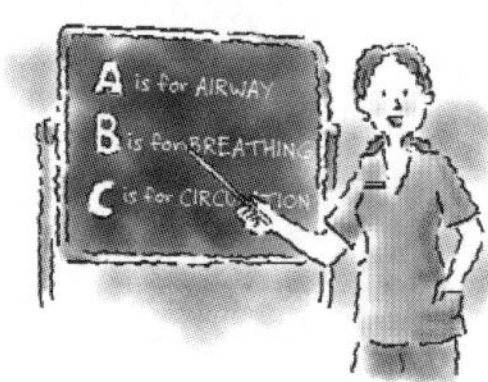
A nurse's responsibility to teach never ends.
A is for AIRWAY
B is for BREATHING

54. Which statement made to a nurse by the parents of a child with idiopathic growth hormone deficiency would indicate the need for further teaching?
1. "This disorder may be familial."
2. "There's no genetic basis for this disorder."
3. "This disorder might be secondary to hypothalamic deficiency."
4. "There may be other disorders related to pituitary hormone deficiencies."

54. 2. The cause of idiopathic growth hormone deficiency is unknown. There's a higher-than-average occurrence of the disorder in some families, which indicates a possible genetic cause. The condition is commonly associated with other pituitary hormone deficiencies, such as deficiencies of thyroid-stimulating hormone and corticotropin, and may be secondary to hypothalamic deficiency.
CN: Psychosocial integrity; CNS: None; CL: Application

55. A nurse is teaching health to a class of fifth graders. Which statement related to growth should be included?
1. "There's nothing that you can do to influence your growth."
2. "Excessive physical activity that begins before puberty might stunt growth."
3. "All children who are short in stature also have parents who are short in stature."
4. "Because this is a time of tremendous growth, being concerned about calorie intake isn't important."

55. 2. Intensive physical activity (greater than 18 hours per week) that begins before puberty may stunt growth so that the child doesn't reach full adult height. Nutrition and environment influence a child's growth. All children who are short in stature don't necessarily have parents who are short in stature. During the school-age years, growth slows and doesn't accelerate again until adolescence.
CN: Health promotion and maintenance; CNS: None; CL: Application

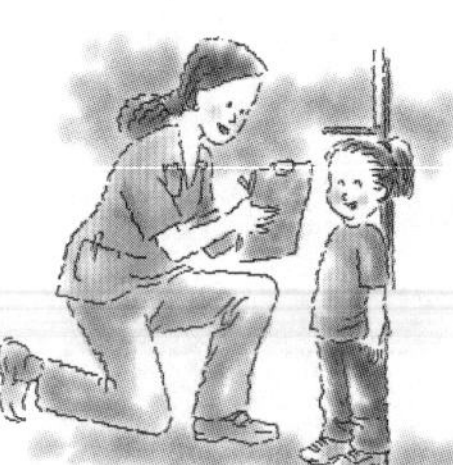
Let's see how you measure up.

56. While teaching the parents of a child with short stature, the nurse discusses familial short stature. Which statement by the nurse about this condition is the most correct?
1. "It occurs in children who are members of a very large family with limited resources."
2. "It occurs in children who have no siblings and who moved a great deal during their early childhood."
3. "It occurs in children with delayed linear growth and skeletal and sexual maturation that's behind that of age mates."
4. "It occurs in children who have ancestors with adult height in the lower percentiles and whose height during childhood is appropriate."

56. 4. Familial short stature refers to otherwise healthy children who have ancestors with adult height in the lower percentiles and whose height during childhood is appropriate for genetic background. Children who are members of very large families with limited resources or who are only children don't fit the description of familial short stature. Children with delayed linear growth and skeletal and sexual maturation that's behind that of age mates are considered to have constitutional growth delay.
CN: Physiological integrity; CNS: Physiological adaptation; CL: Application

57. When assessing a child age 2, which finding would indicate to the nurse the possibility of growth hormone deficiency?

1. The child had normal growth during the first year of life but showed a slowed growth curve below the 3rd percentile for the second year of life.
2. The child fell below the 5th percentile for growth during the first year of life but, at this check-up, falls below only the 50th percentile.
3. There has been a steady decline in growth over the 2 years of this toddler's life that has accelerated during the past 6 months.
4. There was delayed growth below the 5th percentile for the first and second years of life.

57. 1. Children with growth hormone deficiency generally grow normally during the first year and then follow a slowed growth curve that's below the 3rd percentile. If growth is consistently below the 5th percentile, it may be an indication of failure to thrive.

CN: Health promotion and maintenance; CNS: None; CL: Application

58. A nurse is assessing a child with growth hormone deficiency. Which characteristic would the nurse <u>most</u> commonly observe?

1. Decreased weight with no change in height
2. Decreased weight with increased height
3. Increased weight with decreased height
4. Increased weight with increased height

58. 3. Height may be retarded more than weight because, with good nutrition, children with growth hormone deficiency can become overweight or even obese. Their well-nourished appearance is an important diagnostic clue to differentiation from other disorders such as failure to thrive.

CN: Health promotion and maintenance; CNS: None; CL: Application

59. A nurse should find which characteristic in her assessment of a child with growth hormone deficiency?

1. Normal skeletal proportions
2. Abnormal skeletal proportions
3. Child's appearing older than his age
4. Longer than normal upper extremities

59. 1. Skeletal proportions are normal for the age, but these children appear younger than their chronological age. However, later in life, premature aging is evident.

CN: Physiological integrity; CNS: Physiological adaptation; CL: Application

60. When counseling the parents of a child with growth hormone deficiency, the nurse should <u>encourage</u> which sport?

1. Basketball
2. Field hockey
3. Football
4. Gymnastics

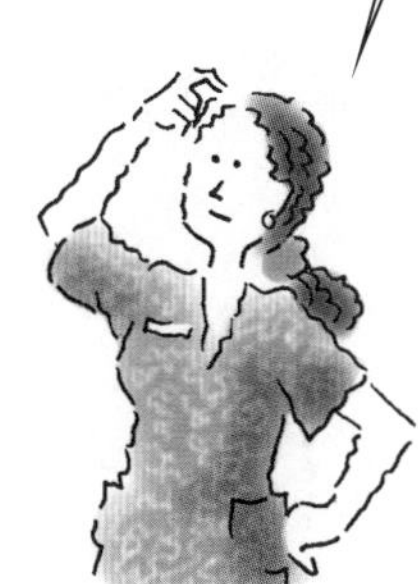
Which of these sports would be best for a child with growth hormone deficiency?

60. 4. Children with growth hormone deficiency can be no less active than other children if directed to size-appropriate sports, such as gymnastics, swimming, wrestling, or soccer.

CN: Health promotion and maintenance; CNS: None; CL: Application

61. In explaining to parents the social behavior of children with hypopituitarism, a nurse should recognize which statement as exhibiting a need for further teaching?

1. "I realize that my child might have school anxiety and a low self-esteem."
2. "Because my child is short in stature, people expect less of him than his peers."
3. "Because of my child's short stature, he may not be pushed to perform at his chronological age by others."
4. "My child's vocabulary is very well developed, so even though he's short in stature, no one will treat him differently."

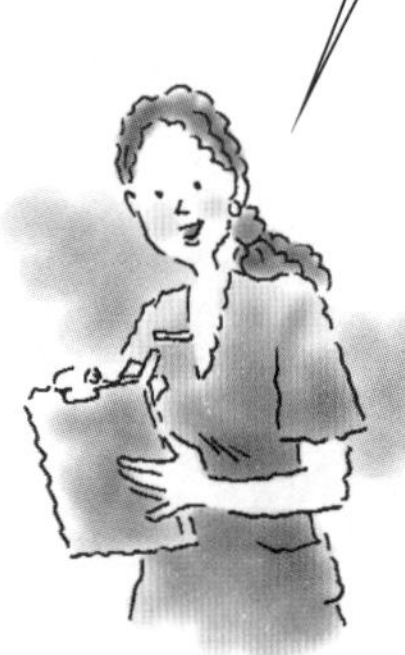

It's important that parents have *realistic* expectations about their child's disorder.

61. 4. Height discrepancy has been significantly correlated with emotional adjustment problems and may be a valuable predictor of the extent to which growth hormone–delayed children will have trouble with anxiety, social skills, and positive self-esteem. Also, academic problems aren't uncommon. These children aren't usually pushed to perform at their chronological age but are commonly subjected to juvenilization (related to in an infantile or childish manner).

CN: Psychosocial integrity; CNS: None; CL: Application

62. The mother of a child diagnosed with hypopituitarism states to the nurse that she feels guilty because she feels that she should have recognized this disorder. Which statement by the nurse about children with hypopituitarism would be the most helpful?"

1. "They're usually large for gestational age at birth."
2. "They're usually small for gestational age at birth."
3. "They usually exhibit signs of this disorder soon after birth."
4. "They're usually of normal size for gestational age at birth."

62. 4. Children with hypopituitarism are usually of normal size for gestational age at birth. Clinical features develop slowly and vary with the severity of the disorder and the number of deficient hormones.

CN: Psychosocial integrity; CNS: None; CL: Application

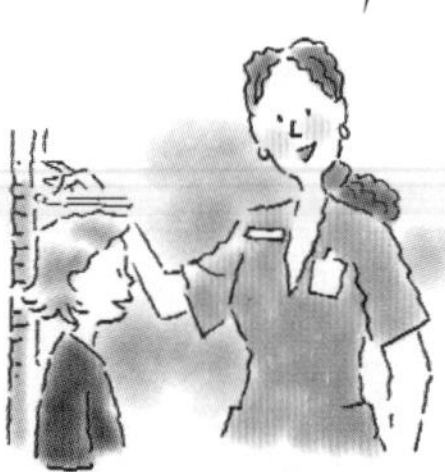

It's important to pay attention to abnormal growth in a child.

63. Which observation when plotting height and weight on a growth chart would indicate that a child age 4 has a growth hormone deficiency?

1. Upward shift of 1 percentile or more
2. Upward shift of 5 percentiles or more
3. Downward shift of 2 percentiles or more
4. Downward shift of 5 percentiles or more

63. 3. When the physician evaluates the results of plotting height and weight, upward or downward shifts of 2 percentiles or more in children older than 3 years may indicate a growth abnormality.

CN: Health promotion and maintenance; CNS: None; CL: Analysis

64. When reviewing the results of radiographic examinations of a child with hypopituitarism, which characteristic should the nurse expect to observe?

1. Bone age near normal
2. Epiphyseal maturation normal
3. Epiphyseal maturation retarded
4. Bone maturation greatly retarded

64. 3. Epiphyseal maturation is retarded in hypopituitarism consistent with retardation in height. This is in contrast to hypothyroidism, in which bone maturation is greatly retarded, or Turner syndrome, in which bone age is near normal.

CN: Health promotion and maintenance; CNS: None; CL: Application

65. A child has been brought to a pediatrician's office for concerns about growth. The physician suspects hypopituitarism. The mother asks the nurse which test will be done to determine the diagnosis. Which response by the nurse would be most accurate?

1. Hypersecretion of thyroid hormone
2. Increased reserves of growth hormone
3. Hyposecretion of antidiuretic hormone (ADH)
4. Decreased reserves of growth hormone

65. 4. Definitive diagnosis is based on absent or subnormal reserves of pituitary growth hormone. ADH and thyroid hormone levels aren't affected.

CN: Health promotion and maintenance; CNS: None; CL: Application

66. The parents of a child who's going through testing for hypopituitarism ask the nurse what type of test results they should expect. The nurse's response should be based on which factor?

1. Measurement of growth hormone will occur only one time.
2. Growth hormone levels are decreased after strenuous exercise.
3. There will be increased overnight urine growth hormone concentration.
4. Growth hormone levels are elevated 45 to 90 minutes following the onset of sleep.

66. 4. Growth hormone levels are elevated 45 to 90 minutes following the onset of sleep. Low growth hormone levels following the onset of sleep would indicate the need for further evaluation. Exercise is a natural and benign stimulus for growth hormone release, and elevated levels can be detected after 20 minutes of strenuous exercise in normal children. Also, growth hormone levels will need to be checked frequently related to the type of therapy instituted.

CN: Physiological integrity; CNS: Physiological adaptation; CL: Application

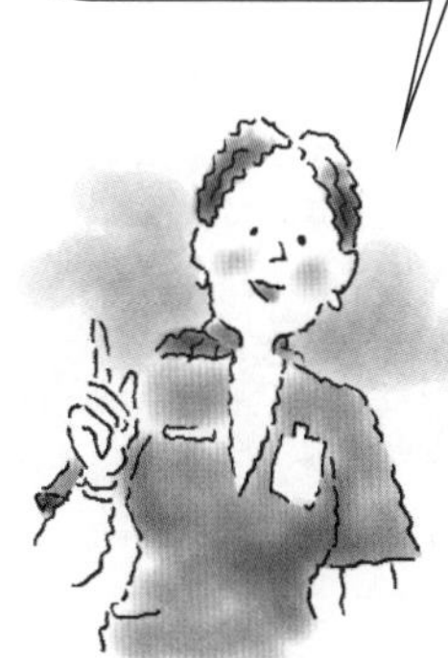

All of these treatments may be used, but only one is definitive.

67. Which method is considered the <u>definitive</u> treatment for hypopituitarism due to growth hormone deficiency?

1. Treatment with desmopressin acetate (DDAVP)
2. Replacement of antidiuretic hormone (ADH)
3. Treatment with testosterone or estrogen
4. Replacement with biosynthetic growth hormone

67. 4. The definitive treatment of growth hormone deficiency is replacement of growth hormone and is successful in 80% of affected children. DDAVP is used to treat diabetes insipidus. ADH deficiency causes diabetes insipidus and isn't related to hypopituitarism. Testosterone or estrogen may be given during adolescence for normal sexual maturation, but neither is the definitive treatment for hypopituitarism.

CN: Physiological integrity; CNS: Pharmacological and parenteral therapies; CL: Application

68. When obtaining information about a child, which comment made by a parent to the nurse would indicate the possibility of hypopituitarism in a child?

1. "I can pass down my child's clothes to his younger brother."
2. "Usually my child wears out his clothes before his size changes."
3. "I have to buy bigger size clothes for my child about every 2 months."
4. "I have to buy larger shirts more frequently than larger pants for my child."

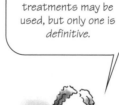

68. 2. Parents of children with hypopituitarism frequently comment that the child wears out clothes before growing out of them or that, if the clothing fits the body, it's commonly too long in the sleeves or legs.

CN: Health promotion and maintenance; CNS: None; CL: Application

69. In helping parents who are planning to give growth hormone at home, a nurse should explain that optimum dosing is achieved when growth hormone is administered at which time?

1. At bedtime
2. After dinner
3. In the middle of the day
4. First thing in the morning

69. 1. Optimum dosing is typically achieved when growth hormone is administered at bedtime. Pituitary release of growth hormone occurs during the first 45 to 90 minutes after the onset of sleep, so normal physiologic release is mimicked with bedtime dosing.

CN: Physiological integrity; CNS: Pharmacological and parenteral therapies; CL: Application

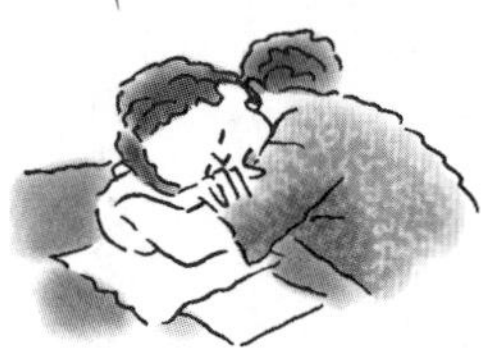
All I can think about is optimum dozing.

70. In educating parents of a child with hypopituitarism about realistic expectations of height for their child who's successfully responding to growth hormone replacement, the nurse should include which statement?

1. "Your child will never reach a normal adult height."
2. "Your child will attain his eventual adult height at a faster rate."
3. "Your child will attain his eventual adult height at a slower rate."
4. "The rate of your child's growth will be the same as children without this disorder."

70. 3. Even when hormone replacement is successful, these children attain their eventual adult height at a slower rate than their peers do; therefore, they need assistance in setting realistic expectations regarding improvement.

CN: Psychosocial integrity; CNS: None; CL: Application

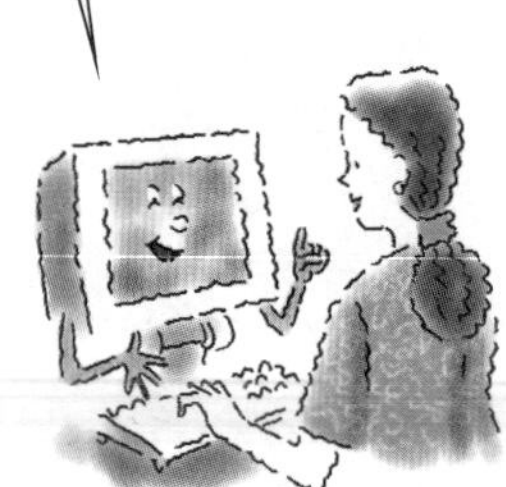
Careful—here's another further teaching question.

71. Which statement made by a parent of a child with short stature would indicate to the nurse the need for further teaching?

1. "Obtaining blood studies won't aid in proper diagnosis."
2. "A history of my child's growth patterns should be discussed."
3. "X-rays should be included in my child's diagnostic procedures."
4. "A family history is important information for me to share with my child's physician."

71. 1. A complete diagnostic evaluation should include a family history, a history of the child's growth patterns and previous health status, physical examination, physical evaluation, radiographic survey, and endocrine studies that may involve blood samples.

CN: Health promotion and maintenance; CNS: None; CL: Application

72. Which signs and symptoms would the health care team most commonly use as a basis for determining appropriate priorities and interventions for a child with type 1 diabetes mellitus? Select all that apply:

1. Polyuria
2. Weakness
3. Abdominal pain
4. Weight loss
5. Postprandial nausea
6. Orthostatic hypertension

72. 1, 2, 4, 5. Polyuria, weakness, weight loss, and postprandial nausea are commonly seen in diabetes mellitus. The healthcare team would plan care to manage these signs and symptoms. Abdominal pain isn't a symptom in this disease, and orthostatic hypotension rather than orthostatic hypertension would be a significant finding.

CN: Safe, effective care environment; CNS: Management of care; CL: Analysis

73. Which metabolic alteration characteristic might be associated with growth hormone deficiency?
1. Galactosemia
2. Homocystinuria
3. Hyperglycemia
4. Hypoglycemia

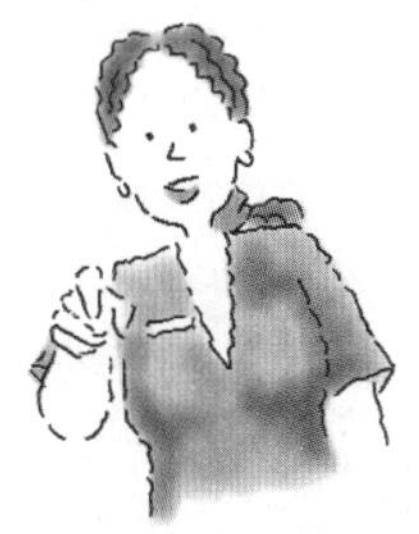

You know the answer to this question. I know you do!

73. 4. The development of hypoglycemia is a characteristic finding related to growth hormone deficiency. Galactosemia is a rare autosomal recessive disorder with an inborn error of carbohydrate metabolism. Homocystinuria is an indication of amino acid transport or metabolism problems. Hyperglycemia isn't a problem in hypopituitarism.

CN: Health promotion and maintenance; CNS: None; CL: Application

74. When providing information to the parents of a child who's receiving growth hormone replacement therapy for hypopituitarism, the nurse should include which intervention?
1. Explaining that growth in height and weight won't begin until puberty
2. Teaching how to perform venipuncture for administration of the growth hormone
3. Helping parents recognize the importance of interacting with the child according to age rather than size
4. Advising parents to hold the child back in school until linear growth begins to approximate the normal patterns

74. 3. To promote self-esteem and healthy development of a child with growth hormone deficiency, parents should be encouraged to interact with the child according to age, not size. Growth in height and weight will begin soon after treatment with growth hormone begins. Growth hormone administration is subcutaneous, and a child shouldn't be held back in school because of his size.

CN: Psychosocial integrity; CNS: None; CL: Application

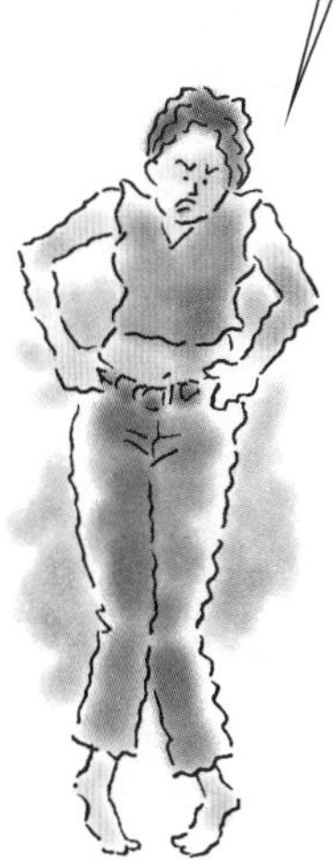

Here's a hint. The answer to question 75 certainly isn't my problem!

75. When assessing a neonate diagnosed with diabetes insipidus, which finding would indicate the need for intervention?
1. Edema
2. Increased head circumference
3. Weight gain
4. Weight loss

75. 4. Diabetes insipidus usually presents gradually. Weight loss from a large loss of fluid occurs. Edema isn't evident in the neonate with diabetes insipidus. There should be an increase in his head circumference with treatment. A normal neonate should gain weight as he grows.

CN: Physiological integrity; CNS: Reduction of risk potential; CL: Application

76. In a client with diabetes insipidus, a nurse could expect which characteristics of the urine?
1. Pale in color; specific gravity less than 1.006
2. Concentrated; specific gravity less than 1.006
3. Concentrated; specific gravity less than 1.03
4. Pale in color; specific gravity more than 1.03

76. 1. With diabetes insipidus, the client has difficulty with excessive urine output; therefore, the urine will be pale in color and the specific gravity will fall below the low normal of 1.01.

CN: Physiological integrity; CNS: Reduction of risk potential; CL: Analysis

77. Which characteristics would most likely be present in the health history of a child with diabetes insipidus?

1. Delayed closure of the fontanels, coarse hair, and hypoglycemia in the morning
2. Gradual onset of personality changes, lethargy, and blurred vision
3. Vomiting early in the morning, headache, and decreased thirst
4. Abrupt onset of polyuria, nocturia, and polydipsia

78. Which condition in a client on fluid restriction for diabetes insipidus diagnostic testing would indicate a need for the nurse to discontinue fluid restriction?

1. Weight gain of 3% to 5%
2. Weight loss of 3% to 5%
3. Increase in urine output
4. Generalized edema

79. When a child with diabetes insipidus has a viral illness that includes congestion, nausea, and vomiting, the nurse should instruct the parents to take which action?

1. Make no changes in the medication regime.
2. Give medications only once per day.
3. Obtain an alternate route for desmopressin acetate (DDAVP) administration.
4. Give medication 1 hour after vomiting has occurred.

80. A nurse is preparing a child with diabetes insipidus who will be taking injectable vasopressin for hospital discharge. Which action is best for the nurse to take when teaching injection techniques?

1. Teach injection techniques to the primary caregiver.
2. Teach injection techniques to anyone who will provide care for the child.
3. Teach injection techniques to anyone who will provide care for the child as well as to the child if he's old enough to understand.
4. Provide information about the nearest home health agency so the parents can arrange for the home health nurse to come and give the injection.

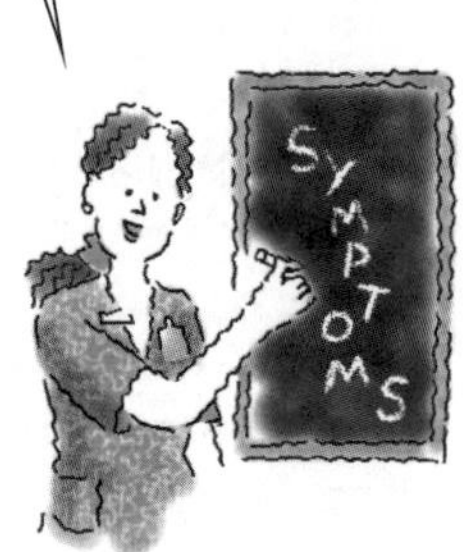

Do you know the symptoms of diabetes insipidus?
SYMPTOMS

77. 4. Diabetes insipidus is characterized by deficient secretion of antidiuretic hormone leading to diuresis. Most children with this disorder experience an abrupt onset of symptoms, including polyuria, nocturia, and polydipsia. The other choices reflect symptoms of pituitary hyperfunction.

CN: Health promotion and maintenance; CNS: None; CL: Application

78. 2. A weight loss between 3% to 5% indicates significant dehydration and requires termination of the fluid restriction. Weight gain would be a good sign. Generalized edema wouldn't occur with fluid restriction, nor would increased urine output.

CN: Physiological integrity; CNS: Physiological adaptation; CL: Analysis

79. 3. An alternate route for administration of DDAVP would be needed for absorption because of nasal congestion. The other options reflect actions that need to be covered by a physician's order.

CN: Health promotion and maintenance; CNS: None; CL: Application

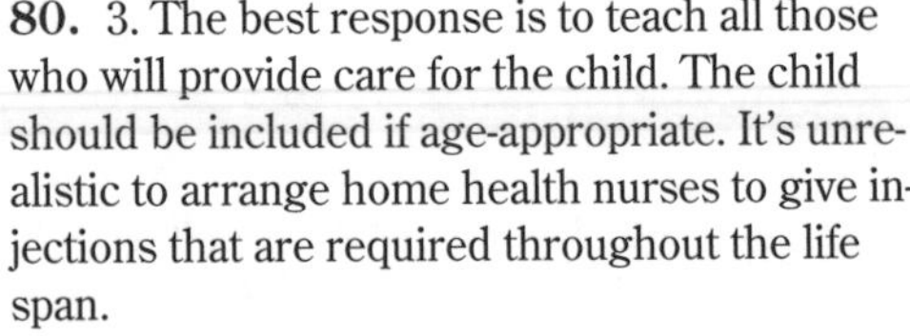

80. 3. The best response is to teach all those who will provide care for the child. The child should be included if age-appropriate. It's unrealistic to arrange home health nurses to give injections that are required throughout the life span.

CN: Physiological integrity; CNS: Pharmacological and parenteral therapies; CL: Application

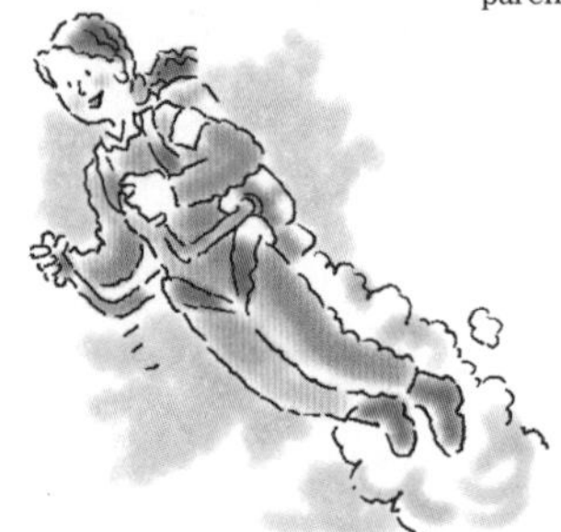

Good work! You're flying through this test!

81. When providing care for a school-age client with diabetes insipidus, the nurse understands that which behavior might be difficult related to this child's growth and development?

1. Taking desmopressin acetate (DDAVP) at school
2. Taking DDAVP before bedtime
3. Letting his mother administer the vasopressin injection
4. Giving himself a vasopressin injection before school starts

82. Which monitoring method would be <u>best</u> for a client newly diagnosed with diabetes insipidus?

1. Measuring abdominal girths every day
2. Measuring intake, output, and urine specific gravity
3. Checking daily weights and measuring intake
4. Checking for pitting edema in the lower extremities

83. A nurse is caring for a neonate with congenital hypothyroidism. Which assessment finding should the nurse anticipate observing in the neonate?

1. Hyperreflexia
2. Long forehead
3. Puffy eyelids
4. Small tongue

84. A child is admitted with complaints of weight loss and lack of energy. The child's ears and cheeks are flushed, and the nurse observes an acetone odor to the child's breath. The child's blood glucose level is 325 mg/dl, his blood pressure is 104/60 mmHg, his pulse is 88 beats/minute, and respirations are 16 breaths/minute. Which does the nurse expect the physician to order <u>first</u>?

1. Subcutaneous administration of glucagon
2. Administration of IV regular insulin by continuous infusion pump
3. Administration of regular insulin subcutaneously every 4 hours as needed by sliding scale insulin
4. Administration of IV fluids in boluses of 20 ml/kg

Question 82 asks
you to rank
monitoring methods
for appropriateness.
I know you can do it!

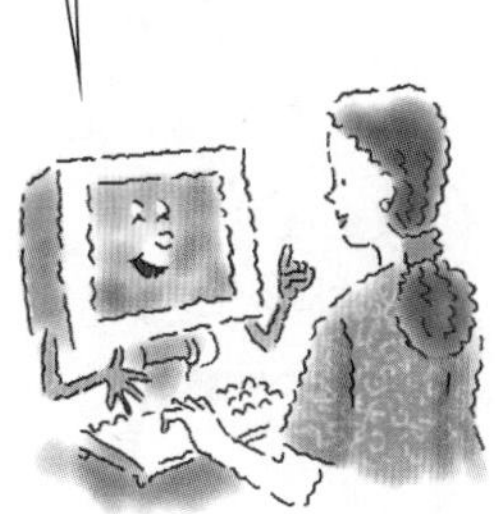

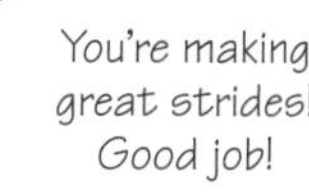
You're making
great strides!
Good job!

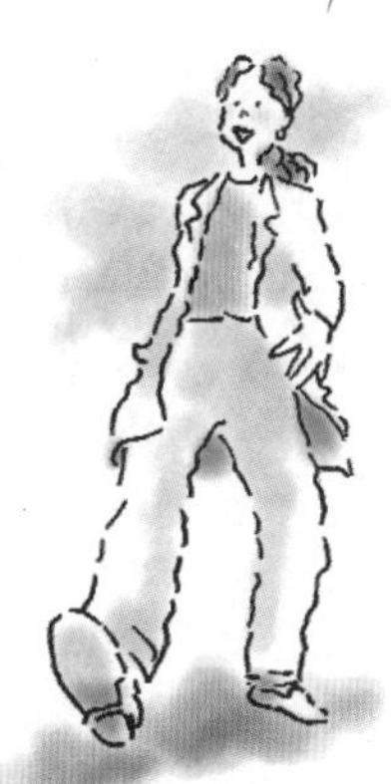

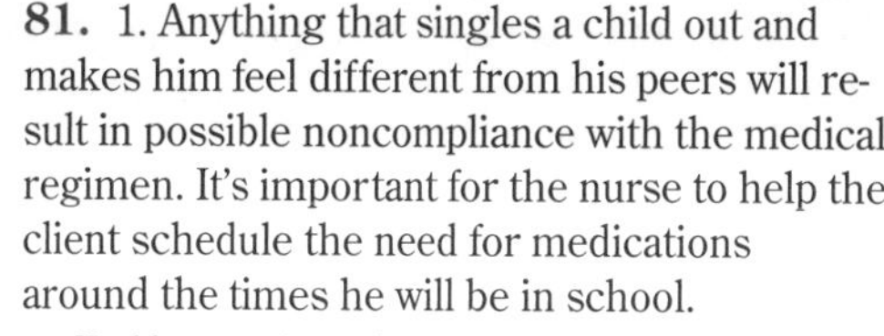

81. 1. Anything that singles a child out and makes him feel different from his peers will result in possible noncompliance with the medical regimen. It's important for the nurse to help the client schedule the need for medications around the times he will be in school.

CN: Health promotion and maintenance; CNS: None; CL: Application

82. 2. Measuring intake and output with related specific gravity results will enable the nurse to closely monitor the client's condition along with daily weights. All of the other options aren't as accurate for a child with diabetes insipidus.

CN: Physiological integrity; CNS: Reduction of risk potential; CL: Application

83. 3. Assessment findings would include depressed nasal bridge, short forehead, puffy eyelids, and large tongue; thick, dry, mottled skin that feels cold to the touch; coarse, dry, lusterless hair; abdominal distention; umbilical hernia; hyporeflexia; bradycardia; hypothermia; hypotension; anemia; and wide cranial sutures.

CN: Physiological integrity; CNS: Physiological adaptation; CL: Application

84. 2. Weight loss, lack of energy, acetone odor to breath, and a blood glucose level of 325 mg/dl indicate diabetic ketoacidosis. Insulin is given IV by continuous infusion pump. Glucagon is administered for mild hypoglycemia. Sliding scale insulin isn't as effective as the administration of insulin by continuous infusion pump. Administration of IV fluids in boluses of 20 ml/kg is recommended for the treatment of shock.

CN: Physiological integrity; CNS: Physiological adaptation; CL: Application

85. Which nursing objective is most important when working with neonates who are suspected of having congenital hypothyroidism?

1. Identifying the disorder early
2. Promoting bonding
3. Allowing rooming in
4. Encouraging fluid intake

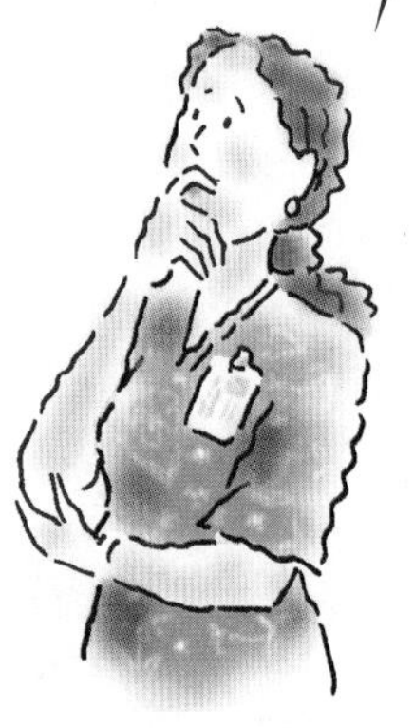
What's the most important nursing objective?

85. 1. The most important nursing objective is early identification of the disorder. Nurses caring for neonates must be certain that screening is performed, especially in neonates who are preterm, discharged early, or born at home. Promoting bonding, allowing rooming in, and encouraging fluid intake are all important but are less important than early identification.

CN: Physiological integrity; CNS: Basic care and comfort; CL: Application

86. When the parents of an infant diagnosed with hypothyroidism have been taught to count the pulse, which intervention should the nurse teach them in case they obtain a high pulse rate?

1. Allow the infant to take a nap, and then give the medication.
2. Withhold the medication and give a double dose the next day.
3. Hold the medication and call the physician.
4. Give the medication and then consult the physician.

86. 3. If parents have been taught to count the infant's pulse, they should be instructed to withhold the dose and consult their physician if the pulse rate is above a certain value.

CN: Health promotion and maintenance; CNS: None; CL: Application

87. In an infant receiving inadequate treatment for congenital hypothyroidism, the nurse should expect to observe which symptom?

1. Irritability and jitteriness
2. Fatigue and sleepiness
3. Increased appetite
4. Diarrhea

87. 2. Signs of inadequate treatment are fatigue, sleepiness, decreased appetite, and constipation.

CN: Health promotion and maintenance; CNS: None; CL: Application

88. When collecting data from a child with Cushing's syndrome, which would the nurse be most likely to find? Select all that apply:

1. Obesity
2. Moon-shaped face
3. Hypotension
4. Emotional instability
5. Quickened healing
6. Loss of hair

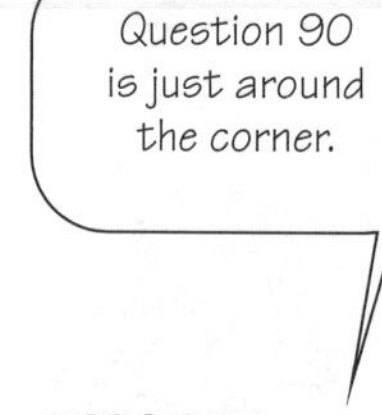
Question 90 is just around the corner.

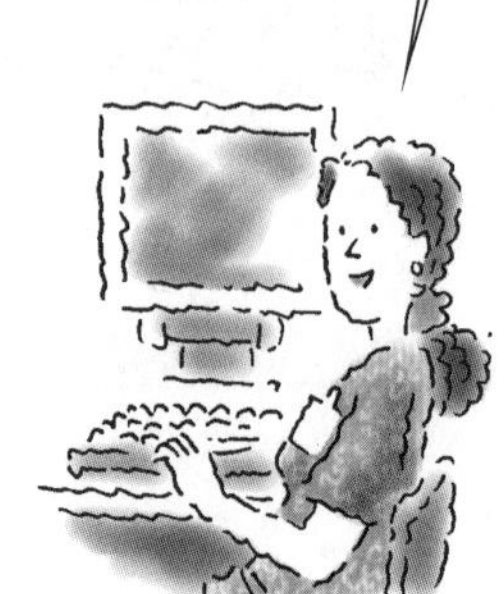

88. 1, 2, 4. Cushing's syndrome occurs as a result of excessive cortisol exposure (through corticosteroid medications or production by the adrenal glands). Common findings include obesity, moon-shaped face, and emotional instability. Hypertension, excessive hair growth, and slower healing are additional findings, making the other options incorrect.

CN: Physiological integrity; CNS: Physiological adaptation; CL: Analysis

CN: Client needs category CNS: Client needs subcategory CL: Cognitive level

89. Which recommendation for preventing hypoglycemia in an adolescent with diabetes type 1 should the nurse make?

1. Limit participation in planned exercise activities that involve competition.
2. Carry crackers or fruit to eat before or during periods of increased activity.
3. Increase the insulin dosage before planned or unplanned strenuous exercise.
4. Check blood sugar before exercising, and eat a protein snack if the level is elevated.

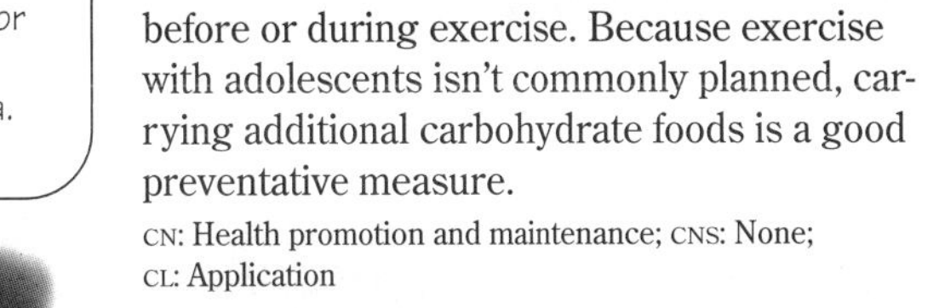

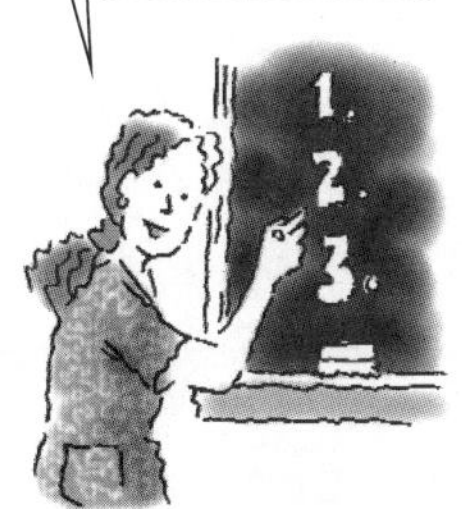
Let's discuss some steps for preventing hypoglycemia.
1.
2.
3.

90. A child with diabetic ketoacidosis is to receive a continuous infusion of insulin for a blood glucose level of 780 mg/dl. Which solution is the most appropriate for the nurse to prepare initially?

1. Normal saline with regular insulin
2. Normal saline with Ultralente insulin
3. 5% dextrose in water with NPH insulin
4. 5% dextrose in water with PZI insulin

91. An adolescent female client is admitted to the hospital with type 1 diabetes and unstable blood glucose levels. Which question is <u>most important</u> to include in her health history?

1. Does she play any team sports?
2. Does she refrigerate her insulin?
3. Is she satisfied with her weight?
4. Does she use recreational drugs?

The answer to this question should be a slam dunk.

92. A 14-year-old male client with type 1 diabetes mellitus plans to join the basketball team at his school. The practices are twice a week with games on Saturdays. He calls the nurse at his clinic for advice. The nurse should respond with which statement?

1. "Delay eating a meal until after practice or a game."
2. "Time your insulin to peak at the time of practice and games."
3. "Monitor your blood sugar before, during, and after exercise."
4. "Increase your daily calorie intake by 10% and up your insulin dose by 10%."

89. 2. Hypoglycemia can usually be prevented if an adolescent with diabetes eats more food before or during exercise. Because exercise with adolescents isn't commonly planned, carrying additional carbohydrate foods is a good preventative measure.

CN: Health promotion and maintenance; CNS: None; CL: Application

90. 1. Short-acting regular insulin is the only insulin that should be used for insulin infusions. Initially, normal saline is used until blood glucose levels are reduced. Then a dextrose solution may be used to prevent hypoglycemia. Ultralente, NPH, and PZI insulins have a longer duration of action and shouldn't be used for continuous infusions.

CN: Physiological integrity; CNS: Pharmacological and parenteral therapies; CL: Application

91. 3. It's important to ascertain the adolescent's feelings about her body, in particular her weight. Some female adolescents skip their insulin because they know doing so will result in weight loss. The other issues of sports, drug use, and technique of administering insulin are all relevant but not as important as knowing what the client is thinking about her own body.

CN: Psychosocial integrity; CNS: None; CL: Application

92. 3. For increases in activity, a client with type 1 diabetes would require a snack before the activity and increased insulin. The amount of insulin is the most difficult determination. Monitoring is required for accurate regulation before, during, and after the activity. The client shouldn't delay eating until afterward because the body needs the calories to provide energy to the muscles and tissues. Extreme hypoglycemia may occur if the insulin peaks without extra calories. There's no standard of 10% increase in calories and insulin; every person would require individualization of the insulin and calories needed.

CN: Health promotion and maintenance; CNS: None; CL: Application

93. A nurse is collecting a health history from the parents of a 12-month-old infant being evaluated for possible hypopituitarism. Which component of this history is important to establish the diagnosis?

1. Did the mother drink alcohol while pregnant?
2. Does the infant receive multivitamins?
3. What's the infant's growth pattern?
4. Was the infant premature?

93. 3. Hypopituitarism presents with a retarded growth pattern, appearance younger than chronological age, and normal skeletal proportions and intelligence. It's related to tumors, irradiation, infection, and head trauma. Therefore, serial growth patterns will be crucial to the diagnosis process. It isn't related to fetal alcoholism, use of multivitamins, or prematurity.
CN: Physiological integrity; CNS: Physiological adaptation; CL: Application

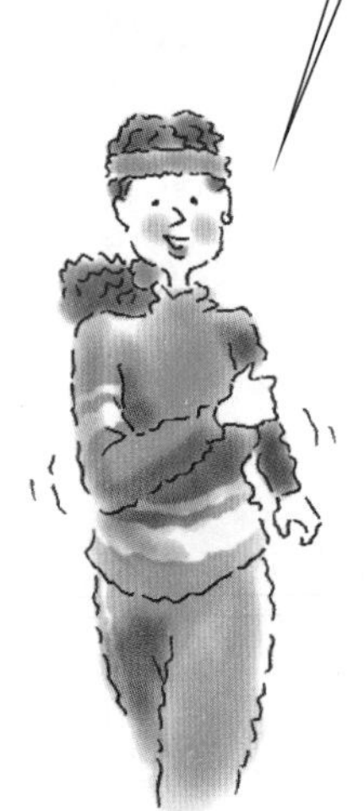
I can see the finish line! You're doing great!

94. A nurse has just completed teaching a family about hypothyroidism. Which actions would indicate the parents understand their child's diagnosis?

1. Providing a diet including whole grains, produce, and water
2. Anticipating their child outgrowing hypothyroidism
3. Providing a white diet for their child
4. Providing a diet high in fat for their child to encourage growth

94. 1. A diet including fruits, vegetables, whole grains, and water will help counteract the trend toward obstinate constipation, the result of a slowed metabolism and hypotonic bowel. Congenital hypothyroidism isn't outgrown, and thyroid replacement is necessary throughout the life span. A white diet involves foods low in fiber, which leads to constipation. Hypothyroid individuals tend to have elevated cholesterol and triglyceride levels; therefore, a diet high in fat is contraindicated.
CN: Health promotion and maintenance; CNS: None; CL: Application

95. A child with diabetes is receiving a continuous insulin infusion for diabetic ketoacidosis. When assessing the child, the nurse should be alert for signs and symptoms of which complication?

1. Hypercalcemia
2. Hyperphosphatemia
3. Hypokalemia
4. Hypernatremia

95. 3. Hypokalemia occurs as insulin causes potassium and glucose to move into the cells. Insulin administration doesn't affect calcium or sodium levels. Insulin administration may lead to hypophosphatemia, not hyperphosphatemia, as phosphorus enters the cells with insulin and potassium.
CN: Physiological integrity; CNS: Physiological adaptation; CL: Analysis

96. A nurse is caring for a client with pheochromocytoma. Which nursing intervention is appropriate for this client?

1. Promoting an environment free from emotional distress
2. Avoiding analgesia administration
3. Advising a low-calorie, high-nutrient diet
4. Avoiding parents rooming in because they make the client less dependent on staff

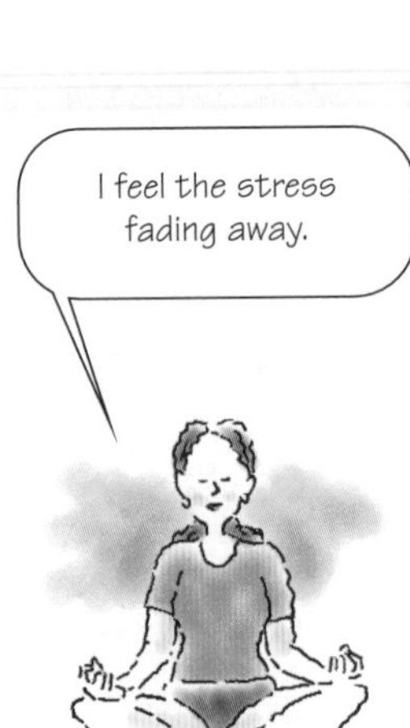
I feel the stress fading away.

96. 1. The child experiencing hyperfunctioning of the adrenal gland, or *pheochromocytoma,* is in a chronic state of "fight or flight" related to excessive exogenous epinephrine. Therefore, the child has an accelerated metabolism. Symptoms include hypertension, headaches, hyperglycemia with weight loss, diaphoresis, and hyperventilation. Through provision of a low-stress environment, analgesia as needed, a high-calorie diet, and supportive parents, the child will be able to prepare for surgery to eliminate the tumor causing the hypersecretion of epinephrine.
CN: Physiological integrity; CNS: Physiological adaptation; CL: Application

97. A nurse is instructing parents about promoting the health of their child with diabetes. Which teaching point should be included?

1. Avoid daily bathing so the skin doesn't become too dry.
2. Cuts and scratches on the playground are of little concern.
3. Children with diabetes need few immunizations.
4. Regular dental care and annual ophthalmologic appointments should be kept.

97. 4. Regular dental care will preserve oral health, and ophthalmologic examinations will ensure visual acuity for reading. Because of their impaired immune system, children with diabetes need to maintain a high level of health to avoid infection. Daily bathing and application of lotion, cleaning minor playground scrapes and applying antibiotic ointments, and keeping immunizations up-to-date are all important.
CN: Health promotion and maintenance; CNS: None; CL: Application

98. A 10-year-old child monitors and adjusts his own insulin. Which response reflects an understanding of appropriate adjustment of insulin dosage when the child has the flu?

1. "I withhold all insulin because I'm not eating."
2. "I'll take my usual dose of regular and NPH insulin."
3. "I'll perform fingerstick blood sugar testing and adjust my insulin according to results."
4. "I'll perform fingerstick blood sugar testing and record the results."

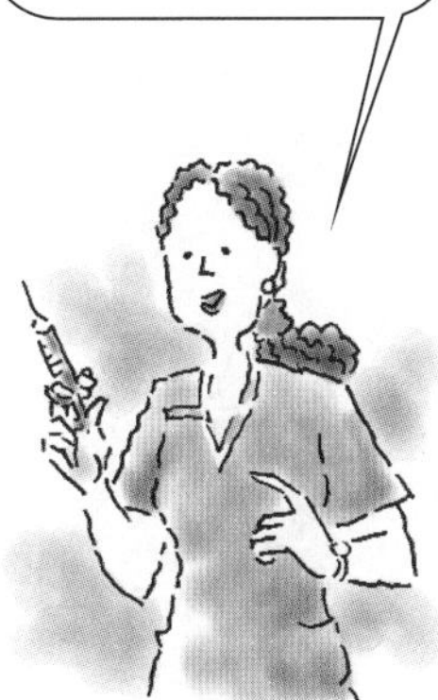

Adjusting insulin reflects that your client understands his disorder.

98. 3. Because of the stress of illness, serum glucose will likely be elevated during an episode of the flu. Appropriate adjustment of insulin dosage will help prevent the child from becoming hypoglycemic or ketoacidotic.
CN: Physiological integrity; CNS: Physiological adaptation; CL: Analysis

99. The nurse is teaching the parents of a child with hypopituitary dwarfism about the diagnosis. Which statement is the most accurate about children with this condition?

1. They're usually low-birth-weight babies.
2. Symptoms aren't apparent until puberty.
3. Symptoms include early primary dentition.
4. They grow normally the first 2 years and then fall below the 3rd percentile.

99. 4. Generally, hypopituitary children are of average birth weight and grow at a normal pace the first 2 or 3 years and then fall behind their peers in height, usually below the 3rd percentile. Dentition of primary teeth is normal; permanent teeth are delayed.
CN: Health promotion and maintenance; CNS: None; CL: Application

100. A client age 10 has been experiencing insatiable thirst and urinating excessively; his serum glucose is <u>normal</u>. Which condition is the client probably experiencing?

1. Type 2 diabetes mellitus
2. Type 1 diabetes mellitus
3. Hyperthyroidism
4. Diabetes insipidus

100. 4. Polydipsia and polyuria with normal serum glucose may be indicative of diabetes insipidus. Interview and laboratory results can determine whether the origin is neurogenic or nephrogenic. Type 1 or 2 diabetes mellitus requires an elevated serum glucose. A child with hyperthyroidism may present as dehydrated from the excessive sweating and rapid respirations that accompany this hypermetabolic state.
CN: Physiological integrity; CNS: Physiological adaptation; CL: Analysis

101. A client age 4½ with diabetes is ordered to receive 25 ml/hour of I.V. solution. The nurse is using a pediatric microdrip chamber to administer the medication. The microdrip chamber should be set for how many drops per minute? Record your answer using a whole number.

____________________ gtt/minute

101. 25. When using a pediatric microdrip chamber, the number of milliliters per hour equals the number of drops per minute. If 25 ml/hour is ordered, the I.V. should infuse at 25 drops/minute.

CN: Physiological integrity; CNS: Pharmacological and parenteral therapies; CL: Application

102. The nurse is preparing to administer I.V. methylprednisolone sodium succinate (Solu-Medrol) to a child who weighs 44 lb. The order is for 0.03 mg/kg I.V. daily. How many milligrams should the nurse prepare? Record your answer using one decimal point.

____________________ milligrams

102. 0.6. To perform this dosage calculation, the nurse should first convert the child's weight to kilograms: 44 lb ÷ 2.2 kg/lb = 20 kg. Then she should use this formula to determine the dose: 20 kg × 0.03 mg/kg = X mg. X = 0.6 mg.

CN: Physiological integrity; CNS: Pharmacological and parenteral therapies; CL: Application

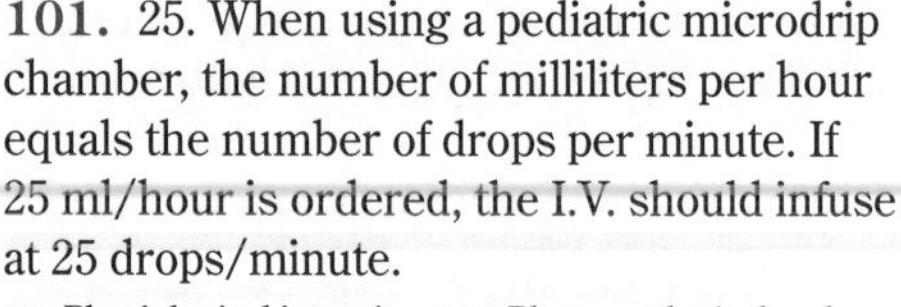
Hooray! Another chapter finished! Good job!

CN: Client needs category CNS: Client needs subcategory CL: Cognitive level

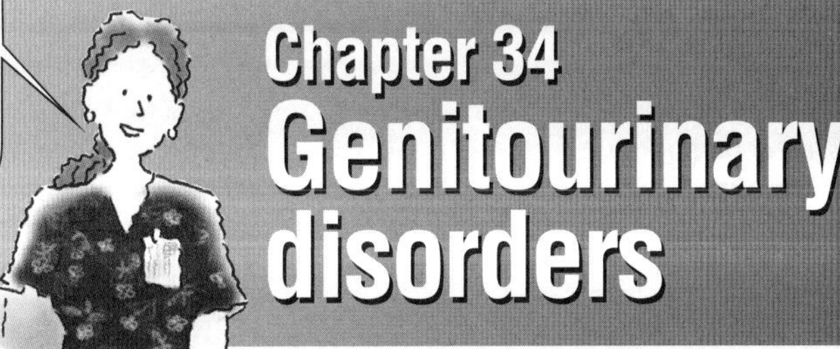

This chapter covers altered patterns of urinary elimination in children and includes glomerulonephritis, hypospadias, and—oh, a whole lot of other conditions. Ready? Let's go!

Chapter 34 Genitourinary disorders

1. A child with acute glomerulonephritis has a nursing diagnosis of *Impaired urinary elimination* related to fluid retention and impaired glomerular filtration. The child should display which expected outcome?
1. Exhibits no evidence of infection
2. Engages in activities appropriate to capabilities
3. Demonstrates no periorbital, facial, or body edema
4. Maintains a fluid intake of more than 2,000 ml in 24 hours

1. 3. The goal of this diagnosis involves interventions, such as decreased fluid and salt intake, designed to minimize or prevent fluid retention and edema. These interventions may be evaluated through observations for edema. The other options are appropriate outcomes for other nursing diagnoses, not the diagnosis in question.
CN: Health promotion and maintenance; CNS: None; CL: Analysis

2. An important nursing intervention to support the therapeutic management of a child with acute glomerulonephritis should include which action?
1. Measuring daily weight
2. Increasing oral fluid intake
3. Providing sodium supplements
4. Monitoring the client for signs of hypokalemia

2. 1. The child with acute glomerulonephritis should be monitored for fluid imbalance, which is done through daily weights. Increasing oral intake, monitoring for hypokalemia, and providing sodium supplements aren't part of the therapeutic management of acute glomerulonephritis.
CN: Physiological integrity; CNS: Basic care and comfort; CL: Application

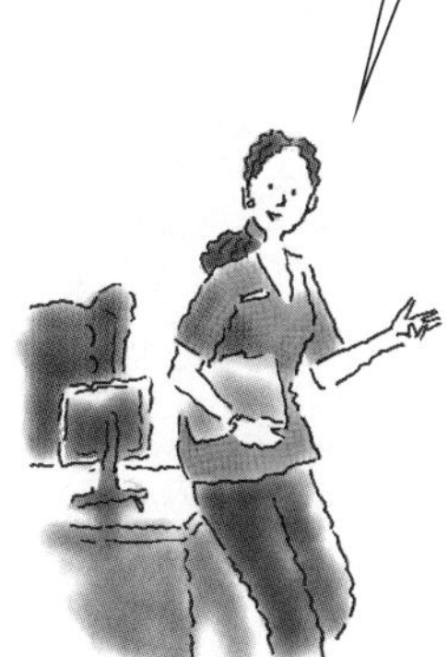

If you're having trouble deciding on an answer, begin by eliminating the ones you *know* are incorrect.

3. A nurse is taking frequent blood pressure readings on a child diagnosed with acute glomerulonephritis. The parents ask the nurse why this is necessary. When implementing nursing care, which teaching statement by the nurse is the most accurate?
1. "Blood pressure fluctuations are a sign that the condition has become chronic."
2. "Blood pressure fluctuations are a common adverse effect of antibiotic therapy."
3. "Hypotension leading to sudden shock can develop at any time."
4. "Acute hypertension must be anticipated and identified."

3. 4. Regular measurement of vital signs, body weight, and intake and output is essential to monitor the progress of the disease and to detect complications that may appear at any time during the course of the disease. Blood pressure fluctuations don't indicate that the condition has become chronic and aren't common adverse reactions to antibiotic therapy. Hypertension is more likely than hypotension to occur with glomerulonephritis.
CN: Physiological integrity; CNS: Physiological adaptation; CL: Application

CN: Client needs category CNS: Client needs subcategory CL: Cognitive level

4. A child has been diagnosed with acute glomerulonephritis. Based on the results of the routine urinalysis below, which component is the most consistent with this diagnosis?

Laboratory results

Urinalysis	
Color:	Straw
Appearance:	Clear
Specific gravity:	1.032
pH:	5.5
Protein:	Negative
Blood:	Negative
RBC casts:	Present
Crystals:	Negative

1. Specific gravity
2. Protein
3. Blood
4. Red blood cell (RBC) casts

4. 4. Urinalysis findings consistent with acute glomerulonephritis would include a specific gravity less than 1.030, proteinuria, hematuria, and the presence of RBC casts. The presence of crystals in the urine typically indicates a congenital metabolic problem.
CN: Physiological integrity; CNS: Physiological adaptation; CL: Application

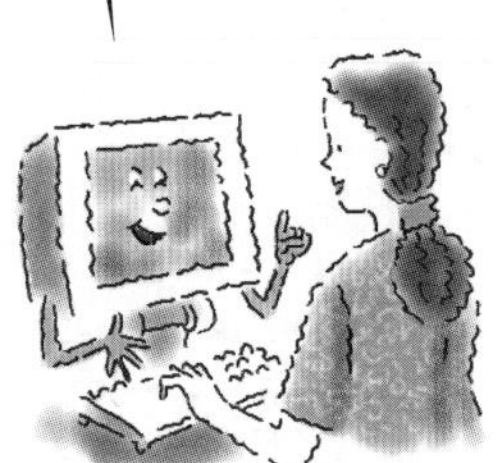

More than one answer may seem correct. It's your job to choose the best answer.

5. When evaluating the urinalysis report of a child with acute glomerulonephritis, the nurse should expect which result?

1. Proteinuria and decreased specific gravity
2. Bacteriuria and increased specific gravity
3. Hematuria and proteinuria
4. Bacteriuria and hematuria

5. 3. Urinalysis during the acute phase of this disease characteristically shows hematuria, proteinuria, and increased specific gravity.
CN: Physiological integrity; CNS: Physiological adaptation; CL: Analysis

6. Which statement by a nurse would be the best response to a mother who wants to know the first indication that her child's acute glomerulonephritis is improving?

1. Urine output will increase.
2. Urine will be free from protein.
3. Blood pressure will stabilize.
4. The child will have more energy.

6. 1. One of the first signs of improvement during the acute phase of glomerulonephritis is an increase in urine output. It will take time for the urine to be free from protein. Antihypertensive drugs may be needed to stabilize the blood pressure. Children generally don't have much energy during the acute phase of this disease.
CN: Health promotion and maintenance; CNS: None; CL: Analysis

7. Which statement regarding acute glomerulonephritis indicates that the parents of a child with this diagnosis understand the teaching provided by the nurse?

1. This disease occurs after a urinary tract infection.
2. This disease is associated with renal vascular disorders.
3. This disease occurs after a streptococcal infection.
4. This disease is associated with structural anomalies of the genitourinary tract.

7. 3. Acute glomerulonephritis is an immune-complex disease that occurs as a by-product of a streptococcal infection. Certain strains of the infection are usually a beta-hemolytic streptococcus.
CN: Health promotion and maintenance; CNS: None; CL: Analysis

8. When obtaining a child's daily weights, the nurse notes that he has lost 6 lb (2.7 kg) after 3 days of hospitalization for acute glomerulonephritis. This is most likely the result of which factor?
1. Poor appetite
2. Reduction of edema
3. Decreased salt intake
4. Restriction to bed rest

8. 2. When there's reduction of edema, the client will lose weight. This should normally occur after treatment for acute glomerulonephritis has been followed for several days. A poor appetite, decreased salt intake, or restriction to bed rest wouldn't lead to such a dramatic weight loss in a child this age.
CN: Physiological integrity; CNS: Basic care and comfort; CL: Application

9. A nurse should make which dietary recommendation to a client who has been newly diagnosed with acute glomerulonephritis?
1. Decrease calories.
2. Increase potassium.
3. Severely restrict sodium.
4. Moderately restrict sodium.

9. 4. Moderate sodium restriction with a diet that has no added salt after cooking is usually effective. Calorie consumption doesn't need to decrease, and potassium consumption shouldn't increase because of the decrease in urinary output. *Severe* sodium restriction isn't needed and will make it more difficult to ensure adequate nutrition. It will also result in hyponatremia.
CN: Physiological integrity; CNS: Basic care and comfort; CL: Application

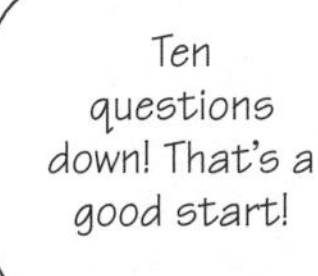
Ten questions down! That's a good start!

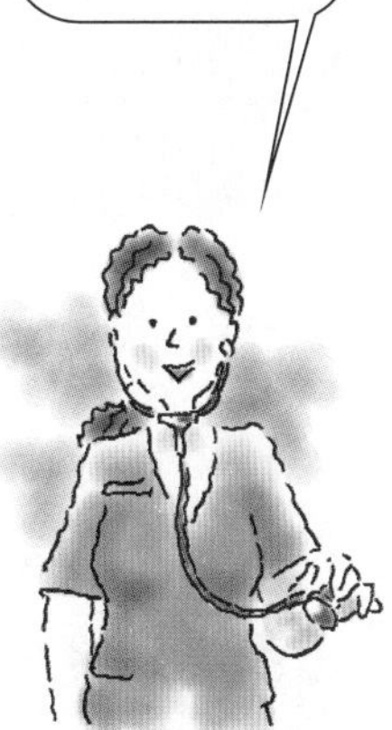

10. A nurse is evaluating a group of children for acute glomerulonephritis. Which client would be most likely to develop the disease?
1. A client who had pneumonia a month ago
2. A client who was bitten by a brown spider
3. A client who shows no signs of periorbital edema
4. A client who had a streptococcal infection 2 weeks ago

10. 4. A latent period of 10 to 14 days occurs between the streptococcal infection of the throat or skin and the onset of clinical manifestations. The peak incidence of disease corresponds to the incidence of streptococcal infections. Pneumonia isn't a precursor to glomerulonephritis, nor is a bite from a brown spider. A sign of periorbital edema would lead the nurse to investigate the possibility of glomerulonephritis, especially if reported to be worse in the morning.
CN: Health promotion and maintenance; CNS: None; CL: Analysis

11. A nurse is questioned by a student nurse about which age group has the highest incidence of acute glomerulonephritis. Which response by the nurse is the most accurate?
1. Ages 1 to 2
2. Ages 6 to 7
3. Ages 12 to 13
4. Ages 18 to 20

11. 2. Acute glomerulonephritis can occur at any age, but it primarily affects early school-age children with a peak age of onset of 6 to 7. It's uncommon in children younger than age 2.
CN: Health promotion and maintenance; CNS: None; CL: Application

12. In understanding the recurrence of glomerulonephritis, a nurse should know which characteristic to be true?
1. Second attacks are quite common.
2. A recessive gene transfers this disease.
3. Multiple cases tend to occur in families.
4. Overcrowding in the schoolroom leads to higher incidence.

12. 3. Multiple cases tend to occur in families. Second attacks are rare. Acute glomerulonephritis isn't transmitted through a recessive gene, and overcrowding in the schoolroom should have no influence on this disease.
CN: Health promotion and maintenance; CNS: None; CL: Application

13. When describing enuresis to a child's parents, which statement would the nurse include in the description? Select all that apply:
1. "Your child may experience involuntary urination after age 5."
2. "Episodes primarily occur when your child is awake and playing."
3. "Your child may suffer deep feelings of shame and may withdraw from peers because of ridicule."
4. "The condition may respond to tricyclic antidepressants and antidiuretics."
5. "The condition may become permanent without appropriate intervention."

14. Which comment made by a parent would indicate to the nurse the need for further education about acute glomerulonephritis complications?
1. "Dizziness is expected, and I should have my child lie down when he feels it."
2. "I should let the nurse know every time my child urinates."
3. "I need to ask my child whether he has a headache."
4. "I should encourage quiet play activities."

15. When teaching an 8-year-old child to obtain a clean-catch urine specimen, which technique should be included?
1. Collect the specimen right after a nap.
2. Never use the first voided specimen of the day.
3. Collect the specimen at the beginning of urination.
4. You don't need to wash your perineal area before collecting the specimen.

16. Which therapy should a nurse expect to incorporate into the care of a child with acute glomerulonephritis?
1. Antibiotic therapy
2. Dialysis therapy
3. Diuretic therapy
4. Play therapy

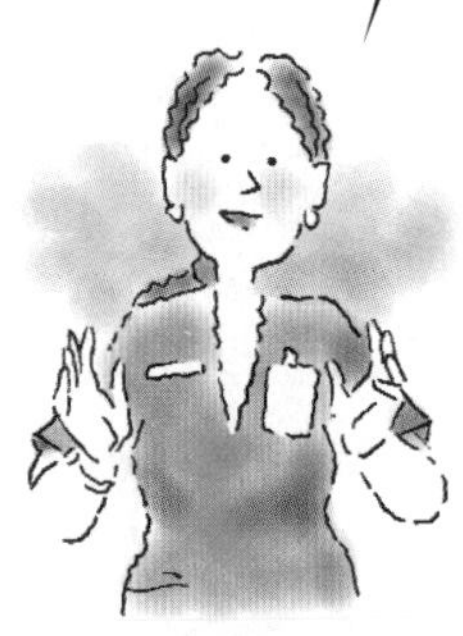

The phrase further education indicates that question 14 is looking for an inaccurate statement.

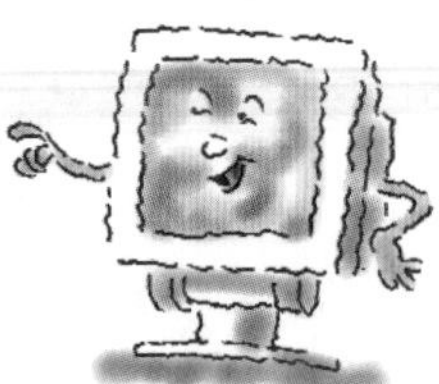

Don't a-void this question. You're doing great!

13. 1, 3, 4. Enuresis is a condition in which there's involuntary urination after age 5. It generally occurs while the child is sleeping. There can be long-lasting emotional trauma resulting from peer ridicule and feelings of shame and embarrassment. The condition may be treated with the use of tricyclic antidepressant and antidiuretics. With support and understanding, the condition generally resolves in time.
CN: Physiological integrity; CNS: Physiological adaptation; CL: Analysis

14. 1. Dizziness and headache are signs of encephalopathy and must be reported to the nurse. Hypertensive encephalopathy, acute cardiac decompensation, and acute renal failure are the major complications that tend to develop during the acute phase of glomerulonephritis. In order to maintain an accurate intake and output record, the parent should let the nurse know when the child urinates. Quiet play is encouraged to avoid overstressing the kidneys.
CN: Physiological integrity; CNS: Reduction of risk potential; CL: Application

15. 2. When collecting a clean-catch urine specimen, the first voided specimen of the day should never be used because of urinary stasis; this also applies after a nap. The specimen should be collected midstream, not at the beginning or end of urination. Washing the perineal area before collecting a specimen is very important to make sure there are no contaminants from the skin in the specimen.
CN: Physiological integrity; CNS: Reduction of risk potential; CL: Application

16. 4. Play therapy is an important aspect of care to help the child understand what's happening to him. Unless the child has the ability to express concerns and fears, he may have night terrors and regress in his stage of growth and development. Antibiotic therapy is indicated for an infectious process. Dialysis therapy is appropriate for renal failure. Diuretic therapy is usually ineffective.
CN: Health promotion and maintenance; CNS: None; CL: Application

17. In explaining treatment for glomerulonephritis, a nurse should include which statement?

1. All children who have signs of glomerulonephritis are hospitalized for approximately 1 week.
2. Parents should expect children to have a normal energy level during the acute phase.
3. Children who have normal blood pressure and a satisfactory urinary output can generally be treated at home.
4. Children with gross hematuria and significant oliguria should be brought to the physician's office about every 2 days for monitoring.

17. 3. Children who have normal blood pressure and a satisfactory urinary output can generally be treated at home. Parents should expect children to have a decrease in energy levels during the acute phase of the disease. Those with gross hematuria and significant oliguria will probably be hospitalized for monitoring.

CN: Health promotion and maintenance; CNS: None; CL: Application

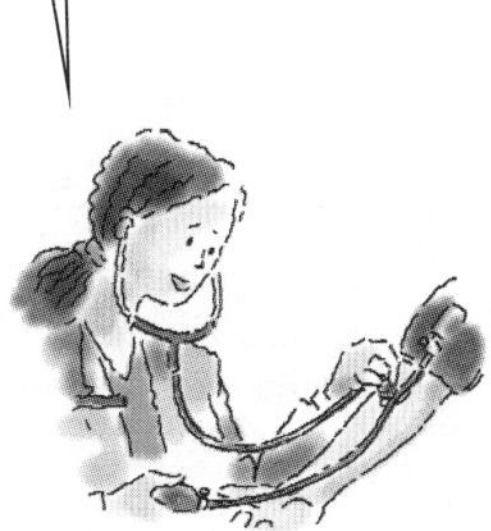
Hypertension is a complication of glomerulonephritis.

18. Which action is a nursing priority for a child with acute glomerulonephritis?

1. Assess blood pressure every 4 hours.
2. Check urine specific gravity every 8 hours.
3. Encourage daily fluid intake of 3,500 L.
4. Provide a 2,500-mg sodium diet.

18. 1. Because hypertension is a complication of acute glomerulonephritis, the nurse should check the child's blood pressure every 4 hours. The urine specific gravity should also be monitored, but it isn't as high a priority as monitoring the blood pressure. The child may be placed on fluid or sodium restrictions.

CN: Physiological integrity; CNS: Reduction of risk potential; CL: Application

19. Which food should a nurse <u>eliminate</u> from the diet of a child who's diagnosed with acute glomerulonephritis?

1. Turkey sandwich with mayonnaise
2. Hot dog with ketchup and mustard
3. Chocolate cake with white icing
4. Apple with peanut butter

19. 2. Foods that are high in sodium content, such as hot dogs, should be eliminated from the child's diet. Snacks such as pretzels and potato chips should also be discouraged. Any other foods that the child likes should be encouraged.

CN: Physiological integrity; CNS: Basic care and comfort; CL: Application

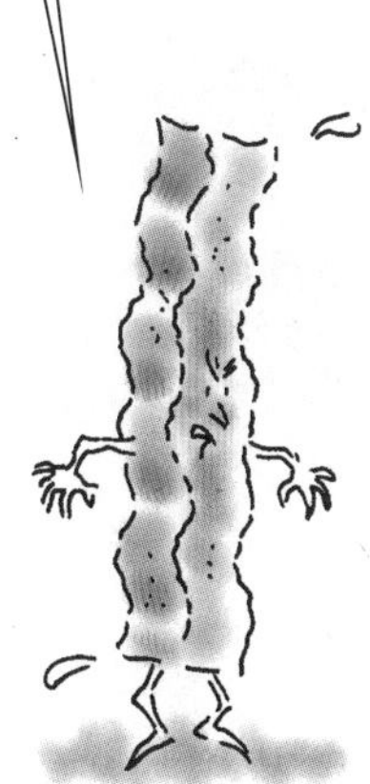
What do you mean I'm being eliminated?

20. A mother of a child with hypospadias asks the nurse what the condition is. The nurse would respond which of the following statements?

1. "It is the absence of a urethral opening."
2. "It is a penis that is shorter than usual for age."
3. "It is an urethral opening along the dorsal surface of the penis."
4. "It is an urethral opening along the ventral surface of the penis."

20. 4. *Hypospadias* refers to a condition in which the urethral opening is located below the glans penis or anywhere along the ventral surface of the penile shaft.

CN: Health promotion and maintenance; CNS: None; CL: Application

21. After the acute phase of glomerulonephritis is over, which discharge instruction should a nurse include?

1. Every 6 months, a cystogram will be needed for evaluation of progress.
2. Weekly visits to the physician may be needed for evaluation.
3. It will be acceptable to keep the regular yearly check-up appointment for the next evaluation.
4. There's no need to worry about further evaluations by the physician related to this disease.

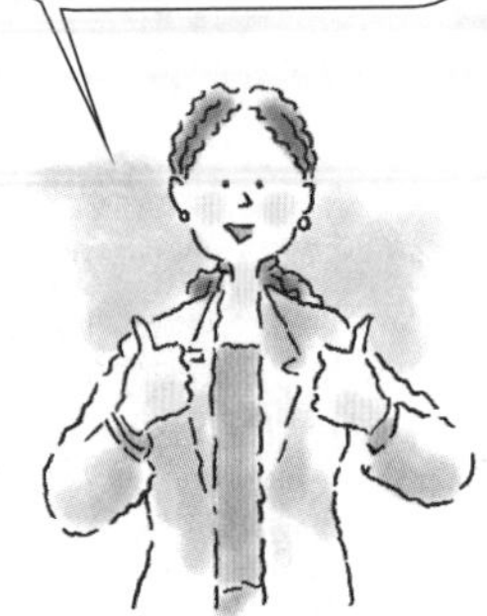

Twenty-one questions done! Keep plugging along!

21. 2. Weekly or monthly visits to the physician will be needed for evaluation of improvement and will usually involve the collection of a urine specimen for urinalysis. A cystogram isn't helpful in determining the progression of this disease; it's used to review the anatomic structures of the urinary tract.

CN: Physiological integrity; CNS: Reduction of risk potential; CL: Application

22. The mother of a newborn tells the nurse that she was told that her infant has chordee. The mother asks the nurse what this condition is. Which response is correct?

1. Ventral curvature of the penis
2. Dorsal curvature of the penis
3. No curvature of the penis
4. Misshapen penis

22. 1. Chordee, or ventral curvature of the penis, results from the replacement of normal skin with a fibrous band of tissue and usually accompanies more severe forms of hypospadias.

CN: Health promotion and maintenance; CNS: None; CL: Application

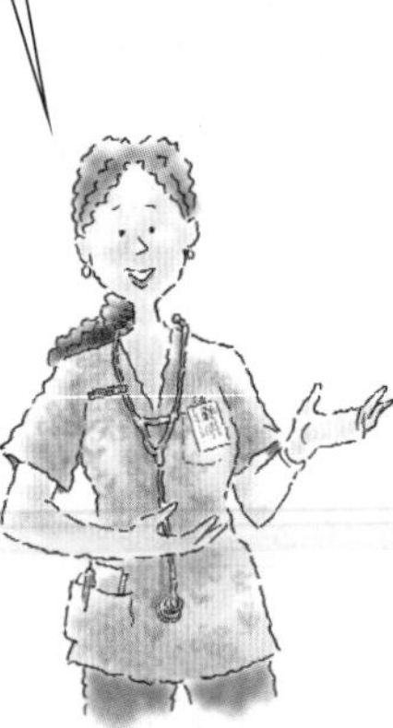

Knowing common accompanying conditions is important for taking the NCLEX.

23. The nurse is caring for an infant with hypospadias. Which anomaly would the nurse assess the infant for that commonly accompanies this condition?

1. Undescended testicles
2. Ambiguous genitalia
3. Umbilical hernias
4. Inguinal hernias

23. 1. Because undescended testes may also be present, the small penis may appear to be an enlarged clitoris. This shouldn't be mistaken for ambiguous genitalia. If there's any doubt, more tests should be performed. Hernias don't generally accompany hypospadias.

CN: Health promotion and maintenance; CNS: None; CL: Application

24. Which reason explains why surgical repair of a hypospadias is done as early as possible?

1. To prevent separation anxiety
2. To prevent urinary complications
3. To promote acceptance of hospitalization
4. To promote development of a normal body image

24. 4. Whenever there are defects of the genitourinary tact, surgery should be performed early to promote development of a normal body image. A child with normal emotional development shows separation anxiety at 7 to 9 months. Within a few months, he understands the mother's permanence, and separation anxiety diminishes. Hypospadias doesn't put the child at a greater risk for urinary complications.

CN: Health promotion and maintenance; CNS: None; CL: Application

25. A nurse should counsel parents to postpone which action until after their son's hypospadias has been repaired?

1. Circumcising the infant
2. Baptizing the infant
3. Getting hepatitis B vaccine
4. Checking blood for inborn errors of metabolism

25. 1. Circumcision shouldn't be performed until after the hypospadias has been repaired. The foreskin might be needed to help in the repair of the hypospadias. None of the other choices has any bearing on the repair of the hypospadias.

CN: Health promotion and maintenance; CNS: None; CL: Application

26. Which statement made about the principal objective of surgical correction by the parents of a child undergoing hypospadias repair implies a need for <u>further teaching</u>?

1. "The purpose is to improve the physical appearance of the genitalia for psychological reasons."
2. "The purpose is to enhance the child's ability to void in the standing position."
3. "The purpose is to decrease the chance of developing urinary tract infections."
4. "The purpose is to preserve a sexually adequate organ."

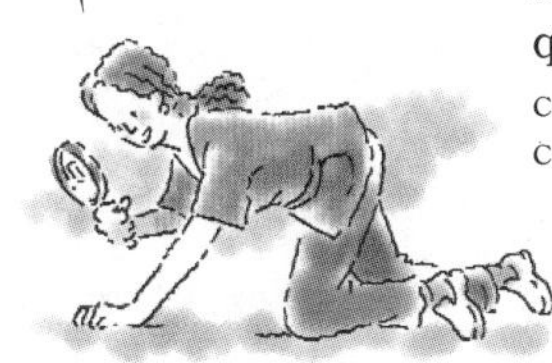

I'm looking for the one *inaccurate* statement.

26. 3. A child with hypospadias isn't at greater risk for urinary tract infections. The principal objectives of surgical corrections are to enhance the child's ability to void in the standing position with a straight stream, to improve the physical appearance of the genitalia for psychological reasons, and to preserve a sexually adequate organ.

CN: Health promotion and maintenance; CNS: None; CL: Application

27. Which nursing intervention should be included in the care plan for a male infant following surgical repair of hypospadias?

1. Sterile dressing changes every 4 hours
2. Frequent assessment of the tip of the penis
3. Removal of the suprapubic catheter on the second postoperative day
4. Urethral catheterization if voiding doesn't occur over an 8-hour period

27. 2. Following hypospadias repair, a pressure dressing is applied to the penis to reduce bleeding and tissue swelling. The penile tip should then be assessed frequently for signs of circulatory impairment. The dressing around the penis shouldn't be changed as frequently as every 4 hours. The physician will determine when the suprapubic catheter will be removed. Urethral catheterization should be avoided after repair of hypospadias to prevent injury to the urethra.

CN: Physiological integrity; CNS: Basic care and comfort; CL: Application

28. The nurse is explaining to the parents of a child with hypospadias the optimum time for repair of this condition. Which response as to the optimum age of choice would be the most accurate?

1. 1 week
2. 6 to 18 months
3. 2 years
4. 4 years

28. 2. The preferred time for surgical repair is 6 to 18 months of age, before the child has developed body image and castration anxiety. Surgical repair of hypospadias as early as 3 months old has been successful but with a high incidence of complications.

CN: Health promotion and maintenance; CNS: None; CL: Application

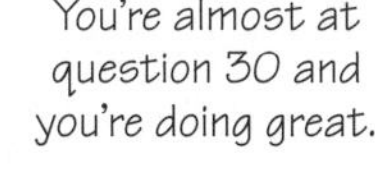

You're almost at question 30 and you're doing great.

29. When providing discharge information to the parents of a child with a hypospadias repair, which instruction would be <u>appropriate</u>?

1. Care of the circumcision
2. Techniques for providing tub baths
3. Care for the indwelling catheter or stent
4. Encouragement of voiding every 2 hours

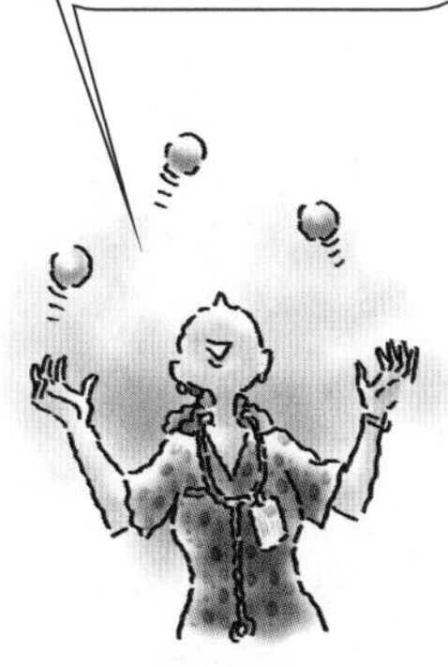

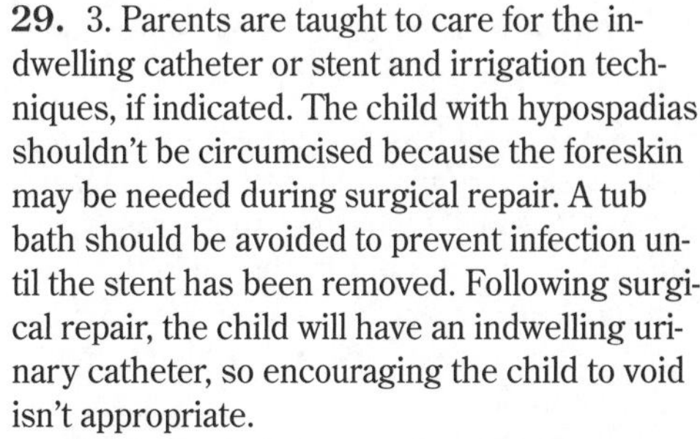

29. 3. Parents are taught to care for the indwelling catheter or stent and irrigation techniques, if indicated. The child with hypospadias shouldn't be circumcised because the foreskin may be needed during surgical repair. A tub bath should be avoided to prevent infection until the stent has been removed. Following surgical repair, the child will have an indwelling urinary catheter, so encouraging the child to void isn't appropriate.

CN: Physiological integrity; CNS: Reduction of risk potential; CL: Analysis

30. When providing discharge instructions to the parents of an older child who has had hypospadias repair, which activity should be encouraged?

1. Riding a bicycle
2. Playing in sandboxes
3. Increased fluid intake
4. Playing with the family pet

30. 3. The family is advised to encourage the child to increase fluid intake. Sandboxes, straddle toys, swimming, and rough activities are avoided until allowed by the surgeon.

CN: Physiological integrity; CNS: Physiological adaptation; CL: Application

31. The mother of a neonate born with hypospadias is sharing her feelings of guilt about this anomaly with a nurse. The nurse should explain which fact about the defect?

1. It occurs around the third month of fetal development.
2. It occurs around the sixth month of fetal development.
3. It's carried by an autosomal recessive gene.
4. It's hereditary.

31. 1. The defect of hypospadias occurs around the end of the third month of fetal development. Many women don't even know that they're pregnant at this time. This defect isn't hereditary, nor is it carried by an autosomal recessive gene.

CN: Health promotion and maintenance; CNS: None; CL: Application

32. A mother reports that her 6-year-old daughter recently began wetting the bed and running a low-grade fever. A urinalysis is positive for bacteria and protein. A diagnosis of a urinary tract infection (UTI) is made, and the child is prescribed antibiotics. Which interventions are appropriate? Select all that apply:

1. Limit fluids for the next few days to decrease the frequency of urination.
2. Assess the mother's understanding of UTI and its causes.
3. Instruct the mother to administer the antibiotic as prescribed—even if the symptoms diminish.
4. Provide instruction solely to the mother, not the child.
5. Discourage the taking of bubble baths.
6. Advise wiping from back to the front after voiding and defecation.

32. 2, 3, 5. Assessing the mother's understanding of UTI and its causes provides the nurse with a baseline for teaching. The full course of antibiotics must be given to eradicate the organism and prevent recurrence, even if the child's signs and symptoms decrease. Bubble baths can irritate the vulva and urethra and contribute to the development of a UTI. Fluids should be encouraged, not limited, in order to prevent urinary stasis and help flush the organism out of the urinary tract. Instructions should be given to the child at her level of understanding to help her better understand the treatment and promote compliance. The child should wipe from front to the back, not back to front, to minimize the risk of contamination after elimination.

CN: Health promotion and maintenance; CNS: None; CL: Application

33. A 3-year-old had a hypospadias repair yesterday; he has a suprapubic catheter in place and an I.V. Which rationale is appropriate for administering propantheline bromide (Pro-Banthine) on an as-needed basis?

1. To decrease the risk of infection at the suture line
2. To decrease the number of organisms in the urine
3. To prevent bladder spasms while the catheter is present
4. To increase urine flow from the kidney to the ureters

33. 3. Propantheline bromide is an antispasmodic that works effectively on children. It isn't an antibiotic and therefore won't decrease the chance of infection or the number of organisms in the urine. The drug has no diuretic effect and won't increase urine flow.

CN: Physiological integrity; CNS: Pharmacological and parenteral therapies; CL: Application

34. Which intervention by a nurse would be most helpful when discussing hypospadias with the parents of an infant with this defect?

1. Refer the parents to a counselor.
2. Be there to listen to the parents' concerns.
3. Notify the physician, and have him talk to the parents.
4. Suggest a support group of other parents who have gone through this experience.

34. 2. The nurse must recognize that parents are going to grieve the loss of the "normal" child when they have a neonate born with a birth defect. Initially, the parents need to have a nurse who will listen to their concerns for their neonate's health. Suggesting a support group or referring the parents to a counselor might be good actions, but not initially. The physician will need to spend time with the parents but, again, the nurse is in the best position to allow the parents to vent their grief and anger.

CN: Psychosocial integrity; CNS: None; CL: Application

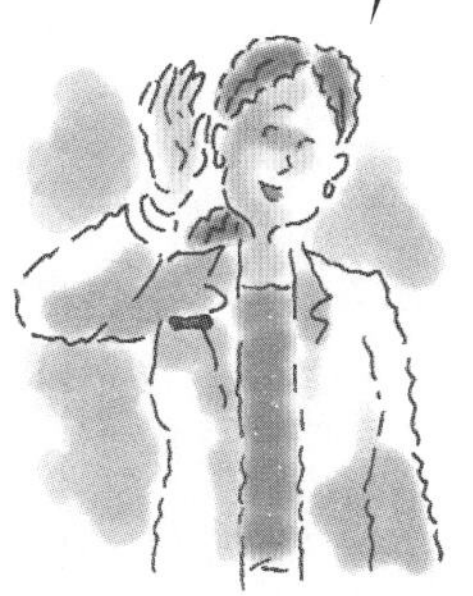

You can almost hear the answer to this question.

35. A nurse should understand that hypospadias defects take the greatest emotional toll on which person?

1. The father
2. The mother
3. The grandfather
4. The grandmother

35. 1. Because the penis is involved, studies have shown that fathers have a great deal of difficulty dealing with a birth defect like hypospadias.

CN: Psychosocial integrity; CNS: None; CL: Application

36. A nurse is questioned by a student nurse about the difference between hypospadias and epispadias. Which response by the nurse is the most accurate?

1. Epispadias defects can only occur in males.
2. The difference between the defects is the length of the urethra.
3. Hypospadias is an abnormal opening on the ventral side of the penis; epispadias is an abnormal opening on the dorsal side.
4. Hypospadias is an abnormal opening on the dorsal side of the penis; epispadias is an abnormal opening on the ventral side.

36. 3. Hypospadias results from the incomplete closure of the urethral folds along the ventral surface of the developing penis. Epispadias results when the urinary meatus is on the dorsal surface of the penis. Epispadias defects can occur in males and females. The difference is where the opening of the urinary meatus is located, not the length of the urethra.

CN: Health promotion and maintenance; CNS: None; CL: Application

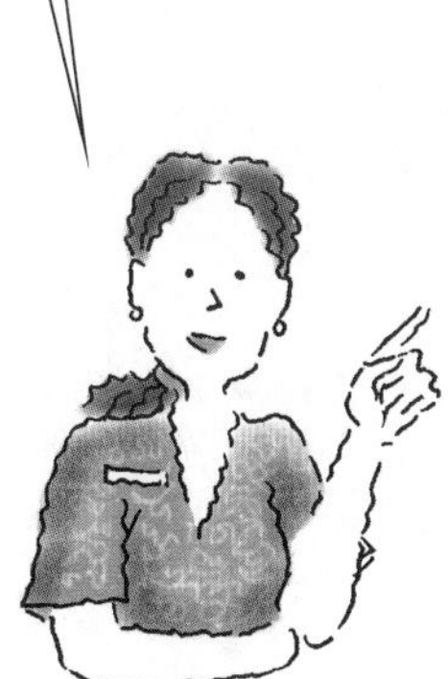

Question 36 is asking you to differentiate between two conditions.

37. Which nursing diagnosis would be most appropriate for a client with hypospadias?

1. *Deficient fluid volume*
2. *Impaired urinary elimination*
3. *Delayed growth and development*
4. *Risk for infection*

37. 2. The most appropriate diagnosis for a client with hypospadias is *Impaired urinary elimination.* A client with hypospadias should have no problems with the ingestion of fluids. The child's growth and development aren't affected with this defect, and he doesn't have any problem with infection until possibly after a repair of the hypospadias is performed.

CN: Health promotion and maintenance; CNS: None; CL: Analysis

38. When a nurse is teaching a parent how to care for the penis after a hypospadias repair with a skin graft, which statement made by the parent would indicate the need for further teaching?

1. "My infant won't be able to take baths until healing has occurred."
2. "I will change the dressing around the penis daily."
3. "I will make sure I change my infant's diaper often."
4. "If there's a color change in the penis, I will notify my child's physician."

38. 2. Dressing changes after a hypospadias repair with a skin graft are generally performed by the physician and aren't performed every day because the skin graft needs time to heal and adhere to the penis. Baths aren't given until postoperative healing has taken place. Changing the infant's diapers typically helps keep the penis dry. If the penis color changes, it might be evidence of circulation problems and should be reported.

CN: Health promotion and maintenance; CNS: None; CL: Analysis

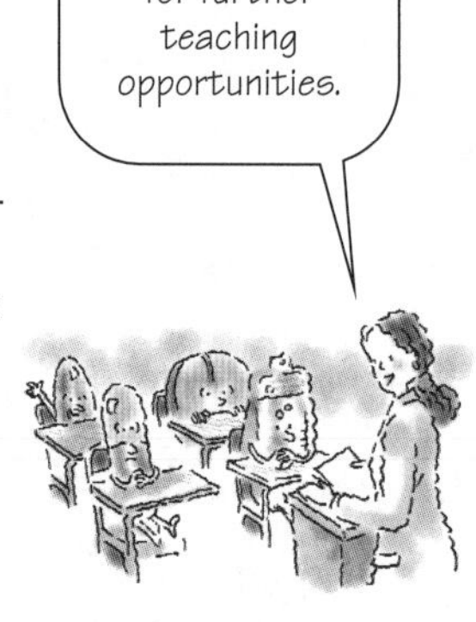
Stay alert for further teaching opportunities.

39. A nurse is preparing the parents of an infant with hypospadias for surgery. Which statement made by a parent indicates the need for further teaching?

1. "Skin grafting might be involved in my infant's repair."
2. "After surgery, my infant's penis will look perfectly normal."
3. "Surgical repair may need to be performed in several stages."
4. "My infant will probably be in some pain after the surgery and might need to take some medication for relief."

39. 2. It's important to stress to the parents that, even after a repair of hypospadias, the outcome isn't a completely "normal-looking" penis. The goals of surgery are to allow the child to void from the tip of his penis, void with a straight stream, and stand up while voiding.

CN: Psychosocial integrity; CNS: None; CL: Application

40. Which piece of assessment data collected by a nurse would indicate to the physician the need for a staged repair of a hypospadias rather than a single repair?

1. There's chordee present with the hypospadias.
2. The urinary meatus opens between the scrotum.
3. The urinary meatus is just below the tip of the penis.
4. The infant had been circumcised before the defect was discovered.

40. 2. Increased surgical experience and improvements in technique have reduced the number of staged procedures applied to hypospadias defects; however, a staged procedure is indicated in particularly severe defects with marked deficits of available skin for mobilization of flaps. Having a chordee present doesn't require a staged hypospadias repair. If an infant has been circumcised but has a relatively minor hypospadias, the repair can still occur in one stage.

CN: Physiological integrity; CNS: Physiological adaptation; CL: Analysis

41. A nurse is planning to teach a female adolescent about pelvic inflammatory disease (PID). Which teaching statement best reflects the focus of preventative teaching needs for this age group?

1. Poor hygiene practices increase the risk of PID.
2. The use of hormonal contraceptives decreases the risk of PID.
3. There are long-term complications related to reproductive tract infections.
4. There are risks of defects in future infants born to adolescents with PID.

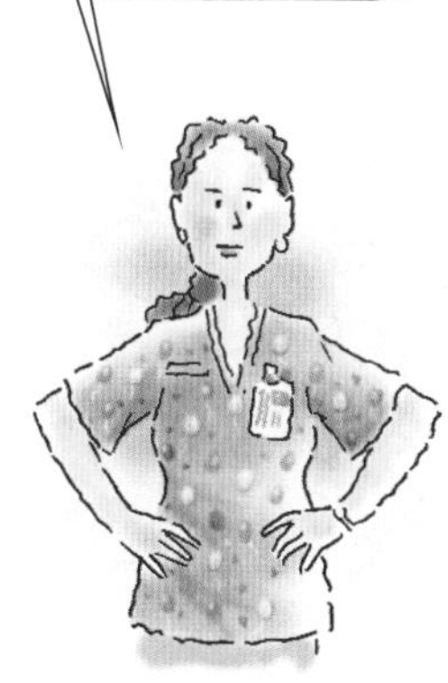

PID untreated can have long-term and serious consequences.

41. 3. Long-term complications of PID include abscess formation in the fallopian tubes and adhesion formation leading to increased risk of ectopic pregnancy or infertility. It isn't prevented by proper personal hygiene or any form of contraception; some forms of contraception, such as the male or female condom, do help to decrease the incidence of it. PID does not increase the risk of birth defects in infants born to adolescents with PID.

CN: Health promotion and maintenance; CNS: None; CL: Application

42. After a nurse has completed discharge teaching, which statement made by a client treated for a sexually transmitted disease (STD) would indicate that discharge instructions were understood?

1. "I don't need condoms because I'm not allergic to penicillin and I'll come for a shot at the first sign of infection."
2. "I will notify my sex partners and not have unprotected sex from now on."
3. "I will be careful not to have intercourse with someone who has an STD."
4. "If you're going to get it, you're going to get it."

42. 2. Goal achievement is indicated by the client's ability to describe preventive behaviors and health practices. The other options indicate that the client doesn't understand the need to take preventive measures.

CN: Health promotion and maintenance; CNS: None; CL: Analysis

43. Which statement regarding chlamydial infections is correct?

1. The treatment of choice is oral penicillin.
2. The treatment of choice is nystatin or miconazole.
3. Clinical manifestations include dysuria and urethral itching in males.
4. Clinical manifestations include small, painful vesicles on genital areas.

43. 3. Clinical manifestations of chlamydia include meatal erythema, tenderness, itching, dysuria, and urethral discharge in the male and mucopurulent cervical exudate with erythema, edema, and congestion in the female. The treatment of choice is doxycycline or azithromycin. Vesicles in the genital area are more consistent with herpes simplex virus.

CN: Health promotion and maintenance; CNS: None; CL: Application

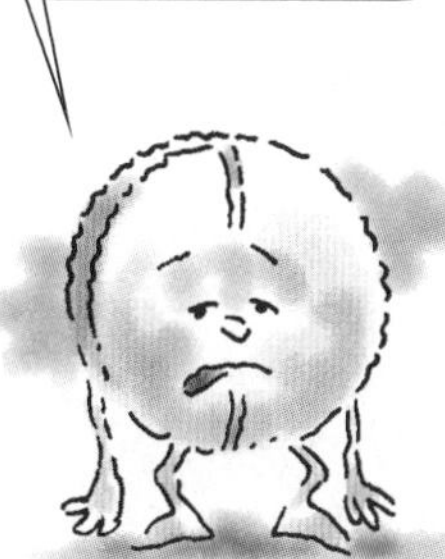

Some people are just hypersensitive— to me, that is.

44. Before a client with syphilis can be treated, the nurse must determine which factor?

1. Portal of entry
2. Size of the chancre
3. Names of sexual contacts
4. Existence of medication allergies

44. 4. The treatment of choice for syphilis is penicillin; clients allergic to penicillin must be given another antibiotic. The other choices aren't necessary before treatment can begin.

CN: Health promotion and maintenance; CNS: None; CL: Application

45. Which technique should a nurse consider when she's discussing sex and sexual activities with adolescents?

1. Break down all the information into scientific terminology.
2. Refer the adolescents to their parents for sexual information.
3. Only answer questions that are asked; don't present any other content.
4. Present sexual information using the proper terminology and in a straightforward manner.

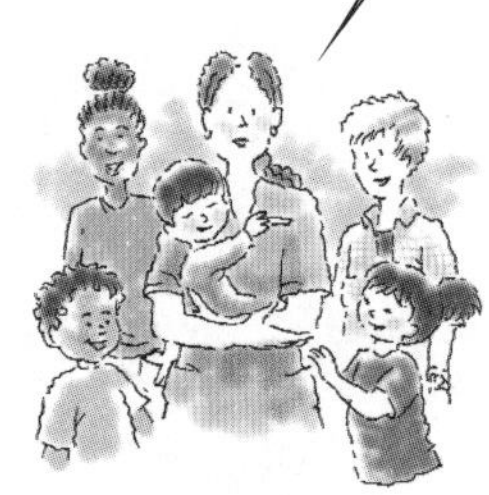

The NCLEX tests your ability to teach clients at different life stages.

45. 4. Although many adolescents have received sex education from parents and school throughout childhood, they aren't always adequately prepared for the impact of puberty. A large portion of their knowledge is acquired from peers, television, movies, and magazines. Consequently, much of the sex information they have is incomplete, inaccurate, riddled with cultural and moral values, and not very helpful. The public perceives nurses as having authoritative information and being willing to take time with parents. To be effective teachers, nurses need to be honest and open with sexual information.

CN: Health promotion and maintenance; CNS: None; CL: Application

46. Without proper treatment, anogenital warts caused by the human papillomavirus (HPV) increases the risk of which illness in adolescent females?

1. Gonorrhea
2. Cervical cancer
3. Chlamydial infections
4. Urinary tract infections (UTIs)

46. 2. All external lesions are treated because of concern regarding the relationship of HPV to cancer. HPV doesn't increase the risk of gonorrhea, chlamydia, or UTIs.

CN: Health promotion and maintenance; CNS: None; CL: Application

47. Which statement should a nurse include when teaching an adolescent about gonorrhea?

1. It's caused by *Treponema pallidum.*
2. Treatment of sexual partners is an essential part of treatment.
3. It's most commonly treated by multidose administration of penicillin.
4. It may be contracted through contact with a contaminated toilet bowl.

47. 2. Adolescents should be taught that treatment is needed for all sexual partners. Gonorrhea is caused by *Neisseria gonorrhoeae.* The medication of choice is a single dose of I.M. ceftriaxone sodium (Rocephin) in males and a single oral dose of cefixime (Suprax) in females. Gonorrhea can't be contracted from a contaminated toilet bowl.

CN: Health promotion and maintenance; CNS: None; CL: Application

48. When planning sex education and contraceptive teaching for adolescents, which factor should a nurse consider?

1. Neither sexual activity nor contraception requires planning.
2. Most teenagers today are knowledgeable about reproduction.
3. Most teenagers use pregnancy as a way to rebel against their parents.
4. Most teenagers are open about contraception but inconsistently use birth control.

48. 4. Most teenagers today are open about discussing contraception and sexuality but may get caught up in the heat of sexuality and forget about birth control measures. Very few teenagers use pregnancy as a way to rebel against their parents. A good deal of the information adolescents have related to reproduction and sexuality may have come from their peers and may not be very reliable.

CN: Health promotion and maintenance; CNS: None; CL: Analysis

49. A sexually active teenager seeks counseling from the school nurse about prevention of sexually transmitted diseases (STDs). Which contraceptive measure should the nurse recommend?

1. Rhythm method
2. Withdrawal method
3. Prophylactic antibiotic use
4. Condom and spermicide use

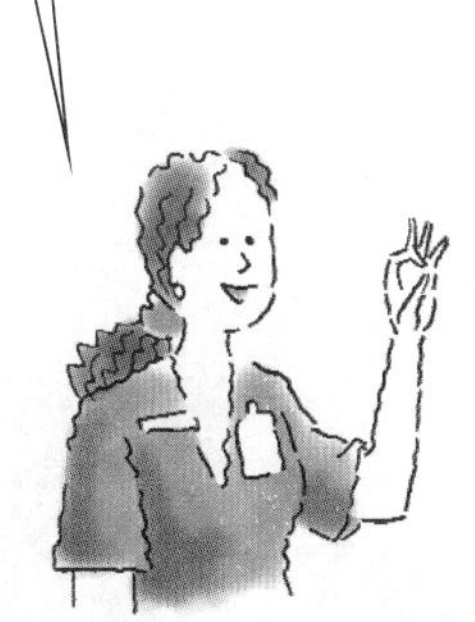

Nice work! You've finished nearly 50 questions already!

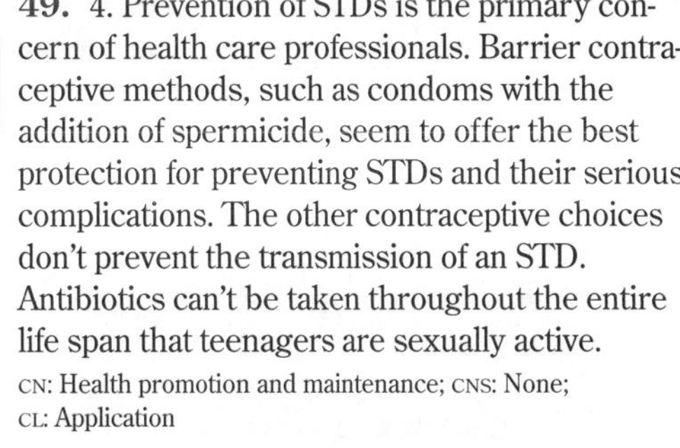

49. 4. Prevention of STDs is the primary concern of health care professionals. Barrier contraceptive methods, such as condoms with the addition of spermicide, seem to offer the best protection for preventing STDs and their serious complications. The other contraceptive choices don't prevent the transmission of an STD. Antibiotics can't be taken throughout the entire life span that teenagers are sexually active.

CN: Health promotion and maintenance; CNS: None; CL: Application

50. A nurse understands that which developmental rationale explains risk-taking behavior in adolescents?

1. Adolescents are concrete thinkers and concentrate only on what's happening at the time.
2. Belief in their own invulnerability persuades adolescents that they can take risks safely.
3. Risk of parents' anger and disappointment usually deters adolescents from risky behavior.
4. Peer pressure usually doesn't play an important part in an adolescent's decision to become sexually active.

50. 2. Understanding the growth and development of adolescents helps the nurse see that they feel they're invulnerable. Adolescents think about the future and can formally operate in their thought process. Peer pressure plays an important role in risk-taking behaviors; more so than fear of parents' anger or disappointment.

CN: Health promotion and maintenance; CNS: None; CL: Analysis

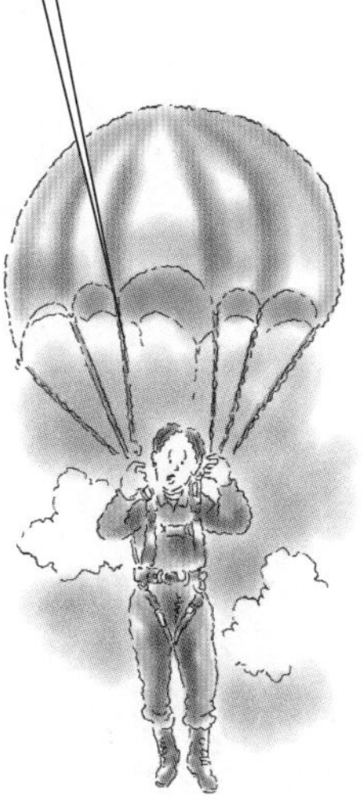

51. Statistics about sexually transmitted diseases (STDs) may not be reliable for which reason?

1. Most adolescents seek out treatment for their STD.
2. Adolescents are usually honest with their parents about their sexual behavior.
3. All sexually transmitted diseases must be reported to the Centers for Disease Control and Prevention (CDC).
4. Chlamydial infections and human papillomavirus (HPV) infections aren't required to be reported to the CDC.

51. 4. Chlamydial infections and HPV infections aren't required to be reported to the CDC. Most teenagers are afraid to seek out health care for sexual diseases or are unaware of the signs and symptoms of STDs. Teenagers find this a very difficult topic to discuss with their parents and will usually seek out a peer or another adult to obtain information.

CN: Safe, effective care environment; CNS: Safety and infection control; CL: Application

52. It's important for a nurse to include which statement in discharge education for the client who's taking metronidazole (Flagyl) to treat trichomoniasis?

1. Sexual intercourse should stop.
2. Alcohol shouldn't be consumed.
3. Milk products should be avoided.
4. Exposure to sunlight should be limited.

52. 2. While taking metronidazole to treat trichomoniasis, clients shouldn't consume alcohol for at least 48 hours following the last dose. The other choices have no effect on the client taking this medication.

CN: Physiological integrity; CNS: Pharmacological and parenteral therapies; CL: Application

53. Which statement by an adolescent should alert the nurse that more education about sexually transmitted diseases (STDs) is needed?

1. "You always know when you've got gonorrhea."
2. "The most common STD in kids my age is chlamydia infection."
3. "Most of the girls who have *Chlamydia* don't even know it."
4. "If you have symptoms of gonorrhea, they can show up a day or a couple of weeks after you got the infection to begin with."

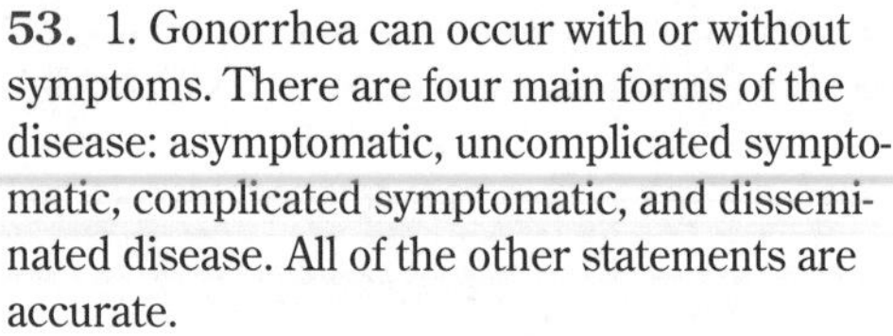
Some sexually transmitted diseases can occur with or without symptoms.

53. 1. Gonorrhea can occur with or without symptoms. There are four main forms of the disease: asymptomatic, uncomplicated symptomatic, complicated symptomatic, and disseminated disease. All of the other statements are accurate.

CN: Health promotion and maintenance; CNS: None; CL: Application

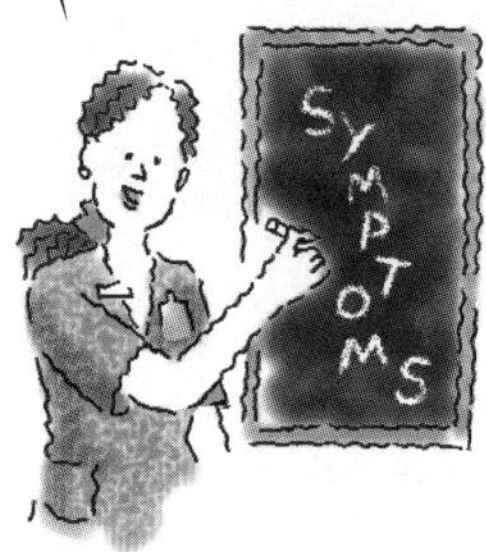
SYMPTOMS

54. Which assessment describes the method of preventing sexually transmitted diseases (STDs) by avoiding exposure?

1. The least accepted and most difficult approach
2. The least expensive and most effective approach
3. The most expensive and least effective approach
4. The most difficult and most time-consuming approach

54. 2. Primary prevention of STDs by avoiding exposure is the least expensive and most effective approach. The nurse can play a role in offering this education to young people before they initiate sexual intercourse.

CN: Safe, effective care environment; CNS: Safety and infection control; CL: Application

55. Which client should a nurse consider to be at greatest risk for developing acquired immunodeficiency syndrome (AIDS)?

1. A client who lives in crowded housing with poor ventilation
2. A young sexually active client with multiple partners
3. An adolescent who's homeless and lives in shelters
4. A young sexually active client with one partner

55. 2. The younger the client when sexual activity begins, the higher the incidence of HIV and AIDS. Also, the more sexual partners he has, the higher the incidence of these diseases. Neither crowded living environments nor homeless environments by themselves lead to an increase in the incidence of AIDS.

CN: Health promotion and maintenance; CNS: None; CL: Analysis

56. When assessing an adolescent for pelvic inflammatory disease (PID), which sign or symptom should the nurse expect to see?

1. A hard, painless, red defined lesion
2. Small vesicles on the genital area with itching
3. Cervical discharge with redness and edema
4. Lower abdominal pain and urinary tract symptoms

Questions about basic assessment skills are common on the NCLEX.

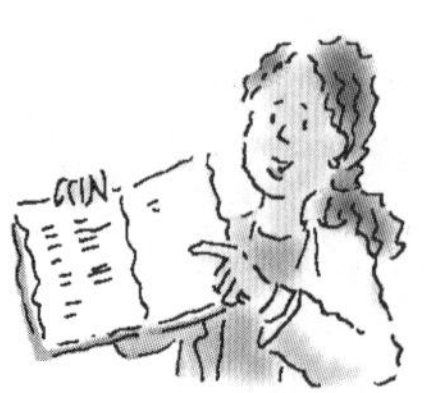

56. 4. PID is an infection of the upper female genital tract most commonly caused by sexually transmitted diseases. Presenting symptoms in the adolescent may be generalized, with fever, abdominal pain, urinary tract symptoms, and vague, influenza-like symptoms. A hard, painless, red defined lesion indicates syphilis. Small vesicles on the genital area with itching indicates herpes genitalis. Cervical discharge with redness and edema indicates chlamydia.

CN: Health promotion and maintenance; CNS: None; CL: Application

57. A nurse should include which fact when teaching an adolescent group about the human immunodeficiency virus (HIV)?

1. The incidence of HIV in the adolescent population has declined since 1995.
2. The virus can be spread through many routes, including sexual contact.
3. Knowledge about HIV spread and transmission has led to a decrease in the spread of the virus among adolescents.
4. About 50% of all new HIV infections in the United States occur in people under age 22.

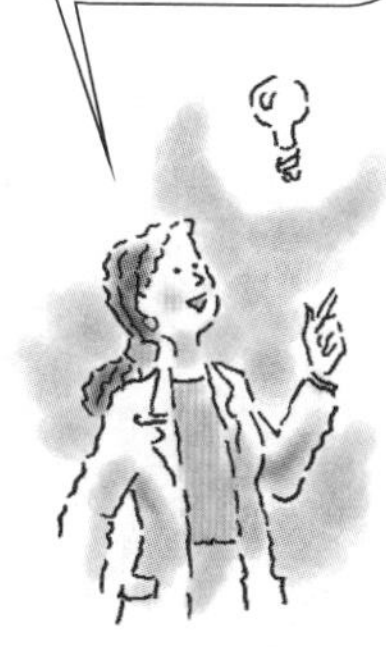

Hey! I think I finally get genitourinary disorders.

57. 2. HIV can be spread through many routes, including sexual contact and contact with infected blood or other body fluids. The incidence of HIV in the adolescent population has *increased* since 1995, even though more information about the virus is targeted to reach the adolescent population. Only about 25% of all new HIV infections in the United States occur in people under age 22.

CN: Health promotion and maintenance; CNS: None; CL: Application

58. When planning a program to teach adolescents about human immunodeficiency virus infection (HIV), which action might lead to better program success?

1. Surveying the community to evaluate the level of education
2. Obtaining peer educators to provide information about HIV
3. Setting up clinics in community centers and having condoms readily available
4. Having primary health care providers host workshops in community centers

58. 2. Peer education programs have noted that teens are more likely to ask questions of peer educators than of adults and that peer education can change personal attitudes and the perception of risk of HIV infection. The other approaches would be helpful but wouldn't necessarily make the outreach program more successful.

CN: Health promotion and maintenance; CNS: None; CL: Analysis

59. After a nurse completes her teaching of an adolescent about syphilis, which statement by the adolescent indicates the need for further teaching?

1. "The disease is divided into four stages: primary, secondary, latent, and tertiary."
2. "Affected persons are most infectious during the first year."
3. "Syphilis is easily treated with penicillin or doxycycline."
4. "Syphilis is rarely transmitted sexually."

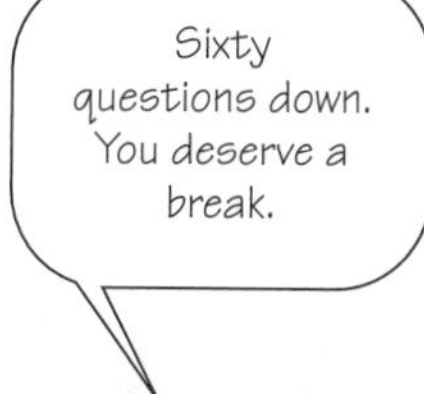

Sixty questions down. You deserve a break.

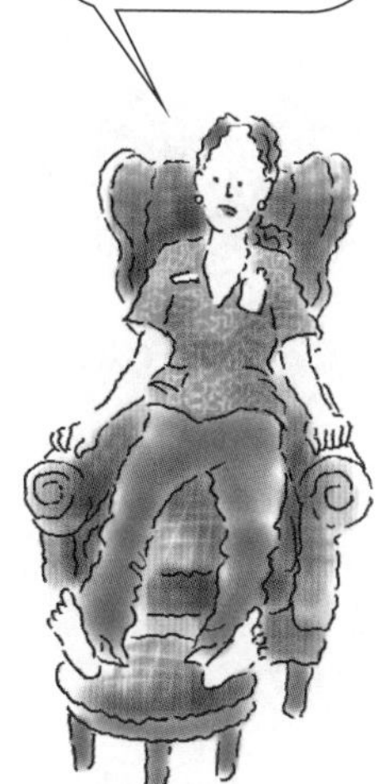

59. 4. About 95% of syphilis cases are transmitted sexually. There are four stages to syphilis, although some people may only experience the first three stages. Affected persons are most contagious in the first year of the disease. The drug of choice for treating syphilis is penicillin or doxycycline.

CN: Health promotion and maintenance; CNS: None; CL: Analysis

60. In teaching a group of parents about monitoring for urinary tract infection (UTI) in preschoolers, which symptom would indicate that a child should be evaluated?

1. Voids only twice in any 6-hour period
2. Exhibits incontinence after being toilet trained
3. Has difficulty sitting still for more than a 30-minute period of time
4. Urine smells strongly of ammonia after standing for more than 2 hours

60. 2. A child who exhibits incontinence after being toilet trained should be evaluated for UTI. Most urine smells strongly of ammonia after standing for more than 2 hours, so this doesn't necessarily indicate UTI. The other options aren't reasons for parents to suspect problems with their child's urinary system.

CN: Health promotion and maintenance; CNS: None; CL: Application

61. Which instruction should a nurse include in the teaching plan for a client receiving co-trimoxazole (Septra) for a repeated urinary tract infection with *Escherichia coli?*

1. "For the drug to be effective, keep your urine acidic by drinking at least a quart of cranberry juice a day."
2. "Take the medication for 10 days even if your symptoms improve in a few days."
3. "Return to the clinic in 3 days for another urine culture."
4. "Take two of the pills a day now, but keep the rest of the pills to take if the symptoms reappear within 2 weeks."

Teaching about medications—that's another common NCLEX subject.

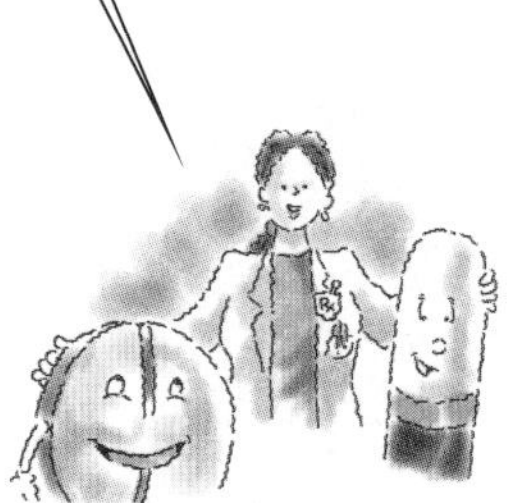

61. 2. Discharge instructions for clients receiving an anti-infective medication should include taking all of the prescribed medication for the prescribed time. Drinking highly acidic juices, such as cranberry juice, may help maintain urinary health but won't get rid of an already present infection. The child won't need to have a culture repeated until the medication is completed.

CN: Physiological integrity; CNS: Pharmacological and parenteral therapies; CL: Application

62. A nurse should include which fact when teaching parents about handling a child with recurrent urinary tract infection (UTI)?

1. Antibiotics should be discontinued 48 hours after symptoms subside.
2. Recurrent symptoms should be treated by renewing the antibiotic prescription.
3. Complicated UTIs are related to poor perineal hygiene practice.
4. Follow-up urine cultures are necessary to detect recurrent infections and antibiotic effectiveness.

62. 4. A routine follow-up urine specimen is usually obtained 2 or 3 days after the completion of the antibiotic treatment. All of the antibiotic should be taken as ordered and not stopped when symptoms disappear. If recurrent symptoms appear, a urine culture should be obtained to see whether the infection is resistant to antibiotics. Simple, not complicated, UTIs are generally caused by poor perineal hygiene.

CN: Health promotion and maintenance; CNS: None; CL: Application

63. A nurse is reviewing a child's clean-voided urine specimen results. The nurse understands that which result indicates a urinary tract infection (UTI)?

1. A specific gravity of 1.020
2. Cloudy color without odor
3. A large amount of casts present
4. 100,000 bacterial colonies per milliliter

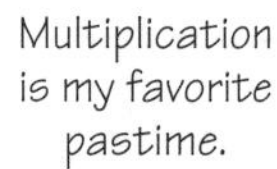
Multiplication
is my favorite
pastime.

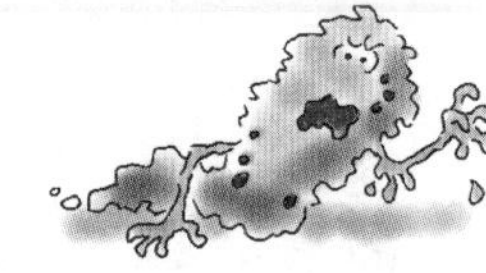

63. 4. The diagnosis of UTI is determined by the detection of bacteria in the urine. Infected urine usually contains more than 100,000 colonies/ml, usually of a single organism. The urine is usually cloudy, hazy, and may have strands of mucus. It also has a foul, fishy odor even when fresh. Casts and increased specific gravity aren't specific to UTI.

CN: Physiological integrity; CNS: Reduction of risk potential; CL: Application

64. The nurse is teaching the parents of a child with a urinary tract infection. Which factor should the nurse recognize as predisposing the urinary tract to infections?

1. Increased fluid intake
2. Short urethra
3. Ingestion of highly acidic juices
4. Frequent emptying of the bladder

64. 2. A short urethra contributes to infection because bacteria have a shorter distance to travel to the urinary tract. The risk of infection is higher in women because women have shorter urethras than men (3/4″ [1.9 cm] in young women, 1″ [3.8 cm] in mature women, 7″ [19.7 cm] in adult men). Increased fluid intake would help flush the urinary tract system and frequent emptying of the bladder would decrease the risk of urinary tract infection. Drinking highly acidic juices, such as cranberry juice, may help maintain urinary health.

CN: Health promotion and maintenance; CNS: None; CL: Application

CN: Client needs category CNS: Client needs subcategory CL: Cognitive level

65. A nurse is assessing a child with vesicoureteral reflux. Which condition should the nurse be alert for as a potential complication?

1. Glomerulonephritis
2. Hemolytic uremia syndrome
3. Nephrotic syndrome
4. Renal infection

65. 4. Reflux of urine into the ureters and then back into the bladder after voiding sets up the client for a urinary tract infection. This can lead to renal damage due to scarring of the parenchyma. Glomerulonephritis is an autoimmune reaction to a beta-hemolytic strep infection. Hemolytic uremia syndrome may be the result of genetic factors. Eighty percent of nephrotic syndrome cases are idiopathic.

CN: Health promotion and maintenance; CNS: None; CL: Analysis

66. The mother of a female child asks the nurse why her child seems to have so many urinary tract infections (UTIs). Which response by the nurse would be the most accurate?

1. Vaginal secretions are too acidic.
2. Girls aren't protected by circumcision.
3. The urethra is in close proximity to the anus.
4. Girls touch their genitalia more often than boys do.

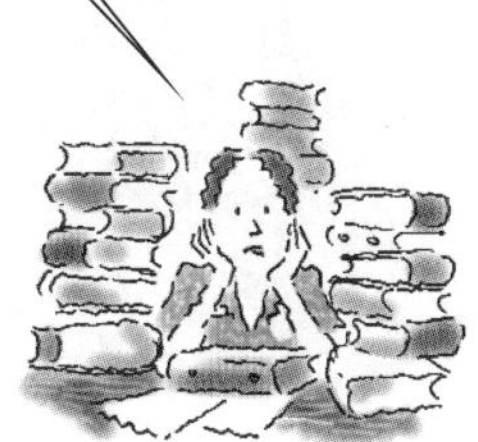

All this studying just to learn that girls are different from boys.

66. 3. Girls are especially at risk for bacterial invasion of the urinary tract because of basic anatomical differences; the urethra is short and in close proximity to the anus. Vaginal secretions are normally acidic, which decreases the risk of infection. Circumcision doesn't protect girls *or* boys from UTIs. There's no documented research that supports that girls touch their genitalia more often than boys do.

CN: Health promotion and maintenance; CNS: None; CL: Application

67. A child has been sent to the school nurse for wetting her pants three times in the past 2 days. The nurse should recommend that this child be evaluated for which complication?

1. School phobia
2. Emotional trauma
3. Urinary tract infection
4. Structural defect of the urinary tract

67. 3. Frequent urinary incontinence should be evaluated by the physician, with the first action being checking the urine for infection. Children exhibit signs of school phobia by complaining of an ailment before school starts and getting better after they're allowed to miss school. After infection, structural defect, and diabetes mellitus have been ruled out, emotional trauma should be investigated.

CN: Health promotion and maintenance; CNS: None; CL: Application

68. When a nurse is teaching parents of children about recurrent urinary tract infections (UTIs), which goal should be included as the <u>most important</u>?

1. Detection
2. Education
3. Prevention
4. Treatment

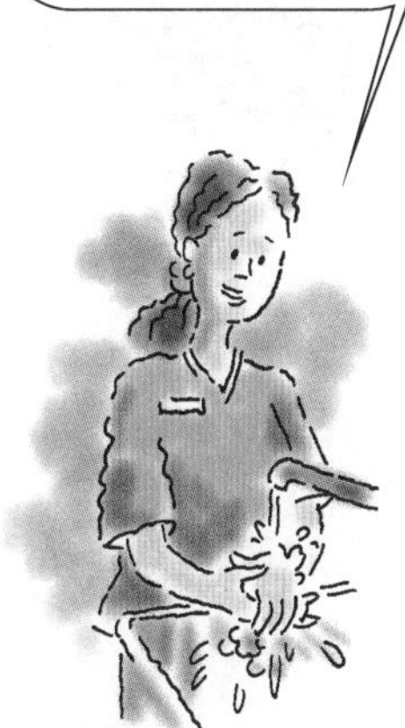

Sometimes simple hygienic habits offer the best preventative measure.

68. 3. Prevention is the most important goal in teaching about primary and recurrent UTIs; most preventive measures are simple, ordinary hygienic habits that should be a routine part of daily care. Treatment, detection, and education are all important, but none is the most important goal.

CN: Physiological integrity; CNS: Reduction of risk potential; CL: Analysis

69. Which intervention should a nurse recommend to parents of young girls to help prevent urinary tract infections (UTIs)?

1. Limit bathing as much as possible.
2. Increase fluids and decrease salt intake.
3. Have the child wear cotton underpants.
4. Have the child clean her perineum from back to front.

69. 3. Cotton is a more breathable fabric and allows for dampness to be absorbed from the perineum. Bathing shouldn't be limited; however, the use of bubble bath or whirlpool baths should. However, if the child has frequent UTIs, taking a bath should be discouraged and taking a shower encouraged. Increasing fluids would be helpful, but decreasing salt isn't necessary. The perineum should always be cleaned from front to back.

CN: Health promotion and maintenance; CNS: None; CL: Application

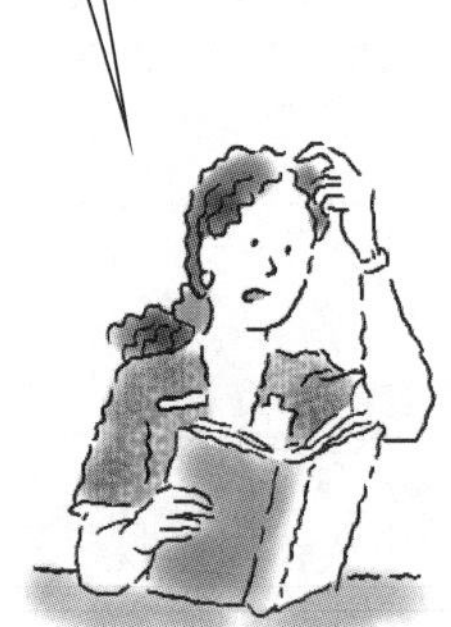

70. A nurse understands that which characteristic is the single most important factor influencing the occurrence of urinary tract infections (UTIs)?

1. Urinary stasis
2. Frequency of baths
3. Uncircumcised penis (in males)
4. Amount of fluid intake

70. 1. Ordinarily, urine is sterile. However, at 98.6° F (37° C), it provides an excellent culture medium. Under normal conditions, the act of completely and repeatedly emptying the bladder flushes away any organisms before they have an opportunity to multiply and invade surrounding tissue. Baths and fluid intake are factors in the development of UTIs, but aren't the most important. There's an increased incidence of UTI in uncircumcised infants under 1 year but not after that age.

CN: Physiological integrity; CNS: Reduction of risk potential; CL: Application

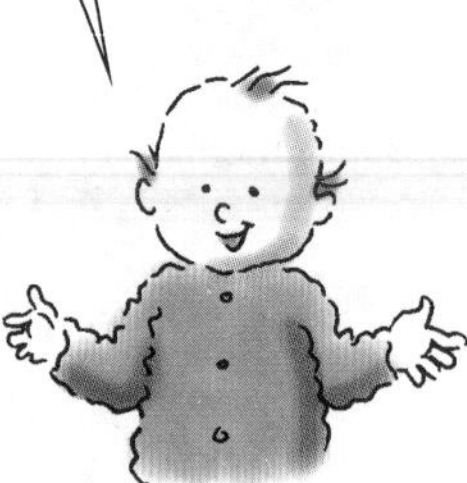

If I'm not eating, something must be wrong!

71. When evaluating infants and young toddlers for signs of urinary tract infections (UTIs), a nurse should know that which symptom would be most common?

1. Abdominal pain
2. Feeding problems
3. Frequency
4. Urgency

71. 2. In infants and children less than 2 years old, the signs are characteristically nonspecific and feeding problems are usually the first indication. Symptoms more nearly resemble GI tract disorders. Abdominal pain, urgency, and frequency are signs that would be observed in the older child with a UTI.

CN: Physiological integrity; CNS: Physiological adaptation; CL: Application

72. When obtaining a urine specimen for culture and sensitivity, a nurse should understand that which method of collection is best?

1. Bagged urine specimen
2. Clean-catch urine specimen
3. First-voided urine specimen
4. Catheterized urine specimen

72. 4. The most accurate tests of bacterial content are suprapubic aspiration (for children less than 2 years old) and properly performed bladder catheterization. The other methods of obtaining a specimen have a high incidence of contamination not related to infection.

CN: Physiological integrity; CNS: Basic care and comfort; CL: Application

CN: Client needs category CNS: Client needs subcategory CL: Cognitive level

73. After collecting a urine specimen, which action by a nurse is the most appropriate?

1. Taking the specimen to the laboratory immediately
2. Sending the specimen to the laboratory on the scheduled run
3. Taking the specimen to the laboratory during the nurse's next break
4. Keeping the specimen in the refrigerator until it can be taken to the laboratory

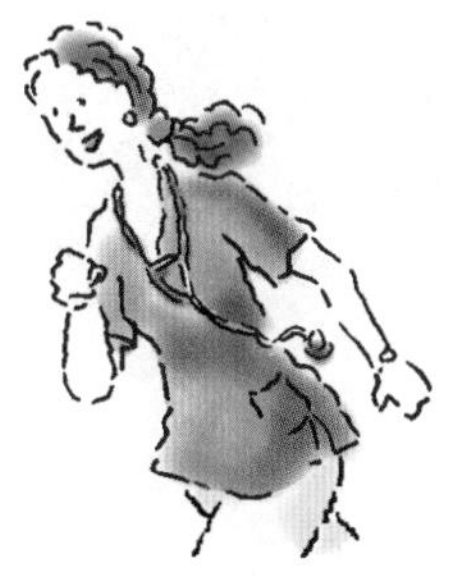

This question calls for immediate action.

73. 1. Care of urine specimens obtained for culture is an important nursing aspect related to diagnosis. Specimens should be taken to the laboratory for culture immediately. If the culture is delayed, the specimen can be placed in the refrigerator, but storage can result in a loss of formed elements, such as blood cells and casts.

CN: Physiological integrity; CNS: Basic care and comfort; CL: Application

74. When teaching parents of a child with a urinary tract infection (UTI) about fluid intake, which statement by a parent would indicate the need for further teaching?

1. "I should encourage my child to drink about 50 ml per pound of body weight daily."
2. "Clear liquids should be the primary liquids that my child should drink."
3. "I should offer my child carbonated beverages about every 2 hours."
4. "My child should avoid drinking caffeinated beverages."

74. 3. Caffeinated or carbonated beverages are avoided because of their potentially irritating effect on the bladder mucosa. Adequate fluid intake is always indicated during an acute UTI. It is recommended that a person drink approximately 50 ml/lb of body weight daily. The client should primarily drink clear liquids.

CN: Physiological integrity; CNS: Basic care and comfort; CL: Analysis

75. Which treatment should a nurse anticipate in a child who has a history of recurrent urinary tract infections (UTIs)?

1. Frequent catheterizations
2. Prophylactic antibiotics
3. Limited activities
4. Surgical intervention

75. 2. Children who experience recurrent UTIs may require antibiotic therapy for months or years. Recurrent UTIs would be investigated for anatomic abnormalities and surgical intervention may be indicated, but the client would also be placed on antibiotics before the tests. The child's activities aren't limited, and frequent catheterization predisposes a child to infection.

CN: Physiological integrity; CNS: Pharmacological and parenteral therapies; CL: Application

76. When teaching parents about giving medications to children for recurrent urinary tract infections (UTIs), which instruction should be included?

1. The medication should be given first thing in the morning.
2. The medication should be given right before bedtime.
3. The medication is generally given four times a day.
4. It doesn't matter when the medication is given.

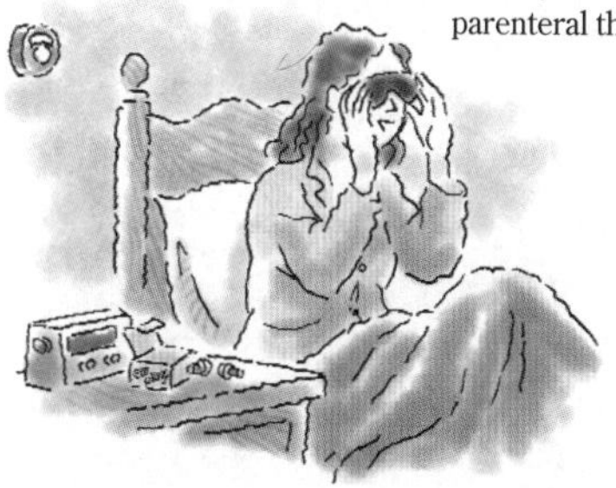

Why do I feel like I'm forgetting something?

76. 2. Medication is commonly administered once a day, and the client and parents are advised to give the antibiotic before sleep because this represents the longest period without voiding.

CN: Physiological integrity; CNS: Pharmacological and parenteral therapies; CL: Application

77. The nurse is providing education to a group of patients about urinary tract infections (UTIs). The nurse knows that teaching has been effective when the patients state that which situation has the greatest impact on the potential for progressive renal injury after UTIs?

1. A school-age child who must get permission to go to the bathroom
2. An adolescent female who has started menstruation
3. Children who compete in competitive sports
4. Young infants and toddlers

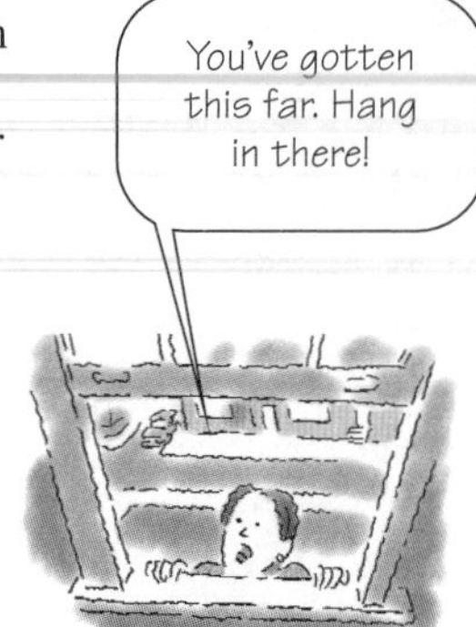

You've gotten this far. Hang in there!

77. 4. The hazard of progressive renal injury is greatest when infection occurs in young children, especially those under 2 years old. The first two options might lead to a simple UTI that would need to be treated. Competitive sports have no bearing on a UTI.

CN: Safe, effective care environment; CNS: Safety and infection control; CL: Application

78. Which statement should a nurse make to help parents understand the recovery period after a child has had surgery to remove a Wilms' tumor?

1. "Children will easily lie in bed and restrict their activities."
2. "Recovery is usually fast in spite of the abdominal incision."
3. "Recovery usually takes a great deal of time because of the large incision."
4. "Parents need to perform activities of daily living for about 2 weeks after surgery."

78. 2. Children generally recover very quickly from surgery to remove a Wilms' tumor, even though they may have a large abdominal incision. Children like to get back into the normalcy of being a child, which is through play. Parents need to encourage their children to do as much for themselves as possible, although some regression is expected.

CN: Psychosocial integrity; CNS: None; CL: Analysis

79. When teaching parents about administering co-trimoxazole (Septra) to a child for treatment of a urinary tract infection (UTI), the nurse should include which instruction?

1. Give the medication with food.
2. Give the medication with water.
3. Give the medication with a cola beverage.
4. Give the medication 2 hours after a meal.

79. 2. When giving co-trimoxazole, the medication should be administered with a full glass of water on an empty stomach. If nausea and vomiting occur, giving the drug with food may decrease gastric distress. Carbonated beverages should be avoided because they irritate the bladder.

CN: Physiological integrity; CNS: Pharmacological and parenteral therapies; CL: Application

80. The nurse is questioned by a student nurse about the incidence of Wilms' tumor. Which response by the nurse is the most accurate?

1. Peak incidence occurs at 10 years of age.
2. It's the least common type of renal cancer.
3. It's the most common type of renal cancer.
4. It has a decreased incidence among siblings.

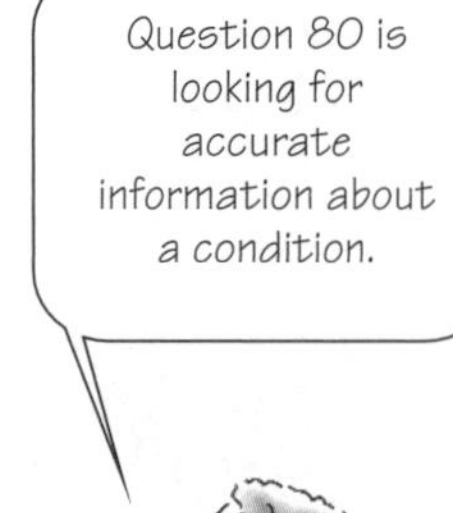

Question 80 is looking for accurate information about a condition.

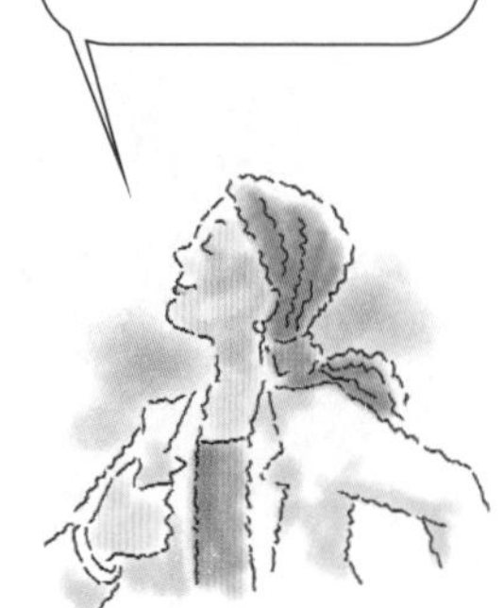

80. 3. Wilms' tumor is the most frequent intra-abdominal tumor of childhood and the most common type of renal cancer. The peak incidence is 3 years, and there's an increased incidence among siblings and identical twins.

CN: Health promotion and maintenance; CNS: None; CL: Application

81. Which presenting sign is most common with Wilms' tumor?

1. Pain in the abdomen
2. Fever greater than 104° F (40° C)
3. Decreased blood pressure
4. Swelling within the abdomen

81. 4. The most common presenting sign is a swelling or mass within the abdomen. The mass is characteristically firm, nontender, confined to one side, and deep within the flank. A high fever isn't a presenting sign for Wilms' tumor. Blood pressure is characteristically increased, not decreased.

CN: Health promotion and maintenance; CNS: None; CL: Application

82. When a nurse is explaining the diagnosis of Wilms' tumor to parents, which statement by a parent would indicate the need for further teaching?

1. "Wilms' tumor usually involves both kidneys."
2. "Wilms' tumor occurs slightly more commonly in the left kidney."
3. "Wilms' tumor is staged during surgery for treatment planning."
4. "Wilms' tumor stays encapsulated for an extended period of time."

82. 1. Wilms' tumor usually involves only one kidney and is usually staged during surgery so that an effective course of treatment can be established. Wilms' tumor has a slightly higher occurrence in the left kidney, and it stays encapsulated for an extended period of time.

CN: Health promotion and maintenance; CNS: None; CL: Application

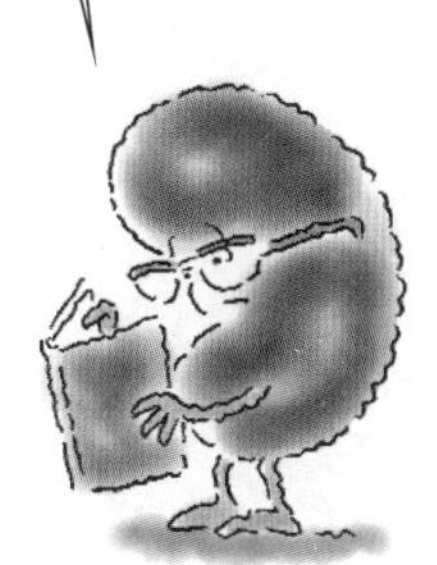

Let me see what I can learn about Wilms' tumor.

83. A parent asks a nurse about the prognosis of her child diagnosed with Wilms' tumor. The nurse should base her response on which factor?

1. Usually children with Wilms' tumor need only surgical intervention.
2. Survival rates for Wilms' tumor are the lowest among childhood cancers.
3. Survival rates for Wilms' tumor are the highest among childhood cancers.
4. Children with localized tumor have only a 30% chance of cure with multimodal therapy.

83. 3. Survival rates for Wilms' tumor are the highest among childhood cancers. Usually children with Wilms' tumor who have stage I or II localized tumor have a 90% chance of cure with multimodal therapy.

CN: Health promotion and maintenance; CNS: None; CL: Application

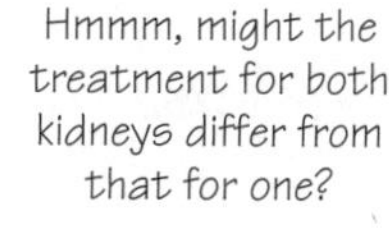

84. If <u>both kidneys</u> are involved in a child with Wilms' tumor, the nurse should understand that treatment prior to surgery might include which method?

1. Peritoneal dialysis
2. Abdominal gavage
3. Radiation and chemotherapy
4. Antibiotics and I.V. fluid therapy

84. 3. If both kidneys are involved, the child may be treated with radiation therapy or chemotherapy preoperatively to shrink the tumor, allowing more conservative therapy. Peritoneal dialysis would be needed only if the kidneys aren't functioning. Abdominal gavage wouldn't be indicated. Antibiotics aren't needed because Wilms' tumor isn't an infection.

CN: Physiological integrity; CNS: Reduction of risk potential; CL: Application

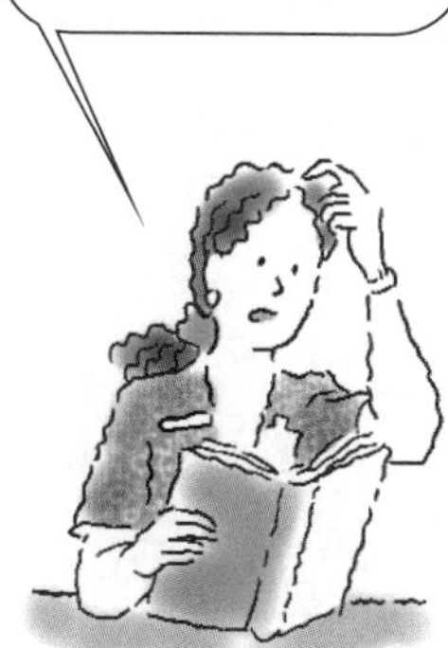

85. When caring for the child with Wilms' tumor preoperatively, which nursing intervention would be most important?

1. Avoid abdominal palpation.
2. Closely monitor arterial blood gas (ABG) levels.
3. Prepare the child and his family for long-term dialysis.
4. Prepare the child and his family for renal transplantation.

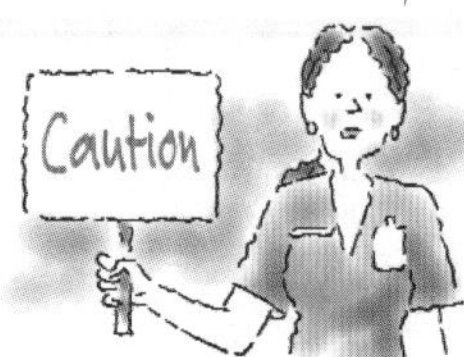

85. 1. After the diagnosis of Wilms' tumor is made, the abdomen shouldn't be palpated. Palpation of the tumor might lead to rupture, which will cause the cancerous cells to spread throughout the abdomen. ABG levels shouldn't be affected. If surgery is successful, there won't be a need for long-term dialysis or renal transplantation.

CN: Physiological integrity; CNS: Reduction of risk potential; CL: Application

86. A child is scheduled for surgery to remove a Wilms' tumor from one kidney. The parents ask the nurse what treatment, if any, they should expect after their child recovers from surgery. Which response would be most accurate?

1. "Chemotherapy may be necessary."
2. "Kidney transplant is indicated eventually."
3. "No additional treatments are usually necessary."
4. "Chemotherapy with or without radiation therapy is indicated."

86. 4. Because radiation therapy and chemotherapy are usually begun immediately after surgery, parents need an explanation of what to expect, such as major benefits and adverse effects. Kidney transplant isn't usually necessary.

CN: Physiological integrity; CNS: Physiological adaptation; CL: Application

87. When assessing the abdomen of a child with a potential diagnosis of Wilms' tumor, which factor might lead to a different diagnosis?

1. The mass is on one side of the abdomen.
2. There is a mass on both sides of the abdomen.
3. The mass crosses the midline of the abdomen.
4. There's no pain associated with palpation of the mass.

87. 3. When an abdominal mass crosses the midline, a neuroblastoma should be suspected—not a Wilms' tumor. A Wilms' tumor arises off the kidneys and can be on one side or both sides of the abdomen but doesn't cross the midline. Pain isn't usually associated with Wilms' tumor.

CN: Health promotion and maintenance; CNS: None; CL: Analysis

88. A parent of a child with Wilms' tumor asks the nurse about surgery. Which statement concerning the nature of surgery for Wilms' tumor is the most accurate?

1. Surgery isn't indicated in children with Wilms' tumor.
2. Surgery is usually performed within 24 to 48 hours of admission.
3. Surgery is the least favorable therapy for the treatment of Wilms' tumor.
4. Surgery will be delayed until the client's overall health status improves.

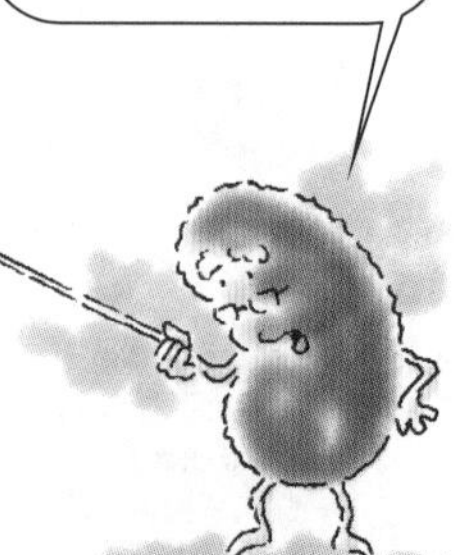

Do you know the preferred treatment for Wilms' tumor?

88. 2. Surgery is the preferred treatment and is scheduled as soon as possible after confirmation of a renal mass, usually within 24 to 48 hours of admission, to be sure the encapsulated tumor remains intact.

CN: Physiological integrity; CNS: Physiological adaptation; CL: Application

89. A 3-year-old child has had surgery to remove a Wilms' tumor. Which action should the nurse take first when the mother asks for pain medication for the child?

1. Get the pain medication ready for administration.
2. Assess the client's pain using a pain scale of 1 to 10.
3. Assess the client's pain using a smiley face pain scale.
4. Check for the last time pain medication was administered.

90. A child has been diagnosed with Wilms' tumor. Because of the parents' religious beliefs, they choose not to treat the child. Which statement by the nurse indicates the need for further discussion?

1. "I know this is a lot of information in a short period of time."
2. "I don't think parents have the legal right to make these kinds of decisions."
3. "These parents just don't understand how easily treated a Wilms' tumor is."
4. "I think the parents are in shock."

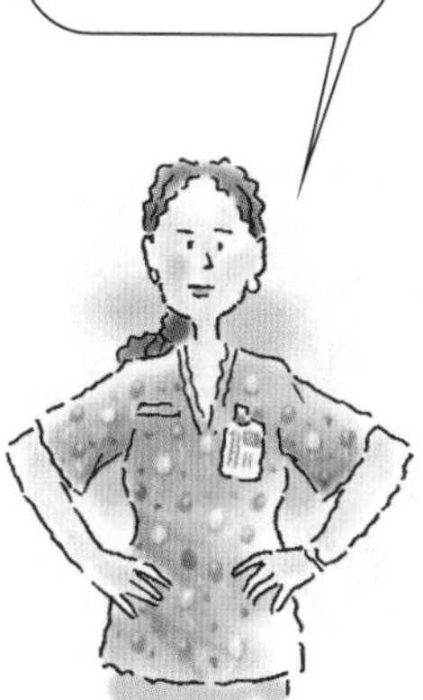
Remember to respect the parents' religious beliefs.

91. A child with a Wilms' tumor has had surgery to remove a kidney and has received chemotherapy. The nurse should include which instruction at discharge?

1. Avoid contact sports.
2. Decrease fluid intake.
3. Decrease sodium intake.
4. Avoid contact with other children.

92. When caring for a child after removal of a Wilms' tumor, which assessment finding would indicate the need to notify the physician?

1. Fever of 101° F (38.3° C)
2. Absence of bowel sounds
3. Slight congestion in the lungs
4. Complaints of pain when moving

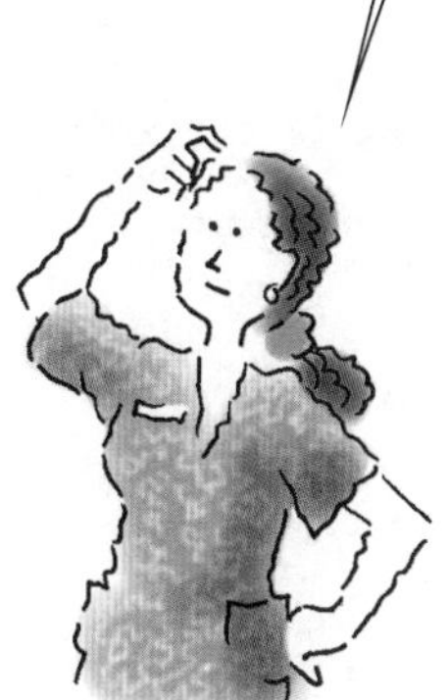
Which finding suggests the need to notify the physician?

89. 3. The first action of the nurse should be to assess the client for pain. A 3-year-old child is too young to use a pain scale from 1 to 10 but can easily use the smiley face pain scale. After assessing the pain, the nurse should then investigate the time the pain medication was last given and administer the medication accordingly.
CN: Physiological integrity; CNS: Pharmacological and parenteral therapies; CL: Application

90. 2. Parents *do* have the legal right to make decisions regarding the health issues for their child. Religion plays an important role in many people's lives, and decisions about surgery and treatment for cancer are sometimes made that scientifically don't make sense to the health care provider. The parents are probably in a state of shock because a lot of information has been given and this is a cancer that requires decisions to be made quickly, especially surgical intervention.
CN: Safe, effective care environment; CNS: Management of care; CL: Analysis

91. 1. Because the child is left with only one kidney, certain precautions, such as avoiding contact sports, are recommended to prevent injury to the remaining kidney. Decreasing fluid intake wouldn't be indicated; fluid intake is essential for renal function. The child's sodium intake shouldn't be reduced. Avoiding other children is unnecessary, will make the child feel self-conscious, and may lead to regressive behavior.
CN: Health promotion and maintenance; CNS: None; CL: Application

92. 2. This child is at risk for intestinal obstruction. GI abnormalities require notification of the physician. A slight fever following surgery isn't uncommon, nor are slight congestion in the lungs and complaints of pain.
CN: Physiological integrity; CNS: Reduction of risk potential; CL: Application

93. Because surgery is performed for a Wilms' tumor within 24 to 48 hours of admission, a nurse must prepare a family and child quickly for procedures. Which statement should guide the nurse in her preparation of the family?

1. Because the parents are in a state of shock, they don't need explanations.
2. Explanations should be kept simple and should be repeated often.
3. Scientific terminology should be used with drawings and models.
4. The play therapist is the best person to prepare this family.

93. 2. Decisions are made rapidly after the diagnosis of Wilms' tumor is made. Parents are typically in shock at this time. Explanations should be kept simple and repeated often. The play therapist might become involved with this family, especially postoperatively. There's generally no time to prepare the play therapist for the role of educator in this situation.

CN: Health promotion and maintenance; CNS: None; CL: Application

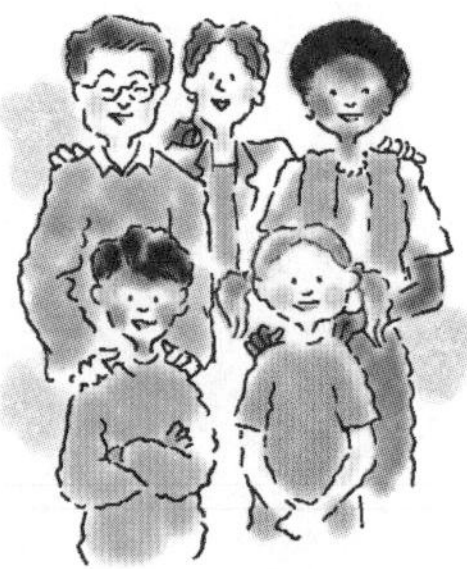

Be sensitive to the needs of a client's family when delivering bad news.

94. Which statement made by the physician to the parents of a child who has had a Wilms' tumor removed would be the most difficult for the parents to hear and might require nursing intervention?

1. "We will start chemotherapy within the next 24 to 48 hours."
2. "The tumor was a stage IV, which indicates other organ involvement."
3. "We were able to remove all of the tumor, but we had to take the kidney as well."
4. "The incision is long, and the dressing will need to be changed daily."

94. 2. Surgery is an anxiety-producing event to parents. It also marks the confirmation of the stage of the tumor. A stage IV tumor has a poor prognosis because other organs are involved. This statement, above all others, would be the most difficult for the parents to hear.

CN: Psychosocial integrity; CNS: None; CL: Analysis

95. In providing psychosocial care to a 6-year-old child who has had abdominal surgery for Wilms' tumor, which activity would be the most appropriate?

1. Allowing the child to watch a 2-hour movie without interruptions
2. Giving the child a puzzle with five pieces to encourage him to move while in bed
3. Telling the child that you can give him enough medication so that he feels no pain
4. Providing the child with puppets and supplies and asking him to draw how he feels

95. 4. A movie is a good diversion, but giving puppets and encouraging the child to draw his feelings is a better outlet. A puzzle with only five pieces is too basic for a 6-year-old child and wouldn't hold his interest. You probably can't give enough pain medication so that a person who has had surgery will feel no pain.

CN: Psychosocial integrity; CNS: None; CL: Application

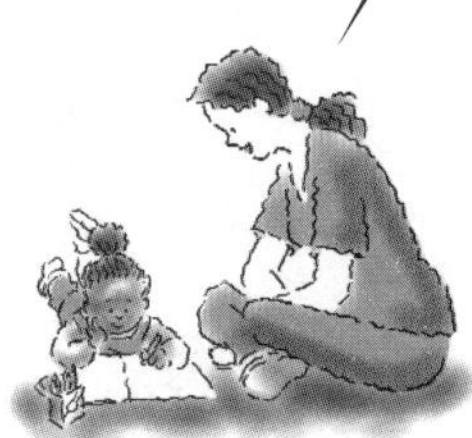

Can you show me how you feel?

96. The nurse is teaching the parents of a child with Wilms' tumor about staging. The nurse knows the teaching has been effective when the parents respond that staging helps determine which parameter?

1. Size of tumor
2. Level of treatment
3. Length of incision
4. Amount of anesthesia

96. 2. Staging of the tumor helps to determine the level of treatment because it provides information about the level of involvement. The other choices are insignificant in staging of the tumor.

CN: Health promotion and maintenance; CNS: None; CL: Application

97. A nurse is educating parents about Wilms' tumor. Which statement made by a parent would indicate the need for further teaching?

1. "My child could have inherited this disease."
2. "Wilms' tumor can be associated with other congenital anomalies."
3. "This disease could have been a result of trauma to the baby in utero."
4. "There's no method of identification of gene carriers of Wilms' tumor."

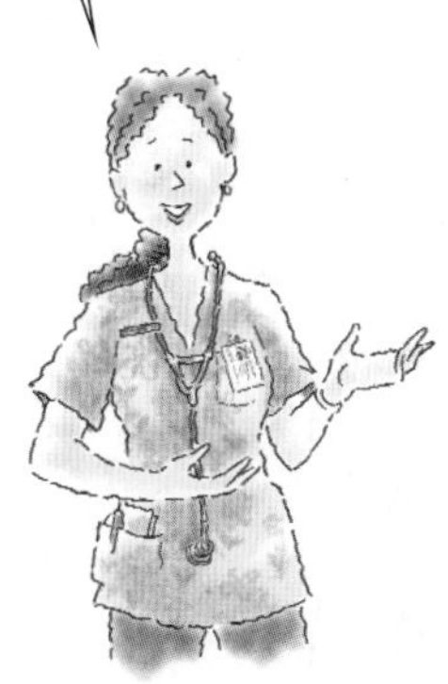

Further teaching is so important that you'll see similar questions more than once.

97. 3. Wilms' tumor isn't a result of trauma to the fetus in utero. Wilms' tumor can be genetically inherited and is associated with other congenital anomalies. However, there's no method for identifying gene carriers of Wilms' tumor at this time.
CN: Health promotion and maintenance; CNS: None; CL: Application

98. Which assessment finding will aid in the differentiation of a Wilms' tumor from the liver when doing an abdominal assessment?

1. The liver moves with respiration.
2. The liver is a more encapsulated organ.
3. A Wilms' tumor isn't as deep as the liver.
4. A Wilms' tumor usually isn't well defined.

98. 1. It's difficult to distinguish a Wilms' tumor from the liver if the tumor is on the right side of the body. One difference is that the liver will move with respirations and a Wilms' tumor won't. A Wilms' tumor is deep in the abdomen and is usually well defined and encapsulated.
CN: Health promotion and maintenance; CNS: None; CL: Application

99. Which action by a nurse would be appropriate to take for a child diagnosed with a Wilms' tumor?

1. Take blood pressure in the right arm only.
2. Offer only clear liquids at room temperature.
3. Post a sign over the bed that reads, "Don't palpate abdomen."
4. Allow the child to participate in group activities in the playroom.

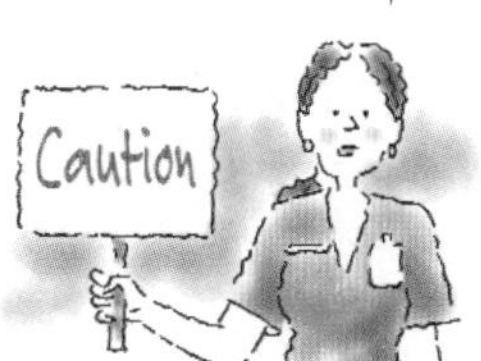

Sometimes you just have to spell it out.
Caution

99. 3. To reinforce the need for caution, it may be necessary to post a sign over the bed that reads, "Don't palpate abdomen." The blood pressure could be taken in any extremity; prior to surgery, there are usually no dietary restrictions. Careful bathing and handling are also important in preventing trauma to the tumor site; thus, group activities should be discouraged.
CN: Health promotion and maintenance; CNS: None; CL: Application

100. Which is the most important instruction for a nurse to tell the parent of a 24-month-old child when the parent asks about starting toilet-training?

1. The child must be developmentally ready.
2. Use a consistent approach.
3. Maintain a positive attitude.
4. Start at the same age siblings were trained.

100. 1. Toilet-training should begin when the child is developmentally ready. After training is started, a consistent approach and a positive attitude should be used. Each child's readiness for toilet-training is individual and the child shouldn't be compared to his siblings.
CN: Health promotion and maintenance; CNS: None; CL: Application

101. A previously toilet-trained 4-year-old child begins wetting the bed after being hospitalized. Which statement should a nurse tell the parents?

1. "Children commonly show regressive behavior when hospitalized."
2. "Your child is just acting out to make you feel bad."
3. "Sometimes 4-year-olds still have accidents."
4. "Let's try cutting back on fluids and see whether that helps."

101. 1. Young children may exhibit regressive behaviors when they're under stress, such as occurs with hospitalization. The child may be acting out, but more likely this is not voluntary bed-wetting. Four-year-olds should be fully toilet-trained. Restricting fluids as a first step in a hospitalized child isn't appropriate; other causes of bed-wetting should be considered first.

CN: Physiological integrity; CNS: None; CL: Application

102. A preschooler is scheduled to have a Wilms' tumor removed. Identify the area of the urinary system where this type of tumor is located.

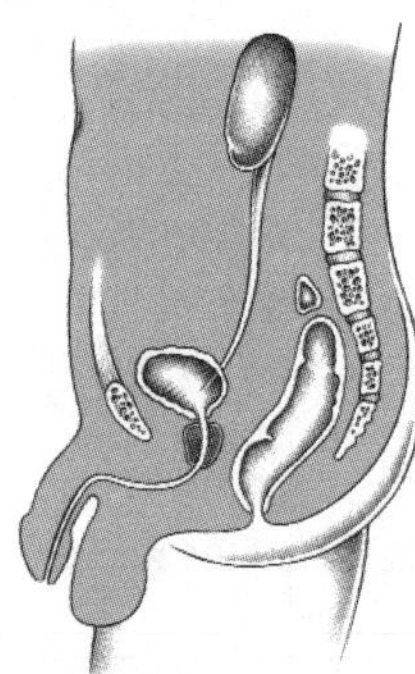

102. Wilms' tumor, also known as *nephroblastoma*, is a tumor located in the kidney. It's most commonly found in children ages 2 to 4.

CN: Physiological integrity; CNS: Physiological adaptation; CL: Application

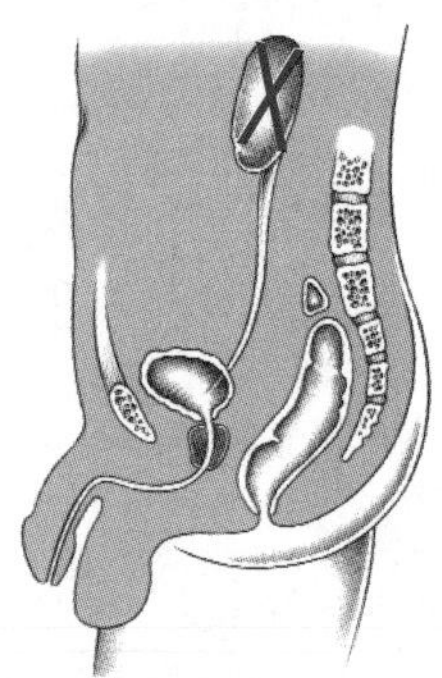

103. A 3-year-old child is to receive 500 ml of dextrose 5% in normal saline solution over 8 hours. At what rate (in ml/hour) should the nurse set the infusion pump? Round your answer to a whole number.

________________ ml/hour

103. 63. To calculate the rate per hour for the infusion, the nurse should divide 500 ml by 8 hours: 500 ml ÷ 8 hours = 62.5 ml/hour, which should be rounded to 63.

CN: Physiological integrity; CNS: Pharmacological and parenteral therapies; CL: Application

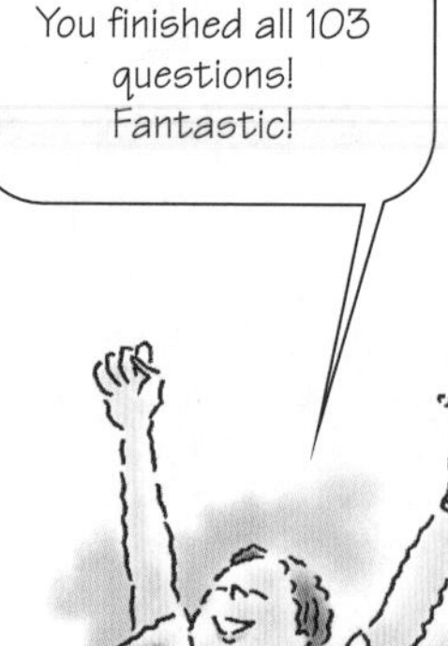
Congratulations! You finished all 103 questions! Fantastic!

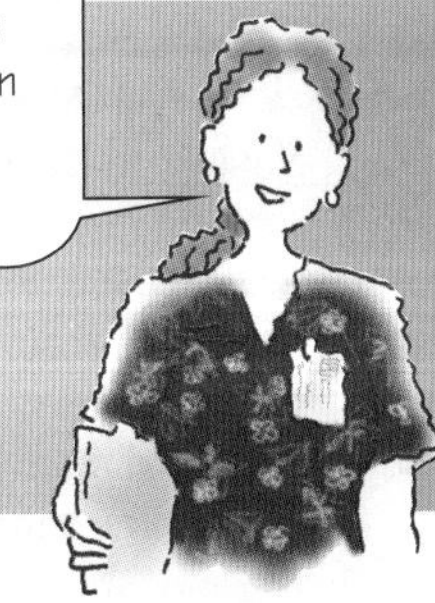

Chapter 35 Integumentary disorders

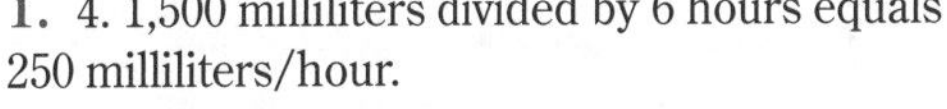

1. A 12-year-old child with burns over 40% of his body is ordered to receive 1,500 ml of I.V. fluid over 6 hours. At what rate should the nurse set the infusion pump?

1. 125 ml/hour
2. 150 ml/hour
3. 175 ml/hour
4. 250 ml/hour

1. 4. 1,500 milliliters divided by 6 hours equals 250 milliliters/hour.

CN: Physiological integrity; CNS: Pharmacological and parenteral therapies; CL: Application

2. Providing adequate nutrition is essential for a burn client. Which statement best describes the nutritional needs of a child who has burns?

1. A child needs 100 cal/kg during hospitalization.
2. The hypermetabolic state after a burn injury leads to poor healing.
3. Caloric needs can be lowered by controlling environmental temperature.
4. Maintaining a hypermetabolic rate will lower the child's risk for infection.

2. 2. A burn injury causes a hypermetabolic state leading to protein and lipid catabolism, which affects wound healing. Caloric intake should be 1½ to 2 times the basal metabolic rate, with a minimum of 1.5 to 2 g/kg of body weight of protein daily. Keeping the temperature within a normal range lets the body function efficiently and use calories for healing and normal physiological processes. If the temperature is too warm or cold, energy must be used for warming or cooling, taking energy away from tissue repair. High metabolic rates increase the risk for infection.

CN: Physiological integrity; CNS: Basic care and comfort; CL: Analysis

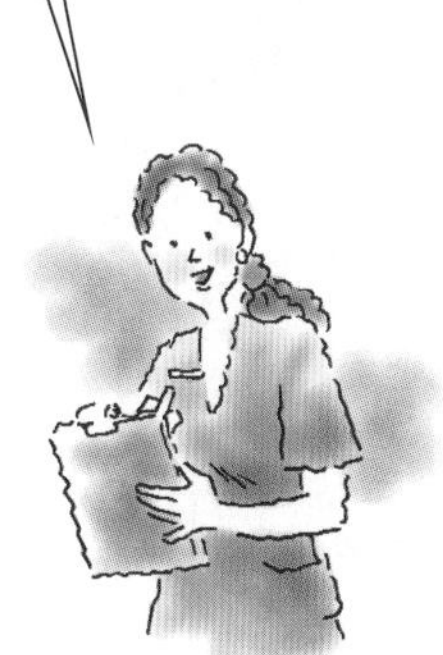

Measuring burns in children is different than measuring burns in adults.

3. A 1-year-old child is treated in the clinic for a burn to the anterior surface of the left hand. Which way to measure burn size would be accurate for this child?

1. The rule of nines
2. Percentage based on the child's weight
3. The child's hand equals 1.25% of the child's body surface area
4. Percentage can't be determined without knowing the type of burn

3. 3. The anterior surface of a child's hand is equal to 1.25% of that child's body surface. The rule of nines is used for children aged 14 years and older. The child's weight is important to calculate fluid replacement for extensive burns, not to estimate total body surface area. Burn type doesn't determine the percentage of body surface involved.

CN: Physiological integrity; CNS: Physiological adaptation; CL: Application

CN: Client needs category CNS: Client needs subcategory CL: Cognitive level

4. An 18-month-old child is admitted to the hospital for full-thickness burns to the anterior chest. The mother asks how the burn will heal. Which statement is accurate about healing for full-thickness burns?

1. Surgical closure and grafting are usually needed.
2. Healing takes 10 to 12 days, with little or no scarring.
3. Pigment in a black client will return to the injured area.
4. Healing can take up to 6 weeks, with a high incidence of scarring.

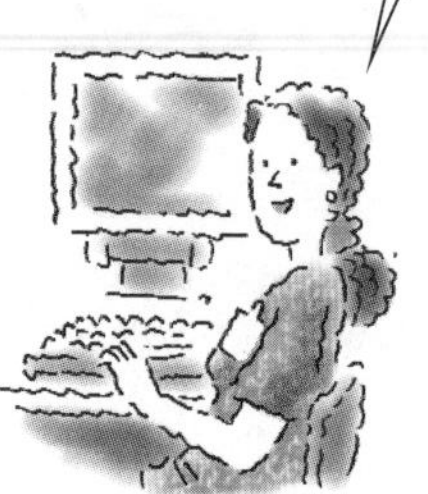

Do you remember what you learned about full-thickness burns?

4. 1. Full-thickness burns usually need surgical closure and grafting for complete healing. Healing in 10 to 12 days with little or no scarring is associated with superficial partial-thickness burns. With superficial partial-thickness burns, pigment is expected to return to the injured area after healing. Deep partial-thickness burns heal in 6 weeks, with scarring.

CN: Physiological integrity; CNS: Physiological adaptation; CL: Analysis

5. A 9-year-old child is admitted to the hospital with deep partial-thickness burns to 25% of his body. Which assessment finding would the nurse associate with a deep partial-thickness burn?

1. Erythema and pain
2. Minimal damage to the epidermis
3. Necrosis through all layers of skin
4. Tissue necrosis through most of the dermis

5. 4. A client with a deep partial-thickness burn will have tissue necrosis to the epidermis and dermis layers. Erythema and pain are characteristic of superficial injury. With deep burns, the nerve fibers are destroyed and the client won't feel pain in the affected area. Superficial burns are characteristic of slight epidermal damage. Necrosis through all skin layers is seen with full-thickness injuries.

CN: Physiological integrity; CNS: Physiological adaptation; CL: Application

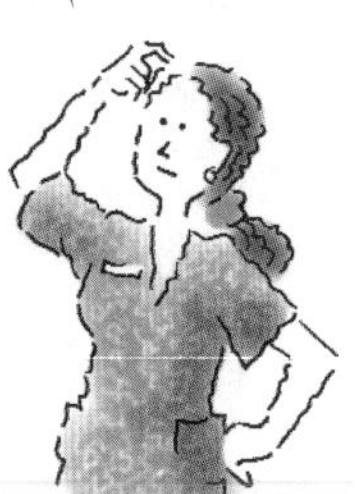

The word circumferential is a clue, right?

6. A 4-year-old child is admitted to the burn unit with a circumferential burn to the left forearm. Which finding should be reported to the physician?

1. Numbness of fingers
2. +2 radial and ulnar pulses
3. Full range of motion (ROM) and no pain
4. Bilateral capillary refill less then 2 seconds

6. 1. Circumferential burns can compromise blood flow to an extremity, causing numbness. +2 Pulses indicate normal circulation. Absence of pain and full ROM implies good tissue oxygenation from intact circulation. Capillary refill less then 2 seconds indicates a normal vascular blood flow.

CN: Physiological integrity; CNS: Physiological adaptation; CL: Application

7. Which fact should be given to the parents of a child with fifth disease?

1. There is a possible reappearance of the rash for up to 1 week.
2. Isolation of high-risk contacts should be avoided for 4 to 10 days.
3. Pregnant clients are at risk for fetal death if infected with fifth disease.
4. Children with fifth disease are contagious only while the rash is present.

7. 3. There's a 3% to 5% risk for fetal death from hydrops fetalis if a pregnant client is exposed during the first trimester. The cutaneous eruption of fifth disease can reappear for up to 4 months. The child should be isolated from pregnant women, immunocompromised clients, and clients with chronic anemia for up to 2 weeks. A child with fifth disease is contagious during the first stage, when symptoms of headache, body aches, fever, and chills are present, not after the rash.

CN: Safe, effective care environment; CNS: Safety and infection control; CL: Application

8. A mother is concerned that her 3-year-old child has been exposed to erythema infectiosum (fifth disease). Which characteristic finding would the nurse incorporate in the response to the mother?

1. A fine, erythematous rash with a sandpaper-like texture
2. Intense redness of both cheeks that may spread to the extremities
3. Low-grade fever, followed by vesicular lesions of the trunk, face, and scalp
4. Three- to 5-day history of sustained fever, followed by a diffuse erythematous maculopapular rash

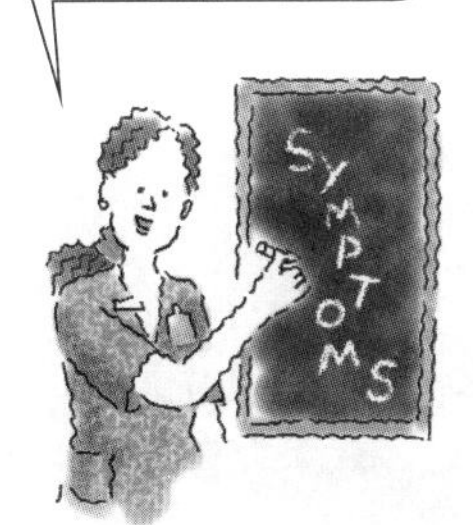
Different symptoms indicate different diagnoses.
SYMPTOMS

8. 2. The classic symptoms of erythema infectiosum begin with intense redness of both cheeks. An erythematous rash with a sandpaper-like texture is associated with scarlet fever, which is a bacterial infection. Children with varicella typically have vesicular lesions of the trunk, face, and scalp after a low-grade fever. An erythematous rash after a fever is characteristic of roseola.

CN: Physiological integrity; CNS: Physiological adaptation; CL: Application

9. A family that recently went camping brings their child to the clinic with a complaint of a rash after a tick bite. Lyme disease is suspected. Which assessment finding would be seen with Lyme disease?

1. Erythematous rash surrounding a necrotic lesion
2. Bright rash with red outer border circling the bite site
3. Onset of a diffuse rash over the entire body 2 months after exposure
4. A linear rash of papules and vesicles that occur 1 to 3 days after exposure

9. 2. A bull's eye rash is a classic symptom of Lyme disease. Necrotic, painful rashes are associated with the bite of a brown recluse spider. In Lyme disease, the rash is located primarily at the site of the bite. A linear, papular, vesicular rash indicates exposure to the leaves of poison ivy.

CN: Physiological integrity; CNS: Physiological adaptation; CL: Application

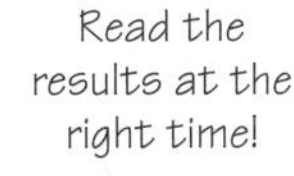
Read the results at the right time!

10. A Mantoux test is ordered for a 6-year-old child. Which action should the nurse take?

1. Read results within 24 hours.
2. Read results 48 to 72 hours later.
3. Use the large muscle of the upper leg.
4. Massage the site to increase absorption.

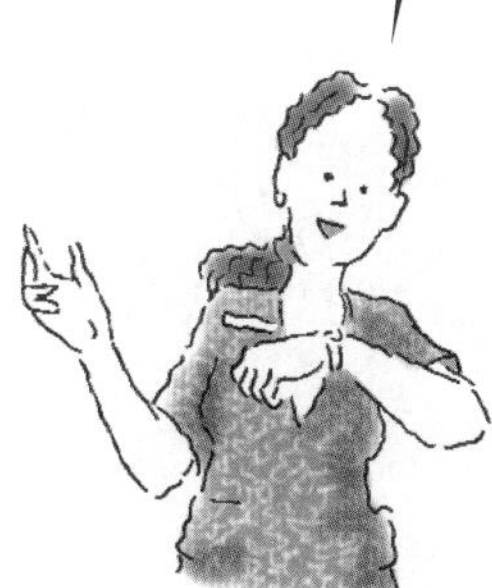

10. 2. The test should be read 48 to 72 hours after placement by measuring the diameter of the induration that develops at the site. The purified protein derivative is injected intradermally on the volar surface of the forearm. Massaging the site could cause leakage from the injection site.

CN: Physiological integrity; CNS: Reduction of risk potential; CL: Application

11. The nurse is teaching the parents of a child with Kawasaki disease. Which statement by the nurse about this condition is the most accurate?

1. "It's a highly contagious condition that requires isolation."
2. "It's an afebrile condition with cardiac involvement."
3. "It usually occurs in children older than 5 years."
4. "Prolonged fever, with peeling of the fingers and toes, is the initial symptom."

11. 4. To be diagnosed with Kawasaki syndrome, the child must have a fever for 5 days or more, plus four of the following five symptoms: bilateral conjunctivitis, changes in the oral mucosa, dermatitis of the peripheral extremities, rash, and lymphadenopathy. The syndrome isn't contagious and doesn't require isolation. Kawasaki syndrome is more likely to occur in children aged younger than 5 years.

CN: Physiological integrity; CNS: Physiological adaptation; CL: Application

12. A 22-lb child is diagnosed with Kawasaki syndrome and started on gamma globulin therapy. The physician orders an I.V. infusion of gamma globulin, 2 g/kg, to run over 12 hours. Which dose is correct?

1. 11 g
2. 20 g
3. 22 g
4. 44 g

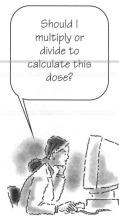

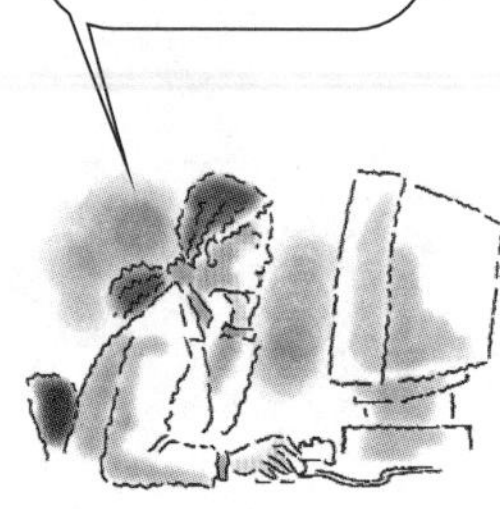

Should I multiply or divide to calculate this dose?

12. 2. First, convert the weight from pounds to kilograms. One kilogram equals 2.2 lb.

Convert the weight using the calculation:

22 (lb) ÷ 2.2 = 10 (kg)

Then, calculate the dose:

2 g × 10 = 20 g

CN: Physiological integrity; CNS: Pharmacological and parenteral therapies; CL: Application

13. A mother is concerned because her child was exposed to varicella in day care. Which statement by the nurse would be the most accurate?

1. "The rash is nonvesicular."
2. "The treatment of choice is aspirin."
3. "Varicella has an incubation period of 5 to 10 days."
4. "A child is no longer contagious once the rash has crusted over."

13. 4. Once every varicella lesion is crusted over, the child is no longer considered contagious. The rash is typically a maculopapular vesicular rash. Use of aspirin has been associated with Reye's syndrome and is contraindicated in varicella. The incubation period is 10 to 20 days.

CN: Physiological integrity; CNS: Physiological adaptation; CL: Application

14. The nurse is discussing with a student nurse the appearance of a rash associated with varicella-zoster virus on a child in the pediatric unit. Which explanation about the rash would be correct?

1. It's diagnostic in the presence of Koplik's spots in the oral mucosa.
2. It's a macular papular rash starting on the scalp and hairline and spreading downward.
3. It's a vesicular macular papular rash that appears abruptly on the trunk, face, and scalp.
4. It appears as yellow ulcers surrounded by red halos on the surface of the hands and feet.

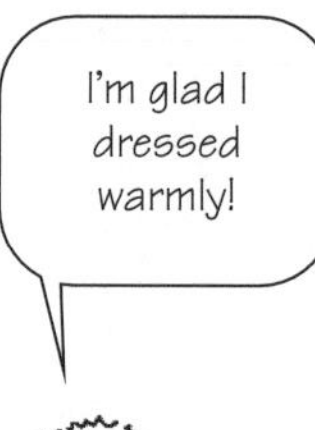

I'm glad I dressed warmly!

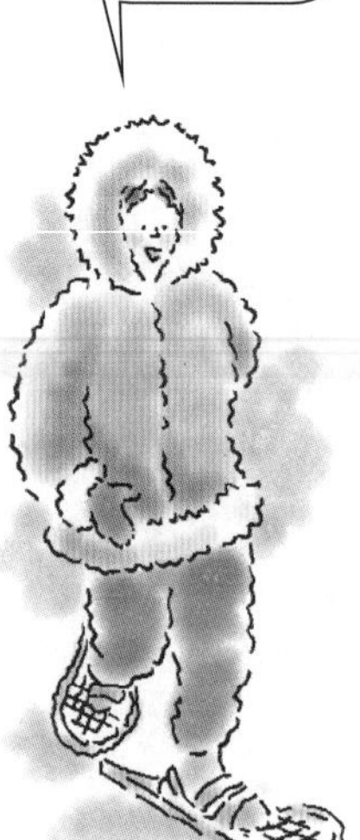

14. 3. Teardrop vesicles on an erythematous base generally begin on the trunk, face, and scalp, with minimal involvement of the extremities. Koplik's spots are diagnostic of rubeola. A descending macular papular rash is characteristic of rubeola. Yellow ulcers of the hands and feet are associated with hand-foot-and-mouth disease caused by the coxsackievirus.

CN: Physiological integrity; CNS: Physiological adaptation; CL: Application

15. A child is brought to the emergency department after an extended period of sledding. Frostbite of the hands is suspected. Which assessment finding should the nurse expect to find?

1. The skin is white.
2. The skin looks deeply flushed and red.
3. The skin is cyanotic.
4. The skin is blistered.

15. 1. Signs and symptoms of frostbite include tingling, numbness, burning sensation, and white skin.

CN: Physiological integrity; CNS: Physiological adaptation; CL: Application

16. A mother brings her child to the physician's office because he complains of pain, redness, and tenderness of the left index finger. The child is diagnosed with a paronychia. Which organism would the nurse suspect to be the most likely cause of this superficial abscess of the cuticle?

1. *Borrelia burgdorferi*
2. *Escherichia coli*
3. *Pseudomonas* species
4. *Staphylococcus* species

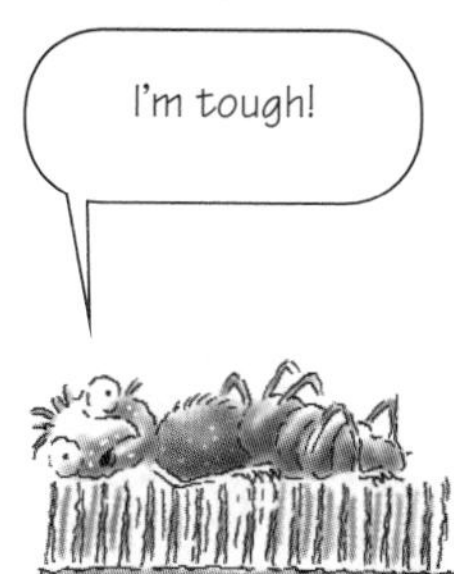
I'm tough!

16. 4. A paronychia is a localized infection of the nail bed caused by either staphylococci or streptococci. *Borrelia burgdorferi* is responsible for Lyme disease. *Escherichia coli* is associated with urinary tract infections. *Pseudomonas* species are associated with ecthyma.
CN: Physiological integrity; CNS: Physiological adaptation; CL: Application

17. Which treatment for paronychia would be the most appropriate?

1. Give warm soaks.
2. Splint and put ice on the affected finger.
3. Allow the infection to resolve without treatment.
4. Admit the child to the hospital for I.V. antibiotic therapy.

17. 1. Giving warm soaks is the treatment of choice for paronychia. Splinting and icing aren't indicated. Untreated, the local abscess can spread beneath the nail bed, called *secondary lymphangitis.* I.V. antibiotic therapy isn't needed if the abscess is kept from spreading.
CN: Physiological integrity; CNS: Physiological adaptation; CL: Analysis

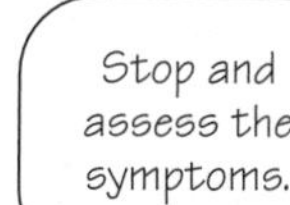
Stop and assess the symptoms.

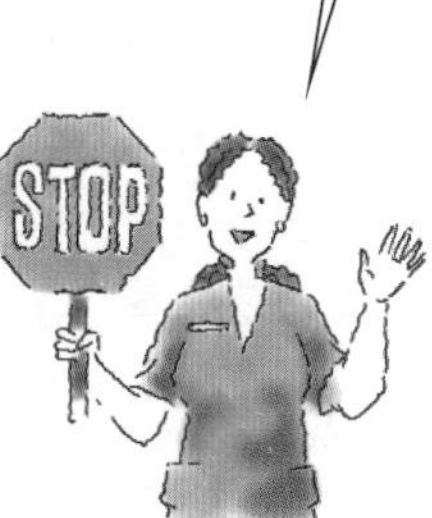
STOP

18. A mother is concerned that her 9-month-old infant has scabies. Which assessment findings are associated with this infestation?

1. Diffuse pruritic wheals
2. Oval white dots stuck to the hair shafts
3. Pain, erythema, and edema with an embedded stinger
4. Pruritic papules, pustules, and linear burrows of the finger and toe webs

18. 4. Pruritic papules, vesicles, and linear burrows are diagnostic for scabies. Diffuse pruritic wheals are associated with an allergic reaction. Nits, seen as white oval dots, are characteristic of head lice. Bites from honeybees are associated with a stinger, pain, and erythema.
CN: Physiological integrity; CNS: Physiological adaptation; CL: Application

19. After treating her 16-month-old child with permethrin (Elimite) for scabies, the mother is concerned the cream didn't work because the child is still scratching. Which explanation or instruction would be correct?

1. Continue the application daily until the rash disappears.
2. Pruritus caused by secondary reactions of the mites can be present for weeks.
3. Stop treatment because the cream is unsafe for children younger than age 2 years.
4. Pruritus caused by permethrin is usually present in children younger than age 5 years.

19. 2. Sensitization of the host is the cause of the intense itching and can last for weeks. Permethrin is the recommended treatment for scabies in infants as young as 2 months. It can safely be repeated after 2 weeks.
CN: Physiological integrity; CNS: Pharmacological and parenteral therapies; CL: Application

20. A mother of a 5-month-old infant is planning a trip to the beach and asks for advice about sunscreen for her child. Which instruction should the nurse give the mother?

1. The sunscreen protection factor (SPF) of the sunscreen should be at least 10.
2. Apply sunscreen to the exposed areas of the skin.
3. Sunscreen shouldn't be applied to infants younger than 6 months of age.
4. Sunscreen needs to be applied heavily only once one half hour before going out in the sun.

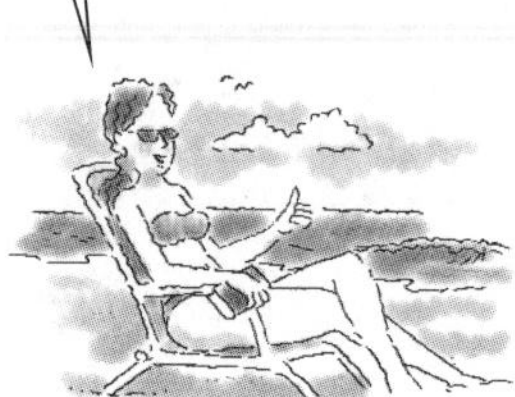

Know the do's and don'ts about sunscreen and its application.

20. 3. Sunscreen isn't recommended for use in infants younger than 6 months of age. These children should be dressed in cool light clothes and kept in the shade. The SPF for children should be 15 or greater. Sunscreen should be applied to all areas of the skin. Sunscreen should be applied evenly throughout the day and each time the child is in the water.

CN: Health promotion and maintenance; CNS: None; CL: Application

21. An infant is being treated with antibiotic therapy for otitis media and develops an erythematous, fine, raised rash in the groin and suprapubic area. Which instruction or explanation will most likely be given to the mother?

1. The infant has candidiasis.
2. Change the brand of diapers.
3. Use an over-the-counter diaper remedy.
4. Stop the antibiotic therapy immediately.

21. 1. Candidiasis, caused by yeast-like fungi, can occur with the use of antibiotics. The treatment for candidiasis is topical nystatin ointment. Changing the brand of diapers or suggesting that the parent use an over-the-counter remedy would be appropriate for treating diaper rash, not candidiasis. Antibiotic therapy shouldn't be stopped.

CN: Physiological integrity; CNS: Physiological adaptation; CL: Analysis

22. The skin in the diaper area of a 6-month-old infant is excoriated and red. Which instructions should the nurse give to the mother?

1. Change the diaper more often.
2. Apply talcum powder with diaper changes.
3. Wash the area vigorously with each diaper change.
4. Decrease the infant's fluid intake to decrease saturating diapers.

22. 1. Simply decreasing the amount of time the skin comes in contact with wet soiled diapers will help heal the irritation. Talc is contraindicated in children because of the risks of inhaling the fine powder. Gentle cleaning of the irritated skin should be encouraged. Infants shouldn't have fluid intake restrictions.

CN: Safe, effective care environment; CNS: Safety and infection control; CL: Application

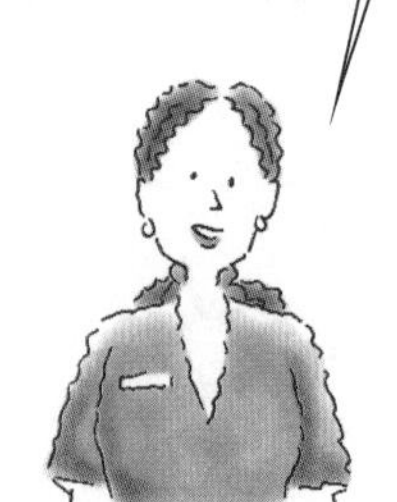

Teaching parents helps keep their children healthy.

23. A 9-year-old child is being discharged from the hospital after severe urticaria caused by an allergy to nuts. Which instruction would be included in discharge teaching for the child's parents?

1. Use emollient lotions and baths.
2. Apply topical steroids to the lesions as needed.
3. Apply over-the-counter products such as diphenhydramine (Benadryl).
4. Instruct the parents and child on how and when to use an epinephrine administration kit (Epi-Pen).

23. 4. Children who have urticaria in response to nuts, seafood, or bee stings should be warned about the possibility of anaphylactic reactions to future exposure. The use of epinephrine pens should be taught to the parents and older children. Other treatment choices, such as diphenhydramine hydrochloride, topical steroids, and emollients, are for the treatment of mild urticaria.

CN: Physiological integrity; CNS: Reduction of risk potential; CL: Application

24. When examining a nursery school-age child, the nurse finds multiple contusions over the body. Child abuse is suspected. Which statement indicates which findings should be documented?

1. Contusions confined to one body area are typically suspicious.
2. All lesions, including location, shape, and color, should be documented.
3. Natural injuries usually have straight linear lines, while injuries from abuse have multiple curved lines.
4. The depth, location, and amount of bleeding that initially occurs is constant, but the sequence of color change is variable.

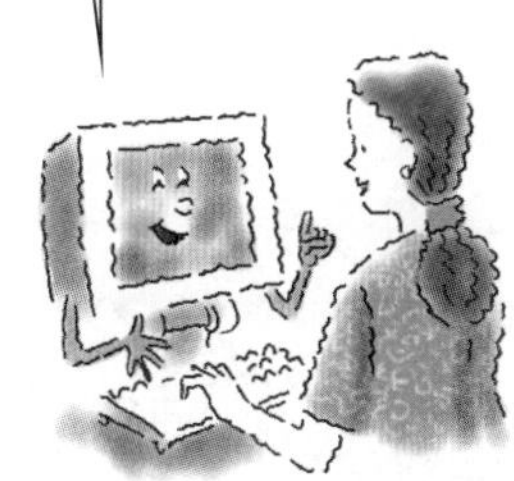

Question 24 already, and you're doing great!

24. 2. An accurate precise examination of all lesions must be properly documented as a legal document. Contusions that result from falls are typically confined to a single body area and are considered a reasonable finding of a child still learning to walk. Injuries from normal falls are usually not linear in nature. The bleeding can cause variations, but the color change is consistent.

CN: Psychosocial integrity; CNS: None; CL: Application

25. A 7-year-old child is diagnosed with head lice. The mother asks what nits are. The nurse states that they represent which part of the louse lifecycle?

1. Adult
2. Empty egg shells
3. Newly laid eggs
4. Nymph

25. 2. The mother is finding empty eggshells in the child's hair. Adults are the last stage of development, living about 30 days. Newly laid eggs are small, translucent, and difficult to see. Nymphs are the newly hatched lice and become adults in 8 to 9 days.

CN: Physiological integrity; CNS: Physiological adaptation; CL: Application

26. The nurse is teaching the mother of a child with lice about treatment options. Which adverse effect would the nurse teach regarding lindane (Kwell) shampoo?

1. Lindane causes alopecia.
2. Lindane causes hypertension.
3. Lindane is associated with seizures.
4. Lindane increases liver function test (LFT) results.

26. 3. Lindane is associated with seizures after absorption with topical use. Alopecia, increased LFT results, and hypertension aren't associated with the use of lindane.

CN: Physiological integrity; CNS: Pharmacological and parenteral therapies; CL: Application

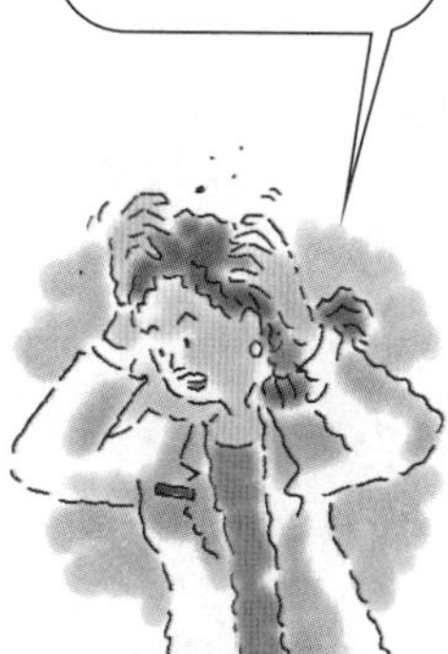

There's nothing nice about head lice.

27. Which instruction should be given to the parents about the treatment of head lice?

1. The treatment should be repeated in 7 to 12 days.
2. Treatment should be repeated every day for 1 week.
3. If treated with a shampoo, combing to remove eggs isn't necessary.
4. All contacts with the infested child should be treated even without evidence of infestation.

27. 1. Treatment should be repeated in 7 to 12 days to ensure that all eggs are killed. Combing the hair thoroughly is necessary to remove the lice eggs. People exposed to head lice should be examined to assess the presence of infestation before treatment.

CN: Physiological integrity; CNS: Physiological adaptation; CL: Application

28. A mother reports that her 4-year-old child has been scratching at his rectum recently. Which infestation or condition should the nurse suspect?

1. Anal fissure
2. Lice
3. Pinworms
4. Scabies

28. 3. The clinical sign of pinworms is perianal itching that increases at night. Anal fissures are associated with rectal bleeding and pain with bowel movements. Lice are infestations of the hair. Scabies are associated with a pruritic rash characterized as linear burrows of the webs of the fingers and toes.

CN: Physiological integrity; CNS: Physiological adaptation; CL: Analysis

29. Diagnosing pinworms by the clear cellophane tape test is preferred. How many tests are necessary to detect infestations at virtually 100% accuracy?

1. One
2. Three
3. Five
4. Ten

29. 3. Detection is virtually 100% accurate with five tests. One test is only 50% accurate. Three tests should detect infestations at about 90% accuracy. Ten tests aren't necessary.

CN: Physiological integrity; CNS: Reduction of risk potential; CL: Application

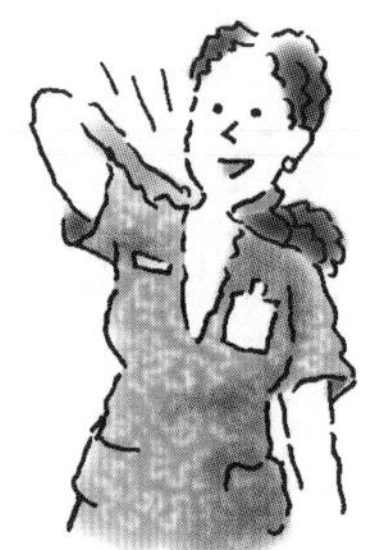

You've finished 30 questions! Good for you!

30. Each member of the family of a child diagnosed with pinworms is prescribed a single dose of pyrantel pamoate (Antiminth). Which statement should the nurse make about pyrantel pamoate?

1. The drug may stain the feces red.
2. The dose may be repeated in 2 weeks.
3. Fever and rash are common adverse effects.
4. The medicine will kill the eggs in about 48 hours.

30. 2. Pyrantel is effective against the adult worms only (not eggs), so treatment can be repeated to eradicate any emerging parasites in 2 weeks. Staining the feces is associated with pyrvinium pamoate. Common adverse effects are headaches and abdominal complaints.

CN: Physiological integrity; CNS: Pharmacological and parenteral therapies; CL: Application

31. A child received a bite to the hand from a large dog. The nurse would expect to assess which type of injury?

1. Abrasion
2. Crush injury
3. Fracture
4. Puncture wound

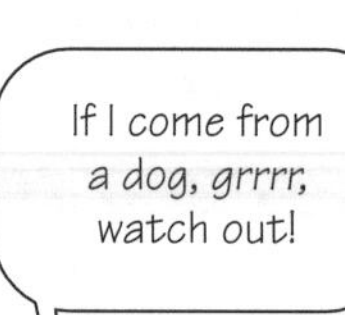

If I come from a dog, grrrr, watch out!

31. 2. Although the bite of a large dog can exert pressure of 150 to 400 pounds per square inch, the bite causes crush injuries, not fractures. Abrasions are associated with friction injuries. Puncture wounds are associated with smaller animals, such as cats.

CN: Physiological integrity; CNS: Physiological adaptation; CL: Application

32. A nurse knows that bites from dogs are at risk for infection. Which intervention should be done to help prevent infection?

1. Give the rabies vaccine.
2. Give antibiotics immediately.
3. Clean and irrigate the wounds.
4. Nothing; bites from dogs have a low incidence of infection.

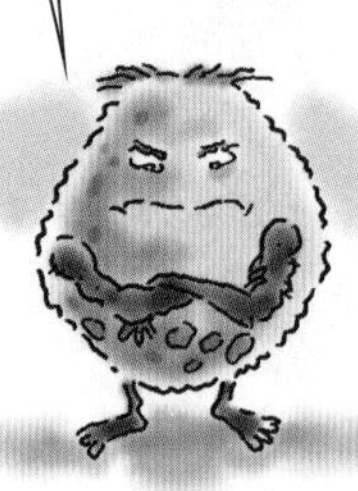

32. 3. Not every dog bite requires antibiotic therapy, but cleaning the wound is necessary for all injuries involving a break in the skin. Rabies vaccine is used if there is a suspicion the dog has rabies. The infection rate for dog bites has been reported to be as high as 50%.

CN: Physiological integrity; CNS: Reduction of risk potential; CL: Application

33. The nurse is reviewing the wound culture report from a child's infected wound caused by a dog bite. Which organism would the nurse suspect to be responsible for the infection?

1. *Escherichia coli*
2. *Francisella tularensis*
3. *Pasteurella multocida*
4. *Rochalimaea henselae*

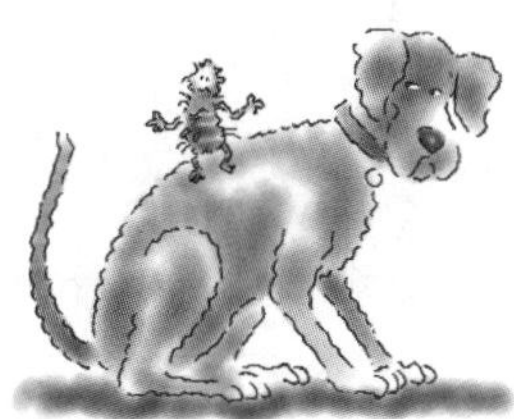

Me and the pooch here are pals.

33. 3. *Pasteurella multocida* is associated with infection in up to 50% of the bites from dogs. *E. coli* is more likely to cause infections of the urinary tract. *Francisella tularensis* is found in such animals as rabbits, hares, and muskrats. *Rochalimaea henselae*, a gram-negative rickettsial bacterium, is associated with cat-scratch disease.

CN: Physiological integrity; CNS: Physiological adaptation; CL: Application

34. A child is brought to a physician's office for multiple scratches and bites from a kitten. Which symptom is primarily found on assessment with cat-scratch disease?

1. Abdominal pain
2. Adenitis
3. Fever
4. Pruritus

34. 2. Adenitis is the primary feature of cat-scratch disease. Although low-grade fever has been associated with cat-scratch disease, it's only present 25% of the time. Pruritus and abdominal pain aren't symptoms of cat-scratch disease.

CN: Physiological integrity; CNS: Physiological adaptation; CL: Analysis

35. The school nurse is discussing giardiasis, a parasitic intestinal infection, with a group of parents. In which population group in the United States is this infection most common?

1. Children riding a school bus
2. Children playing on a playground
3. Children attending a sporting event
4. Children attending group day care or nursery school

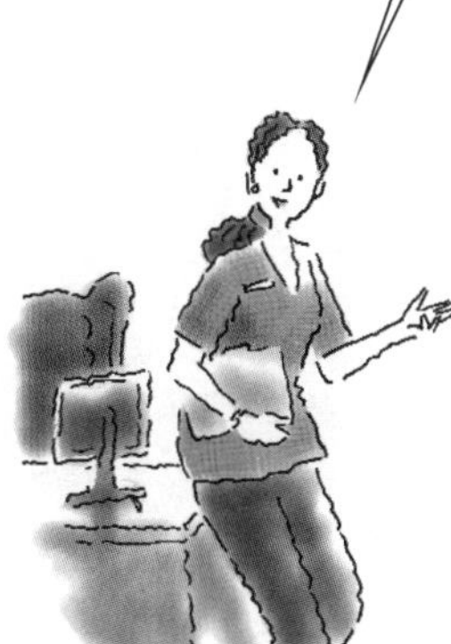

You need to know the correct terms to share information with clients and other health care providers.

35. 4. The most common intestinal parasitic infection in the United States is giardiasis, prevalent among children attending group day care or nursery school. Playgrounds, sporting events, and school buses don't present unusual risk of giardiasis.

CN: Physiological integrity; CNS: Physiological adaptation; CL: Application

36. Which finding should the nurse expect to observe if a child has papules?

1. Palpable elevated masses
2. Loss of the epidermis layer
3. Fluid-filled elevations of the skin
4. Nonpalpable flat changes in skin color

36. 1. Papules are elevated up to 0.5 cm. Nodules and tumors are elevated more than 0.5 cm. Erosions are characterized as loss of the epidermis layer. Fluid-filled lesions are vesicles and pustules. Macules and patches are described as nonpalpable flat changes in skin color.

CN: Health promotion and maintenance; CNS: None; CL: Application

37. A child is diagnosed with impetigo. Pustules are the primary lesions found on this child. Which of the following correctly describes pustules?

1. Lesion filled with pus
2. Superficial area of localized edema
3. Serous-filled lesion less than 0.5 cm
4. Serous-filled lesion greater than 0.5 cm

37. 1. Pustules are pus-filled lesions, such as acne and impetigo. A wheal is a superficial area of localized edema. Vesicles are serous-filled lesions up to 0.5 cm in diameter. Bullae are serous-filled lesions greater than 0.5 cm in diameter.

CN: Physiological integrity; CNS: Physiological adaptation; CL: Application

38. A 3-month-old infant is noted to have café-au-lait spots on examination. The presence of six or more of these lesions with a diameter greater then 1.5 cm is suggestive of which disorder?

1. Meningococcemia
2. Neurofibromatosis
3. Tinea versicolor
4. Vitiligo

39. A child is brought to the physician's office for treatment of a rash. Many petechiae are seen over his entire body. The nurse would suspect which condition?

1. Bleeding disorder
2. Scabies
3. Varicella
4. Vomiting

40. A child fell at camp and sustained a bruise to his thigh. Which description would accurately describe the bruise after 1 week?

1. Resolved
2. Reddish blue
3. Greenish yellow
4. Dark blue to bluish brown

41. Which factor would lead the nurse to suspect child abuse?

1. Multiple contusions of the shins
2. Contusions of the back and buttocks
3. Contusions at the same stages of healing
4. Large contusion and hematoma of the forehead

42. Which statement would the nurse include when teaching a new mother about salmon patches (stork bites)?

1. They're benign and usually fade in adult life.
2. They're usually associated with syndromes of the neonate.
3. They can cause mild hypertrophy of the muscle associated with the lesion.
4. They're treatable with laser pulse surgery in late adolescence and adulthood.

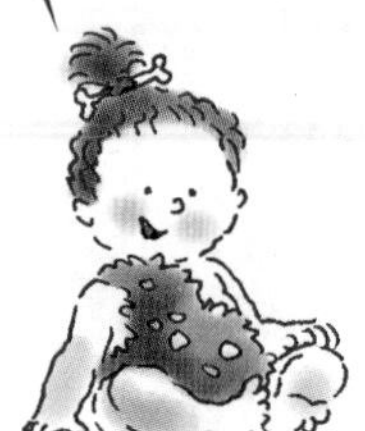
Assessment is an enormously important skill.

38. 2. Six or more uniformly pigmented patches with irregular borders, known as *café-au-lait spots,* with diameters greater then 1.5 cm are associated with neurofibromatosis. Meningococcemia has petechiae, not *café-au-lait spots.* Tinea versicolor is a superficial fungus infection. Depigmented areas are signs of vitiligo.

CN: Health promotion and maintenance; CNS: None; CL: Analysis

39. 1. Petechiae are caused by blood outside a vessel, associated with low platelet counts and bleeding disorders. Petechiae aren't found with varicella disease or scabies. Petechiae can be associated with vomiting, but in that case they'd be present on the face, not the entire body.

CN: Physiological integrity; CNS: Physiological adaptation; CL: Analysis

40. 3. After 7 to 10 days, the bruise becomes greenish yellow. Resolution can take up to 2 weeks. Initially after the fall, there's a reddish blue discoloration followed by a dark blue to bluish brown color at days 1 to 3.

CN: Physiological integrity; CNS: Physiological adaptation; CL: Application

41. 2. Contusions of the back and buttocks are highly suspicious of abuse related to punishment. Contusions at various stages of healing are red flags to potential abuse. Contusions of the shins and forehead are usually related to an active toddler falling and bumping into objects.

CN: Psychosocial integrity; CNS: None; CL: Analysis

42. 1. Salmon patches occur over the back of the neck in 40% of neonates and are harmless, needing no intervention. Port wine stains are associated with syndromes of the neonate such as Sturge-Weber syndrome. Port wine stains found on the face or extremities may be associated with soft tissue and bone hypertrophy. Laser pulse surgery isn't recommended for salmon patches because they typically fade on their own in adulthood.

CN: Health promotion and maintenance; CNS: None; CL: Application

CN: Client needs category CNS: Client needs subcategory CL: Cognitive level

43. A neonate is born with a blue-black macular lesion over the lower lumbar sacral region. Which term should the nurse use when teaching the parents about this lesion?

1. Café-au-lait spots
2. Mongolian spots
3. Nevis of Ota spot
4. Stork bites

43. 2. Mongolian spots are large blue-black macular lesions generally located over the lumbosacral areas, buttocks, and limbs. Café-au-lait spots occur between ages 2 and 16 years, not in infancy. Nevis of Ota is found surrounding the eyes. Stork bites or salmon patches occur at the neck and hairline area.

CN: Health promotion and maintenance; CNS: None; CL: Application

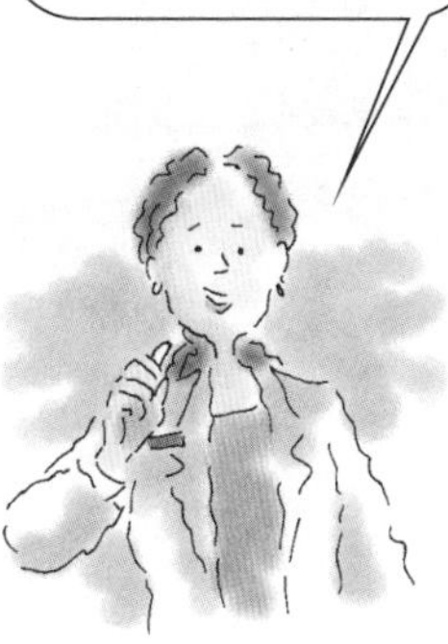

The word severe is a clue to the correct answer.

44. Which finding indicates severe dehydration in a child?

1. Gray skin and decreased tears
2. Capillary refill less than 2 seconds
3. Mottling and tenting of the skin
4. Pale skin with dry mucous membranes

44. 3. Severe dehydration is associated with mottling and tenting of the skin. Malnutrition is characterized by gray skin and tenting of the skin. Capillary refill less then 2 seconds is normal. Pale skin with dry mucous membranes is a sign of mild dehydration.

CN: Health promotion and maintenance; CNS: None; CL: Analysis

45. A client is prescribed isotretinoin (Accutane). Which adverse effect should the nurse include in her teaching?

1. Diarrhea
2. Gram-negative folliculitis
3. Teratogenicity
4. Vaginal candidiasis

45. 3. The use of even small amounts of isotretinoin has been associated with severe birth defects. Most female clients taking this medication are prescribed hormonal contraceptives. Cleocin T (clindamycin), another medicine used in the treatment of acne, is associated with both diarrhea and gram-negative folliculitis. Tetracycline (Achromycin) is associated with yeast infections (vaginal candidiasis).

CN: Physiological integrity; CNS: Pharmacological and parenteral therapies; CL: Application

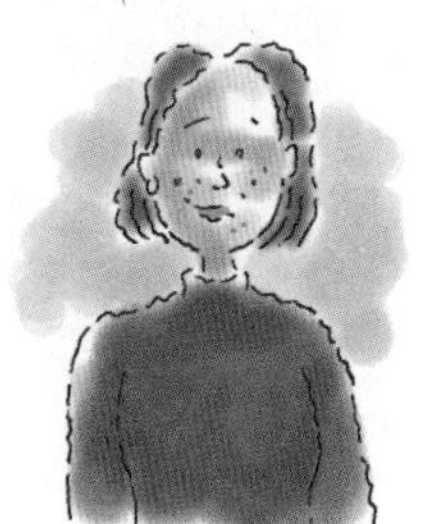

I need to follow the treatment plan.

46. The nurse is developing a teaching plan for adolescents about acne. The nurse incorporates which characteristic as commonly responsible for the failure of treatment of acne in teenagers?

1. Topical treatment
2. Systemic treatment
3. A dominant parent who wants treatment and a passive teenager who doesn't
4. A dominant teenager who wants treatment and a passive uninterested parent

46. 3. The active participation of a teenager is needed for the successful treatment of acne. Systemic and topical therapy are needed in most acne treatment.

CN: Health promotion and maintenance; CNS: None; CL: Application

47. What information should be given to a teenager about acne?

1. Acne is caused by diet.
2. Acne is related to gender.
3. Acne is caused by poor hygiene.
4. Acne is caused by hormonal changes.

47. 4. Acne is caused by hormonal changes in sebaceous gland anatomy and the biochemistry of the glands. These changes lead to a blockage in the follicular canal and cause an inflammatory response. Diet, hygiene, and the client's gender don't cause acne.

CN: Health promotion and maintenance; CNS: None; CL: Application

48. When teaching a client about tetracycline (Achromycin) for severe inflammatory acne, which instruction must be given?
1. Take the drug with or without meals.
2. Take the drug with milk and milk products.
3. Take the drug on an empty stomach with small amounts of water.
4. Take the drug 1 hour before or 2 hours after meals with large amounts of water.

48. 4. Tetracycline must be taken on an empty stomach to increase absorption and with ample water to avoid esophageal irritation. Milk products impede absorption.

CN: Physiological integrity; CNS: Pharmacological and parenteral therapies; CL: Application

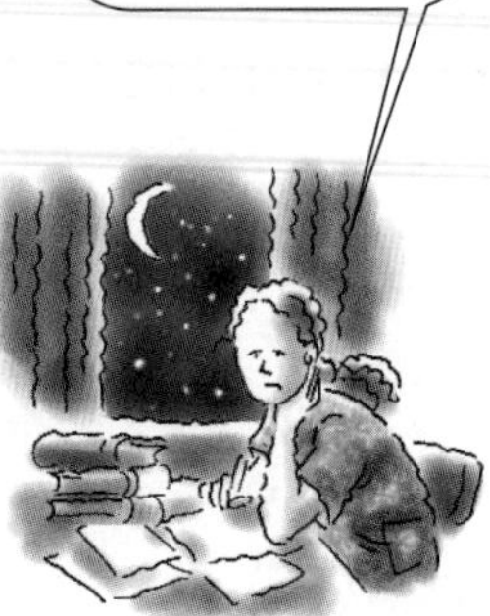

49. When advising parents about the prevention of burns to their child from tap water, which instruction should be given?
1. Set the water-heater temperature at 130° F (54.4° C) or less.
2. Run the hot water first, then adjust the temperature with cold water.
3. Before you put your infant in the tub, first test the water with your hand.
4. Supervise an infant in the bathroom, only leaving him for a few seconds, if needed.

49. 3. Instruct the parents to fill the tub with water first and then test all of the water in the tub with their hand for hot spots. Water heaters should be set at 120° F. The cold water should be run first and then adjusted with hot water. Never leave an infant alone in the bathroom, even for a second.

CN: Health promotion and maintenance; CNS: None; CL: Application

50. While caring for a 2-day-old neonate, a nurse notices the left side of the neonate becomes reddened for 2 to 3 minutes. The nurse interprets this finding as suggestive of:
1. contact dermatitis.
2. environmental conditions.
3. harlequin color change.
4. tet spells.

50. 3. Harlequin color change is a benign disorder related to the immaturity of hypothalamic centers that control the tone of peripheral blood vessels. A new born who has been lying on its side may appear reddened on the dependent side. The color fades on position change. Contact dermatitis isn't short-lived. Changes in environmental conditions can cause diffuse bilateral mottling of the skin. Tet spells are associated with tetralogy of Fallot and cause cyanotic changes.

CN: Health promotion and maintenance; CNS: None; CL: Analysis

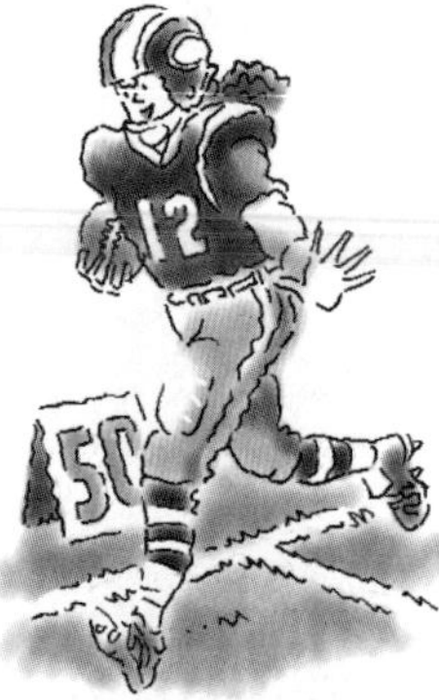

You've reached question 50 and your goal is in sight.
12
50

51. A 15-month-old child is diagnosed with pediculosis of the eyebrows. Which intervention is included in the treatment?
1. Use lindane.
2. Use petroleum jelly.
3. Shave the eyebrows.
4. No treatment is needed.

51. 2. Petroleum jelly should be applied twice daily for 8 days, followed by manual removal of nits. Lindane is contraindicated because of the risk for seizures. The eyebrow should never be shaved because of the uncertainty of hair return.

CN: Physiological integrity; CNS: Physiological adaptation; CL: Analysis

52. A 14-year-old male client is brought to the hospital with smoke inhalation because of a house fire. The nurse's first intervention for this client is to:
1. check the oral mucous membranes.
2. check for any burned areas.
3. obtain a medical history.
4. ensure a patent airway.

52. 4. The nurse's top priority is to make sure the airway is open and the client is breathing. Checking the mucous membranes and burned areas is important but not as vital as maintaining a patent airway. Obtaining a medical history can be pursued after ensuring a patent airway.

CN: Physiological integrity; CNS: Physiological adaptation; CL: Application

53. The nurse is assessing a child suspected of having Kawasaki syndrome. Which changes in the mouth would the nurse observe that would indicate this condition?

1. Koplik's spots
2. Tonsillar exudate
3. Vesicular lesions
4. Strawberry tongue

53. 4. Oral changes associated with Kawasaki syndrome include reddened pharynx, red, dry fissured lips, and strawberry tongue. Koplik's spots are consistent with measles. Tonsillar exudate is consistent with pharyngitis caused by group A beta hemolytic streptococci. Vesicular lesions are associated with coxsackievirus.

CN: Physiological integrity; CNS: Physiological adaptation; CL: Application

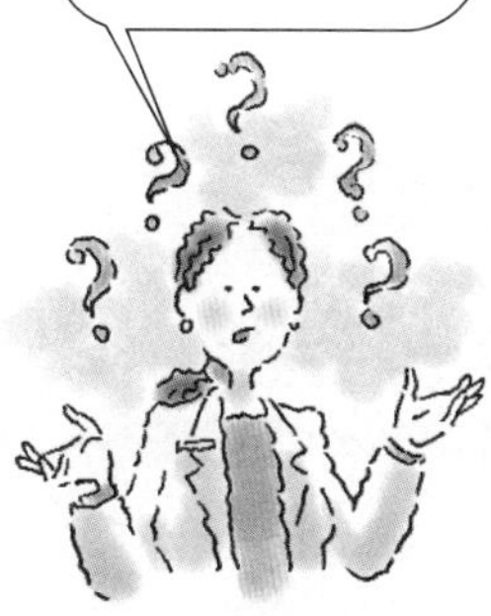

Which symptom goes with which diagnosis?

54. A 3-year-old child has palpable purpura of the buttocks and lower extremities. Which condition would the nurse suspect with these symptoms?

1. Child abuse
2. Henoch-Schönlein purpura (HSP)
3. Idiopathic thrombocytopenic purpura (ITP)
4. Rocky Mountain spotted fever

54. 2. The rash associated with HSP is believed to occur in every client and allows for a definitive diagnosis. It begins as petechiae and progresses to purpuric lesions of the buttocks and lower extremities. The lesions of child abuse are painful and nonraised. Petechiae or purpura associated with ITP are distributed over the entire body. The rash in Rocky Mountain spotted fever is a nonraised macular papular rash spread over the body.

CN: Physiological integrity; CNS: Physiological adaptation; CL: Application

55. Topical treatment with 2.5% hydrocortisone (Cortane) is prescribed for a 6-month-old infant with eczema. The mother is instructed to use the cream for not longer than 1 week. Why is this time limit appropriate?

1. The drug loses its efficacy after prolonged use.
2. This reduces adverse effects, such as skin atrophy and fragility.
3. If no improvement is seen, a stronger concentration will be prescribed.
4. If no improvement is seen after 1 week, an antibiotic will be prescribed.

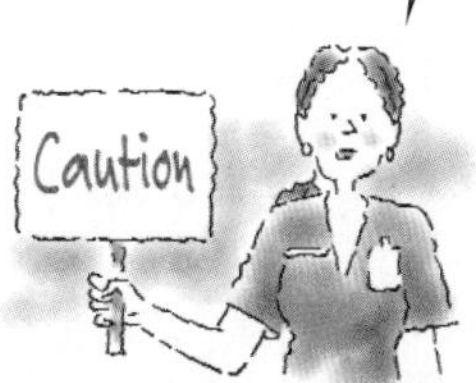

Adverse effects can result from prolonged use of certain medications.
Caution

55. 2. Hydrocortisone cream should be used for brief periods to decrease such adverse effects as atrophy of the skin. The drug doesn't lose efficacy after prolonged use, a stronger concentration may not be prescribed if no improvement is seen, and an antibiotic would be inappropriate in this instance.

CN: Physiological integrity; CNS: Pharmacological and parenteral therapies; CL: Application

56. A 9-year-old child is examined because his mother noticed lesions on his tongue. Painless, slightly depressed, red lesions bordered with white bands are seen on examination. The mother reports the patterns were different yesterday. Which condition would the nurse suspect?

1. Geographic tongue
2. Koplik's spots
3. Scald burns
4. Stomatitis

56. 1. Geographic tongue is a benign disorder caused by loss of filiform papules. The configuration is known to change from day to day. Koplik's spots and stomatitis lesions don't change patterns. Scald burns are painful lesions from hot liquids.

CN: Physiological integrity; CNS: Physiological adaptation; CL: Application

57. A 4-year-old child had a subungual hemorrhage of the toe after a jar fell on his foot. Electrocautery is performed. The nurse explains to the parents that electrocautery is done to:

1. prevent loss of nail growth.
2. prevent spread of the infection.
3. relieve pain and reduce the risk for infection.
4. prevent permanent discoloration of the nail bed.

57. 3. The hematoma is treated with electrocautery to relieve pain and reduce risk for infection. Electrocautery doesn't prevent the loss of the nail. The discoloration seen with subungual hemorrhage is from the collection of blood under the nail bed. It isn't permanent and doesn't affect nail growth.

CN: Physiological integrity; CNS: Physiological adaptation; CL: Application

58. The nurse is caring for a 12-year-old child with a diagnosis of eczema. Which nursing interventions are appropriate for a child with eczema?

1. Administering antibiotics as prescribed
2. Administering antifungals as ordered
3. Administering tepid baths and patting dry or air drying the affected areas
4. Administering hot baths and using moisturizers immediately after the bath

58. 3. Tepid baths and moisturizers are indicated to keep the infected areas clean and minimize itching. Antibiotics are given only when superimposed infection is present. Antifungals aren't usually administered in the treatment of eczema. Hot baths can exacerbate the condition and increase itching.

CN: Physiological integrity; CNS: Physiological adaptation; CL: Application

59. A 9-year-old child is brought to the emergency department with extensive burns received in a restaurant fire. What's the most important aspect of caring for the burned child?

1. Administering antibiotics to prevent superimposed infections
2. Conducting wound management
3. Administering liquids orally to replace fluid
4. Administering frequent small meals to support nutritional requirements

59. 2. The most important aspect of caring for a burned child is wound management. The goals of wound care are to speed debridement, protect granulation tissue and new grafts, and conserve body heat and fluids. Antibiotics aren't always administered prophylactically. Fluids are administered I.V. according to the child's body weight to replace volume. Enteral feedings, rather than meals, are initiated within the first 24 hours after the burn to support the child's increased nutritional requirements.

CN: Physiological integrity; CNS: Physiological adaptation; CL: Application

60. A mother of a 4-month-old infant asks about the strawberry hemangioma on his cheek. What information should the nurse provide to the mother?

1. The lesion will continue to grow for 3 years, then need surgical removal.
2. If the lesion continues to enlarge, referral to a pediatric oncologist is warranted.
3. Surgery is indicated before age 12 months if the diameter of the lesion is greater then 3 cm.
4. The lesion will continue to grow until age 1 year, then begin to resolve by age 2 to 3 years.

60. 4. These rapidly growing vascular lesions reach maximum growth by age 1 year. The growth period is then followed by an involution period of 6 to 12 months. Lesions show complete involution by age 2 or 3 years. These benign lesions don't need surgical or oncologic referrals.

CN: Health promotion and maintenance; CNS: None; CL: Application

61. A 3-year-old child is being discharged from the emergency department after receiving three sutures for a scalp laceration. In how many days should the nurse tell the family to return for suture removal?

1. 1 to 3 days
2. 5 to 7 days
3. 8 to 10 days
4. 10 to 14 days

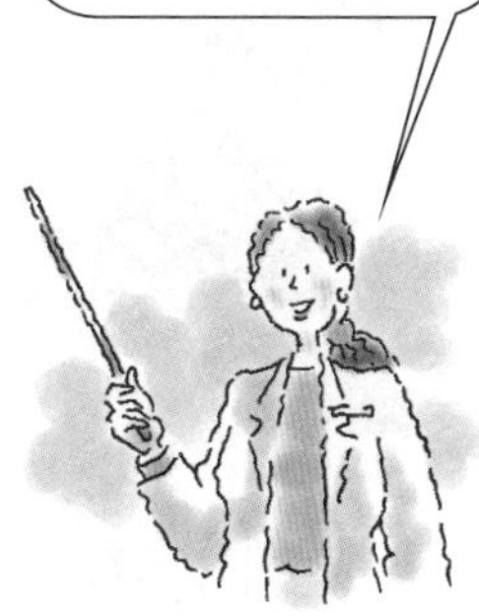

Words with dots
under them point to
the correct answer.

62. Which symptom is an <u>early sign</u> of infection of a laceration?

1. Fever
2. Copious drainage
3. Excessive discomfort
4. Local nodal enlargement

63. The nurse is teaching a 17-year-old client who'll soon be discharged regarding how to change a sterile dressing on the right leg. During the teaching session, the nurse notices redness, swelling, and induration at the wound site, interpreting these as suggesting:

1. infection.
2. dehiscence.
3. hemorrhage.
4. evisceration.

64. A 6-year-old child is diagnosed with herpes zoster of the left anterior chest. Which assessment finding should the nurse expect to find?

1. Bruising and swelling
2. Papulovesicular eruption with complaints of pain and tenderness of the lesion
3. Linear burrows on the fingers and toes
4. Papulovesicular lesions on the chest, trunk, face, and scalp

You made it to question 65. Hang in there.

65. During an examination of a 5-month-old infant, a flat, dull pink, macular lesion is noted on the infant's forehead. The nurse suspects which condition?

1. Cavernous hemangioma
2. Nevus flammeus
3. Salmon patch
4. Strawberry hemangioma

61. 2. The recommended healing time for this type of laceration is 5 to 7 days. Sutures need longer than 1 to 3 days to form an effective bond. Eight to 10 days is needed for sutures of the fingertips and feet, and 10 to 14 days is the recommended time for extensor surfaces of the knees and elbows.

CN: Physiological integrity; CNS: Physiological adaptation; CL: Application

62. 3. The first sign of infection is usually excessive discomfort. Nodal enlargement, fever, and copious drainage are advanced signs of infection.

CN: Health promotion and maintenance; CNS: None; CL: Analysis

63. 1. Infection produces such signs as redness, swelling, induration, warmth, and possible drainage. Dehiscence may cause unexplained fever and tachycardia, unusual wound pain, prolonged paralytic ileus, and separation of the surgical incision. Hemorrhage can result in increased pulse and respiratory rate, decreased blood pressure, restlessness, thirst, and cold, clammy skin. Evisceration produces visible protrusion of organs, usually through an incision.

CN: Physiological integrity; CNS: Physiological adaptation; CL: Analysis

64. 2. Herpes zoster is caused by the varicella-zoster virus. It has papulovesicular lesions that erupt along a dermatome, usually with hyperesthesia, pain, and tenderness. Contusions are present with bruising and swelling. Scabies appear as linear burrows of the fingers and toes caused by a mite. The papulovesicular lesions of varicella are distributed over the entire trunk, face, and scalp and don't follow a dermatome.

CN: Physiological integrity; CNS: Physiological adaptation; CL: Analysis

65. 3. Salmon patches are common vascular lesions in infants. They appear as flat, dull pink, macular lesions in various regions of the face and head. When they appear on the nape of the neck, they're commonly called "stork bites." These lesions fade by the first year of life. Both strawberry and cavernous hemangiomas are raised lesions. Nevus flammeus, or port wine stains, are reddish-purple lesions that don't fade.

CN: Physiological integrity; CNS: Physiological adaptation; CL: Analysis

66. A young child's parents ask for advice on the use of an insect repellent that contains deet. Which statement would be correct?

1. "Spray the child's clothing instead of the skin."
2. "The repellent works better as the temperature increases."
3. "The repellent isn't effective against the ticks responsible for Lyme disease."
4. "Apply insect repellent as you would sunscreen, with frequent applications during the day."

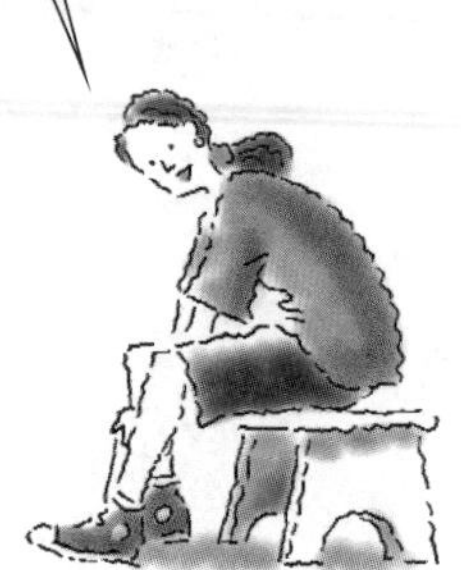

You're almost at question 70. That was quick!

66. 1. Deet spray has been approved for use on children. It should be used sparingly on all skin surfaces. By concentrating spray on clothing and camping equipment, the adverse effects and potential toxic buildup is significantly reduced. Repellent is lost to evaporation, wind, heat, and perspiration. With each 10° F increase in temperature, it leads to as much as a 50% reduction in protection time. Deet is very effective as a tick repellent.

CN: Physiological integrity; CNS: Reduction of risk potential; CL: Application

67. A nurse is teaching a parent about which deet-containing insect repellent to use on his child. Which concentration should she instruct him to use on the child's skin for optimal results?

1. 10%
2. 15%
3. 20%
4. 30%

67. 1. The highest concentration approved by the Food and Drug Administration for children is 10%. Because of thinner skin and greater surface area to mass ratio in children, parents should use deet products sparingly.

CN: Physiological integrity; CNS: Reduction of risk potential; CL: Application

68. Which statement about warts would the nurse incorporate when assisting with a community health teaching program on common skin problems?

1. Cutting the wart is the preferred treatment for children.
2. No treatment exists that specifically kills the wart virus.
3. Warts are caused by a virus affecting the inner layer of skin.
4. Warts are harmless and usually last 2 to 4 years if untreated.

68. 2. The goal of treatment is to kill the skin that contains the wart virus. Cutting the wart is likely to spread the virus. The virus that causes warts affects the outer layer of the skin. Warts are harmless and last 1 to 2 years if untreated.

CN: Health promotion and maintenance; CNS: None; CL: Application

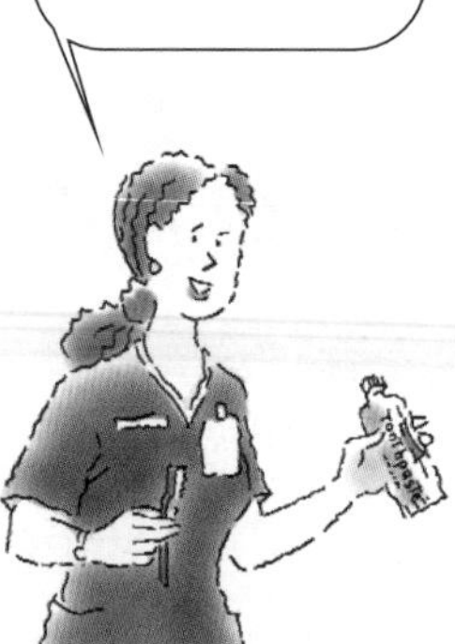

You need to brush those carbs away.

69. The nurse is assisting with a teaching program for new parents that focuses on oral hygiene promotion. Which factor would the nurse include as causing tooth decay and gum disease when allowed to remain on the teeth for prolonged periods?

1. Breast milk
2. Pacifiers
3. Thumb or other fingers
4. Formula

69. 4. Tooth decay and gum disease result when the carbohydrates in formula, cow's milk, and fruit juices are allowed to remain on the teeth for a prolonged period. Studies have shown that breast milk only contributes to dental caries when sugar is already present on the teeth. Breast milk alone actually promotes enamel growth. Pacifiers and fingers don't cause tooth decay and gum disease, although they may contribute to malocclusion.

CN: Health promotion and maintenance; CNS: None; CL: Application

70. A child is suspected of having cellulitis. What classic signs should the nurse expect to see in a child?

1. Pale, irritated, cold to touch
2. Vesicular blisters at the site of the injury
3. Fever, edema, tenderness, warmth at the site
4. Swelling, redness, with well-defined borders

70. 3. Cellulitis is a deep, locally diffuse infection of the skin. It's associated with redness, fever, edema, tenderness, and warmth at the site of the injury. Vesicular blisters suggest impetigo. Cellulitis has no well-defined borders.
CN: Physiological integrity; CNS: Physiological adaptation; CL: Application

71. A 2-year-old child has cellulitis of the finger. Which organism or condition is the most likely cause of the infection?

1. Parainfluenza virus
2. Respiratory syncytial virus
3. *Escherichia coli*
4. *Streptococcus*

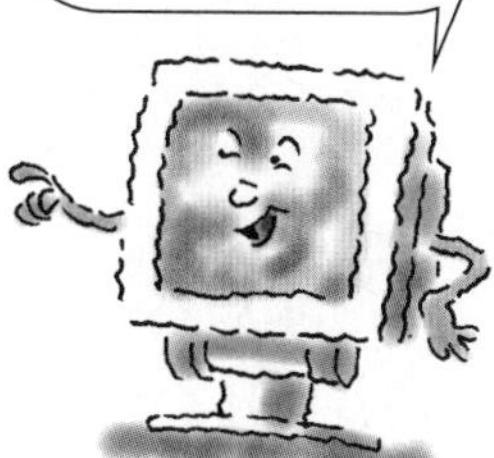
Note that this question asks about the most likely cause, not the only one.

71. 4. *Streptococcus* cause most cases of cellulitis. Parainfluenza and respiratory syncytial virus cause infections of the respiratory tract. *E. coli* is a cause of bladder infections.
CN: Physiological integrity; CNS: Physiological adaptation; CL: Analysis

72. A child has a desquamation rash of the hands and feet. Which additional findings should the nurse expect to observe with this rash?

1. Peeling skin
2. Thin, reddened layers of epidermis
3. Thick skin with deep visible burrows
4. Thinning skin that may appear translucent

72. 1. Desquamation is characteristic in diseases such as Stevens–Johnson syndrome. Scaling is thin, reddened layers of epidermis. Thickening of the skin with burrows is defined as lichenification. Thinning skin is best described as atrophy of the skin.
CN: Physiological integrity; CNS: Physiological adaptation; CL: Application

73. Which instruction would the nurse include for the parents of a child who is to receive nystatin oral solution?

1. Give the solution immediately after feedings.
2. Give the solution immediately before feedings.
3. Mix the solution with small amounts of the feeding.
4. Give half the solution before and half the solution after the feeding.

73. 1. Nystatin oral solution should be swabbed onto the mouth after feedings to allow for optimal contact with mucous membranes. Before meals and with meals doesn't give the best contact with the mucous membranes.
CN: Physiological integrity; CNS: Pharmacological and parenteral therapies; CL: Application

74. An infant is examined and found to have a petechial rash. The nurse documents a description of this rash as:

1. a purple macular lesion larger than 1 cm in diameter.
2. purple to brown bruises, macular or papular, various sizes.
3. a collection of blood from ruptured blood vessels larger than 1 cm in diameter.
4. a pinpoint, pink to purple, nonblanching macular lesion 1 to 3 mm in diameter.

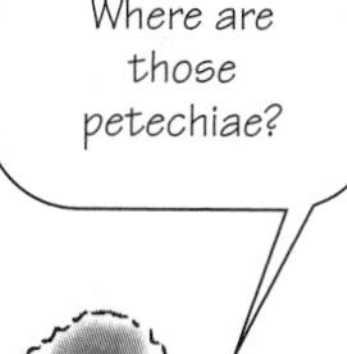
Where are those petechiae?

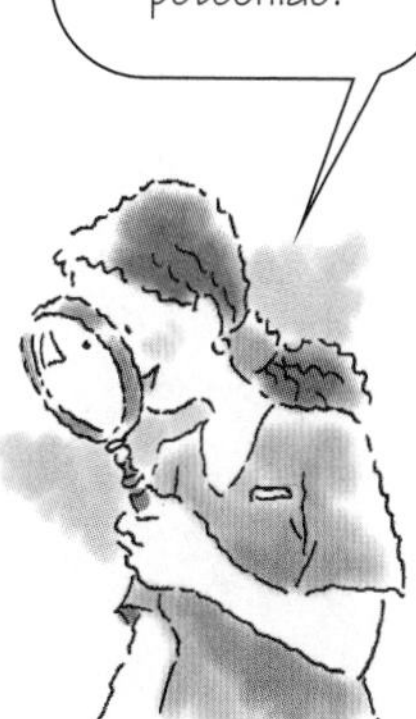

74. 4. Petechiae are small 1- to 3-mm macular lesions. Purple macular lesions greater than 1 cm are defined as purpura. A bruise is defined as ecchymosis. A hematoma is a collection of blood.
CN: Physiological integrity; CNS: Physiological adaptation; CL: Application

75. When inspecting the palms of a child, with which rash would the nurse expect to find no changes?
1. Coxsackie virus
2. Measles
3. Rocky Mountain spotted fever
4. Syphilis

75. 2. The rash in measles occurs on the face, trunk, and extremities. Rocky Mountain spotted fever, syphilis, and coxsackie virus show changes on the palms and soles.

CN: Physiological integrity; CNS: Physiological adaptation; CL: Analysis

76. A mother reports that her teenager is losing hair in small round areas on the scalp. The nurse interprets this as suggesting which condition?
1. Alopecia
2. Amblyopia
3. Exotropia
4. Seborrhea dermatitis

76. 1. Alopecia is the correct term for thinning hair loss. Exotropia and amblyopia are eye disorders. Seborrhea dermatitis is cradle cap and occurs in infants.

CN: Physiological integrity; CNS: Physiological adaptation; CL: Application

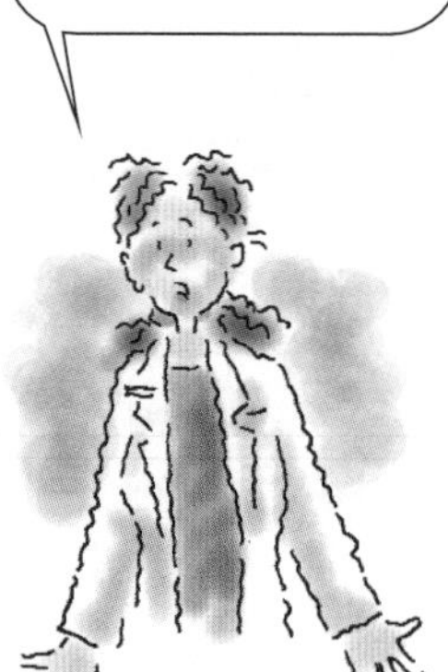
What is the correct term for ready to "pull" your hair out?

77. A topical corticosteroid cream is prescribed for a child with eczema. Which instruction should a nurse give to the mother regarding proper application of the cream?
1. "Apply the cream over the entire body."
2. "Apply the cream in a thin layer to the affected area and rub it in."
3. "Apply the cream to the infected area without washing the area first."
4. "Apply the cream in a thick layer and allow it to absorb."

77. 2. After gently cleansing the affected area, corticosteroid cream should be applied in a thin, not thick layer and rubbed into the area thoroughly. It shouldn't be applied to the entire body.

CN: Physiological integrity; CNS: Pharmacological and parenteral therapies; CL: Analysis

78. A mother of a toddler diagnosed with atopic dermatitis is concerned about how her child acquired the disease. The nurse should explain that the cause of atopic dermatitis is a:
1. fungal infection.
2. hereditary disorder.
3. sex-linked disorder.
4. viral infection.

78. 2. Atopic dermatitis is a hereditary disorder that isn't sex-linked and is associated with a family history of asthma, allergic rhinitis, or atopic dermatitis. Viral and fungal infections don't cause atopic dermatitis.

CN: Physiological integrity; CNS: Physiological adaptation; CL: Application

79. A mother of a 6-month-old infant with atopic dermatitis asks for advice on bathing the child. Which instruction should be given?
1. Bathe the infant twice daily.
2. Bathe the infant every other day.
3. Use bubble baths to decrease itching.
4. The frequency of the infant's baths isn't important in atopic dermatitis.

79. 2. Bathing removes lipoprotein complexes that hold water in the stratum corneum and increase water loss. Decreasing bathing to every other day can help prevent the removal of lipoprotein complexes. Soap and bubble bath should be used sparingly while bathing the child.

CN: Physiological integrity; CNS: Basic care and comfort; CL: Application

CN: Client needs category CNS: Client needs subcategory CL: Cognitive level

80. Discharge instructions for a child with atopic dermatitis include keeping the fingernails cut short. Which rationale should the nurse give for this intervention?

1. To prevent infection of the nail bed
2. To prevent the spread of the disorder
3. To prevent the child from causing a corneal abrasion
4. To reduce breaks in skin from scratching that may lead to secondary bacterial infections

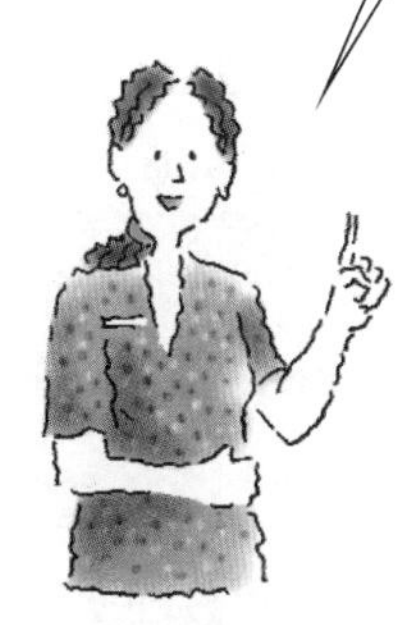

Here's another question pointing out the importance of client teaching.

80. 4. Keeping fingernails cut short will prevent breaks in the skin when a child scratches. Cutting fingernails too short or cutting the skin around the nail can increase the risk of infection. Atopic dermatitis can be found in various areas of the skin, but isn't spread from one area to another. Keeping fingernails short is a good way to reduce corneal abrasions, but doesn't apply to atopic dermatitis.

CN: Physiological integrity; CNS: Physiological adaptation; CL: Application

81. A 10-year-old child being treated for common warts asks about the cause. The nurse would incorporate which virus as the cause?

1. Coxsackievirus
2. Human herpesvirus (HHV)
3. Human immunodeficiency virus (HIV)
4. Human papillomavirus (HPV)

81. 4. HPV is responsible for various forms of warts. Coxsackievirus is associated with hand-foot-mouth disease. HHV is associated with varicella and herpes zoster. HIV infections aren't associated with epithelial tumors known as warts.

CN: Physiological integrity; CNS: Physiological adaptation; CL: Application

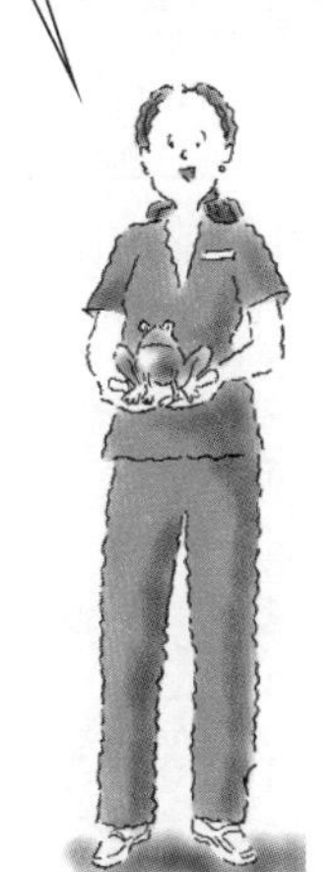

You know what they say about frogs and warts.

82. The nurse is assessing a 6-year-old child with a spiny projection from the skin suspended from a narrow stalk on the forehead. Which condition would the nurse suspect?

1. Filiform wart
2. Flat wart
3. Plantar wart
4. Venereal warts

82. 1. Filiform warts are long spiny projections from the skin surface. Flat warts are flat-topped smooth-surfaced lesions. Plantar warts are rough papules, commonly found on the soles of the feet. Venereal warts appear on the genital mucosa and are confluent papules with rough surfaces.

CN: Physiological integrity; CNS: Physiological adaptation; CL: Application

83. An adolescent says his feet itch, sweat a lot, and have a foul odor. The nurse suspects which condition?

1. Candidiasis
2. Tinea corporis
3. Tinea pedis
4. Molluscum contagiosum

83. 3. Tinea pedis is a superficial fungal infection on the feet, commonly called *athletes' foot.* Candidiasis is a fungal infection of the skin or mucous membranes commonly found in the oral, vaginal, and intestinal mucosal tissue. Tinea corporis, or *ringworm,* is a flat scaling papular lesion with raised borders. Molluscum contagiosum is a viral skin infection with lesions that are small red papules.

CN: Physiological integrity; CNS: Physiological adaptation; CL: Analysis

84. A nurse is explaining treatment to the parents of a child with hypertrophic scarring. Which method would be the best for controlling this condition?

1. Compression garments
2. Moisturizing creams
3. Physiotherapy
4. Splints

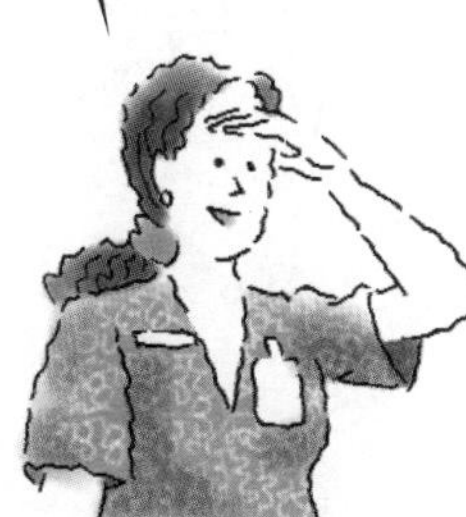

I can almost see the last question.

84. 1. Compression garments are worn for up to 1 year to control hypertrophic scarring. Moisturizing creams help decrease hyperpigmentation. Physiotherapy and splints help keep joints and limbs supple.

CN: Physiological integrity; CNS: Physiological adaptation; CL: Application

85. During a physical examination, a child is noted to have nails with "ice-pick" pits and ridges. The nails are thick and discolored and have splintered hemorrhages easily separated from the nail bed. Which condition would cause this to occur?

1. Paronychia
2. Psoriasis
3. Scabies
4. Seborrhea

85. 2. Psoriasis is a chronic skin disorder with an unknown cause that shows these characteristic skin changes. A paronychia is a bacterial infection of the nail bed. Scabies are mites that burrow under the skin, usually between the webbing of the fingers and toes. Seborrhea is a chronic inflammatory dermatitis or cradle cap.
CN: Physiological integrity; CNS: Physiological adaptation; CL: Application

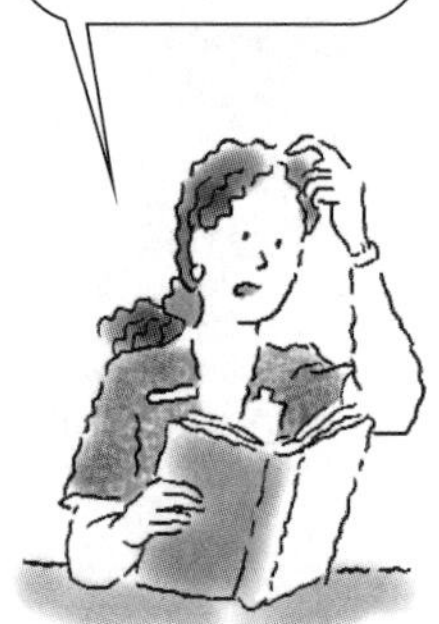
What is the most accurate assessment?

86. A neonate is examined and noted to have bruising on the scalp, along with diffuse swelling of the soft tissue that crosses over the suture line. Which assessment is most accurate?

1. Caput succedaneum
2. Cephalhematoma
3. Craniotabes
4. Hydrocephalus

86. 1. Caput succedaneum originates from trauma to the neonate while descending through the birth canal. It's usually a benign injury that spontaneously resolves over time. Cephalhematoma is a collection of blood in the periosteum of the scalp that doesn't cross over the suture line. Craniotabes is the thinning of the bone of the scalp. Hydrocephalus is an increased volume of cerebrospinal fluid (CSF) or the obstruction of the flow of the CSF and isn't related to soft tissue swelling.
CN: Physiological integrity; CNS: Physiological adaptation; CL: Analysis

87. A child has a healed wound from a traumatic injury. His mother is concerned because a lesion formed over the wound is pink, thickened, smooth, and rubbery in nature. The nurse should use what term to discuss this condition with the mother?

1. Erosion
2. Fissure
3. Keloids
4. Striae

87. 3. Keloids are an exaggerated connective tissue response to skin injury. An erosion is a depressed vesicular lesion. A fissure is a cleavage in the surface of skin. Striae are linear depressions of the skin.
CN: Physiological integrity; CNS: Physiological adaptation; CL: Application

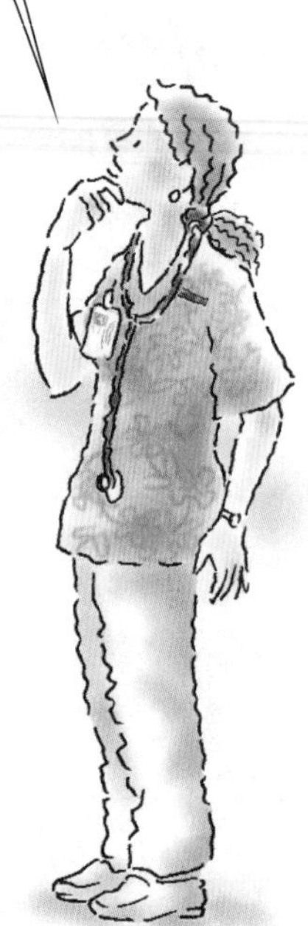
Hmmm, white plaques with an erythematous base. What could that mean?

88. The mother of an infant gives a history of poor feeding for a few days. A complete physical examination shows white plaques in the mouth with an erythematous base. The plaques stick to the mucous membranes tightly and bleed when scraped. The nurse would suspect which condition?

1. Chickenpox
2. Herpes lesions
3. Measles
4. Oral candidiasis

88. 4. Oral candidiasis, or thrush, is a painful inflammation that can affect the tongue, soft and hard palates, and buccal mucosa. Chickenpox, or varicella, causes open ulcerations of the mucous membranes. Herpes lesions are usually vesicular ulcerations of the oral mucosa around the lips. Measles that form Koplik's spots can be identified as pinpoint white elevated lesions.
CN: Physiological integrity; CNS: Physiological adaptation; CL: Application

CN: Client needs category CNS: Client needs subcategory CL: Cognitive level

89. A child was found unconscious at home and brought to the emergency department by the fire and rescue unit. Physical examination showed cherry-red mucous membranes, nail beds, and skin. Which cause is the most likely explanation for the child's condition?

1. Aspirin ingestion
2. Carbon monoxide poisoning
3. Hydrocarbon ingestion
4. Spider bite

90. A 14-year-old diagnosed with acne vulgaris asks what causes it. Which factor should the nurse identify for this client? Select all that apply.

1. Chocolates and sweets
2. Increased hormone levels
3. Growth of anaerobic bacteria
4. Caffeine
5. Heredity
6. Fatty foods

91. Which term describes a fungal infection found on the upper arm?

1. Tinea capitis
2. Tinea corporis
3. Tinea cruris
4. Tinea pedis

92. A 15-kg infant is started on amoxicillin/clavulanate potassium (Augmentin) therapy, 200 mg/5 ml, for cellulitis. The dose is 40 mg/kg over 24 hours given three times daily. How many milliliters would be given for each dose?

1. 2.5 ml
2. 5 ml
3. 15 ml
4. 20 ml

93. A 5-year-old male sustained third-degree burns to the right upper extremity after tipping over a frying pan. Which skin structures would the nurse include when explaining a third-degree burn to the child's mother?

1. Epidermis only
2. Epidermis and dermis
3. All skin layers and nerve endings
4. Skin layers, nerve endings, muscles, tendons, and bones

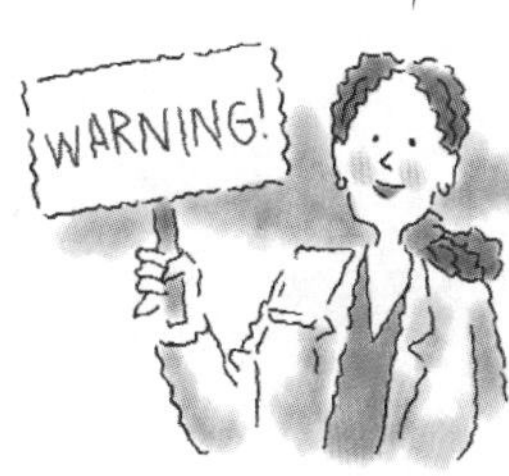

Be careful!
There may be more than one correct answer to this question.
WARNING!

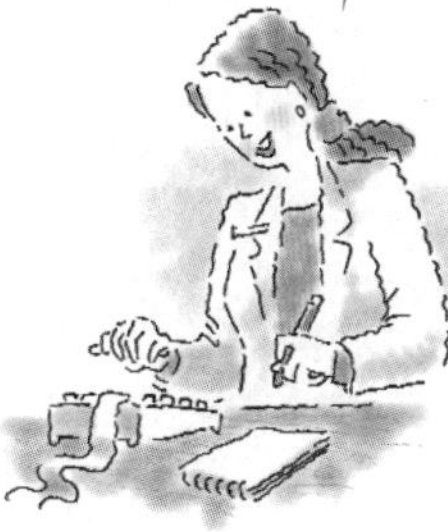

Practice with numbers makes perfect.

89. 2. Cherry-red skin changes are seen when a child has been exposed to high levels of carbon monoxide. Nausea and vomiting and pale skin are symptoms of aspirin ingestion. A hydrocarbon or petroleum ingestion usually results in respiratory symptoms and tachycardia. Spider-bite reactions are usually localized to the area of the bite.

CN: Physiological integrity; CNS: Physiological adaptation; CL: Analysis

90. 2, 3, 5. Acne vulgaris is characterized by the appearance of comedones (blackheads and whiteheads). Comedones develop for various reasons, including increased hormone levels, heredity, irritation or application of irritating substances (such as cosmetics), and growth of anaerobic bacteria. A direct relationship between acne vulgaris and consumption of chocolates, caffeine, or fatty foods hasn't been established.

CN: Physiological integrity; CNS: Physiological adaptation; CL: Application

91. 2. *Tinea corporis* describes fungal infections of the body. *Tinea capitis* describes fungal infections of the scalp. *Tinea cruris* is used to describe fungal infections of the inner thigh and inguinal creases. *Tinea pedis* is the term for fungal infections of the foot.

CN: Physiological integrity; CNS: Physiological adaptation; CL: Application

92. 2. 5 ml should be given. The dose is first calculated by multiplying the weight times the milligrams. It's then divided by three even doses. The milligrams are then used to determine the milliliters based on the concentration of the medicine. 40 mg × 15 kg = 600/3 doses = 200 mg/dose. The concentration is 200 mg in every 5 ml.

CN: Physiological integrity; CNS: Pharmacological and parenteral therapies; CL: Application

93. 3. A third-degree burn involves all of the skin layers and the nerve endings. First-degree burns involve only the epidermis. Second-degree burns affect the epidermis and dermis. Fourth-degree burns involve all skin layers, nerve endings, muscles, tendons, and bone.

CN: Physiological integrity; CNS: Physiological adaptation; CL: Application

94. A 4-year-old child has a tick embedded in the scalp. Which method should the nurse use to remove the tick?

1. Burning the tick at the skin surface
2. Surgically removing the tick
3. Grasping the tick with tweezers and applying slow, outward pressure
4. Grasping the tick with tweezers and quickly pulling the tick out

94. 3. Applying gentle outward pressure prevents injury to the skin and the retention of tick parts. Burning the tick and quickly pulling the tick out may cause injury to the skin and should be avoided. Surgical removal is indicated when tick parts have been retained.

CN: Physiological integrity; CNS: Physiological adaptation; CL: Application

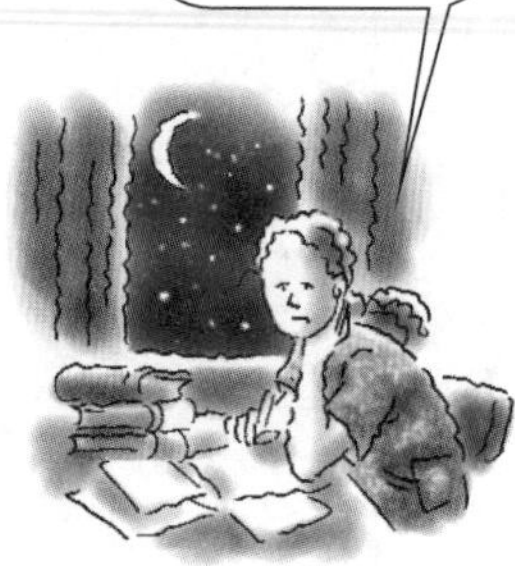

Not another math question!

95. A child with hives is prescribed diphenhydramine (Benadryl) 5 mg/kg over 24 hours in divided doses every 6 hours. The child weighs 8 kg. How many milligrams should be given with each dose?

1. 4.5 mg
2. 10 mg
3. 22 mg
4. 40 mg

95. 2. 10 mg should be given. Multiplying 5 mg by the weight (8 kg) gives the amount of milligrams for 24 hours (40 mg). Divide this by the number of doses per day (4), giving 10 mg/dose. 5 mg × 8 kg = 40 mg/4 doses = 10 mg/dose.

CN: Physiological integrity; CNS: Pharmacological and parenteral therapies; CL: Application

96. An 8-year-old child arrives at the emergency department with chemical burns to both legs. Which treatment should be performed first on this child?

1. Dilute the burns
2. Apply sterile dressings
3. Apply topical antibiotics
4. Debride and graft the burns

96. 1. Diluting the chemical is the first treatment. It will help remove the chemical and stop the burning process. The remaining treatments are initiated after dilution.

CN: Physiological integrity; CNS: Physiological adaptation; CL: Analysis

97. A 12-year-old child with full-thickness, circumferential burns to the chest has difficulty breathing. Which procedure will most likely be performed?

1. Chest tube insertion
2. Escharotomy
3. Intubation
4. Needle thoracocentesis

97. 2. Escharotomy is a surgical incision used to relieve pressure from edema. It's needed with circumferential burns that prevent chest expansion or cause circulatory compromise. Insertion of a chest tube and needle thoracocentesis are performed to relieve a pneumothorax. Intubation is performed to maintain a patent airway.

CN: Physiological integrity; CNS: Physiological adaptation; CL: Analysis

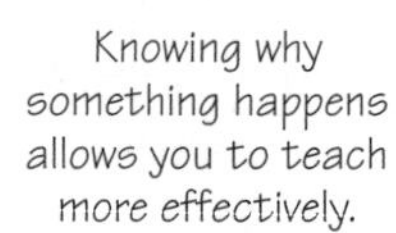

Knowing why something happens allows you to teach more effectively.

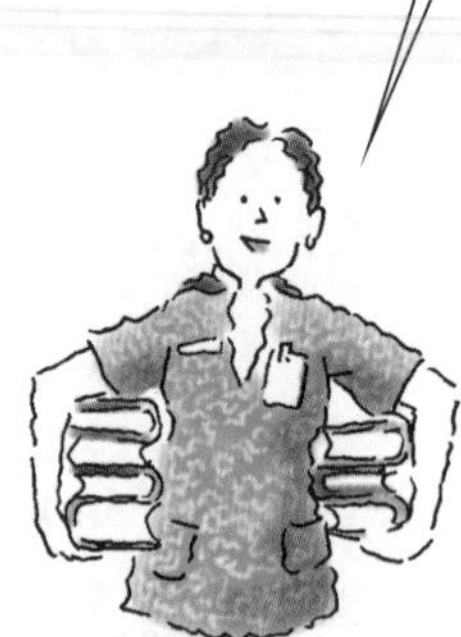

98. A 6-year-old child is evaluated after sustaining burns to his left shoulder. The parents are instructed to use moisturizing cream and protect the burn from sunlight. What's the purpose of this treatment?

1. To avoid keloids
2. To avoid scarring
3. To avoid hypopigmentation
4. To avoid hyperpigmentation

98. 4. Healed or grafted burns would require creams and protection from the sun to decrease hyperpigmentation. Scarring, hypopigmentation, and keloids aren't treated with moisturizing creams and avoidance of sunlight.

CN: Physiological integrity; CNS: Physiological adaptation; CL: Analysis

99. A child arrives in the emergency department 20 minutes after sustaining a major burn injury to 40% of his body. After initiating an I.V. line, which intervention should the nurse perform next?

1. Insert an indwelling catheter.
2. Apply Silvadene cream to the burn.
3. Shave the hair around the burn wound.
4. Obtain cultures from the deepest burn area.

100. A 12-year-old child sustains a moderate burn injury. The mother reports that the child last received a tetanus injection when he was 5 years old. An appropriate nursing intervention would be to administer which immunization?

1. 0.5 ml of tetanus toxoid I.M.
2. 0.5 ml of tetanus toxoid I.V.
3. 250 units of Hyper-Tet I.M.
4. 250 units of Hyper-Tet I.V.

101. A child arrives in the emergency department after sustaining a major burn injury. For which metabolic alterations must the nurse assess during the first 8 hours?

1. Hyponatremia and hypokalemia
2. Hyponatremia and hyperkalemia
3. Hypernatremia and hypokalemia
4. Hypernatremia and hyperkalemia

102. A child weighing 10 kg has a deep partial-thickness burn to 40% of his body surface area. The nurse will titrate this child's I.V. fluids to achieve which hourly urinary outputs?

1. 5 ml
2. 10 ml
3. 30 ml
4. 50 ml

103. A team of nurses is preparing a trauma room for the arrival of a child with partial-thickness burns to both lower extremities and portions of the trunk. Which fluid should be ready for immediate use?

1. Albumin
2. Dextrose 5% and half-normal saline
3. Lactated Ringer's solution
4. Normal saline with 2 mEq KCl/100 ml

What's the magic urinary output number here?

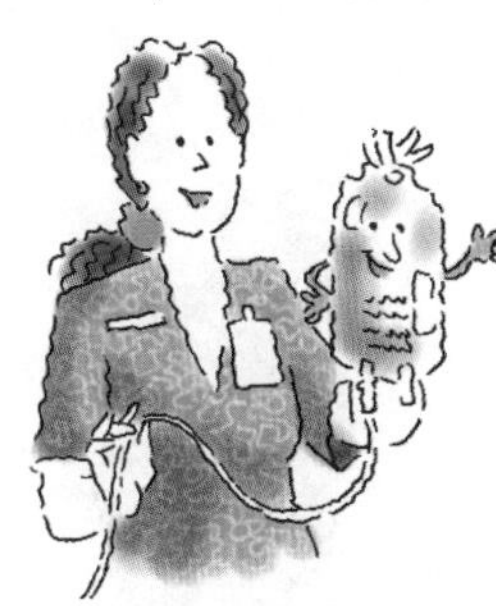

99. 1. I.V. fluids must be started immediately on all children who sustain a major burn injury to prevent the child from going into hypovolemic shock. The fluids are titrated based on urine output. To monitor this output exactly, an indwelling urinary catheter must be inserted. The other interventions will be performed, but not immediately.

CN: Physiological integrity; CNS: Reduction of risk potential; CL: Application

100. 1. Tetanus prophylaxis is given to all clients with moderate to severe burn injuries if it's longer than 5 years since the last immunization or if there is no history of immunization. The correct dosage is 0.5 ml I.M. one time if the child was immunized within 10 years. If it's more than 10 years or the child hasn't received tetanus immunization, the dosage is 250 units of Hyper-Tet one time. There is no I.V. form of tetanus available.

CN: Physiological integrity; CNS: Pharmacological and parenteral therapies; CL: Analysis

101. 2. Capillary permeability increases during the first 48 hours postburn, allowing fluids to shift from the plasma to the interstitial spaces. This fluid is high in sodium, causing the client's serum sodium level to decrease. Potassium also leaks from the cells into the plasma, causing hyperkalemia.

CN: Physiological integrity; CNS: Physiological adaptation; CL: Analysis

102. 2. Fluid resuscitation should be started on all clients with burns over more than 20% of their body surface area. In children, an hourly urine output of 1 to 2 ml/kg of body weight shows adequate kidney perfusion and fluid resuscitation. Adults should have an hourly urine output of 30 to 50 ml.

CN: Physiological integrity; CNS: Physiological adaptation; CL: Application

103. 3. Lactated Ringer's solution is recommended because it replaces the lost sodium and corrects the metabolic acidosis. The use of albumin is controversial. If albumin is given, it's as adjunct therapy and not for primary fluid replacement. The stress from a burn injury affects the glucose metabolism. Dextrose shouldn't be given during the first 24 hours as it can put the client into pseudodiabetes. The client is hyperkalemic from the potassium shift from the intracellular spaces to the plasma, and additional potassium would be detrimental.

CN: Physiological integrity; CNS: Pharmacological and parenteral therapies; CL: Application

104. A mother states that she recently received information that hand-foot-and-mouth disease has been diagnosed in a few of her child's preschool classmates. The nurse should instruct the mother to observe her child for which symptoms?

1. Low-grade fever, followed by vesicular lesions on the trunk, face, and scalp
2. Mild, self-limited eruption of vesicles on the buccal mucosa, tongue, soft palate, hands, and feet
3. Purpuric, maculopapular lesions with GI symptoms and joint pain
4. Bright red rash with a red outer border circling a bite mark

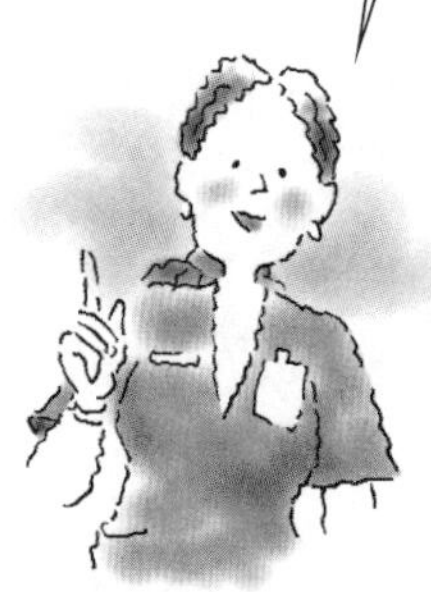

You're being asked about characteristics in question 104.

104. 2. Hand-foot-and-mouth disease is caused by coxsackievirus and usually occurs in preschool children. Vesicular lesions accompanied by a low-grade fever are typically signs of varicella. Purpura, GI symptoms, and joint pain are symptoms of Henoch-Schoenlein purpura. A bright-red bull's eye rash is a classic symptom of Lyme disease.

CN: Physiological integrity; CNS: Physiological adaptation; CL: Application

105. A 27½-lb child is receiving antibiotics for cellulitis. The order reads Pen-Vee K 40 mg/kg/day divided every 6 hours. Which dosage of antibiotics should this child receive with each dose?

1. 225 mg
2. 500 mg
3. 125 mg
4. 12.5 mg

105. 3. The dose is 125 mg. One kilogram equals 2.2 pounds so a 27½-lb child weighs 12.5 kg. 40 mg/kg/day equals a total of 500 mg given every 6 hours or 4 times in 24 hours. 500 mg divided by 4 equals 125 mg.

CN: Physiological integrity; CNS: Pharmacological and parenteral therapies; CL: Application

106. While assessing a 2-year-old child brought into the clinic with an upper respiratory infection, the nurse notes some bruising on his arms, legs, and trunk. Which findings would prompt the nurse to suspect child abuse? Select all that apply:

1. Superficial scrapes on the lower legs
2. Welts or bruises in various stages of healing on the trunk
3. A deep blue-black patch on the buttocks
4. One large bruise on the thigh
5. Circular, symmetrical burns on the lower legs
6. A parent who is hypercritical of the child and pushes the frightened child away

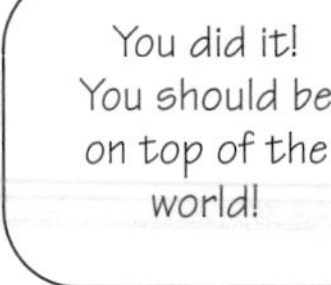

You did it! You should be on top of the world!

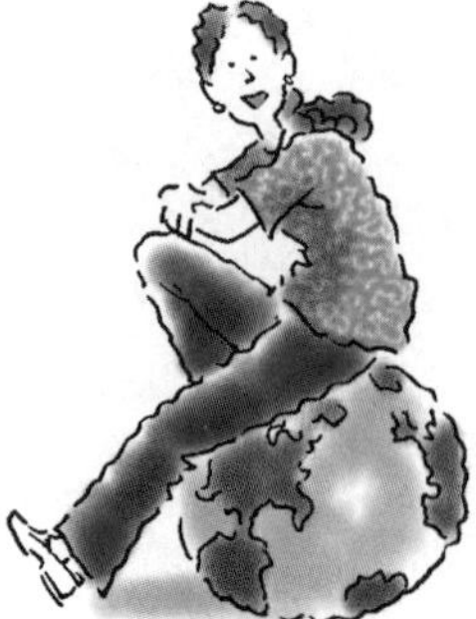

106. 2, 5, 6. Injuries at various stages of healing in protected or padded areas can be signs of inflicted trauma, leading the nurse to suspect abuse. Burns that are bilateral as well as symmetrical are typical of child abuse. The shape of the burn may resemble the item used to create it, such as a cigarette. Pushing away the child and being hypercritical are typical behaviors of abusive parents. Superficial scrapes and bruises on the lower legs are normal in a healthy, active child. A deep blue-black macular patch on the buttocks is more consistent with a Mongolian spot rather than a traumatic injury.

CN: Psychosocial integrity; CNS: None; CL: Analysis

107. A 44-lb preschooler is being treated for inflammation. The physician orders 0.2 mg/kg/day of dexamethasone by mouth to be administered every 6 hours. The elixir comes in a strength of 0.5 mg/5 ml. How many milliliters of dexamethasone should the nurse give this client per dose? Record your answer using a whole number.

______________________ milliliters

107. 10. To perform this dosage calculation, convert the child's weight from pounds to kilograms: 44 lb ÷ 2.2 lb/kg = 20 kg. Then calculate the total daily dose: 20 kg × 0.2 mg/kg/day = 4 mg. Next, calculate the amount to be given at each dose: 4 mg ÷ 4 doses = 1 mg/dose. The elixir contains 0.5 mg of drug per 5 ml. To give 1 mg of drug, administer 10 ml to the child at each dose.

CN: Physiological integrity; CNS: Pharmacological and parenteral therapies; CL: Analysis

Part VI Issues in nursing

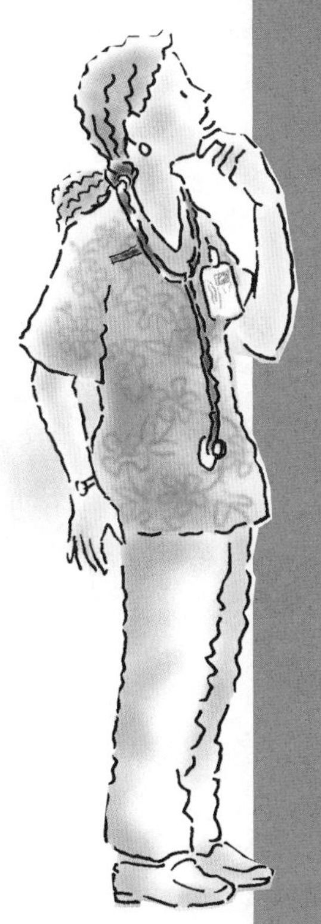

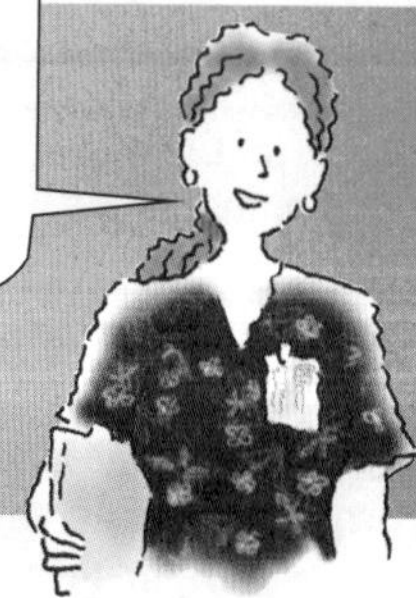

Chapter 36 Management & leadership

1. A nurse-manager of a 20-bed coronary care unit isn't on duty when a staff nurse makes a serious medication error. A client, who received an overdose of medication, nearly dies. Which statement accurately reflects the accountability of the nurse-manager?

1. The nursing supervisor on duty will call the nurse-manager at home and apprise her of the problem.
2. Because the nurse-manager is off duty, she isn't accountable for incidents that occur in her absence. Therefore, the nurse-manager won't be notified.
3. The nurse-manager will be informed of the incident when returning to work on Monday because the nurse-manager was officially off duty when the incident took place.
4. Although the nurse-manager is off duty, the nursing supervisor decides to call the nurse-manager if time permits; the supervisor believes that the manager has no responsibility for what happened during the manager's absence.

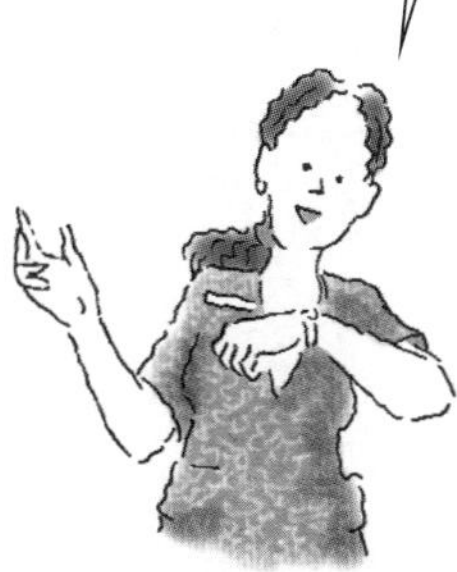

1. 1. The nurse-manager is accountable for what happens on the unit 24 hours per day, 7 days per week. If a serious problem occurs, the nurse-manager should be notified as soon as possible. The other choices don't accurately reflect the accountability of the nurse-manager's position.

CN: Safe, effective care environment; CNS: Safety and infection control; CL: Analysis

2. A community health nurse is working with disaster relief following a flood. As the nurse works with the community in the post-disaster cycle, a variety of prevention measures are employed. Providing counseling and support for families who have lost their homes is an example of which level of prevention?

1. Aggregate care prevention
2. Primary prevention
3. Secondary prevention
4. Tertiary prevention

2. 4. Tertiary prevention involves reducing the degree and quantity of injury, disability, and damage following a disaster or crisis. Aggregate prevention isn't a level of care prevention. Primary prevention focuses on keeping the crisis or disaster from happening. The goal of secondary prevention is to reduce the duration and intensity of the disaster or crisis.

CN: Safe, effective care environment; CNS: Management of care; CL: Application

3. A staff nurse on a busy pediatric unit is an excellent role model for her colleagues. She encourages them to participate in the unit's decision-making process and helps them improve their clinical skills. This nurse is functioning effectively in which role?

1. Manager
2. Autocrat
3. Leader
4. Authority

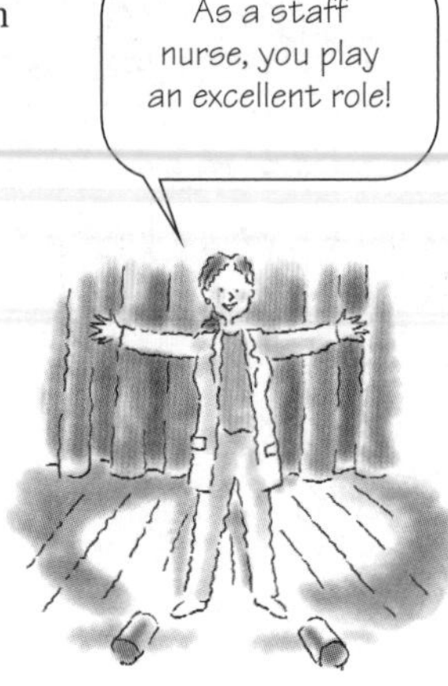

As a staff nurse, you play an excellent role!

3. 3. A leader doesn't always have formal power and authority but influences the success of a unit by being an excellent role model and by guiding, encouraging, and facilitating professional growth and development. A manager has formal power and authority from the status within the organization, and such power and authority is detailed in the manager's job description. An autocrat isn't interested in guiding or encouraging staff or in being an effective role model. Authority, a characteristic of a managerial position, is given by virtue of position within an organization.

CN: Safe, effective care environment; CNS: Management of care; CL: Application

4. The managers of the physical and occupational therapy neurologic departments have expressed concern to a nurse-manager of an adult neurologic rehabilitation unit that clients have been arriving late for therapy. In response, the nursing staff of the rehabilitation unit has complained that therapy schedules don't allow sufficient time for performing nursing interventions. Which action by the nurse-manager is the best solution to this problem?

1. Meet with the managers of physical and occupational therapy and determine how to reschedule clients. The nurse-manager will inform the staff of the changes.
2. Tell the nursing staff that they need to determine how to transport clients to therapy according to the schedules developed by the therapists.
3. Meet with the managers of physical and occupational therapy and identify several possible ways to solve the problem. Ask the adult neurologic rehabilitation staff for input and then make the final decision in conjunction with the therapy managers.
4. Ask several of the nursing leaders in the adult neurologic rehabilitation unit to work with the therapy staff to identify the best way to solve this problem. Ask the rehabilitation staff to solicit input from their colleagues and to keep the nurse-manager informed as they work on this project. Let the rehabilitation staff know that the nurse-manager is available as a resource.

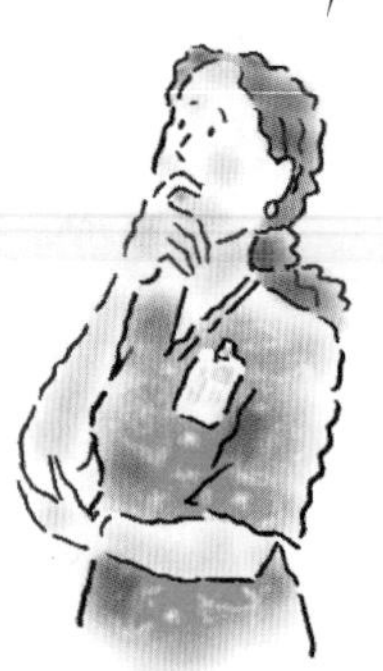

Look! It's your first hint in this chapter!

4. 4. In this situation, functioning as a democratic leader is best. The nursing and therapy staffs who deal with the day-to-day problems of direct client care have the best grasp of the situation and should have autonomy to solve problems. The manager, however, should be available to help. Option 1 reflects the style of an autocratic manager. Without staff input, the nurse-manager won't have the necessary information to identify the best solution. By simply telling the nursing staff to follow the therapists' schedules, the nurse-manager has abdicated responsibility for problem solving (laissez-faire manager), yet the problem still exists. In participative management, the staff is encouraged to share their ideas, but the manager retains the authority to make final decisions. The resentment and frustration comes from the fact that the actual decision made by the manager may not include input from the staff.

CN: Safe, effective care environment; CNS: Management of care; CL: Analysis

5. The staff of an outpatient clinic has formed a task force to develop new procedures for swift, safe evacuation of the unit. The new procedures haven't been reviewed, approved, or shared with all personnel. When the nurse-manager receives word of a bomb threat, the task force members push for evacuating the unit using the new procedures. Which action should the nurse-manager take?

1. Determine that the procedures currently in place must be followed and direct staff to follow them without question.
2. Tell staff members to use whatever procedures they feel are best.
3. Ask staff members to quickly meet among themselves and decide what procedures to follow.
4. Tell staff members to assemble in the staff lounge; there the nurse-manager will quickly gather opinions about evacuation procedures before deciding what to do.

5. 1. In an emergency, such as a bomb scare, the nurse-manager must determine, without hesitation, the best action for the safety and welfare of clients and staff. Allowing staff members to do whatever they think best will cause confusion and inefficient client evacuation, because no one will know how to function effectively as a team during the crisis. Taking time to have staff meet, or gathering opinions about what to do, wastes valuable time.

CN: Safe, effective care environment; CNS: Safety and infection control; CL: Analysis

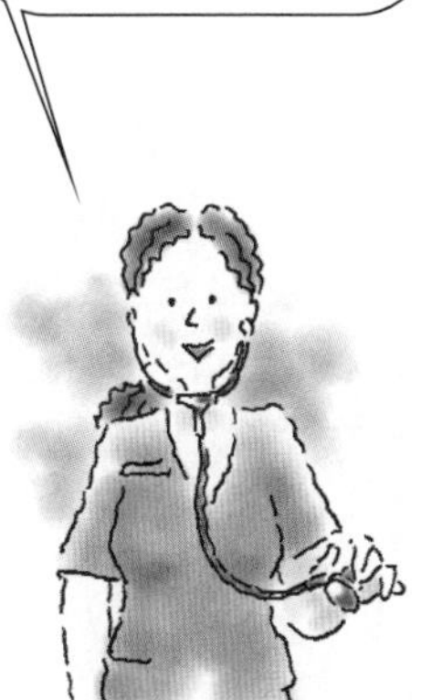

In question 6, it's essential that you know the elements of an NCDS.

6. The selection of a nursing care delivery system (NCDS) is critical to the success of a nursing area. Which factor is <u>essential</u> to the evaluation of an NCDS?

1. Determining how planned absences, such as vacation time, will be scheduled so that all staff are treated fairly
2. Identifying who will be responsible for making client care decisions
3. Deciding what type of dress code will be implemented
4. Identifying salary ranges for various types of staff

6. 2. Determining who has responsibility for making decisions regarding client care is an essential element of all client care delivery systems. Dress code, salary, and scheduling planned staff absences are important to any organization but aren't actually determined by the NCDS.

CN: Safe, effective care environment; CNS: Management of care; CL: Application

7. A nurse-manager on an oncology unit has been informed that she must determine which nursing care delivery system (NCDS) is best for efficient client care, client satisfaction, and cost reduction. Knowing that two or three registered nurses, four licensed practical nurses, and five nursing assistants are generally on duty on each shift, and that the unit environment supports grouping clients together by geographic areas, the nurse-manager and the staff recommend adoption of which NCDS?

1. Functional nursing
2. Case management
3. Team nursing
4. Primary nursing

7. 3. Team nursing is efficient and costs less to implement than primary or case management systems. Because the staff members know each other well, they can function effectively as a team. Although functional nursing is the most cost effective, care is commonly fragmented and client satisfaction decreased. Case management and primary nursing require more registered nurses than are available.

CN: Safe, effective care environment; CNS: Management of care; CL: Analysis

8. On a busy medical-surgical unit, a winter storm has prevented most of the staff members from getting to work. One registered nurse, two licensed practical nurses, and three nursing assistants have been able to get to work. The nurse-manager must decide which nursing care delivery system should be implemented for the best possible client care during this staffing crisis. The nurse-manager directs the staff to implement which delivery system?

1. Team nursing
2. Primary nursing
3. Functional nursing
4. Case management

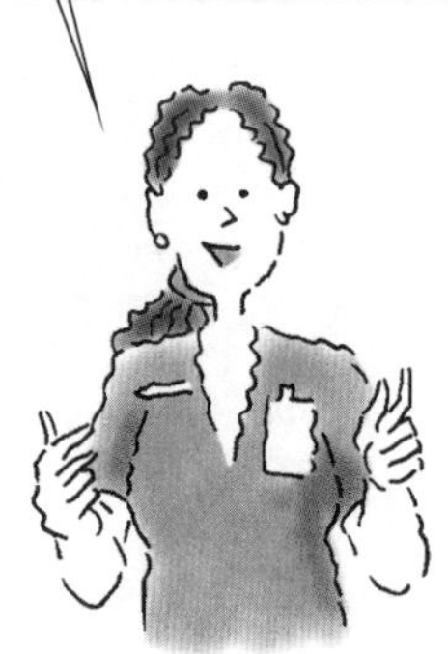

During a crisis, which delivery system functions the best? That's a hint!

8. 3. Functional nursing best uses the skills of all staff in a timely manner during this crisis. This delivery system requires the least staff and delegates tasks to those who can best perform them. Team nursing doesn't allow for the best use of a limited number of staff who must care for a large number of clients. Primary nursing and case management require more registered nurses than are currently available.
CN: Safe, effective care environment; CNS: Management of care; CL: Analysis

9. A nurse-manager in the office of a group of surgeons has received complaints from discharged clients about inadequate instructions for performing home care. Knowing the importance of good, timely client education, the nurse should take which steps?

1. Contact the nurses who work in the facility and tell them that client education should be implemented as soon as the clients are admitted to either the hospital or the outpatient surgical center.
2. Review and revise the way client education is conducted in the surgeons' office.
3. Because no serious damage was done to any of the clients, the nurse-manager can safely ignore their complaints.
4. Work with the surgeons and nursing staff in the hospital and outpatient surgical center to evaluate current client education practices and revise as needed.

9. 4. Client education is the responsibility of all nurses providing care to the client, and the nurses must work together to establish the best methods. The most appropriate response is to contact the nurse-manager, not the nursing staff, at the facility. Evaluating client education in one setting only doesn't consider the entire process and the staff providing it. No complaint should be ignored. Patient education is an important nursing responsibility.
CN: Safe, effective care environment; CNS: Safety and infection control; CL: Application

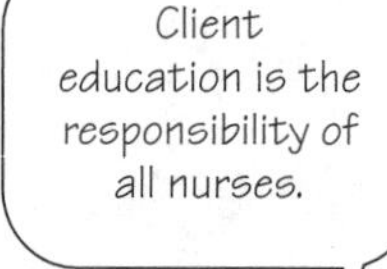

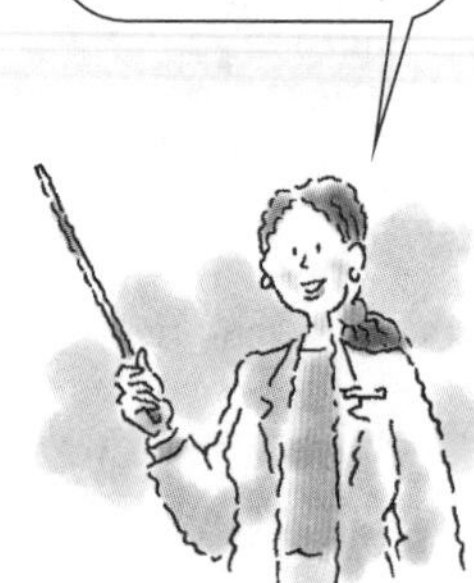

10. A nurse-manager of an intensive care unit (ICU) can't be held legally responsible in a court of law for which action performed by the unit's staff?

1. A nursing assistant administers medications to a client in ICU.
2. A staff nurse refuses to follow a physician's order to administer medication because administering the dosage ordered could seriously harm the client.
3. A nursing assistant attempts to initiate I.V. therapy.
4. A staff nurse fills a client prescription at the hospital pharmacy because the pharmacist on duty is busy.

10. 2. The nurse-manager is legally responsible for actions that fall within the scope of practice of the staff members who perform them. A nurse may not knowingly administer or perform tasks that will harm a client. It's within a nurse's scope of practice to refuse to carry out such orders. Administering medications and initiating I.V. therapy aren't within the scope of practice for nursing assistants. A staff nurse isn't licensed to fill prescriptions.
CN: Safe, effective care environment; CNS: Management of care; CL: Analysis

11. A primary nurse in the unit tells the nurse-manager that a newly hired registered nurse needs an additional week of orientation to function effectively on the staff. Which action is <u>most</u> appropriate for the nurse-manager?

1. Tell the primary nurse that the new nurse must finish orientation in 6 weeks because of a staffing shortage.
2. Meet with the new nurse and the primary nurse and help set up an additional week of orientation.
3. Fire the new nurse because the unit is short-staffed and nurses who can complete the orientation process in the normal length of time are needed.
4. Schedule a staff meeting to find out if there are problems with the orientation process.

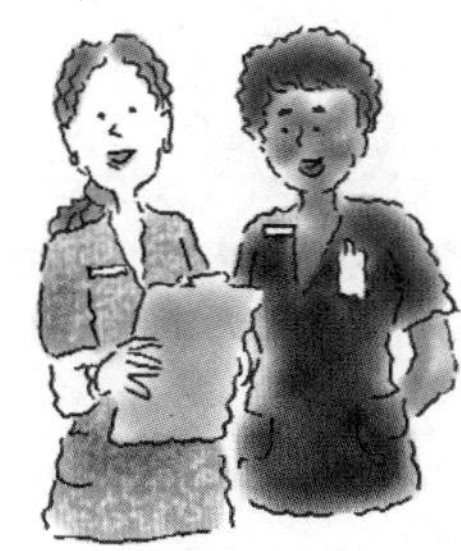

It's important to manage the workload and learn to delegate.

11. 2. The nurse-manager is responsible for adequate orientation of new staff. Needing additional orientation doesn't mean that a nurse isn't competent. However, the new nurse should know what's expected of her and the time frame in which she must accomplish the expectations. Firing the new nurse isn't the answer because she's apparently close to completing orientation and only needs an additional week to function effectively. Periodically reviewing and revising the orientation process is a good idea. However, in this case, the most appropriate course of action is to help the new nurse complete her orientation as efficiently as possible.

CN: Safe, effective care environment; CNS: Management of care; CL: Analysis

12. Delegation is the process of transferring work to subordinates. A nurse-manager can appropriately delegate which task?

1. Scheduling staff assignments for the next month
2. Terminating a nursing assistant for insubordination
3. Deciding on salary increases for licensed practical nurses after they complete orientation
4. Telling a staff nurse to initiate disciplinary action against one of her peers

12. 1. Scheduling may be safely and appropriately delegated. Termination, disciplinary action, and salary increases shouldn't be delegated to staff who don't have the power and authority to take such actions.

CN: Safe, effective care environment; CNS: Management of care; CL: Analysis

13. A nurse-manager appropriately behaves as an autocrat in which situation?

1. Planning vacation time for staff
2. Directing staff activities if a client has a cardiac arrest
3. Evaluating a new medication administration process
4. Identifying the strengths and weaknesses of a client education video

13. 2. In a crisis situation, the nurse-manager should take command for the benefit of the client. Planning vacation time and evaluating procedures and client resources require staff input characteristic of a democratic or participative manager.

CN: Safe, effective care environment; CNS: Management of care; CL: Application

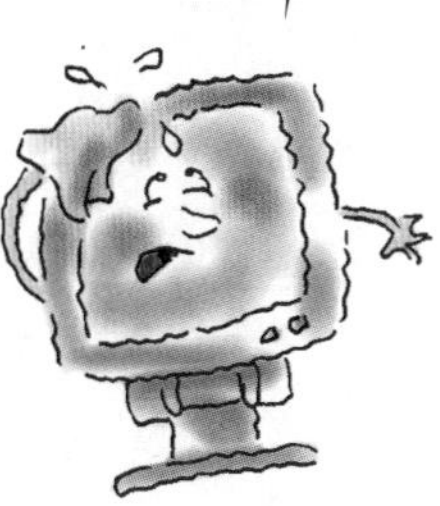

I think I may be on the way out!

14. The nurse-manager is asked to provide a unit budget for the next quarter. In the development of the budget, a variance is projected based on personnel costs. To minimize this variance, the nurse-manager would be advised to:

1. tell the staff that they cannot do any overtime.
2. reduce the use of outside agency personnel.
3. reduce the client census on the unit, thereby reducing the nurse-client ratio.
4. increase the client-to-nurse ratio.

14. 2. Reducing the use of outside agency personnel is the most appropriate way to minimize costs, as there is often an overhead cost of 60% or more for outside agency staff. It is generally less expensive and in the interest of client safety to rearrange staffing patterns for the usual staff to provide coverage, rather than reducing the client census or increasing client-to-nurse ratio.

CN: Safe, effective care environment; CNS: Management of care; CL: Application

15. A nurse-manager delegates responsibility for the review and revision of the surgical unit's client education materials. Which statement illustrates the best method of delegation?

1. Tell the nursing staff they're responsible for the review and revision and that their recommendations for improving the materials are welcome.
2. Ask two of the best staff nurses to form a task force to review and revise client education materials. Explain that they should solicit input from clients and staff members, complete this task within 6 weeks, and submit recommendations in writing.
3. Tell the nursing staff that the education materials aren't satisfactory. Explain that the staff should select people to review them and make recommendations for change. Tell them that the nurse-manager will make the final decisions about changes.
4. Ask the assistant manager to develop a plan for the review and revision of client education materials.

15. 2. Delegation must be done clearly and precisely. The nurse-manager must assign responsibility, identify the task to be accomplished, explain what outcomes are needed, and the time frame for completing the work. The remaining options don't give clear explanations of work to be done, don't clearly assign responsibility or the specific outcomes desired, and don't establish a time frame for completion of the task.

CN: Safe, effective care environment; CNS: Management of care; CL: Application

16. A nurse-manager works for a nonprofit health care corporation in which there has been significant revenue over expenses for the year. The nurse-manager has been told to anticipate which action?

1. Receipt a portion of the revenue to improve client services on the unit.
2. Revenue will be identified as profit.
3. Revenue will be divided among stockholders as dividends.
4. Reduction of operating expenses to help the organization pay taxes on the revenue.

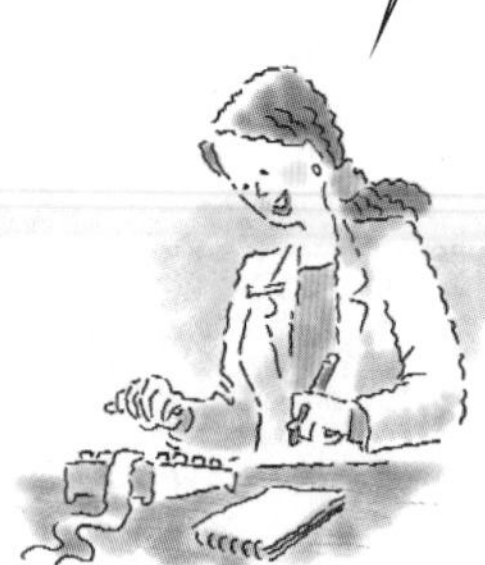

How did we accrue all of this revenue? What shall I do about it?

16. 1. Revenue over expenses in a nonprofit organization is tax-exempt and is usually reinvested in the organization and used to improve services. A for-profit organization calls its revenue over expenses a profit and the revenue can be divided as a dividend among stockholders or reinvested in the organization.

CN: Safe, effective care environment; CNS: Management of care; CL: Application

17. The nurse-manager meets with a staff nurse to evaluate performance after the six-month probationary period. As part of the evaluation process, the nurse-manager would ask the staff nurse to:

1. accept the nurse-manager's evaluation by signing in agreement.
2. contribute a self-evaluation and suggested areas for future growth.
3. have peers vouch for his/her performance.
4. establish a plan for strengthening deficiencies by completing continuing education at the staff nurse's own expense.

17. 2. Performance evaluation is a primary managerial function for nurse managers. Professional growth of staff requires a self-reflective approach and evaluation and goal-setting. A performance evaluation need not be agreed to in full by staff. Peer evaluation is used in some settings, but is done in a systematic way with clear criteria rather than informal "vouching." Staff development is usually the responsibility of the employing institution.

CN: Safe, effective care environment; CNS: Management of care; CL: Application

18. A nurse-manager of an outpatient physical medicine and rehabilitation facility isn't satisfied with the policies and procedures of discharge planning. The manager knows other managers at similar facilities that are regarded as the "best" in the country. As part of a quality-improvement process she decides to take which steps?

1. Contact the nurse-managers at the best facilities and compare their discharge planning policies and procedures with those of her facility. After making the comparison, the nurse-manager will share the information with her staff and together they'll make recommendations.
2. Ask her staff nurses to investigate discharge policies and procedures at other outpatient rehabilitation facilities and provide recommendations for changes. The nurse-manager will present staff findings to administration.
3. Contact the nurse-managers at the best facilities and ask them for copies of their discharge planning policies and procedures. Then the nurse-manager can change her policies and procedures to match those at the best facilities.
4. Ask the staff nurses to form a task force for reviewing and revising the current discharge policies and procedures.

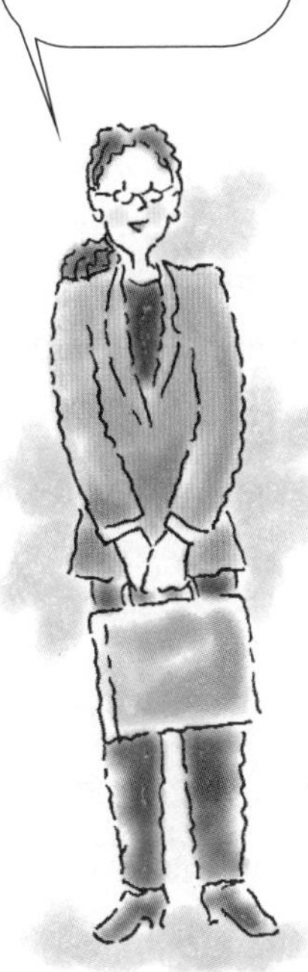
You're
managing this
chapter quite
well.

18. 1. Benchmarking is a good approach for the nurse-manager to take; it's the process of comparing the delivery of client care practices in one organization to those in the best health care organizations. Because the nurse-manager already has contacts at the best facilities, she's the most appropriate person to obtain the necessary information. The nurse-manager, however, shouldn't automatically change her policies and procedures to match those of the best facilities. Instead, she should evaluate the policies to determine which ones might be implemented at her facility, then make recommendations for change in conjunction with her staff. Asking her staff to form a task force is a good idea, but benchmarking is a practice that saves time and effort and allows information to be obtained from excellent resources.

CN: Safe, effective care environment; CNS: Management of care; CL: Application

19. A nurse-manager of a medical-surgical unit reviews this month's risk management data, and notices that a number of incident reports have been completed due to 6 p.m. medications being administered late. Dinner is served between 5:30 p.m. and 6 p.m. Staff take their dinner breaks between 5 p.m. and 6:30 p.m. Based on this information, which is the <u>most</u> appropriate action from the nurse-manager?

1. Terminate the nurses responsible for failing to administer medications on time.
2. Decide that the staff must not take dinner breaks until at least 7 p.m.
3. Decide that the kitchen staff must change the time they deliver supper trays.
4. Review the process of administering medication including the time medications are administered, staff and client dinner times, the number of medications to be administered at 6 p.m., and the number of staff available between 5 and 6 p.m.

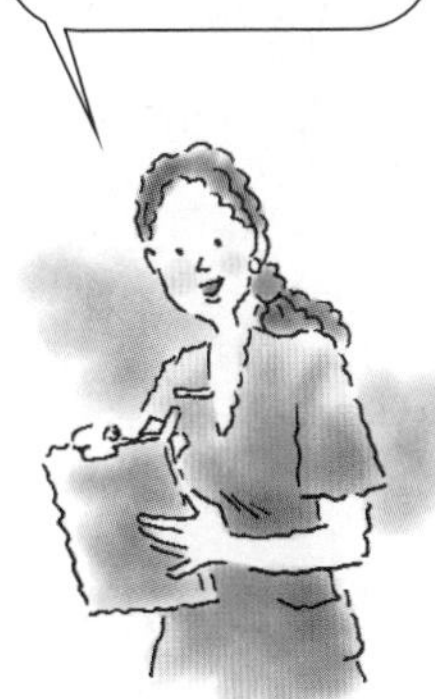
Be sensitive
to time when
evaluating risk
management
findings.

19. 4. An effective nurse-manager knows that to evaluate risk management findings accurately, she must look at the entire process and circumstances surrounding each incident. Terminating staff without such evaluation doesn't resolve all of the factors contributing to the problem. She can't change dinner breaks or kitchen delivery times unless she has evaluated how these factors influence medication administration.

CN: Safe, effective care environment; CNS: Management of care; CL: Analysis

20. Performance improvement is an important component of continuous quality improvement. Which action should an effective nurse-manager take when conducting performance evaluations?

1. Conduct performance evaluations in a group setting so input from peers and subordinates is considered when evaluating a staff member's effectiveness.
2. Provide feedback on strengths as well as areas for improvement and clarify what the staff member is expected to accomplish before the next performance evaluation.
3. Document areas for improvement in writing. Areas of strength don't need to be documented because these areas are complementary and don't describe actions the staff member must take to improve.
4. Delegate responsibility for conducting performance evaluations to primary nurses whenever possible to help them grow professionally.

20. 2. An effective performance evaluation provides recognition of strengths, identifies areas for improvement, and clarifies performance expectations. Performance evaluations should be done in private, not in front of others. All components of a performance evaluation should be documented in writing. Although input from staff members can be useful in preparing performance evaluations, delegating all responsibility to others is inappropriate. The nurse-manager is responsible for the performance of the staff.

CN: Safe, effective care environment; CNS: Management of care; CL: Application

21. The manager of an outpatient clinic is explaining the various health care delivery systems to a client who's interested in joining a system with a reasonable fixed capitation rate. Which organization is the client primarily interested in joining?

1. A preferred provider organization (PPO)
2. A managed-care organization
3. A health-maintenance organization (HMO)
4. A privately funded insurance company

21. 3. An HMO provides comprehensive health services for a fixed rate of payment or capitation. A PPO pays health care expenses for members if they use a provider who's under contract to that PPO. Managed care provides beneficiaries with a variety of services for an established, agreed upon payment. A privately funded insurance company won't offer services for a fixed rate.

CN: Safe, effective care environment; CNS: Management of care; CL: Application

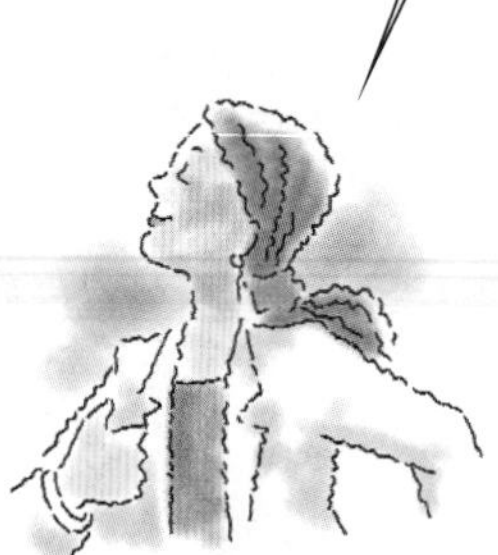

Congratulations! You're finished with this chapter. You're a natural-born leader!

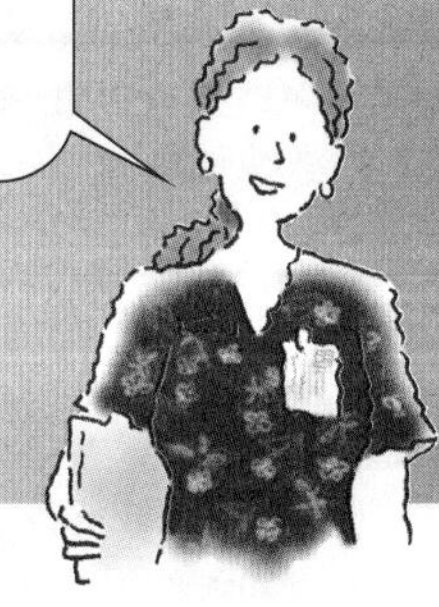

We saved the best, and most challenging, topic for last! Don't stress—you've done an excellent job!

Chapter 37 Ethical & legal issues

1. An elderly client has been admitted to the medical-surgical unit from the postanesthesia care unit. While the nurse is off the floor, the client falls out of bed and fractures his right leg and right wrist. The nurse finding him states that the "side rails were down and the bed was in the high position." Legal charges are filed against the nurse and the hospital. Which charge is the most appropriate for her actions?

1. Collective liability
2. Comparative negligence
3. Battery
4. Negligence

2. A client's attorney can file a lawsuit within which time frame?

1. Discovery rule
2. Statute of limitations
3. Grace period
4. Alternative dispute resolution

3. A client's attorney must prove which elements for a professional negligence action?

1. Duty, breach of duty, damages, and causation
2. Duty, damages, and causation
3. Duty, breach of duty, and damages
4. Breach of duty, damages, and causation

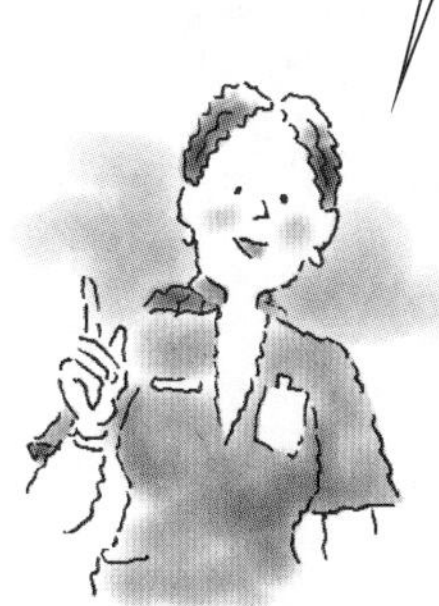

Make sure you choose the most appropriate answer.

1. 4. Negligence is a general term that denotes conduct lacking in due care. Carelessness is interpreted as a deviation from the standard of care that a reasonable person would use in a particular set of circumstances. Collective liability stems from cooperation by several manufacturers in a wrongful activity that by its nature requires group participation. Comparative negligence holds the injured parties accountable for their fault in the injury. Battery involves harmful or unwarranted contact with the client.

CN: Safe, effective care environment; CNS: Safety and infection control; CL: Analysis

2. 2. Statute of limitations is the time period during which a case must be filed or the injured party is barred from bringing the lawsuit. The statute of limitations typically gives clients 1 to 3 years from the date of discovery to file a lawsuit. However, the time may vary from state to state. Discovery rule is the actual term for the client's discovery of the injury. Grace period refers to any period specified in a contract during which payment is permitted, without penalty, beyond the due date of the debt. Alternative dispute resolution refers to any means of settling disputes outside the courtroom setting.

CN: Safe, effective care environment; CNS: Safety and infection control; CL: Application

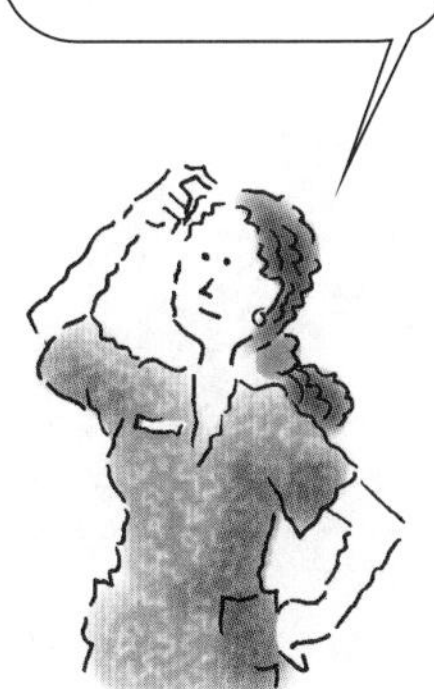

The four D's? Could the first D be for dumb?

3. 1. Any professional negligence action must meet four demands—commonly known as the four D's—to be considered negligence and result in legal action: a **d**uty for the health care professional to provide care to the person making the claim, a **d**ereliction (breach) of that duty, the breach of duty resulted in **d**amages, and the damages were caused by a **d**irect result of the negligence (causation).

CN: Safe, effective care environment; CNS: Management of care; CL: Application

CN: Client needs category CNS: Client needs subcategory CL: Cognitive level

4. Which guidelines define and regulate the scope of the nursing professional practice (that is, set rules on what a nurse can and can't do as a professional)?
1. State legislature
2. Facilities policies and procedures
3. Standards of Care
4. Nurse Practice Act

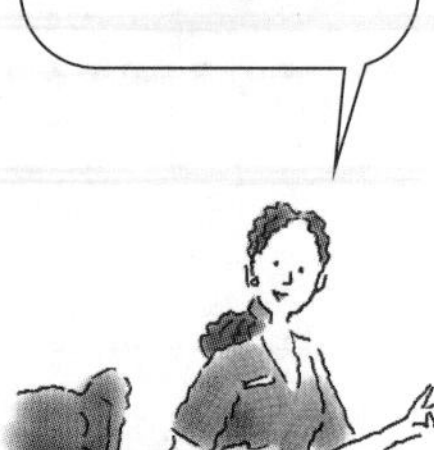
Do you know your state's Nurse Practice Act?

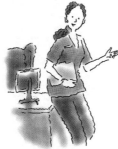

4. 4. The Nurse Practice Act is a series of statutes, enacted by each state legislature, that outline the legal scope of nursing practice within a particular state. The act sets educational requirements for the nurse, distinguishes between nursing practice and medical practice, and defines the scope of nursing practice. State legislatures set acts that create boards of nursing within each state but they don't regulate the scope of nursing. Facility policies and procedures govern the practice in that particular facility. Standards of Care, which are criteria that serve as a basis for comparison when evaluating the quality of nursing practice, are established by federal, accreditation, state, and professional organizations.

CN: Safe, effective care environment; CNS: Management of care; CL: Application

5. A 45-year-old client who's a member of the Jehovah's Witnesses refuses a blood transfusion based on his religious beliefs and practices. The client's decision must be followed based on which ethical principle?
1. The right to die
2. Advance directive
3. The right to refuse treatment
4. Substituted judgment

5. 3. The right to refuse treatment is an ethical principle of respect for the autonomy of the individual. The client can refuse treatment if he's competent and aware of the risks and complications associated with that refusal. The right to die involves whether to initiate or withhold life-sustaining treatment for a client who is irreversibly comatose, vegetative, or suffering with end-stage terminal illness. An advance directive is a document used as a guideline for starting or continuing life-sustaining medical care; the client commonly has a terminal disease or disability and can't indicate his own wishes. Substituted judgment is an ethical principle used when a decision is made for an incapacitated client.

CN: Safe, effective care environment; CNS: Management of care; CL: Application

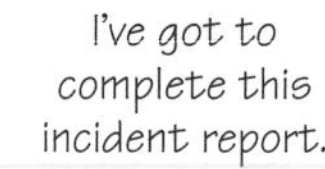
I've got to complete this incident report.

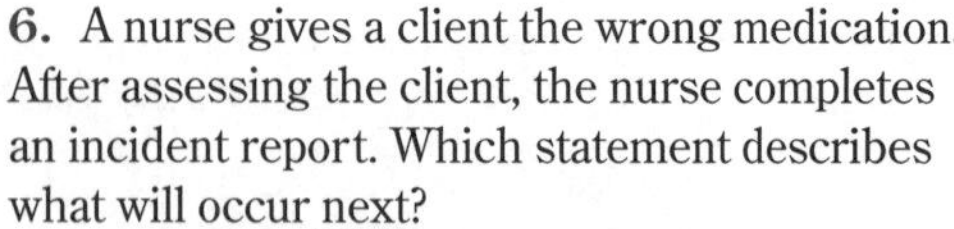

6. A nurse gives a client the wrong medication. After assessing the client, the nurse completes an incident report. Which statement describes what will occur next?
1. The incident will be reported to the state board of nursing for disciplinary action.
2. The incident will be documented in the nurse's personnel file.
3. The medication error will result in the nurse being suspended and, possibly, terminated from employment at the facility.
4. The incident report will be used to promote quality care and risk management.

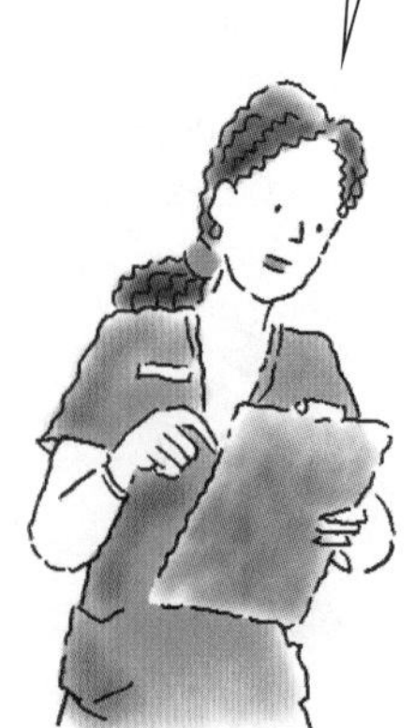

6. 4. Unusual occurrences and deviations from care are documented on incident reports. Incident reports are internal to the facility and are used to evaluate care, determine potential risks, or system problems that could have contributed to the error. This type of error won't result in a report to the state board of nursing or in suspension of the nurse. Some facilities do track the number of errors by a nurse or on particular units; the purpose of tracking errors is to provide appropriate education and to improve the nursing process.

CN: Safe, effective care environment; CNS: Management of care; CL: Analysis

7. While giving change of shift report to the oncoming night shift nurse, the evening shift nurse smells alcohol on the night shift nurse's breath. The evening shift nurse should:

1. immediately report this finding to the nursing supervisor.
2. observe the nurse for other signs of intoxication.
3. leave a note for the nurse-manager when she arrives in the morning.
4. ask the nurse if she has been drinking.

7. 1. The evening shift nurse is liable to report a situation that could cause an unsafe situation for clients. She should immediately report the situation to the nursing supervisor. Observing for other signs of intoxication isn't the nurse's responsibility. The situation requires immediate attention; leaving a note is inappropriate. The evening shift nurse should not confront the night shift nurse; the supervisor should.

CN: Safe, effective care environment; CNS: Management of care; CL: Analysis

8. In which way do nurses play a key role in error prevention?

1. Identifying incorrect dosages or potential interactions of prescribed medications
2. Never questioning the order of a physician because he's ultimately responsible for the client outcome
3. Notifying the Occupational Safety and Health Association (OSHA) of violations in the workplace
4. Informing the client of his bill of rights as a client

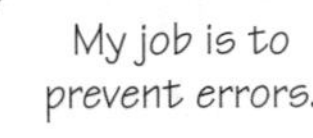
My job is to prevent errors.

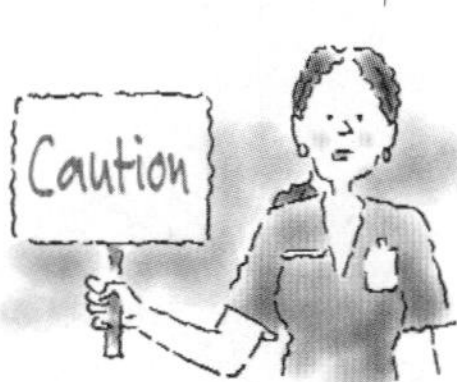
Caution

8. 1. Nurses must be knowledgeable about drug dosages and possible interactions when administering medications; they must follow appropriate policies to correct dosage errors or potential interactions. The nurse is responsible for questioning unclear or ambiguous physician orders and should never carry out an order she feels uncomfortable about. Notifying OSHA doesn't solve medication errors. OSHA establishes comprehensive safety and health standards, inspects workplaces, and requires employers to eliminate safety hazards. The client should be aware of client rights, but that awareness doesn't play a key role in error prevention.

CN: Safe, effective care environment; CNS: Safety and infection control; CL: Application

9. A nurse-attorney is teaching a class of nurses about informed consent. Which statement is true concerning informed consent?

1. Minors are permitted to give informed consent.
2. The professional nurse and physician may both obtain informed consent.
3. The client must be fully informed regarding treatment, tests, surgery, and the risks and benefits prior to giving informed consent.
4. Mentally competent and incompetent clients can legally give informed consent.

9. 3. When the professional nurse is involved in the informed consent process, the nurse is only witnessing the consent process and doesn't actually obtain the consent. Only a minor who is married or emancipated can give informed consent. Obtaining consent is the responsibility of the physician. Legally, the client must be mentally competent to give consent for procedures.

CN: Safe, effective care environment; CNS: Management of care; CL: Application

10. Which statement is correct regarding Section 1138, Title XI, of the Omnibus Reconciliation Act of 1986?

1. All families of clients who are nearing death or have died must be approached with the option of organ and tissue donation.
2. The medical examiner should be notified of all potential organ donors.
3. A request must be made to the family regarding release of the donor's name.
4. Hospitals aren't responsible for establishing designated requesters for donation.

10. 1. The federal Omnibus Reconciliation Act of 1986 mandates that all hospitals establish written protocols for the identification of potential organ and tissue donors. The act sets standards for organ procurement agencies. The medical examiner should be notified if the client is a potential organ or tissue donor only if the medical examiner is involved in the case. Requesters for donation are health care professionals who have received special training on properly approaching family members regarding organ or tissue donation.

CN: Safe, effective care environment; CNS: Management of care; CL: Application

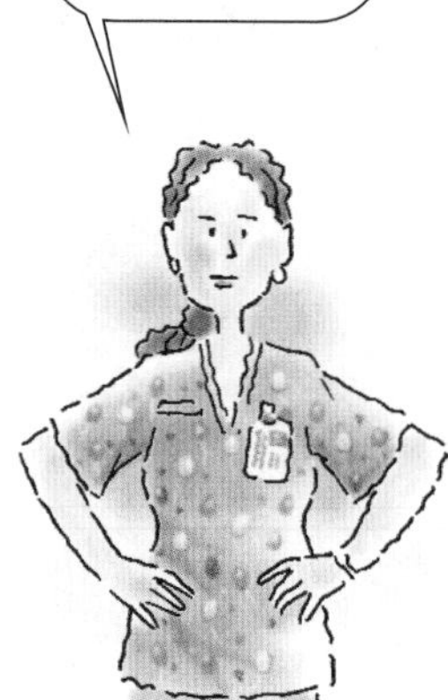

Question 11 brings up a sensitive and serious topic.

11. Which guideline should a nurse keep in mind when approaching a family for organ or tissue donation?

1. Approaching a family is done only with a physician's approval and written order.
2. The requester doesn't have to believe in the benefits of organ donation but should support the process with a positive attitude.
3. The requester is knowledgeable about the basics of organ and tissue donation and is capable of educating the family members about brain death early in the organ donation process.
4. The family is offered an opportunity to speak with an organ procurement coordinator.

11. 4. The family should be offered an opportunity to speak with an organ procurement coordinator. An organ procurement coordinator is knowledgeable about the organ donation process and should have exceptional interpersonal skills for dealing with grieving family members. Physician support in the process is desirable but consent or written orders aren't necessary for a referral to the organ procurement organization. The requestor must believe in the benefits of organ donation and support the process with a positive attitude. The family should be approached about speaking to an organ procurement coordinator only after the family has been made aware of the client's condition and prognosis. Approaching a family member who believes there's still hope for recovery will likely result in a negative outcome.

CN: Safe, effective care environment; CNS: Management of care; CL: Analysis

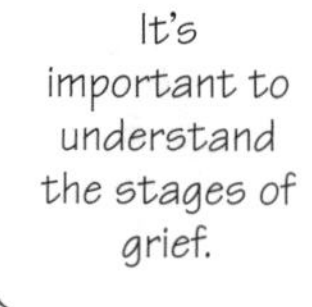

12. A nurse is discussing the stages of grief with family members. Which statement is the most accurate regarding the stages of grief?

1. The stages of grief include acceptance, depression, anger, bargaining, and denial.
2. The stages of grief include denial, anger, decreased interaction, depression, and mourning.
3. The stages of grief include acceptance, anger, denial, and bargaining.
4. The stages of grief include denial, anger, bargaining, depression, and acceptance.

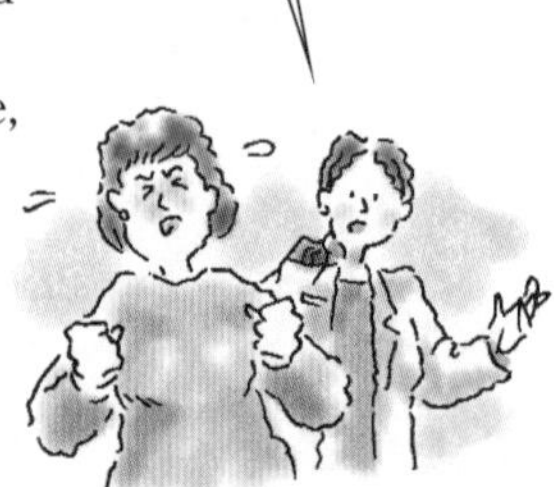

12. 4. Denial is the avoidance of death's inevitability and is the first step of the grieving process. Anger, the most intense grief reaction, arises when people realize that death and loss will actually occur or has occurred for a family member. Bargaining happens when family members attempt to stall or manipulate the outcome or death. Depression is a response to loss that's expressed as profound sadness or deep suffering. Acceptance is the final stage, and it's the ability to overcome the grief and accept what has happened.

CN: Psychosocial integrity; CNS: None; CL: Application

13. While performing an assessment of a 75-year-old client in the emergency department, a nurse notes many bruises in various stages of healing on his body. Which action should the nurse perform first?

1. Notify the nursing supervisor immediately.
2. Notify the physician.
3. Try to obtain more information from the client as to when and how these bruises occurred.
4. Document the findings.

13. 3. The nurse should first try to obtain more information from the client to complete the assessment. Without the information, she shouldn't assume that the bruises are from abuse, and she shouldn't notify her nursing supervisor until she has obtained additional facts. She should, however, inform the physician, so he can examine the client. She should follow the facility's policy and procedure for reporting abuse and document her findings.
CN: Psychosocial integrity; CNS: None; CL: Application

14. Which concept refers to the role of a professional nurse in client advocacy?

1. The nurse makes decisions for clients who can't make decisions for themselves.
2. The nurse follows the basic standards of care and hospital policies and procedures for providing care for clients.
3. The nurse promotes and protects the client's interests and rights.
4. The nurse adapts a paternalistic approach toward the care of clients.

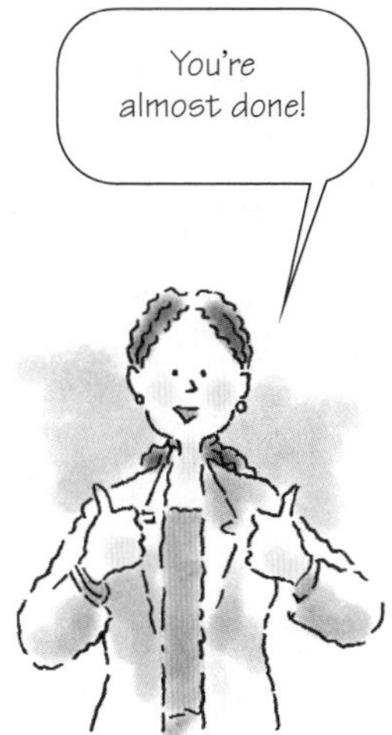

14. 3. The nurse who understands the advocacy role promotes, protects, and, thereby, advocates a client's interests and rights in an effort to make the client well. The nurse doesn't make decisions for clients, but provides care for the acutely ill client with the consent of his significant other, a power of attorney, or his living will. Standards of care are the basis for providing safe competent nursing care and set minimum criteria for proficiency on the job, enabling the nurse and others to judge the quality of care provided. Paternalism violates self-determination and advocacy by acting for another.
CN: Safe, effective care environment; CNS: Management of care; CL: Application

15. A client with a history of heart disease is scheduled for cataract surgery when he tells the nurse that he's experiencing chest discomfort and shortness of breath. The nurse administers a nitroglycerin tablet sublingually as ordered by the admitting physician but fails to notify the physician, surgeon, or anesthesiologist. If the client suffers a massive heart attack during surgery, the nurse could be held liable for which malpractice charge?

1. Failure to act as a client advocate
2. Failure to communicate with the client
3. Failure to assess, monitor, and communicate
4. Failure to protect from harm

15. 3. The nurse has a responsibility to assess, monitor, and communicate a client's status under her care. In this case, the change in the client's status could influence care during surgery and the potential outcomes. Failure to act as a client advocate has been recognized by the courts when the nurse fails to develop and implement nursing diagnoses, and fails to exercise good judgment on the client's behalf. Failure to communicate with the client refers to not adequately educating him about care, procedures, or discharge instructions. Failure to protect from harm occurs when health care providers must protect a client because of the client's vulnerable state and inability to distinguish potentially harmful situations.
CN: Safe, effective care environment; CNS: Management of care; CL: Application

16. In which circumstance may a nurse legally and ethically disclose confidential information about a client?

1. The human immunodeficiency virus (HIV) status of a single male client to his family members.
2. The diagnosis of pancreatic cancer to the client's significant other.
3. The diagnosis of an uncontrolled seizure disorder of a taxi driver to a state agency.
4. The client is 32 weeks pregnant with twins and is legally separated.

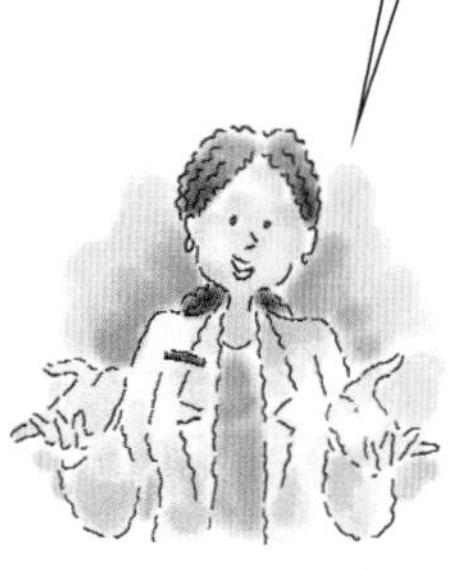

There are legal and ethical issues posed in question 16. Which circumstance can the nurse disclose?

16. 3. The nurse may lawfully disclose confidential information about a client when the welfare of a person is at stake. The physician is required to inform the Department of Motor Vehicles that the taxi driver has an uncontrolled seizure disorder because it's in the best interest of the public's and client's safety. Confidentiality of HIV testing is required, but the client should be encouraged to share the information with others. A positive HIV test can mean the loss of a job, medical insurance, financial security, and even housing because family, friends, and the public may fear the HIV positive person. Options 2 and 4 don't affect the welfare of a person.

CN: Safe, effective care environment; CNS: Management of care; CL: Application

17. A client in a long-term care facility refuses to take his oral medications. The nurse threatens the client and tells him that, if the medication isn't taken, restraints will be applied and the medication will be given by injection. The nurse's statement constitutes which legal tort?

1. Assault
2. Battery
3. Negligence
4. Right to refuse care

17. 1. Assault occurs when a person puts another person in fear of harmful or threatening contact. Battery is the actual contact with one's body. If the nurse actually carried out the threat, battery would also apply. Negligence involves actions below the standard of care. The client has the legal right to refuse care. In this situation, the correct action is to try to calm the client, allow him time to talk, and then determine if he will take the medications. If the client still won't take the medications, the nurse should document his refusal, note the medications, and notify the physician and nursing supervisor.

CN: Safe, effective care environment; CNS: Management of care; CL: Application

18. Entering a client's room to get a neonate for an examination by the physician, the nurse on the maternity unit sees the client holding the crying neonate and slapping his face. Which action is most appropriate?

1. Take the neonate to the nursery, tell the physician so he can examine the neonate for injuries, and notify social services.
2. Leave the room without the neonate and notify the nursing supervisor.
3. Confront the client by asking her what she's doing and why.
4. Take the neonate to the nursery and tell coworkers to observe the client for further incidents.

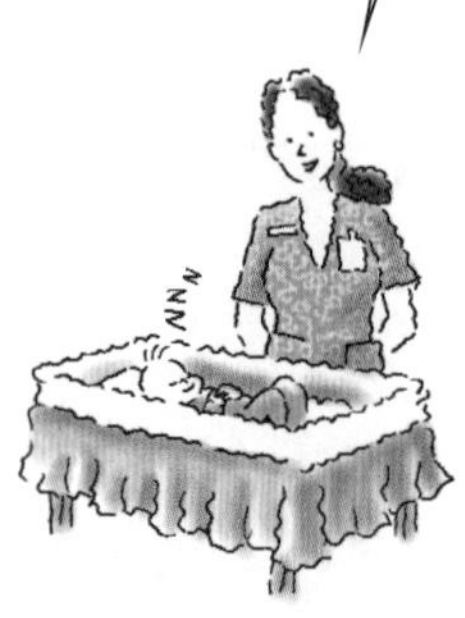

18. 1. The neonate's safety and protection is the first priority. The nurse should immediately take the neonate to the nursery and inform the physician of the abuse. By being the neonate's advocate, the nurse allows the physician to examine him for injuries resulting from the incident. The nurse shouldn't confront the client. Although observing the client for further incidents may be part of the revised care plan, it requires immediate intervention, not simple notification of coworkers.

CN: Psychosocial integrity; CNS: None; CL: Analysis

19. The care plan is revised for a client who has difficulty dealing with a crying neonate. Which strategy should the new care plan include early in the client's hospital stay?
1. Anger management therapy
2. Proper care of a crying infant
3. Proper methods for dealing with stressful situations such as crying infants
4. Assessment of the client's strengths and weaknesses in coping mechanisms and the presence of support systems

19. 4. Assessment of the client's strengths and weaknesses in her coping mechanisms and the presence of support systems is important in the implementation process. Assessment will also help identify situations that the client perceives as stressors. It hasn't been established that the client is angry, so anger management therapy isn't necessary. Proper care of a crying infant is necessary, but assessing the client's coping will help provide the basis for teaching. Providing education about alternatives to expressing feelings and about crisis hotlines and community support systems should also be part of the care plan.

CN: Psychosocial integrity; CNS: None; CL: Analysis

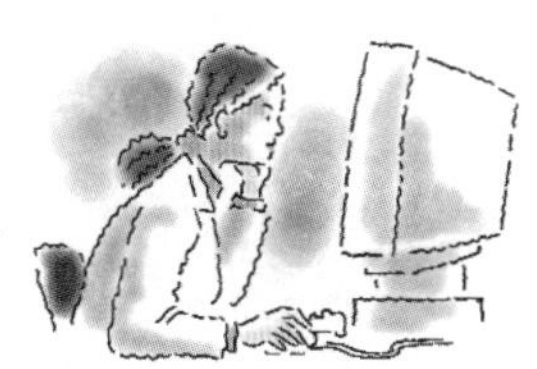
Which provisions should a living will include?

20. Although living will laws vary from state to state, which statement indicates the types of provisions living wills generally include?
1. Instructions on when and how the living will should be executed
2. Who may uphold a living will declaration
3. How long the living will is in effect
4. What will happen to the client's valuables after death

20. 1. Living wills include instructions on how it should be executed, the witness and testator requirements, documentation requirements, and under what circumstances it will take effect. A living will doesn't state who may uphold the declaration or how long it's in effect. A living will doesn't dictate what will happen to the client's valuables.

CN: Safe, effective care environment; CNS: Management of care; CL: Application

21. Which is the role of a nurse in a domestic abuse situation?
1. Document the situation and provide support for the victim.
2. Protect the client's privacy by not documenting the abuse.
3. Provide counseling to the person committing the abuse.
4. Provide counseling for the victim.

21. 1. The nurse must carefully and adequately document the assessment of the abused victim. The documentation must include statements from the victim, physical and psychological assessment findings, and observations relative to the abuse situation. The victim should be provided with local community resources, social agencies, and legal services as necessary to prevent recurrence of physical abuse. The professional nurse isn't qualified to counsel the abuser or the victim. The abuser and victim should be referred for therapy.

CN: Psychosocial integrity; CNS: None; CL: Analysis

22. A nurse is explaining the Bill of Rights for psychiatric patients to a client who has voluntarily sought admission to an inpatient psychiatric facility. Which rights should the nurse include in the discussion? Select all that apply:

1. Right to select health care team members
2. Right to refuse treatment
3. Right to a written treatment plan
4. Right to obtain disability
5. Right to confidentiality
6. Right to personal mail

22. 2, 3, 5, 6. An inpatient client usually receives a copy of the Bill of Rights for psychiatric patients, which includes options 2, 3, 5, and 6. However, a client in an inpatient setting can't select team members. A client may apply for disability as a result of a chronic, incapacitating illness; however, disability is not a patient right, and members of a psychiatric institution don't decide who should receive it.

CN: Psychosocial integrity; CNS: None; CL: Application

23. While providing care to a 26-year-old married female client, a nurse notes multiple ecchymotic areas on her arms and trunk. The color of the ecchymotic areas ranges from blue to purple to yellow. When asked by the nurse how she got these bruises, the client responds, "Oh, I tripped." How should the nurse respond? Select all that apply:

1. Document the client's statement and complete a body map indicating size, color, shape, location, and type of injuries.
2. Report suspicions of abuse to the local authorities.
3. Assist the client in developing a safety plan for times of increased violence.
4. Call the client's husband to discuss the situation.
5. Tell the client that she needs to leave the abusive situation as soon as possible.
6. Provide the client with telephone numbers of local shelters and safe houses.

23. 1, 3, 6. The nurse should objectively document her assessment findings. A detailed description of physical findings of abuse in the medical record is essential if legal action is pursued. All women suspected to be victims of abuse should be counseled on a safety plan, which consists of recognizing escalating violence within the family and formulating a plan to exit quickly. The nurse shouldn't report this suspicion of abuse because the client is a competent adult who has the right to self-determination. Nurses do, however, have a duty to report cases of actual or suspected abuse in children and elderly clients. Contacting the client's husband without her consent violates confidentiality. The nurse should respond to the client in a nonthreatening manner that promotes trust, rather than ordering her to break off her relationship.

CN: Psychosocial integrity; CNS: None; CL: Analysis

You did it! You finished the final chapter! Now, for more fun, try the six comprehensive tests that follow!

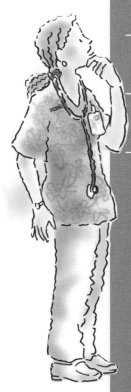

Appendices and index

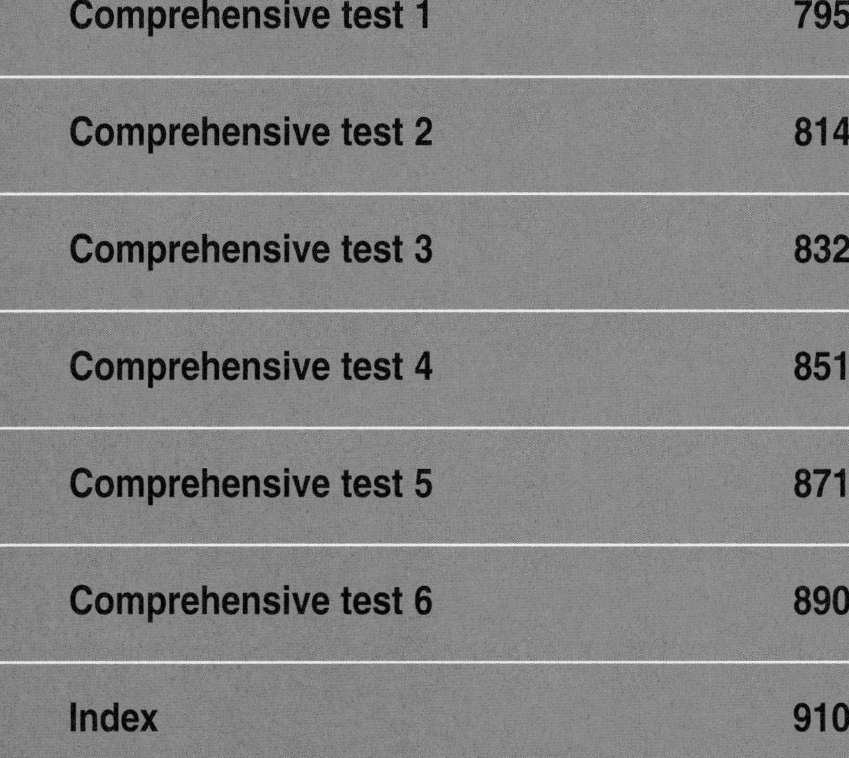

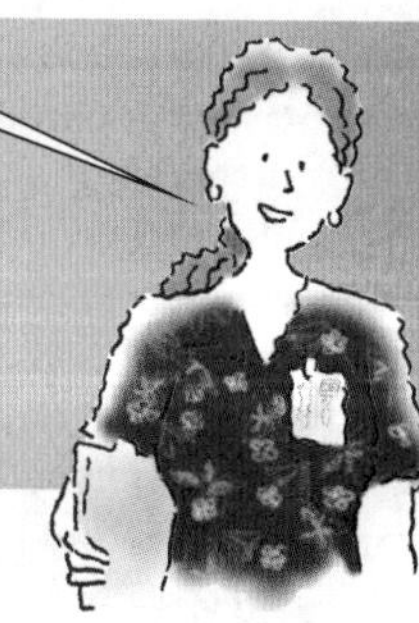

This comprehensive test, the first of six, is just like a real NCLEX test. It's a great way to practice!

COMPREHENSIVE Test 1

1. A 43-year-old client with blunt chest trauma from a motor vehicle collision has sinus tachycardia, is hypotensive, and has developed muffled heart sounds. There are no obvious signs of bleeding. Which condition is suspected?

1. Heart failure
2. Pneumothorax
3. Cardiac tamponade
4. Myocardial infarction (MI)

1. 3. Cardiac tamponade results in signs of obvious shock and muffled heart sounds. Heart failure would result in inspiratory crackles, pulmonary edema, and jugular vein distention. Pneumothorax would result in diminished breath sounds in the affected lung, respiratory distress, and tracheal displacement. In an MI, the client may complain of chest pain. Also, an electrocardiogram could confirm changes consistent with an MI.

CN: Physiological integrity; CNS: Physiological adaptation; CL: Analysis

2. The client is experiencing tamponade. Which type of shock should the nurse expect to observe in the client?

1. Anaphylactic
2. Cardiogenic
3. Hypovolemic
4. Septic

2. 2. Fluid accumulates in the pericardial sac, hindering motion of the heart muscle and causing it to pump inefficiently, resulting in signs of cardiogenic shock. Anaphylactic and septic are types of distributive shock in which fluid is displaced from the capillaries and leaks into surrounding tissues. Hypovolemic shock involves the actual loss of fluid.

CN: Physiological integrity; CNS: Physiological adaptation; CL: Application

3. A nurse asks a nursing assistant to help admit an elderly client diagnosed with pneumonia. Which activity is appropriate for the nurse to ask the assistant to perform?

1. Obtain the client's height and weight.
2. Obtain an arterial blood gas sample.
3. Insert a small-bore feeding tube.
4. Assess lung sounds.

3. 1. Obtaining the client's height and weight are appropriate actions for the nursing assistant to perform. The other options are the responsibility of the registered nurse or other licensed person.

CN: Safe effective care environment; CNS: Management of care; CL: Application

4. The client is experiencing cardiac tamponade. Which intervention or medication should the nurse expect to see prescribed as the most appropriate treatment for this client?

1. Surgery
2. Dopamine
3. Blood transfusion
4. Pericardiocentesis

4. 4. Pericardiocentesis, or needle aspiration of the pericardial cavity, is done to relieve tamponade. An opening is created surgically if the client continues to have recurrent episodes of tamponade. Dopamine is used to restore blood pressure in normovolemic individuals. Blood transfusions may be given if the client is hypovolemic from blood loss.

CN: Physiological integrity; CNS: Physiological adaptation; CL: Application

5. A nurse is teaching a 50-year-old client how to decrease risk factors for coronary artery disease. He's an executive who smokes, has a type A personality, and is hypertensive. Which risk factor is nonmodifiable?

1. Age
2. Hypertension
3. Personality
4. Smoking

5. 1. Age is a risk factor that is nonmodifiable. Type A personality, hypertension, and smoking factors can be controlled.

CN: Health promotion and maintenance; CNS: None; CL: Application

6. A client says he's stressed by his job but enjoys the challenge. Which suggestion is best to help the client?

1. Switch job positions.
2. Take stress management classes.
3. Spend more time with his family.
4. Avoid working from home.

6. 2. Stress management classes will teach the client how to better manage the stress in his life, after identifying the factors that contribute to it. Alternatives may be found to leaving his job, which he enjoys. Not spending enough time with his family and taking his job home with him haven't yet been identified as contributing factors.

CN: Physiological integrity; CNS: Reduction of risk potential; CL: Application

7. A nurse is teaching a client with glaucoma the proper technique for instilling eyedrops. She instructs the client to place the drops:

1. on the cornea.
2. in the outer canthus.
3. near the opening of the lacrimal duct.
4. in the lower conjunctival sac.

7. 4. Eyedrops should be placed in the lower conjunctival sac starting at the inner, not outer canthus. Placing eyedrops on the cornea causes discomfort and should be avoided. Eyedrops shouldn't be placed by the opening of the lacrimal ducts to avoid systemic absorption.

CN: Physiological integrity; CNS: Pharmacological and parenteral therapies; CL: Application

CN: Client needs category CNS: Client needs subcategory CL: Cognitive level

8. A 28-year-old client with human immunodeficiency virus (HIV) is admitted to the hospital with flulike symptoms. He has dyspnea and a cough. He's placed on a 100% nonrebreather mask and arterial blood gases are drawn. Which result indicates the need for intubation?

1. Pa_{O_2}, 90 mm Hg; Pa_{CO_2}, 40 mm Hg
2. Pa_{O_2}, 85 mm Hg; Pa_{CO_2}, 45 mm Hg
3. Pa_{O_2}, 80 mm Hg; Pa_{CO_2}, 45 mm Hg
4. Pa_{O_2}, 70 mm Hg; Pa_{CO_2}, 55 mm Hg

8. 4. An increasing Pa_{CO_2} and decreasing Pa_{O_2} indicate poor oxygen perfusion. Normal Pa_{O_2} levels are 80 to 100 mm Hg and normal Pa_{CO_2} levels are 35 to 45 mm Hg.

CN: Physiological integrity; CNS: Reduction of risk potential; CL: Analysis

9. The nurse is instructing a client regarding transmission of human immunodeficiency virus (HIV). What should the nurse instruct the client as to the most likely route of the virus' transmission?

1. Blood
2. Feces
3. Saliva
4. Urine

9. 1. HIV is transmitted by contact with infected blood. It exists in all body fluids but transmission through saliva, urine, and feces is much less likely to occur than through blood.

CN: Safe, effective care environment; CNS: Safety and infection control; CL: Application

10. A client with acquired immunodeficiency syndrome has developed a protozoa infection. Which opportunistic infection will the client be most likely to develop as a result of the protozoa infection?

1. Tuberculosis (TB)
2. Histoplasmosis
3. Kaposi's sarcoma
4. *Pneumocystis jiroveci* infection

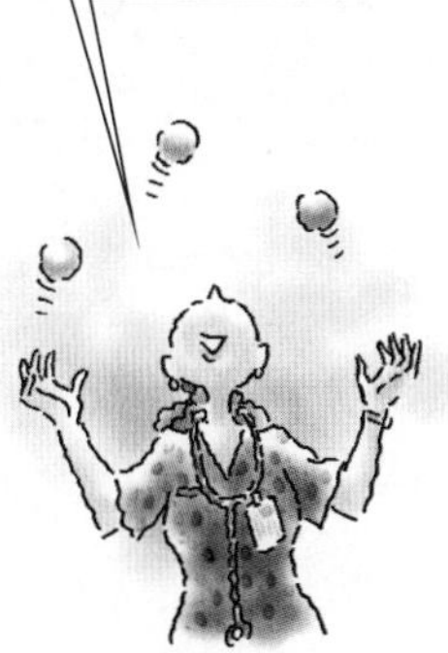

Ten questions done! Are you having fun yet?

10. 4. *P. jiroveci* infection is caused by protozoa. TB is caused by bacteria. Histoplasmosis is a fungal infection. Kaposi's sarcoma is a neoplasm.

CN: Physiological integrity; CNS: Physiological adaptation; CL: Application

11. A client with acquired immunodeficiency syndrome is intubated, leaving him prone to skin breakdown from the endotracheal (ET) tube. Which intervention is best to prevent this?

1. Use lubricant on the lips.
2. Provide oral care every 2 hours.
3. Suction the oral cavity every 2 hours.
4. Reposition the ET tube every 24 hours.

11. 4. Pressure causes skin breakdown. However, repositioning the ET tube from one side of the mouth to the other or to the center of the mouth can relieve pressure in one area for a time. Extreme care must be taken to move the tube only laterally; it must not be pushed in or pulled out. The tape securing the tube must be changed daily. Two nurses should perform this procedure. Oral care, suctioning, and lubricant help keep skin clean and intact and reduce the risk of further infection.

CN: Physiological integrity; CNS: Basic care and comfort; CL: Application

12. A client with acquired immunodeficiency syndrome has developed *Pneumocystis carinii* pneumonia and has begun treatment with pentamidine isethionate (Pentam). Based on the diagnosis and treatment, which medication is most likely to be ordered for the client?
1. Amphotericin B
2. Co-trimoxazole (Bactrim)
3. Fluconazole (Diflucan)
4. Sulfadiazine

12. 2. Co-trimoxazole is given orally or I.V. for *P. carinii* pneumonia. Fluconazole and amphotericin B are used for coccidioidomycosis. Sulfadiazine is used to treat toxoplasmosis.

CN: Physiological integrity; CNS: Pharmacological and parenteral therapies; CL: Application

13. A client is receiving pentamidine isethionate (Pentam). Which parameter will the nurse monitor frequently while the client receives this medication?
1. Heart rate
2. Electrolyte levels
3. Blood sugar levels
4. Complete blood count (CBC)

13. 3. Pentamidine isethionate can cause permanent diabetes mellitus and requires monitoring of blood sugar levels. The client's electrolyte levels, heart rate, and CBC can be monitored less frequently.

CN: Physiological integrity; CNS: Pharmacological and parenteral therapies; CL: Application

14. A nurse caring for a client with acquired immunodeficiency syndrome is working with a nursing student. She notes the student doesn't attempt to suction or assist with care of the client. Which action is appropriate?
1. Talk to the student.
2. Talk to the charge nurse.
3. Address a coworker with the concerns.
4. Seek advice from the student's instructor.

14. 1. The nurse should approach the student to determine her feelings and experience in caring for this client. The charge nurse and coworkers aren't familiar with the student's abilities, but the instructor may be approached if the nurse can't communicate with the student.

CN: Safe, effective care environment; CNS: Management of care; CL: Analysis

15. A client's significant other is tearful over the client's condition and lack of improvement. He says he feels powerless and unable to help his friend. Which response by the nurse is the best?
1. Agree with the person.
2. Tell him there's nothing he can do.
3. State she understands how he must feel.
4. Ask if he would like to help with some comfort measures.

15. 4. The significant other expresses a need to help and the nurse can encourage him to do whatever he feels comfortable with, such as putting lubricant on lips, moist cloth on forehead, or lotion on skin. The nurse may not understand his situation, and agreeing with a person doesn't diminish powerlessness. There are many ways the significant other can help if he wants to.

CN: Psychosocial integrity; CNS: None; CL: Analysis

16. A 31-year-old client is admitted to the hospital with respiratory failure. He's intubated in the emergency department, placed on 100% FIO_2, and is coughing up copious secretions. Which intervention should be done first?

1. Get an X-ray.
2. Suction the client.
3. Restrain the client.
4. Obtain an arterial blood gas (ABG) analysis.

16. 2. Secretions can cut off the oxygen supply to the client and result in hypoxia so suctioning the client is your first priority. X-rays are a priority to check placement of the endotracheal tube. Restraints are warranted if the client is a threat to his safety. After the client has acclimated to his ventilator settings, ABGs can be drawn.

CN: Physiological integrity; CNS: Reduction of risk potential; CL: Analysis

17. A client with an endotracheal (ET) tube has copious, brown-tinged secretions. Which intervention is a priority?

1. Use a trap to obtain a specimen.
2. Instill saline to break up secretions.
3. Culture the specimen with a culturette swab.
4. Obtain an order for a liquefying agent for the sputum.

17. 1. Suspicious secretions should be sent for culture and sensitivity using a sterile technique such as a trap. Saline would dilute the specimen. Swab culturettes are useful for wound cultures — not ET cultures. Various agents are available to help break up secretions, and respiratory therapists can usually help recommend the right agent, but this isn't a priority.

CN: Safe, effective care environment; CNS: Safety and infection control; CL: Analysis

18. An X-ray shows an endotracheal (ET) tube is 2 cm above the carina, and there are nodular lesions and patchy infiltrates in the upper lobe. Which interpretation of the X-ray is accurate?

1. The X-ray is inconclusive.
2. The client has a disease process going on.
3. The ET tube needs to be advanced.
4. The ET tube needs to be pulled back.

18. 2. The X-ray is suggestive of tuberculosis. At 2 cm, the ET tube is at an adequate level in the trachea and doesn't have to be advanced or pulled back.

CN: Physiological integrity; CNS: Reduction of risk potential; CL: Analysis

19. A client has copious secretions. X-ray results indicate tuberculosis (TB). For which intervention should the nurse prepare the client first?

1. Repeat X-ray
2. Tracheostomy
3. Bronchoscopy
4. Arterial blood gas (ABG) analysis

19. 3. Bronchoscopy can help diagnose TB and obtain specimens while clearing the bronchial tree of secretions. X-rays may be repeated periodically to determine lung and endotracheal tube status. Tracheostomy may be done if the client remains on the ventilator for a prolonged period. A change in condition or treatment may require an ABG analysis.

CN: Physiological integrity; CNS: Reduction of risk potential; CL: Application

20. A nurse is aware that family members of a client diagnosed with tuberculosis may have been exposed to the disease. The nurse explains that a tuberculin skin test should be performed on each family member and that this may show:

1. active disease.
2. recent infection.
3. extent of the infection.
4. infection at some point.

21. A client is diagnosed with tuberculosis (TB). In addition to recommending skin testing of the family members, TB should be reported to which individual or agency?

1. Centers for Disease Control and Prevention (CDC)
2. Local health department
3. Infection-control nurse
4. Client's physician

22. A client with tuberculosis (TB) is being treated with isoniazid (INH). Which therapy is most likely to be ordered in conjunction with INH?

1. Theophylline inhaler
2. I.M. penicillin
3. Multiple antibacterial agents
4. Aerosol treatments with pentamidine (Pentam)

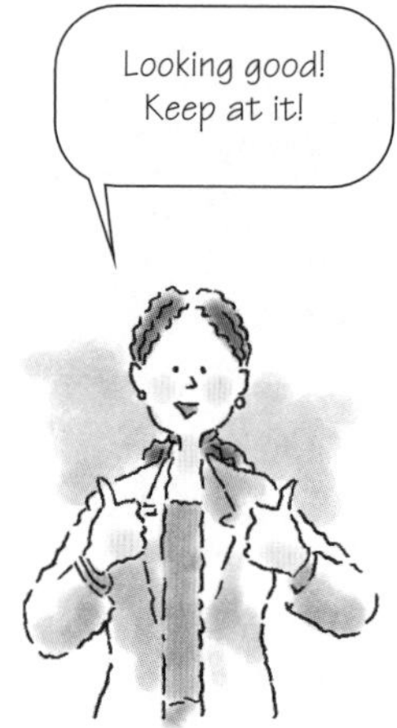

20. 4. A tuberculin skin test shows the presence of infection at some point; a positive skin test doesn't guarantee that an infection is *currently* present, however. Some people have false-positive results. Active disease may be viewed on a chest X-ray. Computed tomography or magnetic resonance imaging can evaluate the extent of lung damage.

CN: Safe, effective care environment; CNS: Safety and infection control; CL: Application

21. 2. The local health department must be informed of an outbreak of TB because it's a reportable disease. They, in turn, inform the CDC. The infection-control nurse or employee health department may request that staff be tested if exposed. Generally, the client's family can inform his physician.

CN: Safe, effective care environment; CNS: Safety and infection control; CL: Application

22. 3. Because TB has become resistant to many antibacterial agents, the initial treatment includes the use of multiple antituberculotic or antibacterial drugs. These may include rifampin, ethambutol hydrochloride, pyrazinamide, cycloserine, clofazimine, and streptomycin. Theophylline is a bronchodilator used to treat asthma and chronic obstructive pulmonary disease. Penicillins are used to treat *Staphylococcus aureus*—not TB. Pentamidine is used in the treatment of pneumonia caused by *Pneumocystis jiroveci*.

CN: Physiological integrity; CNS: Pharmacological and parenteral therapies; CL: Application

23. A nurse is teaching a client with tuberculosis (TB) about his medication treatment. She should explain that most clients receive treatment for TB for:

1. 2 to 4 months.
2. 9 to 12 months.
3. 18 to 24 months.
4. more than 2 years.

23. 2. Treatment for TB is usually continued for at least 9 to 12 months.

CN: Physiological integrity; CNS: Pharmacological and parenteral therapies; CL: Application

24. A nurse teaches a client with tuberculosis that he is still considered infectious after treatment is started for which period of time?

1. 72 hours
2. 1 week
3. 2 weeks
4. 4 weeks

24. 4. After 4 weeks, the disease is no longer infectious but the client must continue to take the medication.

CN: Safe, effective care environment; CNS: Safety and infection control; CL: Application

25. A client tells his nurse that his tuberculosis medications are so expensive that he can't afford to take them. Which intervention by the nurse is best?

1. Refer the client to social services.
2. Tell the client to apply for Medicaid.
3. Refer the client to the local or county health department.
4. Tell the client to follow his insurance rules and regulations.

25. 3. The local and county health departments provide treatment and follow-up free of charge for all residents to ensure proper care. Social services can help seek alternative methods of payment and reimbursement but would probably first refer the client to the local and county health departments. Medicaid or medical assistance is another avenue for the client, *if* he qualifies. Insurance can be an alternative source to help pay for treatment, but the client may not be insured or the policy may not cover prescriptions.

CN: Safe, effective care environment; CNS: Management of care; CL: Analysis

26. A 62-year-old client is admitted to the hospital with pneumonia. He has a history of Parkinson's disease, which his family says is progressively worsening. Which assessment is expected?

1. Impaired speech
2. Muscle flaccidity
3. Pleasant and smiling demeanor
4. Tremors in the fingers that increase with purposeful movement

26. 1. In Parkinson's disease, dysarthria, or impaired speech, is due to a disturbance in muscle control. Muscle rigidity results in resistance to passive muscle stretching. The client may have a masklike appearance. Tremors should decrease with purposeful movement and sleep.

CN: Physiological integrity; CNS: Physiological adaptation; CL: Application

27. Which nursing diagnosis describes a clinical judgment that an individual, family, or community is more vulnerable to developing a certain problem than others in the same or similar situation are?

1. *Risk for compromised human dignity*
2. *Moral distress*
3. *Stress overload*
4. *Readiness for enhanced comfort*

27. 1. *Risk for compromised human dignity* is a risk nursing diagnosis that refers to the vulnerability of a client, family, or community to health problems. *Moral distress* and *Stress overload* are nursing diagnoses that describe a human response to a health problem being manifested. *Readiness for enhanced comfort* is a diagnostic statement describing the human response to levels of wellness in an individual, family, or community that have a potential for enhancement to a higher state.

CN: Safe, effective care environment; CNS: Management of care; CL: Analysis

28. A client is ordered to receive 1,000 ml of 0.45% normal saline with 20 mEq of potassium chloride (KCL) over 6 hours. The infusion set administers 15 gtt/ml. At how many gtt/minute should the nurse set the flow rate?

1. 36
2. 40
3. 42
4. 45

28. 3. The flow rate is determined by the rate of infusion and the number of drops per milliliters of the fluid being administered:
gtt/ml × amount to be infused divided by the number of minutes = the intravenous flow rate.
15 gtt/ml × 1000 ml = 15,000
15,000 ml ÷ 360 minutes = 41.6 gtt/minute
Therefore, the flow rate should be 42 gtt/minute.

CN: Physiological integrity; CNS: Pharmacological and parenteral therapy; CL: Application

29. An 82-year-old male client with Parkinson's disease is frequently incontinent of urine. Which intervention should be done first?

1. Diaper the client.
2. Apply a condom catheter.
3. Insert an indwelling urinary catheter.
4. Provide skin care every 4 hours.

29. 2. A condom catheter uses a condom-type device to drain urine away from the client. Diapering the client may keep urine away from the body but may also be demeaning if the client is alert or the family objects. Because the client with Parkinson's disease is already prone to urinary tract infections, an indwelling urinary catheter should be avoided because it may promote this. Skin care must be provided as soon as the client is incontinent to prevent skin maceration and breakdown.

CN: Physiological integrity; CNS: Basic care and comfort; CL: Analysis

30. Family members report exhaustion and difficulty taking care of a dependent family member. Which approach is in the best interest of the client?

1. Ask the client what he wishes.
2. Have the family members discuss it among themselves.
3. Tell the family the client should go to a nursing care facility.
4. Call a family conference and ask social services for assistance.

30. 4. A family conference with social services can enlighten the family to all prospects of care available to them. The client should supply input if he's able but this may not help solve the problems of exhaustion and care difficulties. The family may not be aware of alternative care measures for the client, so a discussion among themselves may not be helpful. The client may not qualify for a nursing care facility because of stringent criteria.

CN: Safe, effective care environment; CNS: Management of care; CL: Analysis

31. A 30-year-old primagravida in her second trimester tells a nurse her fingers feel tight and sometimes she feels as though her heart skips a beat. She has a history of rheumatic fever. Which assessment indicates the client may be experiencing cardiovascular disease?

1. Clear lungs
2. Sinus tachycardia
3. Increased dyspnea on exertion
4. Runs of paroxysmal atrial tachycardia

31. 3. Increasing dyspnea on exertion should alert the nurse to cardiovascular compromise. Cardiac arrhythmias (other than sinus tachycardia or paroxysmal atrial tachycardia) and persistent crackles at the bases are also symptoms of cardiovascular disease.

CN: Health promotion and maintenance; CNS: None; CL: Analysis

32. Which diagnostic test may be performed to determine the extent of cardiovascular disease during pregnancy?

1. Stress test
2. Chest X-ray
3. Echocardiography
4. Cardiac catheterization

32. 3. Echocardiography is less invasive than X-rays and other methods and provides the information needed to determine cardiovascular disease, especially valvular disorders. Cardiac catheterization and stress tests may be postponed until after delivery.

CN: Physiological integrity; CNS: Physiological adaptation; CL: Analysis

33. A 25-year-old primagravida has been in labor for 20 hours with little progress. The doctor prescribes oxytocin for her. The order reads 10 U oxytocin in 1,000 ml/NSS to infuse via pump at 1 mU/minute for 15 minutes; then increase flow rate to 2 mU/minute. What's the flow rate needed to deliver 1 mU/minute for 15 minutes?

1. 4 ml/hr
2. 6 ml/hr
3. 12 ml/hr
4. 16 ml/hr

33. 2. First, determine the concentration of the solution with 10 U/1,000 ml as the known factor and *X* as the unknown factor:

$$\frac{10\ \text{U}}{1{,}000\ \text{ml}} = \frac{X}{1\ \text{ml}} \quad X = .01\ \text{U/ml}$$

Then, cross-multiply and solve for *X*. Next, convert to mU by multiplying by 1,000.

$$.01 \times 1{,}000 = 10\ \text{mU/ml}$$

Determine flow rate using the following equation:

$$\frac{10\ \text{mU}}{1\ \text{ml}} = \frac{15\ \text{mU}}{X} \quad X = \frac{15\ \text{ml}}{10} = 1.5\ \text{ml}$$

Convert to an hourly rate by multiplying by 4 (60 minutes/15 minutes = 4)

$$1.5\ \text{ml/15 minutes} \times 4 = 6\ \text{ml/hr}$$

CN: Physiological integrity; CNS: Pharmacological and parenteral therapies; CL: Application

34. Which statement by the nurse most accurately reflects subjective data in a nursing assessment?

1. "The client's red blood cell count is elevated."
2. "The client has a positive Babinski sign."
3. "The client's X-ray result showed a fracture present."
4. "The client reported that his pain is a 7 on a 1–10 scale."

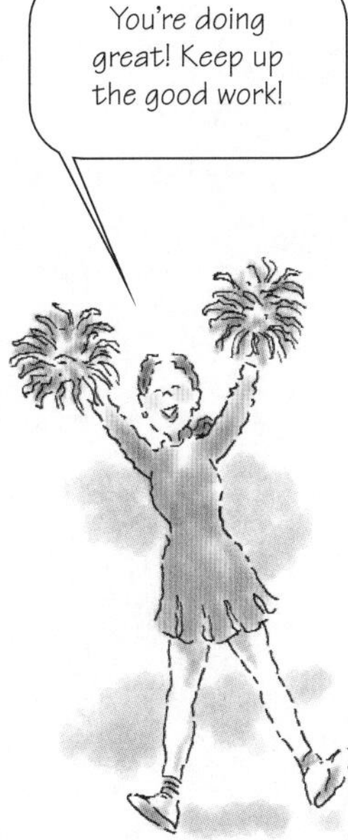
You're doing great! Keep up the good work!

34. 4. Subjective data, also known as *symptoms* or *covert cues,* include the client's own verbatim statements about the health problems. Laboratory study results, physical assessment data, and diagnostic procedure reports are observable, perceptible, and measurable and can be verified and validated by others.

CN: Safe, effective care environment; CNS: Management of care; CL: Application

35. Which classification of medication may be used safely in a pregnant client with cardiovascular disease?

1. Antibiotics
2. Warfarin (Coumadin)
3. Cardiac glycosides
4. Diuretics

35. 3. Cardiac glycosides and common antiarrhythmics, such as procainamide (Procanbid) and quinidine (Quinaglute), may be used. Prophylactic antibiotics are reserved for clients susceptible to endocarditis. If anticoagulants are needed, heparin is the drug of choice—not warfarin. Diuretics should be used with extreme caution, if at all, because of the potential for causing uterine contractions.

CN: Physiological integrity; CNS: Pharmacological and parenteral therapies; CL: Analysis

36. A client arrives at the emergency department in her third trimester with painless vaginal bleeding. Which condition is suspected?

1. Placenta previa
2. Preterm labor
3. Abruptio placentae
4. A sexually transmitted infection (STI)

36. 1. Placenta previa presents with painless vaginal bleeding. Abruptio placentae usually includes vague abdominal discomfort and tenderness. Preterm labor and STIs usually don't cause bleeding.

CN: Health promotion and maintenance; CNS: None; CL: Analysis

37. After assessing vital signs and applying an external monitor, which intervention is a priority for a client with suspected placenta previa?

1. Insert an indwelling urinary catheter.
2. Plan for an immediate cesarean delivery.
3. Place the client in Trendelenburg position.
4. Obtain blood work and start I.V. catheters.

37. 4. Blood for hemoglobin, hematocrit, type, and crossmatch should be collected and I.V. catheters inserted. The nurse shouldn't attempt Trendelenburg positioning or urinary catheterization. The client may be placed on her left side. Depending on the degree of bleeding and fetal maturity, a cesarean delivery may be required.

CN: Physiological integrity; CNS: Reduction of risk potential; CL: Application

38. A pregnant client with vaginal bleeding asks a nurse how the fetus is doing. Which is the best response for the nurse to give?

1. "I don't know for sure."
2. "I can't answer that question."
3. "It's too early to tell anything."
4. "Here's what the monitor shows."

38. 4. The client deserves a truthful answer and the nurse should be objective without giving opinions. Vague answers may be misleading and aren't therapeutic.

CN: Psychosocial integrity; CNS: None; CL: Analysis

39. A client is hospitalized at 35 weeks' gestation with placenta previa and placed on strict bedrest. She states "I lost my last baby at 24 weeks." Which nursing diagnosis would the nurse set as the priority?

1. *Risk for constipation related to immobility*
2. *Anxiety related to unknown fetal outcome*
3. *Impaired physical mobility related to bedrest*
4. *Ineffective coping related to inappropriate thinking*

39. 2. The client's statement reflects concern for her fetus. Therefore the priority diagnosis is *Anxiety related to unknown fetal outcome.* The client may be at risk for constipation and mobility is impaired but these aren't the priority. There's no indication of a disturbed thought process.

CN: Safe, effective care environment; CNS: Management of care; CL: Analysis

40. A neonate requires blood transfusions after birth. Which cannulation site is most preferred?

1. Scalp veins
2. Intraosseous
3. Umbilical cord
4. Subclavian cutdown

40. 3. The umbilical cord may be easily cannulated and is the preferred site. Scalp veins may also be used. Intraosseous cannulation is attempted if two attempts at other sites prove inaccessible. A subclavian cutdown takes a prolonged time and is the least desired.

CN: Health promotion and maintenance; CNS: None; CL: Analysis

41. A nurse working in the triage area of an emergency department sees that several pediatric clients arrive simultaneously. Which client should be treated first?
1. A crying 4-year-old child with a laceration on his scalp
2. A 3-year-old child with a barking cough and flushed appearance
3. A 3-year-old child with Down syndrome who's pale and asleep in his mother's arms
4. A 2-year-old child with stridorous breath sounds, sitting up in his mother's arms and drooling

41. 4. The infant with the airway emergency should be treated first, because of the risk of epiglottitis. The 3-year-old with the barking cough and fever should be suspected of having croup and should be seen promptly, as should the child with the laceration. The nurse would need to gather information about the child with Down syndrome to determine the priority of care.
CN: Safe, effective care environment; CNS: Management of care; CL: Analysis

42. A 2-year-old child is being examined in the emergency department for epiglottitis. Which assessment finding supports this diagnosis?
1. Mild fever
2. Clear speech
3. Tripod position
4. Gradual onset of symptoms

42. 3. The tripod position (sitting up and leaning forward) facilitates breathing. Epiglottitis presents with a sudden onset of symptoms, high fever, and muffled speech. Additional symptoms are inspiratory stridor and drooling.
CN: Physiological integrity; CNS: Physiological adaptation; CL: Application

43. Which method is best when approaching a 2-year-old child to listen to breath sounds?
1. Tell the child it's time to listen to his lungs now.
2. Tell the child to lie down while the nurse listens to his lungs.
3. Ask the caregiver to wait outside while the nurse listens to his lungs.
4. Ask if he would like the nurse to listen to the front or the back of his chest first.

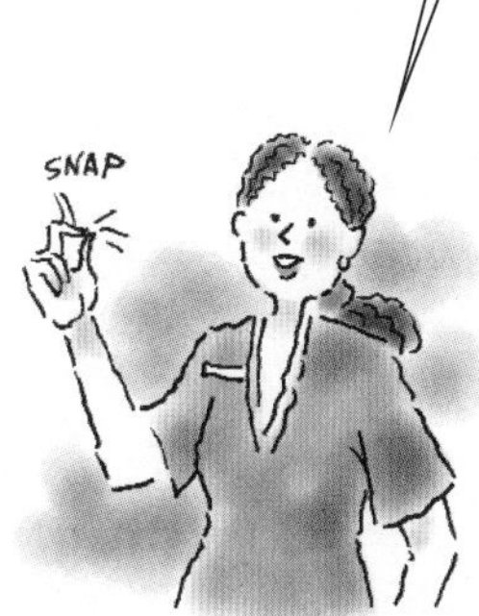

You're more than halfway; the rest should be a snap!
SNAP

43. 4. The 2-year-old child needs to feel in control, and this approach best supports the child's independence. Giving the child no choice may make him uncooperative. The child should be allowed to remain in the tripod position to facilitate breathing. The caregiver should be allowed to remain with the child because fear of separation is common in 2-year-olds.
CN: Health promotion and maintenance; CNS: None; CL: Application

44. A mother says that her 2-year-old child is up to date with his immunizations. The nurse can most accurately determine that the client is up-to-date with his immunizations if his immunizations included:
1. Diptheria-pertussis-tetanus (DTaP), inactivated polio (IPV), measles-mumps-rubella (MMR)
2. DTaP, IPV, MMR, Hemophilus influenza type B (Hib), varicella, pneumococcal, hepatitis B, Rotavirus (Rota)
3. DTaP, hepatitis B, IPV
4. MMR, IPV, hepatitis B

44. 2. By the age of 2, the DTaP, IPV, MMR, Hib, varicella, pneumococcal, hepatitis B and Rotavirus vaccines should have been received. The nurse should clarify this with the mother or caregiver.
CN: Safe, effective care environment; CNS: Safety and infection control; CL: Application

45. Which condition is the biggest threat for a child who has been diagnosed with epiglottitis?

1. Airway obstruction
2. Dehydration
3. Malnutrition
4. Seizures

45. 1. The biggest threat to the child is airway obstruction because of the inflammation and swelling of the epiglottis and surrounding tissue. Dehydration can be prevented with I.V. therapy and seizures averted by decreasing the fever. Malnutrition is least likely to occur because epiglottiditis is a short-lived situation.

CN: Physiological integrity; CNS: Reduction of risk potential; CL: Application

46. What is the most accurate way of diagnosing epiglottitis?

1. Lateral neck X-ray
2. Direct visualization
3. History of sudden onset
4. Presenting signs and symptoms

46. 4. The presenting symptoms are diagnostic of epiglottitis. Lateral neck X-rays aren't necessary. Only an anesthesiologist or physician skilled in intubation should do direct visualization. History of sudden onset helps support the assessment, but a history alone wouldn't be sufficient to make a diagnosis.

CN: Health promotion and maintenance; CNS: None; CL: Application

47. A student nurse working with a registered nurse is assessing a child with epiglottitis. The student tells the client she needs to look at his throat. Which intervention by the registered nurse is best?

1. Hand her a flashlight and tongue blade.
2. Give her a sterile tongue blade and culturette swab.
3. Tell the student that the registered nurse will visualize the child's throat.
4. Tell the student visualization will be done by the anesthesiologist.

47. 4. Direct visualization of the epiglottis can trigger a complete airway obstruction and should only be done in a controlled environment by an anesthesiologist or a physician skilled in pediatric intubation.

CN: Safe, effective care environment; CNS: Management of care; CL: Application

48. The mother of a 2-year-old child with epiglottitis says she needs to pick up her older child from school. The 2-year-old child begins to cry and appears more stridorous. Which intervention by the nurse is best?

1. Ask the mother how long she may be gone.
2. Tell the 2-year-old everything will be all right.
3. Tell the 2-year-old the nurse will stay with him.
4. Ask the mother if there's anyone else who can meet the older child.

48. 4. Increased anxiety and agitation should be avoided in the child to prevent airway obstruction. A 2-year-old child fears separation from parents, so the mother should be encouraged to stay. Other means of picking up the older child need to be found. Telling the child that everything will be all right may not decrease his agitation; the mother is the primary caregiver and important to the child for emotional and security reasons.

CN: Health promotion and maintenance; CNS: None; CL: Analysis

49. A father arrives in a busy emergency department and is upset with his wife for bringing their 2-year-old child with epiglottitis in for treatment. Which intervention by the nurse is best?

1. Leave the room.
2. Call for security.
3. Recognize the father's behavior as his attempt to cope with the situation.
4. Tell both parents to leave because they're upsetting the child.

50. A 40-year-old client is being treated for GI bleeding. On his fifth day of hospitalization, he begins to have tremors, is agitated, and is experiencing hallucinations. These signs suggest which condition?

1. Alcohol withdrawal
2. Allergic response
3. Alzheimer's disease
4. Hypoxia

51. If a nurse suspects a client is experiencing alcohol withdrawal syndrome, which action is appropriate?

1. Verify it with family.
2. Inform social services.
3. Ask the client about his drinking.
4. Tell the client everything will be all right.

52. A client experiencing alcohol withdrawal syndrome says he sees cockroaches on the ceiling. Which response is most appropriate?

1. Ask the client where he sees them.
2. Ask the client if the cockroaches are still there.
3. Tell the client there are no cockroaches on the ceiling.
4. Tell the client it's dim in the room and turn on the overhead lights.

49. 3. Lack of control over his son's situation results in irrational behavior. The nurse should try to calm both parents and let them know they did the right thing due to the seriousness of their child's situation. Calling for security, sending the parents out, or leaving the room won't help the child nor will it reduce frustration or inappropriate behavior.

CN: Safe, effective care environment; CNS: Management of care; CL: Analysis

50. 1. These are signs of alcohol withdrawal syndrome, which can begin 5 to 7 days after the last drink. An allergic reaction would cause difficulty breathing, skin rash, or edema as primary symptoms. Alzheimer's disease occurs in older individuals and has other psychosocial signs, such as a masklike face and altered mentation. Hypoxia would cause symptoms of respiratory distress.

CN: Psychosocial integrity; CNS: None; CL: Analysis

51. 3. Confirming suspicions with the client is the most beneficial way to help in diagnosis and treatment. If the client isn't cooperative, verification can be sought from the family. Social services aren't required at this time but may be helpful in discharge planning. Giving false reassurance isn't therapeutic for the client.

CN: Psychosocial integrity; CNS: None; CL: Application

52. 4. Try to reorient the client to reality and minimize distortions. Don't support the client's hallucinations or place the client on the defensive but try to present reality gently without agitating the client.

CN: Psychosocial integrity; CNS: None; CL: Application

53. A client experiencing alcohol withdrawal syndrome says he's itching everywhere from the bugs on his bed. Which response is appropriate?

1. Examine the client's skin.
2. Ask what kind of bugs he thinks they are.
3. Tell the client there are no bugs on his bed.
4. Tell the client he's having tactile hallucinations.

53. 1. Make sure the client doesn't have a rash, skin allergy, or something on his skin (such as crumbs) causing his discomfort. Reality should then be presented to the client gently without being derogatory. The nurse shouldn't support the client's hallucinations.
CN: Psychosocial integrity; CNS: None; CL: Application

54. A client with alcohol withdrawal syndrome is pulling at his central venous catheter, saying he's swatting the spiders crawling over him. Which intervention is most appropriate?

1. Encourage the client to rest.
2. Protect the client from harm.
3. Tell the client there are no spiders.
4. Tell the client he's pulling the I.V. tubing.

54. 2. During periods of alcohol withdrawal syndrome, the client needs to be protected from harm. If the client dislodges the central venous catheter, he may incur an air embolus, which can be life-threatening. Although reality should be presented to the client, telling him that there are no spiders and that he's pulling the I.V. tubing may not make him stop; therefore, his safety is still at risk. The client may need to be restrained if continued observation during this time isn't available. The client should also be encouraged to rest; however, this intervention doesn't take priority over safety.
CN: Psychosocial integrity; CNS: None; CL: Analysis

55. A client who experienced alcohol withdrawal syndrome is no longer having hallucinations or tremors and says he would like to enter a rehabilitation facility to stop drinking. Which intervention is appropriate?

1. Ask about his insurance.
2. Tell him he should talk with his family.
3. Refer him to Alcoholics Anonymous (AA).
4. Promote participation in a treatment program.

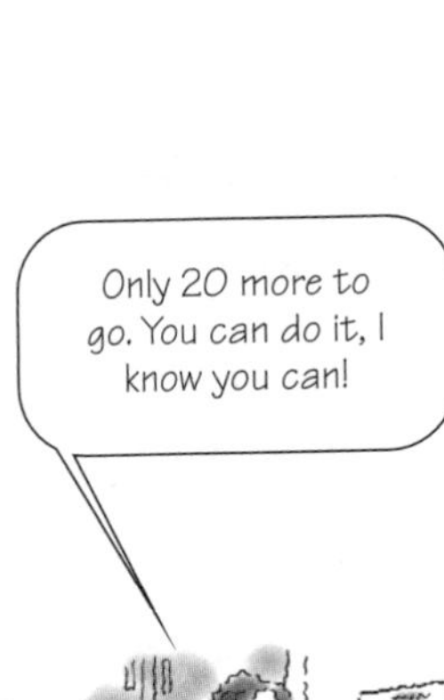

Only 20 more to go. You can do it, I know you can!

55. 4. The client should be encouraged to enter a facility if that's in his best interest. Arrangements that are covered by his insurance can be made and discussed with the social service coordinator and his physician. The client can inform his family, and support should be encouraged. Referral to AA should be considered after rehabilitation takes place.
CN: Psychosocial integrity; CNS: None; CL: Application

56. A 72-year-old man with cirrhosis is admitted to the hospital in a hepatic coma. Based on his condition, which nursing intervention will have the highest priority?

1. Perform a neurologic check.
2. Complete the client admission.
3. Orient the client to his environment.
4. Check airway, breathing, and circulation.

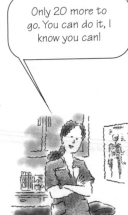

56. 4. Priorities include airway, breathing, and circulation. Once these are ensured, a neurologic check is needed to determine status. General orientation and completing the admission may require the help and affirmation of family members. Depending on the client's alertness, orientation to the environment may need to be kept simple (where he is, date, time).
CN: Physiological integrity; CNS: Reduction of risk potential; CL: Application

57. A client with cirrhosis is restless and at times tries to climb out of bed. Which intervention is best to promote safety?

1. Use leather restraints.
2. Use soft wrist restraints.
3. Use a vest restraint device.
4. Use a sheet tied across the client's chest.

57. 3. The client may require gentle reminders not to get out of bed to prevent a fall. The vest restraint would help in this endeavor. Leather restraints are only warranted for extremely combative and unsafe clients. Soft wrist restraints may not stop the client from sitting up or trying to swing his legs over the bed rails. A sheet tied across the client's chest can hamper breathing or may asphyxiate the client if he slides down in the bed.

CN: Safe, effective care environment; CNS: Management of care; CL: Analysis

58. The nurse is assessing a client with cirrhosis. Which finding is most consistent with late-stage cirrhosis?

1. Constipation
2. Diarrhea
3. Hypoxia
4. Vomiting

58. 3. In late-stage cirrhosis, fluid in the lungs and weak chest expansion can lead to hypoxia. Diarrhea, vomiting, and constipation are early signs and symptoms of cirrhosis.

CN: Physiological integrity; CNS: Physiological adaptation; CL: Application

59. A client with cirrhosis is jaundiced and edematous. He's experiencing severe itching and dryness. Which intervention is best to help the client?

1. Put mitts on his hands.
2. Use alcohol-free body lotion.
3. Lubricate the skin with baby oil.
4. Wash the skin with soap and water.

59. 2. Alcohol-free body lotion applied to the skin can help relieve dryness and is absorbed without oiliness. Mitts may help keep the client from scratching his skin open. Soap dries out the skin. Baby oil doesn't allow excretions through the skin and may block pores.

CN: Physiological integrity; CNS: Basic care and comfort; CL: Application

60. A 20-year-old client with a spinal cord injury sustained in a previous motorcycle collision is hospitalized for renal calculi, or kidney stones. To reduce the client's risk for developing recurrent kidney stones, which instruction is correct?

1. Eat yogurt daily.
2. Drink cranberry juice.
3. Eat more fresh fruits and vegetables.
4. Increase the intake of dairy products.

60. 2. Acid urine decreases the potential for kidney stones. The majority of renal calculi form in alkaline urine. Cranberries, prunes, and plums promote acidic urine. Yogurt helps restore pH balance to secretions in yeast infections. Fruits and vegetables increase fiber in the diet and promote alkaline urine. Dairy products may contribute to the formation of kidney stones.

CN: Physiological integrity; CNS: Reduction of risk potential; CL: Application

61. A client with a spinal cord injury says he has difficulty recognizing the symptoms of urinary tract infection (UTI) before it's too late. Which symptom is an early sign of UTI?

1. Lower back pain
2. Burning on urination
3. Frequency of urination
4. Fever and change in the clarity of urine

61. 4. The client with a spinal cord injury should recognize fever and change in the clarity of urine as early signs of UTI. Lower back pain is a late sign. The client with a spinal cord injury may not have burning or frequency of urination.

CN: Physiological integrity; CNS: Reduction of risk potential; CL: Application

62. A client tells a nurse he boils his urinary catheters to keep them sterile. Which question should the nurse ask the client?

1. "What technique is used for catheterization?"
2. "At what temperature are the catheters boiled?"
3. "Why aren't prepackaged sterile catheters used?"
4. "Are the catheters dried and stored in a clean, dry place?"

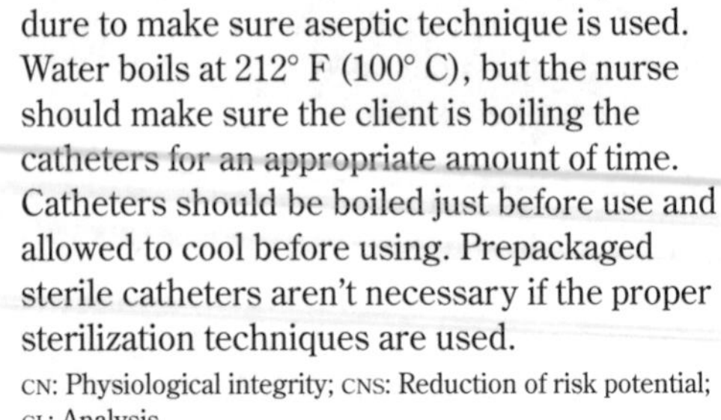

62. 1. The client should describe his procedure to make sure aseptic technique is used. Water boils at 212° F (100° C), but the nurse should make sure the client is boiling the catheters for an appropriate amount of time. Catheters should be boiled just before use and allowed to cool before using. Prepackaged sterile catheters aren't necessary if the proper sterilization techniques are used.

CN: Physiological integrity; CNS: Reduction of risk potential; CL: Analysis

63. A 60-year-old client had a colostomy 4 days ago due to rectal cancer and is having trouble adjusting to it. Which nursing diagnosis would be the most common for the client following this procedure?

1. *Anxiety*
2. *Situational low self-esteem*
3. *Impaired comfort*
4. *Disturbed body image*

63. 4. *Disturbed body image* is most common with a new colostomy and dealing with its care. The client shouldn't have signs of anxiety but he may not be comfortable caring for the colostomy. Low self-esteem may also be a concern for the client, but may not be as common as disturbed body image. The client should be having less discomfort postoperatively.

CN: Safe, effective care environment; CNS: Management of care; CL: Application

64. A nurse approaches a client with a recent colostomy for a routine assessment and finds him tearful. Which action is appropriate?

1. State she'll come back another time.
2. Ask the client if he's having pain or discomfort.
3. Tell the client she needs to perform an assessment.
4. Sit down with the client and ask if he'd like to talk about anything.

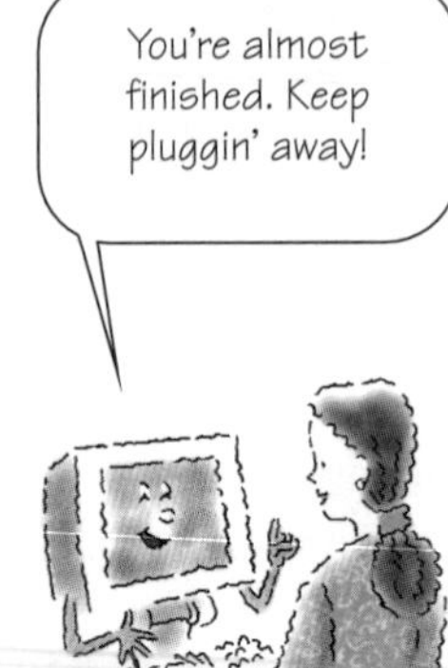
You're almost finished. Keep pluggin' away!

64. 4. Asking open-ended questions and appearing interested in what the client has to say will encourage verbalization of feelings. Leaving the client may make him feel unaccepted. Asking closed-ended questions won't encourage verbalization of feelings. Ignoring the client's present state isn't therapeutic for the client.

CN: Psychosocial integrity; CNS: None; CL: Application

65. After a review of colostomy care, a client says he doesn't know if he'll be able to care for himself at home without help. Which nursing intervention is most appropriate to ensure continuity of care?

1. Review care with the client again.
2. Provide written instructions for the client.
3. Ask the client if there's anyone who can help.
4. Arrange for home health care to visit the client.

65. 4. Although all of these interventions may benefit the patient, arranging for home health care will best ensure continuity of care.

CN: Safe, effective care environment; CNS: Management of care; CL: Application

66. A client is experiencing mild diarrhea through his colostomy. Which instruction is correct to give this client?

1. Eat prunes.
2. Drink apple juice.
3. Increase lettuce intake.
4. Increase intake of bananas.

66. 4. Bananas help make formed stool and aren't irritating to the bowel. Apple juice and prunes can increase the frequency of diarrhea. Lettuce acts as a fiber and can increase the looseness of stools.

CN: Physiological integrity; CNS: Basic care and comfort; CL: Application

67. A client reports a lot of gas in his colostomy bag. Which instruction is best to give this client?

1. Burp the bag.
2. Replace the bag.
3. Put a tiny hole in the top of the bag.
4. Eat less beans.

67. 1. Letting air out of the bag by opening it and burping it is the best solution. Replacing the bag is costly. Putting a hole in the bag will also cause fluids to leak out. The client can be encouraged to note which foods are causing gas and to eat less gas-forming foods.

CN: Physiological integrity; CNS: Basic care and comfort; CL: Application

68. A client at a routine blood glucose screening for diabetes mellitus tells a nurse he has excessive urination and excessive thirst. The nurse should ask about which symptom first?

1. Weakness
2. Weight loss
3. Vision changes
4. Excessive hunger

68. 4. Polyuria, polydipsia, and polyphagia are the three hallmark signs of diabetes mellitus. Weight loss, weakness, and vision changes also occur with diabetes mellitus.

CN: Health promotion and maintenance; CNS: None; CL: Application

69. A client recently diagnosed with prediabetes asks the nurse about the risk factors for developing diabetes mellitus. The nurse identifies which factor as the client's greatest risk for developing diabetes mellitus?

1. Obesity
2. Japanese descent
3. A great-grandparent with diabetes mellitus
4. Delivery of a neonate weighing more than 10 pounds

69. 1. Obesity is a risk factor associated with diabetes mellitus. Delivery of a neonate weighing more than 9 lb, a family history of diabetes mellitus (mother, father, or sibling), and those of Native American, Black, Asian, or Hispanic descent are at high risk for developing diabetes mellitus, but obesity puts the client at greatest risk.

CN: Health promotion and maintenance; CNS: None; CL: Analysis

70. A 52-year-old client had gastric bypass surgery, is on nothing-by-mouth (NPO) status, and is in pain. The nurse gives meperidine (Demerol) 75 mg I.M. as ordered. In 20 minutes, he's feeling nauseous. What would the nurse suspect as the most likely cause?

1. The surgery is causing his nausea.
2. Because he's NPO, the increase in gastric secretions is precipitating this symptom.
3. Meperidine, which was given for his pain, has a tendency to cause nausea.
4. He may be reacting to blood still remaining in his mouth after extubation.

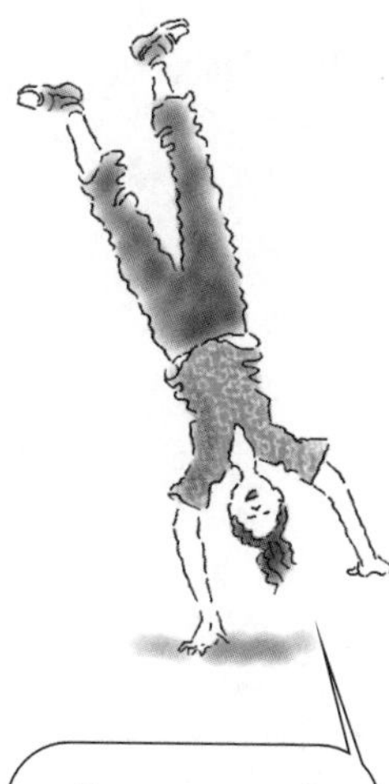

Five more to go! Oooooh, I'm getting excited!

70. 3. Although gastric bypass surgery may precipitate some feelings of nausea, the timing of this symptom after the administration of meperidine is suspicious. Most likely, this client is experiencing a very common adverse effect of the analgesic meperidine. The status of being NPO wouldn't cause an increase in gastric secretions. It's possible that there may be some blood in his mouth after extubation, but the chances of this happening are minimal and less likely to be the cause of the client's complaint.

CN: Physiological integrity; CNS: Pharmacological and parenteral therapies; CL: Analysis

71. A client asks what diabetes mellitus does to the body over time. Which condition should the nurse include in her teaching as a common chronic complication of diabetes mellitus?

1. Multiple sclerosis
2. Diabetic ketoacidosis
3. Cardiovascular disease
4. Hyperosmolar hyperglycemic nonketotic syndrome (HHNS)

71. 3. Cardiovascular disease is a common chronic complication of diabetes mellitus. There's no known relationship between multiple sclerosis and diabetes mellitus. Diabetic ketoacidosis and HHNS are acute complications that can occur.

CN: Health promotion and maintenance; CNS: None; CL: Application

72. A client asks how he might decrease the risk of developing diabetes mellitus, which runs in his family. Which response is appropriate?

1. "Eat only poultry and fish."
2. "Omit carbohydrates from your diet."
3. "Start a moderate exercise program."
4. "Check blood glucose levels every month."

72. 3. Exercise and weight control are the goals in preventing and treating diabetes mellitus. Red meat can be eaten but should be limited because it contributes to cardiovascular disease. Complex carbohydrates account for a large portion of the diabetic diet and shouldn't be omitted. Checking blood glucose levels will help monitor the development of diabetes mellitus but won't prevent or decrease the chance of it occurring.

CN: Physiological integrity; CNS: Reduction of risk potential; CL: Application

73. The nurse is assessing a client's arterial pulses. Which graphic displays the appropriate site for palpating the dorsalis pedis pulse?

1.
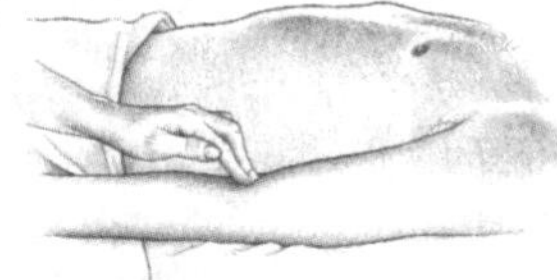

2.
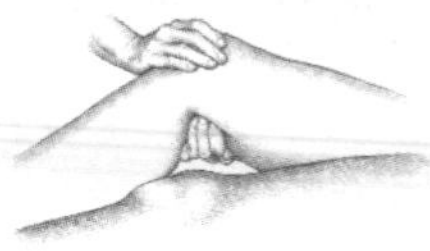

3.
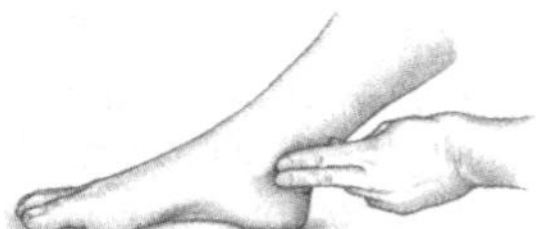

4.
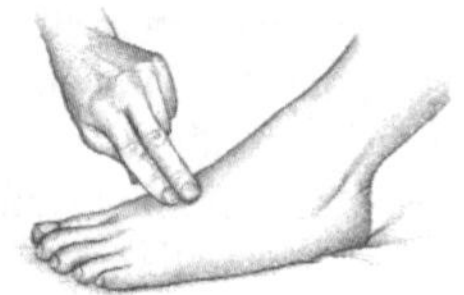

73. 4. To palpate the dorsalis pedis pulse, the nurse places her fingers on the medial dorsum of the foot while the client points his toes down. The first graphic shows palpation of the brachial pulse. This pulse is palpated with the fingers placed medial to the biceps tendon. The second graphic shows palpation of the popliteal pulse in the popliteal fossa of the back of the knee. The third graphic shows palpation of the posterior tibial pulse, slightly below the malleolus of the ankle.

CN: Health promotion and maintenance; CNS: None; CL: Application

74. A nurse is having lunch in the hospital cafeteria when a visitor sitting at the next table begins to choke on his food. According to the American Heart Association (AHA), the nurse should intervene using the actions listed below. List the actions in the sequence in which she should perform them.

1. Administer abdominal thrusts until effective or until the client becomes unresponsive.

2. Activate the emergency response team.

3. Ask the client if he can speak.

4. Start cardiopulmonary resuscitation (CPR).

74.

3. Ask the client if he can speak.

1. Administer abdominal thrusts until effective or until the client becomes unresponsive.

2. Activate the emergency response team.

4. Start cardiopulmonary resuscitation (CPR).

According to the AHA, the nurse should ask the client if he's choking and if he can speak. Next, she should administer abdominal thrusts or chest thrusts (if the client is obese or pregnant). She should continue thrusts until they're effective or until the client becomes unresponsive, at which time she should activate the emergency response team and begin to administer CPR.

CN: Physiological integrity; CNS: Physiological adaptation; CL: Application

75. A nurse is performing a cardiac assessment on a client with a suspected murmur. Identify the area where the nurse should place the stethoscope to auscultate the area referred to as *Erb's point.*

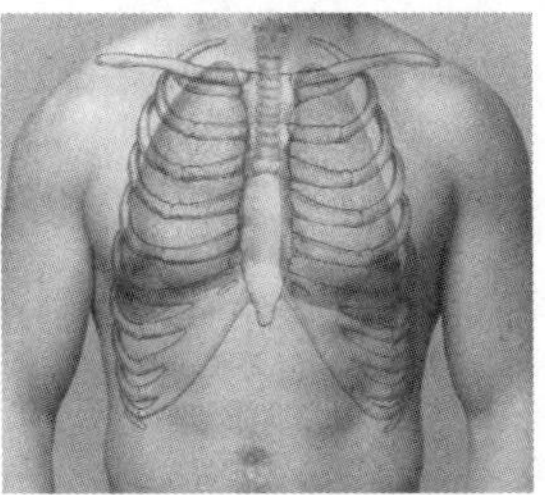

75. Erb's point is located at the third left intercostal space, close to the sternum. Murmurs of both aortic and pulmonic origin may be heard at Erb's point.

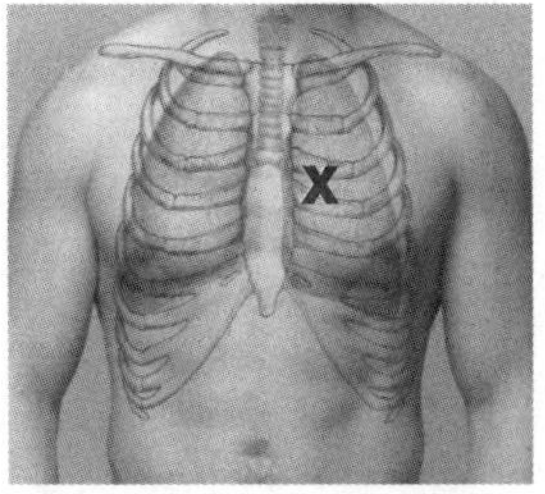

CN: Health promotion and maintenance; CNS: None; CL: Application

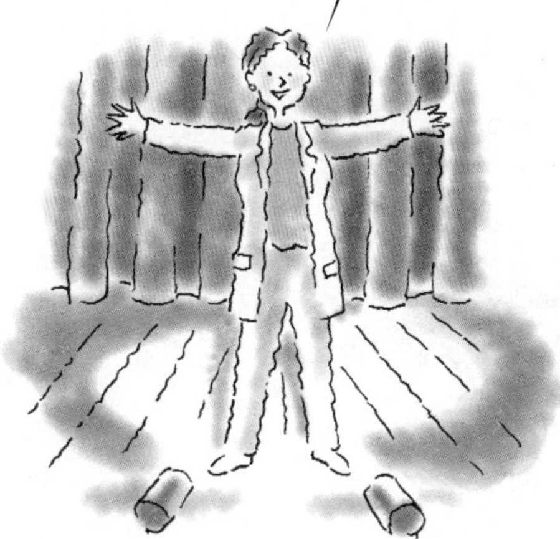

What a performance! For your first comprehensive test, that was outstanding. Congratulations!

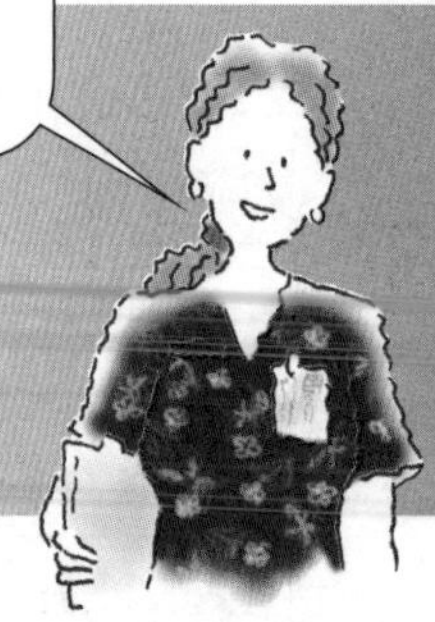
Here's another
comprehensive test to help
you get ready to take the
NCLEX test. Good luck!

COMPREHENSIVE Test 2

1. A newly hired GN is helping the charge nurse admit a client. The charge nurse asks the GN if she understands the facility's rules of ethical conduct. Which statement by the GN indicates the need for further teaching?

1. "I make sure that I do everything in my client's best interest."
2. "I maintain client confidentiality always."
3. "I'll support the Client's Bill of Rights."
4. "I don't discuss advance directives unless the client initiates the conversation."

1. 4. The law mandates that healthcare agencies ask all clients if they have an advance directive. Therefore, the nurse must address this question regardless of whether the client initiates a conversation about it. Nurses always need to act in the best interest of their clients, maintain confidentiality, and support the client's Bill of Rights.

CN: Safe, effective care environment; CNS: Management of care; CL: Analysis

2. Which diagnostic test is performed first to detect transposition of the great vessels (TGV)?

1. Blood cultures
2. Cardiac catheterization
3. Chest X-ray
4. Echocardiogram

2. 3. Chest X-ray would be done first to visualize congenital heart diseases such as TGV. Blood cultures won't diagnose TGV. Cardiac catheterization and an echocardiogram would be done after TGV is seen on the chest X-ray.

CN: Health promotion and maintenance; CNS: None; CL: Application

3. Four 6-month-old children arrive at the clinic for diphtheria-pertussis-tetanus (DTaP) immunization. Which child can safely receive the immunization at this time?

1. The child with a temperature of 103° F (39.4° C)
2. The child with a runny nose
3. The child with uncontrolled epilepsy
4. The child with difficulty breathing after the last immunization

3. 2. Children with mild acute illness without fever can safely receive DTaP immunization. Children with a temperature of more than 102° F (38.9° C), uncontrolled epilepsy, or serious reactions to previous immunizations shouldn't receive DTaP immunization.

CN: Health promotion and maintenance; CNS: None; CL: Analysis

4. A nurse is giving discharge instructions to parents of a child who had a tonsillectomy. Which instruction is the most important?

1. The child should drink extra milk.
2. The child shouldn't drink from straws.
3. Orange juice should be given to provide pain control.
4. The child's mouth should be rinsed with salt water to provide pain relief.

4. 2. Straws and other sharp objects inserted into the mouth could disrupt the clot at the operative site. Extra milk wouldn't promote healing and may encourage mucus production. Drinking orange juice and rinsing with salt water will irritate the tissue at the operative site.

CN: Physiological adaptation; CNS: Reduction of risk potential; CL: Application

CN: Client needs category CNS: Client needs subcategory CL: Cognitive level

5. A 2-year-old child is diagnosed with bronchiolitis caused by respiratory syncytial virus (RSV). The child's family also includes an 8-year-old child. Which statement is correct?

1. RSV isn't highly communicable in infants.
2. RSV isn't communicable to older children and adults.
3. The 2-year-old client must be admitted to the hospital for isolation.
4. The children should be separated to prevent the spread of the infection.

5. 4. Toddlers easily transmit and contract RSV and so they should be separated from other children. RSV is also communicable to older children and adults, but these clients may exhibit only mild symptoms of the disorder. Hospitalization is indicated only for children who need oxygen and I.V. therapy.

CN: Safe, effective care environment; CNS: Safety and infection control; CL: Analysis

6. A child with asthma uses a peak expiratory flowmeter in school. The results indicate his peak flow is in the yellow zone. Which intervention by the school nurse is appropriate?

1. Follow the child's routine asthma treatment plan.
2. Monitor the child for signs and symptoms of an acute attack.
3. Call 911 and prepare for transport to the nearest emergency department.
4. Call the child's mother to take the child to the family physician immediately.

6. 2. The child should be monitored to determine if an asthma attack is imminent. The routine treatment plan may be insufficient when the peak flow is in the yellow zone (50% to 80% of personal best). This isn't an emergency situation. There's no immediate need to see the physician if the child is asymptomatic.

CN: Physiological integrity; CNS: Reduction of risk potential; CL: Application

7. Parents of a child with asthma are trying to identify possible allergens in their household. Which inhaled allergen is the most common?

1. Perfume
2. Dust mites
3. Passive smoke
4. Dog or cat dander

7. 2. The household dust mite is the most commonly inhaled allergen that can cause an asthma attack. Animal dander, passive smoke, and perfume are sometimes allergens causing asthma attacks but aren't as common as dust mites.

CN: Safe, effective care environment; CNS: Safety and infection control; CL: Application

8. A nurse is verifying orders from a physician. Which diet is correct for a child newly diagnosed with celiac disease?

1. Low-fat diet
2. No-gluten diet
3. High-protein diet
4. No-phenylalanine diet

8. 2. The intestinal cells of individuals with celiac disease become inflamed when the child eats products containing gluten, such as wheat, rye, barley, or oats. The child with celiac disease needs normal amounts of fat and protein in the diet for growth and development. Omitting phenylalanine products would be appropriate for the client with phenylketonuria.

CN: Safe, effective care environment; CNS: Safety and infection control; CL: Application

9. A client is undergoing a thoracentesis at the bedside. The nurse assists the client to an upright position with a table and pillow in front of him to support his arms. Which rationale for this intervention is correct?

1. There's easier access to the fluid from this approach.
2. There's less chance to injure lung tissue.
3. It prevents the formation of subcutaneous emphysema.
4. It's less painful for the client in this position.

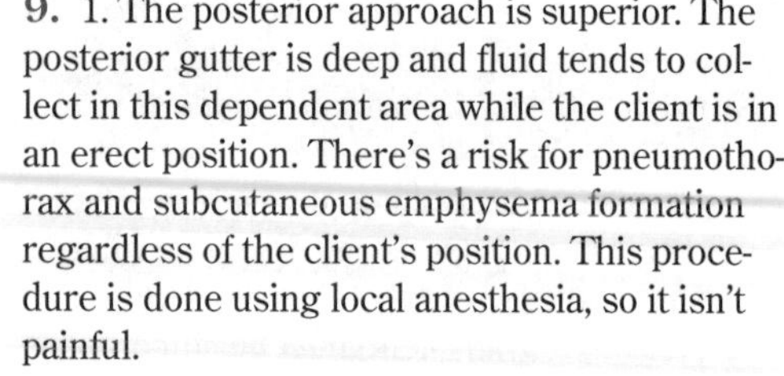

9. 1. The posterior approach is superior. The posterior gutter is deep and fluid tends to collect in this dependent area while the client is in an erect position. There's a risk for pneumothorax and subcutaneous emphysema formation regardless of the client's position. This procedure is done using local anesthesia, so it isn't painful.

CN: Physiological integrity; CNS: Physiological adaptation; CL: Analysis

10. Which leisure activity is recommended for a school-age child with hemophilia?

1. Baseball
2. Cross-country running
3. Football
4. Swimming

10. 4. Swimming is a noncontact sport with low risk for traumatic injury. Baseball, cross-country running, and football all involve a risk for trauma from falling, sliding, or contact.

CN: Physiological integrity; CNS: Physiological adaptation; CL: Application

11. Which assessment is important for an infant in sickle cell crisis?

1. The infant has no bruises.
2. The infant has normal skin turgor.
3. The infant participates in exercise.
4. The infant maintains bladder control.

11. 2. Normal skin turgor indicates the infant isn't severely dehydrated. Dehydration may cause sickle cell crisis or worsen a crisis. Bruising isn't associated with sickle cell crisis. Bed rest is preferable during a sickle cell crisis. Bladder control may be lost when oral or I.V. fluid intake is increased during a sickle cell crisis.

CN: Physiological integrity; CNS: Physiological adaptation; CL: Analysis

12. A client has arterial blood gases drawn. The results are as follows: pH, 7.52; Pao_2, 50 mm Hg; $Paco_2$, 28 mm Hg; HCO_3^-, 24 mEq/L. Which condition is indicated?

1. Metabolic acidosis
2. Metabolic alkalosis
3. Respiratory acidosis
4. Respiratory alkalosis

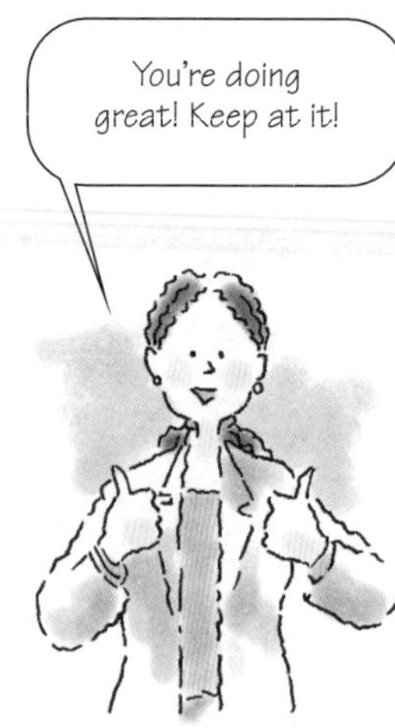
You're doing great! Keep at it!

12. 4. A pH greater than 7.45 and a $Paco_2$ less than 35 mm Hg indicate respiratory alkalosis. A pH less than 7.35 and an HCO_3^- less than 22 mEq/L indicate metabolic acidosis. A pH greater than 7.45 and an HCO_3^- greater than 24 mEq/L indicate metabolic alkalosis. A pH less than 7.35 and a $Paco_2$ greater than 45 mm Hg indicate respiratory acidosis.

CN: Physiological integrity; CNS: Reduction of risk potential; CL: Analysis

13. A client with chronic alcohol abuse is admitted to the hospital for detoxification. Later that day, his blood pressure increases and he's given lorazepam (Ativan) to prevent which complication?

1. Stroke
2. Seizure
3. Fainting
4. Anxiety reaction

13. 2. During detoxification from alcohol, changes in the client's physiologic status, especially an increase in blood pressure, may indicate a possible seizure. Clients are treated with benzodiazepines to prevent this. Stroke, fainting, and anxiety aren't the primary concerns when withdrawing from alcohol.

CN: Physiological integrity; CNS: Pharmacological and parenteral therapies; CL: Application

14. An adolescent client ingests a large number of acetaminophen (Tylenol) tablets in an attempt to commit suicide. Which laboratory result is most consistent with acetaminophen overdose?

1. Metabolic acidosis
2. Elevated liver enzyme levels
3. Increased serum creatinine level
4. Increased white blood cell (WBC) count

14. 2. Elevated liver enzyme levels, which could indicate liver damage, are associated with acetaminophen overdose. Metabolic acidosis isn't associated with acetaminophen overdose. An increased serum creatinine level may indicate renal damage. An increased WBC count indicates infection.

CN: Physiological integrity; CNS: Pharmacological and parenteral therapies; CL: Application

15. A nurse is caring for a client recently diagnosed with acute pancreatitis. Which statement indicates that a short-term goal of nursing care has been met?

1. The client denies abdominal pain.
2. The client doesn't complain of thirst.
3. The client denies pain at McBurney's point.
4. The client swallows liquids without coughing.

15. 1. Pancreatitis is accompanied by acute pain from autodigestion by pancreatic enzymes. When the client denies abdominal pain, the short-term goal of pain control is met. Clients with acute pancreatitis receive I.V. fluids and may not have a sensation of thirst. Pain at McBurney's point accompanies appendicitis. Clients with acute pancreatitis receive nothing by mouth during initial therapy.

CN: Physiological integrity; CNS: Physiological adaptation; CL: Application

16. A client is to take 8 ounces of magnesium sulfate solution. The calibrations on the measuring device are in milliliters. How many milliliters should the nurse give?

1. 8 ml
2. 80 ml
3. 240 ml
4. 480 ml

16. 3. To determine the amount of milliliters to give, use the following equation: One ounce = 30 ml. 8×30 ml = 240 ml.

CN: Physiological integrity; CNS: Pharmacological and parenteral therapies; CL: Application

17. A man stepped on a piece of sharp glass while walking barefoot. He comes to the emergency department with a deep laceration on the bottom of his foot. Which question is the most important for the nurse to ask?

1. "Was the glass dirty?"
2. "Are you immune to tetanus?"
3. "When did you have your last tetanus shot?"
4. "How many diphtheria-pertussis-tetanus (DTaP) shots did you receive as a child?"

17. 3. Questioning the client about the date of his last tetanus immunization is important because the booster immunization should be received every 10 years in adulthood or at the time of the injury if the last booster immunization was given more than 5 years before the injury. Whether the client noticed dirt on the glass is immaterial because all deep lacerations require a tetanus immunization or booster. A client wouldn't know his tetanus immunity status. DTaP immunizations in childhood don't give lifelong immunization to tetanus.

CN: Safe, effective care environment; CNS: Safety and infection control; CL: Application

18. A postmenopausal client asks a nurse how to prevent osteoporosis. Which response is best?

1. "Take a multivitamin daily."
2. "After menopause, there's no way to prevent osteoporosis."
3. "Drink two glasses of milk each day and swim three times a week."
4. "Do weight-bearing exercises regularly."

18. 4. Weight-bearing exercises are recommended for the prevention of osteoporosis. Telling the client that there's no way to prevent osteoporosis would be an incorrect statement. A multivitamin doesn't provide adequate calcium for a post-menopausal woman, and calcium alone won't prevent osteoporosis. Two glasses of milk per day don't provide the daily requirements for adult women, and swimming isn't a weight-bearing exercise.

CN: Health promotion and maintenance; CNS: None; CL: Application

19. A client diagnosed with cardiomyopathy saw a posting on the Internet describing research about a new herbal treatment for the disorder. When the client asks about this research, which response is most appropriate?

1. "Herbs are often used to treat cardiomyopathy."
2. "Cardiomyopathy can be treated only by heart surgery."
3. "The Internet is a reliable source of research, so try this treatment."
4. "Research found on the Internet should be verified with a physician."

19. 4. Although the Internet contains some valid medical research, there's no control over the validity of information posted on it. The research should be discussed with a physician who has access to medical research and can verify the accuracy of the information. Herbs aren't standard treatment for cardiomyopathy. Cardiomyopathy is treatable with drugs or surgery.

CN: Safe, effective care environment; CNS: Management of care; CL: Application

20. A young adult client received her first chemotherapy treatment for breast cancer. Which statement, if made by the client, requires further exploration by the nurse?

1. "I'm thinking about joining a dance club."
2. "I don't think I'm going to work tomorrow."
3. "I don't care about the side effects of drugs."
4. "I want to return to school for a college degree."

20. 3. Adverse effects of chemotherapy may occur after treatment and should be discussed with the client because some can be treated, controlled, or prevented. The nurse needs to explore what the client means by this statement. Joining social clubs is typical behavior for a young adult. The client may feel poorly after chemotherapy and may want to take time off from work until feeling better. Returning to school is also typical of a young adult.

CN: Health promotion and maintenance; CNS: None; CL: Analysis

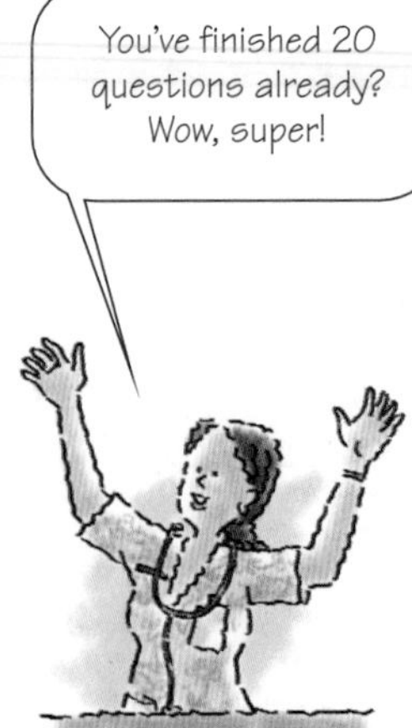

You've finished 20 questions already? Wow, super!

21. A male client has been diagnosed with panhypopituitarism. Which hormone will be given to the client orally?

1. Estrogen
2. Levothyroxine (Synthroid)
3. Serotonin
4. Testosterone

21. 2. Thyroid hormone release depends on the release of thyroid-stimulating hormone (TSH) by the anterior pituitary. TSH is absent from the pituitary when panhypopituitarism exists, so levothyroxine should be given orally. Estrogen isn't indicated for a male client. Serotonin release isn't controlled by the pituitary gland. Testosterone is given by injection or topically by patch.

CN: Physiological integrity; CNS: Pharmacological and parenteral therapies; CL: Application

22. Which nursing intervention is appropriate for an adult client with chronic renal failure?
1. Weigh the client daily before breakfast.
2. Offer foods high in calcium and phosphorous.
3. Serve the client large meals and a bedtime snack.
4. Encourage the client to drink large amounts of fluids.

22. 1. Daily weights are obtained to monitor fluid retention. Calcium intake is encouraged, but clients with chronic renal failure have difficulty excreting phosphorous. Therefore, phosphorous must be restricted. To improve food intake, meals and snacks should be given in small portions. Fluids should be restricted for the client with chronic renal failure.
CN: Physiological integrity; CNS: Physiological adaptation; CL: Application

23. A physician prescribes acetaminophen (Tylenol) gr X (10 grains) as necessary every 4 hours for pain for a client in a long-term care facility. How many milligrams of acetaminophen should the nurse give? Record your answer using a whole number:

______________________ mg.

23. 650 mg. To determine the amount of milligrams to give, use the following equation:

One grain = 65 mg

$$\frac{1 \text{ gr}}{65 \text{ mg}} \times \frac{10 \text{ gr}}{x \text{ mg}}$$

$$X = 65 \times 10$$

$$X = 650 \text{ mg}$$

CN: Physiological integrity; CNS: Pharmacological and parenteral therapies; CL: Application

24. Which assessment finding indicates an increased risk for skin cancer?
1. A deep sunburn
2. A dark mole on the client's back
3. An irregular scar on the client's abdomen
4. White irregular patches on the client's arm

24. 1. A deep sunburn is a risk factor for skin cancer. A dark mole or an irregular scar are benign findings. White irregular patches are abnormal but aren't a risk factor for skin cancer.
CN: Health promotion and maintenance; CNS: None; CL: Application

25. Which behavior is consistent with the diagnosis of conduct disorder in a child?
1. Enuresis
2. Suicidal ideation
3. Cruelty to animals
4. Fear of going to school

25. 3. Cruelty to animals is a symptom of conduct disorder. Enuresis and suicidal ideation aren't usually associated with conduct disorder. Fear of going to school is school phobia.
CN: Psychosocial integrity; CNS: None; CL: Application

26. Which symptom is associated with a genital chlamydia infection?
1. Genital warts
2. No symptoms
3. Purulent discharge
4. Fluid-filled blisters

26. 3. Purulent discharge from the cervix, urethra, or Bartholin's gland is associated with several sexually transmitted diseases, including chlamydia. Genital warts are a sign of human papillomavirus. Although some women with genital chlamydia infection are asymptomatic, this isn't the usual course of this condition. Fluid-filled blisters are a sign of herpes infection.
CN: Health promotion and maintenance; CNS: None; CL: Application

27. Which outcome is appropriate for a client with a diagnosis of depression and attempted suicide?

1. The client will never feel suicidal again.
2. The client will find a group home to live in.
3. The client will remain hospitalized for at least 6 months.
4. The client will verbalize an absence of suicidal ideation, plan, and intent.

27. 4. An appropriate outcome is that the client will verbalize that he no longer feels suicidal. It's unrealistic to ask that he never feels suicidal again. There's no reason for a group home or 6 months of hospitalization.

CN: Psychosocial integrity; CNS: None; CL: Application

28. The nurse is reviewing the proper technique in obtaining a urine specimen from an indwelling urinary catheter. When collecting the urine, which would be the most appropriate technique to use?

1. Collect urine from the drainage collection bag.
2. Disconnect the catheter from the drainage tubing to collect urine.
3. Remove the indwelling catheter and insert a sterile straight catheter to collect urine.
4. Insert a sterile needle with syringe through a tubing drainage port cleaned with alcohol to collect the specimen.

28. 4. Wearing clean gloves, cleaning the port with alcohol, and then obtaining the specimen with a sterile needle and syringe ensures that the specimen and closed drainage system won't be contaminated. A urine specimen must be new urine, and the urine in the drainage collection bag could be several hours' old and growing bacteria. The urinary drainage system must be kept closed to prevent microorganisms from entering. It isn't necessary to remove an indwelling catheter to obtain a sterile urine specimen, unless the physician requests that the system be changed.

CN: Safe, effective care environment; CNS: Safety and infection control; CL: Application

29. A registered nurse (RN) is supervising the care of a licensed practical nurse (LPN). The LPN is caring for a client diagnosed with a terminal illness. Which statement by the LPN should be corrected by the RN?

1. "Some clients write a living will indicating their end-of-life preferences."
2. "The law says you have to write a new living will each time you go to the hospital."
3. "You could designate another person to make end-of-life decisions when you can't make them yourself."
4. "Some people choose to tell their physician they don't want to have cardiopulmonary resuscitation."

29. 2. One living will is sufficient for all hospitalizations unless the client wishes to make changes. A living will explains a person's end-of-life preferences. A durable power of attorney for health care can be written to designate who will make health care decisions for the client in the event the client can't make decisions for himself. The "No-Code" or "Do-Not-Resuscitate" status is discussed with the physician, who then enters this in the client's chart.

CN: Safe, effective care environment; CNS: Management of care; CL: Analysis

30. An elderly client's husband tells a nurse he's concerned because his wife insists on talking about events that happened to her years in the past. The nurse assesses the client and finds her alert, oriented, and answering questions appropriately. Which statement made to the husband is correct?

1. "Your wife is reviewing her life."
2. "A spiritual advisor should be notified."
3. "Your wife should be discouraged from talking about the past."
4. "Your wife is regressing to a more comfortable time in the past."

30. 1. Life review or reminiscing is characteristic of elderly people and the dying. A spiritual advisor might comfort the client but isn't necessary for a life review. Discouraging the client from talking would block communication. Regression occurs when a client returns to behaviors typical of another developmental stage.

CN: Health promotion and maintenance; CNS: None; CL: Application

31. A client with a new colostomy asks a nurse how to avoid leakage from the ostomy bag. Which instruction is correct?

1. Limit fluid intake.
2. Eat more fruits and vegetables.
3. Empty the bag when it's about half full.
4. Tape the end of the bag to the surrounding skin.

31. 3. Emptying the bag when partially full will prevent the bag from becoming heavy and detaching from the skin or skin barrier. Limiting fluids may cause constipation but won't prevent leakage. Increasing fruits and vegetables in the diet will help prevent constipation, not leakage. Taping the bag to the skin will secure the bag to the skin but won't prevent leakage.

CN: Physiological integrity; CNS: Basic care and comfort; CL: Application

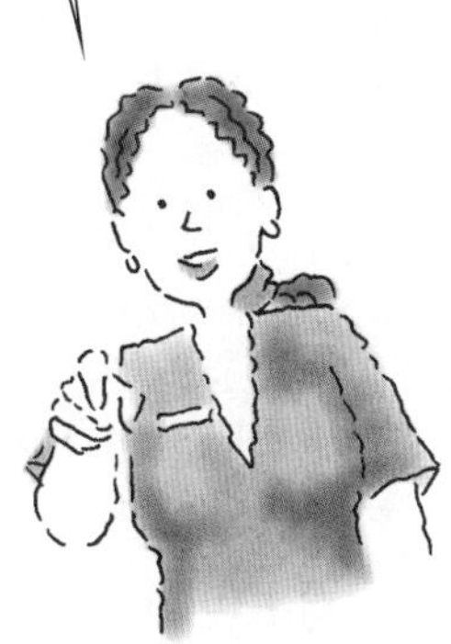

I'm so proud of you. Keep up the good work!

32. A nurse must obtain the blood pressure of a client in airborne isolation. Which method is best to prevent transmission of infection to other clients by the equipment?

1. Dispose of the equipment after each use.
2. Wear gloves while handling the equipment.
3. Use the equipment only with other clients in airborne isolation.
4. Leave the equipment in the room for use only with that client.

32. 4. Leaving equipment in the room is appropriate to avoid organism transmission by inanimate objects. Disposing of equipment after each use prevents the transmission of organisms but isn't cost-effective. Wearing gloves protects the nurse, not other clients. Using equipment for other clients spreads infectious organisms among clients.

CN: Safe, effective care environment; CNS: Safety and infection control; CL: Application

33. To prevent circulatory impairment in an arm when applying an elastic bandage, which method is best?

1. Wrap the bandage around the arm loosely.
2. Apply the bandage while stretching it slightly.
3. Apply heavy pressure with each turn of the bandage.
4. Start applying the bandage at the upper arm and work toward the lower arm.

33. 2. Stretching the bandage slightly maintains uniform tension on the bandage. Wrapping the bandage loosely wouldn't secure the bandage on the arm. Using heavy pressure would cause circulatory impairment. Beginning the wrapping at the upper arm would cause uneven application of the bandage. For example, elastic stockings are applied distal to proximal to promote venous return.

CN: Physiological integrity; CNS: Reduction of risk potential; CL: Application

34. The physician's order reads: 2 grams of cephalexin (Keflex) P.O. daily in equally divided doses of 500 mg each. The nurse would administer this medication at which frequency?

1. 3 times per day
2. 4 times per day
3. 6 times per day
4. 8 times per day

34. 2. 2 grams is equivalent to 2,000 mg (1 gm = 1,000 mg). To give equally divided doses of 500 mg, divide the desired dose of 500 mg into the total daily dose of 2,000 mg. This gives an answer of 4, which is the number of times this dose of medication will be administered per day. This means giving 500 mg every 6 hours, for a total of 4 times per day.

CN: Physiological integrity; CNS: Pharmacological and parenteral therapies; CL: Analysis

35. A client complains of an inability to sleep while on the medical unit. Which intervention should be performed first?

1. Offer a sedative routinely at bedtime.
2. Give the client a backrub before bedtime.
3. Question the client about sleeping habits.
4. Move the client to a bed farthest from the nurses' station.

35. 3. Interviewing the client about sleeping habits may give more information about the causes of the inability to sleep. Sedatives should be given as a last option. A backrub may promote sleep but may not address this client's problem. Moving the client may not address the client's specific problem.

CN: Physiological integrity; CNS: Basic care and comfort; CL: Application

36. In order to assess the function of a client's optic nerve, the nurse would be required to use which equipment?

1. Finger, to test the cardinal fields
2. Flashlight, to test corneal reflexes
3. Snellen's chart, to test visual acuity
4. Piece of cotton, to test corneal sensitivity

36. 3. The Snellen's chart is used to test the function of the optic nerve. Testing the cardinal fields assesses the oculomotor, trochlear, and abducens nerves. Corneal light reflex reflects the function of the oculomotor nerve. Corneal sensitivity is controlled by the trigeminal and facial nerves.

CN: Health promotion and maintenance; CNS: None; CL: Application

37. A nurse is caring for a client following surgery in the post-anesthesia care unit. The nurse observes that the client is gagging on his airway and about to vomit. In which position would the nurse place the client?

1. Prone
2. Trendelenburg
3. Supine
4. Recovery

37. 4. Unless contraindicated, the recovery position, or right- or left-side lying position, should be used. This position is commonly called the recovery position because it is used to prevent aspiration of secretions or vomitus during the postoperative phase. The prone position is face down and not appropriate. Trendelenburg position is used for shock and supine position places the client flat on their back making aspiration possible.

CN: Physiological integrity; CNS: Reduction of risk potential; CL: Application

38. Which intervention is best to prevent bladder infections for a client with an indwelling urinary catheter?

1. Limit fluid intake.
2. Encourage showers rather than tub baths.
3. Open the drainage system to obtain a urine specimen.
4. Irrigate the catheter twice daily with sterile saline solution.

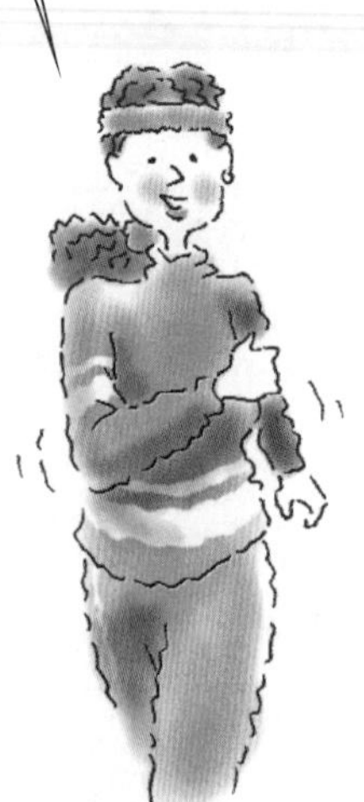

Answer question 38 and you're halfway there.

38. 2. A shower would prevent bacteria in the bath water from sustaining contact with the urinary meatus and the catheter, while a tub bath may allow easier transit of bacteria into the urinary tract. Increased—not limited—fluid intake is recommended for a client with an indwelling urinary catheter. Opening the drainage system would provide a pathway for the entry of bacteria. Catheter irrigation is performed only with an order from the physician to keep the catheter patent.

CN: Physiological integrity; CNS: Reduction of risk potential; CL: Comprehension

39. A nurse wants to use a waist restraint for a client who wanders at night. Which factor or intervention should be considered before applying the restraint?

1. The nurse's convenience
2. The client's reason for getting out of bed
3. A sleeping medication ordered as needed at bedtime
4. The lack of nursing assistants on the night shift

39. 2. The nurse should question the client's reason for getting out of bed because the client may be looking for a bathroom. Lack of adequate staffing and convenience aren't reasons for applying restraints. Sleeping medications are chemical restraints that should be used only if the client is unable to go to sleep and stay asleep.

CN: Safe, effective care environment; CNS: Safety and infection control; CL: Application

40. Six months after the death of her infant son, a client is suspected of dysfunctional grieving. Which assessment would the nurse expect to find in this client?

1. She goes to the infant's grave weekly.
2. She cries when talking about the loss.
3. She's overactive without a sense of loss.
4. She states the infant will always be part of the family.

40. 3. One of the signs of dysfunctional grieving is overactivity without a sense of loss. Including the infant as a part of the family, going to the grave, and crying are all normal responses.

CN: Psychosocial integrity; CNS: None; CL: Application

41. A nurse notices a client has been crying. Which response is most therapeutic?

1. None; this is a private matter.
2. "You seem sad, would you like to talk?"
3. "Why are you crying and upsetting yourself?"
4. "It's hard being in the hospital, but you must keep your chin up."

41. 2. Therapeutic communication is a primary tool of nursing. The nurse must recognize the client's nonverbal behaviors indicate a need to talk. Asking "why" is often interpreted as an accusation. Ignoring the client's nonverbal cues or giving opinions and advice are barriers to communication.

CN: Psychosocial integrity; CNS: None; CL: Application

42. A nurse gives the wrong medication to a client. Another nurse employed by the hospital as a risk manager will expect to receive which communication?

1. Incident report
2. Oral report from the nurse
3. Copy of the medication Kardex
4. Order change signed by the physician

42. 1. Incident reports are tools used by risk managers when a client might be harmed. They're used to determine how future problems can be avoided. An oral report won't serve as legal documentation. A copy of the medication Kardex wouldn't be sent with the incident report to the risk manager. A physician won't change an order to cover the nurse's mistake.

CN: Safe, effective care environment; CNS: Management of care; CL: Application

43. A student nurse wants to know what charge can result from performing a procedure on a client in the absence of informed consent. Which response by the nurse is accurate?

1. Fraud
2. Harassment
3. Assault and battery
4. Breach of confidentiality

43. 3. Performing a procedure on a client without informed consent can be grounds for charges of assault and battery. Fraud is to cheat, harassment means to annoy or disturb, and breach of confidentiality refers to conveying information about the client.

CN: Safe, effective care environment; CNS: Management of care; CL: Application

44. A surgical client newly diagnosed with cancer tells a nurse she knows the laboratory made a mistake about her diagnosis. Which reaction is this client most likely experiencing?

1. Denial
2. Intellectualization
3. Regression
4. Repression

44. 1. Cancer clients often deny this diagnosis when first made. Such a response may benefit the client in that it allows energy for surgical healing. Repression describes not remembering being diagnosed, regression describes childlike behavior, and intellectualization describes speaking of the disease as if reading a textbook.

CN: Psychosocial integrity; CNS: None; CL: Application

45. An unmarried client delivers a premature neonate. Which intervention is included in her treatment plan?

1. An early postpartum physician visit
2. Referral to the health department
3. Request for a social service visit in the hospital
4. Request for a home health visit the day after discharge

45. 3. Due to the client's marital status and premature condition of the neonate, a social service visit is appropriate. The social service visit will determine if there's a need for a referral to the health department. The mother has no physical indications for an early postpartum visit or need for an early home visit.

CN: Safe, effective care environment; CNS: Management of care; CL: Analysis

46. Which statement made by a client about her neonate indicates the need for further teaching?

1. "I'll trim the baby's nails when he's sleeping."
2. "I'll remember to place the baby on his back when he sleeps."
3. "Our infant car seat must be placed in the back seat of the car."
4. "The first thing I'm going to do when we get home is give the baby a tub bath."

46. 4. Neonates shouldn't be placed in a tub bath until after the cord falls off and is completely healed to prevent infection. It's correct to cut his nails while he sleeps, place a neonate on his back, and place the car seat in the back.

CN: Safe, effective care environment; CNS: Safety and infection control; CL: Analysis

47. A client in labor is receiving oxytocin (Pitocin) to augment her labor. A nurse notes a change in her contraction pattern. The fetal heart monitor indicates that her contractions are lasting 2 minutes, with a notable rise in the baseline. Based on this finding, which action is the priority?

1. Notify the physician.
2. Give oxygen through a mask.
3. Turn oxytocin to the lowest level.
4. Turn the client on her left side.

47. 3. The first action must be to lower the oxytocin, to prevent fetal hypoxia or possible rupture of the uterus. The client would then be placed on her left side, given oxygen to prevent fetal hypoxia, and the physician would be notified.

CN: Safe, effective care environment; CNS: Management of care; CL: Analysis

48. A client who just gave birth is concerned about her neonate's Apgar scores of 7 and 8. She says she's been told scores lower than 9 are associated with learning difficulties in later life. Which response is best?

1. "You shouldn't worry so much, your infant is perfectly fine."
2. "You should ask about placing the infant in a follow-up diagnostic program."
3. "You're right in being concerned, but there are good special education programs available."
4. "Apgar scores are used to indicate a need for resuscitation at birth. Scores of 7 and above indicate no problem."

48. 4. Apgar scores don't indicate future learning difficulties; they're for rapid assessment of the need for resuscitation. It's inappropriate to just tell a client not to worry. An Apgar score of 7 and 8 is normal and doesn't indicate a need for intervention.

CN: Health promotion and maintenance; CNS: None; CL: Application

49. After delivering a neonate with a cleft palate and cleft lip, a client has minimal contact with her neonate. She asks the nurse to do most of the neonate's care. Which nursing diagnosis is appropriate?

1. *Anxiety related to fear of harming the neonate*
2. *Deficient knowledge related to neonate's potential*
3. *Risk for impaired parenting related to birth defect*
4. *Ineffective coping related to birth defect*

49. 3. Neonates born with birth defects are at risk for impaired parenting. The parents must work through issues of not producing the perfect child and guilt associated with this. There's nothing in the question that indicates the client felt anxious about caring for the neonate or had ineffective coping problems or a knowledge deficit.

CN: Safe, effective care environment; CNS: Management of care; CL: Application

50. A breast-feeding client asks how she can do breast self-examination (BSE) while nursing. Which response would be the most accurate?

1. "You should do BSE after the infant has emptied the breast."
2. "You don't have to do BSE until after you stop breast-feeding."
3. "You should continue to do BSE the way you did before becoming pregnant."
4. "Your physician will examine your breasts until after you stop breast-feeding."

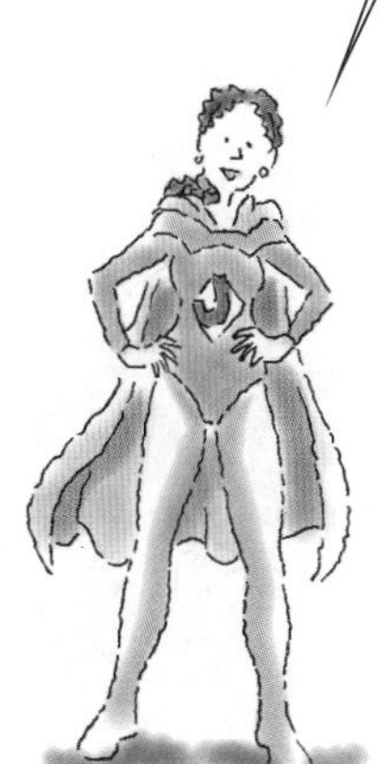

You've now completed 50 questions and are two-thirds finished. Super!

50. 1. During breast-feeding, the client should examine each breast after the neonate has emptied the breast. Women must continue to examine their breasts, even if they're lactating. Contrary to how it's performed before pregnancy, BSE should be done on the same day of the month until the menstrual cycle returns. Breast examination shouldn't be done solely by the physician.

CN: Health promotion and maintenance; CNS: None; CL: Application

51. A prenatal client says she can't believe she has such mixed feelings about being pregnant. She tried for 10 years to become pregnant and now she feels guilty for her conflicting reactions. Which response is best?

1. "You need to talk to your midwife about these feelings."
2. "You're experiencing the normal ambivalence pregnant mothers feel."
3. "These feelings are expected only in women who have had difficulty becoming pregnant."
4. "Let's make an appointment with a counselor."

51. 2. Conflicting, ambivalent feelings regarding pregnancy are normal for all pregnant women. These feelings don't call for counseling or other professional interventions. Ambivalence is felt by most pregnant women, not only mothers who had difficulty becoming pregnant.

CN: Psychosocial integrity; CNS: None; CL: Application

52. A maternity client says her husband is behaving in strange ways since she became pregnant. He's having morning sickness, has put on weight, complains of intestinal pains, and is acting like he's pregnant. Which term describes this reaction?

1. Extreme anxiety
2. Normal couvade
3. Signs of reaction formation
4. Abnormal, needing counseling

52. 2. The father's adjustment may include behaviors referred to as couvade. Historically, there have been different cultural couvades. Today, the term is associated with the father developing pregnancy-like symptoms. Because the behavior is normal and isn't reaction formation or anxiety, there's no need for counseling.

CN: Psychosocial integrity; CNS: None; CL: Analysis

53. Three days after discharge, a client bottle-feeding her neonate calls the postpartum floor, asking what she can do for breast engorgement. Which instruction is correct?

1. Put a tight binder around her breasts.
2. Get under a warm shower and let the water flow on her breasts.
3. Stop drinking milk because it contributes to breast engorgement.
4. Contact her physician; she shouldn't be engorged at this late date.

53. 1. A tight binder is recommended for the client bottle-feeding her neonate to reduce engorgement. A warm shower will stimulate milk production. It's normal to become engorged during the first few days after delivery, and drinking milk isn't the cause.

CN: Physiological integrity; CNS: Basic care and comfort; CL: Application

54. A pregnant client complains of leg cramps that wake her from sleep. Which instruction is correct?

1. Dorsiflex the foot.
2. Elevate the legs at night.
3. Point the toes until the cramp releases.
4. Drink more than 1 quart of milk a day.

54. 1. Dorsiflexion of the foot is the recommended intervention to relieve a leg cramp during pregnancy. Elevating the legs isn't a usual treatment. Drinking more than 1 quart of milk and pointing the toes are associated with causing leg cramps.

CN: Physiological integrity; CNS: Basic care and comfort; CL: Application

55. A client is being treated for premature labor with ritodrine (Yutopar). After receiving this medication for 12 hours, her blood pressure is slightly elevated, her chest is clear, and her pulse is 120 beats/minute. She complains of a little nausea, and the fetal heart rate is 145 beats/minute. Which intervention is correct?

1. Continue routine monitoring.
2. Contact the physician immediately.
3. Turn the client on her left side and give oxygen.
4. Increase the flow rate of the I.V. and give oxygen.

55. 1. These findings are normal adverse effects to the medication and don't call for interventions at this time except to continue routine monitoring. Contacting the physician, placing the client on her left side, changing the I.V. flow rate, and giving oxygen are all interventions for abnormal assessment findings.

CN: Physiological integrity; CNS: Pharmacological and parental therapies; CL: Analysis

56. At 6 cm of dilation, the client in labor receives a lumbar epidural for pain control. Which nursing diagnosis is possible?

1. Risk for injury related to rapid delivery
2. Acute pain related to wearing off of anesthesia
3. Hyperthermia related to effects of anesthesia
4. Ineffective peripheral tissue perfusion related to effects of anesthesia

56. 4. A disadvantage of a lumbar epidural is the risk for hypotension, which can lead to ineffective tissue perfusion. Epidurals are associated with a longer labor and hypothermia. There's no pain involved with the anesthesia wearing off.

CN: Safe, effective care environment; CNS: Management of care; CL: Application

57. When assessing a client who just delivered a neonate, a nurse finds the following: blood pressure, 110/70 mm Hg; pulse, 60 beats/minute; respirations, 16 breaths/minute; lochia, moderate rubra; fundus, above the umbilicus to the right; and negative Homans' sign. Which intervention is correct?

1. Nothing; all findings are normal.
2. Have the client void and recheck the fundus.
3. Turn the client on her left side to decrease the blood pressure.
4. Rub the fundus to decrease lochia flow and prevent hemorrhage.

57. 2. A fundus up and to the right indicates a full bladder. The client should empty her bladder and be reassessed. Lochia flow and blood pressure are normal.

CN: Physiological integrity; CNS: Reduction of risk potential; CL: Analysis

58. A client with diabetes delivers a 9-lb, 6-oz neonate. The neonate is assessed for which condition?

1. Hyperglycemia
2. Hypoglycemia
3. Hyperthermia
4. Hypothermia

58. 2. Neonates of mothers with diabetes and large neonates are at risk for hypoglycemia related to increased production of insulin by the neonate in utero. Hyperglycemia, hypothermia, and hyperthermia aren't primary concerns.

CN: Physiological integrity; CNS: Reduction of risk potential; CL: Application

59. A prenatal client, age 13, asks about getting fat while she's pregnant. A nurse tells her she needs to gain enough weight to be in the upper portions of her recommended weight due to her age to prevent which condition?

1. Delivery of a premature neonate
2. A difficult delivery
3. Delivery of a low birth-weight neonate
4. Gestational hypertension

59. 3. Adolescent girls, especially those younger than age 15, are at higher risk for delivering low birth-weight neonates unless they gain adequate weight during pregnancy. Gaining weight isn't associated with having an easier delivery, risk for gestational hypertension, or risk of delivering a premature neonate.

CN: Physiological integrity; CNS: Reduction of risk potential; CL: Application

60. A mother of a neonate receiving phototherapy asks why her child has developed loose stools. Which response by the nurse would be accurate?

1. They're abnormal and may indicate an infection.
2. They're associated with an adverse reaction to formula.
3. They're common when receiving phototherapy treatments.
4. They're abnormal and phototherapy should be discontinued.

60. 3. While receiving phototherapy, a breakdown of bilirubin often results in loose stools. The neonate must be monitored for diarrhea and dehydration when under the lights. The loose stools wouldn't be considered related to infection or formula at this time.

CN: Physiological integrity; CNS: Physiological adaptation; CL: Application

61. A client at 36 weeks' gestation chokes on her food while eating at a restaurant. Which statement is correct about performing the Heimlich maneuver on a pregnant client?

1. Chest thrusts are used when the client is pregnant.
2. Only back thrusts are used when the client is pregnant.
3. The Heimlich maneuver is performed the same as when not pregnant.
4. The Heimlich maneuver can't be performed on a pregnant client.

61. 1. During pregnancy, chest thrusts are used instead of abdominal thrusts. Abdominal thrusts compress the abdomen, which would harm the fetus. Because of this, the Heimlich is adjusted for the pregnant woman. A fist is made with one hand, placing thumb side against the center of the breastbone. The fist is grabbed with the other hand and thrust inward. Avoid the lower tip of the breastbone. Back thrusts aren't done as they may result in dislodgment of the obstruction, further obstructing the airway.

CN: Physiological integrity; CNS: Reduction of risk potential; CL: Application

62. A nurse is reviewing principles of good body mechanics with a student nurse. Which of the following techniques should be emphasized?

1. Bending from the waist
2. Pulling rather than pushing
3. Stretching to reach an object
4. Using large muscles in the legs for leverage

62. 4. Keeping one's back straight and using the large muscles in the legs will help avoid back injury, as the muscles in one's back are relatively small compared with the larger muscles of the thighs. Bending from the waist can cause stress on the back muscles, causing a potential injury. Pulling isn't the best option and may cause straining. When feasible, one should push an object rather than pull it. Stretching to reach an object increases the risk of injury.

CN: Safe, effective care environment; CNS: Safety and infection control; CL: Application

63. A client with a substance abuse problem is being discharged from the state mental hospital. The client's discharge plans should include which intervention?

1. Referral to Al-Anon
2. Weekly urine testing for drug use
3. Day hospital treatment for 6 months
4. Participation in a support group like Alcoholics Anonymous (AA)

63. 4. AA is a major support group for alcoholics after treatment. Membership in AA is associated with relapse prevention. Al-Anon is a support group for the family of the abuser of alcohol. Weekly urine testing or day hospital treatment isn't usual.

CN: Safe, effective care environment; CNS: Management of care; CL: Application

64. A community mental health nurse visits a client diagnosed with paranoid schizophrenia. When she arrives at his house, he calls her Satan, shouts at her, and tells her to back away. Which intervention should be performed first?

1. Use his phone and call the police.
2. Remain safe by leaving the house.
3. Talk to him in a calm voice to reduce his agitation.
4. Remind him who she is and that he has nothing to fear.

64. 2. Safety is the first priority during any home visit, so the nurse should leave. Attempting to talk with the client, reminding him who she is, or using the phone places the nurse at risk for harm. After the nurse has ensured her safety, arrangements should be made to provide help for the client.

CN: Safe, effective care environment; CNS: Safety and infection control; CL: Analysis

65. A client is scheduled to retire in the next month. He phones his nurse therapist and says he can't cope; his whole world is falling apart. The therapist recognizes this reaction as which condition?

1. Panic reaction
2. Situational crisis
3. Normal separation anxiety
4. Maturational crisis

65. 4. A maturational (developmental) crisis is one that occurs at a predictable milestone during a life span; birth, marriage, and retirement are examples. A panic reaction would also involve physical symptoms. Situational crisis is caused by events such as an earthquake. Separation anxiety is a childhood disorder.

CN: Health promotion and maintenance; CNS: None; CL: Analysis

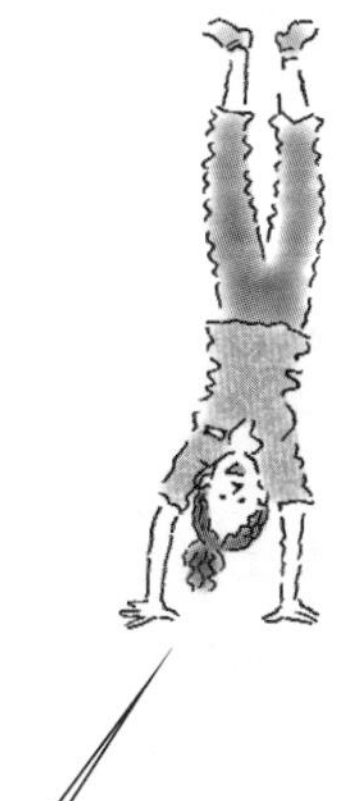

Only 10 more to go! Oh my, I just can't wait!

66. A client with a phobic condition is being treated with behavior modification therapy. Which treatment is expected?

1. Dream analysis
2. Free association
3. Systematic desensitization
4. Electroconvulsive therapy (ECT)

66. 3. Systematic desensitization is a behavior therapy used in the treatment of phobias. Dream analysis and free association are techniques used in psychoanalytic therapy. ECT is used with depression.

CN: Psychosocial integrity; CNS: None; CL: Comprehension

67. A severely depressed client rarely leaves his chair. To prevent physiologic complications associated with psychomotor retardation, which goal is appropriate?

1. Restrict coffee intake.
2. Increase calcium intake.
3. Rest in bed three times per day.
4. Empty the bladder on a schedule.

67. 4. To prevent bladder infections associated with stasis of urine, the client should be encouraged to routinely empty his bladder. Neither calcium nor coffee intake are directly related to the psychological effects associated with this condition. Resting in bed is another form of psychomotor retardation.

CN: Health promotion and maintenance; CNS: None; CL: Application

68. During the termination phase of a therapeutic nurse-client relationship, which intervention is avoided?

1. Refer the client to support groups.
2. Address new issues with the client.
3. Review what has been accomplished during this relationship.
4. Have the client express sadness that the relationship is ending.

68. 2. During the termination phase, new issues shouldn't be explored. It's appropriate to refer the client to support groups. To review what has been accomplished is a goal of this phase. Sadness is a normal response.

CN: Psychosocial integrity; CNS: None; CL: Application

69. The behavior of a client with borderline personality disorder causes a nurse to feel angry toward the client. Which response, if made by the nurse, is the most therapeutic?

1. Ignore the client's irritating behavior.
2. Restrict the client to her room until supper.
3. Report her feelings to the client's physician.
4. Tell the client how her behavior makes the nurse feel.

69. 4. A nursing intervention used with personality disorders is to help the client recognize how her behavior affects others. Restricting the client to her room, ignoring the client, and reporting feelings to the physician aren't appropriate interventions at this time.

CN: Psychosocial integrity; CNS: None; CL: Application

70. During a manic state, a client paced around the dayroom for 3 days. He talked to the furniture, proclaimed he was a king, and refused to partake in unit activities. Which nursing diagnosis has priority?

1. Impaired verbal communication related to hyperactivity
2. Risk for self-directed violence related to manic state
3. Imbalanced nutrition: Less than body requirements related to hyperactivity
4. Ineffective coping related to manic state

70. 3. During a manic state, clients are at risk for malnutrition due to not taking in enough calories for the energy they're expending. The client is not displaying impaired verbal communication. This client isn't showing self-directed violent behavior. Individual coping issues aren't the primary concern at this time.

CN: Safe, effective care environment; CNS: Management of care; CL: Application

71. A client with a panic disorder is having difficulty falling asleep. Which nursing intervention should be performed first?

1. Call the client's psychotherapist.
2. Teach the client progressive relaxation.
3. Allow the client to stay up and watch television.
4. Obtain an order for a sleeping medication as needed.

71. 2. Relaxation techniques work very well with a client showing anxiety. If this doesn't work, then contacting the psychotherapist, diversionary activities, and pharmacological interventions would be in order.

CN: Psychological integrity; CNS: None; CL: Application

72. After electroconvulsive therapy (ECT) which nursing intervention is correct?

1. Assessing the client's vital signs
2. Letting the client sleep undisturbed
3. Allowing the family to visit immediately
4. Restraining the client until completely awake

72. 1. Vital signs are monitored carefully for approximately 1 hour after ECT or until the client is stable. The client shouldn't be restrained or left alone. Visitors should be allowed when the client is awake and ready.

CN: Physiological integrity; CNS: Reduction of risk potential; CL: Application

73. A client diagnosed with bipolar disease is receiving a maintenance dosage of lithium carbonate (Lithobid). His wife calls the community mental health nurse to report that her husband is hyperactive and hyperverbal. Which intervention is appropriate?

1. Mental status examination
2. Measurement of lithium blood levels
3. Evaluation at the local emergency department (ED)
4. Admission to the hospital for observation

73. 2. Increased activity might indicate a need for an increased dose of lithium or that the client isn't taking his medications; blood levels will determine this. The client doesn't need to have a mental status examination, go to the ED, or be admitted to the hospital at this time.

CN: Physiological integrity; CNS: Pharmacological and parenteral therapies; CL: Analysis

74. A nurse is caring for a client with emphysema. Which nursing interventions are appropriate? Select all that apply:

1. Reduce fluid intake to less than 2,500 ml/day.
2. Teach diaphragmatic, pursed-lip breathing.
3. Administer low-flow oxygen.
4. Keep the client in a supine position as much as possible.
5. Encourage alternating activity with rest periods.
6. Teach the use of postural drainage and chest physiotherapy.

74. 2, 3, 5, 6. Diaphragmatic, pursed-lip breathing strengthens respiratory muscles and enhances oxygenation in clients with emphysema. Low-flow oxygen should be administered because a client with emphysema has chronic hypercapnia and a hypoxic respiratory drive. Alternating activity with rest allows the client to perform activities without excessive distress. If the client has copious secretions and has difficulty mobilizing them, the nurse should teach him and his family members how to perform postural drainage and chest physiotherapy. Fluid intake should be increased to 3,000 ml/day, if not contraindicated, to liquefy secretions and facilitate their removal. The client should be placed in high-Fowler's position to improve ventilation.

CN: Physiological integrity; CNS: Basic care and comfort; CL: Application

75. A nurse is assessing the abdomen of a client who was admitted to the emergency department with suspected appendicitis. Identify the area of the abdomen that the nurse should palpate last.

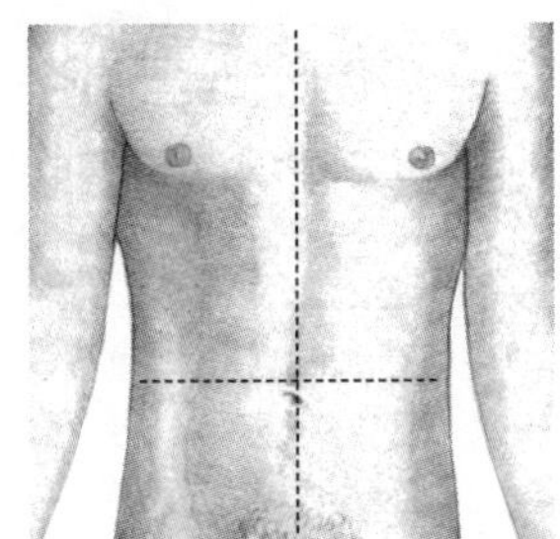

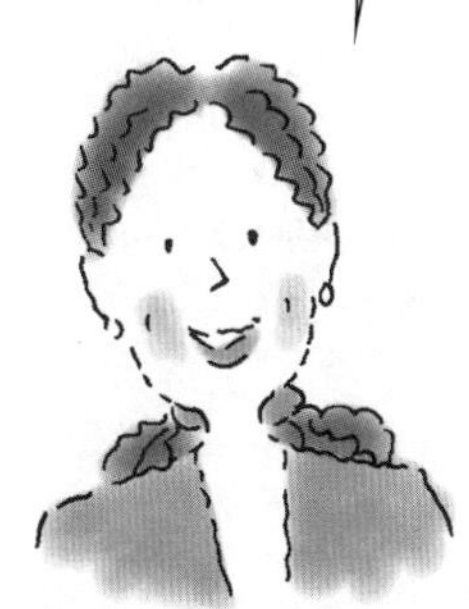

75. An acute attack of appendicitis localizes as pain and tenderness in the lower right quadrant, midway between the umbilicus and the crest of the ilium. This area should be palpated last in order to determine if pain is also present in other areas of the abdomen.

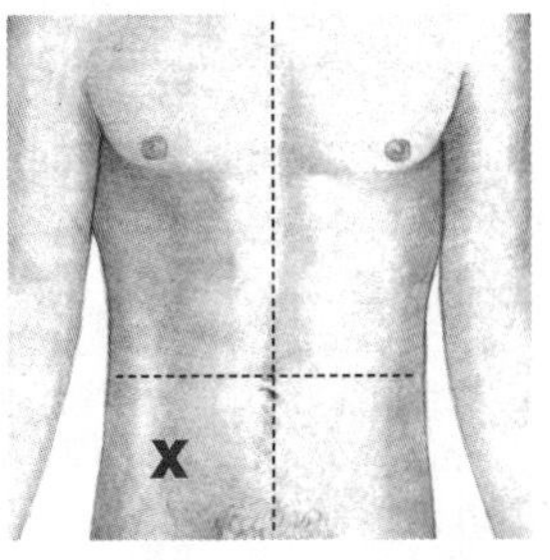

CN: Health promotion and maintenance; CNS: None; CL: Application

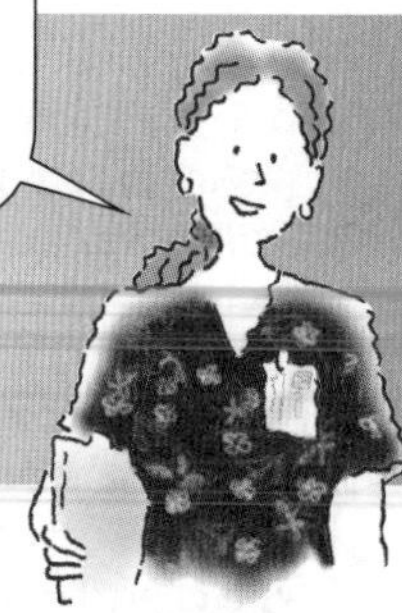

Here's another challenging comprehensive test with a variety of questions like a real NCLEX test. Have a go at it!

COMPREHENSIVE Test 3

1. A client in the postoperative phase of abdominal surgery is to advance his diet as tolerated. The client has tolerated ice chips and a clear liquid diet. Which diet would the nurse expect the client to be given when he advances from this diet?

1. Fluid restricted
2. Full liquids
3. General
4. Soft

1. 2. Clear liquid diets are nutritionally inadequate but minimally irritating to the stomach. Clients are advanced to the full liquid diet next, adding bland and protein foods. A soft diet comes next, which omits foods that are hard to chew or digest. A regular or general diet has no limitations. A fluid restriction is ordered in addition to the diet order for clients in renal failure or congestive heart failure.

CN: Physiological integrity; CNS: Basic care and comfort; CL: Application

2. The following information is recorded on an intake and output record: milk, 180 ml; orange juice, 60 ml; 1 serving scrambled eggs; 1 slice toast; 1 can Ensure oral nutritional supplement, 240 ml; I.V. dextrose 5% in water at 100 ml/hour; 50 ml water after twice daily medications. Medications are given at 9:00 a.m. and 9:00 p.m. What is the client's total intake for the 7 a.m. to 3 p.m. shift?

1. 1,000 ml
2. 1,250 ml
3. 1,330 ml
4. 1,380 ml

2. 3. The client's total intake is 1,330 ml. Use the following equation:
180 + 60 + 240 + 800 + 50 = 1,330.

CN: Physiological integrity; CNS: Basic care and comfort; CL: Analysis

3. A pediatrician writes an order for digoxin (Lanoxin), 2.5 mg, for a neonate. A nurse questions the order with the pharmacist and physician taking the call. Which legal standard is most relevant?

1. American Medical Association
2. American Nurses Association (ANA)
3. American Pharmaceutical Association
4. Nurse Practice Act

3. 4. Each state has a Nurse Practice Act that dictates a nurse's scope of practice. Each nurse must practice competent standards based on her state's Nurse Practice Act. The ANA is an organization of nurses that offers credentialing and nursing education. It doesn't set standards of nursing practice. Physicians and pharmacists must practice competency based on the standards established by their professional organizations.

CN: Safe, effective care environment; CNS: Management of care; CL: Application

CN: Client needs category CNS: Client needs subcategory CL: Cognitive level

4. In checking a client's chart, the nurse notes that there's no record of an opioid being given to the client even though the previous nurse signed for one. The client denies receiving anything for pain since the previous night. Which action should be taken next?

1. Notify the physician that an opioid is missing.
2. Notify the supervisor that the client didn't receive the prescribed pain medication.
3. Notify the pharmacist that the client didn't receive the prescribed pain medication.
4. Approach the nurse who signed out the opioid to seek clarification about the missing drug.

4. 4. The nurse needs to seek clarification in a nonthreatening manner. If the nurse who signed out the opioid can't give a plausible explanation, the nurse who discovered the error must then notify the supervisor. The nurse who signed out the opioid may have a drug problem. The appropriate line of communication is to the hospital supervisor. The physician needs to be notified if the client didn't receive the prescribed medication. The pharmacist needs to be notified of discrepancies in the opioid count.
CN: Safe, effective care environment; CNS: Management of care; CL: Application

5. A client is seen in the emergency department with bruises on her face and back. She has the signs of a domestic abuse victim. Which community resource could provide assistance to the client?

1. Alcoholics Anonymous (AA)
2. Crime Task Force
3. Lifeline Emergency Aid
4. Women's shelter

5. 4. A women's shelter can house women and children who need protection from an abusive partner or parent. AA is a support group for alcoholics and their families. The Crime Task Force and Lifeline Emergency Aid don't provide housing for women or children who want to leave an abusive relationship.
CN: Safe, effective care environment; CNS: Management of care; CL: Application

6. Multidisciplinary team meetings are used frequently as a method of communication among health care disciplines. Which unit uses this method of communication?

1. Hemodialysis
2. Home health care services
3. Labor and delivery units
4. Outpatient surgical units

6. 2. Home health care services and restorative care services (such as rehabilitation units) that use different disciplines are required by The Joint Commission or Medicare to hold multidisciplinary team meetings. This serves as a means of communicating the client's diagnosis, plan of care, and discharge needs, using all disciplines for input. Hemodialysis units, outpatient surgical units, and labor and delivery units use between-shift reporting as a method of communicating and communicate among disciplines on an as needed basis.
CN: Safe, effective care environment; CNS: Management of care; CL: Application

7. A nurse finds a client crying after she was told hemodialysis is needed due to the development of acute renal failure. Which intervention is best?

1. Sit quietly with the client.
2. Refer the client to the hemodialysis team.
3. Remind the client this is a temporary situation.
4. Discuss with the client the other abilities she has.

7. 1. Sitting with the client shows compassion and concern, and may help the nurse establish therapeutic communication. Making a referral doesn't allow the client to explore feelings with the nurse. The nurse can't guarantee the acute renal failure is temporary. Discussing the client's other abilities is diverting the emphasis away from the primary issue for this client.
CN: Psychosocial integrity; CNS: None; CL: Analysis

8. A client was admitted to a mental health ward for hyperexcitability, increasing agitation, and distractibility. Which nursing intervention has priority?

1. Involve the client in a group activity.
2. Be direct, firm, and set rules for the client.
3. Use a quiet room for the client away from others.
4. Channel the client's energy toward a planned activity.

8. 3. Being in a quiet environment away from stimuli facilitates helping the client regain a sense of control. If the nurse attempts to be firm and set rules for this client, it will most likely heighten the agitation. The client is too excited to focus at this time; group activities or other activities may worsen the client's situation.

CN: Psychosocial integrity; CNS: None; CL: Application

9. After maxillofacial surgery, a client, awake and alert, complains of pain, rating it as a 9 on a scale of 1 to 10. He receives meperidine (Demerol) 50 mg and hydroxyzine (Vistaril) 50 mg as ordered, every 4 hours as needed. Twenty minutes after the first dose, he reports his pain as a 6; 2 hours later, it's an 8. What might the nurse suspect is occurring?

1. The hydroxyzine has interfered with the analgesic effect of the meperidine.
2. The client has been moving too much.
3. The client may need a higher dose.
4. The prescription should be changed.

9. 3. It's reasonable to assume that the dose is probably too low for the amount of pain, and it would be prudent to report the client's response to the physician and inquire if the physician feels it's appropriate to increase the dose. The hydroxyzine potentiates the effects of meperidine and doesn't interfere with its effectiveness. There's no evidence to suggest that the client has been moving around too much. It's beyond the nurse's scope of practice to determine that the current medication should be changed.

CN: Physiological integrity; CNS: Pharmacological and parenteral therapies; CL: Analysis

10. A public health nurse visiting a new postpartum client notices that the client has two children under age 4. The nurse notices one infant playing in the cabinet under the sink. Which instruction should the public health nurse give the client?

1. Cover the infant's hands with gloves.
2. Make sure all liquid cleaners are labeled.
3. Tighten all cap tops on the bottles under the sink.
4. Remove all cleaners that could be ingested orally.

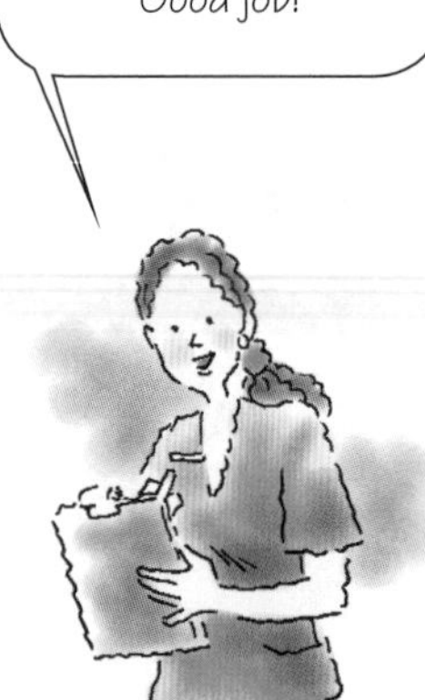

You've finished 10 questions already! Good job!

10. 4. All liquid cleaners must be removed to reduce the risk for poisoning. Safety locks should be placed on cabinets to prevent young children from opening the cabinets or the bottles. Infants can't read danger labels.

CN: Safe, effective care environment; CNS: Safety and infection control; CL: Application

11. A nurse arrives at a motor vehicle collision involving a school bus and a large truck. The school bus is lying on its side. Several people have been thrown from the windows of the school bus. Which victim needs priority care?

1. A girl crying hysterically
2. A boy who's unconscious
3. A boy with a laceration of the scalp
4. A girl with an obvious open fracture

11. 2. The unconscious child should be assessed for breathing and circulation status. An unconscious or unresponsive client always needs assistance first. Once help arrives, emotional support can be given to the girl crying hysterically, pressure can be applied to the laceration of the scalp to stop the bleeding, and the girl's fracture can be stabilized.

CN: Safe, effective care environment; CNS: Management of care; CL: Application

12. Which statement from a newly diagnosed client with diabetes indicates more instruction is needed?

1. "I need to check my feet daily for sores."
2. "I need to store my insulin in the refrigerator."
3. "I can use my plastic insulin syringe more than once."
4. "I need to see my physician for follow-up examinations."

12. 2. Insulin only needs to be stored in the refrigerator if it won't be used within 6 weeks after being opened; it should be at room temperature when given to decrease pain and prevent lipodystrophy. According to a poll by the Juvenile Diabetes Foundation, a very high percentage of diabetics reuse their insulin syringes. However, it's recommended they be carefully recapped and placed in the refrigerator to prevent bacterial growth. The remaining statements show that the client understands his condition and the importance of preventing complications.

CN: Safe, effective care environment; CNS: Safety and infection control; CL: Analysis

13. A client with terminal cancer is receiving large doses of opioids for pain control. He becomes agitated and continues trying to get out of bed but can't stand without two-person assistance. To reduce the risk of falling, which type of restraint is the most beneficial?

1. Leg restraints
2. Chemical restraints
3. Mechanical restraints
4. Tying him in bed with a sheet

13. 2. Antianxiety medication can be used to calm the client. Chemical restraints are effective, especially with highly agitated clients receiving large doses of opioids. Other forms of restraint will only increase the client's agitation and hostility, thus increasing the safety risk.

CN: Safe, effective care environment; CNS: Safety and infection control; CL: Application

14. A client who had a stem cell transplant is in reverse isolation postoperatively. Which explanation for this precaution is correct?

1. To protect the client from his own bacteria
2. To protect the hospital staff from the client
3. To protect the other clients on the nursing unit
4. To protect the client from outside infections from others

14. 4. Immunosuppressed clients need to be protected from infections from others following a stem cell transplant. Infections can occur if strict handwashing techniques aren't observed, especially with hospital staff going from one room to the next. Protective isolation is used to protect the hospital staff and other clients from an infected client.

CN: Safe, effective care environment; CNS: Safety and infection control; CL: Application

15. A physician ordered a sterile dressing tray set up in a client's room to insert a subclavian central venous catheter. Which step is done first to set up the sterile field?

1. Open the tray toward the nurse.
2. Use correct handwashing technique.
3. Put on sterile gloves before opening the tray.
4. Place the sterile dressing tray on an overbed table.

15. 2. Use appropriate handwashing technique before participating in a sterile procedure. Clean the area with an appropriate antiseptic, place the tray in the center of the clean area, and open it away from the nurse. After the dressing tray is opened, put on sterile gloves to assist the physician.

CN: Safe, effective care environment; CNS: Safety and infection control; CL: Application

16. Which action is included in the principles of asepsis?

1. Maintaining a sterile environment
2. Keeping the environment as clean as possible
3. Testing for microorganisms in the environment
4. Cleaning an environment until it's free from germs

16. 2. Asepsis is the process of avoiding contamination from outside sources by keeping the environment clean. A clean environment has a reduced number of microorganisms, but isn't necessarily sterile (the absence of all microorganisms). Testing for microorganisms or culturing isn't indicated in the promotion of asepsis.
CN; Safe, effective care environment; CNS: Safety and infection control; CL: Application

17. A public health nurse is interviewing a young Pakistani client in her home. The nurse notices the client and the infant wear long skirts and coverings over their heads. The home isn't air-conditioned and the room is very warm. The dress code is recognized as part of which characteristic?

1. Culture
2. Economic status
3. Race
4. Socialization

17. 1. Many cultures have specific dress codes. The client's dress, as described, doesn't indicate economic status. Race refers to a group of people with similar physical characteristics such as skin color. Socialization is the process by which individuals learn the ways of a given society to function within that group.
CN: Health promotion and maintenance; CNS: None; CL: Application

18. A nurse is preparing a care plan for a client. Which action should be included in the assessment step of the nursing process?

1. Identify actual or potential health problems specific to the individual client.
2. Judge the effectiveness of nursing interventions that have been implemented.
3. Identify goals and interventions specific to the individualized needs of the client.
4. Systematically collect subjective and objective data with the goal of making a clinical nursing judgment.

18. 4. Assessment involves data collection, organization, and validation. The diagnosis step of the nursing process involves the identification of actual or potential health problems. Evaluation involves judging the effectiveness of nursing interventions and whether the goals of the plan of care have been achieved. The nurse and client work together to identify goals, outcomes, and intervention strategies that will reduce identified client problems in the planning step.
CN: Safe, effective care environment; CNS: Management of care; CL: Application

19. During an interdepartmental team meeting at a hospice, a nurse who practices Catholicism verbalizes concern for the spiritual needs of a terminally ill infant and her non-Catholic family. She suggests the infant be baptized before death. Which recommendation of the multidisciplinary team is most likely?

1. Insist the infant obtain baptism before death occurs.
2. Bathe the infant with special oil to prepare for death.
3. Schedule an appointment with a Catholic priest to see the family.
4. Recognize that not all religions practice infant baptism.

19. 4. Many religious organizations (for example, Baptist, Adventist, Buddhist, Quaker) don't practice baptism or only baptize an individual when he or she is an adult. Hospice organizations use the family's religious leader as a choice for spiritual directions. Deciding whether to baptize the infant isn't the nurse's responsibility. Seventh Day Adventists believe in divine healing and anointing with oil. It's important to honor all customs and religious beliefs of families.
CN: Safe, effective care environment; CNS: Management of care; CL: Application

20. A home health client asks a nurse for information on sources of financial support. The client has an elderly parent who's blind living with her. Which program is the client referred to?

1. Medicare
2. Meals On Wheels
3. Supplemental Security Income
4. Aid to Families with Dependent Children

20. 3. Supplemental Security Income is a governmental subsidy assisting the poor and medically disabled. Medicare is available to elderly individuals age 65 years and older and individuals younger than 65 years with long-term disabilities or end-stage renal disease. Meals On Wheels is a nonprofit organization that delivers food to the poor. Aid to Families with Dependent Children is a state subsidy given to poor families with dependent children.

CN: Safe, effective care environment; CNS: Management of care; CL: Application

21. Giving hearing and vision screening to elementary school children is an example of which type of prevention strategy?

1. Primary
2. Secondary
3. Tertiary
4. None of the above

21. 2. Screening is a major secondary prevention strategy. Secondary prevention is aimed at early detection and treatment of illness. Primary prevention strategies are aimed at preventing the disease from the beginning by avoiding or modifying risk factors. Tertiary prevention strategies focus on rehabilitation and prevention of complications arising from advanced disease.

CN: Health promotion and maintenance; CNS: None; CL: Application

22. Which nursing action is most appropriate in relieving pain related to cancer?

1. Use heat or cold on painful areas.
2. Keep a hard bedroll behind the client's back.
3. Allow the client to stay in one position to prevent pain.
4. Keep bright lights on in the room so the nurse can assess the client more quickly.

22. 1. Using either heat or cold can reduce inflammatory responses, which will reduce pain. Avoid pressure (such as bedrolls) on painful areas. Change the client's position frequently. Coordinate activity with pain medication. Reduce bright lights and noise to prevent anxiety, which can increase pain.

CN: Physiological integrity; CNS: Physiological adaptation; CL: Application

23. A new graduate is assigned to a nursing unit. A nurse manager assesses that the graduate's skills are deficient. Which action is the most appropriate for the nurse manager to take?

1. Talk with the supervisor about terminating the new graduate.
2. Discuss with the graduate that a transfer to another unit is necessary.
3. Work with the graduate and develop a plan to improve the graduate's deficiencies.
4. Counsel the graduate that, if performance doesn't improve, the graduate will be terminated.

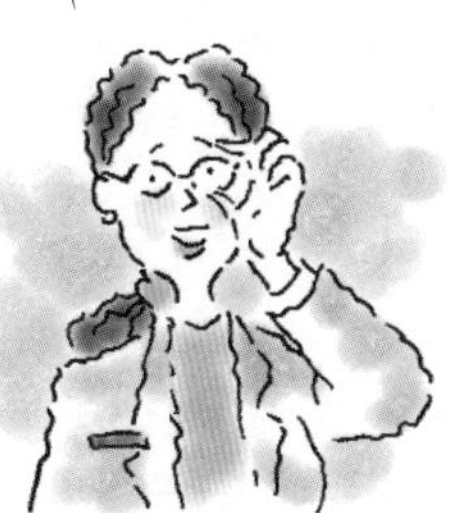

Stay focused, now. You're nearly one-third finished!

23. 3. The leader needs to work with the new graduate and provide opportunities for the graduate to grow and develop. The other responses wouldn't give the new graduate the opportunity and support needed for improvement.

CN: Safe, effective care environment; CNS: Management of care; CL: Application

24. A local community health nurse is asked to speak to a group of adolescent girls on the topic of preventing pregnancy. Which statement indicates the adolescents need more information on this topic?

1. "I can get pregnant even on the first time we have sex."
2. "I can get pregnant even though I don't have sex regularly."
3. "I can't get pregnant because my menstrual cycle isn't regular yet."
4. "I can get pregnant even if my boyfriend withdraws before he comes."

24. 3. Many adolescents have misunderstandings related to risk periods and timing, including periods of susceptibility during the menstrual cycle, age-related susceptibility, and timing of male ejaculation.
CN: Health promotion and maintenance; CNS: None; CL: Analysis

25. Which nursing action is most appropriate in stimulating the appetite of a child with cancer?

1. Use food as a reward system.
2. Serve large meals frequently.
3. Prepare foods appropriate to the age of the child.
4. Place the child on a rigid time schedule for eating.

25. 3. It's important to prepare foods appropriate to children in certain age groups. Involve the child in food preparation and selection. Assess the family's beliefs about food habits. Let the child eat all food that can be tolerated. Take advantage of a hungry period and serve small snacks. Encourage parents to relax pressures placed on eating by stressing the legitimate nature of loss of appetite.
CN: Physiological integrity; CNS: Physiological adaptation; CL: Application

26. A nurse working in a public health clinic is planning tuberculosis (TB) screening. Screening is indicated for which group?

1. All clients coming into the clinic
2. People living in a homeless shelter
3. Clients who haven't received the TB vaccine
4. Clients suspected of having human immunodeficiency virus (HIV)

26. 4. Clients with HIV infection or suspected of having HIV are at greater risk for developing TB. A screening test should be done and, if positive, treatment with isoniazid (Nydrazid) given. Clients coming to the clinic don't need to be tested unless they're at high risk—for example, living with someone infected with TB, abusing I.V. drugs, or suffering from chronic health conditions, such as diabetes mellitus and end-stage renal disease. Clients living in a homeless shelter aren't necessarily at greater risk unless other residents in the shelter have TB. The TB vaccine isn't widely used in the United States.
CN: Health promotion and maintenance; CNS: None; CL: Application

27. A professional nurse should report positive tuberculosis (TB) smears or cultures to the health department within which time period?

1. 12 hours
2. 48 hours
3. 1 week
4. 10 to 14 days

27. 2. A client is considered contagious if he has a positive TB smear or culture, so the results must be reported within 24 to 48 hours. The smear or culture may not have grown an organism in 12 hours. One week or 10 to 14 days is too long to wait.
CN: Safe, effective care environment; CNS: Safety and infection control; CL: Application

28. A 62-year-old female client has been taking vitamin C 500 mg by mouth (P.O.) daily, multivitamins 1 tablet P.O. every day, and aspirin 325 mg every 6 hours as needed for arthritic pain for 4 days. The nurse notices that the client's stool is becoming darker and that a test for occult blood is positive. What would the nurse most likely conclude?

1. The combination of vitamin C and multivitamins are irritating the lining of the intestine.
2. The aspirin should be withheld because it may be causing gastric bleeding.
3. Vitamin C is acidic in nature and may be irritating the GI tissues.
4. From the appearance of the stool, the nurse suspects the client has hemorrhoids.

28. 2. Aspirin is widely known for causing gastric irritation and bleeding. Vitamin C and multivitamins generally don't have an adverse effect in the GI tract. There may be hemorrhoids present, but bleeding from this source would generally be bright red.

CN: Physiological integrity; CNS: Pharmacological and parenteral therapies; CL: Analysis

29. In which nurse-client interaction is a home health nurse demonstrating a secondary intervention as an advocate?

1. Contacting the local church to borrow a walker for the client to use
2. Listening to a client express feelings of frustration over the limitations imposed by his condition
3. Giving I.V. antibiotic therapy every 12 hours with attention to sterile technique and prevention of complications
4. Teaching a client with chronic obstructive pulmonary disease the effect of abdominal distention on breathing and ways to help bowel function

29. 1. Referral to community agencies is an advocacy role for home health nurses. The role of the advocate implies the home care nurse is able to advise clients how to find alternative sources of care. Giving emotional support, giving therapies to clients, and instructing clients about disease processes are direct care activities.

CN: Safe, effective care environment; CNS: Management of care; CL: Application

30. Which action is an example of indirect care function of a home health nurse?

1. Supervising a home health aide
2. Participating in a team conference about a client
3. Showing the home health aide body positioning for the client
4. Teaching the care provider how to read a food label for sodium content

30. 2. Participating in a team conference is an example of indirect care. Direct care is defined as the actual nursing care given to clients in their homes. Direct care may involve assessment of physical or psychosocial status, performance of skilled interventions, supervision of other disciplines, and teaching.

CN: Safe, effective care environment; CNS: Management of care; CL: Application

31. A young pregnant client attending prenatal classes is concerned about her alcohol intake. Which statement indicates the client's child is at high risk of fetal alcohol syndrome (FAS)?

1. "I just snort once or twice a day."
2. "I had one glass of wine with dinner last week."
3. "I drink a six pack of beer daily to settle my nerves."
4. "I smoke marijuana with my boyfriend and his friends."

31. 3. Ingestion of alcohol on a daily basis increases the risk of FAS. Other forms of addictive behavior, such as the ingestion of cocaine and smoking marijuana, increase the risk of fetal abuse—not fetal alcohol syndrome.

CN: Health promotion and maintenance; CNS: None; CL: Analysis

32. According to the Centers for Disease Control and Prevention, which group most likely would need preventive therapy for tuberculosis (TB)?

1. Clients with human immunodeficiency virus (HIV) infection
2. Clients with recent tuberculin skin tests and low risk
3. Persons with no contact with infectious TB clients
4. Clients with abnormal chest X-rays

32. 1. Preventive therapy should be initiated for clients infected with HIV because latent TB can become active if the immune system is weakened. Clients with low risk and negative skin tests are unlikely to be infected with TB or to progress if infected. Clients with no contact with infectious TB cases aren't at high risk for developing TB. Although clients with active TB may have abnormal chest X-rays, many other conditions can cause abnormalities.
CN: Health promotion and maintenance; CNS: None; CL: Application

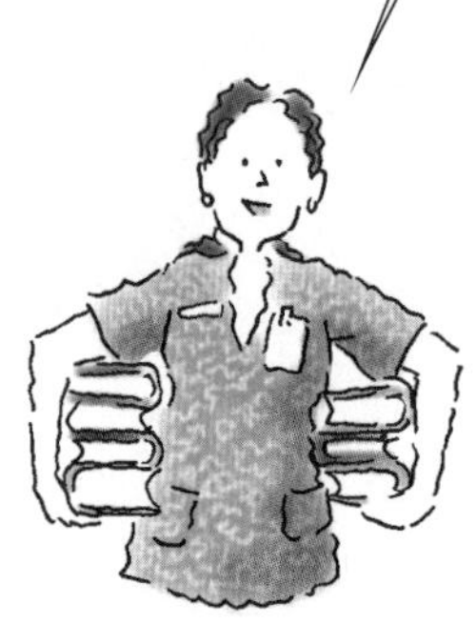

Didn't I tell you all your hard work would pay off?

33. Which psychosocial approach should an emergency department nurse use when dealing with suspected family violence?

1. Punitive
2. Supportive treatment
3. Disgust and avoidance
4. Get the facts at all costs

33. 2. Emotional support is a nonthreatening approach when dealing with suspected family violence. Aggressive, punitive, and disdainful approaches can increase the anxiety of the perpetrator, increasing the risk of more violence.
CN: Psychosocial integrity; CNS: None; CL: Application

34. A concerned client called the school asking that the nurse assess her 13-year-old son for signs of depression. Which symptom should the nurse expect to see?

1. Becomes angry at peers easily
2. Seeks out support from peers
3. Eats several small meals daily
4. Feels he can control everything in his life

34. 1. Adolescents experiencing depression may experience and express anger at peers. Adolescents feel a lack of control over their current situation, so they isolate themselves from their peers. The adolescent often has an intake of nutrients insufficient to meet metabolic needs.
CN: Psychosocial integrity; CNS: None; CL: Analysis

35. A 56-year-old client recently lost his 82-year-old father to lung cancer. In counseling the client, the bereavement nurse expects which sign of grief?

1. Decreased libido
2. Absence of anger and hostility
3. Difficulty crying or controlling crying
4. Clear dreams and imagery of the deceased

35. 4. A grieving client usually has vivid, clear dreams and fantasies. He also has a good capacity for imagery, particularly involving the loss. Difficulty crying or controlling crying, absence of anger and hostility, and decreased libido are signs of depression.
CN: Psychosocial integrity; CNS: None; CL: Analysis

36. A 72-year-old client experienced the death of his wife 1 year ago. He now needs home health services due to severe osteoarthritis. Which statement indicates the client will need further bereavement counseling?

1. "I'm lucky my children live so close."
2. "I really don't have anything to live for."
3. "My health isn't very good, but I can live with it."
4. "I've always had trouble remembering where I placed things."

36. 2. Wishing for death is a sign of depression. Usually after a year, most individuals accept the death of their loved ones and begin restoring their lives. Being grateful for good health and close family ties is a sign of acceptance of a new life that one experiences after the loss of a loved one. Memory loss can be a sign of dementia or depression.
CN: Psychosocial integrity; CNS: None; CL: Analysis

37. A client in the second stage of labor reports strong urges to bear down. The nurse interprets this reflex as:

1. Babinski's reflex
2. Ferguson's reflex
3. Moro's reflex
4. Myerson's reflex

37. 2. Ferguson's reflex is characterized by the strong urge to bear down during the second stage of labor. Babinski's reflex results in dorsiflexion of the big toe and fanning of the other toes when the sole of a client's foot is scraped. Moro's reflex is a normal generalized reflex in an infant when he reacts to a sudden noise, such as when a table next to him is struck. Myerson's reflex results in blinking when the client's forehead, bridge of the nose, or maxilla is tapped.

CN: Physiological integrity; CNS: Physiological adaptation; CL: Analysis

38. Which nursing action is most appropriate for handling chemotherapeutic agents?

1. Wear disposable gloves and protective clothing.
2. Break needles after the infusion is discontinued.
3. Disconnect I.V. tubing with gloved hands.
4. Throw I.V. tubing in the trash after the infusion is discontinued.

38. 1. A nurse must wear disposable gloves and protective clothing to protect skin contact with the chemotherapeutic agent. Don't recap or break needles. Use a sterile gauze pad when priming I.V. tubing, connecting and disconnecting tubing, inserting syringes into vials, breaking glass ampules, or other procedures in which chemotherapeutic agents are being handled. Contaminated needles, syringes, I.V. tubes, and other contaminated equipment must be disposed of in a leak-proof, puncture-resistant container.

CN: Physiological integrity; CNS: Pharmacological and parenteral therapies; CL: Application

39. A client developed oral ulcerations secondary to chemotherapy agents. Which nursing action is most appropriate for reducing pain and irritation in the mouth?

1. Serve a high-fiber diet.
2. Use a toothbrush to clean teeth.
3. Avoid taking oral temperatures.
4. Rinse the mouth with hydrogen peroxide and water.

39. 3. If oral ulcers are present, taking oral temperatures will be painful. Use the axillary region, rectum, or ear as sites for temperature readings. Serving a high-fiber diet won't reduce mouth pain and irritation. Use a soft-sponge toothbrush, cotton-tipped applicator, or gauze-wrapped finger to clean teeth. Give normal saline solution mouthwashes and rinses to reduce pain and inflammation. Hydrogen peroxide mixed with water is too irritating if oral ulcers are present.

CN: Physiological integrity; CNS: Basic care and comfort; CL: Application

40. A client is admitted to the emergency department after being sexually assaulted. Which nursing intervention receives priority?

1. Assisting with medical treatment
2. Collecting and preparing evidence for the police
3. Attempting to reduce the client's anxiety from a panic to a moderate level
4. Providing anticipatory guidance to the client about normal responses to sexual assault

40. 3. Reducing anxiety will help the client participate in medical, forensic, and legal follow-up activities. Medical treatment should begin as soon as the client's anxiety decreases below the panic level. Collecting and preparing evidence and providing anticipatory guidance aren't high-priority interventions.

CN: Psychosocial integrity; CNS: None; CL: Analysis

41. The nurse is caring for an 8-year-old boy diagnosed with attention deficit hyperactivity disorder (ADHD). Which behavior is the nurse most likely to observe in this client?

1. Lethargy
2. Long attention span
3. Short attention span
4. Preoccupation with body parts

41. 3. Short attention span is a common characteristic of ADHD due to difficulty concentrating. These children show hyperexcitability, not lethargy. Children with this disorder are distracted by environmental stimuli, so they won't be concentrating on their body parts.

CN: Psychosocial integrity; CNS: None; CL: Application

42. A client with burns on 50% of his body is receiving total parenteral nutrition (TPN). Which symptom indicates the client is having a complication of TPN?

1. Pain
2. Absent bowel sounds
3. Abdominal cramping
4. Increased urine glucose

42. 4. Glycosuria, increased urine glucose, is associated with high blood glucose levels, a complication of TPN. Pain from major burns is expected. Absent bowel sounds are an indication to begin TPN. Abdominal cramping is associated with diarrhea or constipation.

CN: Physiological integrity; CNS: Basic care and comfort; CL: Application

43. A 35-year-old client is admitted to an inpatient substance abuse unit with a diagnosis of alcohol dependence. Which comment by the client supports this diagnosis?

1. "I don't drink more than two beers when I'm out."
2. "I always remember what happens the next day."
3. "I always ask a friend to drive me home when I'm drinking."
4. "I've had four tickets for driving while intoxicated last month."

43. 4. Driving while intoxicated can be seen as a symptom of alcohol dependence. Designating drivers and limiting alcohol consumption are self-responsible actions, but don't address the underlying problem. The amount one drinks doesn't matter. An alcoholic experiences blackouts, which are periods of amnesia about experiences while intoxicated. By asking someone to drive them home, clients with alcohol dependence rationalize that it's okay to drink if they're responsible.

CN: Psychosocial integrity; CNS: None; CL: Analysis

44. A nurse is working with a client with alcoholism in an acute care mental health unit. The client has been referred to Alcoholics Anonymous (AA). Which statement best indicates that the client is ready to begin the AA program?

1. "I know I'm powerless over alcohol and need help."
2. "I think it will be interesting and helpful to join AA."
3. "I'd like to sponsor another alcoholic with this same problem."
4. "My family is very supportive and will attend meetings with me."

44. 1. In step 1 of AA, a person admits his powerlessness over alcohol and is ready to accept help. This should occur before he begins AA. A supportive family and a desire to help others with the same problem are good for the client, but they don't necessarily indicate readiness to participate in the program.

CN: Psychosocial integrity; CNS: None; CL: Application

45. In planning care for a client diagnosed with paranoid schizophrenia, which action is correct for the psychiatric home health nurse?

1. Confront the client about her hallucinations.
2. Ask the minister to provide spiritual direction.
3. Instruct family members to discourage delusions.
4. Affirm when the client's perceptions and thinking are in touch with reality.

45. 4. The nursing plan of care focuses on reinforcing perceptions and thinking that are in touch with reality. Confronting a client about her hallucinations and delusions isn't effective or therapeutic. Spiritual direction is important, but a client with paranoid schizophrenia may have issues surrounding her religious or spiritual orientation. Therefore, asking a minister to provide spiritual direction may not be effective or therapeutic. Using family members could create distrust between the client and the family.

CN: Psychosocial integrity; CNS: None; CL: Application

46. A psychiatric home health nurse finds a client with bipolar disorder sitting on the porch. The client is wearing a red polka dot dress, large yellow hat, and heavy makeup with large gold jewelry. Which phase of the illness is the client most likely in?

1. Delusional
2. Depressive
3. Manic
4. Suspicious

46. 3. Extreme labile moods are characteristic of clients in the manic phase of bipolar disorder. Hyperactivity, verbosity, and drawing attention to oneself through dress are typical of the manic phase. Delusions and suspiciousness may be seen in bipolar disorder, but are more commonly seen in schizophrenia. In the depressive phase, clients are withdrawn, cry, and may not eat. Visual or auditory hallucinations, delusional thoughts, and extreme suspiciousness are behaviors seen in clients diagnosed with paranoid schizophrenia.

CN: Psychosocial integrity; CNS: None; CL: Analysis

47. A nurse is assessing a 4-week-old neonate for signs of acute pain. Which symptom is expected?

1. Whimpering
2. Eyes opened wide
3. Limp body posture
4. Wanting to breast-feed frequently

47. 1. Crying, whimpering, and groaning are vocal expressions of acute pain in the neonate. Eyes tightly closed, changes in feeding behavior, and fist clenching with rigidity also are signs of acute pain in the neonate.

CN: Health promotion and maintenance; CNS: None; CL: Application

48. A home health nurse is instructing a client about positioning her child, who's diagnosed with juvenile rheumatoid arthritis (JRA). Which position or equipment is needed to maintain posture for a child with JRA?

1. Soft mattress
2. Prone position
3. Large fluffy pillows
4. Semi-Fowler's position

48. 2. Lying in the prone position is encouraged to straighten hips and knees. A firm mattress is needed to maintain good alignment of spine, hips, and knees, and no pillow or a very thin pillow should be used. Semi-Fowler's position increases pressure on the hip joints and should be avoided.

CN: Physiological integrity; CNS: Basic care and comfort; CL: Application

49. Which comfort measure is best to reduce pain and stiffness for a child with juvenile rheumatoid arthritis (JRA)?

1. Hot packs
2. Cool baths
3. Cold compresses
4. Immersion in lukewarm water for 10 minutes

49. 1. Heat is beneficial to children with arthritis. Moist heat is best for relieving pain and stiffness. The most efficient and practical method is in the bathtub. Cold, cool, or lukewarm treatment isn't beneficial in relieving pain or stiffness in children with JRA.

CN: Physiological integrity; CNS: Basic care and comfort; CL: Application

50. While putting an elderly client with an indwelling urinary catheter in bed, the nurse places the tubing in a loop on the bed with the client and makes sure the client won't lie on the tubing. Which rationale explains the nurse's action?

1. To inhibit drainage
2. To allow drainage to occur
3. To allow the urine to collect in the tubing
4. To have the client check the tubing for urine

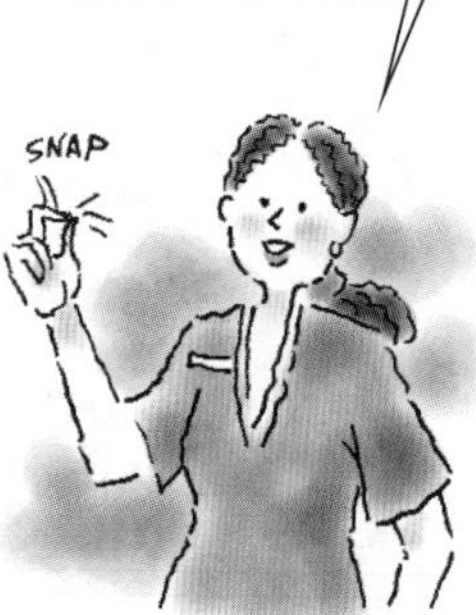

You've finished 50 questions! The remaining 25 should be a snap!
SNAP

50. 2. Catheter tubing shouldn't be allowed to develop dependent loops or kinks because this inhibits proper drainage by requiring the urine to travel against gravity to empty into the bag. Permitting the urine to collect in the tubing increases the risk of infection. Observing the catheter and tubing is the responsibility of the nurse.

CN: Physiological integrity; CNS: Reduction of risk potential; CL: Application

51. A client complains of severe burning on urination. Which instruction is best to give the client?

1. Wear only nylon underwear.
2. Drink coffee to increase urination.
3. Soak in warm water with bubble bath.
4. Drink 2,500 to 3,000 ml of water per day.

51. 4. Drinking large amounts of water will help flush bacteria from the urinary tract. Avoid nylon underwear; wear only cotton undergarments to decrease the warm, moist environment. Avoid tea, coffee, carbonated drinks, and alcoholic beverages because of bladder irritation. Avoid using bubble baths, perfumed soaps, or bath powders in the perineal area. The scent in toiletries can be irritating to the urinary meatus.

CN: Physiological integrity; CNS: Basic care and comfort; CL: Application

52. Which instruction is given to a client with a hearing aid?

1. Clean the hearing aid with baby oil.
2. Wear the hearing aid while sleeping.
3. Keep the hearing aid out of direct sunlight.
4. Leave the hearing aid in place while showering.

52. 3. The hearing aid should be kept out of direct sunlight and away from high temperatures. Solvents or lubricants shouldn't be used on the aid. If there is a detachable ear mold, it can be washed in warm, soapy water and dried with a soft cloth. The hearing aid should be left in place while the client is awake, except when showering.

CN: Physiological integrity; CNS: Basic care and comfort; CL: Application

53. A 72-year-old client is being discharged from same-day surgery after having a cataract removed from his right eye. Which discharge instruction does a nurse give the client?
1. Sleep on the operative side.
2. Resume all activities as before.
3. Don't rub or place pressure on the eyes.
4. Wear an eye shield all day and remove it at night.

53. 3. Rubbing or placing pressure on the eyes increases the risk of accidental injury to ocular structures. The nurse should also caution against lifting objects, straining, strenuous exercise, and sexual activity because such activities can increase intraocular pressure. Caution against sleeping on the operative side to reduce the risk of accidental injury to ocular structures. Glasses or shaded lenses should be worn to protect the eye during waking hours after the eye dressing is removed. An eye shield should be worn at night.

CN: Physiological integrity; CNS: Reduction of risk potential; CL: Application

54. To ensure the safe administration of medications, which action should be performed <u>first</u>?
1. Make sure the client is in the correct room.
2. Check for client allergies.
3. Have the client repeat his name.
4. Open the medications at the client's bedside.

54. 2. Checking for client allergies is the first step in ensuring safe administration of medications. The other actions are important, but not the priority.

CN: Physiological integrity; CNS: Pharmacological and parenteral therapies; CL: Analysis

55. Which instruction is correct for a client taking nortriptyline (Pamelor) for depression?
1. Be aware that this drug can cause hypotension.
2. This drug will work immediately to treat depression.
3. Take this drug in the morning because it causes drowsiness.
4. Wear protective clothing and sunscreen when out in the sun.

55. 4. A common adverse effect of this drug is sensitivity to the sun. Protective clothing and sunscreen are worn in the sun. This drug can cause hypertension. It doesn't work immediately, but takes 2 to 3 weeks to achieve the desired effect. This drug should be taken at bedtime if it causes drowsiness.

CN: Physiological integrity; CNS: Pharmacological and parenteral therapies; CL: Application

56. Which instruction is correct for a client receiving lithium (Eskalith) for bipolar disorder?
1. Avoid drugs containing ibuprofen.
2. Drink at least two cups of coffee daily.
3. Be aware that you may experience increased alertness.
4. It isn't necessary to monitor the blood level of this drug.

56. 1. Avoid drugs that alter the effect of lithium, such as ibuprofen and sodium bicarbonate or other antacids containing sodium. Avoid beverages with caffeine because they increase urination, which may alter the effect of lithium. Lithium can decrease alertness and coordination. Lithium levels may need to be monitored every 2 weeks, especially if adverse effects occur. The dose may need to be regulated.

CN: Physiological integrity; CNS: Pharmacological and parenteral therapies; CL: Application

57. A physician ordered nitroprusside I.V. for a client in cardiogenic shock. Which nursing intervention is needed to give this drug safely?

1. Give only with other drugs.
2. Mix the drug in an alkaline solution.
3. Mix the drug only in normal saline solution.
4. Cover the drug-containing I.V. solution with an opaque wrapper.

57. 4. The nurse should cover the drug-containing I.V. solution with an opaque wrapper because the drug is light-sensitive. Nitroprusside can't be mixed in alkaline solutions, and shouldn't be given with other drugs. Only dilute the drug in dextrose 5% in water; no other fluid should be used.

CN: Physiological integrity; CNS: Pharmacological and parenteral therapies; CL: Application

58. Which nursing intervention is correct for a client receiving total parenteral nutrition (TPN)?

1. Discard TPN solutions after 24 hours.
2. Discard lipid emulsions after 20 hours.
3. Inspect the TPN solution for clearness and visibility.
4. Teach the client to blow out during expiration when the tubing is disconnected.

58. 1. TPN solutions are good media for fungi, so they should be discarded after 24 hours. Lipid emulsions are also good media for fungi and should be discarded after 12 hours. Inspect TPN solutions for cloudiness, cracks, or leaks before hanging. The nurse should teach the client to perform Valsalva's maneuver, taking a deep breath and holding it, when the tubing is disconnected. Valsalva's maneuver increases intrathoracic pressure, which prevents air entry.

CN: Physiological integrity; CNS: Pharmacological and parenteral therapies; CL: Application

59. Which opioid analgesic may be given parenterally to an older client to be more useful?

1. Hydromorphone (Dilaudid)
2. Meperidine (Demerol)
3. Morphine
4. Oxycodone (Percocet)

59. 1. Hydromorphone is a fast-acting drug and is a useful alternative to morphine or meperidine due to its short half-life. Morphine and meperidine can increase the risk of confusion in the elderly. Oxycodone is given only orally or rectally.

CN: Physiological integrity; CNS: Pharmacological and parenteral therapies; CL: Application

60. Which diagnostic test is used to diagnose bacterial endocarditis?

1. Electrolytes
2. Blood cultures
3. Prothrombin time (PT)
4. Venereal Disease Research Laboratory (VDRL)

60. 2. Blood cultures are crucial in diagnosing bacterial endocarditis. Electrolyte levels indicate abnormalities that occur with drug therapy as well as with complications associated with heart failure. PT values are useful in monitoring anticoagulant therapy. A positive VDRL may be evidence of syphilitic heart disease.

CN: Physiological integrity; CNS: Reduction of risk potential; CL: Application

61. In preparing a client for cardiac catheterization, which statement or question is most appropriate?

1. "Are you allergic to contrast dyes or shellfish?"
2. "Have you ever had this kind of procedure before?"
3. "You'll need to fast 24 hours before the procedure."
4. "You'll be given medication to help you sleep during the procedure."

61. 1. The nurse must assess the client for allergies to iodine before the procedure because the dye used during catheterization contains iodine. Knowing the client's history and prior experience with this procedure would be helpful, but knowing the client's allergies is more important. The client is instructed to fast for 6 hours before the procedure. The client will be asked to empty his bladder before the procedure. The client needs to stay awake during the procedure to follow directions, such as taking a deep breath and holding it during injection of the dye, and to report chest, neck, or jaw discomfort.

CN: Physiological integrity; CNS: Reduction of risk potential; CL: Application

62. A 60-year-old male client is suspected of having coronary artery disease. Which noninvasive diagnostic method would the nurse expect to be ordered to evaluate cardiac changes?

1. Cardiac biopsy
2. Cardiac catheterization
3. Magnetic resonance imaging (MRI)
4. Pericardiocentesis

62. 3. MRI is a noninvasive procedure that aids in the diagnosis and detection of thoracic aortic aneurysm and evaluation of coronary artery disease, pericardial disease, and cardiac masses. Cardiac biopsy, cardiac catheterization, and pericardiocentesis are invasive techniques used to evaluate cardiac changes.

CN: Health promotion and maintenance; CNS: None; CL: Application

63. In evaluating an electrocardiogram (ECG) strip in a telemetry unit, a nurse notices a client is having premature ventricular contractions (PVCs). Which criteria is used to evaluate the presence of PVCs on the ECG strip?

1. There's no PR interval.
2. The R-R interval is irregular.
3. Ventricular rate is slower than atrial rate.
4. The QRS complex is followed by a compensatory pause.

63. 4. The QRS complex is followed by a compensatory pause that ends when the underlying rhythm resumes. This is one of the ECG criteria used to evaluate PVCs. The remaining responses are ECG criteria used to evaluate atrial flutter.

CN: Physiological integrity; CNS: Reduction of risk potential; CL: Analysis

64. In evaluating an electrocardiogram (ECG) strip for the presence of a pacemaker, which criteria indicates a malfunction?

1. Short T waves
2. Normal sinus rhythm
3. Pacing spikes appearing at different times during a cardiac cycle
4. Pacing spike followed by a wide QRS complex

64. 3. When pacing spikes appear at different times during a cardiac cycle, it indicates a failure to capture. Failure to capture may result in inappropriate pacing; the ECG would show a pacing spike delivered on time but not followed by a wide QRS complex. Tall T waves or an irregular heart rate indicate a failure-to-sense malfunction.

CN: Physiological integrity; CNS: Reduction of risk potential; CL: Analysis

65. In caring for a client with arterial insufficiency, which instruction is most appropriate for home health teaching?

1. "You may leave your feet open to the air."
2. "It's best to sit and rest for several hours a day."
3. "Avoid crossing your legs at the knees or ankles."
4. "It's best to wear tight socks instead of no socks."

65. 3. Leg crossing should be avoided because it compresses the vessels in the legs. Feet and extremities must be protected to reduce the risk of trauma. Sitting for several hours isn't recommended. Avoid constrictive clothing, such as tight elastic on socks, to prevent compression of vessels in the legs.

CN: Physiological integrity; CNS: Reduction of risk potential; CL: Application

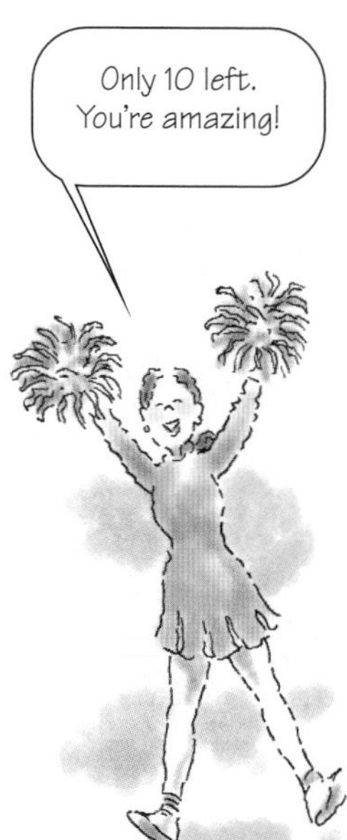
Only 10 left.
You're amazing!

66. Which instruction is correct for home health teaching for a client taking oral anticoagulants?

1. "You may shave with a standard razor."
2. "You may take ibuprofen or aspirin for pain."
3. "Take the anticoagulant at the same time each day."
4. "It's important to eat a large quantity of green, leafy vegetables."

66. 3. It's important to take the anticoagulant at the same time each day to maintain an adequate blood level. An electric razor reduces the risk of cutting the skin. Avoid the use of standard razors. Avoid taking aspirin or ibuprofen because these drugs decrease clotting time. Eating a large amount of green, leafy vegetables, which contain vitamin K, increases the clotting time, thus requiring more anticoagulants.

CN: Physiological integrity; CNS: Pharmacological and parenteral therapies; CL: Application

67. Which action is most appropriate to reduce sensory deprivation for a visually impaired elderly client in the hospital?

1. Keep the lights dimmed.
2. Close the curtains or blinds on windows to reduce glare.
3. Open the hospital door so bright light can shine in the room.
4. Open the curtains during the day so the sun can shine brightly.

67. 2. Closing curtains or blinds on windows can reduce glare and improve vision for the older client. Controlled lighting can help the older client see better in the hospital. Adequate background lighting helps the older client decrease visual accommodation when moving from brightly lit to dimly lit rooms and hallways.

CN: Physiological integrity; CNS: Reduction of risk potential; CL: Application

68. Which action is most appropriate to reduce sensory overload for a hearing-impaired elderly client in the coronary care unit?

1. Keep the overhead light on continuously.
2. Discuss the client's condition at the bedside.
3. Allow all family members to stay with the client.
4. Limit bedside conversation to that directed to the client.

68. 4. Limiting bedside conversation to that directed to the client creates fewer disturbances, thus reducing sensory overload. Turning off or dimming the overhead lights further reduces visual stimulation and facilitates day and night light fluctuations. Although fostering family interaction with the client is necessary, only one or two family members should be allowed to visit with the client at one time. Crowding of people in the client's room may precipitate a loss of privacy and control for the client.

CN: Physiological integrity; CNS: Reduction of risk potential; CL: Application

69. Which instruction is most appropriate in home health teaching for a client with osteoarthritis of the left knee?
1. Use cold on joints.
2. Keep the knee extended.
3. Maintain a healthy weight.
4. Have someone help the client in activities of daily living (ADL).

69. 3. Maintaining a healthy weight decreases joint stress. Local moist heat provides pain relief and will decrease stiffness. The client should perform muscle-strengthening exercises, which help prevent joint stiffness. The nurse should allow the client to perform ADL with less assistance.
CN: Physiological integrity; CNS: Reduction of risk potential; CL: Application

70. A home care aide notified the agency that she found a client lying on the floor. When the home health nurse arrives, the newly diagnosed diabetic client is semicomatose, with a fast heart rate and low blood pressure. The client's skin is warm and dry. Which condition is indicated?
1. Hypoglycemia
2. Cardiogenic shock
3. Diabetic ketoacidosis (DKA)
4. Hyperosmolar hypoglycemic nonketotic syndrome (HHNS)

70. 3. DKA develops as a result of severe insulin deficiency. The incidence of DKA generally results from undiagnosed diabetes and inadequacy of prescribed medication and dietary therapies. Hypoglycemia involves episodes of low blood glucose levels caused by erratic or altered absorption of insulin. In cardiogenic shock, the client has pale, cool, and moist skin. HHNS is a deadly complication of diabetes distinguished by severe hyperglycemia, dehydration, and changed mental status.
CN: Physiological integrity; CNS: Physiological adaptation; CL: Application

71. A nurse is standing next to a person eating fried shrimp at a parade. Suddenly, the man clutches at his throat and is unable to speak, cough, or breathe. The nurse asks the man if he's choking and he nods yes. Which response is most appropriate?
1. Attempt rescue breathing.
2. Perform the Heimlich maneuver.
3. Deliver external chest compressions.
4. Use the head tilt-chin lift maneuver to establish the airway.

71. 2. If a conscious victim acknowledges that he's choking, the best response is to perform the Heimlich maneuver to relieve the airway obstruction. The other options are used for an unresponsive victim with absent heart rate and breathing.
CN: Physiological integrity; CNS: Physiological adaptation; CL: Application

72. Which response is most appropriate to prepare for a cardiopulmonary emergency?
1. Have nasal oxygen ready when needed.
2. Place an oropharyngeal airway at the bedside.
3. Keep the medication cart locked up for safety.
4. Don't start an I.V. line unless necessary.

72. 2. A nurse should learn to anticipate clinical deterioration before overt signs and symptoms are apparent. If a client is having breathing difficulties, the nurse should place an oropharyngeal airway at the bedside while the client is monitored for deterioration. The emergency cart should be placed outside the client's room for easy access. If breathing stops, the client will need to be intubated and placed on a respirator, if necessary. The client should have a stable I.V. line for administration of emergency drugs.
CN: Physiological integrity; CNS: Physiological adaptation; CL: Analysis

73. In preparing for cardioversion, which action is most appropriate?

1. Keep the client awake and alert.
2. Keep the side rails up for client safety.
3. Set the machine on SYNC and charge at 200 watts.
4. Set the machine on DEFIB and charge at 400 watts.

73. 3. If cardioversion is needed, the nurse should set the machine on SYNC and look for a marker on each QRS complex. The nurse should start at a low energy level and increase as needed. The nurse should sedate the client and lower the side rails for easier placement of paddle electrodes.

CN: Physiological integrity; CNS: Physiological adaptation; CL: Application

74. A client who is at 37 weeks' gestation comes to the office for a prenatal visit. The nurse performs Leopold's maneuvers to assess the position of the fetus. After performing the maneuvers, the nurse suspects that the physician will attempt external version. Where did the nurse palpate the head of the fetus?

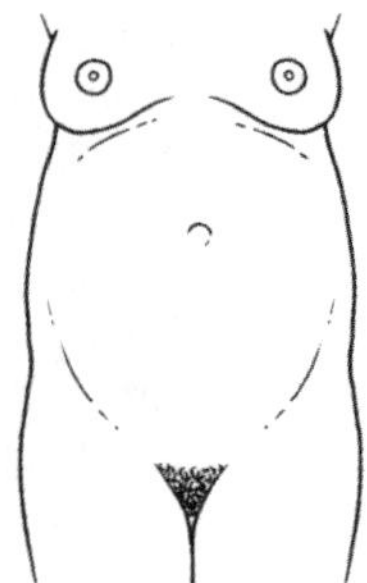

74. If the fetal head is palpated at the top of the uterus, the fetus is in the breech position. The physician may consider external version to convert the fetus to a vertex lie, or head-down position. This is accomplished by applying pressure on the maternal abdomen to turn the infant over, as in a somersault.

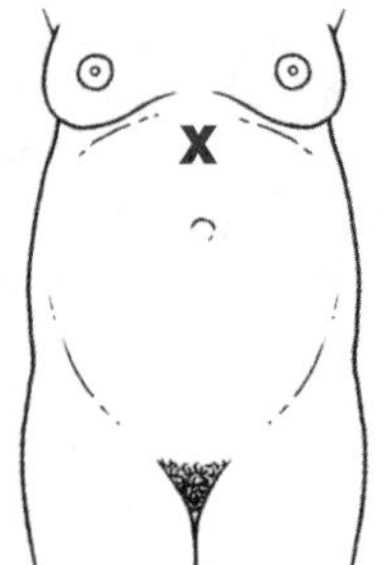

CN: Physiological integrity; CNS: Reduction of risk potential; CL: Analysis

75. A physician orders an I.V. infusion of dextrose 5% in quarter-normal saline solution to be infused at 7 ml/kg/hour for a 10-month-old infant. The infant weighs 22 lb. How many ml/hour of the ordered solution should the nurse infuse? Record your answer using a whole number.

______________________ milliliters/hour

75. 70. To perform this dosage calculation, the nurse should first convert the infant's weight to kilograms: 2.2 lb/kg = 22 lb/X kg; $X = 22 \div 2.2$; $X = 10$ kg. Next, she should multiply the infant's weight by the ordered rate: 10 kg × 7 ml/kg/hour = 70 ml/hour.

CN: Physiological integrity; CNS: Pharmacological and parenteral therapies; CL: Application

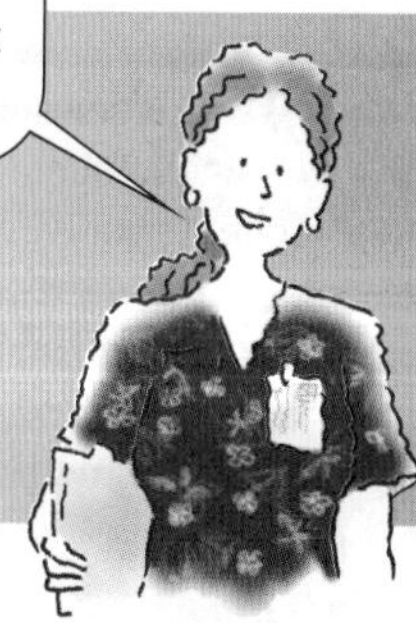
Here's another comprehensive test to practice for the NCLEX. Check it out!

COMPREHENSIVE Test 4

1. A nurse-manager has identified several personal problems with a staff member. Which approach is best for the nurse-manager to take?

1. Map out a plan of action for each problem and discuss it.
2. Begin to solve the first problem and work through the list.
3. Ask the staff member to select the problem she would like to resolve.
4. Prioritize the problems with the staff member and begin to work on them together.

1. 4. It's important for the nurse-manager and staff member to agree on which problem is a priority and work on its resolution together. Mapping out the problem without input from the staff member leaves the possibility that the staff member might not be committed to work on its resolution.

CN: Safe, effective care environment; CNS: Management of care; CL: Application

2. A team leader notes increasing unrest among the staff members. Which action is best for the team leader to take?

1. Discuss the problem with a coworker.
2. Report the problem to the nurse-manager.
3. Bring the group together and discuss the team leader's perception.
4. Ignore the problem and hope the attitude won't interfere with the functioning of the floor.

2. 3. The leader should comment to the group on the observed behavior. This is a firm approach but one that shows concern. Ignoring problems or discussing them with someone else doesn't confront the issue at hand.

CN: Safe, effective care environment; CNS: Management of care; CL: Application

3. A physician ordered a urine specimen for culture and sensitivity stat. Which approach is best for a nurse to use in delegating this task?

1. "We need a stat urine culture on the client in room 101."
2. "Please get the urine for culture for the client in room 101."
3. "A stat urine was ordered for the client in room 101. Would you get it?"
4. "We need a urine for culture stat on the client in room 101. Tell me when you send it to the lab."

3. 4. This option not only delegates the task, but also provides a checkpoint. To effectively delegate, you need to follow up on what someone else is doing. The other options don't provide for feedback, which is essential for communication and delegation.

CN: Safe, effective care environment; CNS: Management of care; CL: Application

CN: Client needs category CNS: Client needs subcategory CL: Cognitive level

4. A 67-year-old client asks the nurse, "Do you think it's wrong to masturbate?" Which response by the nurse is best?

1. "How do you feel about that?"
2. "Do you really want to do that?"
3. "I think you're a little too old for that."
4. "Why don't you ask your physician?"

4. 1. It's essential in communication to find out how the client thinks and feels. Telling the client that he's too old or asking him if he really wants to do that is biased and puts the client down. The last option tells the client the nurse isn't interested. The client might be too uncomfortable to discuss this topic with the physician.

CN: Psychosocial integrity; CNS: None; CL: Analysis

5. A nurse is assisting a client on a clear liquid diet in selecting his menu. Which choice indicates that he needs further teaching?

1. Gelatin dessert
2. Milkshake
3. Popsicle or similar frozen dessert
4. Tea

5. 2. Full-liquid diets contain milk, cereal, gruel, clear liquids, and plain frozen desserts. The clear-liquid diet contains only foods that are clear and liquid at room or body temperature, such as gelatin, fat-free broth, bouillon, popsicles or similar frozen desserts, tea, and regular or decaffeinated coffee.

CN: Physiological integrity; CNS: Basic care and comfort; CL: Analysis

6. Which medication should a nurse withhold from a client 6 hours before a series of pulmonary function tests (PFTs)?

1. Antibiotics
2. Antitussives
3. Bronchodilators
4. Corticosteroids

6. 3. PFTs measure the volume and capacity of air. If a bronchodilator is given, it will improve the bronchial airflow and alter the test results. The other drugs would have no effect on the bronchial tree with regard to PFT results.

CN: Physiological integrity; CNS: Pharmacological and parenteral therapies; CL: Application

7. A client returns to a nursing unit after a bronchoscopy and is expectorating pink-tinged mucus. Which action by the nurse is most appropriate?

1. Notify the physician as soon as possible.
2. Take the client's vital signs, then call the physician.
3. Auscultate the client's lung fields for possible pulmonary edema.
4. Tell the client this is expected after the procedure, but continue to monitor the client.

7. 4. Pink-tinged mucus is an expected outcome after a bronchoscopy due to irritation of the bronchial tree. The client should be told this is common, but that he'll be monitored. The physician doesn't need to be called with this finding. This symptom isn't related to pulmonary edema.

CN: Health promotion and maintenance; CNS: None; CL: Application

8. The assessment of a client on the first day after thoracotomy shows a temperature of 100° F (37.8° C); heart rate, 96 beats/minute; blood pressure, 136/86 mm Hg; and shallow respirations at 24 breaths/minute, with rhonchi at the bases. The client complains of incisional pain. Which nursing action has priority?

1. Medicate the client for pain.
2. Help the client get out of bed.
3. Give ibuprofen (Motrin) as ordered to reduce the fever.
4. Encourage the client to cough and deep-breathe.

8. 1. Although all the interventions are incorporated in this client's care plan, the priority is to relieve pain and make the client comfortable. This would give the client the energy and stamina to achieve the other objectives.

CN: Physiological integrity; CNS: Basic care and comfort; CL: Application

9. Which intervention is most important to include in a nursing care plan for a client with atelectasis?

1. Give oxygen continuously at 3 L/minute.
2. Cough and deep-breathe every 4 hours.
3. Use the incentive spirometer every hour.
4. Get the client out of bed to a chair every day.

9. 3. Incentive spirometry is used to prevent or treat atelectasis. Done every hour, it will produce deep inhalations that help open the collapsed alveoli. Oxygen use doesn't encourage deep inhalation. Coughing and deep breathing is a good intervention, but rarely results in as deep an inspiratory effort as using an incentive spirometer, and should be performed more frequently than every 4 hours. Getting the client out of bed will also help expand the lungs and stimulate deep breathing, but it's done less frequently than incentive spirometry.

CN: Safe, effective care environment; CNS: Management of care; CL: Application

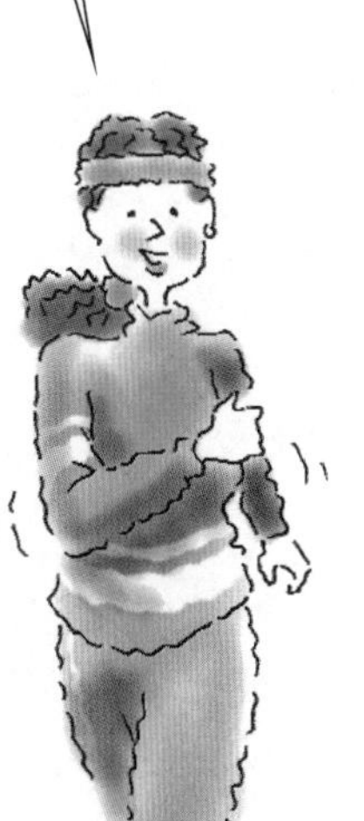

You're off to
a good start!
Keep going!

10. Two hours after submucous resection, a client's nostrils are packed and a drip pad is anchored under the nose. Which assessment alerts the nurse that the surgical site is bleeding?

1. Frequent swallowing
2. Dry mucous membranes
3. Decrease in urine output
4. Temperature elevation

10. 1. Frequent swallowing is a sign of hemorrhage in this surgery. Decreased urine output and dry mucous membranes, as well as temperature elevation, are usually signs of dehydration.

CN: Physiological integrity; CNS: Reduction of risk potential; CL: Analysis

11. A bedridden client develops disuse osteoporosis. Which nursing intervention is most important for this client?

1. Turn, cough, and deep-breathe.
2. Increase fluids to 3,000 ml daily.
3. Promote venous return by elevating the legs.
4. Provide active and passive range-of-motion (ROM) exercises.

11. 4. All the interventions listed are good for a bedridden client. However, active and passive ROM exercises provide the mechanical stresses of weight bearing that are absent and lead to disuse osteoporosis.

CN: Health promotion and maintenance; CNS: None; CL: Application

12. An elderly client on bed rest for a week after a bout of pneumonia is in a negative nitrogen balance. Which complication has highest priority?

1. Constipation
2. Renal calculi
3. Muscle wasting
4. Vitamin B_6 deficiency

12. 3. Negative nitrogen balance leads to muscle wasting. The body breaks down muscle tissue to use as energy. Renal calculi can be a complication of bed rest and demineralization of the bone but treating a negative nitrogen balance takes priority. Constipation and vitamin B_6 deficiency also need to be corrected but aren't of the highest priority.

CN: Physiological integrity; CNS: Physiological adaptation; CL: Application

13. The nurse reviews the arterial blood gas results of a client with asthma. The nurse expects the client's partial pressure of arterial oxygen (Pao_2) result to provide information on which factor?

1. Respiratory status
2. Degree of dyspnea
3. Efficiency of gas exchange
4. Effectiveness of ventilation

13. 3. The Pao_2 reflects the gas exchange ventilation and perfusion. It doesn't measure the respiratory status, degree of dyspnea, or the effectiveness of ventilation.

CN: Physiological integrity; CNS: Reduction of risk potential; CL: Application

14. The nurse prepares to administer morphine to a client with an acute myocardial infarction for which reason?

1. To decrease cardiac output
2. To increase preload and afterload
3. To increase myocardial oxygen demand
4. To decrease myocardial oxygen demand

14. 4. Morphine will calm and relax the client and decrease respiratory rate, anxiety, and stress, thus decreasing myocardial oxygen demand. It doesn't have any affect on cardiac output or preload or afterload.

CN: Physiological integrity; CNS: Pharmacological and parenteral therapies; CL: Application

15. A toddler is ordered 350 mg of amoxicillin (Augmentin) by mouth, four times per day. The pharmacy supplies a bottle of amoxicillin with a concentration of 250 mg/5 ml. How many milliliters would the nurse give for each dose? Record the answer using a whole number:

________________________ml.

15. 7. The nurse would give 7 milliliters for each dose. Use the following equation:

dose on hand/quantity on hand = dose desired/X.

In this example, the equation is:

$250 \text{ mg}/5 \text{ ml} = 350 \text{ mg}/X$.

$X = 7$ ml.

CN: Physiological integrity; CNS: Pharmacological and parenteral therapies; CL: Analysis

16. A nurse is assessing a client and notes an increase in the tactile fremitus. Which condition would the nurse suspect with this client?

1. Atelectasis
2. Emphysema
3. Pneumonia
4. Pneumothorax

16. 3. Pneumonia produces a consolidation of mucus and debris. Mucus causes the lung field to have an increase in tactile fremitus. The other diseases involve air, which would decrease tactile fremitus.

CN: Health promotion and maintenance; CNS: None; CL: Analysis

17. A client with an arm cast complains of severe pain in the affected extremity, and decreased sensation and motion are noted. Swelling in the fingers is also increased. Which intervention has priority?

1. Elevating the arm
2. Removing the cast
3. Giving an analgesic
4. Calling the physician

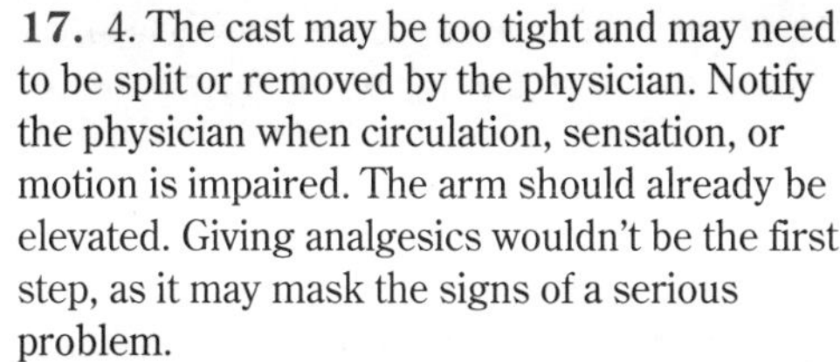

17. 4. The cast may be too tight and may need to be split or removed by the physician. Notify the physician when circulation, sensation, or motion is impaired. The arm should already be elevated. Giving analgesics wouldn't be the first step, as it may mask the signs of a serious problem.

CN: Physiological integrity; CNS: Reduction of risk potential; CL: Application

18. A client is hospitalized for 5 days with mononucleosis. Which assessment finding indicates a possibly serious consequence?

1. Vomiting
2. Dark brown urine
3. Temperature of 101° F (38.3° C)
4. Cervical lymphadenopathy

18. 2. Dark brown urine could indicate the presence of bilirubin and implicate liver involvement. The other answers are typical findings for a client with this diagnosis.

CN: Physiological integrity; CNS: Physiological adaptation; CL: Analysis

19. A nurse is teaching a client about lifestyle changes that need to be made after a myocardial infarction (MI). The diagnosis of *Ineffective coping* is supported when the client is observed in which action?

1. Reading a book about meal planning
2. Pacing the floor of his room on occasion
3. Sitting quietly in his room for a short time
4. Telling his family he didn't have an MI

19. 4. The client is showing the defense mechanism of denial. Reading a book on meal planning is a positive intervention. Pacing the floor on occasion is a form of anxiety that's normal for the client to experience. Sitting quietly is a normal behavior. The client needs time to come to terms with his diagnosis.

CN: Psychosocial integrity; CNS: None; CL: Analysis

20. A client with a history of myasthenia gravis is admitted to the emergency department with complaints of respiratory distress. The client's condition worsens and arterial blood gases are drawn. Which condition is expected?

1. Metabolic acidosis
2. Metabolic alkalosis
3. Respiratory acidosis
4. Respiratory alkalosis

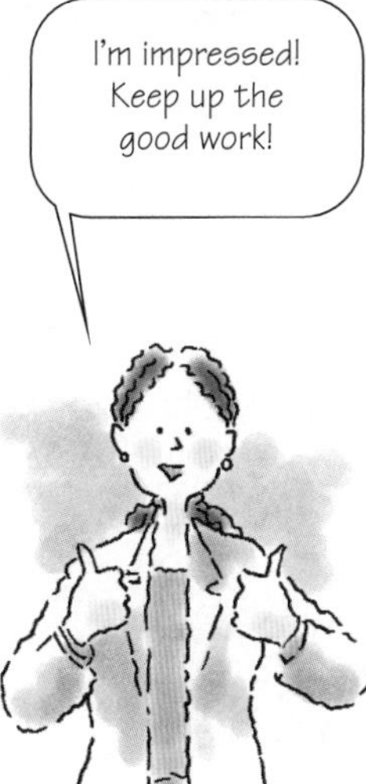
I'm impressed!
Keep up the
good work!

20. 3. The client has a restrictive lung problem because of myasthenia gravis. This is aggravated by respiratory distress. Because of the restrictive problem, the client won't be able to exhale efficiently and carbon dioxide will build up, causing respiratory acidosis. Metabolic acidosis is a metabolic condition that occurs with either accumulation of acids or excessive loss of bases in the body, such as in diarrhea or renal failure. Metabolic alkalosis occurs due to excessive acid loss or base retention, such as from vomiting. Respiratory alkalosis results from a decreased carbon dioxide level, which could occur if the patient were hyperventilating.

CN: Physiological integrity; CNS: Physiological adaptation; CL: Analysis

21. A client who had a thoracotomy is using oxygen and having an arterial blood gas (ABG) analysis. Which statement is correct to tell the client?

1. "The nurse will shave the puncture site before the test."
2. "You need to keep the oxygen mask on for the entire test."
3. "You'll be suctioned immediately before the blood is drawn."
4. "You won't be allowed to drink anything for 2 hours before the blood is drawn."

21. 2. To determine the effectiveness of oxygen therapy, ABGs are drawn with the oxygen in use. This also needs to be written on the test form. No special preparations for the test with regard to skin preparation or diet are needed. Suctioning decreases available oxygen.

CN: Physiological integrity; CNS: Basic care and comfort; CL: Application

22. Which condition causes heart failure after a myocardial infarction (MI)?

1. Increased workload of the heart
2. Increased oxygen demands of the heart
3. Inability of the heart chambers to adequately fill
4. Impairment of contractile function of the damaged myocardium

22. 4. After an MI, the injured myocardium is replaced by scar tissue. This scar tissue causes the ventricle to pump less efficiently. After an MI has resolved, oxygen and workload demands should normalize and the heart's chambers should fill adequately.

CN: Physiological integrity; CNS: Physiological adaptation; CL: Application

23. A client is admitted to the emergency department with severe epistaxis. The physician inserts posterior packing. Later, the client is anxious and says he doesn't feel he's breathing right. Which nursing action is appropriate?

1. Cut the packing strings and remove the packing.
2. Reassure the client that what he's experiencing is normal.
3. Ask the client to fully explain what he means by "right."
4. Use a flashlight and inspect the posterior oral cavity of the client.

23. 4. The nurse must assess the patency of the airway. The packing might have become dislodged. The nurse shouldn't remove the packing or give the client false reassurance. The client is too anxious to explain what he means.

CN: Physiological integrity; CNS: Reduction of risk potential; CL: Analysis

24. The nurse is teaching another nurse about pulmonary capillary wedge pressure. Which response is the most accurate regarding this pressure?

1. "It reflects systemic vascular resistance."
2. "It reflects right ventricular end pressure."
3. "It reflects right atrial presystolic pressure."
4. "It reflects left ventricular end-diastolic pressure."

24. 4. The pulmonary capillary wedge pressure is the reflection of the pressure in the left ventricle at rest, which is end diastole. Wedge pressure doesn't reflect pressures in the right side of the heart or systemic vascular resistance.

CN: Physiological integrity; CNS: Physiological adaptation; CL: Application

25. The nurse is teaching a student nurse about the purpose of diaphragmatic breathing exercises for a client with chronic obstructive pulmonary disease (COPD). Which statement by the nurse is correct?

1. "It dilates the bronchioles."
2. "It decreases vital capacity."
3. "It increases residual volume."
4. "It decreases alveolar ventilation."

25. 1. In COPD, the bronchioles constrict during exhalation due to pressure changes in the lungs. Diaphragmatic breathing exercises keep the bronchioles open during exhalation. These exercises aren't performed for the other reasons stated.

CN: Physiological integrity; CNS: Reduction of risk potential; CL: Application

26. A client with chronic obstructive pulmonary disease (COPD) is being discharged from the hospital. The nurse provided teaching on medications, diet, and exercise. Which statement by the client indicates more teaching is needed?

1. "I'll eat six small meals a day."
2. "I'll get a flu shot every winter."
3. "I'll walk every morning before breakfast."
4. "I'll call my physician if I get cold symptoms."

26. 3. The worst time of the day for a client with COPD is morning. Exercise is important, but should be done later in the day. All other choices are appropriate for the client with COPD.

CN: Physiological integrity; CNS: Basic care and comfort; CL: Application

27. The nurse is caring for a client showing symptoms of bronchial obstruction. Which assessment finding would the nurse expect to find?

1. Hacking cough
2. Diminished breath sounds
3. Production of rust-colored sputum
4. Decreased use of accessory muscles

27. 2. Bronchial obstruction means no passage of air through the bronchi, so diminished or no breath sounds would be heard. A hacking cough is often associated with upper respiratory tract infection and dryness in the upper airways. Rust-colored sputum is a sign of pneumococcal pneumonia. There would be increased use of accessory muscles.

CN: Physiological integrity; CNS: Physiological adaptation; CL: Application

28. A client has just started treatment with Rifampin for tuberculosis. Which statement indicates the client has a good understanding of his medication?

1. "I won't go to family gatherings for 6 months."
2. "My urine will look orange because of the medication."
3. "Now I don't need to cover my mouth or nose when I sneeze or cough."
4. "I told my wife to throw away all the spoons and forks before I come home."

28. 2. Rifampin discolors body fluids, such as urine and tears. The client can go to family functions and eat with normal utensils. The client should cover his mouth and nose when coughing and sneezing until he has been on the medication at least 2 weeks.

CN: Physiological integrity; CNS: Pharmacological and parenteral therapies; CL: Application

29. Before feeding a client with Parkinson's disease, which nursing action is most important?

1. Sit the client upright.
2. Have suction available.
3. Order a clear liquid diet.
4. Have a speech therapist evaluate the client.

29. 4. A speech therapist can evaluate the client's swallowing and make recommendations before the client is fed. Aspiration due to involuntary movement is common. Sitting the client upright and having suction available are helpful when feeding the client, but evaluation of the client's swallowing ability should come first. Clear liquids may be too difficult for the client; semisoft foods may be easier to swallow.

CN: Physiological integrity; CNS: Reduction of risk potential; CL: Analysis

30. The nurse is caring for a pregnant client with cardiovascular disease. Which treatment would the nurse expect for this client?

1. Rest
2. Hospitalization
3. Therapeutic abortion
4. Continuous cardiac monitoring

30. 1. The goal of antepartum management is to prevent complications and minimize the strain on the client. This is done with rest. Hospitalization may be required in older women or those with previous decompensation. Therapeutic abortion is considered in severe dysfunction, especially in the first trimester. Continuous cardiac monitoring isn't necessary.

CN: Physiological integrity; CNS: Reduction of risk potential; CL: Application

31. Which assessment finding most likely indicates a urinary tract infection (UTI) in a 5-year-old child?

1. Incontinence
2. Lack of thirst
3. Concentrated urine
4. Subnormal temperature

31. 1. Incontinence in a toilet-trained child is associated with UTI. Lack of thirst wouldn't be expected in a child with UTI. Concentrated urine is a sign of dehydration. Subnormal temperature isn't a sign of UTI.

CN: Health promotion and maintenance; CNS: None; CL: Application

32. During a home health visit, a nurse assesses a client's medication and notes the client has two prescriptions for fluid retention. One prescription reads "Lasix, 40 mg, one tablet daily." The next prescription reads "Furosemide, 40 mg, one tablet daily." Which instruction is given to the client?

1. Take both medications as ordered.
2. Lasix and furosemide are the same drug.
3. Use Lasix one day and furosemide the next day.
4. Throw away one of the drugs to avoid confusing the client.

32. 2. Using generic names for medications is common, especially for home health clients. It's the responsibility of the nurse to teach the client both brand and generic names of drugs. Setting up medications in a medication tray, using only one pharmacy to dispense medications, and using all medications until the bottle is emptied will reduce medication errors.

CN: Physiological integrity; CNS: Pharmacological and parenteral therapies; CL: Analysis

33. A school nurse is called to assess a preadolescent Vietnamese girl attending a new school. A teacher tells the nurse the student sits in the back of the class and won't speak when spoken to, although her parents confirmed the student speaks English. Which assessment finding is most likely?

1. The student is experiencing cultural shock.
2. The student is developing a peer support system.
3. The student is going through a socialization period.
4. The student is becoming acculturated to the new school.

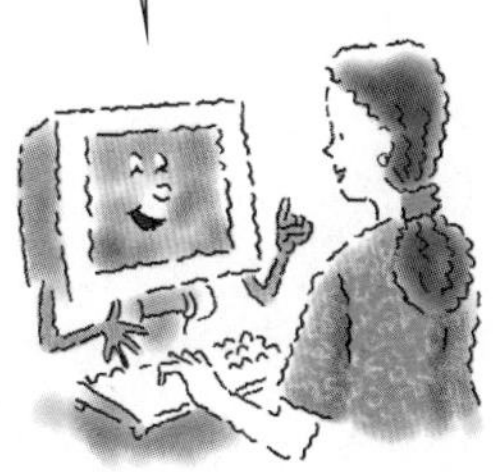

You're doing sensationally! You really know your stuff!

33. 1. Cultural shock is a feeling of helplessness, discomfort, and a state of disorientation when an outsider attempts to comprehend or adapt to a new cultural situation. Peer groups usually develop based on the background, interests, and capabilities of its members. Developing peer cultures is part of the socialization process. Acculturation occurs when there's a blending of cultural or ethnic backgrounds. This process takes time to develop.

CN: Health promotion and maintenance; CNS: None; CL: Application

34. A school nurse is screening for hearing and vision with a group of 11- to 13-year-old students. Which technique is used to communicate effectively with this age group?

1. Give undivided attention to each student.
2. Have the parents present during the screening.
3. Have several adolescents listen to each other's health histories.
4. Use puppets or dolls to show how the screening is going to take place.

34. 1. Give undivided attention to communicate effectively with adolescents. Respect their privacy. The presence of parents and use of puppets or dolls can be used to effectively communicate with younger children.

CN: Health promotion and maintenance; CNS: None; CL: Application

35. A nurse practitioner at a rural health clinic is screening an 18-month-old infant for developmental problems. Which developmental screening test is the most appropriate?

1. Goodenough-Harris Draw-a-Person Test
2. Denver Developmental Screening Test (DDST)
3. McCarthy Scales of Children's Abilities (MSCA)
4. Preschool readiness screening scales

35. 2. The DDST is applicable for children from birth through age 6. The Goodenough-Harris Draw-a-Person Test is used to assess intellectual ability in children ages 3 to 10. The MSCA is a developmental tool for children ages 2½ to 8½. Preschool readiness screening scales are designed for screening 5-year-old children for readiness for school.

CN: Health promotion and maintenance; CNS: None; CL: Application

36. In preparing an educational intervention for college students, a nurse understands that drinking alcoholic beverages is often used to relieve which condition?

1. Fatigue
2. Anxiety
3. Headache
4. Stomach pain

36. 2. Drinking alcoholic beverages is commonly thought to alleviate anxiety. These beverages aren't commonly used to relieve fatigue, headache, or stomach pain.

CN: Psychosocial integrity; CNS: None; CL: Application

37. An educational forum about relaxation techniques is provided for college students preparing for their final exams. Which relaxation technique is most effective to counteract anxiety?

1. Meditation
2. Music therapy
3. Dance therapy
4. Reality orientation

37. 1. Meditation is a relaxation therapy used to counteract anxiety related to stress-inducing internal and external stimuli. Music therapy, dance therapy, and reality orientation are used as adjuncts to psychiatric care.

CN: Psychosocial integrity; CNS: None; CL: Application

38. The parents of a 9-year-old child diagnosed with oppositional defiant disorder (ODD) are discussing treatment options with the nurse. Which action would the nurse expect to have the most positive impact on managing the child's behavior?

1. Daily administration of methylphenidate hydrochloride (Ritalin)
2. Providing praise to the child for positive behaviors
3. Including the child in group therapy with other children diagnosed with ODD
4. Assigning several household chores to the child for weekly completion

38. 2. Children with ODD consistently display negativity, defiance to authority, and hostility. ODD is best managed with consistent parenting and the establishment of a warm, positive home environment. Medication therapies aren't typically used for children with ODD. Methylphenidate is commonly used to manage attention deficit disorder. The focus of treatment for ODD is on the family unit, not on other children with similar problems. The child should be asked to participate in chores, but the parents need to be aware that overwhelming tasks may cause frustration and more defiance.

CN: Psychosocial integrity; CNS: None; CL: Analysis

39. A 40-year-old female client is admitted to a women's shelter after being raped by her estranged husband. The client describes the traumatic event. Which response by the nurse is best?

1. Change the subject to prevent the client from crying.
2. Listen attentively while the client describes the event.
3. Arrange for the client to tell her story in group therapy.
4. Medicate the client with a tranquilizer to prevent hysteria.

39. 2. Retelling the event is part of the healing process. Giving medication and changing the subject don't allow the client to integrate the experience into her life. Group therapy may be helpful, but the best nursing response is to listen and convey empathy.

CN: Psychosocial integrity; CNS: None; CL: Application

40. A nurse is assessing a client with manic-depressive disorder. The client tells the nurse his family physician prescribed lithium. Which symptom indicates the client is developing lithium toxicity?

1. Lethargy
2. Hypertension
3. Hyperexcitability
4. Low urine output

40. 1. Nausea, vomiting, diarrhea, thirst, polyuria, lethargy, slurred speech, hypotension, muscle weakness, and fine hand tremors are signs of lithium toxicity.

CN: Physiological integrity; CNS: Pharmacological and parenteral therapies; CL: Application

41. Which nursing intervention is used during assessment of a pediatric client?

1. Ask the parents to leave the room during health assessment.
2. Position the client on an examination table or bed at all times.
3. Organize the health assessment in the same way for every infant or child.
4. Identify the source (child, parent, caregiver, guardian) and indicate the reliability of the information obtained.

42. Which nursing intervention is used during assessment of an elderly client?

1. Ask the client to change positions quickly.
2. Keep the room temperature cool during health assessment.
3. Speak loudly and quickly to facilitate understanding of directions.
4. Change the height of the examination table or modify the client's position.

43. Which nursing diagnosis is appropriate for a client with chronic obstructive pulmonary disease who is anxious, dyspneic, and hypoxic?

1. *Ineffective breathing pattern related to anxiety*
2. *Risk for aspiration related to absence of protective mechanisms*
3. *Impaired gas exchange related to altered oxygen-carrying capacity of the blood*
4. *Ineffective airway clearance related to presence of tracheobronchial obstruction or secretions*

44. Which statement is a wellness nursing diagnosis?

1. *Readiness for enhanced spiritual well-being*
2. *Risk for activity intolerance related to prolonged bed rest*
3. *Bathing self-care deficit related to fatigue and muscular weakness*
4. *Constipation related to decreased activity and fluid intake as manifested by hard, formed stool every 3 days*

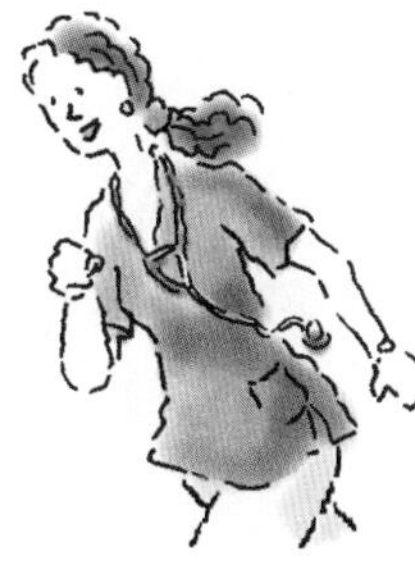
More than halfway home! Excellent!

41. 4. Document the source of information obtained for the nursing assessment of a child. Separation from the parent may cause anxiety and increase the child's fear and distrust. Depending on the child's age, parents may help position and hold the child, facilitating assessment. Organization of the assessment is changed to accommodate the individual child's age and development.

CN: Health promotion and maintenance; CNS: None; CL: Application

42. 4. You may need to change the height of the examination table or use a different position when assessing an elderly client. Physiologically, an older client is prone to falls and dizziness due to decreased ability to respond to sudden movements and position changes. The room temperature should be warm because older clients become hypothermic easily. Speak in a slow, normal tone of voice to facilitate communication.

CN: Health promotion and maintenance; CNS: None; CL: Application

43. 3. The correct nursing diagnosis for this client is based on the impaired oxygenation at the cellular level. The first option applies to a client whose inhalation or exhalation pattern doesn't enable adequate pulmonary inflation or emptying. The second option applies if the client is at risk for aspirating gastric or pharyngeal secretions, food, or fluids into the tracheobronchial passages. The last option is appropriate for a client who's unable to clear secretions or obstructions from the respiratory tract.

CN: Safe, effective care environment; CNS: Management of care; CL: Application

44. 1. Wellness diagnoses are one-part statements containing the label only and begin with "*Readiness for enhanced*," followed by the higher level of wellness desired for the individual or group. The second option is a "risk for" nursing diagnosis. The third option describes a suspected problem for which additional data are needed for confirmation. The last option describes a manifested health problem validated by identifiable major defining characteristics.

CN: Safe, effective care environment; CNS: Management of care; CL: Application

45. A nurse observes that a client with a below-the-knee amputation on the third postoperative day refuses to look at the stump and changes the subject when the nurse attempts to discuss its care. Which nursing diagnosis should the nurse use to address this situation?

1. *Hopelessness*
2. *Impaired physical mobility*
3. *Disturbed body image*
4. *Powerlessness*

45. 3. Refusing to look at the stump is a characteristic of *Disturbed body image.* Other defining characteristics include having a missing body part, hiding a body part, and negative feelings about one's body. The other nursing diagnoses may also be appropriate for this client, but the data presented best reflects *Disturbed body image. Hopelessness* occurs when a person sees limited or no alternatives and is unable to mobilize energy to act. *Impaired physical mobility* may also occur in the client following an amputation, but the data presented doesn't support this diagnosis. With *Powerlessness,* the client doesn't believe his actions will have an effect. Again, the data presented doesn't support this diagnosis.

CN: Safe, effective care environment; CNS: Management of care; CL: Analysis

46. An intake nurse at a mental health facility is admitting a client with psychosis. Which assessment technique is most valuable to use when planning this client's care?

1. Rorschach test
2. Interview with the client
3. Mental Status Examination (MSE)
4. Review old records of the client

46. 3. The MSE is a basis for planning care with a mental health client, especially one who's psychotic. The Rorschach test is used for depression. An interview with a client with psychosis would be unreliable. Review of old records won't assess the current state on which interventions are planned.

CN: Psychosocial integrity; CNS: None; CL: Application

47. Which is a sign that a client with a new diagnosis of breast cancer is having difficulty coping?

1. The client cries when discussing her diagnosis.
2. The client asks questions about treatment.
3. The client is concerned about missing work during chemotherapy.
4. The client changes the topic when treatment is discussed.

47. 4. By changing the topic when breast cancer treatment is discussed, the client may be denying her condition and having difficulty coping. It is normal to cry, ask questions, and be concerned about missing work when discussing a diagnosis such as breast cancer.

CN: Psychosocial integrity; CNS: None; CL: Application

48. Which patient outcome or goal should a nurse identify for a client with the nursing diagnosis *Risk for disuse syndrome?*

1. The client will be free of musculoskeletal complications.
2. The client will experience shorter periods of immobility and inactivity.
3. The nurse will stress the importance of maintaining adequate fluid intake.
4. The nurse will provide holistic care by collaborating with the health care team.

48. 2. This is an appropriate outcome for a client with this nursing diagnosis. Disuse syndrome, a result of prolonged or unavoidable immobility or inactivity, can be prevented. Musculoskeletal complications indicate actual disuse or complications of immobility. Stressing the importance of adequate fluid intake and providing holistic care describe nursing goals, not patient outcomes.

CN: Safe, effective care environment; CNS: Management of care; CL: Application

49. A 42-year-old client who underwent a right modified mastectomy with insertion of a Hemovac drain will be hospitalized overnight because of minor complications. Which goal statement should the nurse include in the plan of care?

1. Teach proper care of the incision site and drain by October 12.
2. The client will know how to care for the incision site and drain by October 12.
3. The client will show the proper care of the incision site and drain by October 12.
4. The client will care for the incision site and contend with psychological loss by October 12.

49. 3. This statement contains a specific measurable verb, clearly identifies the client behavior, and includes a date. Option 1 is a nursing goal as written, not a client-centered goal. The client goal of option 2 isn't measurable as stated. Option 4 includes two goals that need to be addressed separately under the appropriate nursing diagnosis and it contains nonmeasurable verbs.

CN: Physiological integrity; CNS: Basic care and comfort; CL: Application

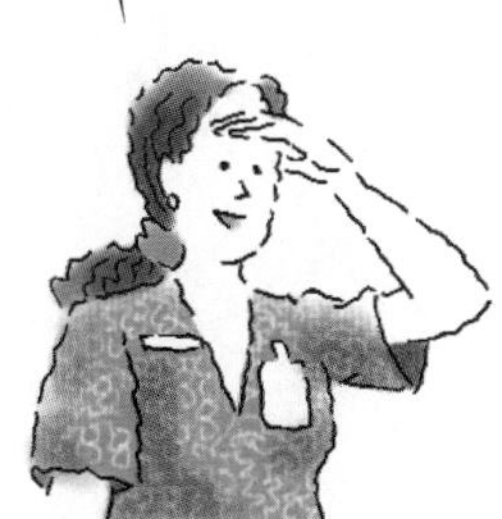

Your goal is in sight. Keep at it!

50. Which expected outcome or goal should a nurse identify for a client with the nursing diagnosis *Risk for injury related to lack of awareness of environmental hazards?*

1. Encourage the client to discuss safety rules with children.
2. Help the client learn safety precautions to take in the home.
3. The client will eliminate safety hazards in his surroundings.
4. The client will contact community resources for more information.

50. 3. This goal is appropriate and measurable as written and focuses on the client. The other options are nursing interventions as written.

CN: Safe, effective care environment; CNS: Management of care; CL: Application

51. What is the best action by a nurse when talking with a client diagnosed with prostate cancer who is tearful and having difficulty talking about his concerns?

1. Ask if he would like to speak with a chaplain.
2. Tell the client that she will be back once he has stopped crying.
3. Sit and ask him if he would like to talk about his concerns.
4. Tell the client that she knows how he is feeling.

51. 3. By sitting down, the nurse shows the client that he is important. Asking if he would like to talk about his concerns lets the client know that the nurse cares about him and wants to help. Calling a chaplain is appropriate after the nurse has assessed the situation and the client has verbalized his concerns. Telling the client that she will return after he stops crying does not show concern for his feelings and does not encourage verbalization. Telling the client that she understands how he feels doesn't help him verbalize his feelings.

CN: Psychosocial integrity; CNS: None; CL: Application

52. A client with heart failure is given furosemide (Lasix) 40 mg I.V. daily. The morning serum potassium level is 2.8 mEq/L. Which nursing action is the most appropriate?

1. Question the physician about the dosage.
2. Give 20 mg of the ordered dose and recheck the laboratory test results.
3. Notify the physician, repeat the potassium as ordered, then give the furosemide.
4. Give the furosemide and get an order for sodium polystyrene sulfonate.

52. 3. Furosemide is a diuretic. As water is lost, so is potassium. Diuresis is a treatment for heart failure. Notifying the physician of the low potassium level and getting an order for potassium chloride is the appropriate action before giving the furosemide. Furosemide, 40 mg, is an appropriate dose for the treatment of heart failure. The nurse shouldn't give half the dose without an order. Giving furosemide and sodium polystyrene sulfonate together would further lower the potassium level.

CN: Physiological integrity; CNS: Pharmacological and parenteral therapies; CL: Application

53. Which client is at greatest risk for developing respiratory alkalosis?

1. A client in labor
2. A client with diabetes
3. A client with renal failure
4. An immediate postoperative client

53. 1. A client's respirations at certain stages of labor increase in volume, causing the $Paco_2$ to decrease, increasing the pH. Diabetes often causes a metabolic imbalance, resulting in metabolic acidosis. In renal failure, the inability of the kidneys to eliminate wastes increases the risk of developing metabolic acidosis. The respirations of a postoperative client are usually shallow after anesthesia and, because of pain, often cause respiratory acidosis.

CN: Physiological integrity; CNS: Physiological adaptation; CL: Analysis

54. Which condition indicates to a nurse that a sterile field has been contaminated?

1. Sterile objects are held above the waist of the nurse.
2. Sterile packages are opened with the first edge away from the nurse.
3. The outer inch of the sterile towel hangs over the side of the table.
4. Wetness on the sterile cloth on top of the nonsterile table has been noted.

54. 4. Moisture outside the sterile package and field contaminates it because fluid can be wicked into the sterile field. Bacteria tend to settle, so there's less contamination above waist level and away from the nurse. The outer inch of the drape is considered contaminated but doesn't indicate that the sterile field itself has been contaminated.

CN: Safe, effective care environment; CNS: Safety and infection control; CL: Application

55. Which intervention should a nurse perform for a client with respiratory alkalosis?

1. Have the client breathe into a paper bag.
2. Give one ampule of bicarbonate as ordered.
3. Give oxygen at 3 L/minute through a nasal cannula.
4. Reposition the client in a high Fowler's position.

55. 1. By breathing into a paper bag, the client will rebreathe some of his own exhaled carbon dioxide and increase the carbon dioxide in his blood, which will correct his respiratory alkalosis. Giving one ampule of bicarbonate will worsen the alkalosis. Giving oxygen won't increase the carbon dioxide to correct the imbalance. Repositioning the client won't help him retain carbon dioxide.

CN: Physiological integrity; CNS: Physiological adaptation; CL: Analysis

56. The nurse is reviewing the laboratory results from a female diabetic client admitted to the acute care facility with dehydration. Which laboratory result is consistent with a diagnosis of dehydration?

1. Serum hematocrit of 40%
2. Urine dipstick specific gravity of 1.035
3. Serum creatinine level of 0.8 mg/dl
4. HbA_{1c} level of 4%

56. 2. Urine specific gravity reflects the ability of the kidneys to concentrate urine. Normal urine specific gravity is 1.005 to 1.030. A higher urine specific gravity indicates that the urine is more concentrated, and this is consistent with dehydration. The normal hematocrit range for a female client is 36% to 48%, so this value is within normal limits. Dehydration would cause an increase in hematocrit. Serum creatinine is used to assess kidney function. The normal range for women is 0.6 to 0.9 mg/dl. HbA_{1c} is used to monitor diabetes treatment and evaluate the average blood glucose over a period of months. The normal range for HbA_{1c} is 4% to 6.7%.

CN: Physiological integrity; CNS: Physiological adaptation; CL: Analysis

57. A client admitted with hypoparathyroidism is being monitored for hypocalcemia. Which finding would the nurse observe with hypocalcemia?

1. Battle's sign
2. Brudzinski's sign
3. Chvostek's sign
4. Homans' sign

57. 3. Hypocalcemia can cause Chvostek's sign, abnormal facial muscle and nerve spasms elicited when the facial nerve is tapped. Battle's sign is bruising over the temporal bone in the presence of a basilar skull fracture. Brudzinski's sign is the flexion of the hips and knees in response to flexion of the head and neck toward the chest, indicating meningeal irritation. A positive Homans' sign indicates deep vein thrombosis.

CN: Physiological integrity; CNS: Reduction of risk potential; CL: Application

58. A client is complaining of pain 1 day after a colostomy. The nurse gives morphine I.M. and, 30 minutes later, finds the respiratory rate at 8 breaths/minute, with the nasal cannula on the floor. Arterial blood gas (ABG) results are pH, 7.23; Pao_2, 58 mm Hg; $Paco_2$, 61 mm Hg; HCO_3^-, 24 mEq/L. Which group of factors contributes most to this client's ABG results?

1. Colostomy, pain, and morphine
2. Morphine, the nasal cannula on the floor, and the colostomy
3. Morphine, respiratory rate of 8 breaths/minute, and the nasal cannula on the floor
4. Pain, respiratory rate of 8 breaths/minute, and the nasal cannula on the floor

58. 3. This client has respiratory acidosis. Opioids can suppress respirations, causing retention of carbon dioxide. A Pao_2 of 58 mm Hg indicates hypoxemia, which is caused by the removal of the client's supplementary oxygen and the decreased respiratory rate. Pain increases—not decreases—the respiratory rate, which causes a decrease in $Paco_2$. Colostomy drainage doesn't start until 2 to 3 days postoperatively, and this drainage would contribute to metabolic alkalosis.

CN: Physiological integrity; CNS: Physiological adaptation; CL: Analysis

59. Which arterial blood gas (ABG) results should a nurse expect to see in a client with emphysema?

1. pH, 7.52; $Paco_2$, 18 mm Hg; HCO_3^-, 22 mEq/L
2. pH, 7.50; $Paco_2$, 38 mm Hg; HCO_3^-, 38 mEq/L
3. pH, 7.30; $Paco_2$, 52 mm Hg; HCO_3^-, 30 mEq/L
4. pH, 7.30; $Paco_2$, 40 mm Hg; HCO_3^-, 18 mEq/L

59. 3. Clients with emphysema retain carbon dioxide due to air trapping, causing an elevated $Paco_2$ and respiratory acidosis. Because emphysema is a chronic disease, the kidneys compensate over time for the increased $Paco_2$ by retaining HCO_3^-, thus attempting to normalize the pH. The other ABG results aren't consistent with results found in a client with emphysema.

CN: Physiological integrity; CNS: Physiological adaptation; CL: Analysis

60. Which factor does a nurse identify as a major cause of metabolic alkalosis in a client who had a colon resection?

1. Hyperventilation
2. Pain management
3. Nasogastric suction
4. I.V. therapy

60. 3. Removing acidic gastric secretions from the stomach is a metabolic cause of alkalinization of the blood pH. Hyperventilation decreases carbon dioxide and increases the pH, causing respiratory alkalosis. Pain management may further decrease the respiratory rate. Most I.V. fluids don't influence pH.

CN: Physiological integrity; CNS: Physiological adaptation; CL: Analysis

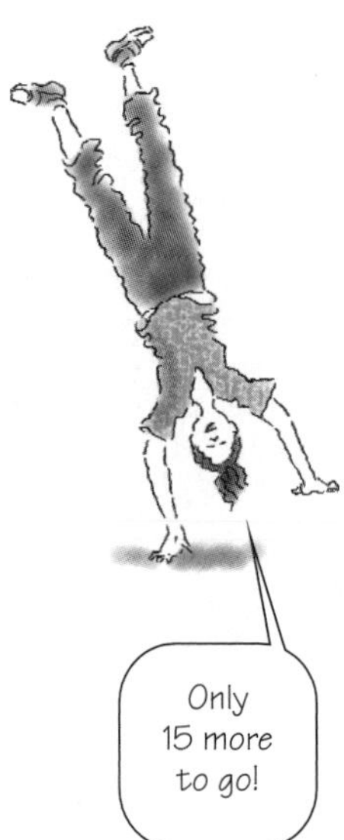

61. Which nursing action should be included in the plan of care to prevent an increase in intracranial pressure (ICP) in a comatose client with a closed head injury?

1. Suction the airway every hour to maintain patency.
2. Elevate the head of the bed 20 degrees.
3. Place in a supine position with the head turned to the side.
4. Provide environmental stimulation.

61. 2. The head of the bed should be elevated between 15 to 30 degrees to promote venous drainage. Suctioning the airway may increase ICP and should only be performed when needed. Turning the head to the side may cause jugular venous compression and an elevation in ICP. Environmental stimulation should be minimized to reduce any rise in ICP.

CN: Physiological integrity; CNS: Reduction in risk potential; CL: Application

62. After making the bed of a client with dementia, which action has priority?

1. Put the bed in the lowest position.
2. Put the call button within the client's reach.
3. Put the top side rails in the upright position.
4. Put soiled linen in a hamper or biohazard bag.

62. 1. To reduce the risk of injury due to falls, the bed should be placed in the lowest position. The call button should be in reach of the client, but the immediate safety of the client comes first. All four side rails should be up to prevent accidental falls and to remind clients to stay in bed. Soiled linens should be placed in a hamper or biohazard bag, but client safety is a priority.

CN: Safe, effective care environment; CNS: Management of care; CL: Application

63. After emptying urine from the bedpan of a client whose urinary output is being monitored, which step should a nurse do next?

1. Wash hands thoroughly.
2. Apply a clean pair of gloves.
3. Report the amount of urine to the nurse in charge right away.
4. Document the amount and characteristics of urine in the chart.

63. 1. After any procedure is completed, the nurse must wash her hands to prevent transmission of microorganisms. The application of gloves is only necessary if the nurse must attend to another item of personal care before documenting urinary output; even so, hands should be washed first. Crucial information is reported to the charge nurse, not routine intake and output. Documentation should take place, but following the handwashing.

CN: Safe, effective care environment; CNS: Safety and infection control; CL: Application

64. Which client should a nurse place in an orthopneic position?

1. A client with edema of the lower legs and ankles
2. A client with a pressure ulcer on the coccyx and buttocks
3. An immobilized client with calf tenderness due to a thrombus
4. An elderly client with difficulty breathing

64. 4. The orthopneic position, which is appropriate for a client with breathing difficulty, is a sitting position with the arms leaning on a bedside table. Sitting with the legs elevated to decrease edema is appropriate for clients with ankle and lower leg swelling. A client with a pressure ulcer will need to be positioned on his side and turned every 2 hours. Fowler's or semi-Fowler's positions are most appropriate for a client on complete bed rest.

CN: Physiological integrity; CNS: Physiological adaptation; CL: Application

65. A client preparing to transfer from the bed to a wheelchair complains of feeling light-headed and dizzy as he rises from a supine to a sitting position. Which action should the nurse take next?

1. Lift the client quickly into the wheelchair.
2. Return the client to the supine position and apply a safety vest.
3. Ask the client to dangle his legs at the bedside while leaving the room for a few seconds to get assistance.
4. Have the client sit at the side of the bed for a few minutes while supporting his back and shoulders.

65. 4. A quick change in position will decrease the blood pressure, causing momentary light-headedness and dizziness. An additional change in position may further reduce the client's blood pressure to a level that may require emergency assistance. This can be avoided by waiting with the client in the sitting position until the blood pressure stabilizes. A safety vest isn't necessary. Leaving the room may put the client in danger if the blood pressure decreases further and the client needs emergency assistance. If the client continues to complain of dizziness and light-headedness, then return the client to bed.

CN: Physiological integrity; CNS: Reduction of risk potential; CL: Application

66. Which nursing action is the most effective infection control measure for preventing the transmission of microorganisms?

1. Change a client's bed linen daily.
2. Wash hands before and after client contact.
3. Wear sterile gloves when touching a client's skin.
4. Wear a mask when in direct contact with infected clients.

66. 2. Typically, the transmission of microorganisms occurs when health care personnel don't wash their hands before and after touching a client or contaminated objects. A daily linen change isn't the most effective method of controlling infection. Sterile gloves and a mask aren't needed during routine client care.

CN: Safe, effective care environment; CNS: Safety and infection control; CL: Application

67. The nurse is teaching a student nurse about standard precautions. Which action by the student nurse indicates that the teaching has been effective?

1. Wear eye goggles while giving a complete bed bath.
2. Recap a needle used for an injection before disposal.
3. Dispose of blood-contaminated materials in a biohazard container.
4. Use alcohol to decontaminate blood-contaminated steel instruments.

67. 3. Blood-contaminated materials are disposed of in a biohazard container. Recapping needles puts the health care provider at risk for sticking himself. Standard precautions needn't be observed during a bath because of the low risk for exposure to blood. Blood-contaminated steel instruments are decontaminated in an autoclave.

CN: Safe, effective care environment; CNS: Safety and infection control; CL: Application

68. A team leader would instruct team members to wear a mask and protective eyewear or a face shield in which situation?

1. When strong odors are emitted from an infected wound
2. When the client has an oral temperature greater than 101° F (38.3° C)
3. If needles or other sharp instruments are to be used in the procedure
4. During a procedure where splashing of blood or body fluid is anticipated

68. 4. Wearing eye goggles or face shields prevents blood or body-fluid splashes into the eyes. Odors don't transmit microorganisms. A client with a fever won't transmit microorganisms into the eyes any more frequently than a client without a fever. The use of needles or other sharp instruments doesn't mandate eye protection.

CN: Safe, effective environment; CNS: Management of care; CL: Application

69. A nurse is caring for a client on neutropenic precautions. At which time should the nurse remove the barrier protection when leaving the room?

1. Within the client's room, just inside the doorway
2. Out of the client's room, just outside the doorway
3. In the hallway, a significant distance from the client's room
4. At the bedside, immediately after completing work with the client

69. 2. Disposing of gowns and gloves just outside the doorway provides sufficient distance from the client for all but airborne microorganisms. The client is protected from infection by airborne pathogens by keeping the door shut as much as possible to decrease the chance of exposure. Disposal of barriers at the bedside or inside the door negates the effectiveness of wearing barriers in the first place. It's unnecessary to wear the barriers away from the doorway as the door should remain closed.

CN: Safe, effective care environment; CNS: Safety and infection control; CL: Application

70. Which timeframe is most appropriate for completing client teaching for a client undergoing an open cholecystectomy?

1. The day of discharge
2. A few weeks before the surgery
3. The first 12 hours after surgery
4. Before discharge, 1 to 2 days after the surgery

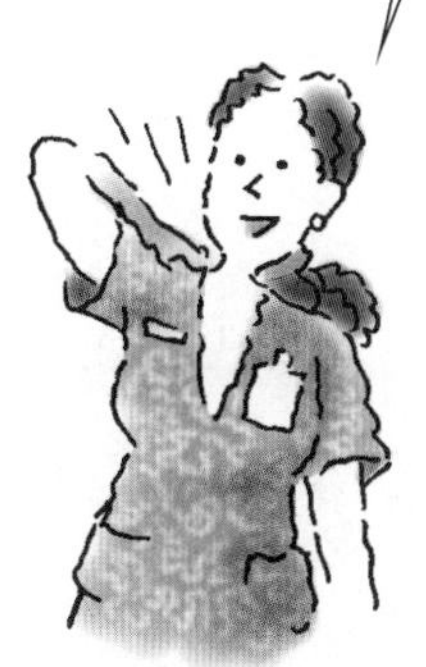
Pat yourself
on the back.
Only five more
to go.

70. 4. Pain levels should have sufficiently subsided 1 to 2 days after the surgical procedure, allowing the client to concentrate on the information. The day of discharge is too late, because it doesn't give the client time to ask questions or practice procedures (such as syringe preparation) that may be necessary. Also, the individual may be anxious about returning home, which may interfere with learning. A few weeks before surgery is generally too early to retain information, and teaching within the first 12 hours after surgery isn't likely to produce retention of information, either.

CN: Physiological integrity; CNS: Physiological adaptation; CL: Application

71. Which technique is appropriate for promoting proper breathing in a client experiencing pain or anxiety?

1. Rapid, light respirations
2. Rapid, deep respirations
3. In through the mouth and out through the nose
4. In through the nose and out through the mouth

71. 4. Air inhaled through the nose is warmed, humidified, and filtered for large particles with the nasal hairs, conditioning the air for delivery to the lungs. Exhaling through the mouth after inhaling through the nose requires some concentration and provides a focus to distract a client experiencing pain and anxiety. This method is used to control respiratory rates when clients are anxious or in pain and optimizes air exchange. Rapid, light, or deep respirations cause the client to lose oxygen exchange time while continuing to blow off carbon dioxide. This leads to hypoxemia and respiratory alkalosis.

CN: Physiological integrity; CNS: Physiological adaptation; CL; Application

72. The nurse is assessing a client who was admitted with a pressure ulcer. The nurse determines that the ulcer is at stage II. Which graphic represents stage II of a pressure ulcer?

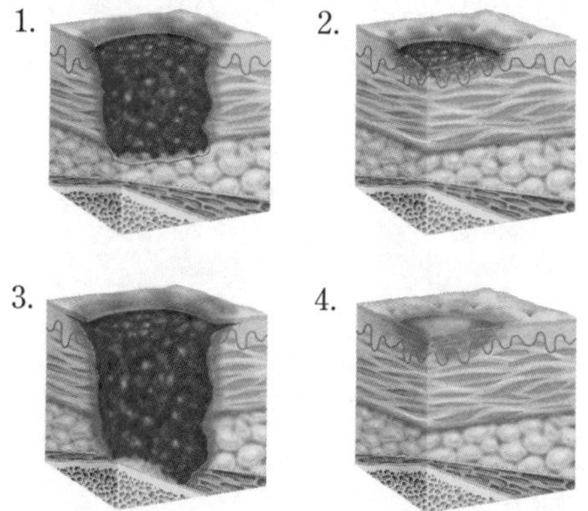

72. 2. Stage II is marked by partial-thickness skin loss that involves the epidermis, dermis, or both, with an abrasion, blister, or shallow crater. The first graphic is stage III, which is a full-thickness wound that appears like a deep crater. The third graphic is of stage IV, which involves all thicknesses and involves the muscle, bone, and supporting structures. The fourth graphic is of stage I, which is a reddened area with intact skin or, in those with dark skin, there may be warmth, edema, discoloration, induration, or hardness.

CN: Physiological integrity; CNS: Physiological adaptation; CL: Analysis

73. A 46-year-old single female client was concerned about her 15-year-old son's behavior. He suddenly decided his mother shouldn't date or have men in the house. He told his mother he was the "man of the house." Which disturbance was occurring in the internal dynamics of the family?

1. Age-appropriate behavior is occurring.
2. The son is powerful in the family system.
3. The son is trying to establish a role reversal.
4. It's culturally acceptable to be the man of the house at age 15.

73. 3. Role reversal occurs when the patterns of expected behavior aren't appropriate to age and ability. Males ages 13 to 17 are developing their identities, and separation from parents becomes necessary for individuation to occur. Males have a better understanding of their roles in relationships and families if they're raised around strong male role models. In healthy families, power is shared appropriate to age until the children are independent.

CN: Psychosocial integrity; CNS: None; CL: Analysis

74. A nurse is reviewing the causes of gastroesophageal reflux disease (GERD) with a client. What area of the GI tract should the nurse identify as the cause of reduced pressure associated with GERD?

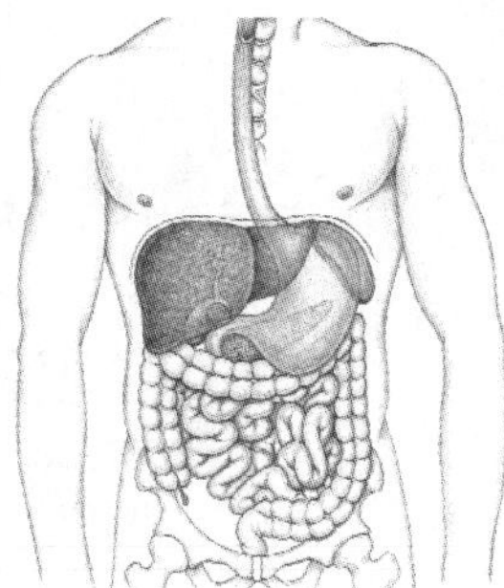

74. Normally, there is enough pressure around the lower esophageal sphincter (LES) to close it. Reflux occurs when LES pressure is deficient or when pressure in the stomach exceeds LES pressure.

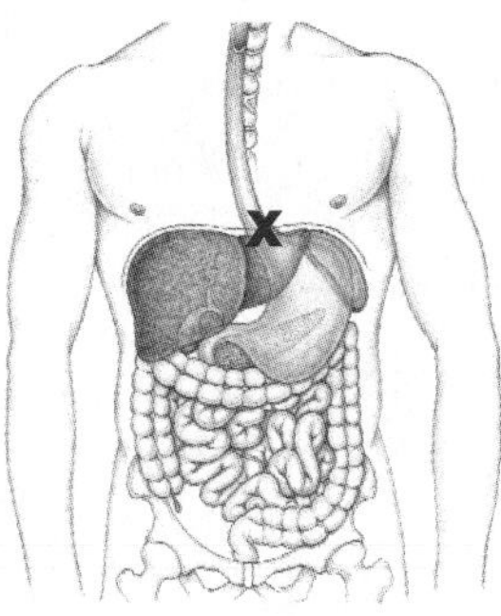

CN: Health promotion and maintenance; CNS: None; CL: Application

75. A nurse is preparing a client with a tracheostomy for discharge. Which statements by the client indicate that he understands the teaching regarding his tracheostomy care?

1. "I will need to cover the opening when I shower."
2. "I can swim as long as I keep my head above water."
3. "I will need to wash my hands after caring for my tracheostomy."
4. "I will need to take antibiotics to prevent infections."

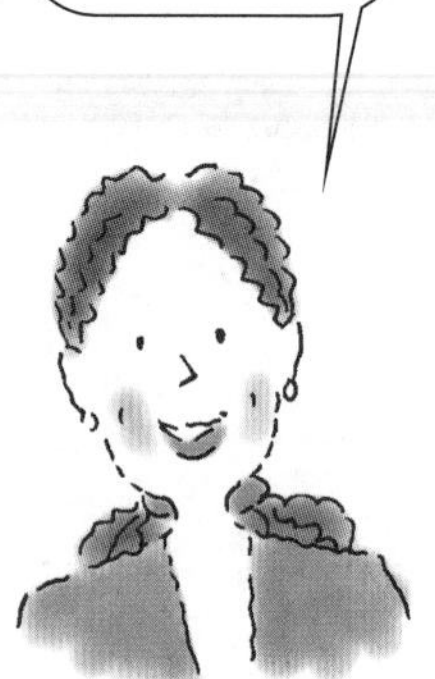

You did a wonderful job! Only two more tests left!

75. 1. The opening will require protection when bathing. Swimming isn't recommended; drowning can occur even if the client's head isn't submerged. It's necessary to wash hands before and after caring for the tracheostomy. Prophylactic antibiotics aren't required for the client with a tracheostomy.

CN: Safe, effective care environment; CNS: Safety and infection control; CL: Application

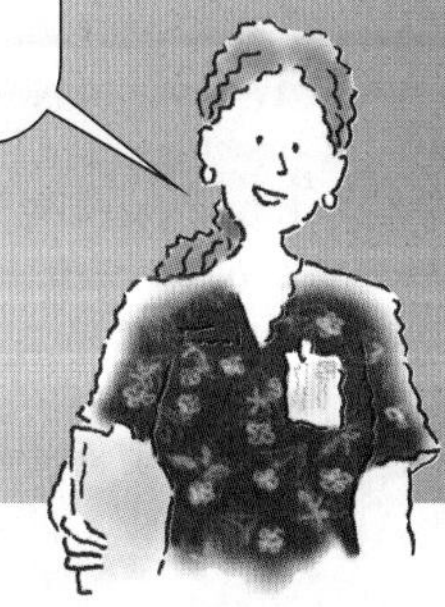

This is the next to last comprehensive test. Go for it, and good luck!

COMPREHENSIVE Test 5

1. Which information about vital signs should a nurse report to the physician?

1. Blood pressure of 120/72 mm Hg in a healthy man
2. Pulse of 110 beats/minute on awakening in the morning
3. Blood pressure of 110/68 mm Hg in a healthy woman
4. Pulse of 120 beats/minute after 30 minutes of aerobic exercise

1. 2. The normal range for a pulse is 60 to 100 beats/minute and, in the morning, the rate is at its lowest. Blood pressures of 120/72 mm Hg for a healthy man and 110/68 mm Hg for a healthy woman are normal. Aerobic exercise increases the heart rate over the normal range of 60 to 100 beats/minute. The formula for maximum aerobic heart rate is: $210 - \text{age} \times 80\%$. A person shouldn't go over the maximum heart rate during aerobic exercise.

CN: Physiological integrity; CNS: Physiological adaptation; CL: Analysis

2. Immediately after a client's cardiac catheterization via the femoral artery, the client is being assessed by the nurse. Which assessment finding would the nurse report immediately to the physician?

1. Apical pulse of 98 beats/minute
2. Dressing with dime-sized red drainage
3. Absence of dorsalis pedis pulse
4. Blood pressure of 105/70 mm Hg

2. 3. The dorsalis pedis is the pulse used to determine peripheral circulation to the lower extremities after a cardiac catheterization. Absence of this pulse should be reported immediately to the physician. An apical pulse of 98 beats/minute and a blood pressure of 105/70 mm Hg are within the normal range. A dressing with dime-sized, red drainage is normal after a catheterization, but should continue to be monitored.

CN: Physiological integrity; CNS: Reduction of risk potential; CL: Application

3. A nurse is preparing to bathe a client who's hospitalized for emphysema. Which nursing intervention is correct?

1. Remove the oxygen and proceed with the bath.
2. Increase the flow of oxygen to 6 L/minute by nasal cannula.
3. Keep the head of the bed slightly elevated during the procedure.
4. Lower the head of the bed and roll the client to his left side to increase oxygenation.

3. 3. The elasticity of the lungs is lost for clients with emphysema, who can't tolerate lying flat because the abdominal organs compress the lungs. The best position is one with the head slightly elevated. The rate of oxygen delivery shouldn't be increased or decreased without an order from the physician. Increasing oxygen flow on a client with emphysema may also suppress the hypoxic drive to breathe. Positioning the client on his left side with the head of the bed flat would decrease oxygenation.

CN: Physiological integrity; CNS: Physiological adaptation; CL: Application

CN: Client needs category CNS: Client needs subcategory CL: Cognitive level

4. A 40-year-old client is scheduled to have elective facial surgery later in the morning. The nurse notes the pulse rate is 130 beats/minute. The nurse suspects which reason best explains the tachycardia?

1. Age
2. Anxiety
3. Exercise
4. Pain

4. 2. Anxiety tends to increase heart rate, temperature, and respirations. The normal heart rate for a client this age is 60 to 100 beats/minute. Exercise will increase the heart rate but most likely won't occur preoperatively. The client shouldn't be in any pain preoperatively.

CN: Physiological integrity; CNS: Physiological adaptation; CL: Application

5. A thin client is sitting up in bed talking on the phone and has a blood pressure of 90/50 mm Hg. Which nursing action is correct?

1. Increase fluids.
2. Call the physician.
3. Consider this a normal variation.
4. Suspect orthostatic hypotension.

5. 3. A thin client can have a blood pressure as low as 88/46 mm Hg and remain asymptomatic. Calling the physician with this information is inappropriate, as is increasing fluids. Orthostatic hypotension is a decrease in blood pressure and increase in heart rate that occur with a sudden change in position from lying to sitting. It might indicate some dehydration, but this client had been sitting up without symptoms for a while.

CN: Health promotion and maintenance; CNS: None; CL: Application

6. Which sign should alert a nurse to a potential problem in a client who has received morphine I.V. for postoperative pain?

1. Heart rate 124 beats/minute
2. Respiratory rate 8 breaths/minute
3. Sleeping, but easily aroused
4. Blood pressure 90/62 mm Hg

6. 2. Since morphine depresses the respiratory center of the brain, the nurse should alert the physician of a respiratory rate less than 10 breaths/minute. While a heart rate of 124 beats/minute is considered tachycardia, the nurse should further assess the client before calling the physician. Morphine shouldn't be given to a client who is sedated and not easily aroused. Morphine can cause hypotension, but the nurse should further assess the client before calling the physician because this may be the client's usual blood pressure.

CN: Physiological integrity; CNS: Pharmacological and parenteral therapies; CL: Analysis

7. The vital signs of a 56-year-old client are: temperature, 98.6° F (37° C) orally; pulse, 80 beats/minute; respirations, 30 breaths/minute; and blood pressure, 118/78 mm Hg. Which interpretation by the nurse is correct?

1. Pulse is above normal range.
2. Temperature is above normal range.
3. Respirations are above normal range.
4. Blood pressure is above normal range.

7. 3. Normal vital signs for an adult client are: temperature, 96.6° to 99° F (36° to 37° C); pulse, 60 to 100 beats/minute; respirations, 16 to 20 breaths/minute; and blood pressure, 90–120/60–80 mm Hg.

CN: Health promotion and maintenance; CNS: None; CL: Analysis

8. A client with type 1 diabetes mellitus is confused, weak, diaphoretic, and has palpitations. What action should the nurse take first?

1. Administer glucagon intramuscularly (I.M.) or subcutaneously (subQ).
2. Give an intravenous (I.V.) bolus of dextrose 50%.
3. Provide 15 to 20 g of a fast-acting oral carbohydrate.
4. Inject 10 units of fast-acting insulin subcutaneously.

8. 3. The client is exhibiting signs of hypoglycemia. Since the client is conscious, the first intervention is to give a fast-acting oral carbohydrate, such as orange juice, hard candy, or honey. If the client becomes unconscious, the nurse would administer I.M. or subQ glucagon or I.V. dextrose 50%. Administering insulin wouldn't be appropriate because the client is experiencing hypoglycemia.

CN: Physiological integrity; CNS: Reduction of risk potential; CL: Analysis

9. Which nursing action is correct for performing tracheal suctioning?

1. Apply suction during insertion of the catheter.
2. Limit suctioning to 10 to 15 seconds' duration.
3. Resterilize the suction catheter in alcohol after use.
4. Repeat suctioning intervals every 15 minutes until clear.

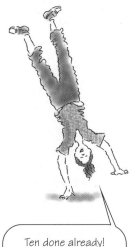

9. 2. The length of time a client should be able to tolerate the suction procedure is 10 to 15 seconds. Any longer may cause hypoxia. Suctioning during insertion can cause trauma to the mucosa and removes oxygen from the respiratory tract. Suctioning intervals with supplemental oxygen between suctions is performed after at least 1-minute intervals to allow the client to rest. Suction catheters are disposed of after each use and are cleansed in normal saline solution after each pass.

CN: Physiological integrity; CNS: Physiological adaptation; CL: Application

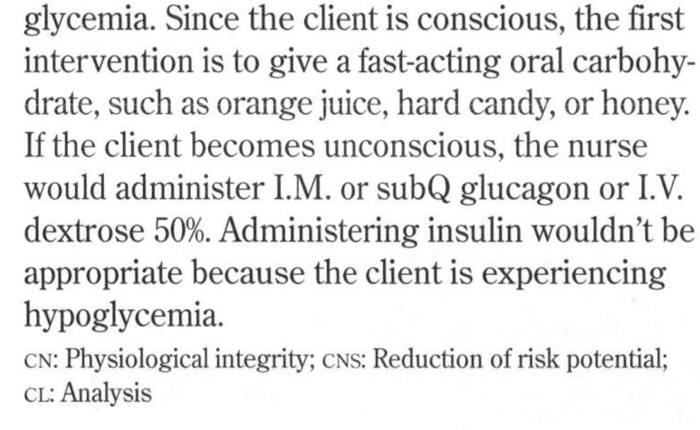
Ten done already!
Good job!

10. While performing nasopharyngeal suction, a nurse notes a client's oxygen saturation reading is 86% by pulse oximeter. Which action should the nurse take?

1. Stop suctioning and give oxygen to the client.
2. Withdraw the suction catheter and tell the client to cough several times.
3. Continue suctioning for 10 to 15 more seconds and then withdraw the suction catheter.
4. Keep the suction catheter inserted and wait a few seconds before beginning suctioning.

10. 1. The pulse oximeter reading indicates the client isn't oxygenating well, so the nurse must stop suctioning and give oxygen to increase the saturation. The normal range for oxygen saturation is 90% to 100%. Suctioning draws air as well as secretions from the lungs, reducing oxygen saturation in the blood. Withdrawing the suction catheter will stop the removal of oxygen, but coughing will delay an increase in saturation. Further suctioning will reduce the oxygen level even more. The suction catheter occupies space in the airway, making it harder for the client to breathe when it's left in place.

CN: Physiological integrity; CNS: Physiological adaptation; CL: Application

11. Two hours after starting total enteral nutrition (TEN) through a nasogastric tube, a client starts to have abdominal distention. Which action should the nurse take first?

1. Aspirate stomach contents.
2. Reposition the tube.
3. Place client in supine position.
4. Stop the feeding.

11. 4. Clients receiving TEN are at risk for abdominal distention due to rapid feeding or delayed emptying of the stomach contents. The first action would be to stop the feeding to prevent further distention and then continue to assess the distention's cause. Aspirating the stomach contents and repositioning the tube may be necessary, but are not the priority. A client receiving a nasogastric tube feeding should be placed in an upright or Fowler's position, not supine, to prevent the risk of aspiration.

CN: Physiological integrity; CNS: Basic care and comfort; CL: Application

12. Which step should a nurse take first when preparing to insert a nasogastric (NG) tube?

1. Wash hands.
2. Apply sterile gloves.
3. Apply a mask and gown.
4. Open all necessary kits and tubing.

12. 1. The first intervention before a procedure is hand washing. Clean gloves are used because the mouth and nasopharynx aren't considered sterile. A mask and gown aren't required. Opening all the equipment is the next step before inserting the NG tube.

CN: Safe, effective care environment; CNS: Safety and infection control; CL: Application

13. As a nurse is inserting a nasogastric tube, the client begins to gag. Which action should the nurse take?

1. Remove the inserted tube and notify the physician of the client's status.
2. Stop the insertion, allow the client to rest, then continue inserting the tube.
3. Encourage the client to take deep breaths through the mouth while the tube is being inserted.
4. Pause until the gagging stops, tell the client to take a few sips of water and swallow as the tube is inserted.

13. 4. Swallowing helps advance the tube by causing the epiglottis to cover the opening of the trachea, thus helping to eliminate gagging and coughing. Removing the tube or stopping the insertion is unnecessary because gagging is an expected response to this procedure. Deep breathing opens the trachea, allowing the tube to possibly advance into the lungs.

CN: Safe, effective care environment; CNS: Safety and infection control; CL: Application

14. Which step, if taken by a nurse after insertion of a nasogastric (NG) tube, could harm the client?

1. Affix the NG tube to the nose with tape.
2. Check tube placement by aspirating stomach contents using a piston syringe.
3. Check tube placement by instilling 100 ml of water into the tube to check for stomach filling.
4. Document in the chart the insertion, method used to check tube placement, and client's response to the procedure.

14. 3. Should the tube be located in the lungs, instilling water would flood the lungs, precipitating choking, coughing, hypoxemia and, possibly, pneumonia. Anchoring the tube after placement to the nose with tape or a manufactured device prevents the tube from becoming dislodged. Withdrawing stomach contents from the NG tube double-checks the correct placement. Documentation is required for any procedure.

CN: Safe, effective care environment; CNS: Management of care; CL: Application

15. A new graduate nurse is assigned to a nursing unit. The nurse-manager notes that the graduate's skills are deficient. Which action is most appropriate for the nurse-manager to take?

1. Talk with the supervisor about terminating the new graduate.
2. Discuss with the graduate that a transfer to another unit is necessary.
3. Work with the graduate and develop a plan to improve the graduate's deficiencies.
4. Counsel the graduate that, if performance doesn't improve, the graduate will be terminated.

15. 3. A principle of leadership involves mastery over ignorance by working with people. The leader needs to work with the new graduate and provide opportunities for the graduate to grow and develop. The other responses wouldn't give the new graduate the opportunity and support needed for improvement.

CN: Safe, effective care environment; CNS: Management of care; CL: Application

16. A client on a cardiac monitor has a heart rate of 170 beats/minute, with frequent premature contractions. Which nursing action is best?

1. Call the client's physician immediately.
2. See the client and make a full assessment.
3. Delegate one of the nurses' assistants to take the client's vital signs.
4. Notify the supervisor about the change in the client's condition.

16. 2. Because a change has occurred in the client's status, the nurse must assess the client first. This shouldn't be delegated to unlicensed personnel. Before the physician or supervisor is notified, a full assessment must be made.

CN: Safe, effective care environment; CNS: Management of care; CL: Application

17. A client is hospitalized with an acute sinus infection. Which assessment made by the nurse indicates serious complications?

1. Orbital edema
2. Nuchal rigidity
3. Fever of 102° F (39° C)
4. Frontal headache

17. 2. Nuchal rigidity indicates neurologic involvement, possibly meningitis. The other symptoms are typical of a sinus infection.

CN: Physiological integrity; CNS: Physiological adaptation; CL: Application

18. Which statement by a client who had nasal surgery indicates to the nurse that the client needs further teaching about postoperative care?

1. "I'll do frequent mouth care."
2. "I'll eat two oranges a day."
3. "I'll eat two bananas a day."
4. "I'll drink at least 8 glasses of fluid a day."

18. 3. After nasal surgery, the client shouldn't strain or bear down as this will increase the risk for bleeding. Bananas can cause severe constipation, which could lead to straining. The other interventions would be appropriate postoperative care for this client.

CN: Physiological integrity; CNS: Reduction of risk potential; CL: Analysis

19. The nurse is collecting a urine specimen from a client's indwelling urinary catheter. Which action should the nurse take?

1. Collect urine from the drainage collection bag.
2. Disconnect the catheter from the drainage tubing to collect urine.
3. Remove the indwelling catheter and insert a sterile straight catheter to collect urine.
4. Insert a sterile needle with syringe through a tubing drainage port cleaned with alcohol to collect the specimen.

19. 4. Wearing clean gloves, cleaning the port with alcohol, and then obtaining the specimen with a sterile needle ensures the specimen and the closed urinary drainage system won't be contaminated. A urine sample must be new urine, and the urine in the bag could be several hours old and growing bacteria. The urinary drainage system must be kept closed to prevent microorganisms from entering. A straight catheter is used to relieve urinary retention, obtain sterile urine specimens, measure the amount of postvoid residual urine, and empty the bladder for certain procedures. It isn't necessary to remove an indwelling catheter to obtain a sterile urine specimen unless the physician requests the whole system be changed.

CN: Safe, effective care environment; CNS: Safety and infection control; CL: Application

20. Which observation indicates to a nurse that a client understands his instructions on crutch walking?

1. The client's axillae rest on the crutches.
2. The client's hands bear the body weight.
3. Crutches are 12″ (30.5 cm) in front of the feet.
4. The client uses long strides when walking.

20. 2. When using crutches, the client should bear weight on his hands. The axillae shouldn't rest on the crutches; there should be 2″ (5 cm) between the crutch and axilla. Crutches should be placed 6″ (15 cm) in front of the feet for stability. A short stride provides maximum safety and mobility.

CN: Physiological integrity; CNS: Basic care and comfort; CL: Application

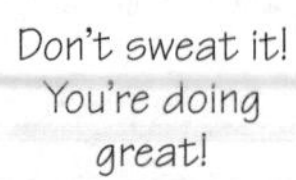
Don't sweat it!
You're doing great!

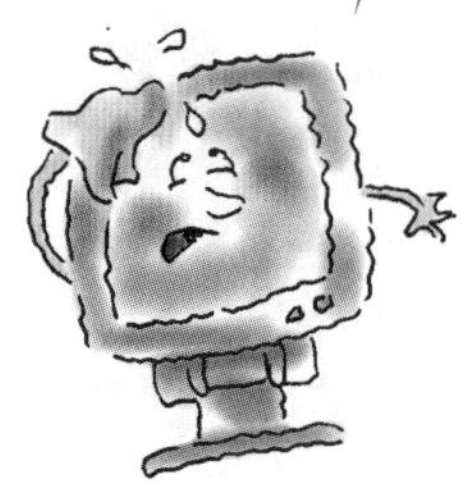

21. A client recovering from a knee replacement has normal saline solution ordered to run at 125 ml/hour I.V. The I.V. bag was hung at 8:00 a.m. It's now 3:00 p.m., and 300 ml have been infused. A nurse has just come on her shift at 3:00 p.m. Which action is correct?

1. Discontinue the I.V. infusion when the bag is complete.
2. Instruct the client to increase his fluid intake.
3. Speed up the rate of the I.V. fluids.
4. Assess the intravenous site.

21. 4. At 125 ml/hour over 7 hours, 875 ml should have been infused. The I.V. fluid is 575 ml behind. The first action would be to make sure the site is not infiltrated before calling the physician for further fluid orders. The physician will determine how the I.V. fluids will be adjusted and will want to know why the client didn't get the prescribed fluids. The order is for I.V. fluids—not oral fluids—and the route change can only be authorized by a physician. Legally, the nurse can't change the rate of I.V. fluids.

CN: Safe, effective care environment; CNS: Management of care; CL: Application

22. A nurse is removing an indwelling urinary catheter from a client. Which action is appropriate?

1. Wear sterile gloves.
2. Cut the lumen of the balloon.
3. Document the time of removal.
4. Position the client on the left side.

22. 3. The client should void within 8 hours of the removal of an indwelling urinary catheter. Documenting the time of removal allows the nurse and physician to verify the duration of elapsed time since removal, thus contributing to continuity of care. Clean, disposable gloves are required because it isn't a sterile procedure. The catheter may retrograde into the bladder, requiring surgical removal, if the balloon is cut from the lumen and the catheter isn't secured. The client should be positioned comfortably on his back, and privacy should be provided.

CN: Safe, effective care environment; CNS: Safety and infection control; CL: Application

23. The nurse obtains a client's stool sample for occult blood. Which of the following diets can cause a false-positive test result?

1. Red meat, horseradish, and turnips
2. Dairy products, canned fruit, and pretzels
3. Cheese, raw fruits, and vegetables
4. Potatoes, orange juice, and decaffeinated coffee

23. 1. Consumption of red meat has caused false-positive readings. The client should also avoid poultry, fish, turnips, and horseradish. Avoid foods that are high in iron. The other foods don't cause false-positive readings.

CN: Physiological integrity; CNS: Basic care and comfort; CL: Application

24. A client complains of excessive flatulence. The nurse teaches the client about foods which, if consumed regularly, may be responsible for flatulence. Which selection of food, if made by the client, would indicate that the teaching has been effective?

1. Cauliflower
2. Ice cream
3. Steak
4. Potatoes

24. 1. Foods that cause flatulence in some people may not produce flatulence in others. It all depends on the amount consumed, but cauliflower is the only food listed that usually results in flatulence.

CN: Physiological integrity; CNS: Basic care and comfort; CL: Application

25. A nurse uses which technique when assisting a client with postoperative coughing and deep-breathing exercises?

1. Splint the incision and cough.
2. Splint the incision, take a deep breath, and then cough.
3. Lie prone, splint the incision, take a deep breath, and then cough.
4. Lie supine, splint the incision, take a deep breath, and then cough.

25. 2. Splinting the incision with a pillow will protect the incision while the client coughs. Taking a deep breath will help open the alveoli, which promotes oxygen exchange and prevents atelectasis. Coughing and deep-breathing exercises are best accomplished in a sitting or semi-sitting position. Expectoration of secretions will be facilitated in a sitting position, as will splinting and taking deep breaths.

CN: Physiological integrity; CNS: Reduction of risk potential; CL: Application

26. Which statement is an appropriate client goal, as written by the nurse?

1. The nurse will perform the client's bath by 3 p.m.
2. The client will bathe with assistance.
3. The nurse will perform the client's bath.
4. The client will bathe with assistance by discharge.

26. 4. All goals should be client focused, allowing the client to understand what needs to be accomplished. Specify a time limit for when this task should be achieved. Be realistic, so the client may be successful in reaching the goal. The goal must be measurable so all staff can evaluate the client's progress. Nurse flexibility is an important attribute and necessary for reassessing needs and approaches for the client's optimal recovery. However, in the actual goal, specific criteria must be identified to allow all staff to work from the same data for achieving client goals.

CN: Safe, effective care environment; CNS: Management of care; CL: Application

27. While helping a cooperative client with a diagnosis of acquired immunodeficiency syndrome with mouth care, the nurse should take which precaution?

1. Wear a mask, gown, and gloves.
2. Wear a gown and gloves.
3. Wear a mask with eye shield and gloves.
4. Wear gloves only.

27. 4. According to standard precautions, the nurse should wear gloves when coming in contact with a client's blood or body fluids. During mouth care with a cooperative client gloves are sufficient to protect the nurse. A mask is worn when airborne droplets of blood or body fluids are anticipated. A gown and mask with eye shield should be worn when splashing of body fluids are expected.

CN: Safe, effective care environment; CNS: Safety and infection control; CL: Application

28. The nurse would perform which action for developmentally-based care?

1. Provide books to a 9-year-old client.
2. Walk a 10-year-old client according to written orders.
3. Provide a pureed diet to a postoperative 13-year-old client.
4. Change a surgical dressing on a 15-year-old client every 4 hours as ordered.

28. 1. Providing books to a 9-year-old client facilitates his reading skills and helps him grow developmentally. Changing a surgical dressing, walking a client, and providing a pureed diet are routine care tasks, which don't necessarily promote further development of the individual.

CN: Health promotion and maintenance; CNS: None; CL: Application

29. A nurse has identified *Ineffective airway clearance* as a nursing diagnosis for a client with pneumonia. Which goal would be appropriate for this client?

1. The client will have clear breath sounds.
2. The client will have a respiratory rate of 32 breaths/minute.
3. The client will be pain-free.
4. The client will have a normal body temperature.

29. 1. Clear breath sounds in a client with pneumonia would indicate the airway is clear. Tachypnea would not indicate clear breath sounds and may occur when the client has difficulty clearing secretions. Being pain-free and having a normal body temperature are appropriate goals for a client with pneumonia but are not an indication that the airway is clear.

CN: Safe, effective care environment; CNS: Management of care; CL: Analysis

You're at question 30 and looking good!

30. A client on complete bed rest complains of excessive flatulence. To best facilitate passage of flatus, the nurse places the client in which position?

1. Fowler's
2. Knee-chest
3. Semi-Fowler's
4. Trendelenburg's

30. 2. Because gas rises, the knee-chest position facilitates the passage of flatus. Semi-Fowler's and Fowler's positions inhibit gas passage. In Trendelenburg's position, the client lies flat with his head lower than his feet.

CN: Physiological integrity; CNS: Basic care and comfort; CL: Application

31. The nurse is assisting with the delivery of a fetus where the mentum is the presenting part. Which graphic illustrates that fetal presentation?

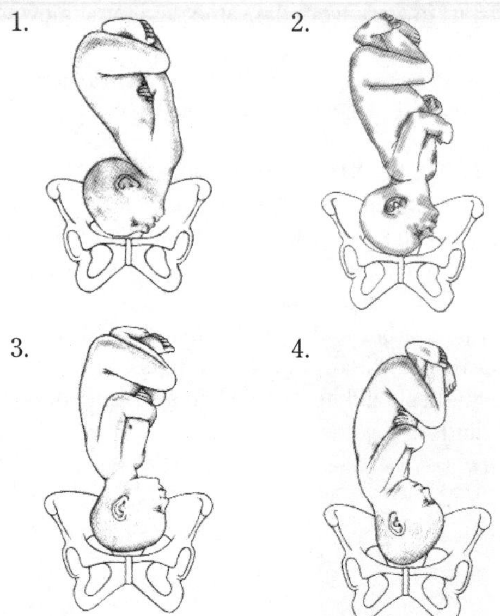

31. 1. In the cephalic, or head-down, presentation, the fetus' position may be classified by the presenting skull landmark: mentum or chin (option 1), brow (option 2), sinciput (option 3), or vertex (option 4).

CN: Health promotion and maintenance; CNS: None; CL: Application

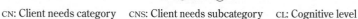

CN: Client needs category CNS: Client needs subcategory CL: Cognitive level

32. In which position should a nurse place a client with pneumonia when performing percussion and postural drainage to the left lower lobe?

1. Supine with the foot of the bed elevated
2. On the left side with the foot of the bed elevated
3. On the left side with the head of the bed elevated
4. Prone with the head of the bed elevated

32. 1. To mobilize secretions from the left lower lobe the client should be positioned supine or on the right side. The foot of the bed should be elevated so that gravity can help mobilize secretions. Placing the client on the left side would put the left lobe in a low or dependent position. Elevating the head of the bed wouldn't use gravity to drain the lower lobes.
CN: Physiological integrity; CNS: Basic care and comfort; CL: Application

33. The client is complaining of moderate pain. Which assessment by the nurse indicates a physiological response to pain?

1. Restlessness
2. Decreased pulse rate
3. Increased blood pressure
4. Protection of the painful area

33. 3. Increased blood pressure is a physiological, or involuntary, response to moderate pain. Restlessness and protection of the painful area are behavioral responses. Decreased pulse rate occurs when pain is severe and deep.
CN: Physiological integrity; CNS: Physiological adaptation; CL: Analysis

34. A client with long-standing rheumatoid arthritis has frequent complaints of joint pain. The nurse's plan of treatment is based on the understanding that chronic pain is most effectively relieved when analgesics are administered in which way?

1. Conservatively
2. I.M.
3. On an as-needed basis
4. At regularly scheduled intervals

34. 4. To control chronic pain and prevent cycled pain, regularly scheduled intervals are most effective. As-needed and conservative methods aren't effective means to manage chronic pain because the pain isn't relieved regularly. I.M. administration isn't practical on a long-term basis.
CN: Physiological integrity; CNS: Pharmacological and parenteral therapies; CL: Application

35. A nurse notes crackles in the lung bases and pedal edema during client assessment. Which factor is a common cause of fluid volume excess?

1. Prolonged fever
2. Hyperventilation
3. Excessive I.V. infusion
4. Fluid volume shifts secondary to vomiting

35. 3. Fluid volume excess can result from excess I.V. fluids, especially in a compromised client. Vomiting, fever, and hyperventilation will result in loss of body fluids, leading to a fluid volume deficit.
CN: Physiological integrity; CNS: Basic care and comfort; CL: Application

36. Which nursing intervention is correct for clients receiving I.V. therapy?

1. Change the tubing every 8 hours.
2. Monitor the flow rate at least every hour.
3. Change the I.V. catheter and entry site daily.
4. Increase the rate to catch up if the correct amount hasn't been infused at the end of the shift.

36. 2. Closely observing the rate of infusion prevents underhydration and overhydration. Tubing is changed according to facility policy but not at the frequency of every 8 hours. The I.V. catheter and entry site should be changed every 48 to 72 hours in most situations. Increasing the rate may lead to fluid overload.
CN: Physiological integrity; CNS: Pharmacological and parenteral therapies; CL: Application

37. A client is given instructions for a low-sodium diet. Which statement best shows the nurse that the client understands the diet instruction?

1. "Meat, fish, and chicken are high in sodium."
2. "I'll miss eating fruits."
3. "I'll enjoy eating at restaurants more often now."
4. "I'll avoid dairy products, potato chips, and carrots."

37. 4. Dairy products, potato chips, carrots, and restaurant food are all high in sodium. Meat, fish, chicken, and fruits aren't.

CN: Physiological integrity; CNS: Basic care and comfort; CL: Application

38. To prevent aspiration in a client with impaired swallowing, the nurse should:

1. provide a straw for drinking liquids.
2. remove dentures before eating.
3. position the client at a 90-degree angle.
4. place food on the paralyzed side of the mouth.

38. 3. When feeding a client with impaired swallowing, the nurse should position the client at a 90-degree angle to reduce the risk of aspiration. Straws shouldn't be used because they increase the risk of aspiration by sending liquids directly to the back of the mouth. Dentures should be well-fitting and in place for eating. If one side of the mouth is paralyzed, food should be placed on the unaffected side.

CN: Physiological integrity; CNS: Basic care and comfort; CL: Application

39. A client must choose a meal that follows his diet orders of a high-calorie, high-protein, low-sodium, and low-potassium diet. Which choice indicates to the nurse that the client understands the dietary guidelines?

1. Halibut, salad, rice, and instant coffee
2. Crab, beets, spinach, and baked potato
3. Salmon, rice, green beans, sourdough bread, coffee, and ice cream
4. Sirloin steak, salad, baked potato with butter, and chocolate ice cream

39. 3. The best choice of these meals is salmon with rice and green beans, which is high in protein, and the sourdough bread and ice cream add calories. Halibut, instant coffee, and potatoes are high in potassium, and beets are high in sodium.

CN: Health promotion and maintenance; CNS: None; CL: Application

40. A client with terminal cancer tells the nurse, "I've given up. I have no hope left. I'm ready to die." Which response is most therapeutic?

1. "You've given up hope?"
2. "We should talk about dying to a social worker."
3. "You should talk to your physician about your fears of dying so soon."
4. "Now, you shouldn't give up hope. There are cures for cancer found every day."

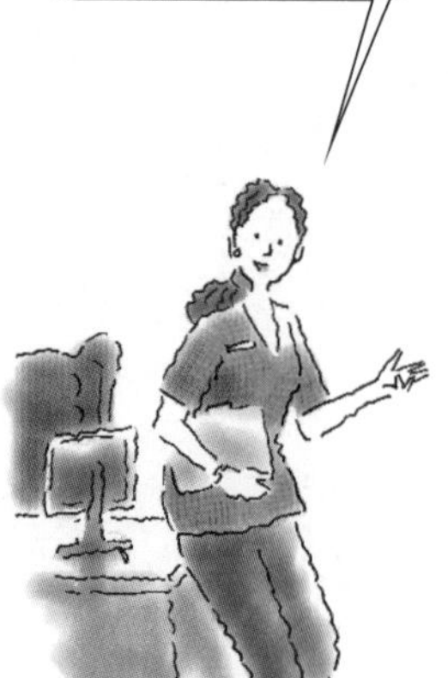

You're more than halfway finished! You're amazing!

40. 1. The use of reflection invites the client to talk more about his concerns. Deferring the conversation to a social worker or physician closes the conversation. Telling the client the cure for cancer is right around the corner gives false hope.

CN: Psychosocial integrity; CNS: None; CL: Analysis

41. Which instruction should a nurse include in the teaching plan for a client with a platelet count of 25,000 mm^3 and petechial rash on the legs, arms, and neck?

1. Take an iron supplement daily.
2. Take acetaminophen rather than aspirin for headache.
3. Stay away from crowds during the flu season.
4. Avoid fresh salads.

41. 2. The client with thrombocytopenia has a low platelet count and should avoid products containing aspirin since they may increase the risk of bleeding. Iron supplements would be helpful in the client with anemia. Staying away from crowds and avoiding fresh salads to reduce the risk of infection would be important for the client with leukopenia.

CN: Physiological integrity; CNS: Reduction of risk potential; CL: Analysis

42. Which laboratory value for a newly diagnosed client with diabetes should the nurse report to the physician?

1. pH, 7.45
2. Sodium, 118 mEq/L
3. Glucose, 120 mg/dl
4. Potassium, 3.9 mEq/L

42. 2. The normal range for sodium is 135 to 145 mEq/L. The rest of the results are within normal limits.

CN: Physiological integrity; CNS: Reduction of risk potential; CL: Analysis

43. A client is 2 days postoperative from a femoral popliteal bypass. The nurse's assessment finds the client's left leg cold and pale. Which action has priority?

1. Check distal pulses.
2. Notify the physician.
3. Elevate the foot of the bed.
4. Wrap the leg in a warm blanket.

43. 1. The client has arterial disease and had vascular surgery. The nurse must assess the client for complications. A potential problem would be a clot at the surgical site, so the nurse must assess circulation by checking for distal pulses. Before the physician is notified, the nurse should determine if distal pulses are present. Elevating the foot of the bed would promote venous return but decrease arterial blood flow and shouldn't be done. The leg can be covered lightly after circulation is assessed.

CN: Physiological integrity; CNS: Physiological adaptation; CL: Application

44. The nurse can administer which mediation through a nasogastric (NG) tube?

1. Enteric coated aspirin
2. Acetaminophen
3. Regular insulin
4. Sublingual nitroglycerine

44. 2. Most oral medications can be given through an NG tube because they're intended for passage into the stomach. Some oral drugs have special coatings intended to keep the pill intact until it passes into the small intestine; these enteric-coated pills shouldn't be crushed and put through an NG tube. Some parenteral medications, such as insulin, may be destroyed by gastric juices. Sublingual means under the tongue and parenteral means I.V., I.M., and subcutaneous.

CN: Physiological integrity; CNS: Pharmacological and parenteral therapies; CL: Application

45. The nurse knows if a client requires oxygen delivery at a FiO_2 of 92%, the appropriate system would be:
1. Face tent
2. Venturi mask
3. Nasal cannula
4. Mask with reservoir bag

45. 4. A mask with a reservoir bag administers 70% to 100% oxygen at flow rates of 8 to 10 L/minute. A face tent maximum delivery is 22% to 34%, the Venturi mask maximum rate is 24% to 55%, and the nasal cannula maximum rate is 44% at 6 L/minute.

CN: Physiological integrity; CNS: Pharmacological and parenteral therapies; CL: Analysis

46. The client has returned from the operating room with the nursing diagnosis of *Acute pain*. The nurse knows that the best means of providing comfort would be to administer:
1. morphine sulfate 10 mg intramuscularly (IM).
2. morphine sulfate 0.2 mg/ml via patient controlled analgesia (PCA).
3. Dilaudid 2 mg intravenously (IV) every 2 hours.
4. Percocet 5 mg orally (PO) every 4–6 hours.

46. 2. Clients who have ready access to an analgesic are more likely to medicate themselves before the pain becomes severe and thus may require reduced amounts of medication. Having control over drug administration also reduces anxiety, which helps to relieve pain.

CN: Physiological integrity; CNS: Pharmacological and parenteral therapies; CL: Application

47. A client with difficulty breathing has a respiratory rate of 34 breaths/minute and seems very anxious. He's refusing all his medications, claiming they're making him worse. Which nursing action is best?
1. Notify the physician of the status of this client.
2. Withhold the medication until the next scheduled dose.
3. Encourage the client to take some of his medications.
4. Put the medicine in applesauce to give it without the client's knowledge.

47. 1. Notifying the physician of the client's condition and his refusal to take his medications allows the physician to decide what alternatives should be instituted. Withholding a medication requires the physician to be notified. Even if the client takes some of the medications, the physician will still need to be notified. It needs to be explored why the client believes the medications are making him worse. Giving medications in applesauce destroys trust between the nurse and client.

CN: Physiological integrity; CNS: Pharmacological and parenteral therapies; CL: Application

48. Which statement is an example of a key element in the nursing care plan?
1. Advance diet to regular as tolerated.
2. Ambulate 30′ (9 m) with walker by discharge.
3. Give furosemide (Lasix) 40 mg I.V. now.
4. Discontinue I.V. fluids when tolerating oral fluids.

48. 2. Ambulating 30′ with a walker by discharge is a measurable expected outcome or goal, a key element of a nursing care plan. Other key elements include nursing diagnoses and interventions. The other options are physician's orders, not key elements of care plans.

CN: Safe, effective care environment; CNS: Management of care; CL: Application

49. A client who was recently hospitalized has a nursing diagnosis of *Constipation related to medical regime*. Which medication may contribute to this problem?
1. Folic acid
2. Iron
3. Potassium
4. Vitamin E

49. 2. Iron may cause constipation when supplements are taken at 100% of the RDA. Folic acid, potassium, and vitamin E don't increase the likelihood of constipation.
CN: Physiological integrity; CNS: Pharmacological and parenteral therapies; CL: Application

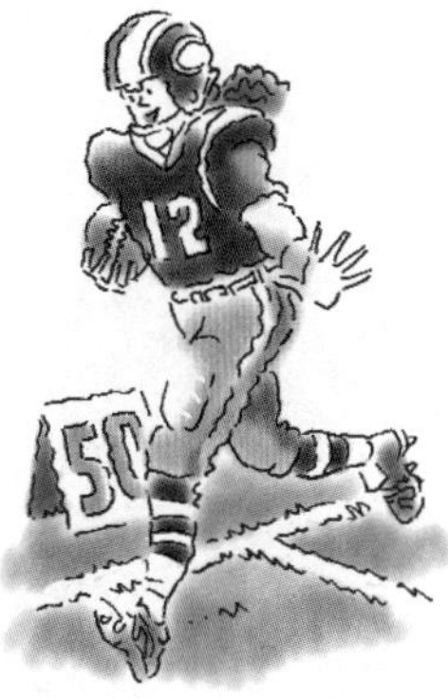

30, 40, 50 down... and only 25 more to go!
12
50

50. A client had an appendectomy 24 hours ago. Which nursing goal is appropriate for this client?
1. The client will be able to walk in the hallway.
2. The client will be able to attend physical therapy.
3. The client will be able to accomplish all activities of daily living.
4. The client will be able to state the rationale for all postoperative medications.

50. 1. A 24-hour postoperative client is expected to be able to walk in the hallway. A client who just had an appendectomy shouldn't need physical therapy unless deconditioning was evident. At 24 hours, a client should begin to assume responsibility for activities of daily living, but shouldn't necessarily be responsible for all activities. It's too early to expect a client to state the rationale for all postoperative medications, especially if the client is elderly.
CN: Physiological integrity; CNS: Basic care and comfort; CL: Application

51. Which nursing discharge instruction has the highest priority for a client going home with a full leg cast?
1. Activity restrictions
2. Proper nutrition
3. Weight-bearing limitations
4. Reporting signs of impaired circulation

51. 4. The nurse should include all these instructions in the teaching plan; however, the highest priority is teaching the signs of impaired circulation to prevent permanent neurovascular damage, including loss of the leg.
CN: Physiological integrity; CNS: Reduction of risk potential; CL: Analysis

52. During an initial nursing assessment, a nurse uses open-ended questions to gather data. Which statement would the nurse make, or which question would the nurse ask?
1. "Tell me how things have been going for you."
2. "Have you been feeling good?"
3. "Tell me what you mean when you say you've been feeling funny."
4. "I'd like to ask you more about your chest pain."

52. 1. "Tell me how things have been going for you" is an open-ended question that encourages the client to speak and express concerns. Asking the client if he feels good is a closed-ended question that only requires a "yes" or "no" response. The third option is seeking clarification of a statement made by the client. The fourth option is a focused question designed to help the nurse collect information on a specific health concern.
CN: Psychosocial integrity; CNS: None; CL: Application

53. A registered nurse (RN) is supervising an unlicensed care provider. Which principle would the nurse follow when delegating tasks?

1. The RN must directly supervise all delegated tasks.
2. After a task is delegated, it's no longer the RN's responsibility.
3. The RN is responsible for delegating tasks to adjunct personnel.
4. Follow-up with a delegated task is necessary only if the assistive personnel are untrustworthy.

53. 3. The RN must delegate tasks that are within the scope of practice of the unlicensed personnel. The RN need not directly supervise all delegated tasks as that would negate the benefits of delegation. Even when the task is delegated, the RN retains responsibility for the successful completion of the task. The RN must always follow up with the assistive personnel to ensure the task was completed appropriately, not only in instances of mistrust.

CN: Safe, effective care environment; CNS: Management of care; CL: Application

54. An elderly client had recent surgery and is on bed rest. When planning care for the client, which nursing intervention is included in the care plan?

1. Daily assessment of the wound site
2. Foot and ankle range-of-motion (ROM) exercises
3. Wound cleaning with hydrogen peroxide
4. Coughing and deep breathing in the prone position

54. 2. Foot and ankle ROM exercises are standard protocol for clients who remain in bed for an extended period of time. ROM exercises promote blood flow to the area, prevent atrophy, and lessen the potential for edema. The wound site should be assessed every shift. Wound cleaning with hydrogen peroxide isn't generally recommended. Coughing and deep breathing aren't generally recommended in the prone position.

CN: Physiological integrity; CNS: Reduction of risk potential; CL: Application

55. A client receiving phenothiazine has become restless and fidgety and has been pacing the hallway continuously for the past hour. This behavior suggests to the nurse that the client may be experiencing which adverse reaction to phenothiazine?

1. Dystonia
2. Akathisia
3. Parkinsonian effects
4. Tardive dyskinesia

55. 2. The client's behavior suggests akathisia—an adverse effect of phenothiazines. Dystonia appears as excessive salivation, difficulty speaking, and involuntary movements of the face, neck, arms and legs. Parkinsonian effects include a shuffling gait, hand tremors, drooling, rigidity, and loose arm movements. Tardive dyskinesia is characterized by odd facial and tongue movements.

CN: Physiological integrity; CNS: Reduction of risk potential; CL: Application

56. A client who had his gallbladder removed 2 days ago now complains of pain in the right calf. Which nursing response has priority?

1. Assess the leg for swelling and redness.
2. Instruct the client to flex his knee and hip.
3. Apply a warm compress and call the physician.
4. Gently massage the calf and notify the physician.

56. 1. Pain in the calf is a symptom of possible deep vein thrombosis. The nurse must assess further. Assessing the client for redness and swelling would be the next intervention. Making the client flex his knee and hip won't help assess for the presence of a clot. Warm compresses may be ordered after a diagnosis of deep vein thrombosis is made. Never massage the calf muscle because the clot could be dislodged.

CN: Physiological integrity; CNS: Reduction of risk potential; CL: Analysis

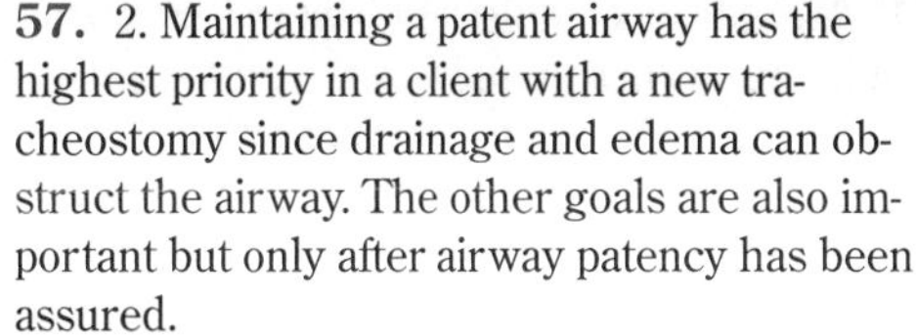

57. Which goal will the nurse make the highest priority in a client with a new tracheostomy?

1. Developing an effective means of communication
2. Maintaining a patent airway
3. Preventing infection
4. Gaining independence in self-care

57. 2. Maintaining a patent airway has the highest priority in a client with a new tracheostomy since drainage and edema can obstruct the airway. The other goals are also important but only after airway patency has been assured.

CN: Physiological integrity; CNS: Reduction of risk potential; CL: Analysis

58. Which statement by a client with chronic arterial disease indicates to the nurse further teaching is needed?

1. "I'm going to stop smoking."
2. "I'm going to have the podiatrist check my feet."
3. "I'm going to keep the heat in my house at 80° F."
4. "I'm going to walk short distances every morning."

58. 3. Clients with peripheral vascular disease need to be at a comfortable temperature because of impaired circulation. Having the heat at 80° F is too warm. The other choices are all appropriate interventions for a client with peripheral vascular disease.

CN: Physiological integrity; CNS: Reduction of risk potential; CL: Application

59. A registered nurse is in charge of eight clients. The nurse has a licensed practical nurse (LPN) and a client care assistant working under her. Which activity should the nurse assign to herself rather than delegate to the staff?

1. Consoling a grieving visitor
2. Assessing a newly admitted client
3. Irrigating a Salem sump to continuous drainage
4. Giving a tap water enema to a preoperative client

59. 2. Assessment of a new admission can't be delegated to an LPN. Consoling a visitor and giving a tap water enema are within the scope of practice of an LPN and client care assistant. Irrigation of a Salem sump is under the scope of practice of an LPN.

CN: Safe, effective care environment; CNS: Management of care; CL: Application

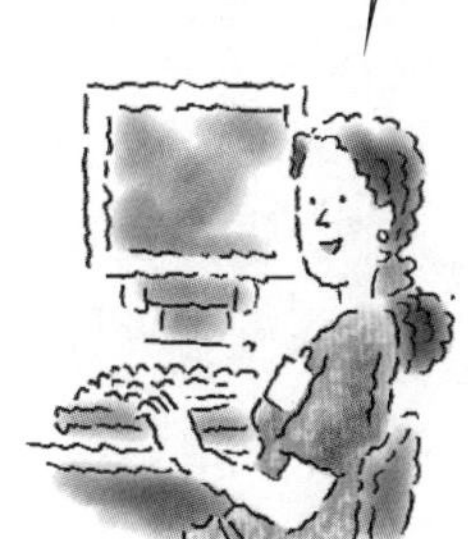
You're almost there! Keep going!

60. A 6-year-old client needs diabetic teaching. Which factor is considered when the nurse plans the teaching?

1. Another child with diabetes can teach the client.
2. The child can teach his parents after the nurse teaches him.
3. The child and parents should be recipients of teaching.
4. Teaching should be directed to the parents, who then can teach the child.

60. 3. The parents and child should participate in the nurse's teaching to ensure accuracy of teaching and that the child has educated adult caregivers. The school-aged child shouldn't be the sole provider of teaching to the parents. Another school-aged child couldn't be entrusted to teach this child, although their input would be valuable. Parents should be included in the teaching plan but shouldn't be responsible for the teaching.

CN: Health promotion and maintenance; CNS: None; CL: Application

61. Parents of a toddler are having problems putting him to bed at night. Which recommendation by a nurse is most appropriate?

1. Stop the afternoon naps.
2. Allow the toddler to have a tantrum for ½ hour.
3. Encourage the parents to develop nighttime rituals.
4. Allow the toddler to have some control over bedtime.

61. 3. Rituals are extremely important for toddlers to feel secure and relaxed. Allowing a toddler to make small decisions, such as choosing the order of the ritual and color of pajamas, will give him the feeling of some control. Stopping the naps may be helpful, depending on the toddler's needs. The toddler must clearly understand that tantrums won't get him what he wants.

CN: Health promotion and maintenance; CNS: None; CL: Application

62. After abdominal surgery for repair of an aortic aneurysm, a client may show maladaptive coping behavior in response to body changes related to the surgery. Which nursing intervention is best?

1. Let the client express his feelings.
2. Explain that a psychological referral would be beneficial.
3. Instruct the client on how to use positive coping strategies.
4. Encourage the client to participate in diversionary activities.

62. 1. Allowing verbalization of feelings is the most therapeutic nursing intervention. Making a referral may help, but initially the client should be allowed to express his feelings. Giving advice may stop therapeutic communication. Providing diversionary activities doesn't foster effective coping.

CN: Psychosocial integrity; CNS: None; CL: Analysis

63. A new nurse graduate has started at the medical center and is assigned to a preceptor. The preceptor and other staff report that the nurse is uncooperative and unwilling to take direction. Which action by the preceptor is appropriate?

1. Explain the behavior won't be tolerated.
2. Ask the nurse why she wants to work here.
3. Reestablish goals with the nurse.
4. Begin the disciplinary process with this nurse.

63. 3. This is a new graduate in orientation and the preceptor should help this nurse learn the responsibilities and routines and reestablish goals. If the behavior continues, the nurse may need career counseling. This person isn't experienced and therefore shouldn't be reprimanded. Asking the nurse "why" in relation to working is inappropriate; it's the behavior that's creating the problem. This nurse shouldn't be disciplined as an initial step.

CN: Safe, effective care environment; CNS: Management of care; CL: Application

64. A client with a history of bipolar disorder rushes into the mental health clinic waiting room scantily dressed and makes loud, obscene remarks to other clients. Which response by the nurse has priority?

1. Encourage the other clients to ignore the behavior.
2. Confront the behavior and make the client take a seat.
3. Tell the client to sit down and stop upsetting the others.
4. Quietly escort the client to a private area and help put on a gown.

64. 4. The client with bipolar disorder is highly excitable. The nurse needs to be firm yet distracting, and this is best done in a private area, which also preserves the client's dignity. Having the others ignore the client won't alter the problem. Confronting the behavior isn't desired as this client lacks judgment and insight. Telling the client to sit down may cause the client to be more resistive and even heighten the behavior.

CN: Psychosocial integrity; CNS: None; CL: Analysis

65. A nurse is reviewing treatment of hypercyanotic spells (tet spells) with the parents of a 4-month-old client being discharged from the hospital. Which discharge instruction is correct?

1. "Calm the baby down by holding her and placing her knees up to her chest."
2. "Call 911 immediately and begin cardiopulmonary resuscitation (CPR) on the baby."
3. "You'll need to administer four back blows to the baby if she begins having a tet spell."
4. "You don't need to worry about these spells yet because the baby is too young. You'll need to watch for them when she becomes more mobile."

65. 1. Tet spells are acute episodes of cyanosis and hypoxia that occur when the infant's oxygen demand exceeds the available supply. They may occur when the infant is crying or eating. Tet spells are emergency situations that require immediate intervention. Begin by calming the infant down and placing the infant in the knee-chest position, which increases systemic vascular resistance by limiting venous return. This decreases the right to left shunting and improves oxygenation. CPR won't calm the infant down or improve oxygenation. Back blows are given to infants who have something lodged in their trachea.

CN: Physiological integrity; CNS: Reduction of risk potential; CL: Application

66. Which nursing intervention should a nurse use when caring for a client with gout?

1. Administer antibiotic.
2. Restrict fluid intake.
3. Encourage a low-purine diet.
4. Administer opioids.

66. 3. A low-purine diet decreases uric acid formation and should be encouraged. Antibiotics aren't used to treat gout. Fluid intake should be encouraged to flush out the uric acid. Anti-inflammatory medications are used during acute phases, but because this is a long-term condition, opioids aren't generally given.

CN: Physiological integrity; CNS: Reduction of risk potential; CL: Application

67. The nurse is evaluating a client who is 2 days post crush injury to his right leg. Which symptom is a late indicator of compartment syndrome?

1. Sudden decrease in pain
2. Swelling in toes or fingers
3. Inability to move fingers or toes
4. Diminished distal pulses

67. 4. Compartment syndrome is a complication of a cast that places pressure on the blood vessels and nerves to the extremity. Symptoms include pain not relieved by analgesics and swelling of the extremity. A late symptom is a change in skin color with diminished distal pulses. After a fracture, some swelling and pain result, but pulses need to be monitored, as well as color, sensation, and movement.

CN: Physiological integrity; CNS: Reduction of risk potential; CL: Analysis

68. A client with an arm cast complains of severe pain in the affected extremity and decreased sensation and motion are noted. Swelling in the fingers is also increased. Which nursing intervention has priority?

1. Elevate the arm.
2. Remove the cast.
3. Give an analgesic.
4. Call the physician.

68. 4. The cast may be too tight and may need to be split or removed by the physician. The arm should already be elevated. Notify the physician when circulation, sensation, or motion is impaired. Giving analgesics wouldn't be the first step as they may mask the signs of a serious problem.

CN: Physiological integrity; CNS: Reduction of risk potential; CL: Application

69. The nurse is performing preoperative teaching on a 4-year-old scheduled for cardiac catheterization. Which characteristic is correct for preoperative teaching?

1. Basic and performed close to the implementation of the procedure
2. Done several days before the procedure so the child will have time to prepare
3. Detailed in regard to the actual procedure so the child will know exactly what to expect
4. Directed at the child's parents because the child is too young to understand the procedure

69. 1. Four-year-old children are in Piaget's cognitive stage of preoperational thought. Their thinking is concrete and tangible, and they're unable to make deductions or generalizations and are egocentric. They don't have a concept for the future so explanations need to be done close to the time of the procedure, not days in advance. They need simple explanations of procedures in relationship to how the procedure will affect them. A 4-year-old child is old enough to understand basic teaching close to the implementation of the procedure.

CN: Health promotion and maintenance; CNS: None; CL: Application

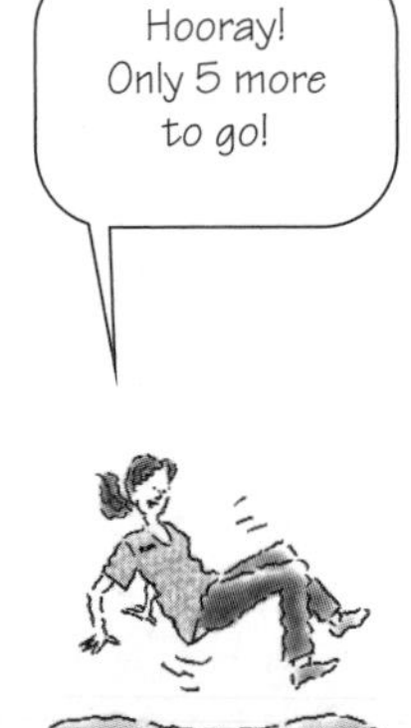

70. A registered nurse is directing unlicensed personnel to draw the morning blood work for a 4-year-old child in the hospital. The nurse emphasizes the procedure is to be done in the treatment room. Which rationale is correct?

1. The procedure will be faster.
2. The child won't fear painful procedures done while he's in his bed.
3. The child can only be restrained on the examination table.
4. The parents won't observe the procedure and upset the child.

70. 2. This implementation is based on the concept of "atraumatic care" and growth and development principles. Small children need to have a safe zone in their beds to relax and rest in their rooms. The treatment room is used instead. It won't be faster to draw blood in the treatment room; it would take the same amount of time regardless of where it's done. The child could be restrained in his room, but it isn't appropriate. Parental support is important and needs to be encouraged during stressful and painful procedures.

CN: Psychosocial integrity; CNS: None; CL: Application

71. A client tells a nurse, "My medical illness is the result of something bad I did to someone in the past." Which response by the nurse is the most appropriate?

1. "What did you do wrong?"
2. "Let's talk about your concerns."
3. "That's silly! Don't believe that!"
4. "You're suffering from a psychiatric delusion. Relax, it will end soon."

71. 2. Asking the client to talk about his concerns allows an opportunity for the nurse to clarify issues. Calling the client silly or asking the client what he did wrong would likely escalate the client's concerns. Telling the client it will end soon gives false reassurance.

CN: Psychosocial integrity; CNS: None; CL: Application

72. A client on a psychiatric unit asks a nurse about the medications another client takes. Which response is best?

1. "How close are the two of you?"
2. "I can't give you that information, I must protect her privacy."
3. "Let me ask her if it's OK for me to tell you about her condition and medications."
4. "The client is taking insulin for her diabetes and digoxin for her heart condition."

72. 2. Revealing one client's medication to another client is violating procedures of client confidentiality. Asking the client the nature of his relationship to the other client won't help the client understand the purpose of protecting confidentiality. Seeking the client's permission to release confidential information is an inappropriate action. Assuring the client that the hospital has an obligation to protect not only his confidentiality but that of others will provide the client with a sense of comfort.

CN: Safe, effective care environment; CNS: Management of care; CL: Application

73. A client's goal is to interact verbally at least once in each group therapy session by a certain date. The client attended the group session, maintained eye contact with the group members, followed the conversation nonverbally as indicated by head nodding, and spoke once to the group leader by giving a one-word answer. Which judgment by a nurse about goal attainment is correct?

1. The goal was partially met.
2. The goal was completely met.
3. The goal was completely unmet.
4. New problems or nursing diagnoses have developed.

73. 1. This goal was partially met because the client must verbally participate more in the group. For a goal to be completely met, the client must show the subjective and objective data indicating the goal has been clearly attained. A completely unmet goal indicates the client's complete lack of behavior change and absence of subjective and objective data to indicate the achievement of the goal. In this case, no new problems or new nursing diagnoses were evident.

CN: Psychosocial integrity; CNS: None; CL: Analysis

74. A client is prescribed heparin 6,000 units subcutaneously every 12 hours for deep vein thrombosis prophylaxis. The pharmacy dispenses a vial containing 10,000 units/ml. How many milliliters of heparin should a nurse administer? Record your answer using one decimal place.

______________________________ milliliters

74. 0.6. The following formula is used to calculate drug dosages: Dose on hand/Quantity on hand = Dose desired/X. The dose dispensed by the pharmacy is 10,000 units/1 ml and the desired dose is 6,000 units. The nurse should use the following equations: 10,000 units/1 ml = 6,000 units/X; 10,000 units (X) = 6,000 units (ml)/10,000 units; X = 0.6 ml.

CN: Physiological integrity; CNS: Pharmacological and parenteral therapies; CL: Analysis

75. A client is prescribed lisinopril (Zestril) for treatment of hypertension. He asks the nurse about possible adverse effects. The nurse should teach him about which common adverse effects of angiotensin converting enzyme (ACE) inhibitors? Select all that apply:

1. Constipation
2. Dizziness
3. Headache
4. Hyperglycemia
5. Hypotension
6. Impotence

75. 2, 3, 5. Dizziness, headache, and hypotension are all common adverse effects of lisinopril and other ACE inhibitors. Lisinopril may cause diarrhea, not constipation. It isn't known to cause hyperglycemia or impotence.

CN: Physiological integrity; CNS: Pharmacological and parenteral therapies; CL: Application

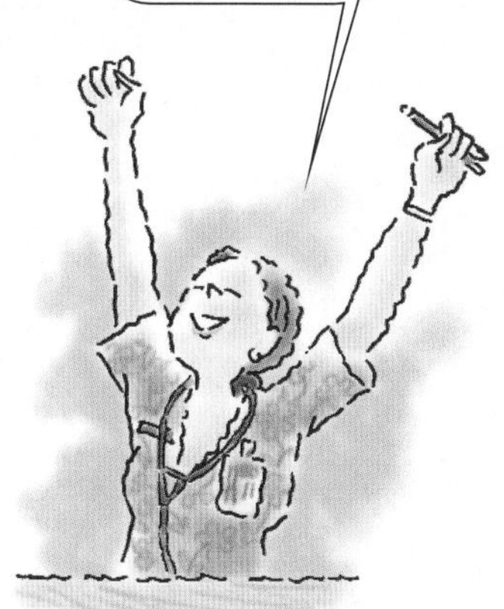

You're terrific! I knew you could do it! Only one more test to take. Go for it!

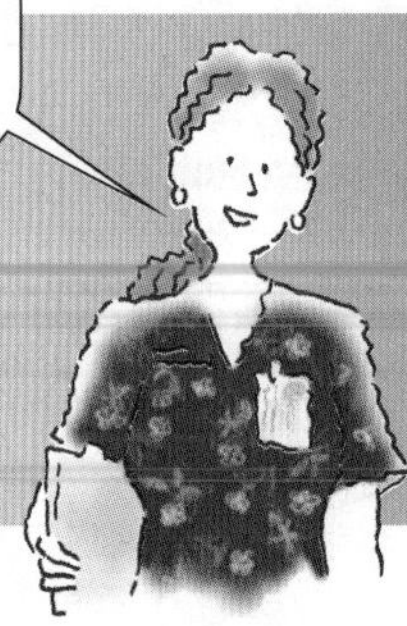

This is the LAST
comprehensive test.
Good luck! I know you're
ready for it.

COMPREHENSIVE Test 6

1. The nurse is teaching clients about hypertension and the importance of risk factors. Which client response identifying a nonmodifiable risk factor indicates that the teaching has been effective?

1. High sodium intake
2. Sedentary lifestyle
3. Tobacco use
4. Family history

1. 4. Family history is a risk factor for hypertension that can't be modified. Risk factors that can be modified include high-sodium intake, sedentary lifestyle, and tobacco use.
CN: Health promotion and maintenance; CNS: None; CL: Application

2. A client experienced an acute inferior myocardial infarction at a community hospital. After antithrombolytic therapy fails, the physician wants to transfer the client to another hospital for emergency cardiac catheterization. Which member of the health care team must accompany the client?

1. Physician
2. Paramedic
3. Registered nurse (RN)
4. Licensed practical nurse (LPN)

2. 3. During transfer, the client must receive the same level of care that he received in the hospital; therefore, an RN must accompany him. It isn't necessary for a physician to accompany the client. A paramedic, although not required, will most likely accompany the nurse. An LPN is below the standard of care for this situation.
CN: Safe, effective care environment; CNS: Management of care; CL: Application

3. A 56-year-old client with heart failure is allergic to sulfa-based medications. Which type of diuretic should be used cautiously?

1. Osmotic diuretics
2. Thiazide and thiazide-like diuretics
3. Potassium-sparing diuretics
4. Carbonic anhydrase inhibitors

3. 2. Thiazide and thiazide-like diuretics are sulfonamide derivatives, so their use should be used cautiously in clients allergic to sulfa-based medications. Osmotic, potassium-sparing, and carbonic anhydrase inhibitor diuretics can be safely administered to these clients.
CN: Physiological integrity; CNS: Pharmacological and parenteral therapies; CL: Application

4. A client with heart failure says he sleeps with two pillows because he experiences difficulty breathing when lying flat. The nurse documents which type of breathing?

1. Bradypnea
2. Dyspnea on exertion
3. Paroxysmal nocturnal dyspnea
4. Orthopnea

4. 4. A client with orthopnea has shortness of breath when lying flat, so he prefers sleeping with the upper body elevated. Bradypnea is decreased but regular breathing. Dyspnea on exertion occurs when the client has difficulty breathing with activity. Paroxysmal nocturnal dyspnea occurs when the client awakens at night and feels short of breath.
CN: Health promotion and maintenance; CNS: None; CL: Application

5. During an initial assessment of a neonate, the nurse notes a respiratory rate of 62 breaths/minute. How should the nurse intervene?

1. Notify the physician immediately.
2. Do nothing; this is a normal respiratory rate for a neonate.
3. Position the isolette so the neonate's head is elevated.
4. Prepare for emergency endotracheal (ET) intubation.

5. 2. A normal respiratory rate for a neonate is 30 to 80 breaths/minute, so notifying the physician or elevating the neonate's head isn't necessary. The nurse should prepare for ET intubation if the neonate has signs of imminent respiratory distress such as an expiratory grunt.

CN: Health promotion and maintenance; CNS: None; CL: Analysis

6. During a neonate's 1-month checkup, the pediatrician flexes the neonate's legs to right angles at the hips and knees, and abducts both hips until the knees touch the table. Which statement describes the purpose of this test?

1. To check the neonate's flexibility
2. To assess leg strength
3. To check for developmental dysplasia of the hip
4. To examine the neonate for a hydrocele

6. 3. This test assesses for developmental dysplasia of the hip. If dysplasia is present, the physician can see, feel, and sometimes hear a click. Although a neonate's flexibility and leg strength may be assessed at age 1 month, the examination techniques differ from those described here. To identify a hydrocele, the physician palpates the neonate's testes.

CN: Physiological integrity; CNS: Physiological adaptation; CL: Analysis

7. At which age should a nurse initially screen for idiopathic juvenile scoliosis?

1. 7 years
2. 10 years
3. 13 years
4. 16 years

7. 2. Children should have initial screening at age 10—immediately before the adolescent growth spurt—when promontory signs of scoliosis may become apparent. By age 13, a child may have significantly developed scoliosis that requires surgery.

CN: Health promotion and maintenance; CNS: None; CL: Application

8. Which position is correct for scoliosis screening of a 10-year-old client?

1. Facing away from the examiner, standing upright with his arms held out straight in front of his body
2. Facing away from the examiner, bending forward in 50% flexion with his arms and head dangling
3. Facing the examiner, standing upright with his arms held straight at his sides
4. Sitting in a chair with feet flat on the floor and his back at a 90-degree angle

8. 2. Assessing a client's back for asymmetry, or a "razorback" hump, is best done with the client bending at the waist in 50% flexion with the arms and head dangling. This assessment can also be done with the arms hanging dependently at the sides so the examiner can check for asymmetry at the shoulders, waist folds, and space between the arms and waist.

CN: Health promotion and maintenance; CNS: None; CL: Application

9. Parents bring their infant to the clinic for a checkup after he was hospitalized with a new onset of type 1 diabetes mellitus. Which statement to the nurse indicates an understanding of their child's current situation?

1. "The physician was wrong about the diagnosis because all of my child's fingersticks have been normal."
2. "My child has experienced a honeymoon period, which could last 1 month to 1 year, and hasn't required any insulin injections."
3. "Nobody in our family has diabetes, so how can my child have it?"
4. "If our child lives a careful, sedentary lifestyle, she won't need as much insulin."

9. 2. A honeymoon phase—in which injected insulin seems to wake up the islet cells and cause them to secrete insulin—is common with type 1 diabetes mellitus. This phase has given many parents false hope that their child has been cured. Type 1 diabetes isn't a genetic trait, and a sedentary lifestyle will increase the secondary effects of diabetes.

CN: Physiological integrity; CNS: Physiological adaptation; CL: Analysis

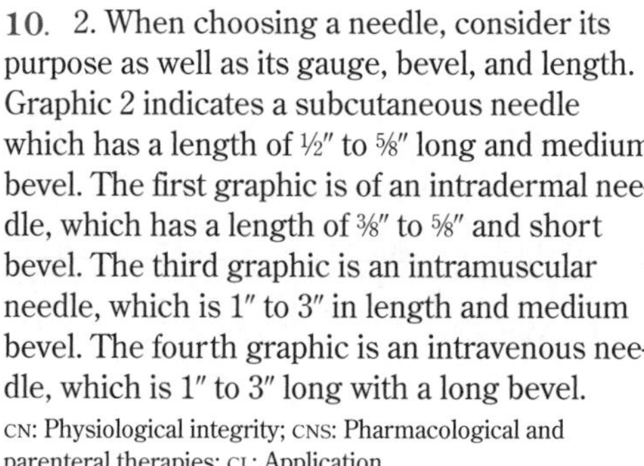
You've finished 10 questions! Cool!

10. The nurse is preparing to administer an injection subcutaneously. Which graphic indicates the appropriate needle selection for this type of injection?

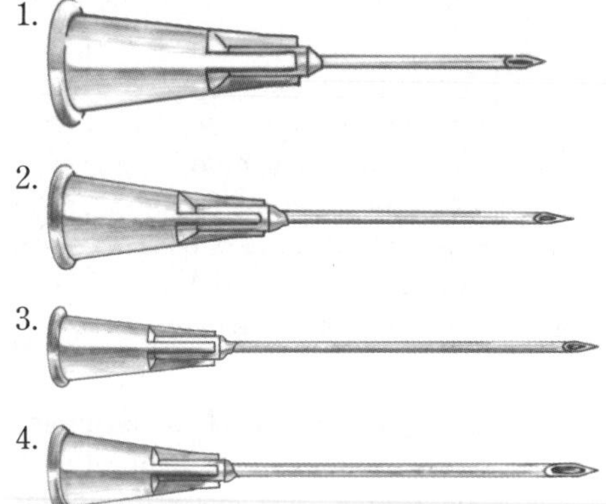
1.
2.
3.
4.

10. 2. When choosing a needle, consider its purpose as well as its gauge, bevel, and length. Graphic 2 indicates a subcutaneous needle which has a length of ½″ to ⅝″ long and medium bevel. The first graphic is of an intradermal needle, which has a length of ⅜″ to ⅝″ and short bevel. The third graphic is an intramuscular needle, which is 1″ to 3″ in length and medium bevel. The fourth graphic is an intravenous needle, which is 1″ to 3″ long with a long bevel.

CN: Physiological integrity; CNS: Pharmacological and parenteral therapies; CL: Application

11. Which intervention should a nurse include in the care plan for a 2-year-old child with Wilms' tumor?

1. Tell the parents that surgery will be within 24 to 48 hours.
2. Palpate the abdomen to monitor tumor size.
3. Massage the abdomen to relieve pain.
4. Place a tight binder around the abdomen for support.

11. 1. The nurse tells the parents that the child will be scheduled for a nephrectomy within 24 to 48 hours because these tumors metastasize quickly. To reduce the risk of dissemination of cancer cells, the abdomen shouldn't be palpated or massaged. A tight binder may put pressure on the tumor, increasing the risk of dissemination and should, therefore, be avoided.

CN: Safe, effective care environment; CNS: Management of care; CL: Application

12. Two days after undergoing a left thoracotomy, a client's temperature reaches 102° F (38.9° C). The nurse notifies the physician who orders two sets of blood cultures. Which amount of blood would the nurse obtain for cultures?

1. 2 ml
2. 5 ml
3. 10 ml
4. 20 ml

12. 3. When an adult client requires blood cultures, the nurse should draw 10 ml of blood; 5 ml should be injected into an anaerobic (without oxygen) bottle and 5 ml injected into an aerobic (with oxygen) bottle.

CN: Physiological integrity; CNS: Reduction of risk potential; CL: Application

13. A charge nurse is developing the client-care assignments for the shift. Which client is most appropriately assigned to a licensed practical nurse (LPN)?

1. A newly admitted client with stroke and do-not-resuscitate (DNR) status
2. A client who underwent cerebral arteriography 1 hour ago
3. A client who underwent carotid endarterectomy 4 hours ago
4. A client who underwent craniotomy 3 days ago and has just been transferred from the intensive care unit (ICU)

13. 1. The most appropriate client to assign to the LPN is the newly admitted client with DNR status; typically, a newly admitted client is assigned to a registered nurse (RN) because the client requires frequent assessments. The client who recently underwent cerebral arteriography and the client who recently underwent carotid endarterectomy require frequent assessments by an RN. The client just transferred from the ICU has the potential for becoming unstable; therefore, an RN should care for this client.

CN: Safe, effective care environment; CNS: Management of care; CL: Analysis

14. A physician prescribes carbamazepine (Tegretol) 1,200 mg P.O. b.i.d. for a client with trigeminal neuralgia. Which action should the nurse take first?

1. Administer the medication with meals.
2. Encourage the client to promptly report unusual bleeding, bruising, fever, or chills.
3. Question the order because the dose exceeds the recommended daily dose.
4. Store the drug in a cool, dry place.

14. 3. The first intervention by the nurse should be to question the order because it exceeds the recommended daily dose. Clients with trigeminal neuralgia should receive no more than 1,200 mg/day. After the nurse obtains an appropriate order, she should encourage the client to take the drug at equally spaced intervals with food to avoid GI distress. The nurse should also encourage the client to promptly report unusual bleeding, bruising, jaundice, dark urine, pale stools, abdominal pain, impotence, fever, chills, sore throat, mouth ulcers, edema, or disturbances in mood, alertness, or coordination. The drug should be stored in a cool, dry place.

CN: Physiological integrity; CNS: Pharmacological and parenteral therapies; CL: Analysis

15. Emergency medical system personnel have used the Cincinnati prehospital stroke scale to assess a client and have alerted the hospital that they're transporting a client with a possible stroke. The nurse plans to administer fibrinolytics within which time period?

1. 4 hours of the onset of symptoms
2. 60 minutes of arrival in the emergency department (ED)
3. 2 hours of arrival in the ED
4. 25 minutes of arrival in the ED

15. 2. The goal for initiating fibrinolytic therapy is within 60 minutes of arrival in the ED. Fibrinolytics must be administered within 3 hours of the onset of symptoms.

CN: Physiological integrity; CNS: Pharmacological and parenteral therapies; CL: Application

16. A client with an above-the-knee amputation visits the orthopedic surgeon for a follow-up. Which comment to the nurse would indicate the client is properly caring for the stump and prosthetic leg?

1. "I inspect the stump weekly to look for signs of redness, blistering, or abrasions."
2. "I put my prosthesis on before I get out of bed."
3. "I wash the stump every day with an antiseptic soap."
4. "I wipe out the socket of my prosthesis with a damp, soapy cloth weekly."

16. 2. The prosthesis should be applied upon rising in the morning. The stump and prosthesis should be inspected daily and cleaned daily with a mild soap. The prosthesis should be kept clean to prevent irritation or pressure areas from dirt or bacteria.

CN: Health promotion and maintenance; CNS: None; CL: Analysis

17. A nurse is caring for a client after a total knee replacement. The extremity was placed in a continuous passive motion (CPM) machine. Which action is one of the nurse's responsibilities?

1. Check the cycle and range-of-motion settings every morning.
2. Increase the degrees of flexion daily guided by client level of tolerance.
3. Decrease the degree of extension daily.
4. Turn the machine off when the client is eating a meal.

17. 4. The CPM machine can be turned off during meals to improve client comfort. The cycle and degrees of flexion should be checked every shift, and either the physician or physical therapist determines how and when the degrees of flexion can be increased. Usually, extension – as well as flexion – is increased, not decreased, on a regular basis.

CN: Physiological integrity; CNS: Basic care and comfort; CL: Application

18. A client has multiple myeloma. Which action should alert the nurse that he may be having difficulty coping with his prognosis?

1. He becomes tearful when discussing his condition.
2. He asks questions about his prognosis.
3. He shows concerns about his family.
4. He avoids any conversation concerning his health.

18. 4. A client who avoids conversation about his health may be denying his condition and not coping well with his prognosis. Crying is a normal response to his disease. Asking questions about his prognosis and showing concern for his family are normal coping responses.

CN: Psychological integrity; CNS: None; CL: Analysis

19. Which client is most likely to develop ankylosing spondylitis?

1. White female, age 16, with knee pain
2. Black male, age 50, with hip pain
3. Asian female, age 70, with chest pain
4. White male, age 23, with back pain

19. 4. Ankylosing spondylitis usually begins between ages 15 to 30 and the prevalence is highest in white males. Back pain is the characteristic feature.

CN: Health promotion and maintenance; CNS: None; CL: Analysis

20. A client with pernicious anemia undergoes gastrectomy. Which route should the nurse use to administer cyanocobalamin (vitamin B_{12}) after the surgery?

1. Buccal route
2. Transdermal route
3. Oral route
4. Parenteral route

20. 4. A client who has undergone gastrectomy is no longer able to produce the intrinsic factor necessary for vitamin B_{12} absorption through the GI tract; therefore, the parenteral route (intramuscular or deep subcutaneous injections) is required. This medication isn't available for buccal or transdermal routes.

CN: Physiological integrity; CNS: Pharmacological and parenteral therapies; CL: Application

21. After a nurse teaches a client with diverticular disease about proper diet, he fills out his lunch menu. Which selection by the client demonstrates the need for further teaching?

1. Tossed salad with tomatoes, sunflower seeds, and tuna
2. Egg salad on whole wheat bread and an apple
3. Cottage cheese with apple, pear, and plum slices
4. Ham salad served with whole wheat crackers and a banana

21. 1. Clients with diverticular disease should avoid high-roughage foods, such as nuts, seeds, popcorn, and raw celery. They should, however, consume high-fiber foods, such as fresh fruit with skins (apples, pears, and plums), bananas, dried fruits, whole wheat bread and crackers, and raw vegetables (lettuce, carrots, and cauliflower).

CN: Physiological integrity; CNS: Basic care and comfort; CL: Application

22. A nurse is teaching nursing students about maintaining a healthy liver. Which measure should the nurse include in her teaching?

1. Take over-the-counter (OTC) medication as needed.
2. Take prescribed medications according to instructions.
3. Add a nutritional supplement to the diet to ensure adequate nutrition.
4. Consume a low-protein diet that contains moderate carbohydrate and fat.

22. 2. Taking these measures will help maintain a healthy liver: take prescribed medications according to instructions; avoid taking unnecessary OTC medications; eat a balanced diet that's moderate to high in protein, moderate in carbohydrate and fat, and adequate in vitamins; and take a nutritional supplement only if advised to do so by a physician.

CN: Health promotion and maintenance; CNS: None; CL: Application

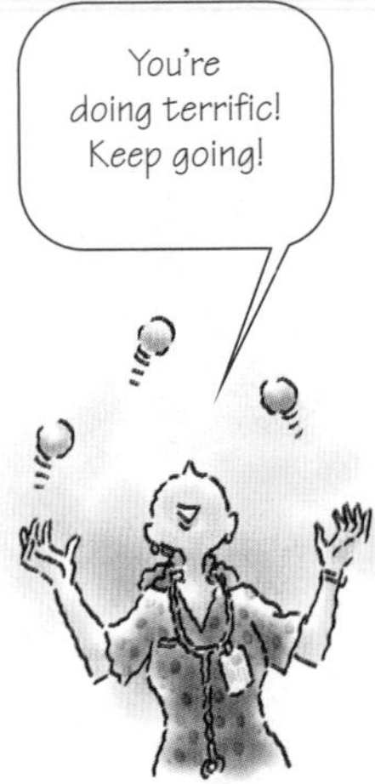
You're
doing terrific!
Keep going!

23. A 28-year-old male client complaining of a racing heart and nervousness is admitted to the telemetry floor. His telemetry shows a heart rate of 130 beats/minute in sinus tachycardia. His skin is very warm, dry, and his eyes appear to be bulging. Which nursing action is the most important upon admission?

1. Inserting a urinary catheter and assessing appearance of urine
2. Observing the client's gait
3. Reaching out and feeling the client's neck
4. Standing behind the client and gently palpating the cricothyroid area

23. 4. The client shows signs of hyperthyroidism, and standing behind him and palpating the cricothyroid area is the correct way to assess for an enlarged thyroid gland. Inserting a catheter isn't necessary; assessing the client's urine, which would be concentrated because of dehydration, can be done after he voids. Observing the client's gait isn't necessary at this time.

CN: Physiological integrity; CNS: Physiological adaptation; CL: Analysis

24. A client is unemployed, has no health insurance, hasn't filled his levothyroxine (Synthroid) prescription for some time, and has been getting "sicker by the day." Which problem is probably related to him not taking his medication?

1 Diarrhea and vomiting
2. Rapid heart rate
3. Warm, dry, flushed skin
4. Rectal temperature of 94° F (34.4° C)

24. 4. Hypothyroidism leads to a hypodynamic state, so a low body temperature is expected after the levothyroxine has been metabolized. Each of the other symptoms is indicative of a hypermetabolic state and, although the client may exhibit these problems, they're probably related to infection and dehydration.

CN: Physiological integrity; CNS: Physiological adaptation; CL: Application

25. A child with chronic renal failure is scheduled for hemodialysis with an external shunt three times per week. As part of the discharge planning, the nurse should tell the family to perform which step?

1. Assess the site daily for symptoms of redness.
2. Wash the serum at the shunt site with normal saline.
3. Assess the child's blood pressure on the same side as the shunt.
4. Keep a clean dressing in place over the shunt site.

25. 1. The child and parents should assess the shunt site for redness daily because a color change may indicate infection. Serum at the shunt site should be washed away with half strength hydrogen peroxide and an antibiotic ointment applied. Blood pressure shouldn't be taken in the arm with the shunt. A sterile dressing should be placed over the shunt site.

CN: Safe, effective care environment; CNS: Safety and infection control; CL: Application

26. A 17-year-old client tells the nurse that she has vulvar itching and a thick, cream-cheese–like vaginal discharge. The nurse anticipates treating the client with which medication?

1. Metronidazole (Flagyl)
2. Erythromycin (Ery-Tab)
3. Miconazole (Monistat)
4. Amoxicillin (Amoxil)

26. 3. The client most likely has *candidiasis,* which produces a thick cream-cheese–like vaginal discharge and is treated with miconazole or nystatin (Mycostatin). Metronidazole is used to treat *Trichomonas vaginalis.* Erythromycin, amoxicillin, or other antibiotic therapy can contribute to *candidiasis* infections and isn't used to treat this infection.

CN: Physiological integrity; CNS: Pharmacological and parenteral therapies; CL: Application

27. When assessing a 5-hour-old neonate, which finding would prompt a nurse to call a physician?

1. Color is dusky, axillary temperature is 96.8° F (37° C), and the baby is spitting up mucus.
2. Hands and feet are cyanotic, abdomen is rounded, and the infant hasn't voided or passed meconium.
3. Anterior fontanel is ¾″ (2 cm) wide, head is molded, and sutures are overriding.
4. Irregular abdominal respirations and intermittent tremors in the extremities.

27. 1. Skin color should be pink tinged or ruddy and saliva should be scant. The normal axillary temperature ranges from 97.7° to 98.6° F (36.5° to 37° C). Acrocyanosis may be present for 2 to 6 hours. The neonate should pass meconium and void within 24 hours. Overriding sutures and molding, when present, may persist for a few days. Neonatal tremors are normal in the neonate; however, they must be evaluated to differentiate them from seizures.

CN: Safe, effective care environment; CNS: Management of care; CL: Application

28. A mother calls the pediatrician because there's an outbreak of scabies at her child's school. The nurse would teach the mother to check for which finding?

1. Pain, erythema, and edema at the site of the bite
2. Oval white dots that adhere to hair shafts
3. Diffuse pruritic wheals
4. Pruritic papules, vesicles, and linear burrows on the finger and toe webs

28. 4. The mother should check her child for pruritic papules, vesicles, and linear burrows on the finger and toe webs. Oval white dots that adhere to the hair shaft can indicate head lice.

CN: Safe, effective care environment; CNS: Safety and infection control; CL: Application

29. The school nurse assesses a young child with a rash that's raised and has circumscribed areas filled with fluid. The nurse documents this finding as which type of rash?

1. Vesicular rash
2. Papular rash
3. Macular rash
4. Petechial rash

29. 1. A vesicular rash contains small, raised, circumscribed lesions filled with clear fluid. A papular rash contains raised solid lesions with color changes in circumscribed areas. A macular rash is flat with color changes in circumscribed areas. Petechiae are pinpoint purple or red spots on the skin caused by multiple hemorrhages.

CN: Safe, effective care environment; CNS: Safety and infection control; CL: Application

30. A 20-month-old toddler has been treated with permethrin (Nix) for scabies. Because he continues to scratch, his mother wonders whether the drug is working. Which response by a nurse is most appropriate?

1. "Stop treatment because the drug isn't safe for children under age 2."
2. "Pruritus can be present for weeks after treatment."
3. "Apply the drug every day until the rash and itching disappears."
4. "Pruritus is common in children under age 5 treated with permethrin."

30. 2. Pruritus may be present for weeks in a child treated with permethrin for scabies. The drug is safe for use in infants as young as age 2 months. Treatment with permethrin can be safely repeated in 2 weeks. Pruritus is caused by secondary reactions of the mites.

CN: Physiological integrity; CNS: Pharmacological and parenteral therapies; CL: Application

31. An 8-year-old child was sent home after the school reported the presence of head lice. Which information is most helpful to the parents?

1. The child should remain isolated for 1 week after treatment.
2. Lindane (Kwell) is the treatment of choice for head lice.
3. Treatment with a pediculicide followed by combing the hair with a fine-tooth comb will usually kill all lice and remove the nits. Retreatment in 7 to 10 days may be necessary to kill newly hatched lice.
4. The only way to get rid of head lice is to cut the hair.

31. 3. Treatment with a pediculicide followed by combing the hair with a fine-tooth comb will usually kill all lice and remove the nits. Retreatment in 7 to 10 days may be necessary to kill newly hatched lice. After the infestation has been appropriately treated, there's no reason to isolate the child. Lindane isn't the drug of choice because of its potential for neurotoxicity. The hair should be cut in severe cases only.

CN: Safe, effective care environment; CNS: Safety and infection control; CL: Application

32. Which assessment should a nurse do prior to administering disulfiram (Anatabuse) to a client with a history of alcohol abuse?

1. Assess the client's commitment to attend Alcoholics Anonymous (AA) meetings.
2. Assess whether the client admits to a problem with alcohol.
3. Assess when the client's last alcoholic beverage was consumed.
4. Assess the client's nutritional status.

32. 3. The client must be alcohol-free for 12 hours before starting therapy with disulfiram. Assessing the client's commitment to attend AA meetings, the client's perception of his problem, and nutritional status are all important interventions, but they aren't necessary prior to starting disulfiram.

CN: Physiological integrity; CNS: Pharmacological and parenteral therapies; CL: Application

33. The nurse is assessing a client with schizophrenia who exhibits negativism, rigidity, excitement, stupor, or posturing. The nurse suspects that the client has which type of schizophrenia?

1. Catatonic
2. Undifferentiated
3. Disorganized
4. Paranoid

33. 1. Catatonic schizophrenia is a state of psychologically induced immobilization, which is, at times, interrupted by episodes of extreme agitation, such as negativism, rigidity, excitement, stupor, or posturing. Undifferentiated schizophrenia occurs when no single clinical presentation dominates (paranoid, disorganized, or catatonic). Disorganized schizophrenia is characterized by disorganized speech, disorganized behavior, and inappropriate affect. The dominant theme in paranoid schizophrenia is one of delusions and hallucinations.

CN: Psychosocial integrity; CNS: None; CL: Application

34. Which statement is an example of a key element in a nursing care plan?

1. Advance diet to regular as tolerated.
2. Ambulate 30′ (9.1 m) with walker by discharge.
3. Give furosemide (Lasix) 40 mg I.V. now.
4. Discontinue I.V. fluids when tolerating oral fluids.

34. 2. Option 2 is a measurable expected outcome or goal, a key element of a nursing care plan. Other key elements include nursing diagnoses and interventions. The other options are physician's orders, not key elements of nursing care plans.

CN: Safe, effective care environment; CNS: Management of care; CL: Application

35. A client complains of chronic lower back pain and fatigue and has seen multiple care providers without relief of symptoms. The client insists that something is "terribly wrong." Which action should the nurse take first?

1. Refer the client for a psychiatric evaluation.
2. Initiate group therapy for behavior modification.
3. Obtain a thorough health assessment to rule out physical illnesses.
4. Refer the client to physical therapy.

35. 3. The first action by the nurse should be to take a thorough health assessment including laboratory studies to rule out physical illnesses. The other actions aren't appropriate until a diagnosis is made.

CN: Safe, effective care environment; CNS: Management of care; CL: Application

36. Which sign alerts a nurse to a possible mild toxic reaction in a client receiving lithium for manic episodes of manic-depressive illness?

1. Vomiting and diarrhea
2. Hypertension
3. Seizures
4. Increased appetite

36. 1. Vomiting and diarrhea are signs of mild to moderate lithium toxicity. Hypotension, not hypertension, and seizures occur with moderate to severe toxic reactions. Anorexia occurs with mild toxic reactions.

CN: Physiological integrity; CNS: Pharmacological and parenteral therapies; CL: Application

37. A client with bipolar disorder is taking lithium and tells the nurse, "I can stop taking the medicine when I feel better." Which response by the nurse is best?

1. "That's correct. When you feel better, you can stop taking the medication."
2. "Take the medication for 1 week after you feel better to be sure there's enough medication in your system."
3. "Bipolar disorders may require lithium indefinitely to prevent relapses."
4. "This medication is given as needed. That means that you can take it when you feel that you need it."

37. 3. Lithium, which helps clients with bipolar disorder stabilize their mood swings, is a long-term treatment. Blood measurements are taken regularly to monitor lithium levels in the client's body. He shouldn't stop taking lithium when he feels better because the therapeutic blood level will decrease. Stopping the medication 1 week after he feels better or taking it as needed will also decrease the therapeutic blood level of lithium.

CN: Physiological integrity; CNS: Pharmacological and parenteral therapies; CL: Analysis

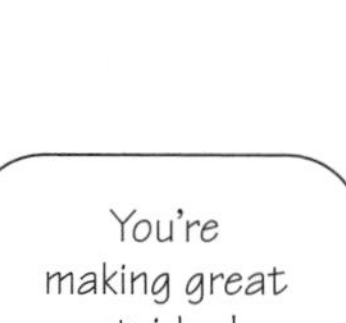
You're
making great
strides!

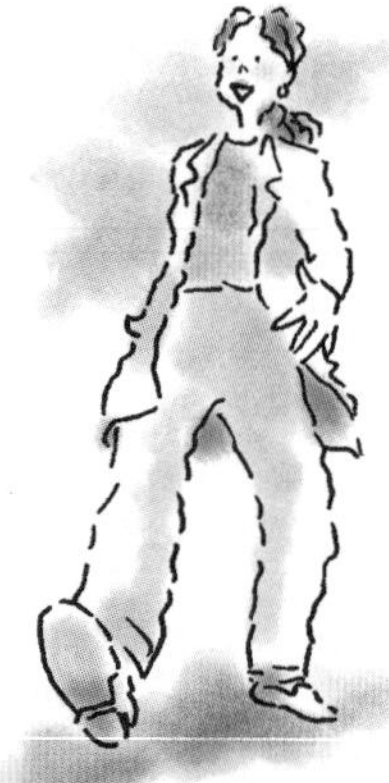

38. A client's condition is becoming stabilized after an episode of substance-induced delirium. During the initial recovery period, the nurse should assess the client for which psychosocial health problem?

1. Flashbacks
2. Depression
3. Nightmares
4. Dissociation

38. 2. Depression and anxiety are common mental health problems seen immediately after substance withdrawal. Flashbacks and nightmares are commonly observed in clients with posttraumatic stress disorder. Dissociation occurs when a client undergoes prolonged physical and sexual abuse.

CN: Psychosocial integrity; CNS: None; CL: Analysis

39. A client with a history of depression demonstrates some inconsistent symptoms of cognitive impairment. The nurse should expect which situation when the depression is treated?

1. Delusional thinking ceases
2. Recognition of objects improves
3. Memory problems resolve
4. Suicidal ideation is no longer a problem

39. 3. In a condition called *pseudodementia,* a client treated for depression will have a dramatic improvement in memory. Delusional thinking and object-recognition problems aren't characteristic of pseudodementia. The nurse must assess all clients with depression for suicidal ideation because they're at some degree of risk for suicide.

CN: Psychosocial integrity; CNS: None; CL: Application

40. A client with borderline personality disorder has extreme views of himself and his situation. Which behavior indicates that the client is a candidate for medication?

1. Disorientation
2. Hyperactivity
3. Regression
4. Mood swings

40. 4. Medications aren't typically given to clients with personality disorders. However, clients with mood swings, hallucinations, or psychotic behaviors are appropriate candidates for medications. Disorientation, hyperactivity and regression aren't necessarily seen in clients with borderline personality disorders.

CN: Psychosocial integrity; CNS: None; CL: Application

41. A client has traits of an avoidant personality disorder. Which family intervention should the nurse give the highest priority in the care plan?

1. Explaining that the family should teach the client social skills.
2. Recommending that the family recognize the client's high sensitivity to criticism.
3. Exploring ways for the family to help the client express true feelings.
4. Asking the family to keep a daily log of the client's adjustment difficulties.

41. 2. A client with traits of an avoidant personality disorder is very sensitive to criticism and disapproval but doesn't typically have learning or social skills problems. Such a client may have difficulty expressing feelings and may have few friends or only family members for interaction. Having the family keep a log of the client's adjustment difficulties isn't an appropriate intervention; the list may be interpreted as a statement of rejection.

CN: Safe, effective care environment; CNS: Management of care; CL: Analysis

42. A client with a substance abuse disorder says the problem doesn't really exist. Which intervention should be the nurse's initial one?

1. Educating about the principles of mental health
2. Examining the use of defense mechanisms
3. Recognizing and discussing feelings of resentment
4. Discussing the need for a caretaker while in recovery

42. 2. Defense mechanisms contribute to the client's denial. Education won't be well received unless the client recognizes the problem and determines that the nurse's teaching would be useful. The client can't recognize and discuss feelings of resentment when denying that a problem exists. The client needs to become responsible for his own behavior and take care of himself.

CN: Psychosocial integrity; CNS: None; CL: Application

43. A nurse is evaluating drug therapy effectiveness in a client undergoing alcohol detoxification. Which finding indicates that drug therapy needs to be adjusted?

1. There are signs of toxicity from the drug.
2. The drug prevents the occurrence of further problems.
3. During the course of treatment, the dosage has increased.
4. The drug facilitates the client's interactions with staff.

43. 1. If signs of toxicity from drug therapy occur during the detoxification period, the drug therapy needs to be adjusted. The medication is working if it prevents further problems. Sometimes, the dosage must be adjusted to obtain the maximum benefit. If the drug enables the client to have therapeutic interactions with the staff, the client is benefiting from the therapy.

CN: Physiological integrity; CNS: Pharmacological and parenteral therapies; CL: Application

44. A nurse explains the unit's rules to a client with bulimia nervosa. Which action by the client indicates that learning has occurred?

1. The client asks to be accompanied to the bathroom after lunch.
2. The client writes down every food item eaten in the past 24 hours.
3. The client decides to help the dietitian plan the unit's meals.
4. The client discusses current problems with the nurse before mealtime.

44. 1. When the client asks to be accompanied to the bathroom after a meal, the client is following protocol for restoring healthy eating and promoting adequate nutrition. This action indicates the client's commitment to not purging after a meal. Recording the food eaten in a 24-hour period would be appropriate for a client with anorexia nervosa, not a client with bulimia nervosa. It's inappropriate for a client to plan meals for the unit's clients. The client can discuss problems any time, not just before mealtimes.

CN: Psychosocial integrity; CNS: None; CL: Analysis

45. A nurse is teaching a client with an eating disorder about cues that trigger unhealthy eating behaviors. Which example explains social cues?
1. Diet advertisements
2. Troublesome memories
3. Interpersonal conflict
4. Frustration fatigue

45. 3. Social cues that trigger maladaptive behavior include feelings of isolation and conflict with family or friends. Diet advertisements are considered situational cues. Troublesome memories are psychological cues. Frustration fatigue is an example of a physiological cue.
CN: Psychosocial integrity; CNS: None; CL: Application

46. A schizophrenic client states, "The voices keep talking to me. They're telling me that I have to leave here and that I shouldn't talk to you. Don't you hear what they're saying?" Which response is best?
1. "You didn't take your medicine this morning, did you?"
2. "The voices aren't real. You're sick and they're part of your illness."
3. "Are you hearing voices again?"
4." I don't hear the voices, but I see that you are upset."

46. 4. The nurse should be honest and tell the client that she doesn't hear the voices while acknowledging the client's feelings. Asking if the client took his medication or explaining his illness doesn't allow the client to feel valued by the nurse. Asking him if he hears voices makes him feel that the nurse wasn't listening.
CN: Psychosocial integrity; CNS: None; CL: Application

47. The nurse is teaching caregivers about the signs and symptoms of schizophrenia relapse. Which response by the caregivers about the signs and symptoms to report to a mental health professional indicates that the teaching has been effective?
1. Changes in appetite resulting in weight loss or gain
2. Loss of interest in sexual activities
3. Increased socialization
4. Feelings of tenseness and difficulty sleeping

47. 4. Signs and symptoms of schizophrenia relapse include difficulty concentrating and sleeping, feelings of tenseness, and increased bizarre thinking and withdrawal. The other choices aren't signs and symptoms of schizophrenia.
CN: Psychosocial integrity; CNS: None; CL: Analysis

48. A client with schizophrenia has been prescribed risperidone (Risperdal). The client's symptoms include hallucinations, delusions, and withdrawal. A nurse explains that the medication will help improve which symptoms?
1. Negative symptoms
2. Positive symptoms
3. Negative and positive symptoms
4. Paranoid symptoms

48. 3. Risperidone targets both negative and positive symptoms. Positive symptoms include delusions, hallucinations, and bizarre behaviors. Negative symptoms indicate a loss or lack of normal functioning such as lack of motivation and social withdrawal.
CN: Physiological integrity; CNS: Pharmacological and parenteral therapies; CL: Application

49. A newly graduated nurse is caring for a client recently diagnosed with dissociative identity disorder. The nurse asks the preceptor about discussing a client's traumatic childhood with the client. Which advice from the preceptor is best?

1. "Ask pointed questions and demand specific answers."
2. "If the client begins talking about it, just listen and be supportive."
3. "Tell the client that you suspect that much of his memory is exaggerated."
4. "Tell the client that those issues can be discussed with a physician only."

49. 2. If the subject is painful, the client will discuss it when he feels comfortable and ready. Forcing him to talk about the subject will cause severe anxiety and result in distrust. The other choices don't facilitate a trusting relationship between the nurse and the client.

CN: Safe, effective care environment; CNS: Management of care; CL: Application

50. A client with dissociative identity disorder frequently switches from one personality to another. The nurse can identify the switch by which finding?

1. Episodes of orthostatic hypotension
2. Blinking or rolling the eyes frequently
3. Dystonic reactions
4. Episodes of tachycardia

50. 2. Switching from one personality to another is manifested in a number of ways including blinking, facial movements, and changes in voice. Changes in blood pressure or pulse or dystonic reactions aren't indicative of switching from one personality to another.

CN: Psychosocial integrity; CNS: None; CL: Application

51. A 38-year-old female client is scheduled to have a hysterectomy and is concerned about no longer being a "whole woman." Which intervention by the nurse is best?

1. Tell her to talk to her husband about the permanent changes that will be taking place with her body.
2. Refer her to group therapy.
3. Encourage her to discuss her concerns and feelings.
4. Give her information to read and leave the room.

51. 3. The nurse should encourage the client to express her feelings. Telling her to talk to her husband will cause the client added concern and anxiety. Referring her to group therapy isn't an appropriate intervention at this time. Giving her information and leaving the room doesn't allow her to ask questions and express concerns.

CN: Psychosocial integrity; CNS: None; CL: Analysis

52. A 23-year-old female client is seen in the emergency department for rape. The woman is very calm and appears emotionally unaffected by the event. Which assessment of the client's behavior is appropriate?

1. The client probably isn't telling the truth but is trying to get the perpetrator in trouble.
2. The client was a willing partner.
3. The client's initially deceptive calm may be masking distress, denial, or emotional shock.
4. The client is pregnant and is trying to blame the pregnancy on a rape.

52. 3. One of the immediate consequences of rape is deceptive calmness. This behavior usually masks emotional shock, denial, or distress. The other responses are judgmental opinions. Nurses are to remain nonjudgmental in providing care.

CN: Psychosocial integrity; CNS: None; CL: Analysis

53. A full-term neonate was just admitted to the transitional nursery. He has a large meningomyelocele covered by an intact sac. The nurse knows immediately to place this neonate on his stomach with hips slightly elevated. Which statement describes the rationale for this position?

1. To prevent the sac covering the defect from rupturing
2. To preserve urine and bowel control
3. To assess neurologic functioning more easily
4. To prevent further neurologic damage

53. 1. The sac covering the defect is the only barrier preventing bacteria from directly entering the neonate's central nervous system and causing meningitis and encephalitis. A large defect will result in loss of urine and bowel control. The nurse can assess neurologic functioning when the child is on his back or stomach. The damage to the neurologic system happened in utero, and the nurse should prevent further damage by placing the infant on his stomach until after surgery. Preventing neurologic damage isn't the priority.

CN: Physiological integrity; CNS: Reduction of risk potential; CL: Analysis

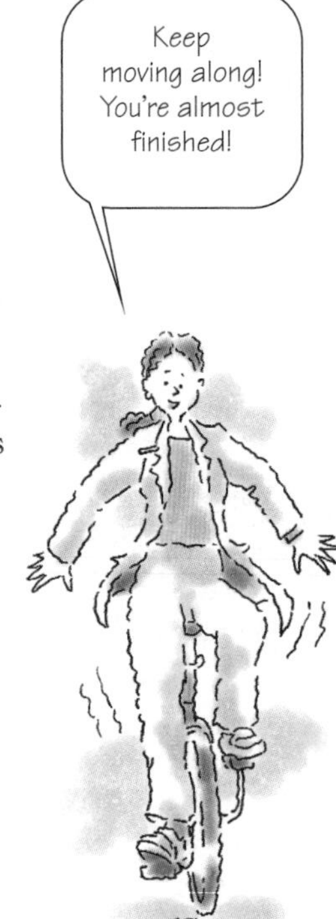
Keep moving along! You're almost finished!

54. A nurse is teaching the mother of a neonate with a cleft palate how to feed him. Which instruction should the nurse give the mother?

1. Feed the neonate in a semi-reclining position with his head resting on the mother's curved elbow.
2. Feed the neonate in an upright position.
3. Feed the neonate lying on his stomach with his head turned toward his mother.
4. Feed the neonate in any position that the mother and child are comfortable.

54. 2. Feed the neonate with a cleft palate in an upright position. Incorrect feeding can allow formula to slip through the palate opening, enter the upper respiratory tract and lungs, and cause aspiration pneumonia. Any of the other positions is placing the neonate at risk for aspiration pneumonia.

CN: Physiological integrity; CNS: Reduction of risk potential; CL: Analysis

55. A nurse observes school-age children playing. Which activity is typical of this age-group?

1. Barbie dolls
2. Monopoly
3. Sony Play Station video games
4. Hot Wheels cars

55. 2. School-age children engage in competitive play with established rules and goals. Monopoly is an excellent example of play that pulls these elements together. Playing with Barbie dolls is an example of associative play, which preschoolers engage in. Solitary play of video games is seen in adolescents. Playing with Hot Wheels cars is more indicative of toddlers' parallel play.

CN: Health promotion and maintenance; CNS: None; CL: Application

56. A nurse is assessing an infant's growth and development. Which action by the nurse indicates the best understanding of a 4-month-old's stage of growth and development?

1. Eliciting a social smile
2. Allowing the infant to hold his own bottle
3. Playing peek-a-boo with the infant
4. Letting the infant sit without support

56. 1. A social smile should be seen in a 4-month-old. An infant can't hold his own bottle until age 6 to 7 months, and he'll engage in peek-a-boo activity at age 10 to 12 months. He can sit without support at about age 8 months.

CN: Health promotion and maintenance; CNS: None; CL: Application

57. The nurse is caring for an 11-year-old client with cerebral palsy who has a pressure ulcer on the sacrum. When teaching the client's mother about dietary intake, which foods should the nurse plan to emphasize?

1. Legumes and cheese
2. Whole grain products
3. Fruits and vegetables
4. Lean meats and low fat milk

57. 4. Although the client should eat a balanced diet with foods from all food groups, the diet should emphasize foods that supply complete protein, such as lean meats and low-fat milk. Protein helps build and repair body tissue, which promotes healing. Legumes provide incomplete protein. Cheese contains complete protein but also fat, which should be limited to 30% or less of caloric intake. Whole grain products supply incomplete proteins and carbohydrates. Fruits and vegetables mainly provide carbohydrates.

CN: Physiological integrity; CNS: Basic care and comfort; CL: Application

58. A client is diagnosed with pneumonia. Which nursing diagnosis would take priority for this client?

1. *Excess fluid volume*
2. *Ineffective airway clearance*
3. *Activity intolerance*
4. *Deficient knowledge*

58. 2. Pneumonia refers to inflammation of the lungs, and can produce copious amounts of tracheobronchial secretions. These secretions interfere with airway patency and gas exchange. Therefore, airway clearance is a priority. The client may experience a decrease in fluid volume, not an excess, due to increased temperature and respiratory rate. The client also may experience activity intolerance and deficient knowledge, but neither is the priority diagnosis.

CN: Safe, effective care environment: CNS: Management of care; CL: Analysis

59. A nurse is caring for a client in active labor. Which observation would cause the nurse to suspect fetal distress?

1. Fetal heart rate of 144 beats/minute
2. Accelerations of the fetal heart rate with contractions
3. Fetal scalp pH of 7.14
4. Presence of long-term variability

59. 3. A scalp pH below 7.25 indicates acidosis and fetal hypoxia. A fetal heart rate of 144 beats/minute, acceleration of the fetal heartbeat with contractions, and the presence of long-term variability with contractions are normal responses of a healthy fetus to labor.

CN: Health promotion and maintenance; CNS: None; CL: Application

60. During a routine examination, the mother of a 3-month-old child asks the nurse, "How soon will she have her first tooth?" Which response by the nurse would be the most accurate as to the age by which the first tooth usually erupts?

1. 4 months
2. 5 months
3. 6 months
4. 7 months

60. 3. The first tooth typically erupts at age 6 months, although some infants do get their first tooth when a little younger or older.

CN: Health promotion and maintenance; CNS: None; CL: Application

61. A nurse assesses an 18-month-old toddler. Which activity would indicate to the nurse that the child is exhibiting normal growth and development patterns?

1. Running and jumping in place
2. Jumping down from a chair
3. Naming a specific color
4. Saying his full name

61. 1. An 18-month-old child should be able to run and jump in place. Typically, a child of 30 months is able to jump down from a chair, can name one color, and knows his full name.

CN: Health promotion and maintenance; CNS: None; CL: Application

62. A mother was diagnosed with polyhydramnios during her pregnancy and just delivered a preterm male neonate. In which manner should the nurse assess a neonate for tracheoesophageal fistula?

1. Observing the neonate during the first formula feeding
2. Determining if cyanosis is present at birth
3. Inserting a catheter through the esophagus to the stomach
4. Assessing lung sounds to determine if possible pneumonia is present

62. 3. Tracheoesophageal fistula is present if a catheter can't be passed through the neonate's esophagus to the stomach. A barium swallow or a bronchial endoscopy examination will reveal the blind-end esophagus. The condition should be diagnosed before the infant is fed; otherwise, the infant will cough and may become cyanotic during feeding. Immediately after birth, pneumonia shouldn't be present with a tracheoesophageal fistula. Emergency surgery is essential to prevent pneumonia caused by the stomach's contents leaking into the lungs.

CN: Health promotion and maintenance; CNS: None; CL: Analysis

63. Which instruction should be included in the care plan for a client following total hip replacement?

1. Keeping the legs adducted
2. Not bending at the hip more than 90 degrees
3. Keeping the hips lower than the knees when seated
4. Teaching how to bend forward to put on socks and shoes

63. 2. Following a total hip replacement, the client should be instructed not to bend more than 90 degrees at the hip. The legs should be kept abducted to prevent dislocation of the prosthesis. The hips should be kept higher than the knees when seated to minimize hip flexion. The client should be instructed not to bend forward at the hip to put on shoes and socks. Assistive devices can be used to help the client safely dress below the waist.

CN: Physiological integrity; CNS: Reduction of risk potential; CL: Application

64. Which cause of myocarditis is the most common?

1. Bacteria
2. Parasite
3. Fungus
4. Virus

64. 4. Myocarditis (inflammation of the myocardium) is usually caused by a virus. Of all the viruses, coxsackieviruses and echoviruses are the most common agents. Bacteria, parasites, and fungi may cause myocarditis, but they aren't the most common causes.

CN: Physiological integrity; CNS: Physiological adaptation; CL: Analysis

65. A nurse is caring for a 7-year-old client receiving cyclophosphamide (Cytoxan). In addition to administering mesna (Mesnex), which action should the nurse take?

1. Transfusing platelets before administering the drug
2. Giving the child cranberry juice to drink
3. Encouraging the child to void frequently
4. Limiting the child's fluid intake

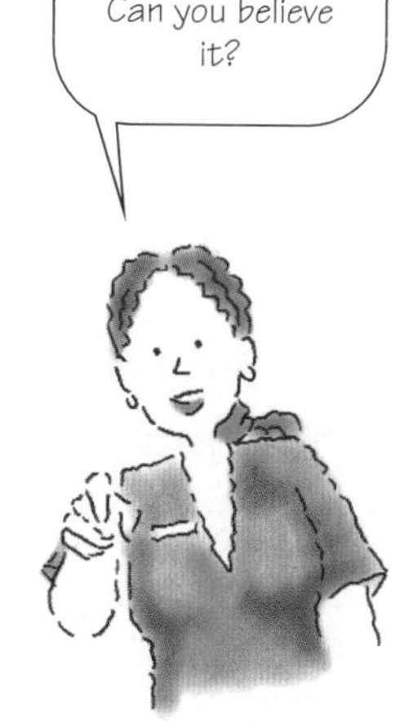
Only 10
more questions.
Can you believe
it?

65. 3. Hemorrhagic cystitis can result when the by-products of cyclophosphamide metabolism remain in the bladder; therefore, emptying the bladder at least every 2 hours when the child is awake can help prevent this painful condition. The child should be encouraged to void as soon as the urge is felt. Bacteria or low platelets don't cause the condition, so transfusing platelets and giving cranberry juice aren't correct. Limiting fluid is contraindicated. Instead, the child will be given fluids liberally, usually by I.V. infusion, and encouraged to drink; a high intake of fluids will increase elimination of the drug's toxic by-products.

CN: Physiological integrity; CNS: Pharmacological and parenteral therapies; CL: Analysis

66. When protective isolation isn't indicated, a nurse plans which activity for a child receiving chemotherapy?

1. Bed rest
2. Activity as tolerated
3. Walk to bathroom only
4. Out of bed for brief periods

66. 2. Children receiving chemotherapy should be able to engage in activities of interest and maintain as much independence and autonomy as possible; they'll limit their activity when they feel tired or ill. Limiting their activities to bed rest, walking to bathroom only, or only out of bed for brief periods isn't necessary and restricts activity unnecessarily. Whenever possible, include children in planning their care. These children should avoid adults and other children with infections.

CN: Health promotion and maintenance; CNS: None; CL: Application

67. A child is intubated and placed on a ventilator after a near drowning. The physician's order is to suction every 3 to 4 hours. The child's parents ask the nurse why the suctioning is necessary. Which response by the nurse is the most accurate?

1. To keep the client free of infection
2. To keep the client from experiencing cardiac arrhythmias
3. To keep the client's airway patent
4. To maintain fluid and electrolyte balance

67. 3. Because of the increased secretions from drowning, the airway is more prone to obstruction, and suctioning is essential for maintaining patency. Suctioning won't prevent infection and may even cause it. Suctioning can cause bradycardia; therefore, preoxygenation is essential to prevent arrhythmias. Suctioning doesn't affect fluid and electrolyte balance.

CN: Physiological integrity; CNS: Reduction of risk potential; CL: Application

68. A child with cystic fibrosis has a bronchodilator, steroids ordered by metered-dose inhaler, and chest physiotherapy. In which order should these medications and treatments be administered?

1. Perform chest physiotherapy first.
2. Administer the bronchodilator first.
3. Administer the steroid first.
4. Let the client eat lunch first and then perform chest physiotherapy.

68. 2. Administer the bronchodilator to dilate the bronchi. The steroid can then reach further down the respiratory tract. After each medication is given, perform chest physiotherapy to expectorate secretions in the lower airways. Administer the medications and chest physiotherapy before meals to prevent aspiration.

CN: Physiological integrity; CNS: Pharmacological and parental therapies; CL: Application

69. A nurse is teaching a student nurse about ketogenic diet. Which condition would the nurse state is a ketogenic diet sometimes used to treat?

1. Anorexia nervosa
2. Nephrotic syndrome
3. Epilepsy
4. Ulcerative colitis

69. 3. A ketogenic diet is typically suggested as a method of treatment for epilepsy. Anorexia nervosa is treated with counseling and slowly reintroducing food. Children with nephrotic syndrome are usually on a low-sodium diet. Ulcerative colitis is treated with a low-residue diet.

CN: Physiological integrity; CNS: Reduction of risk potential; CL: Application

70. A child is unable to walk without assistance because of decreased oxygen at birth. Which disorder is characterized by a malfunction of the brain's motor center from hypoxia?

1. Down syndrome
2. Cerebral palsy
3. Sickle cell anemia
4. Osteogenesis imperfecta

70. 2. Cerebral palsy affects the motor center of the brain and is usually caused by brain trauma. Down syndrome is a chromosomal abnormality. Sickle cell anemia is a genetic disorder of red blood cells. Osteogenesis imperfecta is a congenital anomaly involving decreased calcium in the bones and leads to multiple fractures at birth.

CN: Physiological integrity; CNS: Physiological adaptation; CL: Application

71. A 17-year-old client who injured his right knee during a basketball game is scheduled for an arthroscopy. The nurse teaches the client about the procedure. Which response by the nurse regarding arthroscopy would be accurate?

1. An X-ray using a contrast media
2. Visualization of the joint with a small instrument
3. Inserting a needle and withdrawing fluid for biopsy
4. Aspirating synovial fluid from the bursa

71. 2. After a small incision is made in the knee, a small tube-shaped instrument is inserted for viewing the knee and surrounding cartilage, tendon, and ligaments. Contrast media is typically used for X-rays of joints. Biopsies are taken if cancer is a concern. Synovial fluid is collected for culture if an infection or inflammation is a concern.

CN: Physiological integrity; CNS: Physiological adaptation; CL: Application

72. A nurse is assessing a 13-year-old child 12 hours after surgery for a compound-fracture repair of the right arm. Which finding requires immediate attention?

1. Bruising of the fingers
2. Capillary refill of 3 seconds
3. Pallor of the nail beds
4. Edema of the extremity

72. 3. Pallor suggests a decrease in circulation to the extremity, and the surgeon should be notified. Bruising can be expected with a compound fracture. The fingers should be observed for further discoloration indicating decreased circulation. Capillary refill of 3 seconds is normal. Edema is expected but should be watched; increased edema might impair circulation.

CN: Physiological integrity; CNS: Reduction of risk potential; CL: Application

73. A 3-year-old child has diarrhea, and the pediatrician has recommended a BRAT diet for the next 24 hours. The nurse teaches the parents about the diet. Which response by the parents about the diet indicates the teaching has been effective? "The diet consists of:

1. bran, rice crispies, apple juice, and tomato juice."
2. beans, red meat, apples, and tomatoes."
3. bananas, rice, applesauce, and toast."
4. broccoli, red ice pops, apple butter, and tacos."

73. 3. BRAT stands for bananas, rice, applesauce, and toast. This diet is commonly used for children with diarrhea because these foods add some form to the stool without further irritating the bowel. The other diet choices can cause gas, irritation, and inflammation in the already inflamed bowel.

CN: Physiological integrity; CNS: Basic care and comfort; CL: Application

74. After undergoing small-bowel resection, a client is prescribed metronidazole (Flagyl) 500 mg I.V. The mixed I.V. solution contains 100 ml. A nurse is to run the drug over 30 minutes. The drip factor of the available I.V. tubing is 15 gtt/ml. What is the drip rate? Record your answer usng a whole number.

______________________ gtt/minute

74. 50. Use the following equation: 100 ml/30 minutes × 15 gtt/1 ml = 49.9 gtt/minute (50 gtt/minute).

CN: Physiological integrity; CNS: Pharmacological and parenteral therapies; CL: Application

75. A nurse is caring for a client whose cultural background is different from her own. Which actions are appropriate? Select all that apply:

1. Consider that nonverbal cues, such as eye contact, may have different meanings in different cultures.
2. Respect the client's cultural beliefs.
3. Ask the client if he has cultural or religious requirements that should be considered in his care.
4. Explain your beliefs so that the client will understand the differences.
5. Understand that all cultures experience pain in the same way.

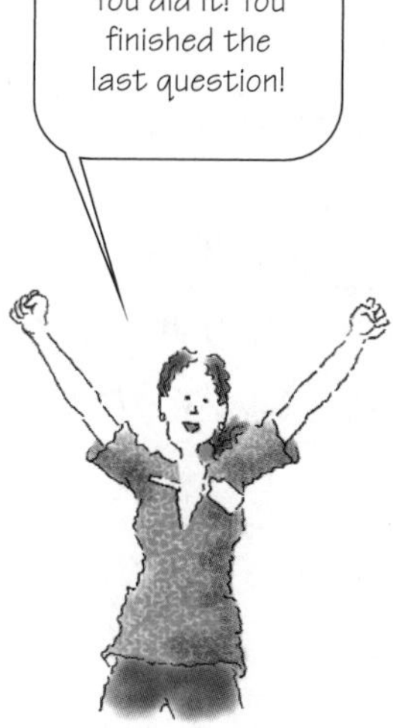

Congrats! You did it! You finished the last question!

75. 1, 2, 3. Nonverbal cues may have different meanings in different cultures. In one culture, eye contact is a sign of disrespect; in another, eye contact shows respect and attentiveness. The nurse should always respect the client's cultural beliefs and ask if he has cultural or religious requirements. This may include food choices or restrictions, body coverings, or time for prayer. The nurse should attempt to understand the client's culture; it isn't the client's responsibility to understand the nurse's culture. The nurse should never impose her own beliefs on her clients. Culture influences a client's experience of pain. For example, in one culture pain may be openly expressed, whereas in another culture it may be quietly endured.

CN: Psychosocial integrity; CNS: None; CL: Analysis

Index

B

C

D

E

I

J

K

L

M

N

Q

R

S

T

U

V

W

X Y

Z

RRS1004